ADVANCED DIAGNOSTIC METHODS IN

Pathology

ADVANCED DIAGNOSTIC METHODS IN

Pathology

Principles, Practice, and Protocols

TIMOTHY J. O'LEARY, MD

Chairman, Department of Cellular Pathology and Genetics
Armed Forces Institute of Pathology
Washington, D.C.

SAUNDERS

An Imprint of Elsevier Science

Philadelphia London New York St. Louis Sydney Toronto

SAUNDERS
An Imprint of Elsevier Science

The Curtis Center
Independence Square West
Philadelphia, Pennsylvania 19106

Library of Congress Cataloging-in-Publication Data

O'Leary, Timothy J.
Advanced diagnostic methods in pathology: principles, practice, and protocols/Timothy J. O'Leary.
p. cm.
ISBN 0-7216-4976-9
1. Cytodiagnosis. 2. Histology, Pathological.
I. Title

RB43. O477 2002
616.07′582-dc21 2002-019196

Acquisitions Editor: Natasha Andjelkovic
Editorial Assistant: Danielle Burke
Publishing Services Manager: Frank Polizzano
Project Manager: Marian A. Bellus
Book Designer: Lynn Foulk

ADVANCED DIAGNOSTIC METHODS IN PATHOLOGY:
PRINCIPLES, PRACTICE, and PROTOCOLS ISBN 0-7216-4976-9

Disclaimer
For chapters written by authors affiliated with the Armed Forces Institute of Pathology, the opinions and assertions contained therein are the private views of the authors and are not to be construed as official or reflecting the views of the Department of Defense.

Please note that Chapters 5, 6, 7, 10, 15, 16, and 17 are in the public domain.

Printed in the United States of America
Last digit is the print number: 9 8 7 6 5 4 3 2 1

To my wife Dianne,
my children Theresa, Thomas, and Brendan,
and my parents Kathleen and Timothy

CONTRIBUTORS

Susan L. Abbondanzo, MD
Chair, Department of Hematopathology
Armed Forces Institute of Pathology
Washington, DC

Nadine S. I. Aguilera, MD
Assistant Chair, Department of Hematopathology
Armed Forces Institute of Pathology
Washington, DC

José Costa, MD
Professor of Pathology and Biology
Yale University School of Medicine
Director of Anatomical Pathology
Vice-Chairman, Department of Pathology
Yale-New Haven Hospital
Deputy Director, Yale Cancer Center
New Haven, Connecticut

Deborah Dillon, MD
Associate Research Scientist
Yale University School of Medicine
Attending Pathologist
Molecular and Surgical Pathology
Yale-New Haven Hospital
New Haven, Connecticut

Agnes Fogo, MD
Professor of Pathology, Medicine and Pediatrics
Vanderbilt University Medical Center
Director, Renal/Electron Microscopy Laboratory
Vanderbilt University Medical Center
Nashville, Tennessee

Dennis M. Frisman, MD
Staff Pathologist
Affiliated Pathologists Medical Group
Torrance, California

Alan E. Hubbs, PhD
Research Cytologist
Department of Cellular Pathology and Genetics
Armed Forces Institute of Pathology
Washington, DC

Mary B. Kenny-Moynihan, MD
Metropolitan Pathologists
Denver, Colorado

Michael N. Koss, MD
Professor of Pathology
Keck School of Medicine
University of Southern California
Pulmonary and Renal Pathologist
USC University Hospital, Norris Cancer Center
Los Angeles County Medical Center
Los Angeles, California

Jack H. Lichy, MD, PhD
Staff Pathologist and Director of Molecular Diagnostics Laboratory
Department of Cellular Pathology and Genetics
Armed Forces Institute of Pathology
Rockville, Maryland

Irina A. Lubensky, MD
Molecular Pathogenesis Unit SNB, NINDS
National Institutes of Health
Bethesda, Maryland

Timothy J. O'Leary, MD
Chairman, Department of Cellular Pathology and Genetics,
Armed Forces Institute of Pathology
Washington, DC

Ronald M. Przygodzki, MD
Medical Genetic and Clinical Research Pathologist
Armed Forces Institute of Pathology
Department of Cellular Pathology and Genetics
Rockville, Maryland

Ann H. Reid, MA
Research Biologist
Department of Cellular Pathology
Armed Forces Institute of Pathology
Rockville, Maryland

Liliane Striker, MD
Professor of Medicine
University of Miami
Miami, Florida

Jeffery K. Taubenberger, MD, PhD
Chief, Division of Molecular Pathology,
Department of Cellular Pathology and Genetics,
Armed Forces Institute of Pathology
Rockville, Maryland

Elizabeth R. Unger, PhD, MD*
Associate Professor, Department of Pathology and Laboratory Medicine*
Emory University School of Medicine
Atlanta, Georgia

Cynthia F. Wright, PhD
Associate Professor
Department of Pathology and Laboratory Medicine
Medical University of South Carolina
Charleston, South Carolina

*Current Affiliation:
Centers for Disease Control and Prevention
Atlanta, Georgia

PREFACE

When begun, this book was envisioned as a reference that would bring together current information on newer techniques in biology and medicine that find use in diagnostic pathology and that would put this information together, in context. While this remains a goal, it is a goal that is only partially achieved, because the evolution of new technologies applicable to diagnostic pathology occurs at a rate surpassing that of those who would capture them in book form. The attempt to integrate these modalities has forced greater attention on the molecular pathogenesis of disease, however. Thus, we attempt to provide some insight not only about how specialized techniques can be used to assist in pathologic examination but also about how the use of these methods has provided insights into pathogenesis. Such insights are currently guiding the development of "targeted therapeutics," such as trastuzumab and imatinib mesylate, and are stimulating the development of diagnostic products intended solely to guide therapy. It seems likely that in the next few years it will be at least as important to the patient to understand from a molecular perspective the characteristics of his or her disease as it is to make a traditional pathologic diagnosis. We hope that this book will help pathologists, clinicians, and researchers to develop insights that allow them to integrate "classical" histologic information with that provided by these newer diagnostic modalities.

A book such as this necessarily owes much to countless writers and editors who have previously helped synthesize information in review articles and books. These sources undoubtedly have provided much insight beyond those cited. Several Internet-based tools have proven to be particularly valuable: the web resources provided by the National Center for Biotechnology Information—especially OMIM (Online Mendelian Inheritance in Man)—and Entrez Structure, which was used to construct the molecular models. ImmunoQuery, a web-accessible immunohistochemical database maintained by Dennis Frisman, was used to construct most of the tables of immunoreactivity appearing in this book. The Genew3 search tool was used to search the nomenclature database maintained by the Human Genome Organization (HUGO). It was this tool that made it possible to use a "standard" gene nomenclature that provides a framework for choosing a single gene symbol for use in the text, where several synonyms appear in the literature.

This work could not have been completed without the guidance and assistance of numerous professional colleagues. Particular thanks are due to Walter Gander of the Eidgenössische Technische Hochschule Zürich and his wife Heidi, whose hospitality enabled me to concentrate on this book during a six-month stay in Switzerland. My colleagues at the Armed Forces Institute of Pathology—Robert Becker, Florabel Mullick, Myra Washington, Michael Dickerson, and Glenn Wagner, provided encouragement and the administrative support that enabled me to focus on this work. Allen Burke and Renu Virmani provided valuable critiques of the chapter on cardiovascular disease. The chapter authors contributed not only their time but also their patience, often through several updates. My editor at Elsevier, Natasha Andjelkovic, the copyeditor, Jeanne Carper, and the project manager, Marian Bellus have worked tirelessly to make certain that the book makes sense and to make certain that the project continued to move forward. Final thanks are due to my wife Dianne, and my children, Theresa, Thomas, and Brendan. Their encouragement kept me going when things were not going well; their patience allowed me to spend many nights, holidays, and weekends writing and editing. Without their support, this work would never have been completed.

Timothy J. O'Leary, M.D.

CONTENTS

ADVANCED DIAGNOSTIC METHODS IN

Pathology

COLOR FIGURES

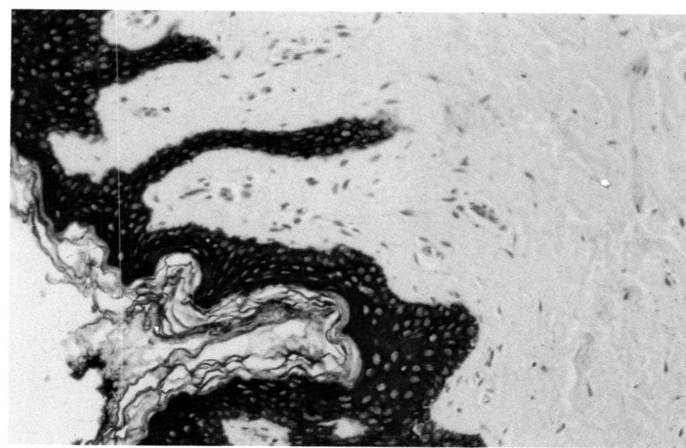

FIGURE 2–1
Section of skin immunohistochemically stained with a pancytokeratin antibody (×200).

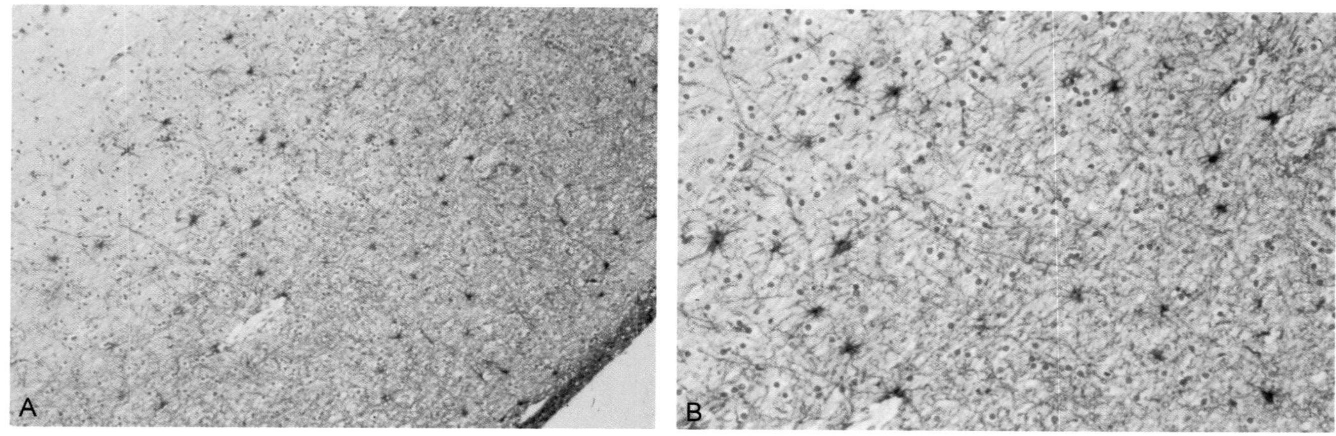

FIGURE 2–2
Section of brain immunohistochemically stained for glial fibrillary acidic protein (GFAP), ×100 (*A*) and ×200 (*B*).

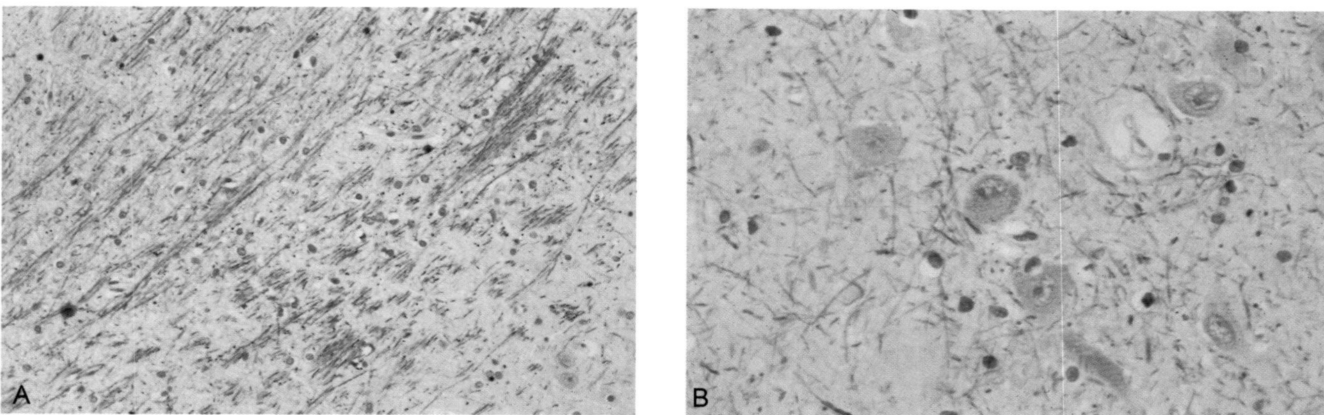

FIGURE 2–3
Section of brain immunohistochemically stained for neurofilament protein (NFP), ×200 (*A*) and ×400 (*B*).

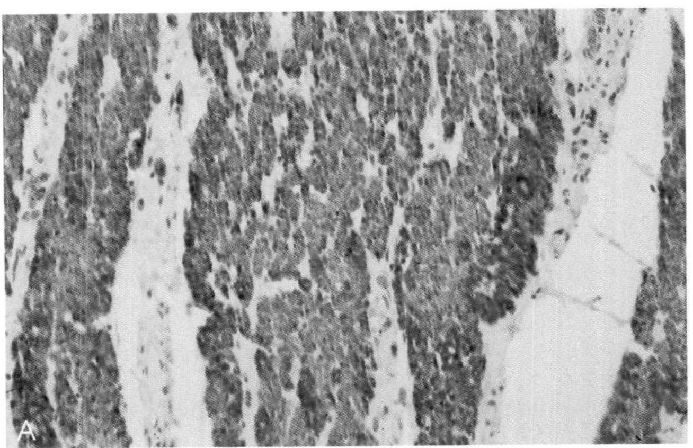

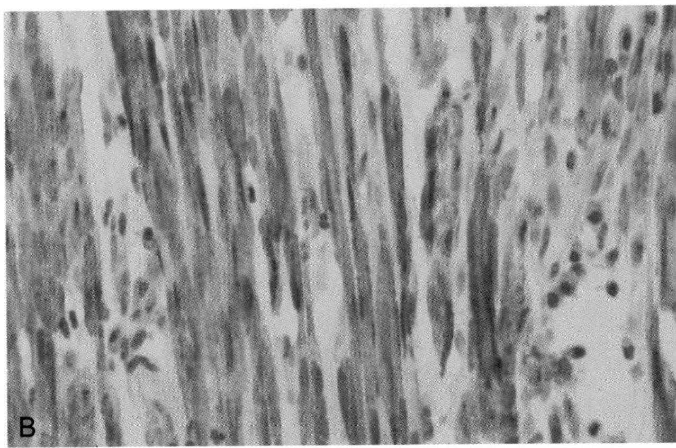

FIGURE 2–4
A and *B*, Two sections of colonic wall immunohistochemically stained for desmin (×200).

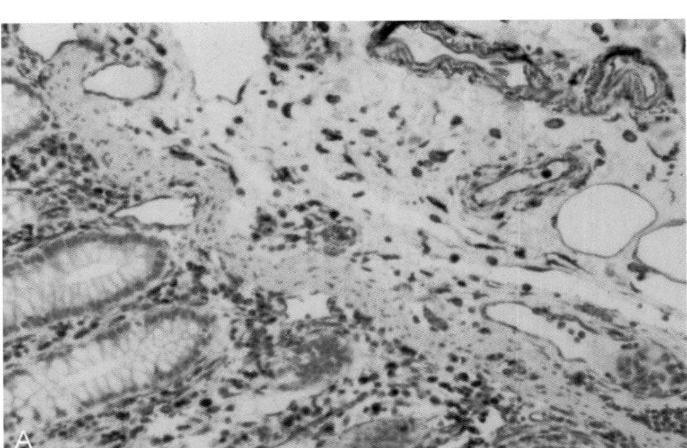

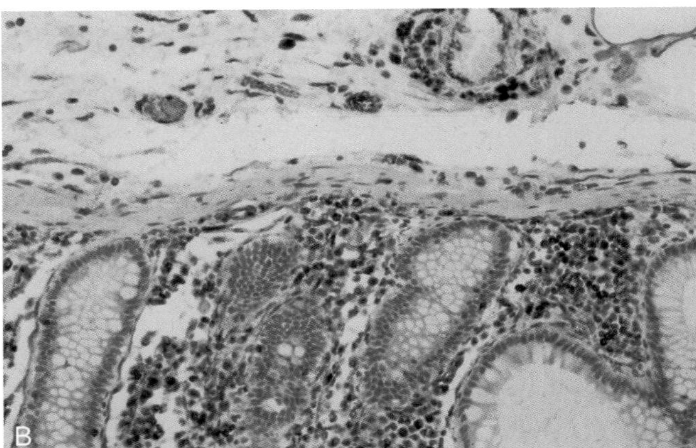

FIGURE 2–5
Sections of colon immunohistochemically stained for vimentin, ×200 (*A*) and ×400 (*B*).

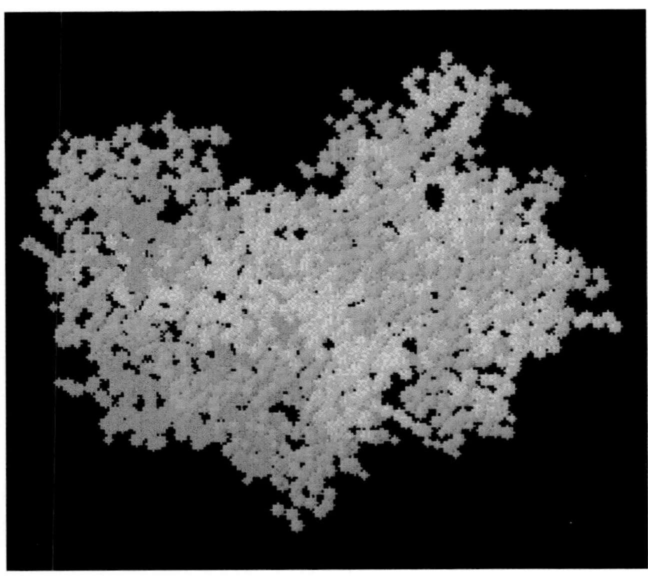

FIGURE 2–6
Space-filling structure model of α_1-antitrypsin, generated using Cn3D and Brookhaven Protein Structure Data Base data.[78] Helical regions are shown in *green*, and regions of β-pleated sheet are shown in *orange*.

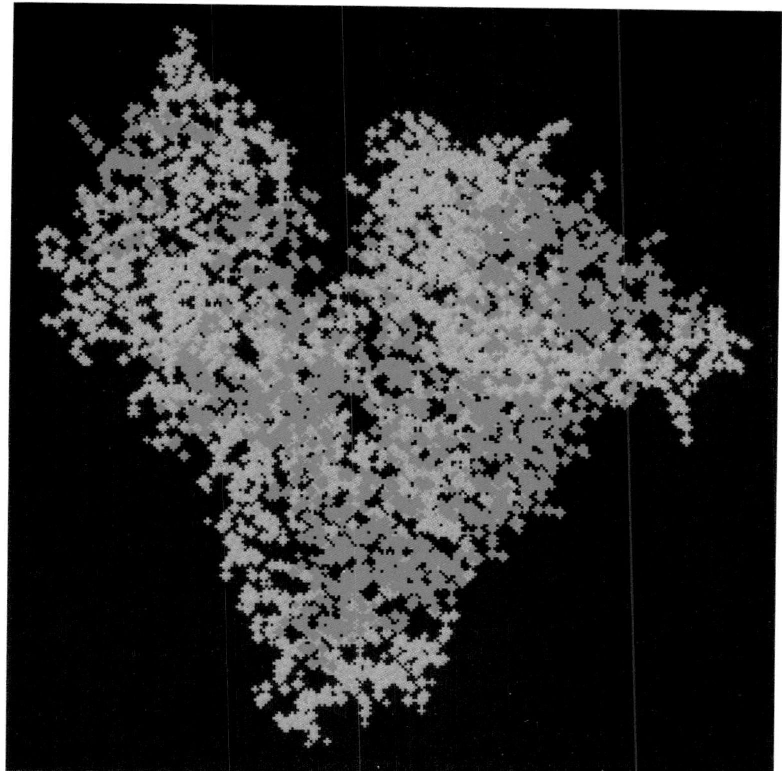

FIGURE 2–7
Space-filling structure model of albumin, generated using Cn3D and Brookhaven Protein Structure Data Base data.[97] Helical regions are shown in *green*.

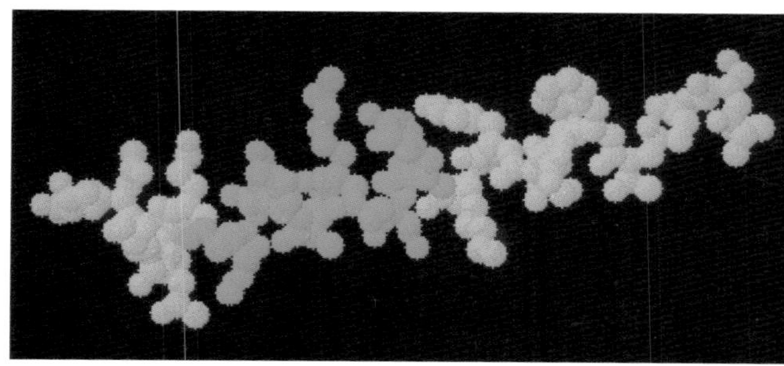

FIGURE 2–8
Space-filling structure model of glucagon, generated using Cn3D and Brookhaven Protein Structure Data Base data.[97] Helical regions are shown in *green*.

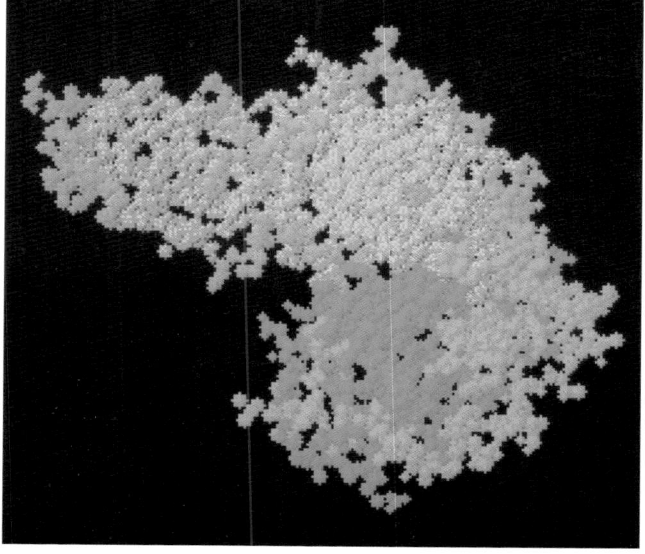

FIGURE 2–9
Space-filling model of human growth hormone, generated using Cn3D and Brookhaven Protein Structure Data Base data.[554] Helical regions are shown in *green*, and β-pleated sheets are shown in *orange*.

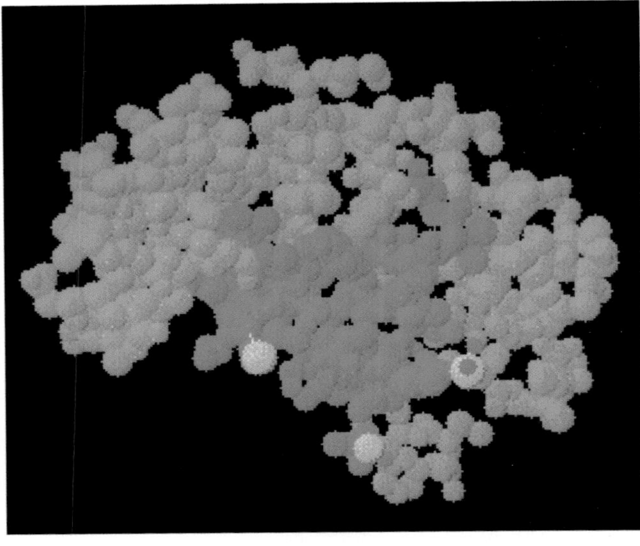

FIGURE 2–10
Space-filling structure model of insulin, generated using Cn3D and Brookhaven Protein Structure Data Base data.[215] Helical regions are shown in *green*.

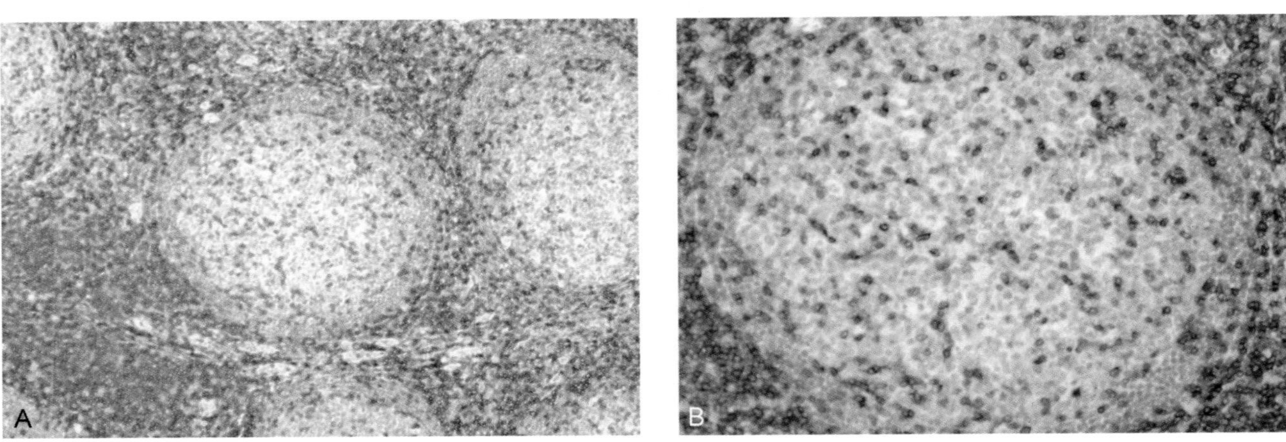

FIGURE 2–11
Section of tonsil immunohistochemically stained for CD3, ×100 (*A*) and ×200 (*B*).

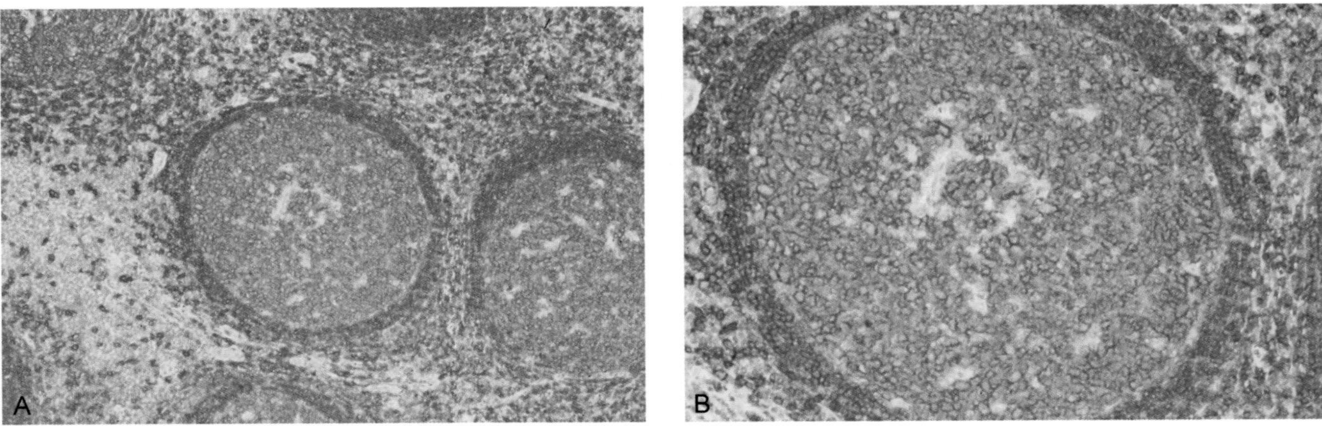

FIGURE 2–12
Section of tonsil immunohistochemically stained for CD20, ×100 (*A*) and ×200 (*B*).

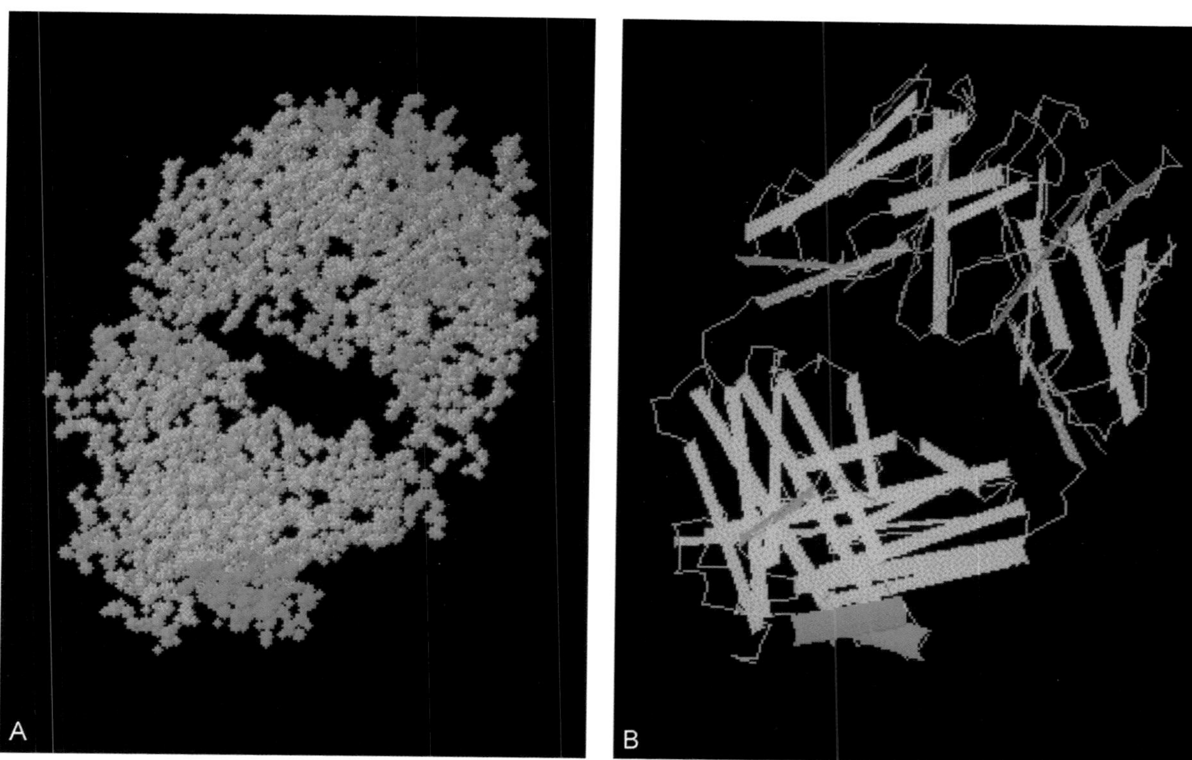

FIGURE 2–13
Space-filling (*A*) and secondary structure (*B*) models looking "end-on" at an immunoglobulin FAB fragment. Models were generated using Cn3D and Brookhaven Protein Structure Data Base data.[555, 556]

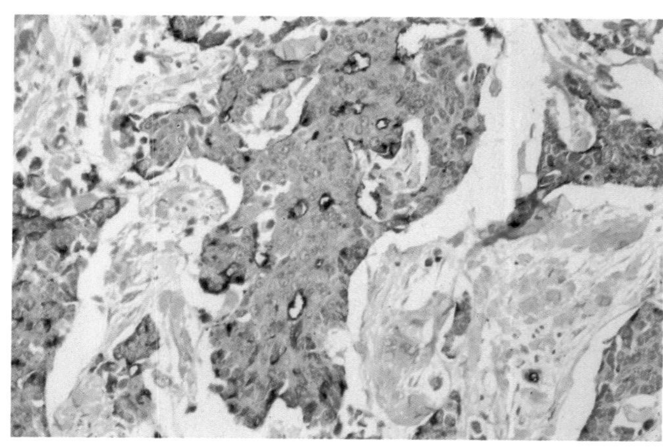

FIGURE 2–14
Section of breast carcinoma stained immunohistochemically with the monoclonal antibody B72.3 (×200).

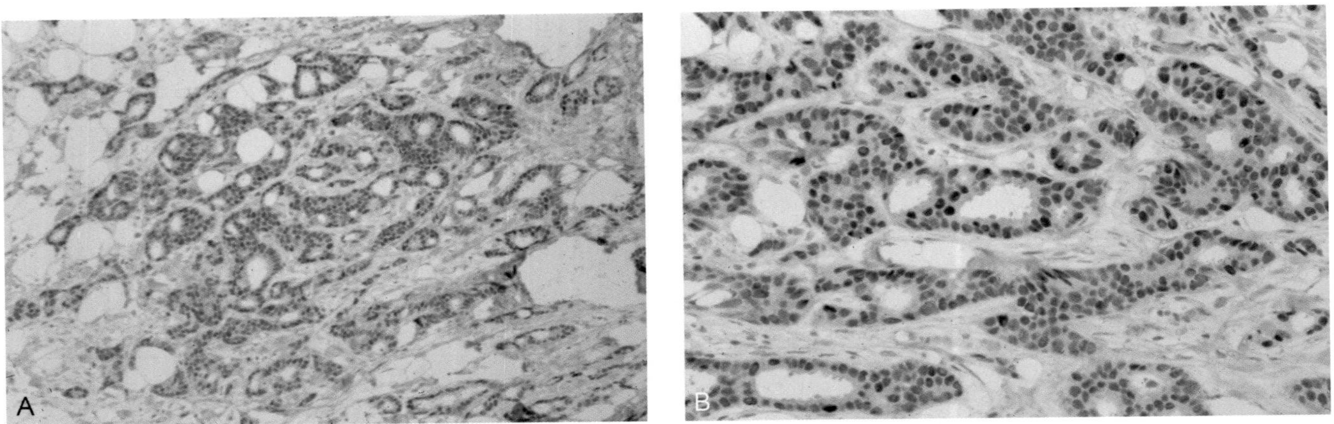

FIGURE 2–15
Section of tubular carcinoma of breast immunohistochemically stained for estrogen receptor protein, ×100 (*A*) and ×200 (*B*).

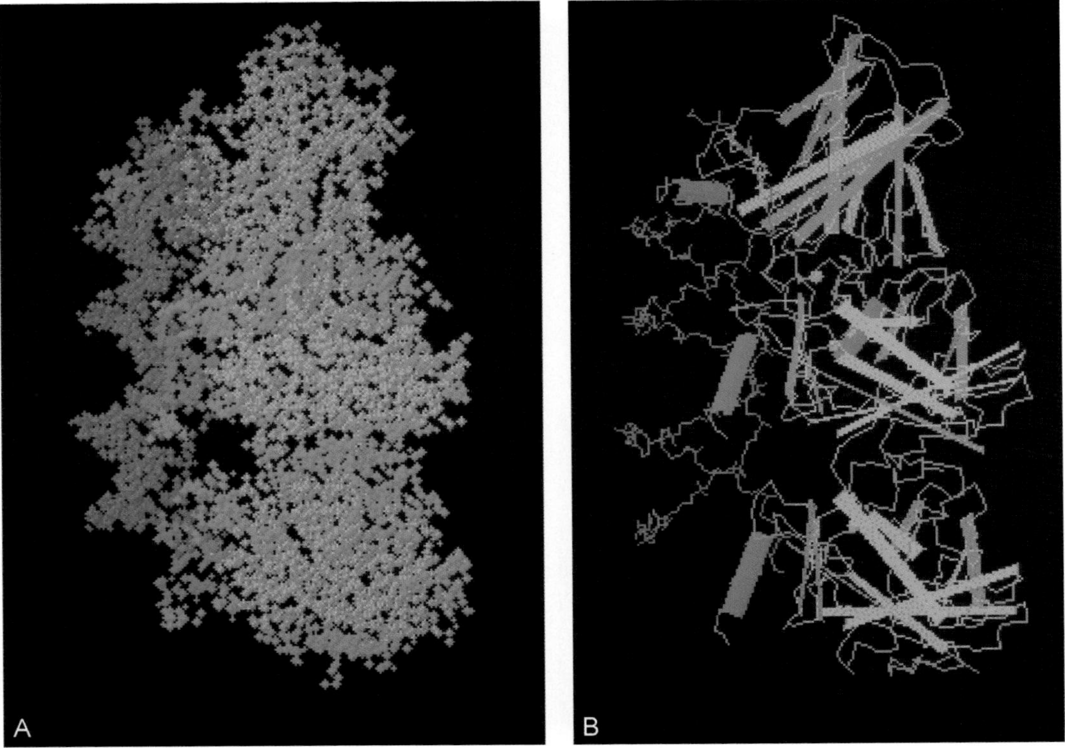

FIGURE 2–16
Space-filling (*A*) and secondary structure (*B*) models showing p53 bound to DNA. The models were generated using Cn3D and Brookhaven Protein Structure Data Base data.[518] Helical regions are shown in *green*, and β-sheets are shown in *orange*.

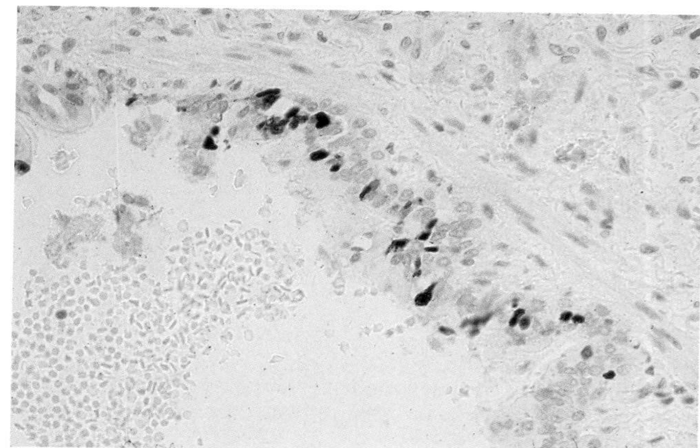

FIGURE 6–1
Immunohistochemical demonstration of adenovirus species in airway tissue (×200).

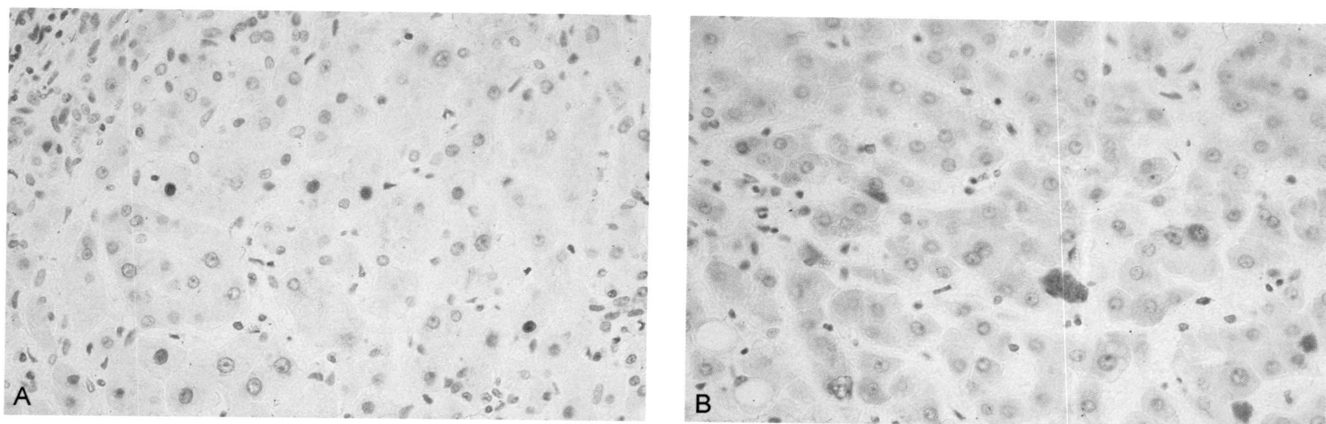

FIGURE 6–2
Immunohistochemical demonstration of *(A)* hepatitis B core antigen (×200) and *(B)* hepatitis B surface antigen (×400) in liver tissue.

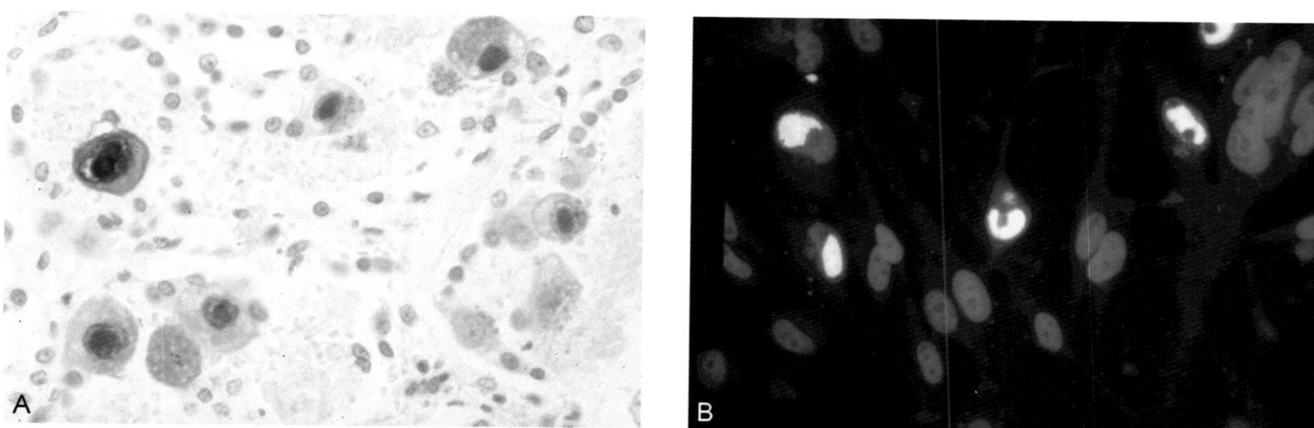

FIGURE 6–3
A, Immunohistochemical demonstration of cytomegalovirus in lung tissue (×400). *B,* Demonstration of fluorescent in situ hybridization of a cytomegalovirus genome in cultured fibroblasts (×400).

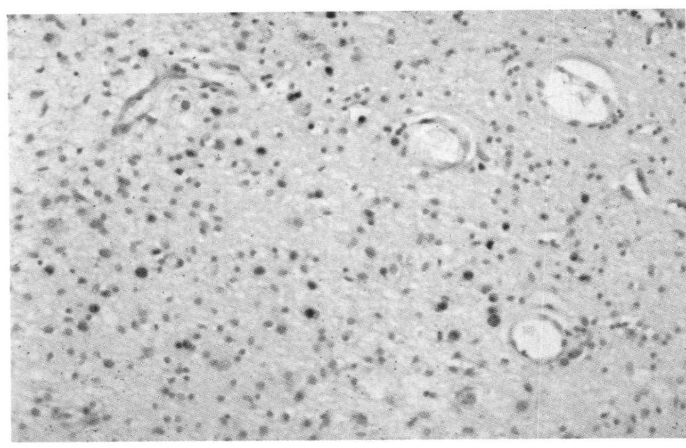

FIGURE 6–4
Demonstration of a JC virus genome by in situ hybridization in brain tissue from a patient with progressive multifocal leukoencephalopathy (×100).

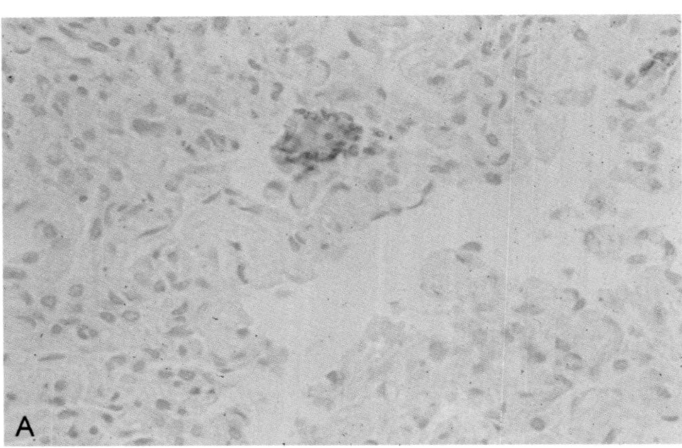

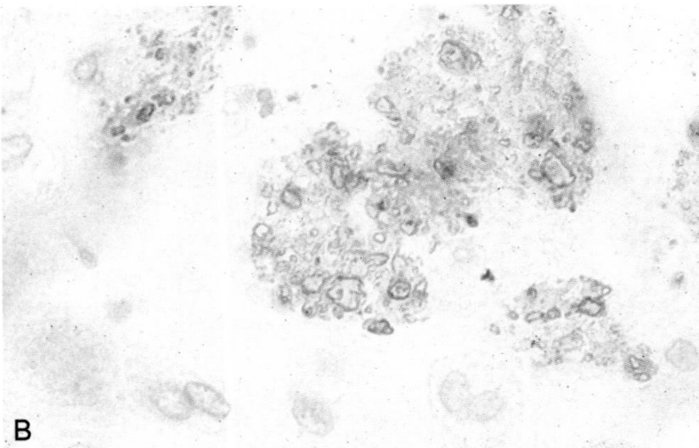

FIGURE 6–5
Immunohistochemical demonstration of *Pneumocystis carinii* in the "foamy exudate" of lung tissue, seen at ×100 *(A)* and at ×400 *(B)*.

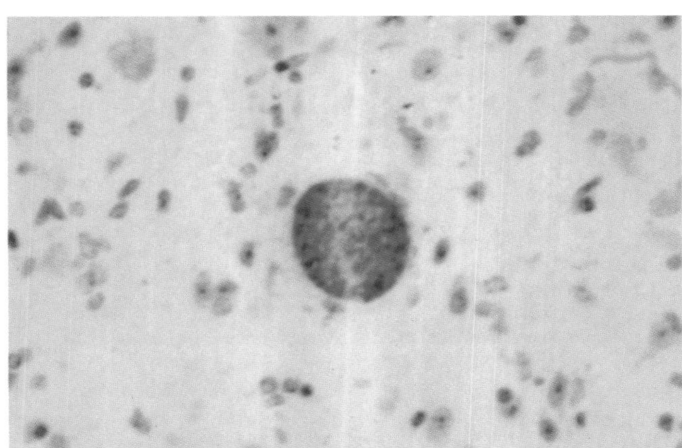

FIGURE 6–6
Immunohistochemical demonstration of a *Toxoplasma gondii* cyst in brain tissue of a patient with acquired immunodeficiency syndrome (×400).

I

ADVANCED DIAGNOSTIC METHODS

Principles

JACK H. LICHY

1

Oncogenes and Tumor Suppressor Genes

The oncogenes and tumor suppressor genes are the genes directly involved in the pathogenesis of cancer. The discovery and characterization of such genes has provided an understanding of cancer at the molecular level that presents new opportunities for the prevention and diagnosis of cancer and new tools for the management of the cancer patient. The aim of this chapter is to present the broad spectrum of oncogene and tumor suppressor gene biology in a manner that emphasizes the clinical relevance of the findings of basic research. The focus of the discussion is on those genes frequently altered in human malignancies. Less emphasis has been placed on the large number of genes that display transforming activity in experimental systems but do not yet have demonstrable functions in human cancer.

DEFINITIONS OF ONCOGENE AND TUMOR SUPPRESSOR GENE

Cancer cells uniformly suffer from a defect in one of the pathways that regulate cell growth. Cell growth regulation involves complex regulatory networks, including proteins and cofactors that regulate responses to extracellular signals, passage through the cell cycle, and the repair and replication of DNA. In addition to the regulation of cell growth, it has become evident in recent years that specific pathways exist for the regulation of cell death. Aberrations in the regulatory pathways that permit normal programmed cell death, or apoptosis, can contribute to the malignant phenotype. The genes that participate in these cellular regulatory pathways are the oncogenes and tumor suppressor genes.

Oncogenes

The term *oncogene* derived from work on the transforming retroviruses. These viruses were found, in experimental cell culture systems, to have the capacity to confer aspects of the malignant or "transformed" phenotype onto the infected cells.[1–3] Examples of such viruses include the Moloney murine sarcoma virus and the avian sarcoma virus. Extensive genetic analysis of these viruses identified a single gene responsible for the transforming activity. Because these viruses were associated with sarcomas in the infected animal, these genes were initially named "Src."[2] Expression of such a gene in a cell growing in culture conferred growth properties characteristic of cancer cells. These properties include anchorage-independent growth (the ability to grow in the absence of attachment to a surface), a reduced requirement for growth factors, usually supplied by serum in the culture medium, and the ability to grow to a higher density than untransformed cells and to form transformed foci of densely packed cells on a tissue culture plate. The transformed cells also had altered cellular morphology characterized by cytoskeletal changes resulting in an increase in refractility when viewed by phase contrast microscopy, a change from a polygonal cell morphology to a spindly, fusiform structure with an apparent reduction in cytoplasmic volume. Thus, the evidence suggested that a single gene could influence multiple aspects of cellular behavior. These were the first oncogenes.

The importance of the discoveries in the area of retrovirus research became clear with the key observation that the retroviral oncogenes were variant forms of normal cellular genes.[4] The normal cellular homologues of the viral oncogenes were designated "proto-oncogenes." In the case of animals that developed sarcomas after infection by an oncogene containing retrovirus, the presence of the oncogene was sufficient to override the effects of the proto-oncogene present in the same cell. In other words, these oncogenes acted in a dominant fashion. With these observations, the hypothesis was developed that a proto-oncogene in a human cell could mutate into an oncogene, resulting in malignant transformation. Evidence that this was in fact the case came initially with the discovery of a gene from the bladder carcinoma designated EJ with the ability to transform NIH3T3 cells in culture. The sequence of the transforming gene revealed it to be a mutated form of the proto-oncogene now known as *HRAS*.[3] Furthermore, the mutation was recognized immediately, because the same sequence alteration, a conversion of a glycine residue at position 12 to a valine, had previously been identified in the transforming oncogene from the Harvey rat sarcoma virus. This finding was of enormous importance because it gave credence to the idea that the oncogenes of retroviruses represented modified forms of genes normally present in the human genome and that similar activating mutations of these genes can occur in human cancers.

The seminal observations made with the *HRAS* gene gave rise to the current view of the definition of an oncogene. In general, an oncogene is a gene whose protein product activates some cellular growth regulatory pathway to contribute to the malignant phenotype. This activation is abnormal in that it does not respond to the normal inhibitory influences that keep cell growth in check. The ability to act in a dominant fashion is a hallmark of oncogenes: in a diploid cell, two copies of each gene including the proto-oncogenes are present; activation of one copy to the oncogene form, even with continued expression of the normal gene, is sufficient to confer abnormalities in growth regulation.

Tumor Suppressor Genes

While investigations into the transforming genes of retroviruses were leading to the identification of the oncogenes, other lines of inquiry were demonstrating that a distinct variety of abnormality was also present in human cancers. Epidemiologic studies of the ocular tumor retinoblastoma, which was known to occur in both familial and sporadic forms, led to the "two-hit hypothesis" first proposed by Alfred Knudson.[5, 6] Whereas sporadic cases of retinoblastoma typically present as a solitary tumor affecting adults, the familial form, transmitted in an autosomal dominant manner, typically occurs in children and is often multicentric or bilateral. Devised to explain the differences between the familial and sporadic forms of the disease, the two-hit hypothesis proposed that two genetic mutations—"hits"—are required to cause a retinoblastoma. In the familial form, individuals would inherit one hit from the affected parent, and therefore only one additional mutation would be sufficient to cause a tumor. Each cell in the affected individual's body would already have one hit. The random occurrence of the second hit would lead immediately to tumor development, and the frequency of this second hit was sufficient to result in multiple tumors presenting at an early age. Although the frequency of such hits was proposed to be the same in the sporadic disease, tumors would only develop when two hits affected the same cell. The relative rarity of developing the two required hits as somatic mutations accounted for the later age at onset of sporadic retinoblastoma and the usual presentation of a single tumor rather than multiple tumors.

It was further proposed as the simplest realization of the two-hit model that the two hits represented inactivating mutations in the two copies of the same gene, presumably a gene involved in the negative regulation of cell growth. It was envisioned that one normal copy of such a gene would be sufficient to provide the normal function of the gene product that was in some way to suppress tumor formation. Thus, the proposed gene was considered to be a "tumor suppressor gene."

As a result of extensive genetic linkage analysis in familial retinoblastoma families, a gene associated with the disease was mapped to the chromosomal locus 13q14. The gene was eventually cloned and analyzed in both familial and sporadic cases.[7, 8] This analysis confirmed the major predictions of the two-hit hypothesis. In familial retinoblastoma, mutations were in fact found in one allele of the gene in unaffected tissue. In tumors, the second allele was either lost completely from the genome or was affected by a mutation. In sporadic tumors, both copies of the gene were found to be abnormal, often with complete loss of one copy combined with a point mutation in the other. The pattern of a mutation in one allele of a tumor suppressor gene with loss of the other allele has become almost a defining feature of a tumor suppressor gene and is discussed later under "Loss of Heterozygosity."

Another line of research that gave rise to evidence for the existence of tumor suppressor genes involved the study of somatic cell hybrids. This experimental approach involved methods of physically fusing two distinct cell lines with each other and isolating, through the use of selectable genetic markers, hybrid cell lines that contained at least some of the genetic material from each of the two fusion partners. One of the questions addressed by this approach was whether the properties of the malignant phenotype were dominant or recessive: If a cell line with benign properties were fused with a cell line from a cancer, which phenotype would be dominant, the benign or the malignant? If the major determinant of malignancy were a dominant oncogene such as those identified in the retroviruses, then it would be expected that the hybrids would demonstrate the malignant phenotype. However, in several experimental situations the opposite situation was found to prevail: the hybrids had lost certain aspects of the malignant phenotype. Therefore, the results with the hybrids provided evidence for the existence of genes capable of suppressing the malignant phenotype.[9, 10]

Loss of Heterozygosity

As a general definition, a tumor suppressor gene encodes a protein involved in the negative regulation of cell growth. Inactivation of the gene contributes to the abnormal growth properties that characterize a malignant cell. In contrast to oncogenes, one normal copy of a tumor suppressor gene usually suffices to provide the essential functions of the gene product; inactivation of gene function requires inactivation of both copies of the gene. As was noted in the analysis of retinoblastoma specimens, one of the inactivation events often involves physical loss of one copy of the gene while the mutationally inactivated copy remains in the genome. The genome of normal diploid cells contains two copies of each genetic locus. If one copy is deleted, as often happens in the progressive steps that lead toward malignancy, then that locus demonstrates "loss of heterozygosity" (LOH).

LOH may be detected at any site in the genome containing a polymorphic locus. A polymorphic genetic locus is one with multiple alleles that differ by subtle variations in sequence sufficient to allow them to be distinguished by standard molecular biologic methods, such as polymerase chain reaction (PCR) followed by gel electrophoresis, or restriction enzyme digestion followed by Southern blot. The most common type of polymorphism currently employed for LOH analysis is the short tandem repeat (STR). An STR, also known as a microsatellite, consists of a short sequence unit, usually two to four nucleotides in length, repeated in tandem a variable number of times (Fig. 1–1*A*). Microsatellites with a basic repeat unit consisting of the dinucleotide G-T occur very commonly throughout the human genome; over 5000 instances of this type of polymorphism have been identified.[11] Microsatellites tend to be highly polymorphic: the number of repeats is found to vary over a fairly wide range when multiple chromosomes from multiple individuals are examined. However, within an individual the number of repeats almost always remains constant during cell division. Therefore, normal diploid somatic tissues, having two copies of each chromosome per cell, will all have the same two alleles of each microsatellite. Detection of these alleles involves PCR amplification of the region containing the repeated motif. This is accomplished by using PCR primers designed to recognize unique, single copy sequence in the regions on either side of the repeat. When the PCR products are analyzed by gel electrophoresis, the size of the band detected reflects the number of repeats. Thus, diploid tissues will give either one or two bands, depending on whether the specimen is homozygous (both alleles having the same number of repeats) or heterozygous at the locus analyzed. If the normal tissue is heterozygous, loss of one allele in tumor DNA is readily detected by comparing results obtained with tumor relative to normal DNA from the same individual. An example of LOH in a tumor specimen detected by this method is presented in Figure 1–1*B*.

It has been observed that loci that harbor tumor suppressor genes show LOH in tumor specimens much more frequently that those that do not. Many studies directed toward the identification of novel tumor suppressor genes have been performed based on the converse assumption, namely, that the observation of high-frequency LOH at a specific genetic locus suggests the presence of a tumor suppressor gene.[12–14] By analyzing multiple closely linked polymorphic loci on a particular chromosome, the extent of the deleted segment can be

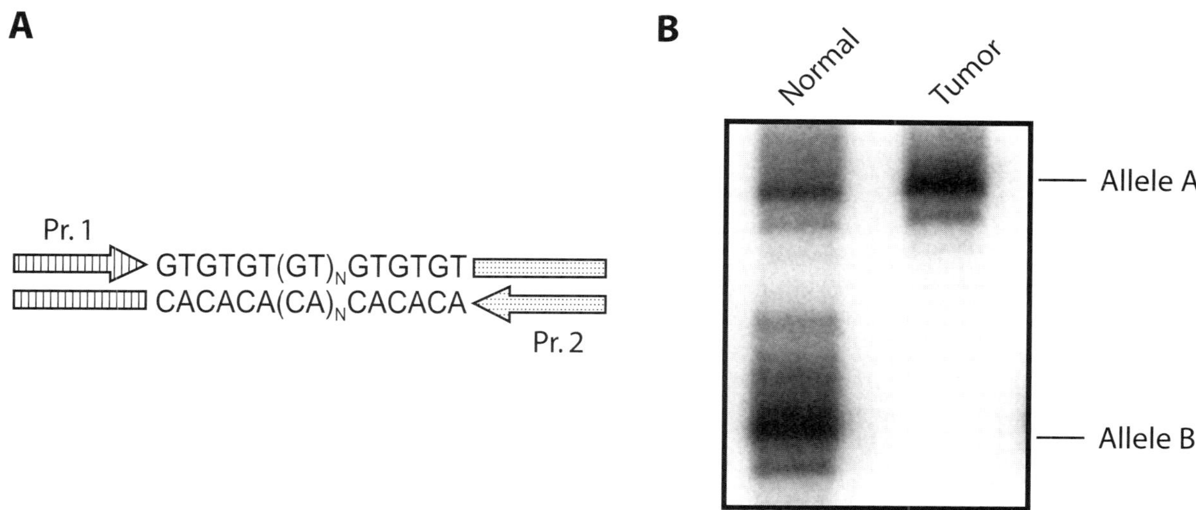

FIGURE 1–1
Detection of loss of heterozygosity (LOH) by polymerase chain reaction (PCR) at a dinucleotide repeat polymorphism. *A,* Primers (Pr. 1 and Pr. 2) are designed to recognize unique sequence on either side of the polymorphic G-T repeat. *B,* Primers specific for one microsatellite, in this case the G-T polymorphism D13S263 located near the *BRCA2* gene on chromosome 13q12, were used to amplify DNA extracted from benign tissue and a breast carcinoma from the same patient. The PCR products were analyzed by denaturing polyacrylamide gel electrophoresis. The tumor demonstrates LOH for allele B (the smaller allele). Minor bands present below the major PCR products result from slippage, or "stuttering," of the DNA polymerase along the (GT)N repeats during PCR amplification.

determined for each tumor analyzed. Assuming that the deletions in all or most tumors must include the tumor suppressor gene, the deletions can be compared to determine a minimal region of overlap, thereby localizing a putative tumor suppressor gene to a short segment of the chromosome. Once localized, other methods can be employed to clone the specific gene involved.

PATHWAYS OF ONCOGENE AND TUMOR SUPPRESSOR GENE ACTION

As a means of organizing information about a large number of individual genes and their products into a comprehensible format, the following discussion classifies the oncogenes and tumor suppressor genes by function. Four categories are considered: (1) mitogenic signal transduction; (2) cell cycle regulation; (3) DNA replication and repair; and (4) apoptosis. It will become apparent that this classification is something of an oversimplification and that the categories, in fact, overlap substantially. For example, a principal function of the mitogenic signaling pathways is to activate the machinery that moves the cell through the cell cycle, which in turn involves activation of DNA replication and suppression of apoptotic mechanisms.[15] Nevertheless, this classification reflects the organization of research efforts directed at understanding the oncogenes and tumor suppressor genes and provides a framework for organizing a very complicated puzzle into smaller pieces that can be understood more readily.

Mitogenic Signal Transduction Pathways

Among the pathways that regulate cell growth are those involved in responding to extracellular signals. The response to such signals has obvious importance in embryonic development, in which growth and differentiation must occur under a strictly regulated program. In the mature organism, extracellular signals are involved in two types of processes. In some circumstances, such as wound healing, normally quiescent or slowly replicating cells must be signaled to enter the cell cycle or to increase their rate of replication. In other situations, a population of replicating cells must be present continuously to replace cells with a limited lifetime in tissues. Examples of the latter include the cells of the hematopoietic system, the liver, and the epithelial cells of the gut. In either case, the pathways must be subject to efficient growth regulatory mechanisms to prevent abnormal proliferation. The regulatory pathways that convey the extracellular signal to intracellular components that cause the cell to respond are collectively termed the *mitogenic signal transduction pathways.* The term *transduction* refers to the alteration in form of the signal as it passes through the cell. As is discussed later, the signal typically initiates in the form of a growth factor, usually a protein, binding to a receptor expressed as a transmembrane protein with both extracellular and intracellular domains. As the signal moves toward the various subcellular compartments, it may take the form of a phosphorylated amino acid, a guanine nucleotide bound to a protein, or a change in cellular localization of a component of the signaling pathway.

Many of the known proto-oncogenes, including those commonly altered in human cancers as well as those defined by the ability to transform murine fibroblasts, participate in mitogenic signal transduction pathways. As a general rule, the conversion of such a proto-oncogene into an oncogene results in constitutive activation of the associated signal transduction pathway. That is, the pathway in which the oncogene acts becomes resistant to the normal influences that inhibit the signal. To illustrate the types of proteins involved and the kinds of alterations that may occur to generate an oncogene, the pathway leading from stimulation by epidermal growth factor (EGF) is presented in detail.

A diagram illustrating the major participants in this pathway is presented in Figure 1–2.[16] The EGF molecule is a small protein of about 6 kd cleaved from a larger precursor transmembrane protein.[17] EGF is thought to play a role both in normal development and in wound healing. The pathway initiates with the binding of the EGF polypeptide to its receptor, a transmembrane protein of 175 kd. The receptor molecule contains an endogenous protein tyrosine kinase activity. This enzymatic activity transfers the terminal (gamma-) phosphate from adenosine triphosphate (ATP) to a tyrosine residue within the protein substrate recognized by the enzyme. Dimerization of the receptor molecule in response to binding

A. Activation of RAS by EGF

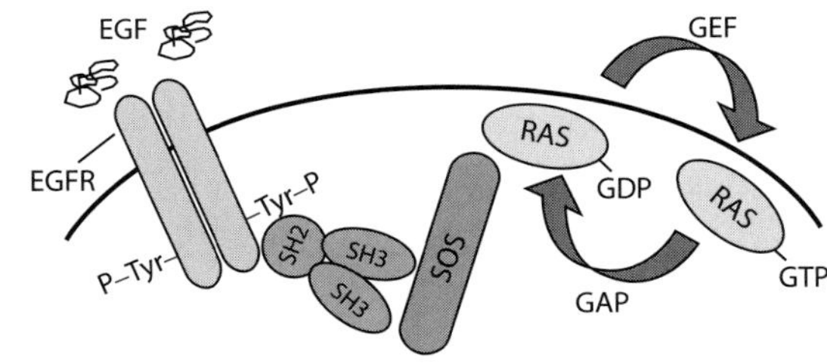

B. Kinase Cascades

Raf
MEK Kinase
MAP Kinase Kinase Kinase
MEK
MAP Kinase Kinase
ERK
MAP Kinase

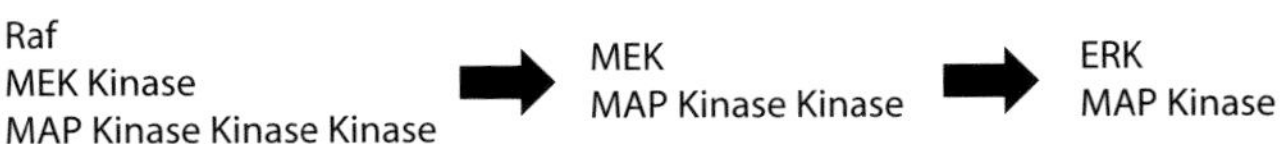

FIGURE 1–2
The RAS/MAP kinase signal transduction pathway. *A,* Binding of EGF to its receptor decreases guanosine diphosphate (GDP)-bound and increases guanosine triphosphate (GTP)-bound RAS. *B,* RAS-GTP activates a cascade of kinases culminating in the activation of MAP kinase. Alternative names for kinases at each level are indicated.

of the EGF ligand plays a crucial role in activation of the tyrosine kinase activity. The major target of the EGF receptor tyrosine kinase appears to be the receptor molecule itself. Thus, the binding of EGF to the receptor results in the autophosphorylation of the intracellular portion of the receptor molecule on a specific tyrosine residue.

SRC HOMOLOGY DOMAINS

The signal at this point has been transduced into a phosphotyrosine residue within the EGF receptor molecule, localized to the inner surface of the plasma membrane. This phosphotyrosine residue together with its surrounding amino acids form a high affinity binding site for the next components of the signaling pathway. These proteins serve as adapter molecules, linking the growth factor receptor to the downstream components of the pathway. Specific structural domains within the adapter proteins mediate protein-protein interactions in signaling pathways. Among the most common of the adapter domains are those that show sequence homology to the Src protein. One of the first oncogenes described, *src* was discovered as the transforming gene of the Rous sarcoma virus. Subsequent characterization identified Src as a tyrosine kinase. However, unlike the EGF receptor, which also possesses tyrosine kinase activity, Src does not contain a transmembrane domain and does not serve as a growth factor receptor. Src is now known to be a representative of a class of molecules known as the "nonreceptor" tyrosine kinases. These proteins participate in signal transduction pathways affecting a wide range of cellular functions. Analysis of the structure of Src and related proteins identified three domains, now termed Src homology regions 1, 2, and 3, or SH1, SH2, and SH3 domains, which were homologous to segments of the amino acid sequences of a large number of proteins. The SH1 domain contains the tyrosine kinase activity of the protein. The SH2 and SH3 domains are not required for enzymatic activity but function as binding domains involved in interactions with other proteins.[18] SH2 domains interact with polypeptides containing phosphotyrosine residues. Although similar in amino acid sequence, the differences in sequence among different SH2 domains determine their binding specificity. SH3 domains also serve as sequence-specific binding domains that mediate interactions with other proteins. SH3 domains bind to proline-rich sequences. Individual SH3 domains vary in their affinities for different proline-rich sequences, explaining, at least in part, the specificity of an SH3 domain for particular proteins.[19, 20]

In the signaling pathway depicted in Figure 1–2, the autophosphorylation of the EGF receptor on a tyrosine residue creates a binding site for an SH2 domain. The protein that interacts at this site is GRB2.[21–26] This protein was originally identified by screening an expression library with a phosphotyrosine-containing peptide corresponding to the predicted binding site on the EGF receptor. The proteins identified thereby were designated growth factor receptor binding, or GRB, proteins. In addition to the SH2 domain, the GRB2 protein contains two SH3 domains. In contrast to the Src molecule, however, GRB2 lacks a kinase domain and consists essentially entirely of the single SH2 and two SH3 domains. In response to the phosphorylation of the EGF receptor, GRB2 binds to its recognition sequence by means of the SH2 domain, resulting in a translocation of the protein from the cytoplasm to the membrane.

GUANINE NUCLEOTIDE EXCHANGE FACTORS

With the translocation of GRB2, a protein bound to GRB2 through its SH3 domains also translocates to the membrane.[22–25, 27] This protein is SOS, a name derived from the designation "son of sevenless," the name given to a genetically identified gene of *Drosophila melanogaster*. The SOS protein catalyzes the activation of the next protein in the sequence, RAS. RAS proteins comprise a family of proteins, closely related in sequence and having a molecular weight of approximately 21 kd, that bind the guanine nucleotides guanosine diphosphate (GDP) and guanosine triphosphate (GTP). The specific guanine nucleotide bound to RAS determines whether the signal will be passed farther downstream in the pathway: association with GTP activates, whereas association with GDP inhibits, signaling. In a quiescent cell in vivo, or in serum-starved cells in culture, most of the RAS protein exists in the GDP-bound form. Activation of the pathway requires dissociation of RAS from GDP and binding to GTP. This guanine nucleotide exchange is catalyzed by the SOS protein, a member of a family of guanine nucleotide exchange factors (GEFs). Thus, translocation of SOS to the membrane results in the accumulation of RAS-GTP, which favors activation of downstream components of the pathway.

In addition to the positive regulatory influence of the GEFs on RAS, a family of negative regulatory proteins exists that serves to convert RAS-GTP to the inactive GDP-bound form. These inhibitory proteins, the GTPase activator proteins (GAPs), function by stimulating hydrolysis of the RAS-bound GTP molecule.[28] Although the actual GTPase enzymatic activity involved in this reaction is intrinsic to the RAS molecule, and RAS-GTP will spontaneously hydrolyze its associated GTP to GDP, the reaction is markedly accelerated by the GAP proteins.

KINASE CASCADES

The activated RAS molecule transmits the signal to a cascade of protein kinases. The cascade involves three levels of kinases that act sequentially to amplify the signal and transmit it to the final targets of the pathway.[29–31] The kinases were given different names by different investigators. A major target of the pathway is the enzyme

MAP kinase. This protein was originally named "microtubule-associated protein kinase,"[32] because of its ability to phosphorylate microtubule associated proteins, and "mitogen-activated protein kinase" because of its activation in response to growth-promoting agents. The same enzyme was identified by investigators attempting to identify kinases activated by extracellular signals and was given the alternative name extracellular signal regulated kinase (ERK). Two forms of the enzyme encoded by different genes have been identified, designated ERK1 and ERK2.

The other proteins in the kinase cascade were named based on their location in the pathway relative to MAP kinase. The enzyme that phosphorylates MAP kinase is designated either MKK (for MAP kinase kinase) or MEK (for *M*AP or *E*RK *K*inase). The proteins that phosphorylate MKK are designated MKKK (MAP kinase kinase kinase) or MEKK (MEK kinase). One specific example of a MEK kinase, which had been independently identified as an oncogene of a transforming retrovirus, is the protein RAF.

Activated RAS leads by an as yet poorly understood mechanism to activation of the first level of the kinase cascade, the MEK kinases. These activate MEK by means of phosphorylation, and the MEK proteins likewise activate MAP kinase. The protein kinases recognize specific target amino acid sequences in their substrates and phosphorylate specific amino acids within the target sequence. Some kinases phosphorylate the structurally similar amino acids serine (Ser) and threonine (Thr), whereas others phosphorylate tyrosine (Tyr) residues. In the EGF pathway, the kinase intrinsic to the receptor molecule is a tyrosine kinase. The kinase cascade downstream of RAS involves Ser/Thr kinases at the top and bottom levels, represented by the proteins MEKK and MAP kinase. In contrast, MEK is a dual-specificity kinase, meaning that this enzyme phosphorylates its substrates on both Ser/Thr and Tyr residues. The target sequence for MEK takes the form Ser/Thr-X-Tyr, where X = any amino acid.

Once the signal has been transmitted down the kinase cascade, MAP kinase has become activated, owing to phosphorylation on specific threonine and tyrosine residues. The activated MAP kinase phosphorylates multiple proteins, resulting in the activation of multiple mechanisms that stimulate cell proliferation. The activated MAP kinase molecule undergoes dimerization, a step that appears to be important in permitting the subsequent translocation of the protein to the nucleus, where many of its key substrates are located.[33] The optimum recognition sequence for MAP kinase has been shown to be Pro-X-Ser/Thr-Pro, a sequence that often occurs multiple times in MAP kinase substrates.

Among the targets of MAP kinase are transcription factors, sequence-specific DNA binding proteins involved in regulating transcription. Transcription factors act by binding to specific DNA sequences present in the promoter regions of target genes, resulting either in activation or repression of gene expression. In many transcription factors the segment of the protein involved in transcriptional activation is a physically distinct structural domain from the segment involved in DNA binding. This modular architecture of transcription factors has important consequences in cancer biology. A major mechanism by which transcription factors become constitutively activated to become oncogenic involves a pathologic shuffling of domains as a result of a chromosome translocation, resulting in a fusion protein that can continue to function as a transcription regulator but can no longer respond to the regulatory influences that control the wild-type protein.

RECURRING THEMES IN SIGNAL TRANSDUCTION

Several basic concepts, or themes, appear repeatedly in the signal transduction literature. First, research studies aimed at the identification and characterization of protein-protein interactions have provided many key insights into the pathways in which specific signaling proteins function and in the position in the pathway at which they act. For example, the discovery of the GRB2 protein resulted from a search for proteins that would physically associate with the tyrosine phosphorylated EGF receptor. In the analysis of adenovirus-mediated transformation, a major breakthrough in the understanding of the E1A transcription factor, which had properties of an oncogene in experimental systems, came with the identification of proteins that physically associated with E1A, as demonstrated in this case by co-precipitation experiments. In the EGF pathway, several important protein-protein interactions occur, including those between phosphotyrosine and SH2 domains, between proline-rich sequences and SH3 domains, and between activated RAS and the MEK kinases.

Second, many signaling proteins have a modular architecture. Domains such as SH2 and SH3, originally identified in the Src protein, occur in many other proteins in the mitogenic signaling pathways. Two other types of domains occur frequently in signaling proteins. One, the Pleckstrin homology (PH) domain, appears to mediate interactions with phosphoinositides, which serve as second messengers in some signaling pathways.[34] The other, the DBL-homology (DH) domain, may mediate interactions with G protein subunits.[35] Such domains demonstrate substantial homology at the level of amino acid sequence. Crystallographic studies have shown that this homology extends to the level of three-dimensional structure. Currently available bioinformatics tools available through the Internet, such as the BLAST program provided by the National Center for Biotechnology Information (http://www.ncbi.nlm.nih.gov), readily identify these common domains based on amino acid sequence alone. The dissection of an amino acid sequence into structural domains often provides insight into the function of the protein. As an example, the proteins CRK, GRB2, and NCK all consist of combinations of SH2 and SH3 domains with variations in number of each domain and order of occurrence. This structure strongly suggests a role as adapter proteins that serve to connect components of signal transduction pathways while lacking intrinsic enzymatic activity themselves. Another area in which the modular architecture comes into play is in the transcription factors, in which DNA binding and transcriptional activation domains often exist as distinct structural domains of the protein. Such domains can become physically separated from one another but still retain their biologic activity by processes both physiologic, such as alternative RNA splicing, or pathologic, such as chromosome translocation.

Third, several signal transduction pathways have an overall architecture that parallels the EGF-MAP kinase pathway. The elucidation of the EGF-MAP kinase signaling pathway resulted from investigations into widely divergent biologic phenomena. Key contributions came from studies of organisms amenable to genetic manipulation, including yeast, the fruit fly *Drosophila melanogaster*, and the nematode *Caenorhabditis elegans*. In the fly, genetic analysis of the "sevenless" phenotype, characterized by developmental failure of the R7 cell in the multicellular photoreceptor unit of the compound eye, resulted in the identification of the genes *sevenless* and *son-of-sevenless* (SOS) as necessary components of the pathway.[36] Genetic analysis demonstrated that these genes were necessary and that *sevenless* acted upstream of SOS.[37] Further studies showed that *sevenless* encoded a transmembrane receptor on the R7 cell that responded to interaction with another transmembrane protein, BOSS (bride of sevenless) on the adjacent R8 photoreceptor cell.[38–40] The SOS protein was shown to encode a GEF, initially by sequence homology to the cdc25 protein of the yeast *Saccharomyces cerevisiae*.[41] In *C. elegans*, an analogous pathway was defined genetically in studies focused on characterization of development of the vulva. In this system the receptor gene *LET23*, the *RAS*-like gene *LET60*, and a gene encoding an adapter protein, *SEM5*, were identified, shown to be necessary for vulvar development, and placed in their order of activity in the pathway.[42] The findings with these model systems pointed the way for biochemical studies in mammalian systems not amenable to genetic manipulation and lent credence to the proposed functions of the analogous proteins identified in such systems.

A final general theme that emerges is the redundancy and complexity of signaling pathways. The EGF pathway is one example of multiple pathways with a similar overall architecture. Even within this one pathway, multiple proteins can function at each level. The EGF receptor is one product of a multi-gene family with at least five, and probably a total of seven, members. Four different MEK kinases have been identified. Similarly, multiple variants of MEK and MAP kinase are now known. In addition to this level of complexity within this pathway, parallel pathways, each with their own participants from the receptor to the final kinase, have been identified. Briefly, one pathway appears to mediate the principal response of the cell to certain types of stress. Important components in this pathway include the small GTP-binding proteins RAC and RHO, which function in a manner analogous to RAS, and the major kinase targeted by the pathway, the JUN N-terminal kinase (JNK), also known as stress-activated protein kinase (SAPK). Other parallel pathways direct signals toward other protein kinases, of which approximately seven thought to function analogously to MAP kinase have been identified. In addition to redundancy within each pathway and the existence of multiple parallel pathways, it has become clear that the pathways interact with one another, introducing a further level of complexity to the system.

ONCOGENES AND TUMOR SUPPRESSOR GENES IN THE SIGNALING PATHWAYS

Dissection of the mitogenic signaling pathways has been and continues to be a formidable task for the research community. This section focuses on those aspects of the signal transduction pathways that have clinical relevance to the diagnosis, treatment, and management of cancer. In principle, any component of a growth regulatory pathway has the potential to be a proto-oncogene. However, numerous studies focusing on many individual types of cancer have provided strong evidence that oncogenes and tumor suppressor genes in human malignancies, as opposed to experimental systems, occur only at a limited number of points in the pathway. These sites are at the level of the receptor, the RAS protein, the GAP protein, and the transcription factor. Studies looking for mutations in other components of the pathway have been performed; however, such mutations can be identified only rarely, if at all, and the clinical significance of even such rare mutations remains unclear. Specific examples of particular importance are presented in Table 1–1 and discussed in the following paragraphs.

Receptors as Oncogenes

The EGF receptor can become an oncoprotein. The mechanism of activation is through overexpression rather than alteration in the primary structure of the protein. Overexpression of the EGF receptor results in abnormal activation of the signaling pathway in the absence of EGF stimulation. The mechanism by which overexpression of the protein occurs may involve gene amplification or transcriptional activation by mechanisms that usually cannot be defined precisely in a specific

TABLE 1–1

Oncogenes and Tumor Suppressor Genes in Signal Transduction Pathways

Oncogene	Mechanism of Activation/ Inactivation	Associated Tumors	Genetic Syndrome
EGF receptor	Gene amplification	Lung, esophagus, others	
ERBB2 (HER2/neu)	Gene amplification	Breast, ovarian, lung, stomach, others	
PDGF receptor (*c-sis*)	Overexpression	Astrocytoma, osteosarcoma	
CSF1 receptor (*c-fms*)	Overexpression	Leukemia	
KIT	Activating in-frame deletions and point mutations	Gastrointestinal stromal tumors	
RET	Point mutation, translocation	Medullary carcinoma of thyroid	MEN 2A, 2B, FMTC
RAS, (*HRAS*, *KRAS*, *NRAS*)	Point mutation	Many	
NF1	Deletions, point mutations	Neurofibromas	Neurofibromatosis
APC	Deletions, point mutations associated with protein truncation	Colorectal carcinoma	Familial adenomatous polyposis
PTEN	Deletions, point mutations	Hamartomas, breast, kidney, prostate, melanoma, glioblastoma, endometrial	Cowden syndrome Bannayan-Zonana syndrome
VHL	Deletions, point mutations	Hemangioblastoma Renal cell carcionoma	von Hippel-Lindau syndrome

FMTC, familial medullary thyroid carcinoma; MEN, multiple endocrine neoplasia.

tumor. Overexpression of the EGF receptor has been observed in carcinomas of the lung, breast, and bladder and in glioblastoma.[43–46]

ERBB2

The protein now commonly designated HER2/neu, a member of the EGF receptor family, plays an important role in breast cancer.[46] The protein was described independently by several investigators as HER2,[47] neu,[48] and ERBB2.[49] The *ERBB2* gene product is a 185-kd glycoprotein homologous to the EGF receptor. The protein is overexpressed in approximately 30% of breast carcinomas. Overexpression is associated with poor prognosis in breast cancer.[46, 50, 51] Overexpression also occurs commonly in carcinomas of the lung, ovary, stomach, and salivary glands. The usual mechanism of overexpression is gene amplification, although transcriptional mechanisms have also been reported. The *ERBB2* protein has assumed greater importance with the introduction of Herceptin, a humanized monoclonal antibody directed against the ERBB2 protein, as a therapy for breast cancer.[52] Because this therapy depends on expression of the ERBB2 protein for effectiveness, quantitation of ERBB2 expression levels in tumor specimens is an important laboratory test in the management of breast cancer.

BCR/ABL

The *BCR/ABL* oncogene formed as a result of the t(9;22) translocation (the Philadelphia chromosome) fuses the *BCR* gene on chromosome 22q11 to the *ABL* gene on chromosome 9q34. The *ABL* proto-oncogene contains an endogenous tyrosine kinase activity, plus single SH2 and SH3 domains. Fusion of *BCR* with *ABL* results in constitutive activation of the *ABL* tyrosine kinase activity. The fusion protein recruits GRB2/SOS to the plasma membrane, thereby activating the RAS-MAP kinase pathway in a manner analogous to the activated EGF receptor.[53, 54] The fusion protein also functions to inhibit apoptosis.[55] The *BCR/ABL* messenger RNA (mRNA) is readily detectable by RT-PCR assays, which have clinical use in diagnosis and management of leukemias having this translocation. The *BCR/ABL* fusion is found in most cases of chronic myelogenous leukemia, in 3% to 5% of cases of juvenile acute lymphoblastic leukemia, and in approximately 25% of adult acute lymphoblastic leukemia. The characteristic acute lymphoblastic leukemia fusion incorporates a smaller segment of the BCR protein than the fusion associated with chronic myelogenous leukemia. The fusion proteins are designated by their molecular weights, P210 in chronic myelogenous leukemia and P190 in acute lymphoblastic leukemia. The presence of the Philadelphia chromosome in childhood acute lymphoblastic leukemia correlates strongly with poor prognosis.[56]

The *RET* Proto-Oncogene

The *RET* proto-oncogene encodes a transmembrane receptor tyrosine kinase. The gene maps to the peri-centromeric region of chromosome 10. Germline mutations are responsible for multiple endocrine neoplasia (MEN) types 2A and 2B and familial medullary thyroid carcinoma. The mutations in these syndromes are of the missense variety and result in constitutive activation of signaling. As a result, one abnormal gene suffices to cause the syndrome and inheritance is autosomal dominant. MEN 2A is characterized by medullary thyroid carcinoma, pheochromocytoma, and parathyroid adenoma. The mutations involved in MEN 2A cluster in exons 10 and 11, which encode part of the extracellular domain of the receptor molecule. In MEN 2B, associated with neuromas or ganglioneuromas in addition to medullary thyroid cancer and pheochromocytoma, mutations in the cytoplasmic domain of the protein result in abnormal activation of the receptor tyrosine kinase activity. The genomic segment containing exons 10 and 11 is small enough to permit amplification in a single PCR reaction. Therefore, mutations can be readily detected by PCR followed by DNA sequencing. The gene is also commonly mutated in sporadic medullary thyroid carcinomas. In papillary carcinomas of the thyroid, especially those associated with exposure to radiation, a chromosomal translocation commonly occurs that results in the fusion of the *RET* gene with one of at least three other genes designated *PTC1*, *PTC2*, and *PTC3* (where PTC stands for papillary thyroid carcinoma).[57, 58]

The *KIT* Proto-Oncogene

The *KIT* oncogene encodes a transmembrane receptor molecule with intrinsic tyrosine kinase activity. Mutations have been described in gastrointestinal stromal tumors (GISTs).[59] The KIT protein serves as the receptor for stem cell factor (SCF).[60] Mutations take the form of in-frame deletions of the coding sequence, resulting in the deletion of several amino acids from the juxtamembrane domain of the receptor extending from lysine at position 550 to valine at position 560. These deletions result in constitutive activation of receptor activity and activation of the RAS-MAP kinase pathway.[61, 62]

The presence of a *KIT* mutation can be detected by amplification of exon 11 by PCR followed by size analysis or DNA sequencing. The presence of a mutation is a poor prognostic factor in GISTs.[63, 64] The presence of a mutation is also an independent prognostic indicator and therefore may have clinical utility in the management of patients with these tumors.[65]

RAS Mutations in Cancer

Mutation of one of the *RAS* proto-oncogenes is one of the most common findings in a wide variety of human cancers. Of the multiple *RAS* genes, *HRAS* and *KRAS* genes are the most commonly involved by mutation. Mutations in cancers almost always affect one of four codons in the amino acid sequence, numbers 12, 13, 59, and 61. These mutations render the RAS protein resistant to the inhibitory action of the GTPase activator proteins and consequently result in constitutive activation of RAS. The most common mutation converts the glycine at position 12 to a valine residue. This is the mutation that was originally present in the *ras* gene cloned from the Harvey rat sarcoma virus and subsequently found in the transforming oncogene cloned from the EJ cell line derived from a human bladder carcinoma.[3] The frequency of occurrence of *RAS* mutations varies significantly in different tumors (see Table 1–1). The frequency is notably high in cancers of the pancreas, where 80% to 90% of tumors have been reported to contain a *KRAS* mutation.[66–68]

GAP Proteins as Tumor Suppressors

The gene responsible for the autosomal dominant syndrome familial neurofibromatosis, *NF1*, has been noted to have homology to GAP proteins.[69] The *NF1* gene maps to chromosome 17q. The gene encodes a large protein of 2818 amino acids believed to function like GAP to inactivate a mitogenic signaling pathway. In support of this concept, biochemical analysis of RAS proteins in neurofibroma tissue has demonstrated an increase in the activated, GTP-bound form of the RAS protein.[70, 71]

Transcription Factors as Oncoproteins and Tumor Suppressors

In experimental systems, many transcription factors, including MYC, MYB, ETS, JUN, and FOS, demonstrate transforming activity either in their wild type or mutated form. The following discussion concentrates on the subset of transcription factors believed to play an important role in human cancer. Some examples of this large group of proteins are listed in Table 1–2.

The MYC protein, encoded by a gene on chromosome 8q24, functions as an oncogene in a variety of human cancers.[72] The mechanism of activation usually involves overexpression of the gene product. In addition, mutations of the gene are common in Burkitt's lymphoma, with the mutations tending to cluster in the amino-terminal transactivation domain.[73, 74] Overexpression often results from translocation of the gene to a trancriptionally active region in close proximity to the immunoglobulin heavy chain locus (14q32) or one of the light chain loci. The 48-kd protein contains a basic region followed by helix-loop-helix (HLH) and leucine zipper (LZ) domains, structural elements found in a family of transcription factors designated the bHLH-ZIP family. The protein can bind to the DNA sequence $CA^{T}/_{C}GTG$ in the promoter regions of target genes.[75] Transcriptional activation by the MYC protein depends on its association with another bHLH-ZIP protein, MAX.[76–79] Whereas MYC has a short half-life in cells, with increased levels in proliferating cells, the MAX protein is stable and maintained at fairly constant levels in quiescent or cycling cells.[78] In addition to MYC, the MAX protein also binds to a family of four bHLH-ZIP proteins related to its first identified member, MAD.[80] The MAD-MAX complex opposes the transcriptional activation induced by the MYC-MAX complex. Accumulation of MAD-MAX accompanying a reduction in MYC-MAX levels has been observed during differentiation in several experimental systems including monoblasts, myeloblasts, and keratinocytes.[81, 82] Experiments with transgenic mice support the concept that MAD family members antagonize MYC in differentiation.[83–85]

Numerous altered transcription factors representing fusion proteins derived by chromosome translocation have been described in a variety of cancers. Many of these are associated with specific leukemias. These include the AML/ETO fusion—t(8;21) (q22;q22)—of acute myelogenous leukemia M2, the CBFβ-MYH11 fusion—inv (16) (p13q22)—of AML M1, M2, and M4Eo, the PML-RARA translocation—t (15;17) (q22;q21)—of AML M3, and at least 12 distinct translocations involving the *MLL* gene on chromosome 11q23.[86] In sarcomas, characteristic translocations result in the t (1;13) PAX7/FOXO1A(FKHR) and t (2;13) PAX3/FOXO1A fusion proteins found in alveolar rhabdomyosarcoma.[87–89] In peripheral neuroectodermal tumors, the t(11;22) translocation fuses the *EWS* gene on chromosome 22 to the FLI1 transcription factor, a member of the *ETS* family of transcription factors.[83–85] Interestingly, in some sarcomas, the *EWS* gene is found fused with another transcription factor gene, *ERG*, on chromosome 21.[90] Still another fusion partner for *EWS* results from the characteristic t(11;22) translocation of desmoplastic small round cell tumors; however, the chromosome 11 fusion partner is not *FLI1*, which maps to 11q24, but *WT1* on 11p13, the gene responsible for familial Wilms' tumor, discussed next.[91] Although a large number of transcription factor fusion proteins have now been described, this diverse group of proteins represents variations on a common theme, in that the fusion protein retains the DNA binding specificity of the parent transcription factor but has lost the ability to respond to the normal regulatory mechanisms that govern its activity.

The Wilms' Tumor Gene *WT1*

The product of the *WT1* gene on chromosome 11p13 is a sequence specific DNA binding protein that functions as a transcription factor.[92] The gene product is a protein with several isoforms ranging in size from 46 to 49 kd that shows homology to the transcription factors EGR1 and EGR2 and binds to the same sequence as these proteins.[93] Germline mutations in the gene result in a familial variant of Wilms' tumor. Mutations in familial Wilms' tumor usually take the form of small intragenic deletions. In some affected families, the deletions span several genes and result in a syndrome that includes aniridia, genitourinary tract abnormalities, and mental retardation in addition to Wilms' tumor.[94] The genome of the tumors has usually lost the second allele of the *WT1* gene, suggesting that *WT1* behaves as a tumor suppressor gene. The gene is normally expressed predominantly in the kidney, spleen, gonads, and uterus.[95] Transgenic mice lacking the gene show multiple developmental abnormalities, including complete absence of the kidney and gonads, and die between day 13.5 and 15.5 of embryonic life.[96] The DNA binding

TABLE 1–2

Some Examples of Transcription Factors as Oncogenes and Tumor Suppressor Genes

Gene	Mechanism of Activation/Inactivation	Associated Tumors	Associated Genetic Syndrome
MYC	Gene amplification, translocation, point mutation	Burkitt's lymphoma, many others	
WT1	Deletions, point mutations, translocation	Wilms' tumor, desmoplastic small round cell tumor	Familial Wilms' tumor
PML/RARA	t(15;17)(q22;q21)	Acute myelogenous leukemia M3	
AML/ETO	t(8;21)(q22;q22)	Acute myelogenous leukemia M2	
PAX3/FOXO1A, PAX7/FOXO1A	t(2;13), t(1;13)	Alveolar rhabdomyosarcoma	
EWS/FLI1	t(11;22)	Ewing's sarcoma, peripheral neuroectodermal tumor	

domain of the same gene is involved in the t(11;22) translocation of desmoplastic small round cell tumor.

The *APC* Tumor Suppressor Gene and β-catenin

The *APC* gene functions in a signal transduction pathway related to the WNT/β-catenin family of pathways.[97] The pathway is illustrated in Figure 1–3. These pathways respond to an extracellular signal provided by WNT proteins, a group of homologous proteins sharing a conserved motif of 23 to 24 cysteine residues. These pathways may also respond to signals resulting from cell-cell or cell-matrix interactions involving the cadherins and the integrins. Reception of the WNT signal at the cell membrane appears to involve a complex of proteins, including glypican, a heparan sulfate proteoglycan, and products of a multi-gene family related to the *Frizzled* gene of *Drosophila*. These proteins contain seven hydrophobic membrane spanning domains, placing them within the larger group of "seven-transmembrane" receptors. The extracellular portion of the receptor contains a cysteine-rich domain capable of high-affinity interactions with WNT proteins.

From the receptor, the signal passes to β-catenin, and it is at this site in the pathway that the APC suppressor protein appears to function. The activation state of the pathway is determined by the stability of the β-catenin molecule. In the unactivated state, β-catenin is rapidly degraded by means of the ubiquitin-proteasome pathway. Activation of the pathway blocks ubiquitination of β-catenin, thereby stabilizing the protein and increasing levels of the protein in the cell. The β-catenin then translocates to the nucleus, where it acts by forming a complex

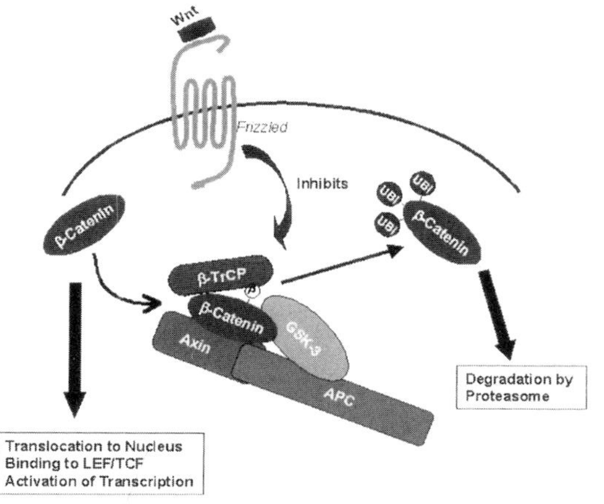

FIGURE 1–3
Role of adenomatous polyposis gene product APC in WNT/β-catenin pathway. Activation of WNT receptor leads to inactivation of the β-catenin destruction complex, which contains APC. Inhibition of destruction complex allows β-catenin to translocate to the nucleus and activate transcription. The active destruction complex phosphorylates β-catenin, providing a signal for ubiquitination (Ubi) and degradation by the proteasome.

with members of the TCF/LEF family of transcription factors. This interaction activates the transcription of target genes involved in promoting cell proliferation. These target genes include those encoding the growth-promoting proteins MYC and cyclin D1.

The adenomatous polyposis coli (APC) protein participates in a multiprotein complex that promotes the degradation of β-catenin. APC interacts with the three proteins, glycogen synthase kinase 3 (GSK-3), axin, and the β-transducin repeat containing protein (β-TrCP), to form the "destruction complex" that destabilizes β-catenin in the absence of WNT signaling. Axin and APC serve as scaffolds that bind β-catenin and GSK-3. GSK-3 phosphorylates β-catenin on serine and threonine residues near its amino terminus. The protein β-TrCP, a component of the E3-ubiquitin ligase complex SCF, recognizes the phosphorylated β-catenin, leading to its ubiquitination and degradation in the proteasome. The mechanism by which WNT binding to its receptor leads to inactivation of the destruction complex is not yet clear. Ther is evidence that supports the roles for decreased phosphorylation of axin and physical disassembly of the destruction complex as mechanisms for its inactivation

The *APC* gene maps to chromosome 5q21.[98] Germline mutations are responsible for familial adenomatous polyposis, and somatic mutations occur in a high percentage of sporadic colon cancers.[99] Most germline mutations are deletions or nonsense mutations, resulting in protein truncation.[100] These truncated proteins lack a region in the central third of the molecule that is required for binding to β-catenin and Axin. Consequently, they fail to form a functional destruction complex, leading to marked elevation in steady-state β-catenin levels and constitutive activation of the WNT/β-catenin signaling pathway. Experiments with transgenic mice have demonstrated that knockout of the gene results in embryonic lethality before the eighth day of gestation. Mice heterozygous for the *APC* mutation develop a syndrome similar to familial adenomatous polyposis, characterized by large numbers of intestinal tumors.

Although the size of the *APC* gene and the lack of clustering of mutations makes screening by direct DNA sequencing impractical, mutations can often be detected by means of the protein truncation test.[101, 102] Because nonsense and frameshift mutations constitute more than 95% of all APC alterations, this test has a high degree of sensitivity. The test involves PCR amplification of either genomic APC sequence or reverse transcribed APC mRNA. The PCR product is then subjected to in vitro transcription and translation, followed by separation of the proteins by gel electrophoresis. The presence of a nonsense or frameshift mutation results in premature termination of protein synthesis, resulting in a smaller in vitro translation product than expected from the wild-type sequence.

The identification of β-catenin as a focal point of signal transduction and as the putative target of the APC protein raised the theoretical possibility that mutations that rendered β-catenin resistant to the destruction complex could contribute to the malignant phenotype. Such mutations have in fact been identified.[103–105] The β-catenin mutations cluster at the four sites of phosphorylation targeted by GSK3, namely the serines at positions 33 and 37 and threonines at 41 and 45. Other mutations that have been identified include missense mutations at positions 31 and 34, which flank one of the phosphorylation sites, and deletion of exon 3. Mutations in β-catenin have been identified in about 13% of cases of colorectal carcinoma, 14% of endometrial carcinoma, 20% of hepatocellular carcinoma, and 15% of ovarian carcinoma.

The *PTEN* Tumor Suppressor Gene

The *PTEN* gene (alternative names *MMAC1* and *TEP1*) was identified as a tumor suppressor gene through several lines of investigation. Analysis of homozygous deletions at chromosome 10q23 in a variety of cancer cell lines identified the novel gene in a region where the deletions overlapped.[106] Homozygous deletions at this locus had been identified in a high percentage of cases of glioblastoma multiforme.[107] The gene encodes a 5.5-kb mRNA. Sequence analysis of the predicted gene product revealed a domain homologous to protein tyrosine phosphatases and to tensin, a protein that links actin filaments to focal adhesions at the plasma membrane. The gene was found to be mutated in breast, kidney, and prostate cancer cell lines and in primary glioblastomas. Germline mutations in the gene result in Cowden disease, an autosomal dominant multiple hamartoma syndrome associated with a predisposition to skin, breast, and thyroid cancer.[108, 109] Another genetic hamartoma syndrome, named either the Bannayan-Zonana or the Rubalcalva-Riley-Smith syndrome, is also usually associated with mutations in the *PTEN* gene. In the genetic diseases, mutations can be missense, nonsense, insertions, deletions, or splice site mutations. These mutations are scattered throughout the gene, with a hot spot in exon 5, which encodes the phosphatase domain.[110] Mutations in the gene in breast cancer are rare except in association with Cowden's disease.[111–115] A study of the gene in 35 melanoma cell lines revealed deletions of the *PTEN* gene, either partial or complete, in nine cases (26%) and a mutation combined with loss of the second allele in another six cases (17%).[116] An analysis of 34 glioblastomas found mutations in 15 cases (44%). In the manner of a classic tumor suppressor gene, all of the mutations detected were associated with LOH at the *PTEN* locus. Conversely, of 25 (74%) of the cases demonstrating LOH, mutations were identified in 15 cases (60%).[117] In gynecologic malignancies, the gene has been reported to be mutated frequently in endometrial carcinoma, but not in cervical or ovarian cancers.[118–120] A study of 60 adenocarcinomas of the prostate found homozygous deletions in eight cases but no point mutations or internal deletions.[121] Mutations of the gene were found to be rare in head and neck squamous cell carcinoma, non–small cell lung cancer, bladder cancer, renal cell carcinomas, adenocarcinoma of the pancreas; and non-Hodgkin's lymphoma.[122–126]

The discovery of the PTEN phosphatase confirmed the prediction that naturally occurring antagonists to the tyrosine kinases that activate signal transduction pathways would exist, could function by dephosphorylation of activated signaling molecules, and would function as tumor suppressors.[127] Although the PTEN phosphatase has demonstrable activity on protein substrates, biochemical analysis of the protein suggests that its physiologically more important function may be as a lipid phosphatase.[128] The protein can dephosphorylate phosphatidylinositol 3,4,6-trisphosphate (PIP3) at position 3 on the inositol ring.[129, 130] The dephosphorylation of PIP3 may inactivate the protein kinase B (PKB, or AKT) signaling pathway.[131–134] In keeping with this concept, glioblastoma cell lines containing mutated PTEN have been shown to have increased PKB/Akt activity.[135] Activation of this pathway is believed to protect cells from apoptosis. In further support of the importance of the lipid phosphatase activity of PTEN, a point mutation, G129E, identified in a Cowden disease family, specifically inhibited the activity of the protein on lipid substrates.[136] In transfection experiments, overexpression of wild-type PTEN inhibited focal adhesion formation and cell spreading and the protein associated with the focal adhesion kinase (FAK).[137] The ability of the gene to function as a tumor suppressor has been demonstrated directly in a glioblastoma cell line by adenovirus mediated gene transfer.[138] Expression of the gene inhibited anchorage-independent cell growth and tumorigenicity in nude mice.

The *VHL* Tumor Suppressor Gene

The von Hippel-Lindau syndrome is an autosomal dominant tumor syndrome characterized by hemangioblastomas of the cerebellum, vascular lesions of the central nervous system and retina, renal cell carcinoma, pheochromocytoma, pancreatic islet cell tumors, and endolymphatic sac tumors. The syndrome results from mutations in a gene on chromosome 3p25.5 designated *VHL*.[139–141] Tumors in von Hippel-Lindau syndrome show loss of the second allele of the gene, in accordance with the two-hit model for tumor suppressor genes.[142] Mutations of *VHL* are common in sporadic renal cell carcinomas and hemangioblastomas but have not been identified in sporadic tumors other than those associated with the von Hippel-Lindau syndrome.[143]

The product of the *VHL* gene is a protein of approximately 30 kd localized predominantly to the cytoplasm.[144–146] The protein inhibits expression of a group of genes that share the property of being inducible by hypoxia, including the gene for vascular endothelial growth factor (VEGF). This regulation may occur post-transcriptionally, at the level of mRNA stability.[147] Because the hypoxia-induced genes tend to induce blood vessel formation, the absence of normal repression of such genes resulting from mutational inactivation of the *VHL* gene leads to abnormal angiogenesis, accounting for the vascular nature of the tumors associated with the syndrome. The protein forms a complex with the proteins elongin B, elongin C, and cullin 2.[102, 148] Many of the germline mutations in the gene result in a protein that is unable to bind to this multiprotein complex. The proteins elongin C and cullin 2 are homologous to the yeast proteins Skp1 and Cdc53, which function to target specific proteins for degradation through ubiquitination. This homology has led to the proposal that the VHL protein may be involved in activating the degradation of proteins involved in stabilizing hypoxia-induced mRNAs.[149, 150]

Identification of mutations in the gene has clinical use in identifying affected family members so that surveillance for associated tumors can begin at an early age.[151] About half of the germline lesions are missense or nonsense mutations that can be identified by amplifying each of the three exons containing coding sequence by PCR and sequencing the products. In about 20% of cases, the syndrome results from a germline deletion that can be detected by Southern blot analysis but may be missed by PCR. These methods fail to detect a *VHL* mutation in about 20% of families with von-Hippel-Lindau syndrome.[152] The nature of the mutation has been associated with the phenotypic expression of the syndrome: missense mutations account for 96% of mutations in von Hippel-Lindau syndrome type 2 (with pheochromocytoma) whereas truncating mutations, including deletions, insertions, or nonsense mutations, have been found in 56% of von-Hippel-Lindau syndrome type 1 (without pheochromocytoma).[153]

Cell Cycle Regulation

Several oncogenes and tumor suppressor genes can best be categorized as regulators of the cell cycle (Table 1–3). These include the gene responsible for familial retinoblastoma, *RB1*, and the tumor suppressor gene *TP53*, which is found mutated in a wide variety of human cancers. The oncogenes of the DNA tumor viruses, including the human papillomaviruses (HPVs) important in the pathogenesis of cervical carcinoma, also fall into this category. As in mitogenic signal transduction, a series of protein kinases act in the pathway: their activators have the capacity to function as oncoproteins, whereas their inhibitors can act as tumor suppressors.

Replicating cells pass progressively through phases of the cell cycle designated G_1, S, G_2, and M, where S represents the period of replicative DNA synthesis, M indicates mitosis, and G_1 and G_2 refer to the "gaps" before and after DNA synthesis, respectively. Many of the proteins involved in progression through the cycle have now been identified.[154] Overall, the scheme of progression and regulation of the cell cycle may be depicted as a circle representing the successive phases of the cycle with controls on progression radiating from the center, meeting the circle near the junctions between phases (Fig. 1–4). The negative regulatory pathways radiating from the center of this diagram represent the mechanisms by which the cell imposes certain conditions that must be met before the cell can advance to the subsequent phase. Before DNA synthesis can begin, the cell checks for and senses DNA damage. If detected, the pathway directs a signal to the cell cycle progression machinery that blocks progression into S phase. The points in the cell cycle at which the regulatory pathways impinge on the mechanisms moving the cell cycle forward are referred to as cell cycle checkpoints. The checkpoint that has received the most attention in studies of the pathogenesis of cancer regulates the progression from G_1 to S phase, although increasing attention has been focused on the role of the oncogenes and tumor suppressor genes, particularly *TP53* and *ATM* (the latter being the gene responsible for ataxia-telangiectasia), in regulating mitotic and G_2 checkpoints.[155] Some of the key participants in these checkpoints are indicated in Figure 1–4.

A family of proteins known collectively as the *cyclins* constitute an important part of the mechanism that drives the cell through the cell cycle. As originally defined, a cyclin is a protein expressed at a specific phase of the cell cycle. The cyclin family consists of cyclins A through E, plus several subtypes designated numerically, such as cyclins D1 through D4. Each cyclin shows marked variation in expression throughout the cell cycle and has a characteristic peak expression at a specific phase of the cycle. Cyclin A shows peak expression in late G_1 and early S phase. Maximum expression of cyclin B occurs in G_2. Cyclins C, D, and E peak in early to mid G_1. At the end of the expression peak, cyclins are removed from the cell by proteolytic degradation through the ubiquitin-proteasome pathway. In this pathway, the cyclin becomes covalently modified by the addition of multiple copies of the small 6-kd molecule ubiquitin, which targets the protein for degradation.

The cyclins do not have any known intrinsic enzymatic activity but rather function as cofactors that bind to and activate a group of Ser/Thr protein kinases, the *cyclin-dependent kinases*, or CDKs. These kinases specifically phosphorylate proteins that cause the cell to advance to the next phase of the cell cycle. For example, the CDK1/Cyclin B (CCNB1) complex controls the $G_2 \rightarrow M$ transition.[156] In early G1, synthesis of the D type cyclins activates CDK4 and CDK6. Later in G1, cyclin E expression increases, resulting in activation of CDK2. The three activated CDK complexes, cyclin D with CDKs 4 and 6 and cyclin E/CDK2, phosphorylate proteins required for the cell to advance to S phase. One of the most

TABLE 1–3

Cell Cycle Regulators as Oncogenes and Tumor Suppressor Genes

Gene	Mechanism of Activation/Inactivation	Associated Tumors	Associated Genetic Syndrome
Cyclin D1 (*CCND1*)	Overexpression	Breast, esophagus, liver, parathyroid adenoma, mantle cell lymphoma	
CDK4	Overexpression	Melanoma, sarcoma, glioblastoma	Familial melanoma
CDKN2A *ARF*	Deletion, point mutation	Many	Familial melanoma
RB1	Inactivation by point mutations, deletions	Retinoblastoma osteosarcoma	Familial retinoblastoma, osteosarcoma
TP53	Inactivation by point mutations, deletions	Many	Li-Fraumeni syndrome
ATM	Deletions, point mutations; protein truncations common	Leukemias and lymphomas, others	Ataxia-telangiectasia
HPV E6, E7	Viral infection	Cervical cancer	

important of these is the product of the retinoblastoma tumor suppressor gene *RB1*.[157–159]

Phosphorylation of the RB1 protein results in the transcriptional activation of the proteins required for DNA replication, including the DNA polymerases. In its unphosphorylated state, the 105-kd RB1 protein binds to the E2F family of transcription factors and prevents them from functioning as transcriptional activators. As a result of phosphorylation of RB1, the E2F proteins are released and activate transcription by binding to specific target sequences.

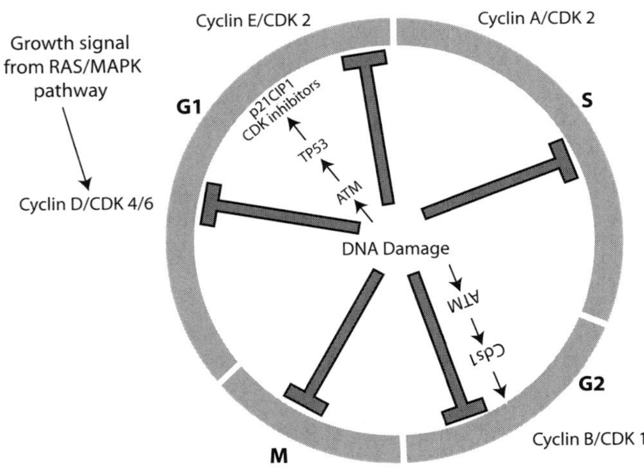

FIGURE 1–4
Regulators of the cell cycle. Growth signals from the RAS/MAP kinase and other pathways communicate with the cell cycle regulatory mechanisms in part by activating transcription of cyclin D. Different cyclin/CDK complexes activate progression through the successive stages of the cell cycle. Checkpoint regulatory pathways respond to DNA damage by sending inhibitory signals that act at various points in the cell cycle.

Normal cells will undergo growth arrest at the G_1-S checkpoint in the cell cycle after DNA damage or nutritional deprivation. Growth stimulatory signals transmitted down the RAS/MAP kinase pathway activate the cell cycle machinery. In response to such a signal, transcription factors activated by MAP kinase activate transcription of the cyclin D gene, leading to increased levels of the cyclin D/CDK4/6 complex, hyperphosphorylation of RB1, and, consequently, progression to S phase.

Opposing these events, which advance the cell from G_1 to S phase, is the $G_1 \rightarrow S$ checkpoint. This checkpoint comprises a group of proteins that functions to sense when DNA replication should not occur. For example, the checkpoint becomes activated in the presence of damaged DNA, which could be present after exposure to ultraviolet irradiation or a chemical carcinogen. The temporary halt in cell cycle progression allows the DNA repair machinery to act before the process of DNA replication induces permanent deleterious changes, such as point mutations, deletions, or translocations, into the genome.

The $G_1 \rightarrow S$ checkpoint involves several proteins of great importance to the pathogenesis of cancer, including the CDK inhibitors CDKN2A and P19ARF, the products of *TP53* and *RB1*, and the product of the *ATM* gene. The CDK inhibitors function in direct opposition to the cyclins, which are CDK activators. The expression of at least one CDK inhibitor, CDKN1A, is directly regulated by p53 in its role as a transcription factor. The gene encoding a CDK4-specific inhibitor, *CDKN2A*, is a frequent target of mutations in a variety of tumors, an observation that led to its alternative designation as *MTS*, for multiple tumor suppressor.[160] Characterization of the *CDKN2A* gene has revealed that this locus encodes three distinct proteins involved in cell cycle regulation. This segment of chromosome 9p encodes two CDK4 inhibitors, CDKN2A and CDKN2B. In addition, a protein encoded by a gene that overlaps the *CDKN2A* coding sequence but is translated in a different reading frame encodes the protein P19ARF.[161] The P19ARF protein functions as an inhibitor of MDM2-mediated degradation of p53; therefore, expression of this protein stabilizes p53 in the cell.[162–164] Deletion of this single locus therefore results in loss of both p53 and CDK4 inhibitors, severely compromising $G_1 \rightarrow S$ checkpoint regulation.

Current evidence supports the checkpoint pathway shown in Figure 1–4, linking ATM through p53 to the CDK inhibitors.[165–168] The protein product of the *ATM* gene is a protein Ser/Thr kinase with sequence homology to a family of PI3K-related kinases.[169] Another member of this family is a DNA-dependent protein kinase, which may be involved in the response to DNA damage in a manner similar to ATM.[170] The ATM protein may specifically bind to and become activated by double-stranded breaks in DNA, thereby serving as the first protein to respond to DNA damage.[171]

The activated ATM protein can bind to and phosphorylate p53 at a key regulatory site, serine-15, an event that eventually leads to elevated p53 protein levels in the cell.[172–176] The mechanism by which this occurs involves another p53 regulatory protein, MDM2. The MDM2 protein binds to p53 through its amino terminus, blocks its transactivation function, and targets it for destruction through the ubiquitin-proteasome pathway.[177–179] Once phosphorylated at critical sites, which include serines at positions 15 and 20, the p53 molecule has a reduced affinity for MDM2.[180, 181] As a result, the rate of destruction of the protein decreases and increased levels of the protein accumulate in the cell.

The regulatory pathway controlling the $G_1 \rightarrow S$ transition includes the products of the oncogenes cyclin D1 and *CDK4* and the tumor suppressor genes *RB1*, *TP53*, and *ATM*.

CYCLIN D1 (*CCND1*)

The cyclin D1 protein is frequently overexpressed in carcinomas of the breast, esophagus, and liver. Overexpression in carcinomas usually is a result of gene amplification. In two specific neoplasms, overexpression of cyclin D1 results from a specific chromosomal translocation. In parathyroid adenomas, a pericentric inversion of chromosome 11 places the cyclin D1 gene on 11q32 close to the parathyroid hormone (PTH) gene on 11p15.[182–184] As a result, the cyclin D1 gene falls under the influence of the transcriptional regulatory mechanisms of PTH, resulting in cyclin D1 overexpression. This translocation led to the original identification of the cyclin D1 gene as "parathyroid adenoma 1," or *PRAD1*. A similar mechanism results in transcriptional activation of the cyclin D1 gene in the t(11;14) translocation of mantle cell lymphoma. This translocation places the cyclin D1 gene on chromosome 11 adjacent to the immunoglobulin heavy chain locus on 14q32. The initial work to analyze the chromosome 11 breakpoints involved in this translocation found that the 11q13 breakpoints tended to cluster within a small segment of DNA a few thousand nucleotides in length.[185, 186] This region was designated BCL1, for "breakpoint cluster locus 1." Hence the cyclin D1 gene is sometimes referred to as the *BCL1* oncogene.[187]

Diagnostically, detection of cyclin D1 overexpression has substantial utility in distinguishing mantle cell lymphoma from other lymphomas, because the cyclin D1 gene rarely shows significant levels of expression in other types of lymphoma. A PCR-based method has been described with high sensitivity and specificity for this purpose.[188] The t(11;14) translocation can be detected by Southern blot analysis of tumor DNA or by PCR-based methods; however, the sensitivity of PCR is low for detection of this translocation, owing to the variability of the 11q13 breakpoints.[188, 189]

CDK4

Overexpression of CDK4 due to gene amplification has been reported in melanomas, sarcomas, and glioblastoma. Rare cases of familial melanoma have been associated with mutations in the *CDK4* gene.[190–192]

CDKN2A

Mutations of the locus encoding both CDKN2A proteins occur frequently in multiple tumor types. Mutations take the form of deletions, often encompassing the entire gene. Germline mutations have been identified in approximately 20% of cases of familial melanoma.[190–193] Functional analysis of the mutant proteins usually demonstrates deficiencies in ability to bind CDK4, to inhibit the kinase activity, or to induce cell cycle arrest after transfection into cultured cells.

RB1

The 105-kd RB1 protein[8] participates in cell cycle regulation through the interaction with other proteins, including the E2F transcription factor family, which now includes at least six members. Protein-protein interactions occur through a region of the RB1 molecule termed the *pocket domain*.[158] A conserved sequence motif, LXCXE, is present in several RB1 ligands and forms a key element of the interaction site. A nine amino acid peptide from the papillomavirus E7 protein bound to the pocket of RB1 has been crystallized and its structure determined.[194] The structure revealed direct interactions between the LXCXE motif and a groove in the domain within the pocket termed the *B box*. A second domain, the *A box*, serves to stabilize the structure of the B box. Two proteins containing regions homologous to the pocket domain of RB1 have been identified, RBL1 (P107) and RBL2 (P130). Although these proteins can interact with many of the same proteins as RB1, they have not been found to be the target of mutations in cancers and are not considered to be tumor suppressor genes. The three pocket-containing proteins differ in their relative affinities for the different E2F family members and their level of expression at different phases of the cell cycle.[195]

Despite the key role of RB1 in cell cycle regulation, studies with transgenic mice have demonstrated that cells can divide and begin the differentiation sequence in the complete absence of RB1 but fail to complete the differentiation process.[196] Embryos of RB1 knockout mice die between 13 and 15 days of gestation. These embryos show marked defects in development of the hematopoietic and nervous systems. Increased apoptosis was noted in tissues of the central and peripheral nervous system, as was evidence of deficiencies in maintaining cells in a noncycling, quiescent state. Thus the RB1 protein has an important function in inhibiting progression through the cell cycle. In addition, the protein seems to play an important role in the induction of terminal differentiation. In several experimental systems of cell differentiation, cells deficient in RB1 expression can be induced to express early markers of differentiation but not later ones.[197, 198]

Germline mutations in the *RB1* gene on chromosome 13q14 result in familial retinoblastoma.[8] The familial syndrome is also associated with a high incidence of osteosarcoma. Routine detection of mutations in the gene is not practical at this time because the gene is large and mutations may occur over a wide region.

p53

The p53 protein plays a role in a wide variety of human cancers.[199] The crucial role of p53 in cell cycle checkpoint regulation has led to its designation as the "guardian of the genome"[200] and the "gatekeeper for growth and division."[201] Mutation of *TP53*, one of the most common genetic abnormalities in human cancers, leads to defects in checkpoint control and genetic instability in cancer cells. The p53 protein also appears to play a pivotal role in directing cells toward programmed cell death, or apoptosis.[202] Several specific functions have been assigned to the p53 protein.

Many of the biologic properties of p53 are thought to emanate from its role as a transcription factor, in which the protein binds to specific DNA sequences and activates specific genes. Mutations of p53 in cancers almost always abrogate this transactivation function of the protein. Studies of the DNA binding specificity of p53 have identified the motif 5′-PuPuPuGA/T as the target sequence recognized by the protein. The protein exists as a tetramer that recognizes sites containing four copies of this motif. The amino terminus of the protein contains a transcriptional activation domain. In addition to binding to a specific DNA sequence, the protein contains a domain near the carboxyl terminus that binds specifically to a component of the basal transcriptional apparatus, the TATA-binding protein TBP.[203] Searches for proteins related to p53 have identified two proteins, p73 and p63, which have similar transcriptional activity but are not mutated in cancer.[204]

The first gene convincingly demonstrated to be regulated by p53 was that encoding the CDK inhibitor CDKN1A, alternatively named *WAF1*.[205] A broader search for genes induced by p53 has been conducted in an experimental system by serial analysis of gene expression (SAGE).[206] This method involves the conversion of each mRNA present in a cell extract into a 9-nt sequence, or "tag." The tags are concatenated, amplified by PCR, and analyzed by DNA sequencing. Tabulation of the frequency with which each tag occurs reflects the relative level of expression of that tag, and therefore the corresponding mRNA, in the original specimen. Through the use of an inducible p53 expression system developed in the colorectal carcinoma cell line DLD-1, gene expression patterns were compared before and 9 hours after induction of p53 induction. Analysis of more than 50,000 tags from each of the two specimens, corresponding to 9,954 distinct individual genes, revealed 34 tags represented in at least 10-fold greater abundance after p53 induction, approximately half of which corresponded to known genes. Among these were the CDKN1A inhibitor previously identified as a p53 target, the *JUNB* proto-oncogene, a tyrosine kinase, and the gene for thrombospondin 1, an extracellular protein implicated in tumor suppression. Other genes that had previously been reported to be regulated by p53 include *BAX*, *PIG3*, *14-3-3σ*, *MDM2*, *GADD45*, *cyclin G1*, *FAS*, and *cathepsin D1*.[207] The expression of candidate p53 inducible genes was studied in five additional cell lines. Only eight genes were consistently induced in all five lines (*Caveolin*, *DR5*, *GPC*, *14-3-3σ*, *CDKN1A*, *HO1*, *EPHB4*, and *BAX*). The response of the other genes tested showed marked variability among cell lines.

Treatment with the chemotherapeutic agents doxorubicin and 5-fluorouracil induces increased levels of p53 expression. Examination of the response of the candidate p53 inducible genes to treatment of cell lines with these agents revealed that many of the 34 genes tested were induced by treatment with one or both of these agents. However, there was substantial heterogeneity in the response of two cell lines tested. Surprisingly, most of the genes responded equally well to chemotherapeutic agents even in cells lacking p53. Only three genes (*CDKN1A*, *PIG3*, and *MDM2*) showed a marked reduction in response to doxorubicin or 5-fluorouracil in p53-negative cells. Therefore, the results of this extensive analysis suggest that the total number of genes that respond to p53 at the level of transcription is actually quite small and that of these genes only a subset are dependent on p53 for induction in response to exposure to 5-fluorouracil or doxorubicin.

Mutations of *TP53* in Human Cancer. The spectrum of *TP53* mutations has been analyzed in a wide variety of human malignancies.[208–212] The specific type of mutation, and in some cases even a specific mutation, has been interpreted as evidence for a specific carcinogen. In lung cancer, three "hot spots," at amino acids 157, 248, and 273, account for a high percentage of mutations.[213] These sites correspond to genomic sites most likely to be modified by chemical carcinogens in cigarette smoke. One specific mutation, a codon 249 G→T transversion, has been identified in more than 50% of hepatocellular carcinomas from areas of Africa and India with high levels of aflatoxin exposure.[214] Other mutations are characteristic of ultraviolet light–induced skin cancers. Whereas transversions (purine→pyrimidine or pyrimidine→purine) predominate in carcinomas of the lung and liver, transitions (pyrimidine→pyrimidine or purine→purine) predominate in cancers of the colon, brain, and hematopoietic system.[215]

The Li-Fraumeni Syndrome. Li-Fraumeni syndrome refers to a familial predisposition to develop multiple cancers, including breast cancer, sarcomas, and brain tumors, at an early age.[216, 217] In 80% of these cases, the syndrome results from a germline mutation in *TP53*. Most mutations are missense, but splice site and nonsense mutations have also been observed.[218, 219]

ATM

The *ATM* gene, located on chromosome 11q23, encodes the gene responsible for ataxia-telangiectasia, an autosomal recessive syndrome characterized by radiation sensitivity, immunodeficiency, cerebellar ataxia, cutaneous telangiectasia, and a predisposition to lymphoid malignancy.[220–222] The carrier frequency for mutations in the *ATM* gene has been estimated as approximately 1%.

The *ATM* gene contains 66 exons spanning approximately 150 kb of genomic DNA.[166, 223] Mutations are widespread throughout the gene, with more than 70% resulting in truncation of the gene product. Because of the large size of the gene, screening for mutations is not practical at the present time.

ONCOGENES OF DNA TUMOR VIRUSES

The oncoproteins of the DNA tumor viruses promote cell growth at least in part through their interference with the G_1/S cell cycle checkpoint. The current understanding of these proteins derives from basic research into the biology of the simian papovavirus SV40 and the adenoviruses. These viruses made suitable models for laboratory studies because they are easily propagated in tissue culture, can be readily purified, and are amenable to both genetic and biochemical analysis. The insights derived through the use of these model systems provided the basis for experimental approaches that have revealed the transforming mechanism of the HPVs, which play an important role in human cancer.[224–226] Specific segments of the viral genome were identified as having transforming activity in experimental systems. Molecular dissection of this transforming activity led to the conclusion that the critical genes for the transforming activity of the viruses were the large T antigen of SV40 and the two genes designated E1A and E1B of the adenoviruses. Biochemical analysis of these viral oncoproteins resulted in the identification of two proteins that later proved to be tumor suppressors of great importance in human cancers: p53 and RB1. The SV40 large T antigen was found to be complexed with a 53-kd protein, the level of which was highly elevated in SV40 transformed fibroblasts. Therefore, it was initially thought that this protein, p53, was a transforming protein. Subsequent studies eventually favored the interpretation that the interaction with large T antigen actually inactivated the suppressor activity of p53 rather than activating it. A similar interaction with p53 was observed in the adenovirus system with the transforming protein E1B.

Biochemical analysis of the adenovirus E1A protein identified several specific proteins that co-precipitated with E1A from crude lysates of infected cells.[227] One of these proteins proved to be RB1, the product of the retinoblastoma tumor suppressor gene *RB1* that had been identified only 2 years previously.[228] A similar interaction with RB1 was subsequently identified in the SV40 system. In SV40, the large T antigen was found to form a complex with RB1.[229] The observations with SV40 and adenovirus suggested that the DNA tumor viruses might share a common mechanism of cell transformation involving interaction with the tumor suppressor proteins p53 and RB1. Subsequent studies demonstrated that the transforming proteins encoded by the oncogenic papillomaviruses act in a similar fashion.[230]

Whereas neither SV40 nor the adenoviruses have been implicated in human cancers, the knowledge derived from these systems formed the basis for an understanding of the transforming genes of the HPVs, which have an etiologic role in cancer of the cervix.[231] In contrast to the viruses favored for early experimental studies, the HPVs cannot be propagated efficiently in tissue culture. Genetic analysis of the HPVs has generally involved transfection of cloned segments of the viral genome into cells growing in culture. This type of genetic analysis led to the demonstration that two early genes, *E6* and *E7*, were necessary and in some cases sufficient for immortalization of primary human keratinocytes and transformation of primary cultures of rat embryo fibroblasts.[232–234] The transforming and transactivating activities of E7 were noted to bear several similarities to those of the adenovirus E1A protein.[224] With the discovery of the E1A-RB1 interaction, it was noted that the E7 protein contained sequences similar to the RB1 binding sequences of E1A. The E7 protein was then shown to have the ability to bind to RB1 in vitro.[235, 236]

The parallels between the HPVs and the other DNA tumor viruses were extended with the demonstration that the E6 protein binds to p53.[225] Thus, the oncoproteins of SV40, adenovirus, and the HPVs share the ability to bind to the tumor suppressor proteins RB1 and p53 (Fig. 1–5). However, cells experimentally transformed by HPV as well as several HPV-containing cell lines, including the HeLa cell line used extensively in research laboratories, were found to contain little or no detectable p53 protein by immunoblot analysis. This contrasted sharply to observations made with SV40 large T antigen expressing cells, which expressed very large amounts of p53. When RNA levels were examined, it was found that p53 RNA was readily detectable in the HPV transformed cell lines. It was therefore proposed that the result of the E6-p53 interaction might be a destabilization of p53. Destabilization of p53 by E6 was first demonstrated in vitro in a series of experiments that implicated the ubiquitin-proteasome pathway in the proteolytic destruction of p53 mediated by E6.[237] The ability of E6 to induce p53 degradation in vivo was demonstrated by expressing cloned complementary DNAs for the E6 and p53 proteins into a p53-negative cell line.[238]

If the HPV oncogenes act by blocking the suppressor activities of p53 and RB1, then it might be expected that mutations of these tumor suppressor genes in HPV-containing tumors would be uncommon. This concept has been supported by several studies. Analysis of the *TP53* sequence of five HPV-positive cervical cancer cell lines revealed only the wild-type sequence, whereas mutations were identified in two HPV-negative cervical cancer cell lines.[239] Studies of primary cervical carcinomas containing oncogenic HPV types confirm that *TP53* mutation occurs only rarely in this kind of tumor.[240, 241]

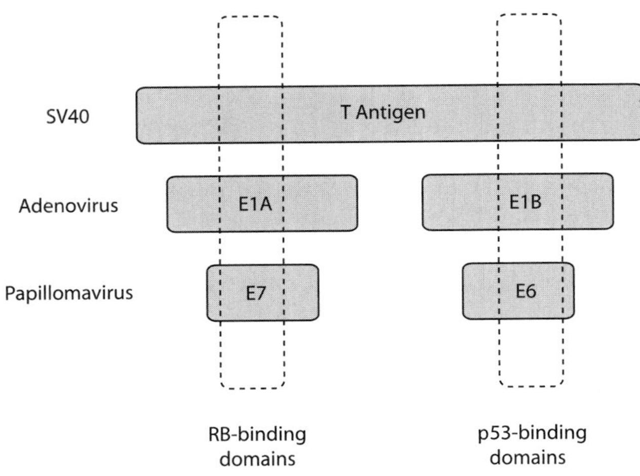

FIGURE 1–5
Viral oncogenes of SV40, adenovirus, and human papillomavirus function by binding to and inactivating the tumor suppressor gene products p53 and RB1.

DNA Replication and Repair

The group of genes encoding the proteins involved in maintaining genomic integrity constitutes a distinct class of oncogenes and tumor suppressor genes. This class includes the mismatch repair genes involved in hereditary nonpolyposis colon cancer (HNPCC), the enzyme telomerase that maintains the length of telomeres during cell division, and the genes *BRCA1* and *BRCA2*, which are mutated in familial breast cancer (Table 1–4).

MISMATCH REPAIR GENES

The importance of mismatch repair genes in human cancer became apparent with the identification of the genetic basis for hereditary nonpolyposis colon cancer (HNPCC). This familial predisposition to cancer accounts for 5% to 8% of all cases of colorectal carcinoma.[242] Genetic analysis of tumors occurring in patients with this syndrome revealed that the large majority demonstrated the property of microsatellite instability. As described earlier in the discussion of loss of heterozygosity, a microsatellite is a short segment of genomic DNA consisting of multiple tandem repeats of a simple DNA sequence, usually a di-, tri-, or tetranucleotide, with an allele pattern that is identical throughout the benign diploid somatic tissues of an individual. Analysis of tumor DNA sometimes reveals a novel allele not present in the benign somatic tissues of the same individual. This finding, which results from an error in DNA replication consisting of either the insertion of extra repeat units or the deletion of such units from a microsatellite, is called microsatellite instability (MSI). If enough loci are examined, isolated examples of MSI can be identified in many tumors. However, some tumors demonstrate MSI with a very high frequency. These are considered to have a specific phenotype associated with high-frequency MSI, now commonly referred to as the "replication error," or "RER+" phenotype. This phenotype is a property of tumors in HNPCC and has also been associated with about 10% of sporadic colorectal cancers.[99]

The genes responsible for the RER+ phenotype have been identified and cloned. These DNA mismatch repair genes include *MSH2*, *MLH1*, *PMS1*, and *PMS2*. Mutations in these genes account for most cases of HNPCC. One review has summarized the reported prevalence of mutations by gene as 50% for *MSH2*, 30% for *MLH1*, 5% for *PMS1*, and 5% for *PMS2*.[243]

TELOMERASE

The ends of chromosomes consist of specialized structures called telomeres. In humans, telomeres consist almost entirely of tandem repeats of the hexanucleotide TTAGGG. Telomeres in other species similarly consist of repeating units of 5 to 8 nucleotides, with the exact

TABLE 1–4

Oncogenes and Tumor Suppressor Genes in DNA Replication and Repair Pathways

Oncogene/Gene	Mechanism of Activation/Inactivation	Associated Tumors	Genetic Syndrome
BRCA1	Point mutations, deletions	Breast, ovarian cancer	Familial breast and ovarian cancer
BRCA2	Point mutations, deletions	Breast cancer	Familial breast and ovarian cancer
MSH2, MLH1, PMS1, PMS2	Point mutation	Colorectal cancer	Hereditary nonpolypomatous colon cancer
Telomerase	Transcriptional activation	Activated in most malignant tumors	

sequence depending on the species. The replication of telomeres presents special problems in biochemistry because of a fundamental property of DNA polymerases recognized since the first such enzymes were discovered in bacteria. This property is the dependence of the enzyme on a primer; a DNA polymerase can elongate a DNA strand base paired to a template but cannot initiate a strand de novo. At any site except the termini of a linear double-stranded DNA molecule, specialized enzymes exist to generate primers, in the form of short RNA molecules, which then allow the DNA polymerase to proceed with synthesis of the complementary DNA strand. Completion of the progeny DNA strand requires removal of the primer, leaving a gap in the daughter DNA strand, followed by repair of the gap by extension of the upstream DNA strand. This mechanism fails at the extreme ends of DNA molecules because there is nothing upstream of the gap created by removing the primer. In the absence of a specialized replication mechanism, each round of replication will result in loss of terminal sequence and a shortening of the molecule. The enzyme that overcomes this problem is telomerase.

The shortening of telomeres in replicating somatic cells not expressing telomerase appears to place a limitation on the life span of the cell. The property of immortalization observed in tissue culture cells, and considered to represent an important step on the road to malignant transformation, requires activation of telomerase. Expression of the enzyme is seen in a very high percentage of malignant tumors and immortalized cell lines but not in benign tissues other than germ cells or in nonimmortalized cell lines. The expression of telomerase together with SV40 large T antigen and an activated *RAS* oncogene by transfection suffices to immortalize and confer the property of tumorigenicity on primary human fibroblasts and epithelial cells.[244, 245] The ability of telomerase to cooperate with oncogenes in transforming primary mammalian cells underscores the importance of telomerase expression in malignant transformation.

Telomerase functions as a terminal transferase, a specialized form of DNA polymerase that can extend the 3′-end of a single-stranded DNA molecule but does not require a template strand to copy. Despite the absence of the usual kind of template, the enzyme adds only the specific sequence corresponding to the species specific telomere unit. The sequence specificity of telomerase is determined by a short RNA molecule associated with the telomerase complex. This RNA molecule contains a sequence complementary to the telomere repeat and serves as the template for synthesis of DNA by the enzyme. Because the enzyme copies RNA into DNA, the enzyme is also an example of a reverse transcriptase.

The detection of telomerase may become an important diagnostic test for the identification of cancer cells. Two types of assays to detect telomerase activity have been described. The telomerase repeat amplification protocol (TRAP) assay depends on enzymatically active telomerase in the specimen.[246] Consequently, this assay is applicable only to fresh or frozen tissue. Active enzyme is not present in formalin-fixed or paraffin-embedded material. In the TRAP assay, the specimen is incubated with an oligonucleotide under optimal conditions for telomerase enzymatic activity. The products of this reaction are then subjected to PCR amplification with a second oligonucleotide designed to bind to the telomere repeat unit. The products are separated on a polyacrylamide gel. The presence of telomerase in the specimen results in a ladder of bands resulting from the addition of different multiples of the hexameric telomere repeat to the primer. With the use of the TRAP assay, telomerase activity has been detected in a wide variety of tumors with high frequency. A 1995 review reported that of the data published at that time, which was based on the TRAP assay, 84.8% of tumors but only 4.2% of benign tissues tested positive for telomerase.[247]

A second type of assay directly detects the mRNA that codes for one of the two protein subunits of the telomerase ribonucleoprotein. This protein has been designated TERT, for human telomerase reverse transcriptase. The regulation of this subunit determines telomerase activity, whereas the other protein subunit, TEP, can be expressed by cells lacking the active enzyme.[248] The promoter for the *TERT* gene has been cloned and characterized for the presence of transcriptional regulatory elements.[249–251] These studies revealed a consensus binding site for the MYC protein in a region critical for regulation of gene expression and demonstrated transcriptional activation by MYC in transfection experiments. Therefore, *TERT* may be a direct target of MYC in vivo.

In contrast to the TRAP protocol, the assay for TERT expression does not require active enzyme and therefore has the potential for application to fixed and embedded tissues, assuming that RNA of adequate quality can be recovered. In this assay, a standard reverse transcriptase-PCR reaction is performed using primers specific for the TERT sequence. The PCR product can be detected by electrophoresis or by one of several real-time PCR product detection methodologies currently available.[252] This assay has been applied to urine samples as a diagnostic test for bladder cancer, with a reported sensitivity of approximately 80% and a specificity of greater than 90%.[253] Similar methods have been applied to fine-needle aspirates of thyroid nodules,[254] demonstrating sensitive and specific detection of papillary and follicular carcinoma in such specimens. A real-time quantitative PCR assay for TERT was applied to a series of breast cancer cases.[252] This study demonstrated correlations between TERT expression and reduced survival, higher histologic grade, and estrogen and progesterone receptor negativity. A significant correlation was also observed between MYC overexpression and TERT positivity, a result consistent with the idea that the MYC protein may directly regulate TERT.

BRCA1 AND *BRCA2*

The identification of families with an inherited predisposition to breast cancer led to the search for and discovery of two breast cancer susceptibility genes, *BRCA1* and *BRCA2*.[255, 256] Extensive genetic characterization of the affected families progressively narrowed the candidate genetic loci, on 17q12-21 for *BRCA1* and on 13q12 for *BRCA2*, until a specific target region containing only a few genes remained.[257–260] Sequencing of the candidate region identified unique genes at each locus that consistently demonstrated mutations in affected family members. Furthermore, these mutations consistently segregated with the cancer predisposition phenotype in pedigrees, further supporting the identification of these genes as the ones responsible for the syndrome. Familial breast cancer is estimated to represent approximately 10% of all breast cancer. The *BRCA1* and *BRCA2* genes together are believed to account for more than 80% of cases of familial breast cancer.[261]

Progress in understanding the function of the proteins encoded by these positionally cloned genes has been slow, due to the lack of functional assays and to the lack of significant homologies to known proteins. Significant insight into the function of these proteins has come from transgenic mouse models, the characterization of protein-protein interactions, and the development of functional assays. The evidence now supports a role for these proteins in DNA repair.[262, 263] Interestingly, although the proteins do not share homologous amino acid sequences, they function in similar pathways, participate in the same multiprotein complexes, and share certain similarities in the overall structure of their genes. Both genes have a total length of approximately 80 kb and contain a large exon containing more than half of the total coding sequence. The proteins encoded by these genes are large: 1843 amino acids for *BRCA1* and 3418 for *BRCA2*. The amino terminus of *BRCA1* contains a motif known as a RING finger, a cysteine- and histidine-rich domain involved in protein-protein and protein-DNA interactions.[264] This motif appears to target proteins for ubiquitin-mediated degradation.

Several transgenic mouse models of *BRCA1* and *BRCA2* mutation have been reported. Homozygous deletion of either gene results in embryonic lethality between 5.5 and 13.5 days of gestation. Heterozygosity for such a deletion yields mice that develop normally and show no increased susceptibility to tumor development. A transgenic mouse engineered to delete *BRCA1* exon 11 specifically in the ductal epithelium of the breast showed abnormalities in breast development, including small size and abnormal branching of ducts.[265] Approximately 20% of these mice developed tumors of the breast, both benign and malignant, confirming the ability of the gene product to control breast tumorigenesis. These tumors were aneuploid, showed a high frequency of chromosomal rearrangements, and contained mutations in other genes, including *TP53*. The deletion of a *TP53* allele in these mice increased the rate of tumor formation.

Biochemical studies aimed at identifying binding partners for *BRCA1* and *BRCA2* have identified numerous candidates, including the products of the tumor suppressor genes *RB1*, *TP53*, and *ATM;* components of the transcriptional apparatus including RNA helicase A; the P300/CBP histone deacetylase complex; and proteins involved in homologous recombination and DNA repair.[266] One complex of particular importance contains the two BRCA proteins and RAD51, a protein involved in recombination and double-strand break repair. These three proteins relocalize to sites of DNA synthesis after exposure of cells to ionizing radiation or hydroxyurea. BRCA1 has also been identified in a multiprotein complex of DNA repair proteins, including RAD50, MRE11, and NBS1.[267] Expression of BRCA1 in a cell line lacking the protein has been shown to reduce the sensitivity of the cell to ionizing radiation and increase the efficiency of repair of radiation-induced double-strand DNA breaks.[268] Mutant forms of the protein failed to demonstrate these activities. These results provide functional evidence for a role of BRCA1 in DNA repair.

The BRCA1 protein becomes phosphorylated in response to DNA damage. The *ATM* gene product has been implicated as a protein kinase involved in this phosphorylation event. In one study, cell lines deficient in ATM were found to lack the ability to phosphorylate BRCA1 in response to ionizing radiation.[269] This study also presents evidence for a physical association between the BRCA1 and ATM proteins and demonstrates that the ATM protein can phosphorylate the BRCA1 protein on specific serine residues in the motif S-Q (serine-glutamine) near the carboxyl terminus of the molecule. Although BRCA1 also becomes phosphorylated in response to other DNA-damaging agents, such as ultraviolet light, methylmethane sulfonate, and hydroxyurea, the phosphorylation induced by these agents appears to be ATM independent. Another family of kinases, represented by the protein CHEK2 (CDS1), first identified as mediators of the DNA damage response in yeast, may play an important role in phosphorylating BRCA1 at serine 988 in response to ionizing radiation.[270] BRCA1 has also been reported to associate with RB1.[271] The ability of BRCA1 to suppress growth upon transfection into cell lines has been found to require functional RB1. BRCA1 also interacts with pathways involving p53. Transfection of BRCA1 has been shown to transactivate p53-dependent promoter sequences in the presence but not the absence of p53.[272] In this study, BRCA1 was shown to coprecipitate with p53, raising the possibility of direct physical interaction between the two proteins.

Mutations associated with an increased risk of cancer are distributed over the full length of the coding sequence. Therefore, screening for the presence of a mutation requires extensive analysis, currently involving the determination of the sequence of each exon individually.[273] This type of analysis is expensive and can only be offered by highly specialized laboratories. The indications for such an analysis have been the subject of much discussion and continue to be in a state of rapid evolution.[273–276]

Apoptosis

As a result of studies of the growth rate of cancer cells, it has become evident that for some cancers it is not only the rate of cell growth that matters but also the rate of cell removal. Deficiencies in the mechanisms regulating programmed cell death, or apoptosis, can contribute to the malignant phenotype.[277] In this section, the overall architecture of the apoptosis regulatory pathway is reviewed and the specific components implicated in the pathogenesis of cancer are discussed.

As a normal physiologic process, apoptosis plays a role in embryonic development, in tissue remodeling in the adult, and in the regulation of the immune response. Cells may also undergo apoptosis in response to DNA damaging agents, such as radiation and chemical carcinogens. Like cell cycle checkpoint regulation, the apoptotic response constitutes a mechanism by which the cell responds to damage without producing abnormal, and possibly malignant, progeny. Apoptosis may be induced by growth factor withdrawal or by exposure to a family of polypeptides including tumor necrosis factor (TNF), FAS ligand, and the TNF-related protein TNFSF10 (TRAIL).[278–282]

The apoptotic response may help protect cells from the transforming influences of activated oncogenes. Thus, there are seemingly paradoxical responses to oncogene activation that have been reported under certain experimental conditions. For example, activation of a *RAS* proto-oncogene, which might be expected to be growth promoting, can in some circumstances drive cells toward apoptosis.[283, 284] In NIH3T3 cells, a standard immortalized cell line used for studies of the transforming activity associated with *RAS* signaling, expression of *RAS* does in fact promote cell growth. In contrast, expression of an activated RAS protein in primary cultures of mouse embryonic fibroblasts induces apoptosis.[285, 286]

As with the *RAS* signaling pathway, elucidation of the mechanisms involved in regulating apoptosis has profited immensely from the use of model systems amenable to genetic manipulation. The key players in the pathway include a series of cysteine proteases, the proteins that regulate their activity, and a deoxyribonuclease (DNase) that degrades nuclear DNA. In *C. elegans*, genetic analysis identified three loci involved in regulation of the cell death pathway: CED3, CED4, and CED9. CED3 acts as an initiator protease in the pathway. Activation of CED3 requires interaction with CED4. CED9 inhibits the ability of CED4 to activate CED3. The mammalian counterpart of CED3 is the cysteine protease caspase 8. The activation of caspase 8 occurs through interactions with death effector domains of other proteins. One of the best characterized systems in apoptosis research is the pathway initiated by the interaction of the transmembrane receptor FAS with the peptide hormone designated FAS ligand, illustrated in Figure 1–6. In response to ligand binding, the FAS molecule undergoes trimerization. The intracellular portion of FAS then binds to the adapter protein FADD. FADD binds to the initiator cysteine protease caspase 8. Caspase 8 activates a variety of effector caspases via specific proteolytic cleavages.

Caspases 3 and 7, the effector caspases, are activated by caspase 8 and by binding to the apoptotic protease activating factor-1 (APAF1) protein, which is a homologue of CED4. APAF1 becomes activated by dimerization, which is dependent on the release of cytochrome C from the mitochondria and requires dATP. Activated APAF1 binds to caspase 9, another initiator caspase. Caspase 9 can then activate caspases 3 and 7 by proteolysis.

One hallmark of apoptosis, the distinctive pattern of degradation of nuclear DNA into a nucleosomal pattern, is caused by the activity of the deoxyribonuclease CAD.[287–289] This enzyme is present normally in a complex with an inhibitor, I^{CAD}, in the cytoplasm. Activation

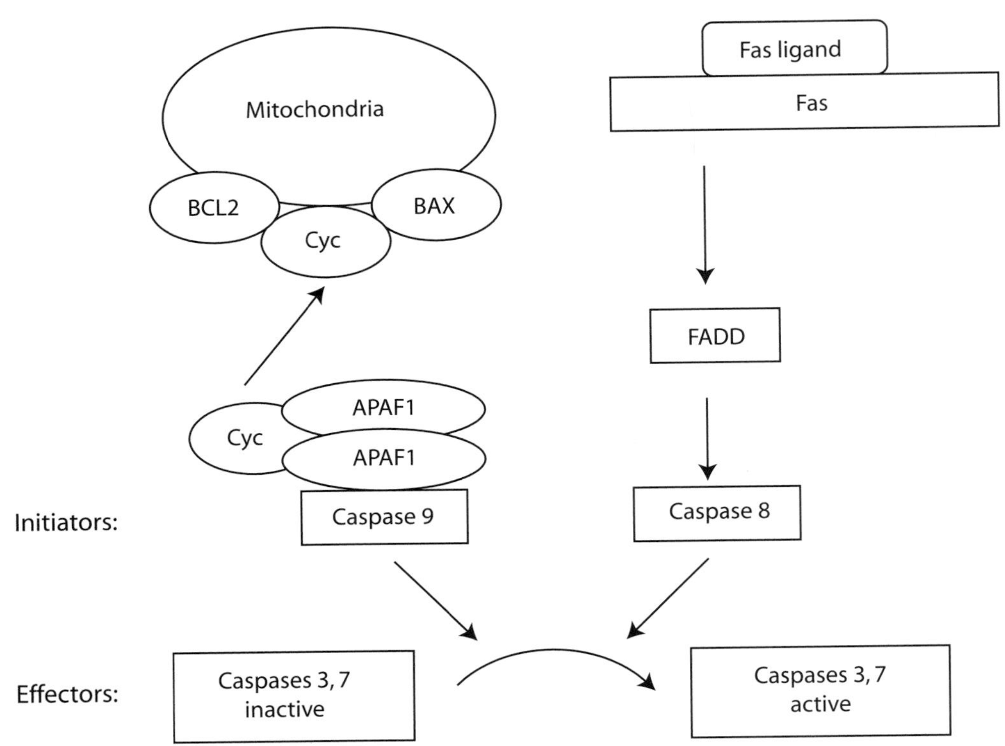

FIGURE 1–6
Activation of caspases by apoptotic signals. Extracellular polypeptides, such as Fas ligand, bind to specific receptors, leading through "death domain" interactions to activation of initiator caspases, which then activate effector caspases 3 and 7. In the mitochondria, the balance of the pro-apoptotic BAX family of proteins and the anti-apoptotic BCL2 proteins regulate release of cytochrome C (CyC), which complexes with APAF1 and either ATP or dATP to activate initiator caspase 9. Caspase 9 activates effector caspases 3 and 7.

of the nuclease results from cleavage of I^{CAD} by the effector caspases, which then permits the activated CAD to migrate to the nucleus.[290, 291]

THE BCL2 FAMILY OF PROTEINS

The translocation t(14;18), present in a high percentage of follicular lymphomas and a smaller percentage of large cell lymphomas, results in the overexpression of the BCL2 protein. Overexpression in this case results from the proximity of the translocated *BCL2* gene from chromosome 18 to the transcriptional enhancer of the immunoglobulin heavy-chain gene on chromosome 14q32. The mechanism is analogous to that resulting in overexpression of the cyclin D1 gene in mantle cell lymphoma and parathyroid adenoma. The gene for *BCL2* was first identified through cloning of the breakpoints of the t(14;18) translocation. The BCL2 protein functions as an oncoprotein by inhibiting apoptosis. The protein is a member of a larger family of antiapoptotic proteins sharing certain structural features, including domains designated BH1, BH2, BH3, and BH4. In addition to these domains, the proteins share a hydrophobic segment that serves to anchor them to the outer mitochondrial membrane.[292, 293]

A closely related family of proteins shares common structural features with the BCL2 family but serves the opposite function: the promotion of apoptosis. The group includes the BAX protein[294] and the BAX family of proteins, in which individual members have been named BAK, BOK, BIK, BAD, and BID.[295]

The BCL2 and BAX family of proteins function by regulating the release of cytochrome C from the mitochondria. The BCL2 proteins inhibit this release, whereas the BAX proteins promote it. The balance between BCL2 and BAX activities therefore appears to be an important mechanism regulating the decision between cell survival and cell death.[296] Overexpression of BCL2 pushes the balance in the direction of survival, thereby contributing to the growth abnormalities that constitute the malignant phenotype in follicular lymphoma and other tumors that may overexpress this gene.

Clinically, detection of the t(14;18) translocation has use in the diagnosis of follicular lymphoma. Because the translocation is not normally present in human tissue, the detection of the translocation has potential use in the detection of minimal residual disease. However, the clinical significance of residual t(14;18) positive cells has been a matter of controversy, with some studies not finding evidence for a correlation between minimal residual disease and prognosis.[297]

p53 and Apoptosis

The p53 tumor suppressor protein, discussed earlier as a transcription factor and cell cycle checkpoint regulator, contributes to the regulation of apoptosis[298] and is considered a focal point of several pathways that ultimately determine whether the cell will undergo apoptosis or growth arrest without cell death.[202] In some experimental systems, the ability to undergo apoptosis depends on the presence of normal p53. Using a temperature-sensitive p53 mutant, it was shown that expression of wild-type p53 can induce apoptosis in myeloid leukemia cells. Hematopoietic cells deficient in p53 either due to mutation or genetic manipulation are relatively resistant to radiation-induced apoptosis. In murine fibroblasts transformed by the adenovirus E1A protein plus activated ras, a variety of agents, including radiation, doxorubicin, 5-fluorouracil, and etoposide will induce apoptosis in the presence of p53 but not in its absence. As with the cell cycle checkpoint function of p53 discussed earlier, phosphorylation of p53 on the serines at positions 15 and 20 regulates the ability of the protein to induce apoptosis by blocking its ability to bind to the MDM2 protein, which enhances its degradation.[180, 181] The mechanism by which p53 induces apoptosis may involve its ability to induce transcription of the pro-apoptotic BAX protein,[299] although this pathway remains to be fully dissected.

PROSPECTS FOR NEW CLINICAL APPLICATIONS

This chapter has provided a summary of a wide spectrum of individual genes and metabolic pathways that regulate cell growth, survival, and death. Alterations in these pathways constitute the basic molecular abnormalities in cancer. Through applications of the techniques of molecular biology, including the polymerase chain reaction, methods of DNA sequencing, and techniques for quantitative determination of gene expression levels, it is now possible for the pathologist to analyze a tumor at the molecular level. In specific cases, particularly in the area of hematopathology, the determination of a molecular abnormality already plays an important role in diagnosis and management of the cancer patient. Specific examples include the determination of cyclin D1 overexpression in the diagnosis of mantle cell lymphoma and the detection of the *BCR-ABL* translocation to determine the presence of minimal residual disease in chronic myelogenous leukemia. Until recently, however, the complexity of the technology involved made it seem unlikely that extensive characterization of tumor specimens to determine the specific oncogene and tumor suppressor gene mutations present would become a part of routine pathologic analysis. New developments in the technology of gene expression analysis now raise the possibility that more detailed molecular characterization of tumor specimens could become a standard part of tumor analysis in the near future. These new approaches include the use of robotic and micro-manufacturing technologies to generate arrays that permit the analysis of thousands of genes at a time. Active research efforts are underway to develop a molecular classification of tumors.[300–302] It is to be hoped that the ability to define specific molecular abnormalities will enhance the value of the pathologist's contribution to patient care by providing information important to diagnosis, to the early detection of primary and recurrent disease, and to determining the course of treatment most likely to result in a favorable outcome for patients suffering from these devastating diseases.

REFERENCES

1. Huebner RJ, Todaro GJ: Oncogenes of RNA tumor viruses as determinants of cancer. Proc Natl Acad Sci USA 1969;64:1087–1094.
2. Levinson AD, Oppermann H, Levintow L, et al: Evidence that the transforming gene of avian sarcoma virus encodes a protein kinase associated with a phosphoprotein. Cell 1978;15:561–572.
3. Parada LF, Tabin CJ, Shih C, Weinberg RA: Human EJ bladder carcinoma oncogene is homologue of Harvey sarcoma virus ras gene. Nature 1982;297:474–478.
4. Stehelin D, Varmus HE, Bishop JM, Vogt PK: DNA related to the transforming gene(s) of avian sarcoma viruses is present in normal avian DNA. Nature 1976; 260:170–173.
5. Knudson AG: Mutation and cancer: Statistical study of retinoblastoma. Proc Natl Acad Sci USA 1971;68: 820–824.
6. Knudson AG: Hereditary cancer: Two hits revisited. J Cancer Res Clin Oncol 1996;122:135–140.
7. Dryja TP, Rapaport JM, Joyce JM, Petersen RA: Molecular detection of deletions involving band q14 of chromosome 13 in retinoblastomas. Proc Natl Acad Sci USA 1986;83:7391–7394.
8. Friend SH, Bernards R, Rogelj S, et al: A human DNA segment with properties of the gene that predisposes to retinoblastoma and osteosarcoma. Nature 1986;323: 643–646.
9. Harris H: The biology of tumour suppression. Ciba Found Symp 1989;142:199–208; discussion 208–213.
10. Stanbridge EJ: Suppression of malignancy in human cells. Nature 1976;260:17–20.
11. Dib C, Faure S, Fizames C, et al: A comprehensive genetic map of the human genome based on 5,264 microsatellites. Nature 1996;380:152–154.
12. Aldaz CM, Chen T, Sahin A, et al: Comparative allelotype of in situ and invasive human breast cancer: high frequency of microsatellite instability in lobular breast carcinomas. Cancer Res 1995;55:3976–3981.
13. Boland CR, Sato J, Appelman HD, et al: Microallelotyping defines the sequence and tempo of allelic losses at tumour suppressor gene loci during colorectal cancer progression. Nat Med 1995;1:902–909.
14. Weston A, Willey JC, Modali R, et al: Differential DNA sequence deletions from chromosomes 3, 11, 13, and 17

in squamous-cell carcinoma, large-cell carcinoma, and adenocarcinoma of the human lung. Proc Natl Acad Sci USA 1989;86:5099–5103.
15. Hunter T: Oncoprotein networks. Cell 1997;88:333–346.
16. Davis RJ: The mitogen-activated protein kinase signal transduction pathway. J Biol Chem 1993;268: 14553–14556.
17. Mroczkowski B, Reich M, Chen K, et al: Recombinant human epidermal growth factor precursor is a glycosylated membrane protein with biological activity. Mol Cell Biol 1989;9:2771–2778.
18. Koch CA, Anderson D, Moran MF, et al: SH2 and SH3 domains: Elements that control interactions of cytoplasmic signaling proteins. Science 1991;252:668–674.
19. Alexandropoulos K, Cheng G, Baltimore D: Proline-rich sequences that bind to Src homology 3 domains with individual specificities. Proc Natl Acad Sci USA 1995;92:3110–3114.
20. Ren R, Mayer BJ, Cicchetti P, Baltimore D: Identification of a ten amino acid proline-rich SH3 binding site. Science 1993;259:1157–1161.
21. Gale NW, Kaplan S, Lowenstein EJ, et al: Grb2 mediates the EGF-dependent activation of guanine nucleotide exchange on Ras. Nature 1993;363:88–92.
22. Rozakis-Adcock M, Fernley R, Wade J, et al: The SH2 and SH3 domains of mammalian Grb2 couple the EGF receptor to the Ras activator mSos1. Nature 1993;363: 83–85.
23. Li N, Batzer A, Daly R, et al: Guanine-nucleotide-releasing factor hSos1 binds to Grb2 and links receptor tyrosine kinases to Ras signaling. Nature 1993;363:85–88.
24. Egan SE, Giddings BW, Brooks MW, et al: Association of Sos Ras exchange protein with Grb2 is implicated in tryrosine kinase signal transduction and transformation. Nature 1993;363:45–51.
25. Buday L, Downward J: Epidermal growth factor regulates $p21^{ras}$ through the formation of a complex of receptor, Grb2 adapter protein, and sos nucleotide exchange factor. Cell 1993;73:611–620.
26. Lowenstein EJ, Daly RJ, Batzer AG, et al: The SH2 and SH3 domain-containing protein GRB2 links receptor tyrosine kinases to ras signaling. Cell 1992;70:431–442.
27. Chardin P, Camonis JH, Gale NW, et al: Human Sos1: A guanine nucleotide exchange factor for ras that binds to GRB2. Science 1993;260:1338–1343.
28. McCormick F: ras GTPase activating protein: Signal transmitter and signal terminator. Cell 1989;56:5–8.
29. Ahn NG: The MAP kinase cascade: Discovery of a new signal transduction pathway. Mol Cell Biochem 1993; 127–128:201–209.
30. Brunet A, Pouyssegur J: Mammalian MAP kinase modules: How to transduce specific signals. Essays Biochem 1997;32:1–16.
31. Karandikar M, Cobb MH: Scaffolding and protein interactions in MAP kinase modules. Cell Calcium 1999;26:219–226.
32. Ahn NG, Seger R, Bratlien RL, Krebs EG: Growth factor–stimulated phosphorylation cascades: Activation of growth factor-stimulated MAP kinase. Ciba Found Symp 1992;164:113–126.
33. Cobb MH, Goldsmith EJ: Dimerization in MAP-kinase signaling. Trends Biochem Sci 2000;25:7–9.
34. Saraste M, Hyvonen M: Pleckstrin homology domains: A fact file. Curr Opin Struct Biol 1995;5:403–408.
35. Cerione RA, Zheng Y: The Dbl family of oncogenes. Curr Opin Cell Biol 1996;8:216–222.
36. Dickson B, Sprenger F, Morrison D, Hafen E: Raf functions downstream of Ras1 in the Sevenless signal transduction pathway. Nature 1992;360:600–603.
37. Rogge RD, Karlovich CA, Banerjee U: Genetic dissection of a neurodevelopmental pathway: Son of sevenless functions downstream of the sevenless and EGF receptor tyrosine kinases. Cell 1991;64:39–48.
38. Kramer H, Cagan RL, Zipursky SL: Interaction of bride of sevenless membrane-bound ligand and the sevenless tyrosine-kinase receptor. Nature 1991;352:207–212.
39. Zipursky SL, Rubin GM: Determination of neuronal cell fate: Lessons from the R7 neuron of *Drosophila*. Annu Rev Neurosci 1994;17:373–397.
40. Reinke R, Zipursky SL. Cell-cell interaction in the *Drosophila* retina: The bride of sevenless gene is required in photoreceptor cell R8 for R7 cell development. Cell 1988;55:321–330.
41. Bonfini L, Karlovich CA, Dasgupta C, Banerjee U: The Son of sevenless gene product: A putative activator of Ras. Science 1992;255:603–606.
42. Clark SG, Stern MJ, Horvitz HR: *C. elegans* cell-signalling gene sem-5 encodes a protein with SH2 and SH3 domains. Nature 1992;356:340–344.
43. Veale D, Kerr N, Gibson GJ, Harris AL: Characterization of epidermal growth factor receptor in primary human non-small cell lung cancer. Cancer Res 1989; 49:1313–1317.
44. Libermann TA, Razon N, Bartal AD, et al: Expression of epidermal growth factor receptors in human brain tumors. Cancer Res 1984;44:753–760.
45. Ozanne B, Richards CS, Hendler F, et al: Over-expression of the EGF receptor is a hallmark of squamous cell carcinomas. J Pathol 1986;149:9–14.
46. Gullick WJ: The role of the epidermal growth factor receptor and the c-erbB-2 protein in breast cancer. Int J Cancer Suppl 1990;5:55–61.
47. Hudziak RM, Schlessinger J, Ullrich A: Increased expression of the putative growth factor receptor p185HER2 causes transformation and tumorigenesis of NIH 3T3 cells. Proc Natl Acad Sci USA 1987;84: 7159–7163.
48. Schechter AL, Stern DF, Vaidyanathan L, et al: The *neu* oncogene: An erb-B–related gene encoding a 185,000-Mr tumour antigen. Nature 1984;312:513–516.
49. Fukushige S, Matsubara K, Yoshida M, et al: Localization of a novel v-erbB-related gene, c-erbB-2, on human chromosome 17 and its amplification in a gastric cancer cell line. Mol Cell Biol 1986;6:955–958.
50. Wright C, Angus B, Nicholson S, et al: Expression of c-erbB-2 oncoprotein: A prognostic indicator in human breast cancer. Cancer Res 1989;49:2087–2090.
51. Slamon DJ, Godolphin W, Jones LA, et al: Studies of the HER-2/neu proto-oncogene in human breast and ovarian cancer. Science 1989;244:707–712.
52. Cobleigh MA, Vogel CL, Tripathy D, et al: Multinational study of the efficacy and safety of humanized anti-HER2 monoclonal antibody in women who have HER2-overexpressing metastatic breast cancer that has

progressed after chemotherapy for metastatic disease. J Clin Oncol 1999;17:2639–2648.

53. Pendergast AM, Quilliam LA, Cripe LD, et al: BCR-ABL–induced oncogenesis is mediated by direct interaction with the SH2 domain of the GRB-2 adaptor protein. Cell 1993;75:175–185.
54. Cortez D, Reuther G, Pendergast AM: The Bcr-Abl tyrosine kinase activates mitogenic signaling pathways and stimulates G1-to-S phase transition in hematopoietic cells. Oncogene 1997;15:2333–2342.
55. Gotoh A, Broxmeyer HE: The function of BCR/ABL and related proto-oncogenes. Curr Opin Hematol 1997;4:3–11.
56. Pui CH, Crist WM, Look AT: Biology and clinical significance of cytogenetic abnormalities in childhood acute lymphoblastic leukemia. Blood 1990;76:1449–1463.
57. Komminoth P: The RET proto-oncogene in medullary and papillary thyroid carcinoma: Molecular features, pathophysiology and clinical implications. Virchows Arch 1997;431:1–9.
58. Santoro M, Melillo RM, Carlomagno F, et al: Molecular biology of the *MEN2* gene. J Intern Med 1998;243:505–508.
59. Nakahara M, Isozaki K, Hirota S, et al: A novel gain-of-function mutation of c-*kit* gene in gastrointestinal stromal tumors. Gastroenterology 1998;115:1090–1095.
60. Linnekin D: Early signaling pathways activated by c-Kit in hematopoietic cells. Int J Biochem Cell Biol 1999;31:1053–1074.
61. Lam LP, Chow RY, Berger SA: A transforming mutation enhances the activity of the c-Kit soluble tyrosine kinase domain. Biochem J 1999;338(Pt 1):131–138.
62. Lennartsson J, Blume-Jensen P, Hermanson M, et al: Phosphorylation of Shc by Src family kinases is necessary for stem cell factor receptor/c-*kit* mediated activation of the Ras/MAP kinase pathway and c-*fos* induction. Oncogene 1999;18:5546–5553.
63. Ernst SI, Hubbs AE, Przygodzki RM, et al: KIT mutation portends poor prognosis in gastrointestinal stromal/smooth muscle tumors. Lab Invest 1998;78:1633–1636.
64. Lasota J, Jasinski M, Sarlomo-Rikala M, Miettinen M: Mutations in exon 11 of c-Kit occur preferentially in malignant versus benign gastrointestinal stromal tumors and do not occur in leiomyomas or leiomyosarcomas. Am J Pathol 1999;154:53–60.
65. Taniguchi M, Nishida T, Hirota S, et al: Effect of c-*kit* mutation on prognosis of gastrointestinal stromal tumors. Cancer Res 1999;59:4297–4300.
66. Howe JR, Conlon KC: The molecular genetics of pancreatic cancer. Surg Oncol 1997;6:1–18.
67. Friess H, Kleeff J, Gumbs A, Buchler MW: Molecular versus conventional markers in pancreatic cancer. Digestion 1997;58:557–563.
68. Kimura W, Zhao B, Futakawa N, et al: Significance of K-*ras* codon 12 point mutation in pancreatic juice in the diagnosis of carcinoma of the pancreas. Hepatogastroenterology 1999;46:532–539.
69. Shen MH, Harper PS, Upadhyaya M: Molecular genetics of neurofibromatosis type 1 (NF1). J Med Genet 1996;33:2–17.
70. Zwarthoff EC: Neurofibromatosis and associated tumour suppressor genes. Pathol Res Pract 1996;192:647–657.
71. Weiss B, Bollag G, Shannon K: Hyperactive Ras as a therapeutic target in neurofibromatosis type 1. Am J Med Genet 1999;89:14–22.
72. Nesbit CE, Tersak JM, Prochownik EV: MYC oncogenes and human neoplastic disease. Oncogene 1999;18:3004–3016.
73. Bhatia K, Huppi K, Spangler G, et al: Point mutations in the c-Myc transactivation domain are common in Burkitt's lymphoma and mouse plasmacytomas. Nat Genet 1993;5:56–61.
74. Albert T, Urlbauer B, Kohlhuber F, et al: Ongoing mutations in the N-terminal domain of c-Myc affect transactivation in Burkitt's lymphoma cell lines. Oncogene 1994;9:759–763.
75. Blackwell TK, Kretzner L, Blackwood EM, et al: Sequence-specific DNA binding by the c-Myc protein. Science 1990;250:1149–1151.
76. Blackwood EM, Luscher B, Kretzner L, Eisenman RN: The Myc:Max protein complex and cell growth regulation. Cold Spring Harb Symp Quant Biol 1991;56:109–117.
77. Blackwood EM, Eisenman RN: Max: A helix-loop-helix zipper protein that forms a sequence-specific DNA-binding complex with Myc. Science 1991;251:1211–1217.
78. Blackwood EM, Luscher B, Eisenman RN: Myc and Max associate in vivo. Genes Dev 1992;6:71–80.
79. Kretzner L, Blackwood EM, Eisenman RN: Myc and Max proteins possess distinct transcriptional activities. Nature 1992;359:426–429.
80. Ayer DE, Kretzner L, Eisenman RN: Mad: A heterodimeric partner for Max that antagonizes Myc transcriptional activity. Cell 1993;72:211–222.
81. Hurlin PJ, Ayer DE, Grandori C, Eisenman RN: The Max transcription factor network: Involvement of Mad in differentiation and an approach to identification of target genes. Cold Spring Harb Symp Quant Biol 1994;59:109–116.
82. Ayer DE, Eisenman RN: A switch from Myc:Max to Mad:Max heterocomplexes accompanies monocyte/macrophage differentiation. Genes Dev 1993;7:2110–2119.
83. Foley KP, McArthur GA, Queva C, et al: Targeted disruption of the MYC antagonist MAD1 inhibits cell cycle exit during granulocyte differentiation. Embo J 1998;17:774–785.
84. Queva C, Hurlin PJ, Foley KP, Eisenman RN: Sequential expression of the MAD family of transcriptional repressors during differentiation and development. Oncogene 1998;16:967–977.
85. Foley KP, Eisenman RN: Two MAD tails: What the recent knockouts of Mad1 and Mxi1 tell us about the MYC/MAX/MAD network. Biochim Biophys Acta 1999;1423:M37–M47.
86. Downing JR: Molecular genetics of acute myeloid leukemia. *In* Pui C-H (ed): Childhood Leukemias. Cambridge, England, Cambridge University Press, 1999.
87. Galili N, Davis RJ, Fredericks WJ, et al: Fusion of a fork head domain gene to *PAX3* in the solid tumour alveolar rhabdomyosarcoma [published erratum appears in Nat Genet 1994;6:214]. Nat Genet 1993;5:230–235.
88. Shapiro DN, Sublett JE, Li B, et al: Fusion of *PAX3* to a member of the forkhead family of transcription factors in

human alveolar rhabdomyosarcoma. Cancer Res 1993; 53:5108–5112.

89. Davis RJ, D'Cruz CM, Lovell MA, et al: Fusion of *PAX7* to *FKHR* by the variant t(1;13)(p36;q14) translocation in alveolar rhabdomyosarcoma. Cancer Res 1994;54: 2869–2872.
90. Sorensen PH, Lessnick SL, Lopez-Terrada D, et al: A second Ewing's sarcoma translocation, t(21;22) fuses the *EWS* gene to another ETS-family transcription factor, ERG. Nat Genet 1994;6:146–151.
91. Ladanyi M, Gerald W: Fusion of the *EWS* and *WT1* genes in the desmoplastic small round cell tumor. Cancer Res 1994;54:2837–2840.
92. Call KM, Glaser T, Ito CY, et al: Isolation and characterization of a zinc finger polypeptide gene at the human chromosome 11 Wilms' tumor locus. Cell 1990;60: 509–520.
93. Rauscher FJ, Morris JF, Tournay OE, et al: Binding of the Wilms' tumor locus zinc finger protein to the EGR-1 consensus sequence. Science 1990;250:1259–1262.
94. Riccardi VM, Sujansky E, Smith AC, Francke U: Chromosomal imbalance in the Aniridia-Wilms' tumor association: 11p interstitial deletion. Pediatrics 1978;61: 604–610.
95. Pritchard-Jones K, Fleming S, Davidson D, et al: The candidate Wilms' tumour gene is involved in genitourinary development. Nature 1990;346:194–197.
96. Herzer U, Crocoll A, Barton D, et al: The Wilms tumor suppressor gene *wt1* is required for development of the spleen. Curr Biol 1999;9:837–840.
97. Miller JR, Hocking AM, Brown JD, Moon RT: Mechanism and function of signal transduction by the Wnt/beta-catenin and Wnt/Ca^{2+} pathways. Oncogene 1999;18: 7860–7872.
98. Groden J, Thliveris A, Samowitz W, et al: Identification and characterization of the familial adenomatous polyposis coli gene. Cell 1991;66:589–600.
99. Gryfe R, Swallow C, Bapat B, et al: Molecular biology of colorectal cancer. Curr Probl Cancer 1997;21:233–300.
100. Nakamura Y, Nishisho I, Kinzler KW, et al: Mutations of the adenomatous polyposis coli gene in familial polyposis coli patients and sporadic colorectal tumors. Princess Takamatsu Symp 1991;22:285–292.
101. Kirchgesser M, Albers A, Vossen R, et al: Optimized non-radioactive protein truncation test for mutation analysis of the adenomatous polyposis coli (APC) gene. Clin Chem Lab Med 1998;36:567–570.
102. O'Sullivan MJ, McCarthy TV, Doyle CT: Familial adenomatous polyposis: From bedside to benchside. Am J Clin Pathol 1998;109:521–526.
103. Polakis P: The oncogenic activation of beta-catenin. Curr Opin Genet Dev 1999;9:15–21.
104. Morin PJ: Beta-catenin signaling and cancer. Bioessays 1999;21:1021–1030.
105. Behrens J: Cadherins and catenins: Role in signal transduction and tumor progression. Cancer Metastasis Rev 1999;18:15–30.
106. Li J, Yen C, Liaw D, et al: *PTEN*, a putative protein tyrosine phosphatase gene mutated in human brain, breast, and prostate cancer. Science 1997;275:1943–1947.
107. Steck PA, Pershouse MA, Jasser SA, et al: Identification of a candidate tumour suppressor gene, *MMAC1*, at chromosome 10q23.3 that is mutated in multiple advanced cancers. Nat Genet 1997;15:356–362.
108. Liaw D, Marsh DJ, Li J, et al: Germline mutations of the *PTEN* gene in Cowden disease, an inherited breast and thyroid cancer syndrome. Nat Genet 1997;16:64–67.
109. Nelen MR, van Staveren WC, Peeters EA, et al: Germline mutations in the *PTEN/MMAC1* gene in patients with Cowden disease. Hum Mol Genet 1997;6:1383–1387.
110. Marsh DJ, et al: Mutation spectrum and genotype-phenotype analyses in Cowden disease and Bannayan-Zonana syndrome, two hamartoma syndromes with germline PTEN mutation. Hum Mol Genet 1998;7:507–515.
111. Rhei E, Kang L, Bogomolniy F, et al: Mutation analysis of the putative tumor suppressor gene *PTEN/MMAC1* in primary breast carcinomas. Cancer Res 1997;57: 3657–3659.
112. Tsou HC, Teng DH, Ping XL, et al: The role of *MMAC1* mutations in early-onset breast cancer: Causative in association with Cowden syndrome and excluded in *BRCA1*-negative cases. Am J Hum Genet 1997;61:1036–1043.
113. Lynch ED, Ostermeyer EA, Lee MK, et al: Inherited mutations in *PTEN* that are associated with breast cancer, Cowden disease, and juvenile polyposis. Am J Hum Genet 1997;61:1254–1260.
114. Ueda K, Nishijima M, Inui H, et al: Infrequent mutations in the *PTEN/MMAC1* gene among primary breast cancers. Jpn J Cancer Res 1998;89:17–21.
115. FitzGerald MG, Marsh DJ, Wahrer D, et al: Germline mutations in *PTEN* are an infrequent cause of genetic predisposition to breast cancer. Oncogene 1998;17:727–731.
116. Guldberg P, thor Straten P, Birck A, et al: Disruption of the *MMAC1/PTEN* gene by deletion or mutation is a frequent event in malignant melanoma. Cancer Res 1997;57:3660–3663.
117. Wang SI, Puc J, Li J, et al: Somatic mutations of *PTEN* in glioblastoma multiforme. Cancer Res 1997;57: 4183–4186.
118. Tashiro H, Blazes MS, Wu R, et al: Mutations in *PTEN* are frequent in endometrial carcinoma but rare in other common gynecological malignancies. Cancer Res 1997; 57:3935–3940.
119. Risinger JI, Hayes AK, Berchuck A, Barrett JC: *PTEN/MMAC1* mutations in endometrial cancers. Cancer Res 1997;57:4736–4738.
120. Obata K, Morland SJ, Watson RH, et al: Frequent *PTEN/MMAC* mutations in endometrioid but not serous or mucinous epithelial ovarian tumors. Cancer Res 1998;58:2095–2097.
121. Wang SI, Parsons R, Ittmann M: Homozygous deletion of the *PTEN* tumor suppressor gene in a subset of prostate adenocarcinomas. Clin Cancer Res 1998;4: 811–815.
122. Okami K, Wu L, Riggins G, et al: Analysis of *PTEN/MMAC1* alterations in aerodigestive tract tumors. Cancer Res 1998;58:509–511.
123. Kohno T, Takahashi M, Manda R, Yokota J: Inactivation of the *PTEN/MMAC1/TEP1* gene in human lung cancers. Genes Chromosomes Cancer 1998;22:152–156.
124. Cairns P, Evron E, Okami K, et al: Point mutation and homozygous deletion of *PTEN/MMAC1* in primary bladder cancers. Oncogene 1998;16:3215–3218.

125. Shao X, Tandon R, Samara G, et al: Mutational analysis of the *PTEN* gene in head and neck squamous cell carcinoma [published erratum appears in Int J Cancer 1999;80:636]. Int J Cancer 1998;77:684–688.
126. Nakahara Y, Nagai H, Kinoshita T, et al: Mutational analysis of the *PTEN/MMAC1* gene in non-Hodgkin's lymphoma. Leukemia 1998;12:1277–1280.
127. Parsons R: Phosphatases and tumorigenesis. Curr Opin Oncol 1998;10:88–91.
128. Hopkin K: A surprising function for the *PTEN* tumor suppressor [news]. Science 1998;282:1027, 1029–1030.
129. Maehama T, Dixon JE: The tumor suppressor, *PTEN/MMAC1*, dephosphorylates the lipid second messenger, phosphatidylinositol 3,4,5-trisphosphate. J Biol Chem 1998;273:13375–13378.
130. Wu X, Senechal K, Neshat MS, et al: The *PTEN/MMAC1* tumor suppressor phosphatase functions as a negative regulator of the phosphoinositide 3-kinase/Akt pathway. Proc Natl Acad Sci USA 1998;95:15587–15591.
131. Stambolic V, Suzuki A, de la Pompa JL, et al: Negative regulation of PKB/Akt-dependent cell survival by the tumor suppressor *PTEN*. Cell 1998;95:29–39.
132. Li J, Simpson L, Takahashi M, et al: The *PTEN/MMAC1* tumor suppressor induces cell death that is rescued by the AKT/protein kinase B oncogene. Cancer Res 1998;58:5667–5672.
133. Cantley LC, Neel BG: New insights into tumor suppression: *PTEN* suppresses tumor formation by restraining the phosphoinositide 3-kinase/AKT pathway. Proc Natl Acad Sci USA 1999;96:4240–4245.
134. Maehama T, Dixon JE: PTEN: A tumour suppressor that functions as a phospholipid phosphatase. Trends Cell Biol 1999;9:125–128.
135. Haas-Kogan D, Shalev N, Wong M, et al: Protein kinase B (PKB/Akt) activity is elevated in glioblastoma cells due to mutation of the tumor suppressor *PTEN/MMAC*. Curr Biol 1998;8:1195–1198.
136. Myers MP, Pass I, Batty IH, et al: The lipid phosphatase activity of *PTEN* is critical for its tumor supressor function. Proc Natl Acad Sci USA 1998;95:13513–13518.
137. Tamura M, Gu J, Matsumoto K, et al: Inhibition of cell migration, spreading, and focal adhesions by tumor suppressor *PTEN*. Science 1998;280:1614–1617.
138. Cheney IW, Johnson DE, Vaillancourt MT, et al: Suppression of tumorigenicity of glioblastoma cells by adenovirus-mediated *MMAC1/PTEN* gene transfer. Cancer Res 1998;58:2331–2334.
139. Aguilo F, Tamayo N, Vazquez-Quintana E, et al: Pheochromocytoma: A twenty year experience at the University Hospital [published erratum appears in P R Health Sci J 1992;11:6]. P R Health Sci J 1991;10:135–142.
140. Gnarra JR, et al: Molecular cloning of the von Hippel-Lindau tumor suppressor gene and its role in renal carcinoma. Biochim Biophys Acta 1996;1242:201–210.
141. Latif F, Tory K, Gnarra J, et al: Identification of the von Hippel-Lindau disease tumor suppressor gene. Science 1993;260:1317–1320.
142. Kaelin WG Jr, Maher ER: The VHL tumour-suppressor gene paradigm. Trends Genet 1998;14:423–426.
143. Gnarra JR, Lerman MI, Zbar B, Linehan WM: Genetics of renal-cell carcinoma and evidence for a critical role for von Hippel-Lindau in renal tumorigenesis. Semin Oncol 1995;22:3–8.
144. Bertherat J: Von Hippel-Lindau tumor suppressor protein and transcription elongation: New insights into regulation of gene expression. Eur J Endocrinol 1996;134:157, 159.
145. Maher ER, Kaelin WG Jr: von Hippel-Lindau disease. Medicine (Baltimore) 1997;76:381–391.
146. Shilatifard A: Factors regulating the transcriptional elongation activity of RNA polymerase II. Faseb J 1998;12:1437–1446.
147. Gnarra JR, Zhou S, Merrill MJ, et al: Post-transcriptional regulation of vascular endothelial growth factor mRNA by the product of the VHL tumor suppressor gene. Proc Natl Acad Sci USA 1996;93:10589–10594.
148. Conaway JW, Kamura T, Conaway RC: The Elongin BC complex and the von Hippel-Lindau tumor suppressor protein. Biochim Biophys Acta 1998;1377:M49–M54.
149. Kaelin WG, Iliopoulos O, Lonergan KM, Ohh M: Functions of the von Hippel-Lindau tumour suppressor protein. J Intern Med 1998;243:535–539.
150. Liakopoulos D, Busgen T, Brychzy A, et al: Conjugation of the ubiquitin-like protein NEDD8 to cullin-2 is linked to von Hippel-Lindau tumor suppressor function. Proc Natl Acad Sci USA 1999;96:5510–5515.
151. Richards FM, Webster AR, McMahon R, et al: Molecular genetic analysis of von Hippel-Lindau disease. J Intern Med 1998;243:527–533.
152. Friedrich CA: Von Hippel-Lindau syndrome: A pleomorphic condition. Cancer 1999;86(11 Suppl):2478–2482.
153. Chen F, Kishida T, Yao M, et al: Germline mutations in the von Hippel-Lindau disease tumor suppressor gene: Correlations with phenotype. Hum Mutat 1995;5:66–75.
154. Kohn KW: Molecular interaction map of the mammalian cell cycle control and DNA repair systems. Mol Biol Cell 1999;10:2703–2734.
155. Laird AD, Shalloway D: Oncoprotein signalling and mitosis. Cell Signal 1997;9:249–255.
156. Kaufmann WK: Human topoisomerase II function, tyrosine phosphorylation and cell cycle checkpoints. Proc Soc Exp Biol Med 1998;217:327–334.
157. Weinberg RA: The retinoblastoma protein and cell cycle control. Cell 1995;81:323–330.
158. Grana X, Garriga J, Mayol X: Role of the retinoblastoma protein family, pRB, p107 and p130 in the negative control of cell growth. Oncogene 1998;17:3365–3383.
159. Palmero I, Peters G: Perturbation of cell cycle regulators in human cancer. Cancer Surv 1996;27:351–367.
160. Kamb A, Gruis NA, Weaver-Feldhaus J, et al: A cell cycle regulator potentially involved in genesis of many tumor types [see comments]. Science 1994;264:436–440.
161. Quelle DE, Zindy F, Ashmun RA, Sherr CJ: Alternative reading frames of the *INK4a* tumor suppressor gene encode two unrelated proteins capable of inducing cell cycle arrest. Cell 1995;83:993–1000.
162. Pomerantz J, Schreiber-Agus N, Liegeois NJ, et al: The *Ink4a* tumor suppressor gene product, p19Arf, interacts with MDM2 and neutralizes MDM2's inhibition of p53. Cell 1998;92:713–723.

163. Zhang Y, Xiong Y, Yarbrough WG: ARF promotes MDM2 degradation and stabilizes p53: ARF-INK4a locus deletion impairs both the Rb and p53 tumor suppression pathways. Cell 1998;92:725–734.
164. Kamijo T, Weber JD, Zambetti G, et al: Functional and physical interactions of the ARF tumor suppressor with p53 and Mdm2. Proc Natl Acad Sci USA 1998;95: 8292–8297.
165. Morgan SE, Kastan MB: p53 and ATM: Cell cycle, cell death, and cancer. Adv Cancer Res 1997;71:1–25.
166. Rotman G, Shiloh Y: The ATM gene and protein: Possible roles in genome surveillance, checkpoint controls and cellular defence against oxidative stress. Cancer Surv 1997;29:285–304.
167. Rotman G, Shiloh Y: Ataxia-telangiectasia: Is ATM a sensor of oxidative damage and stress? Bioessays 1997; 19:911–917.
168. Westphal CH: Cell-cycle signaling: Atm displays its many talents. Curr Biol 1997;7:R789–R792.
169. Lavin MF: ATM: The product of the gene mutated in ataxia-telangiectasia. Int J Biochem Cell Biol 1999;31: 735–740.
170. Smith GC, Divecha N, Lakin ND, Jackson SP: DNA-dependent protein kinase and related proteins. Biochem Soc Symp 1999;64:91–104.
171. Suzuki K, Kodama S, Watanabe M: Recruitment of ATM protein to double strand DNA irradiated with ionizing radiation. J Biol Chem 1999;274:25571–25575.
172. Nakagawa K, Taya Y, Tamai K, Yamaizumi M: Requirement of ATM in phosphorylation of the human p53 protein at serine 15 following DNA double-strand breaks. Mol Cell Biol 1999;19:2828–2834.
173. Khanna KK, Keating KE, Kozlov S, et al: ATM associates with and phosphorylates p53: Mapping the region of interaction. Nat Genet 1998;20:398–400.
174. Nakamura Y: ATM: The p53 booster. Nat Med 1998;4: 1231–1232.
175. Banin S, Moyal L, Shieh S, et al: Enhanced phosphorylation of p53 by ATM in response to DNA damage. Science 1998;281:1674–1677.
176. Lakin ND, Jackson SP: Regulation of p53 in response to DNA damage. Oncogene 1999;18:7644–7655.
177. Chen J, Lin J, Levine AJ: Regulation of transcription functions of the p53 tumor suppressor by the mdm-2 oncogene. Mol Med 1995;1:142–152.
178. Freedman DA, Levine AJ: Nuclear export is required for degradation of endogenous p53 by MDM2 and human papillomavirus E6. Mol Cell Biol 1998;18: 7288–7293.
179. Ashcroft M, Vousden KH: Regulation of p53 stability. Oncogene 1999;18:7637–7643.
180. Unger T, Sionov RV, Moallem E, et al: Mutations in serines 15 and 20 of human p53 impair its apoptotic activity. Oncogene 1999;18:3205–3212.
181. Unger T, Juven-Gershon T, Moallem E, et al: Critical role for Ser20 of human p53 in the negative regulation of p53 by Mdm2. Embo J 1999;18:1805–1814.
182. Motokura T, Bloom T, Kim HG, et al: A novel cyclin encoded by a bcl1-linked candidate oncogene. Nature 1991;350:512–515.
183. Arnold A, Motokura T, Bloom T, et al: The putative oncogene PRAD1 encodes a novel cyclin. Cold Spring Harb Symp Quant Biol 1991;56:93–97.
184. Arnold A, Motokura T, Bloom T, et al: *PRAD1* (cyclin D1): A parathyroid neoplasia gene on 11q13. Henry Ford Hosp Med J 1992;40:177–180.
185. Williams ME, Swerdlow SH, Meeker TC: Chromosome t(11;14)(q13;q32) breakpoints in centrocytic lymphoma are highly localized at the bcl-1 major translocation cluster. Leukemia 1993;7:1437–1440.
186. Williams ME, Meeker TC, Swerdlow SH: Rearrangement of the chromosome 11 bcl-1 locus in centrocytic lymphoma: Analysis with multiple breakpoint probes. Blood 1991;78:493–498.
187. Withers DA, Harvey RC, Faust JB, et al: Characterization of a candidate *bcl-1* gene. Mol Cell Biol 1991;11: 4846–4853.
188. Aguilera NS, Bijwaard KE, Duncan B, et al: Differential expression of cyclin D1 in mantle cell lymphoma and other non-Hodgkin's lymphomas. Am J Pathol 1998; 153:1969–1976.
189. Fan H, Gulley ML, Gascoyne RD, et al: Molecular methods for detecting t(11;14) translocations in mantle-cell lymphomas. Diagn Mol Pathol 1998;7:209–214.
190. Castellano M, Parmiani G: Genes involved in melanoma: An overview of INK4a and other loci. Melanoma Res 1999;9:421–432.
191. Greene MH: The genetics of hereditary melanoma and nevi: 1998 Update. Cancer 1999;86:2464–2477.
192. Newton Bishop JA, Harland M, Bennett DC, et al: Mutation testing in melanoma families: *INK4A*, *CDK4* and *INK4D*. Br J Cancer 1999;80:295–300.
193. Kamb A, Shattuck-Eidens D, Eeles R, et al: Analysis of the p16 gene *(CDKN2)* as a candidate for the chromosome 9p melanoma susceptibility locus. Nat Genet 1994;8: 23–26.
194. Lee JO, Russo AA, Pavletich NP: Structure of the retinoblastoma tumour-suppressor pocket domain bound to a peptide from HPV E7. Nature 1998;391:859–865.
195. Mulligan G, Jacks T: The retinoblastoma gene family: Cousins with overlapping interests. Trends Genet 1998;14:223–229.
196. Lipinski MM, Jacks T: The retinoblastoma gene family in differentiation and development. Oncogene 1999;18: 7873–7882.
197. Chen PL, Riley DJ, Chen Y, Lee WH: Retinoblastoma protein positively regulates terminal adipocyte differentiation through direct interaction with C/EBPs. Genes Dev 1996;10:2794–2804.
198. Novitch BG, Mulligan GJ, Jacks T, Lassar AB: Skeletal muscle cells lacking the retinoblastoma protein display defects in muscle gene expression and accumulate in S and G2 phases of the cell cycle. J Cell Biol 1996;135: 441–456.
199. May P, May E: Twenty years of p53 research: Structural and functional aspects of the p53 protein. Oncogene 1999;18:7621–7636.
200. Lane DP: Cancer: p53, guardian of the genome [news; comment] [see comments]. Nature 1992;358:15–16.
201. Levine AJ: p53, the cellular gatekeeper for growth and division. Cell 1997;88:323–331.

202. Sionov RV, Haupt Y: The cellular response to p53: The decision between life and death. Oncogene 1999;18: 6145–6157.
203. Horikoshi N, Usheva A, Chen J, et al: Two domains of p53 interact with the TATA-binding protein, and the adenovirus 13S E1A protein disrupts the association, relieving p53-mediated transcriptional repression. Mol Cell Biol 1995;15:227–234.
204. Kaelin WG Jr: The p53 gene family. Oncogene 1999; 18:7701–7705.
205. el-Deiry WS, Tokino T, Velculescu VE, et al: *WAF1*, a potential mediator of p53 tumor suppression. Cell 1993; 75:817–825.
206. Yu J, Zhang L, Hwang PM, et al: Identification and classification of p53-regulated genes. Proc Natl Acad Sci U S A 1999;96:14517–14522.
207. el-Deiry WS: Regulation of *p53* downstream genes. Semin Cancer Biol 1998;8:345–357.
208. Nigro JM, Baker SJ, Preisinger AC, et al: Mutations in the *p53* gene occur in diverse human tumour types. Nature 1989;342:705–708.
209. Harris CC: *p53* tumor suppressor gene: At the crossroads of molecular carcinogenesis, molecular epidemiology, and cancer risk assessment. Environ Health Perspect 1996;104(Suppl 3):435–439.
210. Greenblatt MS, Bennett WP, Hollstein M, Harris CC: Mutations in the *p53* tumor suppressor gene: Clues to cancer etiology and molecular pathogenesis. Cancer Res 1994;54:4855–4878.
211. Hainaut P, Hernandez T, Robinson A, et al: IARC Database of *p53* gene mutations in human tumors and cell lines: Updated compilation, revised formats and new visualisation tools. Nucleic Acids Res 1998;26:205–213.
212. Levine AJ, Wu MC, Chang A, et al: The spectrum of mutations at the *p53* locus: Evidence for tissue-specific mutagenesis, selection of mutant alleles, and a "gain of function" phenotype. Ann NY Acad Sci 1995;768: 111–128.
213. Brambilla E, Brambilla C: *p53* and lung cancer. Pathol Biol (Paris) 1997;45:852–863.
214. Shen HM, Ong CN: Mutations of the *p53* tumor suppressor gene and *ras* oncogenes in aflatoxin hepatocarcinogenesis. Mutat Res 1996;366:23–44.
215. Hollstein M, Sidransky D, Vogelstein B, Harris CC: *p53* mutations in human cancers. Science 1991;253:49–53.
216. Li FP, Fraumeni JF Jr, Mulvihill JJ, et al: A cancer family syndrome in twenty-four kindreds. Cancer Res 1988;48:5358–5362.
217. Li FP, Fraumeni JF Jr: Prospective study of a family cancer syndrome. JAMA 1982;247:2692–2694.
218. Frebourg T, Barbier N, Yan YX, et al: Germ-line *p53* mutations in 15 families with Li-Fraumeni syndrome. Am J Hum Genet 1995;56:608–615.
219. Frebourg T, Friend SH: Cancer risks from germline *p53* mutations. J Clin Invest 1992;90:1637–1641.
220. Lavin MF, Shiloh Y: Ataxia-telangiectasia: A multifaceted genetic disorder associated with defective signal transduction. Curr Opin Immunol 1996;8:459–464.
221. Lavin MF, Shiloh Y: The genetic defect in ataxia-telangiectasia. Annu Rev Immunol 1997;15:177–202.
222. Canman CE, Lim DS: The role of ATM in DNA damage responses and cancer. Oncogene 1998;17:3301–3308.
223. Concannon P, Gatti RA: Diversity of ATM gene mutations detected in patients with ataxia-telangiectasia. Hum Mutat 1997;10:100–107.
224. Phelps WC, Yee CL, Munger K, Howley PM: The human papillomavirus type 16 E7 gene encodes transactivation and transformation functions similar to those of adenovirus E1A. Cell 1988;53:539–547.
225. Werness BA, Levine AJ, Howley PM: Association of human papillomavirus types 16 and 18 E6 proteins with p53. Science 1990;248:76–79.
226. Stoler MH: Human papillomaviruses and cervical neoplasia: A model for carcinogenesis. Int J Gynecol Pathol 2000;19:16–28.
227. Harlow E, Whyte P, Franza BR Jr, Schley C: Association of adenovirus early-region 1A proteins with cellular polypeptides. Mol Cell Biol 1986;6:1579–1589.
228. Whyte P, Buchkovich KJ, Horowitz JM, et al: Association between an oncogene and an anti-oncogene: The adenovirus E1A proteins bind to the retinoblastoma gene product. Nature 1988;334:124–129.
229. DeCaprio JA, Ludlow JW, Figge J, et al: SV40 large tumor antigen forms a specific complex with the product of the retinoblastoma susceptibility gene. Cell 1988;54: 275–283.
230. Howley PM, Scheffner M, Huibregtse J, Munger K: Oncoproteins encoded by the cancer-associated human papillomaviruses target the products of the retinoblastoma and *p53* tumor suppressor genes. Cold Spring Harb Symp Quant Biol 1991;56:149–155.
231. zur Hausen H: Papillomaviruses in human cancers. Proc Assoc Am Physicians 1999;111:581–587.
232. Barbosa MS, Vass WC, Lowy DR, Schiller JT: In vitro biological activities of the E6 and E7 genes vary among human papillomaviruses of different oncogenic potential. J Virol 1991;65:292–298.
233. Hudson JB, Bedell MA, McCance DJ, Laiminis LA: Immortalization and altered differentiation of human keratinocytes in vitro by the E6 and E7 open reading frames of human papillomavirus type 18. J Virol 1990; 64:519–526.
234. Munger K, Phelps WC, Bubb V, et al: The E6 and E7 genes of the human papillomavirus type 16 together are necessary and sufficient for transformation of primary human keratinocytes. J Virol 1989;63:4417–4421.
235. Dyson N, Howley PM, Munger K, Harlow E: The human papilloma virus-16 E7 oncoprotein is able to bind to the retinoblastoma gene product. Science 1989; 243:934–937.
236. Munger K, Werness BA, Dyson N, et al: Complex formation of human papillomavirus E7 proteins with the retinoblastoma tumor suppressor gene product. Embo J 1989;8:4099–4105.
237. Scheffner M, Werness BA, Huibregtse JM, et al: The E6 oncoprotein encoded by human papillomavirus types 16 and 18 promotes the degradation of p53. Cell 1990;63: 1129–1136.
238. Mietz JA, Unger T, Huibregtse JM, Howley PM: The transcriptional transactivation function of wild-type p53 is inhibited by SV40 large T-antigen and by HPV-16 E6 oncoprotein. Embo J 1992;11:5013–5020.
239. Scheffner M, Munger K, Byrne JC, Howley PM: The state of the *p53* and retinoblastoma genes in human cer-

vical carcinoma cell lines. Proc Natl Acad Sci USA 1991; 88:5523–5527.

240. Fujita M, Inoue M, Tanizawa O, et al: Alterations of the *p53* gene in human primary cervical carcinoma with and without human papillomavirus infection. Cancer Res 1992;52:5323–5328.

241. Crook T, Wrede D, Tidy JA, et al: Clonal *p53* mutation in primary cervical cancer: Association with human-papillomavirus-negative tumours. Lancet 1992;339: 1070–1073.

242. Lynch HT, de la Chapelle A: Genetic susceptibility to non-polyposis colorectal cancer. J Med Genet 1999;36: 801–818.

243. Craanen ME, Blok P, Offerhaus GJ, Tytgat GN: Recent developments in hereditary nonpolyposis colorectal cancer. Scand J Gastroenterol Suppl 1996;218: 92–97.

244. Hahn WC, Counter CM, Lundberg AS, et al: Creation of human tumour cells with defined genetic elements [see comments]. Nature 1999;400:464–468.

245. Dickson MA, Hahn WC, Ino Y, et al: Human keratinocytes that express hTERT and also bypass a p16(INK4a)-enforced mechanism that limits life span become immortal yet retain normal growth and differentiation characteristics. Mol Cell Biol 2000;20:1436–1447.

246. Kim NW, Piatyszek MA, Prowse KR, et al: Specific association of human telomerase activity with immortal cells and cancer. Science 1994;266: 2011–2015.

247. Rhyu MS: Telomeres, telomerase, and immortality [see comments]. J Natl Cancer Inst 1995;87:884–894.

248. Uchida N, Otsuka T, Shigematsu H, et al: Differential gene expression of human telomerase-associated protein hTERT and TEP1 in human hematopoietic cells. Leuk Res 1999;23:1127–1132.

249. Cong YS, Wen J, Bacchetti S: The human telomerase catalytic subunit hTERT: Organization of the gene and characterization of the promoter. Hum Mol Genet 1999;8:137–142.

250. Takakura M, Kyo S, Kanaya T, et al: Cloning of human telomerase catalytic subunit (hTERT) gene promoter and identification of proximal core promoter sequences essential for transcriptional activation in immortalized and cancer cells. Cancer Res 1999;59:551–557.

251. Kyo S, Takakura M, Taira T, et al: Sp1 cooperates with c-Myc to activate transcription of the human telomerase reverse transcriptase gene (hTERT). Nucleic Acids Res 2000;28:669–677.

252. Bieche I, Nogues C, Paradis V, et al: Quantitation of *hTERT* gene expression in sporadic breast tumors with a real-time reverse transcription-polymerase chain reaction assay. Clin Cancer Res 2000;6:452–459.

253. Ito H, Kyo S, Kanaya T, et al: Detection of human telomerase reverse transcriptase messenger RNA in voided urine samples as a useful diagnostic tool for bladder cancer. Clin Cancer Res 1998;4:2807–2810.

254. Zeiger MA, Smallridge RC, Clark DP, et al: Human telomerase reverse transcriptase *(hTERT)* gene expression in FNA samples from thyroid neoplasms. Surgery 1999; 126:1195–1198; discussion 1198–1199.

255. Hall JM, Friedman L, Guenther C, et al: Closing in on a breast cancer gene on chromosome 17q. Am J Hum Genet 1992;50:1235–1242.

256. Hall JM, Lee MK, Newman B, et al: Linkage of early-onset familial breast cancer to chromosome 17q21. Science 1990;250:1684–1689.

257. Friedman LS, Ostermeyer EA, Szabo CI, et al: Confirmation of *BRCA1* by analysis of germline mutations linked to breast and ovarian cancer in ten families. Nat Genet 1994;8:399–404.

258. Miki Y, Swensen J, Shattuck-Eidens D, et al: A strong candidate for the breast and ovarian cancer susceptibility gene *BRCA1*. Science 1994;266:66–71.

259. Wooster R, Bignell G, Lancaster J, et al: Identification of the breast cancer susceptibility gene *BRCA2* [see comments] [published erratum appears in Nature 1996;379: 749]. Nature 1995;378:789–792.

260. Goldgar DE, Neuhausen SL, Steele L, et al: A 45-year follow-up of kindred 107 and the search for BRCA2. J Natl Cancer Inst Monogr 1995;17:15–19.

261. Duncan JA, Reeves JR, Cooke TG: BRCA1 and BRCA2 proteins: Roles in health and disease. Mol Pathol 1998; 51:237–247.

262. Chen Y, Lee WH, Chew HK: Emerging roles of *BRCA1* in transcriptional regulation and DNA repair. J Cell Physiol 1999;181:385–392.

263. Dasika GK, Lin SC, Zhao S, et al: DNA damage-induced cell cycle checkpoints and DNA strand break repair in development and tumorigenesis. Oncogene 1999;18: 7883–7899.

264. Borden KL: RING fingers and B-boxes: Zinc-binding protein-protein interaction domains. Biochem Cell Biol 1998;76:351–358.

265. Xu X, Wagner KU, Larson D, et al: Conditional mutation of *Brca1* in mammary epithelial cells results in blunted ductal morphogenesis and tumour formation [see comments]. Nat Genet 1999;22:37–43.

266. Irminger-Finger I, Siegel BD, Leung WC: The functions of breast cancer susceptibility gene 1 *(BRCA1)* product and its associated proteins. Biol Chem 1999;380:117–128.

267. Zhong Q, Chen CF, Li S, et al: Association of *BRCA1* with the hRad50-hMre11-p95 complex and the DNA damage response. Science 1999;285:747–750.

268. Scully R, Ganesan S, Vlasakova K, et al: Genetic analysis of *BRCA1* function in a defined tumor cell line. Mol Cell 1999;4:1093–1099.

269. Cortez D, Wang Y, Qin J, Elledge SJ: Requirement of ATM-dependent phosphorylation of brca1 in the DNA damage response to double-strand breaks [see comments]. Science 1999;286:1162–1166.

270. Lee JS, Collins KM, Brown AL, et al: hCds1-mediated phosphorylation of BRCA1 regulates the DNA damage response. Nature 2000;404:201–204.

271. Aprelikova ON, Fang BS, Meissner EG, et al: *BRCA1*-associated growth arrest is RB-dependent. Proc Natl Acad Sci USA 1999;96:11866–11871.

272. Ouchi T, Monteiro AN, August A, et al: *BRCA1* regulates p53-dependent gene expression. Proc Natl Acad Sci USA 1998;95:2302–2306.

273. Frank TS: Laboratory determination of hereditary susceptibility to breast and ovarian cancer. Arch Pathol Lab Med 1999;123:1023–1026.

274. Gauthier-Villars M, Gad S, Caux V, et al: Genetic testing for breast cancer predisposition. Surg Clin North Am 1999;79:1171–1187, xxi.

275. Pharoah PD, Stratton JF, Mackay J: Screening for breast and ovarian cancer: The relevance of family history. Br Med Bull 1998;54:823–838.
276. Frank TS, Braverman AM: The pros and cons of genetic testing for breast and ovarian cancer risk. Int J Fertil Womens Med 1999;44:139–145.
277. Ashwell JD, Berger NA, Cidlowski JA, et al: Coming to terms with death: Apoptosis in cancer and immune development. Immunol Today 1994;15:147–151.
278. Itoh N, Yonehara S, Ishii A, et al: The polypeptide encoded by the cDNA for human cell surface antigen Fas can mediate apoptosis. Cell 1991;66:233–243.
279. Nagata S, Golstein P: The Fas death factor. Science 1995;267:1449–1456.
280. Gruss HJ: Molecular, structural, and biological characteristics of the tumor necrosis factor ligand superfamily. Int J Clin Lab Res 1996;26:143–159.
281. Griffith TS, Lynch DH: TRAIL: A molecule with multiple receptors and control mechanisms. Curr Opin Immunol 1998;10:559–563.
282. Schulze-Osthoff K, Ferrari D, Los M, et al: Apoptosis signaling by death receptors. Eur J Biochem 1998;254: 439–459.
283. Blagosklonny MV: A node between proliferation, apoptosis, and growth arrest. Bioessays 1999;21:704–709.
284. Perez-Sala D, Rebollo A: Novel aspects of Ras proteins biology: Regulation and implications. Cell Death Differ 1999;6:722–728.
285. Tanaka N, Ishihara M, Kitagawa M, et al: Cellular commitment to oncogene-induced transformation or apoptosis is dependent on the transcription factor IRF-1. Cell 1994;77:829–839.
286. Downward J: Ras signalling and apoptosis. Curr Opin Genet Dev 1998;8:49–54.
287. Enari M, Sakahira H, Yokoyama H, et al: A caspase-activated DNase that degrades DNA during apoptosis, and its inhibitor ICAD [see comments] [published erratum appears in Nature 1998;393:396]. Nature 1998;391: 43–50.
288. McIlroy D, Sakahira H, Talanian RV, Nagata S: Involvement of caspase 3-activated DNase in internucleosomal DNA cleavage induced by diverse apoptotic stimuli. Oncogene 1999;18:4401–4408.
289. Mukae N, Enari M, Sakahira H, et al: Molecular cloning and characterization of human caspase-activated DNase. Proc Natl Acad Sci USA 1998;95:9123–9128.
290. Sakahira H, Enari M, Nagata S: Functional differences of two forms of the inhibitor of caspase-activated DNase, ICAD-L, and ICAD-S. J Biol Chem 1999;274: 15740–15744.
291. Sakahira H, Enari M, Nagata S: Cleavage of CAD inhibitor in CAD activation and DNA degradation during apoptosis. Nature 1998;391:96–99.
292. Korsmeyer SJ: Regulators of cell death. Trends Genet 1995;11:101–105.
293. Yin XM, Oltvai ZN, Veis-Novack DJ, et al: *Bcl-2* gene family and the regulation of programmed cell death. Cold Spring Harb Symp Quant Biol 1994;59:387–393.
294. Oltvai ZN, Milliman CL, Korsmeyer SJ: *Bcl-2* heterodimerizes in vivo with a conserved homolog, Bax, that accelerates programmed cell death. Cell 1993;74: 609–619.
295. Chao DT, Korsmeyer SJ: *BCL-2* family: Regulators of cell death. Annu Rev Immunol 1998;16:395–419.
296. Korsmeyer SJ: *BCL-2* gene family and the regulation of programmed cell death. Cancer Res 1999;59(7 Suppl): 1693s–1700s.
297. Sharp JG, Chan WC: Detection and relevance of minimal disease in lymphomas. Cancer Metastasis Rev 1999; 18:127–142.
298. Sheikh MS, Fornace AJ Jr: Role of p53 family members in apoptosis. J Cell Physiol 2000;182:171–181.
299. Miyashita T, Reed JC: Tumor suppressor *p53* is a direct transcriptional activator of the human *bax* gene. Cell 1995;80:293–299.
300. Golub TR, Slonim DK, Tamayo P, et al: Molecular classification of cancer: Class discovery and class prediction by gene expression monitoring. Science 1999;286: 531–537.
301. McManus AP, Gusterson BA, Pinkerton CR, Shipley JM: The molecular pathology of small round-cell tumours—relevance to diagnosis, prognosis, and classification. J Pathol 1996;178:116–121.
302. Carey FA: Pulmonary adenocarcinoma: Classification and molecular biology. J Pathol 1998;184:229–230.

TIMOTHY J. O'LEARY
DENNIS M. FRISMAN

2

Antigens

Immunohistochemical demonstration of differentiation antigens is a routine adjunct to light microscopy in tumor diagnosis and is increasingly advocated for assessment of tumor prognosis. Many excellent monographs detail the use of "immunomicroscopy" in diagnostic pathology.[1–3] Although the diagnostic utility of the antigens is well described in these references, their biologic structure and their physiologic significance often are not. In the hope that pathologists will find the structure and function of these antigens to be both interesting and useful, we present here an overview not only of the diagnostic utility but also of the genetic, physiologic, and structural characteristics of many of the tumor differentiation antigens and certain prognostic markers.

Several invaluable reference sources have allowed identification of pertinent literature. The Online Mendelian Inheritance in Man is an invaluable source of information on the molecular biology, function, and clinical genetics of many proteins. CN3D, an Internet interface to the Brookhaven Protein Structure Data Bank, provides an easy-to-use utility for demonstration of the macromolecular structures that have been characterized by nuclear magnetic resonance or x-ray diffraction techniques.[4, 5] Finally, the *Extracellular Matrix FactsBook*,[6] the *Leukocyte Antigen FactsBook*,[7] and the *Adhesion Molecule FactsBook*[8] provide succinct sources of molecular biologic, nucleic acid sequence, and functional data for several of the antigens discussed in this chapter.

THE INTERMEDIATE FILAMENTS

The intermediate filaments are 8- to 12-nm unbranched filaments that constitute the cytoskeletal matrix of most cells. Thus, the intermediate filaments help to maintain both cell shape and internal organization. Although the expression of intermediate filaments is not absolutely tissue specific (e.g., most epithelial cells express small amounts of vimentin), cytoplasmic immunohistochemical staining of intermediate filament proteins may be used to differentiate epithelial cells from mesenchymal and lymphoid cells and to differentiate among the various classes of mesenchymal cells. Immunohistochemical demonstration of keratins generally reflects epithelial differentiation, whereas expression of vimentin is seen in mesenchymal cells, desmin in muscle cells, glial filaments (predominantly glial fibrillary acidic protein [GFAP]) in glial cells, and neurofilaments in neuronal cells. The significant sequence homologies among the five major classes of intermediate filaments may result in immunologic cross-reactivity, particularly when antibodies that have been raised against the "core" domains of the intermediate filaments are employed. Further complications arise because the demonstration of all intermediate filament proteins varies both with the primary antibody that is employed and also with the fixation and embedding of the specimen.

Keratins

The expression of keratin proteins is, in general, a hallmark of epithelial differentiation (Fig. 2–1). Immunohistochemical identification of keratin is used to identify epithelial tumors, as well as to characterize subsets of mesenchymal tumors, such as epithelioid sarcoma and synovial sarcoma. Immunohistochemical demonstration of keratin proteins is often facilitated by protease digestion; overdigestion may give rise to an artifact in which staining is observed in both nucleus and cytoplasm of affected cells. Antigen retrieval techniques may also enhance immunohistochemical reactivity.

The 20 to 30 different keratin proteins[9] belong to two families—acidic (type I), with pI of 4.5 to 5.5 and molecular weights of 40 to 57 kd, and basic (type II), with pH of 5.5 to 7.5 and molecular weights of 53 to 67 kd.[10] The 10 known acidic keratins include keratins 9 through 19; the basic keratins include keratins 1 through 8. The acidic keratins, which display little homology with the basic keratins, are coded by genes clustered on chromosome 17 (except for keratin 18); the basic keratins are coded by genes clustered on chromosome 12.

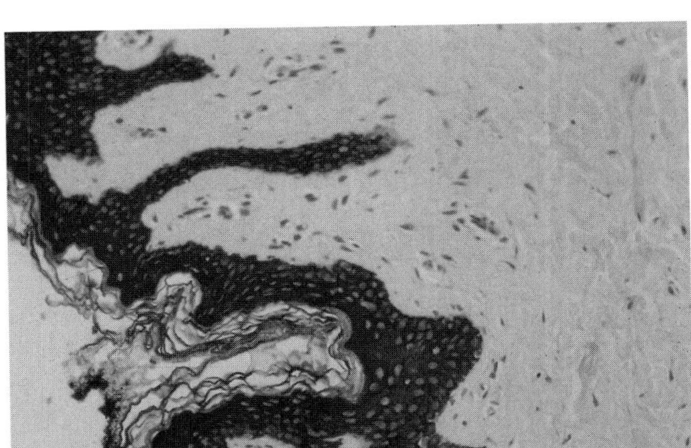

FIGURE 2–1
Section of skin immunohistochemically stained with a pancytokeratin antibody (×200). (See also Color Fig. 2–1.)

Although, in vitro, any acidic keratin may associate with any basic keratin, the composition of the keratin pairs found in vivo is different. For the most part, keratin pairs are highly specific; they are synthesized so that at least one acidic and one basic keratin protein is expressed in each epithelial cell. Keratins 5 and 14 are observed in epidermal basal cells. In the lower spinous layer, expression of keratins 1 and 10 is seen, whereas in the upper spinous layer of the palm and sole, keratins 2e and 9 are found. Keratins 6 and 14 are normally expressed in the outer root sheath of the hair follicle and in the epidermis of palms and soles. Keratins 6 and 16 are found in hyperproliferative cells. Keratins 3 and 12 are expressed in the cornea. Thus, immunohistochemical detection of specific keratins can be used to help assess tissue differentiation. Few, if any, commercially available antibodies react with all keratins. Immunohistochemical interpretation thus depends on a knowledge of specific patterns of reactivity. AE1, for example, reacts only with acidic keratins, whereas AE3 reacts with the basic keratins. Although each reacts with both high- and low-molecular-weight keratins, the AE1/AE3 cocktail in common use demonstrates simple epithelia more effectively than it does complex stratified squamous epithelia.

All keratins demonstrate a conserved 300 to 330 amino acid central rod of coiled-coil α helices flanked by head and tail regions of varying size. Sequence homology is limited to the central core.

KERATIN 1

Keratin 1, a 67-kd keratin of hair and epidermis, is coded by a gene that maps to the type II keratin gene cluster at 12q11–q13, and is coexpressed with keratin 10.[11] Mutations of keratin may be responsible for some cases of epidermolytic hyperkeratosis.[12] Keratin 1 immunoreactivity is observed on most cases of Bowen's disease and most syringomas.

KERATIN 2E

Keratin 2e is a basic 65.8-kd protein encoded by a 2.6-kb messenger RNA (mRNA) species[13]; the gene locus is as yet undetermined. Keratin 2e is specific to epidermal upper spinous cells of the palms and soles and is coexpressed with keratin 9. Mutations in the keratin 2e gene have been observed in patients with ichthyosis bullosa of Siemens.[14]

KERATIN 3

Keratin 3 (KRT3), a 64-kd basic protein, is coexpressed with keratin 12 during differentiation of the corneal epithelium.[15] The keratin 3 gene is localized to 12q12-13[16] and expresses a 6.5-kb mRNA.

KERATIN 4

The suprabasal cells of nonkeratinizing squamous epithelia coexpress keratins 4 and 13. Keratin 4 is coded by a gene localized to 12p11.2-q11.[17] There are two codominant alleles to the keratin 4 gene. There is no current diagnostic use for keratin 4 immunohistochemistry.

KERATIN 5

Keratin 5, a 58-kd protein, is coexpressed with keratin 14 in stratified squamous epithelia. The gene for keratin 5, which has been cloned[18] and localized to chromosome 12q11-13,[19] may develop point mutations responsible for epidermolysis bullosa simplex.[20, 21]

KERATINS 6A AND 6B

Keratin 6a is a low-molecular-weight basic keratin coded at low levels by a gene on chromosome 12q12-14[22]; keratin 6b is coded by a gene localized nearby on chromosome 12. Expression of keratin 6, which is typically coexpressed with keratin 16, is usually found only in hyperproliferating cells.

KERATIN 7

Keratin 7 is a low-molecular-weight keratin expressed by simple epithelia and coded by a gene found on 12q12-14.[22] It is strongly expressed in neoplasms originating in such epithelia, as seen in Table 2–1.

TABLE 2–1

Immunoreactivity of Selected Neoplasms for Keratin 7

Diagnosis	Percentage of Cases Demonstrating Immunoreactivity
Adenocarcinoma, endometrium	87–100
Adenocarcinoma, gallbladder	100
Adenocarcinoma, lung	90–99
Adenocarcinoma, pancreas	68–94
Adenocarcinoma, stomach	52–80
Bronchioloalveolar carcinoma	100
Cholangiocarcinoma	100
Combined hepatocellular carcinoma/cholangiocarcinoma	100
Infiltrating ductal carcinoma, breast	92–100
Mesothelioma	61–84
Paget's disease (extramammary)	100

KERATIN 8

Keratin 8 is a low-molecular-weight basic keratin coded by a gene localized to 12q13.2-24.1[23] and coexpressed with keratin 18 in simple epithelia. Keratin 8 is the only basic keratin expressed in normal hepatocytes.

KERATIN 10

Keratin 10 is a 56.5-kd acidic keratin that is coded by a gene that maps to 17q12-q21.[11] Keratin 10 is coexpressed with keratin 1 in terminally differentiated epidermal cells. The gene has been cloned, and the nucleotide and amino acid sequences have been determined.[24, 25] Mutations in the keratin 10 gene cause epidermolytic hyperkeratosis, as can mutations in the keratin 1 gene.[12, 26, 27]

KERATIN 14

Keratin 14, which is coexpressed with keratin 5 in epidermal basal cells, is coded by a gene that maps to 17p11-12.[22] Mutations in the keratin 14 gene give rise to degeneration of the keratin network, associated with epidermal cytolysis, resulting in clinical manifestations of epidermolysis bullosa simplex.[19, 28]

KERATIN 15

Keratin 15 is a basic keratin coded by a gene that maps to 17q21-q23.[17]

KERATIN 16

Keratin 16 is an acidic keratin coded by a gene that localizes to 17q12-q21.[22] It is generally observed in hyperproliferating cells.

TABLE 2–2

Immunoreactivity of Selected Neoplasms for Keratin 18

Diagnosis	Percentage of Cases Demonstrating Immunoreactivity
Adenocarcinoma, lung	100
Adenocarcinoma, pancreas	55–100
Adenoma, thyroid	100
Follicular carcinoma, thyroid	100
Mesothelioma	100
Papillary carcinoma, thyroid	100

KERATIN 17

Keratin 17 is normally expressed in the basal cells of complex epithelia but not in stratified or simple epithelia. The gene coding keratin 17 is localized to the keratin type I gene cluster on chromosome 17[29]; two pseudogenes for keratin 17 are localized nearby.

KERATIN 18

Keratin 18 is a low-molecular-weight acidic keratin coexpressed with keratin 8 by simple epithelium. It is coded by a 3.8-kb gene[30] that localizes to 17p11-p12.[31] Keratin 18 is the only acidic keratin expressed in normal hepatocytes. Selected neoplasms demonstrating frequent reactivity for keratin 18 are shown in Table 2–2.

KERATIN 19

Keratin 19 is a 40-kd acidic keratin coded by a completely sequenced gene that maps to 17q21-q23.[32–34] This keratin is found in the periderm, an embryologic superficial layer, and in some carcinomas.

Glial Fibrillary Acidic Protein

Glial fibrillary acidic protein (GFAP) is a 59-kd intermediate-filament protein first identified in plaques of multiple sclerosis.[35, 36] It is found predominantly in cells of glial origin and thus forms a useful immunohistochemical marker for cells of astrocytic/glial origin (Fig. 2–2), but it may also be seen in a variety of nonglial tumors ranging from pleomorphic adenomas of the salivary gland to pheochromocytomas (Table 2–3). GFAP is coded by a single gene localized to chromosome 17q21.[37, 38] The *GFAP* gene has been sequenced[39]; strong sequence homologies between GFAP, desmin, and vimentin suggest structural similarities between the central rod and carboxyl-terminal domain of these intermediate filaments. This is supported by circular dichroism measurements demonstrating the presence of helical structures.[40]

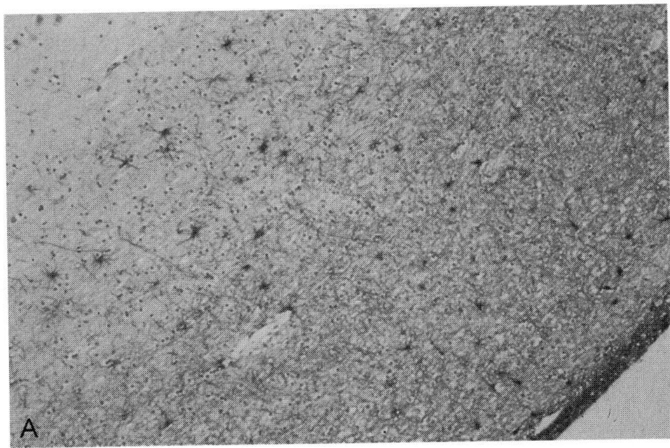

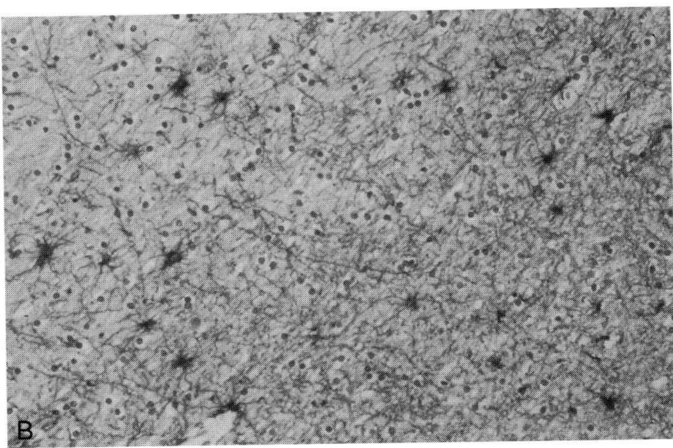

FIGURE 2–2
Section of brain immunohistochemically stained for glial fibrillary acidic protein (GFAP), ×100 (*A*) and ×200 (*B*). (See also Color Fig. 2–2.)

TABLE 2–3

Immunoreactivity of Selected Neoplasms for Glial Fibrillary Acidic Protein

Diagnosis	Percentage of Cases Demonstrating Immunoreactivity
Astrocytoma	100
Ganglioglioma	100
Hemangioblastoma, cerebellar	26–55
Paraganglioma, parasympathetic	67–100
Pheochromocytoma	34–74
Pleomorphic adenoma, salivary gland	69–93
Primitive neuroectodermal tumor, central	87–100

There are many more GFAP mRNA transcripts in white matter than in gray matter.[36] GFAP forms bundles within cell bodies and cytoplasmic processes of differentiated astrocytes, particularly fibrous astrocytes. Reactive gliosis results in increased GFAP expression; ingestion of GFAP by reactive macrophages can result in diagnostic confusion.

Demonstration of GFAP is often facilitated by enzymatic digestion or antigen retrieval techniques.

Neurofilament Protein

Although the Bodian stain was classically employed to demonstrate neurofilaments, immunohistochemical identification of neurofilament proteins (Fig. 2–3) is now more often used to identify neuronal and neuroectodermal tumors (Table 2–4). Neurofilament protein may also be observed in pulmonary carcinoids and small cell carcinomas and in Merkel cell tumors. Demonstration of neurofilaments is often facilitated by enzymatic digestion and is frequently better in B5-fixed tissues than in formalin-fixed tissues.

There are three different neurofilament proteins (NFPs), which are distinguished on the basis of molecular weight—NFL (or NF68, 68 kd), NFM (or NF125, 125 kd),[41] and NFH (or NF200, 200 kd).[42] Estimates for the relative percentage of each of these components within the neurofilament vary. NFL is coded by a gene that localizes to chromosome 8p21.[43, 44] Cloned NFP gene sequences[45] demonstrate that, like desmin and vimentin, NFP contains

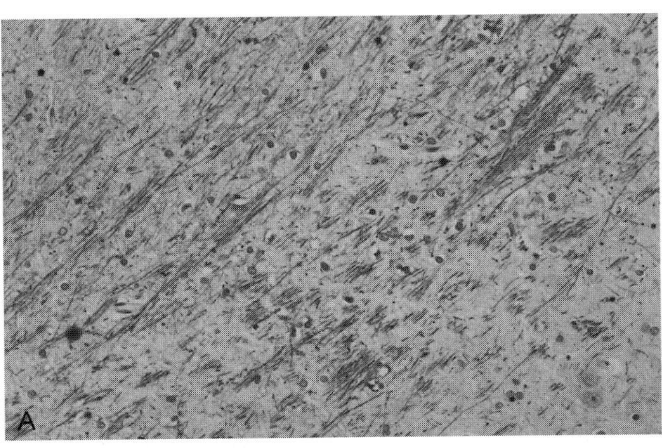

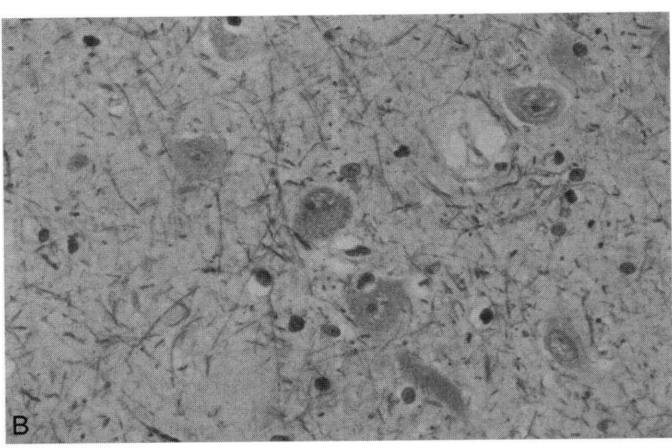

FIGURE 2–3
Section of brain immunohistochemically stained for neurofilament protein (NFP), ×200 (*A*) and ×400 (*B*). (See also Color Fig. 2–3.)

TABLE 2–4

Immunoreactivity of Selected Neoplasms for Neurofilament Protein

Diagnosis	Percentage of Cases Demonstrating Immunoreactivity
Ganglioglioma	82–97
Ganglioneuroma	100
Ganglioneuroblastoma	100
Medullary carcinoma, thyroid	62–100
Merkel cell carcinoma	30–70
Neuroblastoma	63–86
Neurofibroma	28–65
Pheochromocytoma	85–98
Primitive neuroectodermal tumor, central	54–91

an α-helical domain capable of forming coiled coils; the NFL gene differs from other intermediate filaments in that, rather than eight introns, it only contains three.

The *NFH* gene is localized to chromosome 22q12.1-q13.1,[46] at or near the site of a gene for neurofibromatosis type 2.[47]

Neurofilaments are among the major cytoskeletal constituents in many nerves; they are frequently the predominant structural element within the axon and are found more sparsely within dendrites. Typically, neurofilaments are packaged as small bundles that lie along a portion of an axon. There is little direct information available regarding the conformation of NFPs; amino acid sequence homologies suggest structures similar to those of vimentin and desmin.

The NFPs have a high concentration of glutamic acid (approximately 20% of total amino acid content in each). There are three separate regions—the amino (N) terminus, which is about 80 amino acids long and which is very basic; the rod domain (approximately 310 residues consisting of a 7 amino acid repeat); and the carboxyl (C) terminal extension, in which nearly half the residues are glutamic acid. The carboxyl-terminal regions of the three polypeptides are radically different in length. The amino-terminal is predicted to be sheet, the rod, α helix, and the carboxyl-terminal, random coil. The rod segment is 80% helix. Between the rod segment and the carboxyl-terminal is a sequence with high proline content. The NFM and NFH proteins contain carboxyl-terminal mull-tiphosphorylation repeat regions; during the course of neuronal maturation, the degree of phosphorylation increases.[48] Binding of aluminum or calcium to this region results in the formation of β-sheet structures; this may be relevant to the formation of amyloid in Alzheimer's disease.[49, 50] Theoretical analyses predict that, like all other all intermediate filament proteins, NFPs have a rod domain consisting of four α-helix–rich segments that intertwine with similar segments from a second polypeptide, giving rise to a two-stranded rope.[51]

Most anti-NFP antibodies bind an epitope near the carboxyl-terminal end of the rod.

The function of NFP is only partially understood. It appears to play both a structural and a transport role in neuronal cells and their extensions. Links between microtubules and neurofilaments have been observed. Both microtubule-associated proteins and microtubules themselves seem to be transported in a fashion coordinated with NFP movement within the cell.

Desmin

Smooth muscle cells contain an axial bundle of 10-nm filaments that extends the length of the cell and is associated with clusters of mitochondria near the nucleus.[52] These 10-nm filaments contain a 53-kd protein, desmin; vascular tissue smooth muscle cells also contain another 54-kd intermediate filament, vimentin.[53] Desmin is coded by a gene localized at 2q35,[54] and it is highly homologous with vimentin. It appears to play a role in differentiation of muscle cells and maintenance of their shape; desmin abnormalities may be associated with several types of myopathy.[55–57] Immunohistochemical demonstration of desmin (Fig. 2–4) is useful in establishing the presence of muscle cell differentiation (Table 2–5). Although enzymatic digestion may (or may not) improve immunohistochemical detection of desmin, antigen retrieval procedures have not proven useful in our laboratory.

Circular dichroism studies show that desmin has a secondary structure that is about 45% α helix,[58] similar to vimentin. Desmin exhibits three major domains—an amino-terminal 70-residue headpiece, a middle rod portion consisting of three α-helical segments connected by short, non–α-helical spacers, and a carboxyl-terminal nonhelical tailpiece of about 50 residues.[59] The rod segment demonstrates a peptide repeat pattern of hydrophobic amino acids that is necessary to form the interchain coiled-coil packed α-helical pattern seen in the intermediate filaments.

Vimentin

Vimentin is an intermediate filament that is expressed primarily in mesenchymal tissue; immunohistochemical demonstration of vimentin is useful in establishing the mesenchymal derivation of a tumor (Table 2–6). In addition, because cells that express vimentin may be found in virtually any tissue section, immunohistochemical assessment of vimentin is a useful internal control for preservation of immunohistochemical reactivity (Fig. 2–5). Although demonstration of vimentin may be improved by antigen-retrieval techniques, their use is seldom necessary.

Vimentin is coded by a single gene[60, 61] that maps to 10p13.[61] Sequencing demonstrates that the gene is

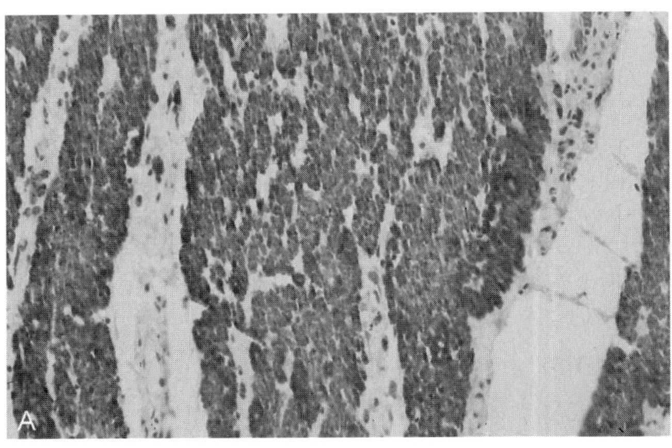

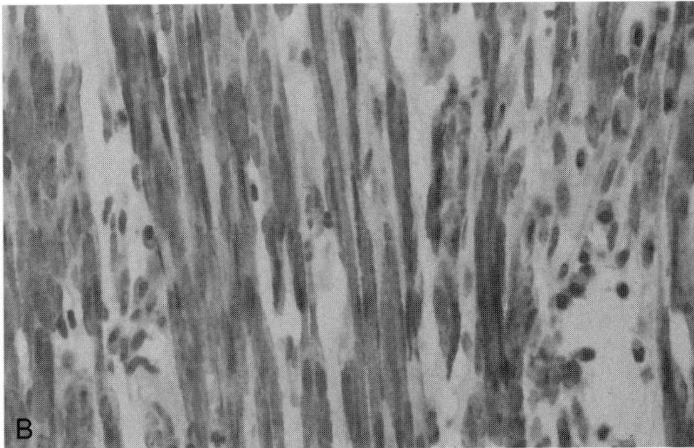

FIGURE 2–4
A and *B,* Two sections of colonic wall immunohistochemically stained for desmin (×200). (See also Color Fig. 2–4.)

TABLE 2–5
Immunoreactivity of Selected Neoplasms for Desmin

Diagnosis	Percentage of Cases Demonstrating Immunoreactivity
Inflammatory pseudotumor	41–60
Intra-abdominal desmoplastic small cell tumor	92–100
Leiomyoma	100
Leiomyosarcoma	62–74
Rhabdomyosarcoma, alveolar	100
Rhabdomyosarcoma, NOS	86–95
Sarcoma botryoides	100
Wilms' tumor	65–100

NOS, not otherwise specified.

TABLE 2–6
Immunoreactivity of Selected Neoplasms for Vimentin

Diagnosis	Percentage of Cases Demonstrating Immunoreactivity
Adrenal cortical carcinoma	48–81
Ameloblastoma	100
Atypical fibroxanthoma	100
Chondrosarcoma	94–100
Chordoma	100
Dermatofibroma	100
Dermatofibrosarcoma protuberans	100
Ewing's sarcoma	80–93
Fibosarcoma	100
Gastrointestinal stromal tumor (GIST)	94–99
Granular cell tumor	100
Granulosa cell tumor	98–100
Hemangiopericytoma	100
Hodgkin's disease	100
Malignant fibrous histiocytoma	94–100
Malignant melanoma	95–100
Neurilemoma	100
Neurofibroma	100
Non-Hodgkins's lymphoma	54–76
Osteogenic sarcoma	100

highly conserved across species.[62] Vimentin and desmin share significant homology; care must be taken to ensure that immunohistochemical assays differentiate between these two antigens.

Chemical studies have demonstrated that whereas vimentin, like the other intermediate filaments, has large helical regions, both thze non–α-helical, amino-terminal head and carboxyl-terminal tail regions are essential for formation and stability of vimentin filaments. Binding between vimentin molecules associates nonhelical regions of one molecule with helical regions of another, giving rise to an antiparallel arrangement.[63, 64]

PLASMA PROTEINS

α_1-Antichymotrypsin

α_1-Antichymotrypsin (AACT) is a marker for histiocytes, monocytes, and liver cells, particularly those of hepatocellular carcinoma (Table 2–7). Immunohistochemical identification of this cytoplasmically localized antigen is facilitated by enzymatic digestion.

AACT is a 374 amino acid protein that, like α_1-antitrypsin (AAT), is a member of the serpin serine protease inhibitor family.[65] Deficiency of AACT, like deficiency of AAT, can lead to severe liver and lung disease. It is coded by a 12-kb gene residing with a serpin gene cluster at 14q32.1, which also contains coding sequences for AAT, corticosteroid-binding globulin, and protein C.[66, 67] Forty-five percent of the AACT amino acid sequence is identical with that of AAT.[68]

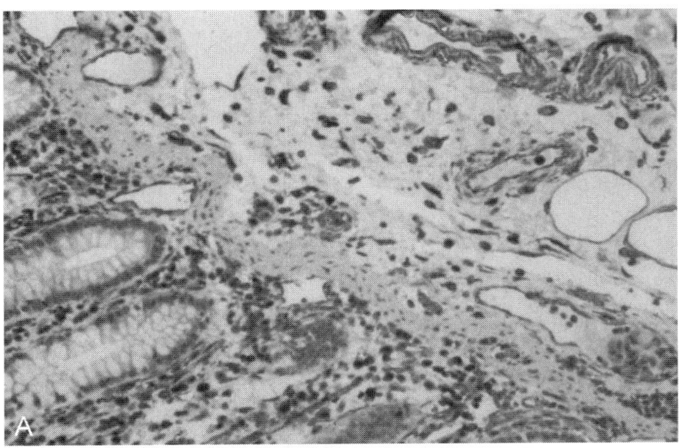

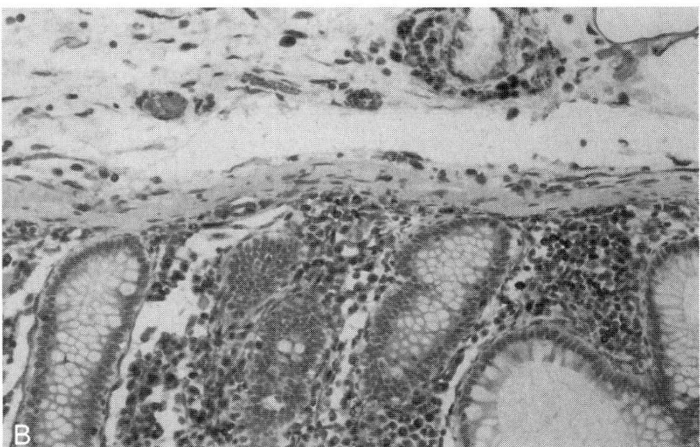

FIGURE 2–5
Sections of colon immunohistochemically stained for vimentin, ×200 (*A*) and ×400 (*B*). (See also Color Fig. 2–5.)

AACT may exist in three distinct conformations: (1) the native form, a fully active protein with the reactive site loop intact; (2) the proteolytically modified form in which inhibitory capacity is abolished; and (3) the proteinase-complexed form, a stable equimolar complex between the inhibitor and a target proteinase.[69] Of these, the cleaved form appears to be most conformationally stable.[70] The cleaved form has been characterized by x-ray diffraction techniques; the structure is similar to that of the cleaved form of AAT,[71] as is the conformational rearrangement triggered by enzymatic cleavage.[72]

TABLE 2–7

Selected Tumors Displaying Immunoreactivity for α_1-Antichymotrypsin

Diagnosis	Percentage of Cases Demonstrating Immunoreactivity
Acute myeloid leukemia	31–63
Atypical fibroxanthoma	48–80
Anaplastic carcinoma, thyroid	30–64
Dermatofibroma	8–32
Epithelioid sarcoma	29–77
Granular cell tumor	49–88
Kaposi's sarcoma	86–100
Leiomyosarcoma	10–30
Liposarcoma	36–69
Malignant fibrous histiocytoma	78–89
Malignant melanoma	43–82
Malignant mesenchymoma	38–100
Meningioma, secretory	63–92
Neurofibrosarcoma	8–51
Osteogenic sarcoma	61–97
Rhabdomyosarcoma, NOS	20–53

NOS, not otherwise specified.

α_1-Antitrypsin

α_1-Antitrypsin is a cytoplasmic marker for monocytes, histiocytes, liver cells, and nonseminomatous germ cell (particularly yolk sac) tumors (Table 2–8). Although enzymatic digestion improves immunohistochemical demonstration of AAT, some antigen retrieval techniques may decrease immunostaining.[73]

AAT is a member of a highly conserved family (the serpins) of serine proteinase inhibitors found in plants, birds, mammals, and viruses.[65] Abnormal secretion of AAT is associated with pulmonary emphysema and liver disease. AAT is coded by a gene that is part of a cluster of serine protease inhibitor genes localized at chromosome 14q32.1.[74] The cluster also includes genes coding for AACT, protein C inhibitor (PCI), and corticosteroid-binding globulin (CBG) genes and the AAT-like pseudogene *PIL*.[74] Human liver cDNA sequences for AAT reveal a precursor molecule that contains a 24 amino acid signal peptide and 394 amino acids present in the mature polypeptide chain.[75]

Although AAT is primarily secreted by liver, it is also expressed in blood monocytes. It appears that there are three macrophage-specific transcriptional initiation sites approximately 2 kb upstream from a single hepatocyte-specific transcriptional initiation site. Macrophages use these sites during basal and modulated expression. Hepatocytes use the hepatocyte-specific transcriptional initiation site during basal and modulated expression but may also use transcription from the upstream macrophage transcriptional initiation sites when stimulated.[76]

The conformation of AAT has been investigated by both spectroscopic[77] and x-ray diffraction[78] techniques (Fig. 2–6). Circular dichroism studies reveal the protein to be approximately 50% α helix, 25% β sheet, and 10% β turn.[77] Serpins have a proteolytically sensitive reactive-site loop that, when cleaved, relaxes from an unstable stressed native protein to a more stable relaxed cleaved

TABLE 2–8

Selected Tumors Demonstrating Immunoreactivity for α_1-Antitrypsin

Diagnosis	Percentage of Cases Demonstrating Immunoreactivity
Acinar cell carcinoma	39–84
Acute myeloid leukemia, NOS (M0)	15–65
Anaplastic carcinoma, thyroid	18–51
Atypical fibroxanthoma	49–79
Carcinoma, spindle cell	80–100
Choriocarcinoma, NOS	14–52
Endodermal sinus tumor	20–64
Epithelioid sarcoma	30–75
Fibrohistiocytic tumor, NOS	91–100
Fibroma, nonossifying	79–100
Hepatocellular carcinoma	19–68
Histiocytic lymphoma (true)	62–100
Malignant fibrous histiocytoma	64–79
Malignant histiocytosis	8–51
Malignant mixed müllerian tumor	87–100
Meningioma, secretory	68–94
Osteogenic sarcoma	54–100
Xanthogranuloma	31–69

NOS, not otherwise specified.

molecule. This results from secondary structure alterations,[70, 79] including a 7-nm movement of the newly generated carboxyl terminus to the opposite pole of the molecule. Inhibitory activity of AAT may depend on this mobility in the extended α-helical reactive site loop.[79] AAT has three oligosaccharide side chains attached to three different asparagine residues by *N*-glycosyl linkages.[80] The functions of these carbohydrate moieties are unknown.

α-Fetoprotein

Immunohistochemical identification of α-fetoprotein (AFP) is useful predominantly in the identification of germ cell tumors and hepatocellular carcinoma (Table 2–9). Cytoplasmic demonstration of AFP is frequently improved by antigen retrieval techniques.

AFP is coded by a gene on chromosome 4q11-22, in the same region as the albumin gene.[81] There is extensive sequence homology between AFP and serum albumin.[82] Considerable homology between albumin, AFP, and the human vitamin D–binding protein (hDBP) is also observed.[83] The genes for albumin and AFP are present in tandem, in the same transcriptional orientation, with the gene for albumin 14.5 kb upstream of the gene for AFP.[84] The gene for AFP codes for a 19 amino acid signal sequence, followed by a 590 amino acid structure characterized by 15 regularly spaced disulfide bridges within three repeating domains.[85, 86] Similar secondary structures are predicted for serum albumin and AFP.[87] AFP has a hydrophilic exposed surface at neutral pH and possesses extensive hydrophobic binding sites located in crevices, similar to serum albumin; as with albumin, there is a high α-helix content (approximately 70%). Hence, physical measurements confirm the molecular similarities between AFP and albumin.[88]

AFP is produced in the yolk sac and liver of the fetus, where it serves as a major plasma protein; it appears to be the fetal counterpart to albumin.

Albumin

Serum albumin is used immunohistochemically as a marker for hepatocellular carcinoma. Special care must be taken in the interpretation of apparently positive

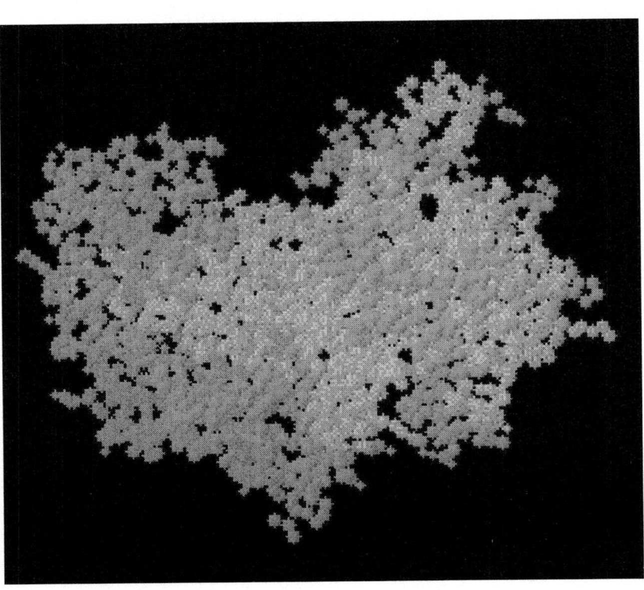

FIGURE 2–6
Space-filling structure model of α_1-antitrypsin, generated using Cn3D and Brookhaven Protein Structure Data Base data. (See also Color Fig. 2–6.)

TABLE 2–9
Selected Tumors Demonstrating Immunoreactivity for α_1-Fetoprotein

Diagnosis	Percentage of Cases Demonstrating Immunoreactivity
Cholangiocarcinoma	3–20
Embryonal carcinoma	21–46
Endodermal sinus tumor	70–95
Hepatocellular carcinoma	52–66

cytoplasmic staining, because necrotic cells of any tissue derivation may take up albumin (or other high-concentration circulating proteins) from the serum, giving rise to a misleading result. Immunohistochemical demonstration of albumin is enhanced by trypsin or protease digestion.

Albumin is a soluble, 65-kd unglycosylated polypeptide that comprises about one half of the blood serum protein. The protein is coded by a 17-kb gene that colocalizes with that of AFP to a cluster at 4q11-13.[84, 89, 90] The gene consists of 15 exons split into three domains that are believed to have arisen by triplication of a single "primordial domain." This three-domain structure is found in both albumin and AFP from all mammals; nevertheless, the amino acid sequences of various albumins are quite variable. Albumin is synthesized in the liver as preproalbumin, an amino-terminal peptide that is removed before the protein is released from the rough endoplasmic reticulum; the proalbumin product is further cleaved in the Golgi apparatus.

Albumin functions as a carrier protein for steroids, fatty acids, and thyroid hormones; it also binds the human immunodeficiency virus GP41 protein.[91] It assists in stabilizing both serum pH and extracellular fluid volume. Albumin is not an essential protein, however, because hereditary albuminuria produces small clinical effects and allelic variants are relatively common.[92, 93] In addition to analbuminuria, these genetic variants include hyposecretion and various mutated proteins with altered electrophoretic mobility. Abnormalities of thyroid hormone binding can give rise to a syndrome of "familial dysalbuminemic hyperthyroxinemia," which manifests itself as elevated serum thyroxine and free-thyroxine index in a euthyroid individual.[94]

Although it is possible that the allelic variants of albumin structure may affect immunohistochemical reactivity of the protein, such an effect has not been reported.

Albumin has been studied by spectroscopic and x-ray diffraction techniques. The structure is predominantly α-helical[95, 96]; three separate lobes, corresponding to the three domains of the albumin gene, assemble to form a heart-shaped molecule.[97] This three-lobed structure is observed in albumins ranging from hen egg albumin (Fig. 2–7) to human serum albumin. Each domain is a product of two subdomains that possess common structural motifs. The ligand-binding regions are found in hydrophobic cavities in two subdomains.[97] Considerable conformational alteration is observed with changes in pH or on binding of drugs[98, 99]; although the helix content of human serum albumin is nearly 70% at physiologic pH, it is reduced to approximately 50% at pH 2.[88]

Fibrinogen

Fibrinogen is a plasma glycoprotein synthesized in the liver. Immunohistochemical identification of fibrinogen in the cytoplasm may be useful in the recognition of hepatocellular differentiation[100] and in the characterization of renal glomerular diseases.[101, 102] Fibrinogen is most easily demonstrated in sections that have been enzymatically digested.

The fibrinogen molecule is a dimer, each half of which is composed of three structurally distinct subunits—α, β, and γ. The two halves of the dimer are connected by three disulfide bonds in an antiparallel orientation,[103] forming a central globular domain. Two additional globular regions are connected to this central core by thin rod domains, which resemble the coiled-coil rod domain of laminin.[104] The two large end dómains are constructed from the carboxyl terminus of a β chain and γ chain, respectively. The carboxyl terminus of the one α chain forms an additional central domain. Thus, the carboxyl-terminal region of each of the chains is folded into an independent globular domain.[105] The fibrinogen assembly is approximately 40% α helix[106]; reduction of disulfide bonds reduces the helix content to approximately 30%. The coiled-coil portion of the molecule is approximately 70% α helix; the globular portions are rich in β-sheet structures.[107] Binding of fibrinogen to platelet membrane glycoproteins results in conformational alteration,[108] as does change in calcium concentration.[109]

Thrombin catalyzes cleavage of α and β chains of fibrinogen, releasing fibrinopeptides A and B. Cleavage occurs at arginine-glycine bonds and leaves glycine as the amino-terminal amino acid on both chains. Thrombin also activates factor XIII (fibrin stabilizing factor). All three fibrinogen genes localize to a single cluster at 4q31[110] in the order γ–α–β.[111] The three genes, although clustered, are transcribed as separate mRNAs[112] whose transcription is coordinately regulated.[113] The fibrinogen α chain is coded as a polypeptide composed of a 19 amino acid signal sequence and a 625 amino acid circulating form.[114, 115] Subsequent proteolysis reduces the circulating form to 610 amino acids. The fibrinogen γ gene consists of 10 exons that code for the 411 amino acid mature protein and a signal sequence of 26 amino acids.[116–118] The γ chain occurs in two forms (A and B), differing only in their carboxyl termini, which arise from alternative

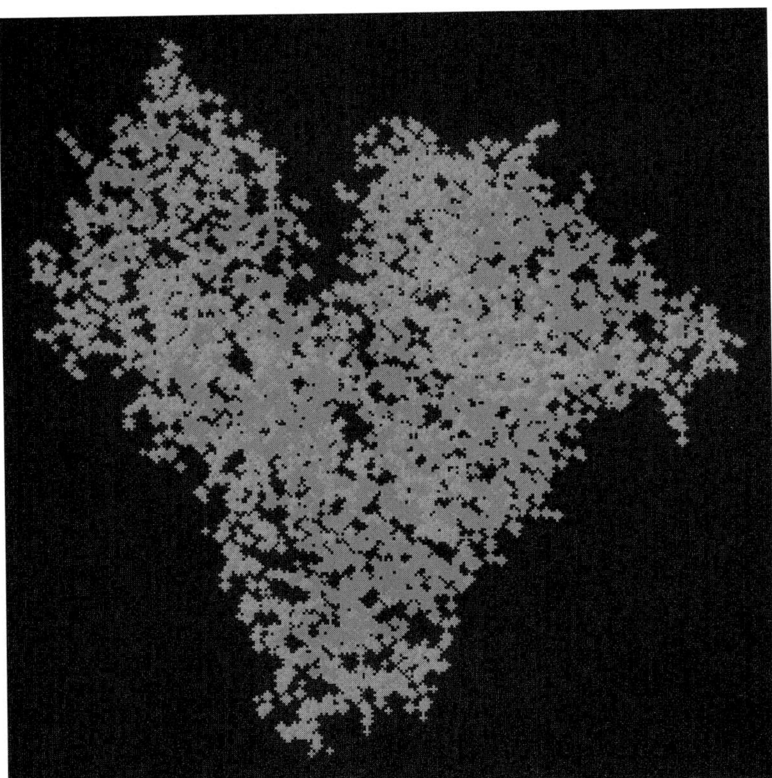

FIGURE 2–7
Space-filling structure model of albumin, generated using Cn3D and Brookhaven Protein Structure Data Base data. (See also Color Fig. 2–7.)

splicing.[119–121] The γ chains of fibrinogen carry the main sites of platelet receptor interaction; the structure of these sites has been determined by x-ray diffraction.[122] The fibrinogen β chain gene codes for a signal sequence of 16 to 30 amino acids, followed by a mature polypeptide of 461 amino acids.[117]

Defects in fibrinogen structure may result in thrombosis (when more rapidly clotting forms are produced) or bleeding.[123]

Von Willebrand Factor

Immunohistochemical demonstration of the von Willebrand factor (factor VIII related antigen, vWF) is useful in the identification of endothelial cells (Fig. 2–8). Thus, staining for this factor can assist in diagnosis of vascular tumors (Table 2–10) and in the identification of neovascularization in tumors (which may serve as a prognostic factor). vWF is most easily demonstrated in enzymatically digested sections.

vWF is a glycoprotein that is synthesized by endothelial cells, megakaryocytes and platelets, and that has a basic molecular weight of 220 kd. In the endothelial cell, vWF is found in the Weibel-Palade bodies. Polymerization gives rise to a factor VIII complex weight of 1000 to 20,000 kd. vWF binds blood vessels that have lost their endothelial lining; platelets adhere to this vWF-coated surface.

vWF is coded by a single 178-kb gene at 12p13[124, 125] that has been cloned and sequenced.[126] The protein has 24% α-helix and 18% β-pleated sheet structure and appears to contain ordered conformational domains, including an amphipathic, α-helix platelet receptor adhesion site, linked by regions of random polypeptide chain.[127, 128] It assembles with factor VIII into complexes consisting of flexible filaments ranging from 50 to 1150 nm long that contain small, irregularly spaced nodules.[129] Mutation of the vWF gene causes von Willebrand

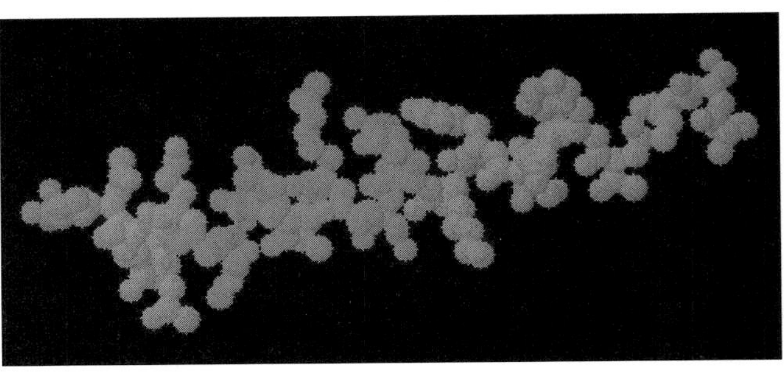

FIGURE 2–8
Space-filling structure model of glucagon, generated using Cn3D and Brookhaven Protein Structure Data Base data. (See also Color Fig. 2–8.)

TABLE 2–10

Selected Tumors Demonstrating Immunoreactivity for Factor VIIIRA

Diagnosis	Percentage of Cases Demonstrating Immunoreactivity
Angiosarcoma, epithelioid	83–100
Hemangioendothelioma, epithelioid	91–97
Hemangioma, capillary	93–100
Hemangioma, NOS	94–100
Hemangiosarcoma	65–80
Kaposi's sarcoma	42–63
Lymphangioma, NOS	84–100
Myxoma, NOS	51–74

NOS, not otherwise specified.

disease,[130] a disorder characterized by skin ecchymoses, hemorrhage, and prolonged bleeding time.

Factor XIII

Immunohistochemical identification of factor XIII is useful in the identification of certain dermal fibrohistiocytic tumors (Table 2–11). Although factor XIII is synthesized by megakaryocytes, highly homologous transglutaminases are also produced in many other tissues, including keratinocytes[131]; immunohistochemical cross-reactivity presumably accounts for some of the staining seen in the dermis and elsewhere. Use of antigen retrieval or enzymatic digestion techniques generally improves demonstration of this antigen.

Factor XIII, the last enzyme in the blood coagulation cascade, is the zymogen for fibrinoligase, an enzyme that forms intramolecular γ-glutamyl-ε-lysine cross-links between fibrin molecules. These cross-links stabilize the clot, with little change in the spatial organization of the fibrinogen aggregates. Cross-linking also accelerates the assembly of the fibrinogen aggregate.[132] Mutations in the factor XIII gene give rise to bleeding disorders similar to those of hemophilia A.[133, 134]

Factor XIII is composed of two A subunits, which have catalytic function, and two B subunits, which do not. Factor XIII is activated by the cleavage of a small peptide from the A subunit by thrombin. Factor XIIIA is encoded by a 160-kb gene,[135] which localizes to 6p25-p24.[136] X-ray crystallographic secondary structure analysis shows that each A chain of the factor XIII protein is folded into four sequential domains and that a catalytic site is found in the core domain.[137]

TABLE 2–11

Selected Tumors Demonstrating Immunoreactivity for Factor XIIIA

Diagnosis	Percentage of Cases Demonstrating Immunoreactivity
Dermatofibroma	82–96
Dermatofibrosarcoma protuberans	13–37
Hepatocellular carcinoma	88–98
Kaposi's sarcoma	25–66
Malignant fibrous histiocytoma, NOS	38–72
Malignant fibrous histiocytoma, myxoid	0–7
Meningioma, fibrous	44–86
Meningioma, hemangioblastic	62–93
Meningioma, secretory	0
Xanthogranuloma, NOS	100

NOS, not otherwise specified.

Factor XIIIB

The B subunit of factor XIII is composed of 10 short consensus repeats (SCRs) similar to that of complement system regulatory proteins. The B subunits of factor XIII have no enzymatic activity and may serve as plasma carrier molecules. Factor XIIIB maps to 1q31.2-q31.3[138] and is not generally employed as an immunohistochemical marker.

POLYPEPTIDE HORMONES

Immunohistochemical identification of polypeptide hormones is useful in the identification and characterization of a number of secretory tumors, particularly those demonstrating neuroendocrine differentiation. The polypeptide hormones localize immunohistochemically to the cytoplasm but may show an apparent increase in staining near the membrane as a result of lipid insertion by amphipathic helices.

Adrenocorticotropic Hormone

Immunocytochemical assessment of adrenocorticotropic hormone (ACTH) is used primarily for identification of small and/or fragmented adenomas associated with Cushing's disease. ACTH-secreting cells are located in the "wedge" of the anterior pituitary, where they constitute 15% to 20% of the cells. ACTH stimulates adrenal cortical cells to secrete greatly increased quantities of glucocorticoids and slightly increased amounts of aldosterone and adrenal androgens. ACTH may also be secreted ectopically, particularly by pulmonary tumors (Table 2–12). Immunohistochemical demonstration of ACTH is not improved by enzymatic digestion but may be improved by antigen retrieval methods.

ACTH is a 39 amino acid long polypeptide that is a member of a family of biologically related peptides, including melanotropin, lipotropin, the endorphins, and met- and leu-enkephalin.[142] All the members of this

TABLE 2–12

Selected Tumors Demonstrating Immunohistochemical Reactivity for Adrenocorticotropic Hormone

Diagnosis	Percentage of Cases Demonstrating Immunoreactivity
Carcinoid, NOS	8–23
Carcinoma, large cell neuroendocrine	3–24
Carcinoma, small cell, lung	8–42
Sclerosing hemangioma, lung	81–100

NOS, not otherwise specified.

family are coded for by a single gene on chromosome 2p23-25, called the pro-opiomelanocortin (POMC) gene, which codes for a 31-kd (241 amino acid) precursor peptide.[139–141] During preprocessing, it is cleaved to a glycosylated amino-terminal fragment of 11 kd, a 16-kd carboxyl-terminal fragment (β-lipotropin), and a central 4.5-kd fragment (ACTH). β-Lipotropin can further be cleaved to form the melanocyte-stimulating hormones and β-endorphin. Pituitary adenomas may demonstrate increased POMC/ACTH expression, increased transcription with normal levels of ACTH expression, or decreased transcription and translation.[143] The secondary structure of ACTH is controversial; circular dichroism spectra have been interpreted as showing a left-helical conformation of the poly-L-proline II type.[144]

There are two pituitary-specific promoters that confine most secretion to the anterior pituitary gland,[145] although POMC and its cleavage products have also been found in the pineal gland, placenta, ovaries, testes (Leydig cells), epididymis, and gastrointestinal tract.[146] Both POMC and the ACTH fragment are highly conserved among species.

Gastrin-Releasing Peptide (Bombesin)

Gastrin-releasing peptide has been used in the characterization of neuroendocrine tumors throughout the body but most particularly in small cell carcinoma of the lung, in which it is frequently demonstrated (Table 2–13). Gastrin-releasing peptide is the 27 amino acid long human homologue of bombesin, a 14 amino acid peptide that was first isolated from frog skin.[147] The carboxyl-terminal seven amino acids of bombesin are identical to those of gastrin-releasing peptide, which gives rise to the immunologic cross-reactivity among antibodies derived against these two antigens. A 10-kb gene on chromosome 18q21[148–150] codes for the polypeptide, which is secreted as a preprohormone. In solution, gastrin-releasing peptide exists as random coil type conformers with perhaps a β turn between residues 14 and 19.[151] Gastrin-releasing peptide increases plasma levels of gastrin, pancreatic polypeptide, glucagon, gastric inhibitory peptide, and insulin.[150] It is produced in large quantities by small cell lung cancer and appears to be a growth factor for these cells.[152]

TABLE 2–13

Immunohistochemical Reactivity of Selected Tumors for Gastrin-Releasing Peptide

Diagnosis	Percentage of Cases Demonstrating Immunoreactivity
Atypical carcinoid	0–83
Carcinoid, NOS	20-48
Large cell neuroendocrine carcinoma	35–88
Merkel cell carcinoma	14–56
Paraganglioma	0
Small cell carcinoma, lung	23–67

NOS, not otherwise specified.

Gastrin-releasing peptide is found not only in small cell lung cancer but also in nerves and endocrine cells of the gastric antrum and the duodenum.[142, 146] High levels of reactivity for gastrin-releasing peptide have also been observed in C cells of the thyroid gland.[153] In spite of the wide variety of pharmacologic actions, the physiologic role of gastrin-releasing peptide is not well established.

Calcitonin

Immunohistochemical assessment of calcitonin is used for the identification of medullary carcinoma of the thyroid and the identification of nests of hyperplastic C cells. Ectopic secretion is not uncommon, however (Table 2–14). Enzymatic digestion and antigen retrieval methods generally degrade the immunohistochemical demonstration of calcitonin.

Calcitonin, a highly conserved 32 amino acid member of the parathyroid hormone/calcitonin family, is coded

TABLE 2–14

Selected Tumors Demonstrating Immunohistochemical Reactivity for Calcitonin

Diagnosis	Percentage of Cases Demonstrating Immunoreactivity
Carcinoid, NOS	14–32
Carcinoma, large cell neuroendocrine	22–48
Carcinoma, Merkel cell	1–24
Medullary carcinoma, thyroid	98–100
Pheochromocytoma, NOS	6–37
Sclerosing hemangioma, lung	51–96

NOS, not otherwise specified.

by a gene localized to 11p15.1-15.2.[154, 155] This gene is normally expressed in thyroid C cells (where it codes for calcitonin) and in a restricted population of cells in the central and peripheral nerve system,[156] where it codes for a second peptide, calcitonin gene–related peptide (CGRP), a potent vasodilator.[157] The different peptides are synthesized by alternative processing of RNA transcripts, which allows the calcitonin gene to yield mRNAs that encode either calcitonin or CGRP. The calcitonin mRNA predominates in the thyroid whereas the CGRP-specific mRNA is expressed in the hypothalamus and in medullary carcinoma of the thyroid.[146, 158, 159] Both calcitonin and CGRP are secreted as prohormones.[146] Nuclear magnetic resonance spectroscopy suggests that, in solution, calcitonin exists predominantly in an extended random structure[160]; in organic solvents, such as biologic membranes, it readily forms an amphipathic helix.[161–164]

Calcitonin decreases plasma calcium levels by stimulating osteoblastic activity. Although predominantly localized in the C cells, calcitonin has also been found in brain, hypothalamus, pituitary gland, lungs, thymus, liver, gastrointestinal tract, adrenals, muscle, parathyroid gland, cerebrospinal fluid, seminal fluid, and breast milk.[146]

Cholecystokinin

Cholecystokinin (pancreozymin, CCK) is coded by a 7-kb gene located at 3q12-3pter[165] and is formed as a pre-pro-CCK, which is cleaved to form peptides containing 58, 39, 33, 22, 12, 8, 5, and 4 amino acids. The 33 amino acid moiety is identical to the 39 amino acid form, except that it lacks six amino-terminal amino acids; these two forms predominate. The last 5 residues are identical to those of gastrin, giving rise to immunohistochemical cross-reactivity.[142] CCK is normally synthesized in the brain, small intestine, and (occasionally) pancreas[146] and stimulates the secretion of pancreatic amylase. The carboxyl-terminal portion of the peptide (which exhibits biologic activity) demonstrates a high degree of folding, possibly stabilized by hydrogen bonds[166, 167]; it is not clear whether this conformation is required for biologic activity.

Passage of fat into the small intestine results in CCK release; CCK, in turn, stimulates rhythmic contraction of the gallbladder.

Follicle-Stimulating Hormone

Immunocytochemical demonstration of follicle-stimulating hormone (FSH), which stimulates growth of the ovarian follicles, is useful in the identification of gonadotrophic adenomas of the pituitary. Gonadotrophic cells normally make up about 10% of the anterior pituitary gland and are scattered throughout.

FSH is a two-subunit glycoprotein secreted by the pituitary gland that is closely related to thyroid-stimulating hormone (TSH) and human chorionic gonadotropin (HCG).[168] The α subunit, a 92 amino acid polypeptide chain that demonstrates five disulfide bonds[146, 169] and two carbohydrate moieties, is coded by a gene on chromosome 6.[170] The β subunit, which is noncovalently linked to the α chain, coded by a gene on 11p13,[171] is species-specific.[168] Neither the α nor the β subunit of FSH, HCG, or TSH, all of which have identical α subunits, has any biologic activity individually.[146, 169, 172] Approximately two thirds of commercial monoclonal antibodies react against the α subunit; the remainder are directed against the β subunit, which is relatively uniform from species to species.[168] Because the α subunits are identical, antibodies raised against either whole FSH, HCG, or TSH or the α subunits may be expected to cross-react. The interaction between FSH and its receptor have been extensively characterized. FSH amino acids 33 to 53 are sufficient to bind to the receptor[172] and are also involved in formation of the α/β heterodimer.[173] Bound FSH demonstrates antiparallel β-pleated sheet, turns including a β turn, other structures, and a small amount of α helix.[173] It appears that some amino acids within the FSH β amino acid 33 to 53 region are surface oriented, whereas others, found at the ends of this region, bind to the α subunit.[174]

Gastrin

Immunohistochemical demonstration of gastrin is useful in the characterization of the islet cell tumors, gastrin-secreting tumors of the stomach and small intestine, and G cell hyperplasias associated with Zollinger-Ellison syndrome. Assessment of gastrin may also be useful in defining certain gastrointestinal carcinoid tumors.

Gastrin is the most important hormone involved in regulation of gastric acid secretion.[175] The gene for gastrin, located on 17q12-21,[165, 176] codes for a 101 amino acid peptide containing within it the structure of "big gastrin" (G34) and a carboxyl-terminal extension. Post-translational processing of this pre-progastrin gives rise to the active peptides G34 and G17 (a 17 amino acid gastrin). G17, in turn, exists in two forms, I and II, which differ by the presence of a sulfate ester on Tyr12.[142, 146] Three less common biologically active forms of gastrin, G14 ("mini-gastrin"), G6, and G5, are also found. When any form of gastrin binds its receptor on the parietal cell, an inositol pathway is activated, giving rise to acid secretion.[175]

The carboxyl-terminal pentapeptide of gastrin is identical with that of CCK, giving rise to immunohistochemical cross-reactivity with some antibodies.[142, 146] Biologic cross-reactivity is avoided by means of conformational differences.[177, 178] The biologically active conformation of receptor-bound gastrin is partly helical, with the indole of tryptophan and the aromatic ring of phenylalanine close to one another and the methionine and aspartic acid side chains pointing in the opposite direction. In contrast, the receptor-bound conformation of CCK-7 is a β bend. There appears to be little conformational difference between gastrin I and II.[178] In addition to the homology between gastrin and CCK, there is also structural similarity between gastrin and the transformation protein of polyomavirus.[146]

In addition to the G cells of the antral, pyloric, and duodenal mucosa, gastrin has also been found in the normal pituitary gland, pancreas, and vagus nerve.[146]

Glucagon

Approximately 15% of the pancreatic islet cells secrete glucagon. Immunohistochemical assessment of glucagon is useful in defining the biologic behavior of islet cell tumors.

Glucagon is a 29 amino acid member of the family that includes secretin, vasoactive inhibitory peptide (VIP), gastric inhibitory peptide, and growth hormone-releasing factor (GHRF). It is secreted by pancreatic alpha cells.[179] Glucagon's most important target organ is the liver, where it stimulates formation of glucose from glycogen and ketone bodies from amino acids.[146] The gene, a 9.4-kb sequence that localizes to 2q36-7,[180, 181] codes for a large polypeptide, pre-proglucagon, which contains glucagon and two glucagon-like polypeptides that are highly conserved among species. Proglucagon is expressed at high levels in the A cells of the pancreatic islets and the L cells of the intestine, indicating that tissue-specific transcription factors regulate glucagon expression.[182] Glucagon arises by cleavage from the prohormone within the A cells of the pancreatic islets but in the intestine remains as part of a partially processed precursor.[183] Thus, processing of pre-proglucagon is governed by a complex, tissue-specific mechanism. Glucagon-like peptide I (GLP-I, insulinotropin) stimulates insulin release from the pancreas, suggesting that it serves as part of a glucagon/insulin feedback loop system.[184]

The structural conformational requirements for glucagon activity have been extensively investigated but not yet well defined.[185–187] Although glucagon has been crystallized and examined by x-ray diffraction techniques (see Fig. 2–8), the relationship between x-ray diffraction results and solution structure is often tenuous for such small molecules.[188]

Growth Hormone

Growth hormone (GH)–secreting cells (somatotrophs) make up about half the cells of the anterior pituitary and are concentrated in the lateral wings. Immunocytochemical assessment of GH is useful in characterization of both acidophilic and chromophobic adenomas of the pituitary. GH increases the rate of protein synthesis in all cells, decreases the rate of carbohydrate utilization, and mobilizes fats. It stimulates growth and division of all cells capable of either through a receptor dimerization mechanism.

GH is a member of the secretin family,[146] which includes placental lactogen (with which it is about 90% homologous),[189] prolactin, and VIP. There is also amino acid homology between GH (amino acids 30–38), gastrin, and the carboxyl-terminal end of the insulin β chain.[146] GH is coded by a gene at 17q22-24, near that of human placental lactogen.[81, 190] Although the two hormones share extensive homology, they differ in their 3′ flanking regions, which suggests that they are regulated differently. Evolutionary analysis suggests that the growth hormone/placental lactogen gene cluster evolved quite recently and that the mechanism of gene duplication involved homologous exchange between repetitive elements of the Alu family.[189]

GH is a 191 amino acid protein[146] that is originally synthesized as a prohormone. The final product is secreted as a single amino acid chain with two intramolecular disulfide bonds,[142] which occur in monomers, dimers, and oligomers. The structure of both porcine and human GH has been completely determined at high resolution by x-ray crystallography.[191, 192] The protein is predominantly helical and consists mainly of four antiparallel α helices arranged in a left-twisted helical bundle (Fig. 2–9). Comparison of amino acid sequences of various GHs demonstrates that the residues within these helices are invariant and probably necessary for structural and functional integrity.[193]

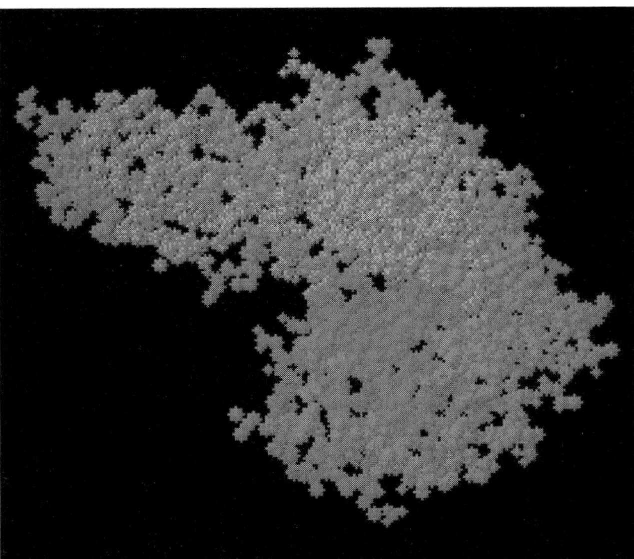

FIGURE 2–9
Space-filling model of human growth hormone, generated using Cn3D and Brookhaven Protein Structure Data Base data. (See also Color Fig. 2–9.)

Human Chorionic Gonadotropin

Human chorionic gonadotropin (HCG) is useful in differentiating between gestational choriocarcinoma and placental trophoblastic tumors, in identifying trophoblastic elements in curettage specimens, and in the differentiation of various ovarian, testicular, and mediastinal germ cell tumors (Tables 2–15 and 2–16). HCG prevents involution of the corpus luteum and stimulates secretion of progesterone and estrogens.

HCG is a two-subunit glycoprotein hormone; the subunits are noncovalently linked and coded by separate genes. The α subunit, a 92 amino acid polypeptide chain that demonstrates five disulfide bonds[146] and two carbohydrate moieties, is coded by a gene on chromosome 6.[170] The 145 amino acid β subunit differs from that of luteinizing hormone (LH) by only about 20% of residues[146] and is localized to a family of six genes/pseudogenes near the coding region for LH on chromosome 19.[194] It is the β subunit that confers unique biologic activity on the protein; the various β-HCG gene products are not expressed to the same extent in the developing placenta; it appears that differential expression may reflect differential methylation.[195]

Chemical and spectroscopic studies provide many details of the requirements for HCG to have biologic activity.[196] The agonist and receptor-binding regions are physically distinct.[197] His-94 is believed to be part of the receptor-binding region of the hormone, and an His-83 is thought to be an active site residue. The 38 to 57 amino acid region of the β subunit is exposed on the surface and is part of the receptor-binding domain; an amphipathic-helical structure in the 38 to 57 amino acid sequence may promote hormone-receptor interactions.[198] Asparagine-linked carbohydrate chains are attached to the subunits, and β-chain serine moieties are O-glycosylated. The carbohydrates are essential for full biologic activity[199]; it appears that deglycosylation results in protein conformational changes, which account, at least in part, for loss of biologic activity.[200] X-ray diffraction studies show that each of the two HCG subunits has a similar topology and that the heterodimer is stabilized by a segment of the β subunit that wraps around the α subunit and is covalently linked like a seat belt by a disulfide bond. This feature may be essential for receptor binding.[201]

The structural similarities between HCG, TSH, and LH give rise to difficulties in raising antibodies that are specifically directed to any of these hormones.[202, 203] Great care must be taken in the immunohistochemistry laboratory to guarantee specificity. Demonstration of HCG may be improved by antigen retrieval methods.

TABLE 2–15

Immunohistochemical Reactivity of Selected Tumors of the α Subunit of Human Chorionic Gonadotropin

Diagnosis	Percentage of Cases Demonstrating Immunoreactivity
Carcinoid, NOS	25–40
Islet cell tumor	26–39
Large cell neuroendocrine carcinoma	16–56
Medullary carcinoma, thyroid	30–62

NOS, not otherwise specified.

TABLE 2–16

Immunohistochemical Reactivity of Selected Tumors of the β Subunit of Human Chorionic Gonadotropin

Diagnosis	Percentage of Cases Demonstrating Immunoreactivity
Adenocarcinoma, gallbladder	7–46
Choriocarcinoma, NOS	100
Embryonal carcinoma	10–32
Endodermal sinus tumor	0
Epidermoid carcinoma, NOS	15–59
Seminoma, NOS	0–9

NOS, not otherwise specified.

Human Pancreatic Polypeptide

Pancreatic polypeptide is a 36 amino acid protein[146] that inhibits pancreatic exocrine function. Although pancreatic polypeptide secreting cells are found predominantly in islets in the head of the pancreas, they may occasionally be found in pancreatic ducts, exocrine pancreas, gastric mucosa, and intestines.[142]

Pancreatic polypeptide is coded by a gene localized to 17q21.[204] Although its amino acid sequence is unrelated to that of glucagon or other gastrointestinal hormones, it shares 18 of 36 residues with neuropeptide Y, suggesting common ancestral origins. The neuropeptide Y gene is found on chromosome 7q, however.[205] Pancreatic polypeptide cDNA is 465 bp long and encodes 95 amino acids. The pancreatic polypeptide sequence is flanked by a 29 amino acid amino-terminal leader sequence, a connecting tripeptide, and a 27 amino acid peptide at the carboxyl terminus. This precursor, pre-propancreatic polypeptide, is cleaved to produce pancreatic polypeptide, an icosapeptide, and a smaller peptide; each of these peptides appears to be encoded by a separate exon.[206]

The secondary structure of pancreatic polypeptide has been determined by x-ray diffraction techniques. The peptide forms a stable globular structure stabilized by hydrophobic interactions between a polyproline-like helix and an α helix.[207] This interaction appears to be important not only for molecular function but also for immunochemical reactivity.[208]

Human Placental Lactogen (Chorionic Somatotropin)

Human placental lactogen (HPL, chorionic somatotropin) is useful in the identification of trophoblastic tumors, but it may be found in other types of neoplasms (Table 2–17). HPL is relatively specific to placental trophoblast; it is not normally expressed elsewhere in the body.

HPL is a 191 amino acid polypeptide with a molecular weight of about 21 kd and two internal disulfide bridges. It is a member of the secretin family,[146] which includes growth hormone (with which it is about 90% homologous),[189] prolactin, and vasoactive intestinal polypeptide. It is coded by a gene cluster at 17q22-24, which includes the gene coding for human GH.[81, 190] Although the two hormones share extensive homology, they differ in their 3′ flanking regions, which suggests that they are regulated differently. Evolutionary analysis suggests that the GH/HPL gene cluster evolved quite recently and that the mechanism of gene duplication involved homologous exchange between repetitive elements of the Alu family.[189] Although the genes for GH, HPL, and prolactin are closely related, tissue-specific promoters result in expression in different cell types[209]; this tissue-specific expression seems to be under the regulation of an upstream promoter.[210] In addition, there seems to be one or more placenta-specific enhancers downstream from one of the coding sequences.[211] Like other polypeptide hormones, HPL is synthesized as a pre-prohormone and processed in the rough endoplasmic reticulum. Its biologic role is unclear, although it clearly is related to mammary growth and lactation.

Details of the HPL tertiary structure have not been defined. Like GHs and prolactins, HPL is 50% to 60% α helix.[142] It also is a glycoprotein that has N-linked and O-linked carbohydrate side chains.[212] Although HPL is 85% identical to human GH hormone it binds 2300-fold more weakly than GH to the GH receptor; nevertheless, these two hormones have similar affinities for prolactin receptors.[213] Both prolactin and GH require zinc for tight binding to the extracellular domain of the human prolactin receptor and contain virtually identical receptor-binding determinants and zinc ligands.

TABLE 2–17

Immunohistochemical Reactivity of Selected Tumors for Human Placental Lactogen

Diagnosis	Percentage of Cases Demonstrating Immunoreactivity
Adenocarcinoma, lung	5–31
Choriocarcinoma, NOS	100
Large cell carcinoma, lung	32–31
Placental trophoblastic tumor	83–100
Squamous cell carcinoma, lung	5–52

NOS, not otherwise specified.

Insulin

Insulin-secreting cells constitute approximately 70% of the pancreatic islet; immunohistochemical assessment of insulin is important in the characterization of islet cell tumors, as well as identification of nesidioblastosis and other islet cell hyperplasias.

Insulin is a member of a family of polypeptide hormones that includes secretin, glucagon, somatotropin, prolactin, and somatostatin.[146] Insulin is synthesized in the pancreatic islet β cell by means of two intermediates—pre-proinsulin and proinsulin—which are cleaved to yield the final configuration of two polypeptide chains that are linked by two disulfide intramolecular bonds. The nucleotide sequence for human insulin has been established,[214] and it has been reported that sequence abnormalities are found in the flanking regions for some persons with diabetes mellitus.

The crystal structure of insulin has been determined; the molecule contains an α-helical core surrounded by coil structures (Fig. 2–10).[215]

Leucine Enkephalin

Pre-proenkephalin-B cleavage gives rise to leu-enkephalin, a hormone that is widely distributed in the body and that is found in brain, gastrointestinal tract, adrenal cortex, corpus luteum, heart, and germ cells.[146] Leu-enkephalin, only 5 amino acids long, differs from met-enkephalin by a single amino acid. The hormone inhibits transmitter release from presynaptic nerve terminal in both central and peripheral nervous systems and binds to δ receptors, resulting in a central analgesic effect. Leu-enkephalin also modulates both endocrine and exocrine pancreatic secretion.

Enkephalins have been extensively studied spectroscopically. These small molecules are characterized by a very high conformational flexibility and thus a large number of different conformations in solution.[216, 217] When exposed to a lipid environment, the molecule folds into an intramolecularly hydrogen-bonded β-turn structure.[218]

Luteinizing Hormone

Luteinizing hormone, which is secreted in the pituitary, consists of two chains. The α chain is identical to

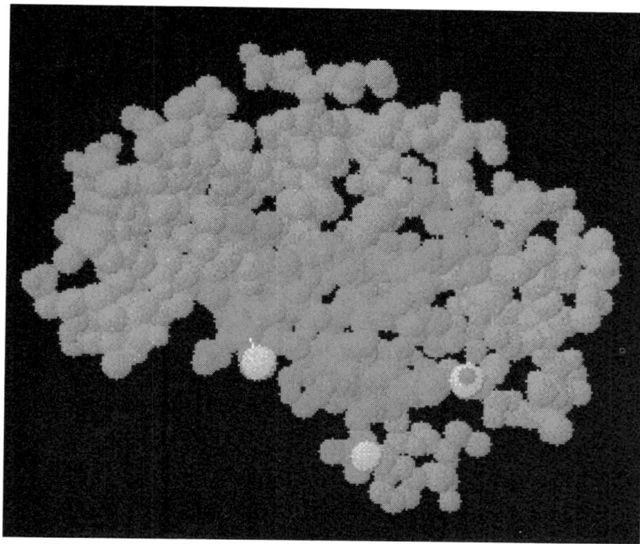

FIGURE 2–10
Space-filling structure model of insulin, generated using Cn3D and Brookhaven Protein Structure Data Base data.[215] (See also Color Fig. 2–10.)

that of FSH and HCG. The unique β chain, coded by a gene on 19q13.2,[219, 220] is 121 amino acids long.[146] The β subunits of TSH, LH, and FSH are identical at about 40% of all residues. The positions of the six disulfide bridges are completely conserved, as are proline residues, and contain three carbohydrate moieties.[142] The sequences of β-HCG and LH are 80% identical, except at the carboxyl terminus. These findings suggest that the secondary and tertiary structures of LH are very similar to those of GH.

In the ovaries, LH stimulates cyclic adenosine monophosphate and inositol triphosphate. In the male, spermatogenesis can only occur if both LH and FSH are present.

Prolactin

Prolactin is a 198 amino acid protein that is coded by a gene localized to chromosome 6p21.3-6p22.2.[221, 222] Although the hormone is primarily synthesized in acidophilic cells of the pituitary, it is also found in placenta, myometrium, ovaries, and the hypothalamus.[146] Like most polypeptide hormones, prolactin is synthesized as pre-prolactin, with a signal peptide attached to the amino terminus. After processing in the rough endoplasmic reticulum and the Golgi apparatus, it is stored as large irregular membrane-bound granules.

Although the genes for GH, HPL, and prolactin are closely related, tissue-specific promoters result in expression in different cell types[209]; this tissue-specific expression seems to be under the regulation of an upstream promoter.[210] Prolactin receptors are found in mammary gland, liver, kidneys, brain, prostate, testes, ovaries, and lymphocytes. Prolactin increases production of milk, initiates maternal behavior, increases dopaminergic tone, stimulates synthesis of progesterone, inhibits estradiol and testosterone, and increases blood pressure.[146]

Although conformational analysis of prolactin is incomplete, it is apparent that several structural features must be preserved for biologic activity. Circular dichroism spectra demonstrate that prolactin is conformationally 60% to 70% α helix.[223] Disruption of an apparently helical region of the hormone results in almost complete loss of biologic activity.[224] Analysis of prolactins from several species demonstrates 32 common amino acid residues.[225] Eight of these residues, including four cysteines, are conserved by other members of the GH family. Thirteen other residues are almost completely conserved in the prolactins, suggesting that these residues are indispensable for receptor-specific binding.

Somatostatin

Somatostatin, a 14 residue peptide hormone coded by a gene on 3q28,[141] is formed in the stomach and pancreatic δ cells as a pre-prosomatostatin. It is found to a lesser extent in cells of the gastrointestinal mucosa, thymus, tongue, extrahepatic bile ducts, C-cells of the thyroid gland, and ovaries;[146] similar substances are found in the hypothalamus, central and peripheral nervous system.[142] Somatostatin is released in the gastric antrum in response to fasting and operates with growth hormone releasing factor to regulated the secretion of growth hormone and thyroid stimulating hormone. Somatostatin receptors are found in the brain.

Thyroid-Stimulating Hormone

Thyroid-stimulating hormone, sometimes known as thyrotropin, is secreted by the anterior pituitary gland and stimulates the formation of the thyroid hormones triiodothyronine (T_3) and thyroxine (T_4). These hormones, in turn, inhibit release of TSH. TSH, LH, and FSH belong to a family of hormones that consists of two glycoproteins in a noncovalent association—an α chain and a β chain. TSH and the gonadotropins, LH and FSH, have an identical α chain. The TSH β chain is coded by a gene localizing at chromosome 1p22.[170]

Vasoactive Intestinal Polypeptide

Vasoactive intestinal polypeptide is a 28 amino acid hormone that is useful in the characterization of neuroblastoma and of pheochromocytomas associated with the watery diarrhea and hypokalemia syndrome. VIP-secreting cells are found in neural tissue, as well as in gastrointestinal epithelium and neural tissue from the stomach to the rectum.

VIP is coded by an 8-kb single-copy gene localized to chromosome 6q26-27.[226–228] Gene transcription depends on a 17-bp DNA element located 70 bp upward from the transcription initiation site.[229] Like most of the other polypeptide hormones, VIP is synthesized as part of a polyprotein, pre-proVIP. Pre-proVIP generates, in addition to VIP, an additional bioactive peptide known as PHM.[230]

Although the conformation of VIP has not been determined crystallographically, its secondary structure in solution has been highly investigated by spectroscopic methods. In methanol/water solution, VIP is largely helical.[231] A π helix is believed to occur when the hormone is bound to membrane receptors.[232, 233]

LEUKOCYTE DIFFERENTIATION ANTIGENS

CD1 (Leu6)

CD1 is a surface-bound member of the immunoglobulin superfamily, with an immunoglobulin-type constant-region structure similar to that of major histocompatibility complex (MHC) class I proteins, and is coded for by five genes located on chromosome 1q22-23.[234] CD1 antigens are expressed on cortical thymocytes, where expression is inversely correlated with the T-cell receptor (TcR), as well as on dendritic reticular cells. CD1C is expressed on B cells, and CD1D is expressed on intestinal epithelium.[7] An antigen-presentation function has been postulated based on the structural similarities with the MHC class I proteins.[7]

Immunohistochemical staining with CD1A is useful for the identification of histiocytosis X.

CD2 (Sheep Erythrocyte Rosette Receptor, Leu5)

The membrane-associated CD2 antigen, found on virtually all T cells and natural killer (NK) cells, is a member of the immunoglobulin gene superfamily and is coded for by a 28-kb sequence found on chromosome 1p13.[7, 235] CD2 interacts through its amino-terminal domain with CD58 to form an adhesion pair; signal transduction by means of this mechanism resembles that of the TcR-CD3 complex.[236] The secondary structure of the amino-terminal domain has been established by nuclear magnetic resonance spectroscopy[237] and is similar to that of the immunoglobulin variable region.

CD3 Antigens and the T-Cell Receptor Complex

The CD3 antigens are membrane-associated antigens that, in association with the TcR, form part of the CD3/TcR complex.[7] The CD3 antigens (Fig. 2–11) are expressed during thymopoiesis and on peripheral T cells (Table 2–18). Immunohistochemical demonstration requires proteolytic digestion or antigen retrieval.

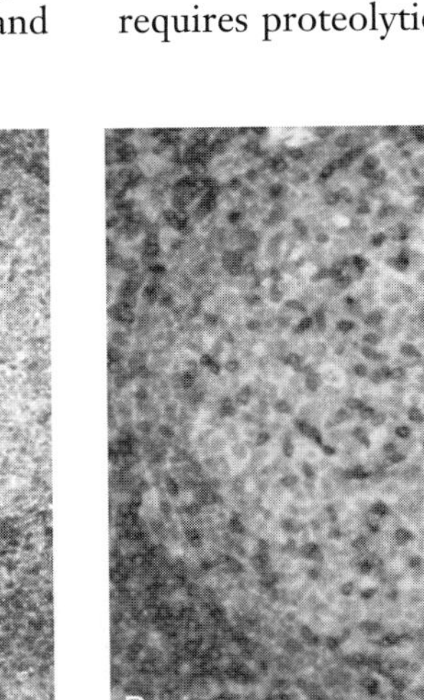

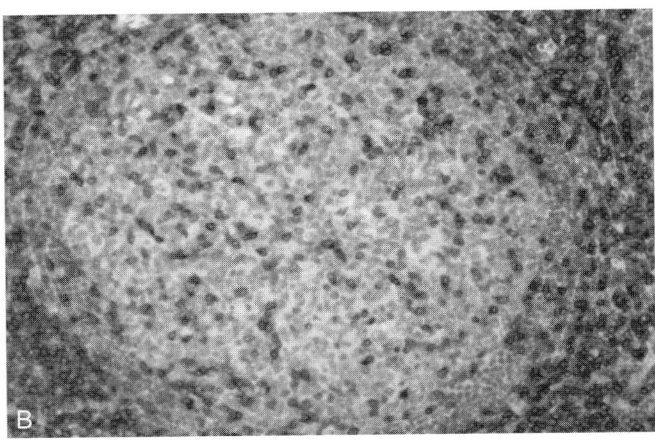

FIGURE 2–11
Section of tonsil immunohistochemically stained for CD3, ×100 (*A*) and ×200 (*B*). (See also Color Fig. 2–11.)

TABLE 2–18

Immunoreactivity of Selected Neoplasms for CD3

Diagnosis	Percentage of Cases Demonstrating Immunoreactivity
Ki-1 lymphoma	27–45
T-cell lymphoma	92–100
Mycosis fungoides	92–100

Three different CD3 chains, γ, δ, and ε, are coded for by genes 9, 3.7, and 13 kb long, respectively, located on chromosome 11q23.[238–240] Two TcR chains, α, and β, are coded for by 800- and 600-kb genes located on chromosomes 14q11.2 and 7q35, respectively.[241] The large size of these genes results from the need to encode immunoglobulin-like variable regions, which recombine during differentiation, with immunoglobulin-like constant, joining, and diversity regions. Two additional TcR genes, γ (160 kb) and δ (195 kb), are encoded by genes found on chromosomes 7p15 and 14q11.2, respectively.[242–244] The γ/δ receptor complex demonstrates relatively limited receptor diversity and is expressed on fewer than 10% of human peripheral T cells.

After recognition of peptide antigens bound to MHC antigens, the invariant CD3 chains mediate a signal transduction process that appears to involve tyrosine kinase and phospholipase C activation and the phosphatidylinositol pathway.[245, 246]

The precise stoichiometry of the CD3/TcR complex is not known. Amino acid sequence analysis suggests that all three CD3 chains will have conformations similar to that of an immunoglobulin constant region. Similarly, the TcR complex is expected to structurally resemble an immunoglobulin G complex.

CD4 (Leu3)

CD4, an antigen that is expressed on most thymocytes and approximately two thirds of human peripheral T cells,[7] assists in the recognition of foreign molecules in association with MHC class II antigens.[247] During T-cell activation, the cytoplasmic domain of the CD4 molecule is phosphorylated, enabling interaction with a tyrosine kinase CDKL2 $(p56)^{lck}$.[248, 249] The CD4 molecule serves as a receptor for human immunodeficiency virus, by means of binding of the CD4 amino terminus to HIV gp120.[250] The CD4 gene is 32 kb long and is located on 12pter-12p12.[251] It consists of two variable and two constant regions, arranged V1–C1–V2–C2, which are anchored to the cell membrane. The secondary structure of these domains is expected to be similar to that of the corresponding immunoglobulin regions.

CD5 (OKT1, Leu1)

CD5 and CD6, unlike most hematopoietic differentiation antigens, are members of the scavenger receptor superfamily. Although sequence homology has been established among members of this molecular family, including the macrophage scavenger receptor and a complement control protein, secondary and tertiary structure are not yet established. The CD5 antigen is coded by a gene localized on chromosome 11q13 and is expressed on all mature T cells, most thymocytes, and a subset of mature B cells.[7] The function of CD5 has not yet been completely elucidated, although it is known that CD72 is a ligand for CD5. The secondary structure of the scavenger receptor proteins has not been elucidated.

Although CD5 may be identified immunohistochemically in frozen sections, it is not reliably demonstrated in formalin-fixed, paraffin-embedded material.

CD6 (OKT17)

CD6 is another member of the scavenger receptor superfamily and is expressed on peripheral blood T cells, mostly thymocytes, and B-cell chromic lymphocyte leukemia cells. The antigen is postulated to function in signal transduction.[7] Demonstration of this antigen by immunohistochemical methods requires the use of frozen sections.

CD7 (Leu9)

CD7 is one of the earliest expressed T-cell markers and is expressed on multipotential hematopoietic cells, T-cell precursors, and most human thymocytes and peripheral blood T cells.[7] Demonstration requires the use of frozen sections. The protein, coded by a 3-kb gene on chromosome 17,[252] consists of an immunoglobulin-like variable region separated from a transmembrane helix by an unusual sequence consisting largely of proline, serine, and threonine residues. The function of the CD7 protein is unknown.

CD10 (CALLA)

The common acute lymphoblastic leukemia antigen (CD10, CALLA) is coded by an 80-kb gene localized to chromosome 3q21-3q27.[253] Immunohistochemical demonstration of CD10 requires the use of frozen sections. The CD10 antigen is an integral membrane protein that serves as an endopeptidase, cleaving a variety of biologically active peptides, including angiotensin I and II, enkephalins, bradykinin, neurotensin, oxytocin, and substance P.[7, 254] In keeping with this range of enzymatic activity, it is expressed not only on B- and T-cell precursors, B-blasts, granulocytes, and bone marrow stromal cells, but also on the brush borders of kidney and intestines, brain, and myoepithelial cells.[7] CD10 is structurally similar to the Kell blood group antigen.[255]

CD15 (LeuM1)

CD15, the Lewis X antigen, is expressed by neutrophils, eosinophils, basophils, monocytes, embryonic tissues, adenocarcinomas, myeloid leukemias, and the Reed-Sternberg cells of Hodgkin's disease.[2, 7, 256] It may be demonstrated in formalin-fixed, paraffin-embedded tissue. Unlike most of the leukocyte antigens, it is a branched carbohydrate (pentasaccharide) antigen that is found on various molecules of the integrin superfamily. The function of CD15 is unknown.

Some representative tumors demonstrating frequent CD15 immunoreactivity are shown in Table 2–19.

CD19 (B4)

CD19 is a membrane-associated member of the immunoglobulin superfamily that is expressed on all human B cells and many B-cell precursors.[7] It may be demonstrated in frozen tissue. The protein, coded for by a 8-kb gene[257] that has not yet been localized to a chromosome, consists of two constant region domains that form eight-stranded β- barrels and a cytoplasmic domain that contains several serine/threonine/tyrosine phosphorylation sites.[258] It appears to assist in regulation of B-cell proliferation by forming a signal-transduction complex with several other B-cell membrane proteins.[259]

CD20 (L26)

CD20 is an unglycosylated phosphoprotein that is expressed on B cells (Fig. 2–12) and dendritic reticulum cells. It is particularly useful for the immunohistochemical identification of B cells in formalin-fixed, paraffin-embedded tissue (Table 2–20); demonstration is often enhanced by the use of antigen retrieval techniques. The 16-kb gene, localized to chromosome 11q12-11q13.1,[260] codes for a 35-kd polypeptide chain[261] that spans the membrane with four probably α-helical channels; this type of structure is typically seen in molecules regulating ion conductance,[7] and it appears that CD20 directly regulates a transmembrane calcium flux.[262] CD20 is thought to assist in regulating B-cell activation and proliferation.[7]

TABLE 2–19

Immunoreactivity of Selected Neoplasms for CD15

Diagnosis	Percentage of Cases Demonstrating Immunoreactivity
Adenocarcinoma, lung	68–76
Adenocarcinoma, breast	44–95
Cystadenocarcinoma, ovary	59–80
Hodgkin's disease, lymphocyte-predominant	27–40
Hodgkin's disease, mixed cellularity	80–87
Hodgkin's disease, nodular sclerosis	86–91
Intra-abdominal desmoplastic small cell tumor	51–87

CD21 (B2)

CD21 is a membrane-associated protein consisting of 15 or 16 complement-control domains, coded for by a 30-kb gene located on chromosome 1q32.[263] The protein is expressed on mature B cells, dendritic reticulum cells, a subset of thymocytes, and mucosal epithelium, such as that of the uterine cervix and the nasopharynx.[7] Immunohistochemical staining is found in about half of all marginal zone lymphomas. In addition to serving as a receptor for the C3d complement fragment[264] and possibly interferon,[265] it may also attach Epstein-Barr virus.[264]

CD21 associates with surface immunoglobulin and with CD35 and CD19. It appears to be involved in regulation of B-cell activation and proliferation. Immunohistochemical demonstration is limited to frozen tissue. Complement control protein domains consist of stacked β-sheet domains,[7] with no helical structure.

CD22 (Leu14)

CD22 is the designation given to either of two immunoglobulin superfamily proteins found on a subset of B cells before B-cell activation. These antigens can be demonstrated immunohistochemically only in frozen sections. The α form consists of a single variable and four constant region domains[7, 266]; the β form has two additional constant domains and a slightly longer cytoplasmic domain[267, 268]; the sequence is similar to that of myelin-associated glycoprotein.[266, 267] The α form mediates adhesion of transfected cells to monocytes and erythrocytes[266]; the β form mediates adhesion of B cells and CD4-bearing T cells.[7, 267, 268] CD45RO and CD75 serve as ligands for CD22β.[267]

CD23 (Blast-2)

CD23 is an integral membrane protein, coded by a 13-kb gene on 19p13.3, which serves as a low affinity receptor for IgE[7, 269] and mediates IgE-dependent cytotoxicity by macrophages and eosinophils.

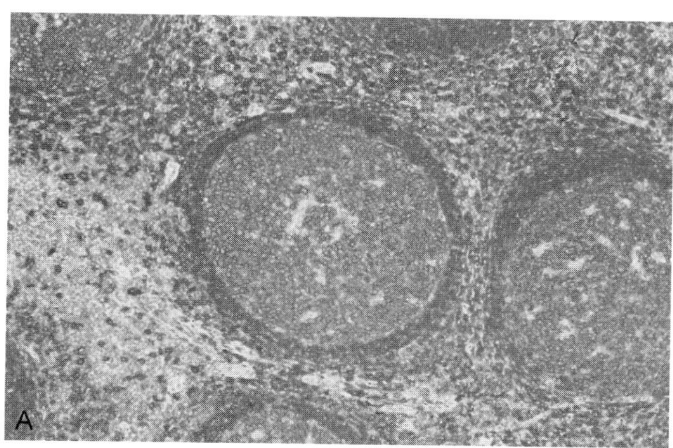

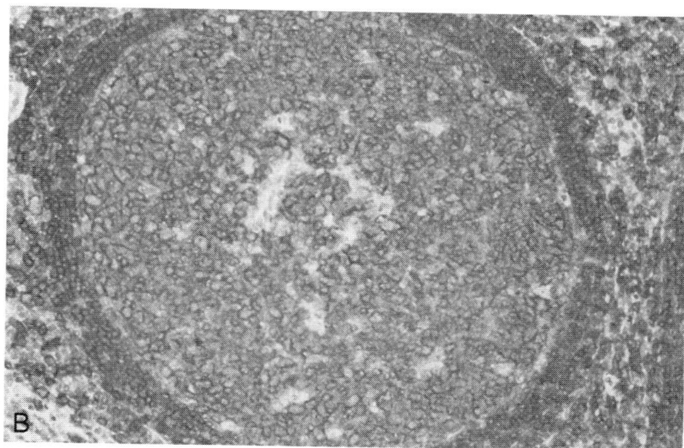

FIGURE 2–12
Section of tonsil immunohistochemically stained for CD20, ×100 (*A*) and ×200 (*B*). (See also Color Fig. 2–12.)

Two alternatively spliced forms, FceRIIa and FCeRIIb, are expressed on mature B cells; the antigen is demonstrated immunohistochemically on 79% to 96% of well-differentiated lymphomas. In contrast, FceRIIb is also found on monocytes, macrophages, eosinophils, platelets, and dendritic reticulum cells.[7]

CD30 (BerH2, Ki-1)

CD30 is an antigen of unknown function that is expressed on activated T and B cells,[7, 270, 271] including the Reed-Sternberg cells of Hodgkin's disease and the cells of large cell anaplastic (Ki-1) lymphoma (Table 2–21). CD30 is a member of the nerve-growth factor receptor superfamily.[272] Like other members of this family, including the tumor necrosis factor receptor, the molecule expresses multiple (in the case of CD30—five) cysteine-rich repeats in the amino-terminal extracellular region. The gene has been sequenced and localized to chromosome 1p36.[272]

TABLE 2–20
Immunoreactivity of Selected Neoplasms for CD20

Diagnosis	Percentage of Cases Demonstrating Immunoreactivity
Hodgkin's disease, lymphocyte-predominant	83–100
Leukemia, hairy cell	79–100
Malignant lymphoma, B-cell	94–98
Malignant lymphoma, HIV-related	51–97
Malignant lymphoma, lymphocytic, well-differentiated	100
Malignant lymphoma, marginal zone	100
Malignant lymphoma, T-cell rich B-cell type	100

CD43 (MT1, Leu22)

CD43 is the major sialoglycoprotein of thymocytes and mature T cells. It is also expressed on granulocytes, monocytes, NK cells, platelets, activated B cells, plasma cells, and bone marrow hematopoietic stem cells.[7] The 4.6-kB gene, which is located on chromosome 16p11.2,[273] codes for a 239 amino acid extracellular domain that binds intracellular adhesion molecule-1 (ICAM-1).[274] Nevertheless, the precise function of CD43 is unknown. Two antibodies that bind CD43 are in widespread use—Leu22 and MT1. Although both stain predominantly T cells and T-cell lymphomas (Table 2–22), they do not always stain each tissue identically.

The CD45 (LCA) Protein Family

CD45 proteins are found on all hematopoietic cells except erythrocytes.[7] CD45 proteins are coded by a 120-kb gene found on chromosome 1q31-1q32.[275] The extracellular domain of CD45 varies from 391 to 552

TABLE 2–21
Immunoreactivity of Selected Neoplasms for CD30

Diagnosis	Percentage of Cases Demonstrating Immunoreactivity
Anaplastic large cell lymphoma	93–100
Carcinoma, embryonal	74–95
Fibroadenoma	100
Hodgkin's disease, lymphocyte-predominant	13–33
Hodgkin's disease, mixed cellularity	86–93
Hodgkin's disease, nodular sclerosis	7–92
Mixed germ cell tumor	67–100

TABLE 2–22

Immunoreactivity of Selected Neoplasms for CD43

Diagnosis	Percentage of Cases Demonstrating Immunoreactivity
Anaplastic large cell lymphoma	36–66
Chloroma	80–99
Leukemia, lymphoid, acute, precursor B cell	87–100
Leukemia, myeloid, acute, NOS (M0)	68–93
Malignant lymphoma, cutaneous T-cell	82–95
Malignant lymphoma, high-grade T-cell	82–96
Malignant lymphoma, lymphoblastic, B-cell	56–87
Malignant lymphoma, lymphoblastic, T-cell	78–97
Malignant lymphoma, lymphocytic, well-differentiated, diffuse	92–100
Malignant lymphoma, mantle cell	70–85
Malignant lymphoma, peripheral T-cell	84–91
Malignant lymphoma, small lymphocytic, B-cell	43–51
Malignant lymphoma, T-cell, NOS	69–83

NOS, not otherwise specified.

amino acids and has about a dozen amino-linked carbohydrate attachment sites. The 700 amino acid cytoplasmic domain demonstrates phosphotyrosine phosphatase activity. Expression of CD45 is necessary for signaling through the TcR.

Different isoforms of CD45 may be formed by alternative splicing of three exons that can be inserted immediately after a preserved eight amino acid amino-terminal sequence. Of eight possible isoforms, seven have been found.[276] The various isoforms are expressed on different lymphoid cell types, giving rise to the various patterns of immunoreactivity with various anti-CD45 antibodies. This restricted expression is useful in differentiating cell lineage. In addition, antibodies directed against the preserved amino-terminal sequence identify all nonerythroid hematopoietic cells. Some commonly used anti-CD45 antibodies, the epitopes against which they are directed, and their patterns of discrimination are shown in Table 2–23; patterns of tumor immunoreactivity are shown in Tables 2–24—2–26.

CD57 (HNK-1, Leu7)

This antigen is present on virtually all NK cells, some B and T cells, some monocytes, and some neural tissues. Although the antigen is known to be a polysaccharide, the details of its structure and function are unknown.[7]

CD68 (Kp1)

CD68 belongs to a family of highly acidic lysosomal glycoproteins. Although these are the major protein components of the lysosomal membrane, their function is unknown. It is expressed primarily in macrophages. Although partial sequences for the gene are available, the complete sequence is unknown, as is its chromosomal localization.[7]

We have found Kp1 particularly useful in identifying reactive histiocytes in effusions; it may also prove useful in diagnosis of a limited number of tumors (Table 2–27).

CD74 (LN2)

The CD74 molecule is an MHC class II–associated integral membrane glycoprotein that is expressed in MHC class II–positive cells. CD74 associates with both the α and β chains of MHC class II molecules and may prevent the binding of endogenous peptides to these molecules in the endoplasmic reticulum.[7] Expression of CD74 appears to be coregulated with that of MHC class II α and β chains. There is some surface expression seen in both B cells and on monocytes, as well as a subset of activated T cells and some epithelial cells (Table 2–28). This integral membrane glycoprotein consists of four distinct forms encoded by alternative splicing schemes.[277] The amino acid sequence for the gene has

TABLE 2–23

Reactivity of Various Anti-CD45 Antibodies

Cluster Designation	Common Antigen Name	Blood Elements Stained
CD45 (N-terminus)	LCA	All nonerythroid
CD45RA	MB1	B cells, suppressor-inducer T cells
CD45RA	MT2	Mantle and marginal B cells, suppressor-inducer T cells
CD45RO	UCHL1	T cells, monocytes

TABLE 2–24

Immunoreactivity of Selected Neoplasms for CD45

Diagnosis	Percentage of Cases Demonstrating Immunoreactivity
Chloroma	63–90
Hodgkin's disease, lymphocyte-predominant	59–85
Hodgkin's disease, mixed cellularity	9–25
Hodgkin's disease, nodular sclerosis	2–10
Anaplastic large cell lymphoma	69–84
Malignant lymphoma, B-cell, NOS	95–98
Malignant lymphoma, T-cell, NOS	85–95
Plasmacytoma	45–83

NOS, not otherwise specified.

TABLE 2–25

Immunoreactivity of B- and T-Cell Lymphomas for CD45RA

Diagnosis	Percentage of Cases Demonstrating Immunoreactivity
Lymphoma, NOS	68–73
Lymphoma, B-cell, NOS	71–76
Lymphoma, T-cell, NOS	7–13

NOS, not otherwise specified.

TABLE 2–26

Immunoreactivity of B- and T-Cell Lymphomas for CD45RO

Diagnosis	Percentage of Cases Demonstrating Immunoreactivity
Anaplastic large cell lymphoma	34–64
Malignant lymphoma, B-cell, NOS	2–5
Malignant lymphoma, T-cell, NOS	72–80

NOS, not otherwise specified.

been determined,[277–279] and the localization of this 12-kb gene to chromosome 5q31-33 has been established.[278]

CDw75 (LN1)

The CDw75 antigen is expressed on mature B cells and on a fraction of T cells; B-cell activation increases its expression. This antigen is also expressed in several epithelial cell types and on erythroid series precursors. A cDNA has been cloned[280, 281]; the sequence shows the molecule to be a galactoside α-2,6-sialotransferase, which seems to be confined to the Golgi apparatus. Its biologic function is unknown, as is its chromosomal localization.

TABLE 2–27

Immunoreactivity Selected Neoplasms for CD68 (Kp1)

Diagnosis	Percentage of Cases Demonstrating Immunoreactivity
Malignant lymphoma, histiocytic	100
Giant cell tumor of bone	90–100
Chloroma	79–94
Malignant melanoma	70–83
Atypical fibroxanthoma	46–70
Malignant fibrous histiocytoma	39–54
Leiomyosarcoma	30–48
Inflammatory pseudotumor	100

NOS, not otherwise specified.

Immunoglobulins

Immunohistochemical assessment of immunoglobulin chains is used to assess clonality and lineage in lymphoid proliferations, thus assisting in the diagnosis of lymphoma and myeloma. Nine different classes of immunoglobulin heavy chain combine with two classes of light chain and (for IgA and IgM) a J chain to constitute four classes of IgG, two of IgA, and one each of IgD, IgE, and IgM. These immunoglobulin heavy and light chains are coded by different genes localized to several chromosomes.

TABLE 2–28

Immunoreactivity of Selected Neoplasms for CD74

Diagnosis	Percentage of Cases Demonstrating Immunoreactivity
Adenocarcinoma, NOS	82–99
Hodgkin's disease, lymphocyte-predominant	49–81
Hodgkin's disease, mixed cellularity	31–59
Hodgkin's disease, nodular sclerosis	49–81
Leukemia, hairy cell	90–100
Malignant lymphoma, B-cell, NOS	64–78
Malignant lymphoma, T-cell, NOS	0–12

NOS, not otherwise specified.

Immunoglobulins are among the most notable exceptions to the "one gene, one polypeptide," rule, because rearrangements involving variable region foci and a common region focus can give rise to a multiplicity of different chains. In particular, one of about 120 different variable regions combines with one of the four IgG heavy-chain regions, a "D" (or "diversity") segment and a "J" (or "joining") region to create a rearranged gene from which an mRNA transcript can be made. Detection of the gene rearrangements that make this possible is a mainstay of diagnostic molecular hematopathology; the mechanism of gene rearrangement is discussed in greater detail in Chapter 14.

The structure of a typical FAB fragment is shown in Figure 2–13. The chains fold into a distinctive array of β sheets connected by β turns[282]; this basic functional structure is observed in all immunoglobulins of all classes. The two different immunoglobulin binding sites formed by the two heavy- and light-chain pairs are well removed from one another, allowing independent binding to different antigens.

IMMUNOGLOBULIN G

Immunoglobulin G is the major circulating immunoglobulin. It is composed of two heavy chains (γ_1–γ_4) and two light chains (κ or λ). The gene for the first IgG heavy chain (γ_1) localizes to chromosome 14q32.33.[283] The other heavy-chain constant-region genes lie nearby, in a span of about 3 Mb.[284] Although most of the variable region genes are also clustered in this area, V(H) segments have been localized to chromosomes 15q11.2 and 16p11.2; a cluster of D segments is also found on chromosome 15q11.2.[285] Only chromosome 14 contains J segments. The κ and λ light chains are about half as long as the immunoglobulin heavy chains and are joined to the heavy chains by disulfide bonds. There are 25 to 50 κ variable region genes; these genes cluster at chromosome 2p12.[286–288] The λ light chain cluster is localized to chromosome 22q11 and contains 7 genes, each preceded by a single J region, arranged tandemly on a 50-kb segment.[289] Of these seven genes, only four are transcriptionally active.

IMMUNOGLOBULIN A

IgA is the predominant immunoglobulin in such body secretions as saliva, tears, respiratory and digestive mucosal secretions, prostatic fluid, and vaginal secretions. There are two different genes coding for IgA heavy chains—α_1 and α_2. IgA molecules can consist of monomers (each consisting of two heavy and two light chains), dimers joined by a J peptide, or higher-order multimers. The genes coding IgA heavy chains are localized to the heavy-chain gene cluster on chromosome 14,

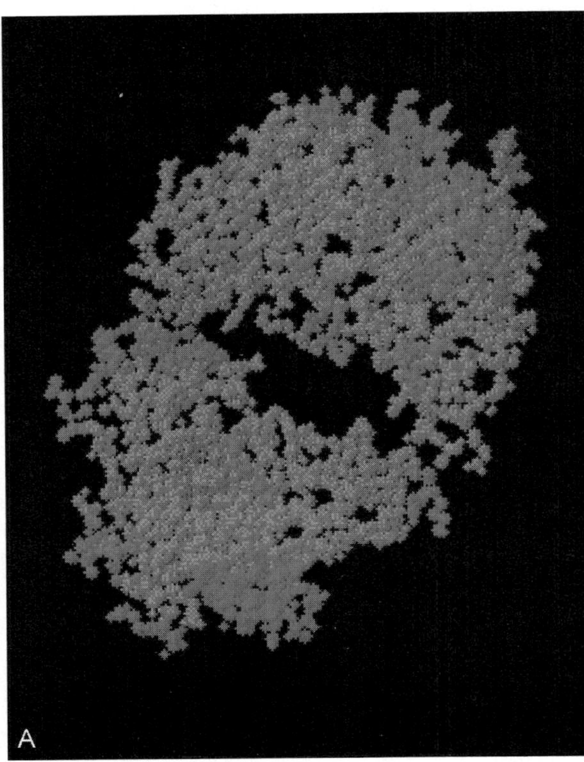

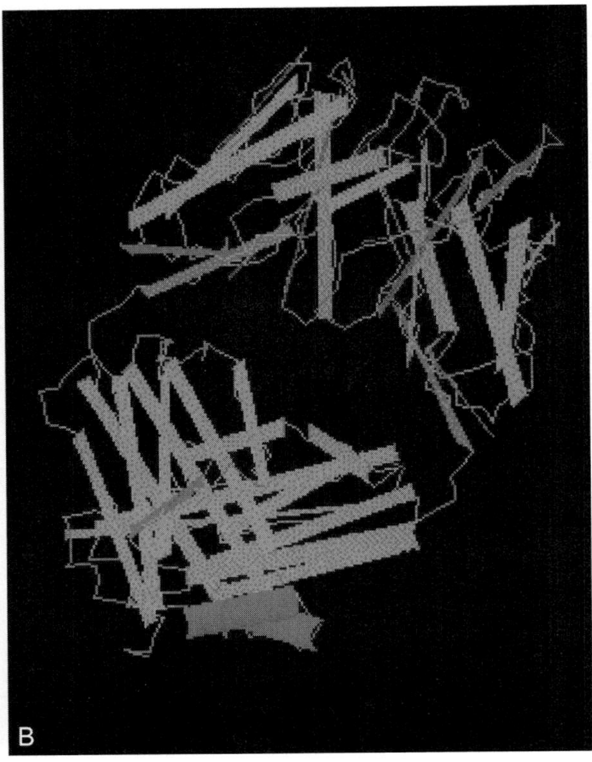

FIGURE 2–13
Space-filling (*A*) and secondary structure (*B*) models looking "end-on" at an immunoglobulin FAB fragment. Models were generated using Cn3D and Brookhaven Protein Structure Data Base data. (See also Color Fig. 2–13.)

as are the genes coding for the heavy chains of all immunoglobulin molecules. The κ and λ polypeptides are coded by the same genes in all immunoglobulin classes.

IMMUNOGLOBULIN M

Immunoglobulin M is responsible for much of the "early response." It is the major B cell surface immunoglobulin and is typically coexpressed with IgD. Immunoglobulin M molecules are composed of five subunits, each of which contains two μ heavy chains and two light chains. The subunits are connected in a pentameric arrangement by J chains.

IMMUNOGLOBULIN D

Immunoglobulin D constitutes one of the two major surface immunoglobulins of B lymphocytes and is typically coexpressed with immunoglobulin M. The heavy chain for immunoglobulin D is known as δ.[290]

IMMUNOGLOBULIN E

Immunoglobulin E mediates the acute allergic response seen in allergies. The ε chain is the heavy chain of IgE. There are several different constant regions genes for ε, which have been cloned and sequenced.[291]

J CHAIN

The J chain is a 137-amino acid protein coded by a gene localized to chromosome 4q21. J chain is synthesized in B lymphocytes and both links immunoglobulin monomers (IgM to pentamers IgA to dimers) and binds immunoglobulins to secretory component.[292]

Lysozyme

Lysozyme is a glycosidase present in histiocytes, some epithelial cells, and cells of myeloid lineage. Immunohistochemical assessment is most frequently employed in the differentiation of hematopoietic tumors. Lysozyme is coded by a 5-kb gene on chromosome 12 and gives rise to a 1.5-kb mRNA. The gene contains four exons; the base sequence is highly homologous to both the egg lysozymes and human α-lactalbumin.[293] Gene expression results in a mature lysozyme preceded by an 18 amino acid signal peptide.[294]

The conformation of lysozyme from a variety of sources has been extensively studied by spectroscopic, x-ray diffraction, and theoretical techniques.[295–301] The protein consists of approximately 40% α helix, 25% β sheet, and 35% disordered structures[295]; binding of substrate or inhibitor to the active site results in substantial conformational changes.[300] This enzyme was one of the first whose structure and mechanism of action were defined in detail; both have long been presented in standard biochemistry texts.[301]

MARKERS FOR GLANDULAR DIFFERENTIATION

The identification of glandular differentiation is an important use for immunohistochemistry. Sometimes general assays for glandular differentiation, such as those offered by carcinoembryonic antigen (CEA), tumor-associated glycoprotein-72 (TAG-72), BER-EP4, epithelial membrane antigen (EMA) and CD15 (LeuM1), prove useful. Organ-specific antigens, such as prostate-specific antigen, prostatic acid phosphatase, amylase, and thyroglobulin, establish not only glandular differentiation, but specific tissue type.

Thyroglobulin

Thyroglobulin is a 2750 amino acid glycoprotein synthesized only in the thyroid, which is cleaved to form the thyroid hormones thyroxine (T_4) and triiodothyronine (T_3). It is coded by a 300-kb gene that yields an 8301 nucleotide mRNA and localizes to chromosome 8q24.2-24.3.[302–305] The protein has a 19 amino acid amino-terminal signal peptide, followed by a long (1190 residue) repetitive amino-terminal region and a carboxyl-terminal region demonstrating significant homology with both acetylcholinesterase and the invariant chain of the Ia class II histocompatibility antigen.[305, 306] The signal peptide mediates assembly in the rough endoplasmic reticulum and transport to the Golgi apparatus; the acetylcholinesterase-like region may be involved in binding to the cell membrane. Thyroid hormone synthesis can occur at sites that are clustered at both ends of the thyroglobulin monomer. Glycosylation sites are scattered along the polypeptide chain.[305]

The thyroglobulin gene is expressed only in differentiated thyroid cells under the positive control of the pituitary hormone TSH by means of a cyclic adenosine monophosphate–dependent pathway. Regulation appears to be mediated by a *trans*-acting factor, expressed only in thyroid cells, which binds a highly conserved promoter element approximately 100 bp upstream of the transcription initiation site.[307] Tissue-specific expression is further assured by methylation of the gene that occurs in non-thyroid, but not thyroid, tissues.[308]

Surprisingly, it does not appear that the secondary structure of thyroglobulin has been completely elucidated. Based on theoretical considerations and homology to acetylcholinesterase, the C-terminal region is expected to be approximately 20% α helix, 30% β structure, and 17% β turns.[309] The precise conformation appears to depend on calcium binding.[310, 311] Immunologic reactivity with certain antibodies is dependent on macromolecular conformation and/or glycosylation[312]

TABLE 2–29

Thyroglobulin Immunoreactivity of Various Thyroid Tumors

Diagnosis	Percentage of Cases Demonstrating Immunoreactivity
Anaplastic carcinoma	4–16
Follicular carcinoma	82–98
Medullary carcinoma	1–10
Mucoepidermoid carcinoma	54–100
Oxyphilic carcinoma	100
Papillary carcinoma	89–100

and may change in various disease states.[313] This may eventually prove useful in pathologic diagnosis.[314]

Although immunohistochemical demonstration of thyroid hormone in the cytoplasm of a tumor is strong evidence of thyroid derivation, anaplastic and medullary carcinomas of the thyroid seldom demonstrate the protein (Table 2–29).

Carcinoembryonic Antigen

Carcinoembryonic antigen is used immunohistochemically to identify cells originating in glandular epithelium (Table 2–30). This 70-kd protein, coded by a 24-kb gene that contains seven immunoglobulin-like domains, localizes to chromosome 19q13.1-13.3.[315] CEA is a member of the immunoglobulin gene superfamily and appears to be involved in intercellular adhesion.[8] The gene encoding CEA has been cloned and sequenced. *N*-Glycosylation has been identified at 3 of 28 possible glycosylation sites; CEA is anchored to the cell membrane through linkage to a glycosyl phosphatidylinositol moiety.

Assessment of anti-CEA staining in tissue must consider the possible presence of nonspecific cross-reacting antigens that are found in granulocytes and normal tissues. Most polyclonal anti-CEA antisera react with these antigens, which do not reflect glandular differentiation. Monoclonal antisera may or may not react with nonspecific cross-reacting antigens.

TABLE 2–30

Carcinoembryonic Antigen (Polyclonal) Immunoreactivity of Various Tumors

Diagnosis	Percentage of Cases Demonstrating Immunoreactivity
Adenocarcinoma, breast	13–30
Adenocarcinoma, bladder	60–95
Adenocarcinoma, colorectal	78–91
Adenocarcinoma, endometrial	5–16
Adenocarcinoma, lung	83–89
Adenocarcinoma, pancreas	54–86
Adenocarcinoma, stomach	33–71
Adenocarcinoma, NOS	69–80
Anaplastic carcinoma, thyroid	6–22
Basal cell carcinoma	0
Brenner tumor	66–98
Carcinoid, goblet cell	100
Carcinoid, insular	2–21
Carcinoid, mixed	9–48
Carcinoid, NOS	27–40
Carcinoma in situ, cervix	19–31
Cholangiocarcinoma	78–100
Chondrosarcoma	0
Chordoma	28–52
Choriocarcinoma	5–33
Cystadenocarcinoma, mucinous, ovary	23–44
Cystadenocarcinoma, serous, ovary	0–2
Cystadenoma, hepatobiliary	100
Cystadenoma, serous, ovary	0
Embryonal carcinoma, NOS	0–8
Endodermal sinus tumor	10–39
Endometrioid carcinoma, ovary	25–66
Follicular carcinoma, thyroid	21–47
Granulosa cell tumor	0
Hepatocellular carcinoma	52–68
Lymphoma, NOS	0–15
Malignant melanoma, NOS	26–58
Medullary carcinoma, thyroid	80–96
Mesothelial proliferation, NOS	0–6
Mesothelioma, epithelioid	0
Mesothelioma, NOS	3–7
Paget's disease, breast	14–56
Paget's disease, extramammary	100
Papillary carcinoma, thyroid	28–56
Seminoma, NOS	0
Synovial sarcoma	2–32
Small cell carcinoma, lung	58–80
Squamous cell carcinoma, cervix	25–42
Squamous cell carcinoma, lung	12–36
Teratoma, NOS	8–44
Thecoma	0
Transitional cell carcinoma, NOS	1–20

NOS, not otherwise specified.

TAG-72

The tumor associated glycoprotein-72 (TAG-72), recognized by the monoclonal antibody B72.3,[316] is useful in pathology as an immunohistochemical marker of glandular differentiation (Table 2–31). The antigen name is misleading, because TAG-72 is expressed by a variety of non-neoplastic tissues.[317] The antigen (Fig. 2–14) is a glycoprotein of molecular weight 72 kd; although its distribution appears to be that of a mucin, little is known about the genetics or biochemistry of this molecule.

BER-EP4

BER-EP4 is monoclonal antibody directed against an epitope on the protein moiety of two 34-kd and 39-kd glycopolypeptides on human epithelial cells.[318] It is useful as a marker of epithelial (particularly glandular)

TABLE 2–31
Immunoreactivity of Selected Tumors with Monoclonal Antibody B72.3

Diagnosis	Percentage of Cases Demonstrating Immunoreactivity
Adenocarcinoma, breast	60–91
Adenocarcinoma, lung	84–90
Adenocarcinoma, NOS	77–86
Adenocarcinoma, pancreas	65–87
Adenocarcinoma, prostate	61–80
Angiosarcoma, epithelioid	57–100
Apocrine carcinoma, breast	84–100
Apocrine metaplasia, NOS	88–100
Benign prostatic hypertrophy	85–100
Cystadenocarcinoma, ovary	71–87
Hepatocellular carcinoma	3–19
Mesothelioma, epithelioid	0–3
Mesothelioma, NOS	10–17
Prostatic intraepithelial neoplasia	73–100

NOS, not otherwise specified.

differentiation (Table 2–32) and has been found useful in identification of epithelial cells in effusions[319–321] and differentiation of adenocarcinoma from mesothelioma.[322, 323] The gene coding for these proteins has not been identified, nor has the antigen been structurally characterized.

Prostate-Specific Antigen

Prostate-specific antigen (PSA) is utilized in the immunohistochemical identification of prostate cells. Together with PAP, it is one of very few nearly organ-specific immunoassays available to the pathologist (Table 2–33). Assessment of serum PSA levels may be useful in detection and management of adenocarcinoma of the prostate.

PSA is a kallikrein-like protease coded by a 6-kb gene[324] that localizes to 19q13.2-13.4,[325] as do the tissue kallikrein (KLK1), and human glandular kallikrein-1 (hGK-1 or KLK2) genes.[326] Variant transcripts may arise by means of alternative splicing. The gene has been cloned and sequenced.[327, 328]

PSA is glycosylated and is thought to assist in liquefaction of seminal coagulum. The secondary structure of the protein has not been determined.

Prostatic Acid Phosphatase

Immunohistochemical assessment of prostatic acid phosphatase (PAP) is used to determine whether a cell population is of prostate origin (Table 2–34). PAP is coded by a 40-kb gene[329] that localizes to chromosome 3q21-23.[330] The gene gives rise to a 354 amino acid product that is 50% homologous to lysosomal acid phosphatase.[331] Although the predicted weight of PAP is approximately 50 kd, the actual weight is approximately 89 kd, owing to extensive glycosylation.[332] The protein contains 38 to 41 carbohydrate residues, of which 3 are fucose, 4 are galactose, 11 are mannose, 15 are glucosamine, and 7 to 8 are sialic acid. Circular dichroism experiments suggest an α-helix content of about 30%. Rat PAP has been crystallized and characterized by x-ray diffraction analysis.[333]

PAP consists of two domains, an α/β domain consisting of a seven-stranded mixed β-pleated sheet with helices on both sides of the sheet and a smaller α domain. A dimer is formed through interactions of the two subunits that effectively extends the β-pleated sheet from 7 to 14 strands. The active site is at the carboxyl end of the parallel strands of the α/β domain. The overall structure of the enzyme remains unchanged on binding of the metal oxyanions.[334]

α-Amylase

The α-amylases are a multigene family whose members function as digestive proteins secreted by

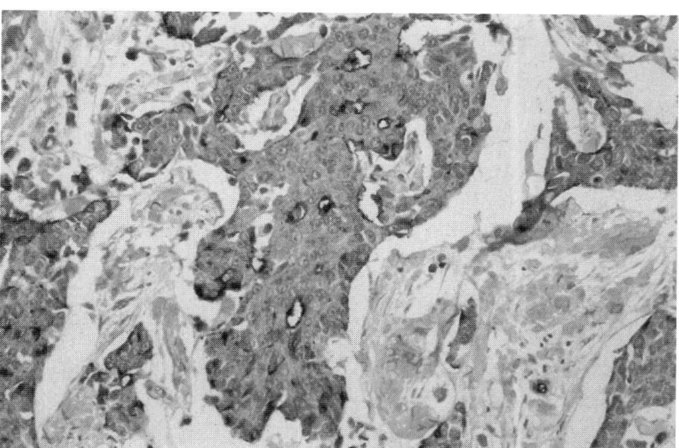

FIGURE 2–14
Section of breast carcinoma stained immunohistochemically with the monoclonal antibody B72.3 (×200). (See also Color Fig. 2–14.)

TABLE 2–32

Selected Neoplasms Demonstrating Immunoreactivity for BER-EP4

Diagnosis	Percentage of Cases Demonstrating Immunoreactivity
Adenocarcinoma, colon and rectum	100
Adenocarcinoma, lung	88–95
Adenocarcinoma, NOS	58–70
Adenocarcinoma, stomach	86–100
Cystadenocarcinoma, ovary	87–100
Hepatocellular carcinoma	23–48
Infiltrating ductal carcinoma, breast	74–95
Mesothelioma, biphasic	2–34
Mesothelioma, epithelioid	6–15
Mesothelioma, NOS	2–7
Small cell carcinoma, lung	100

NOS, not otherwise specified.

TABLE 2–33

Selected Neoplasms Demonstrating Immunoreactivity for Prostate-Specific Antigen

Diagnosis	Percentage of Cases Demonstrating Immunoreactivity
Adenocarcinoma, bladder	0
Adenocarcinoma, colorectal	0
Adenocarcinoma, prostate, metastatic	87–100
Adenocarcinoma, prostate, primary	89–100

TABLE 2–34

Selected Neoplasms Demonstrating Immunoreactivity for Prostatic Acid Phosphatase

Diagnosis	Percentage of Cases Demonstrating Immunoreactivity
Carcinoid, NOS	3–18
Adenocarcinoma, prostate, metastatic	100
Adenocarcinoma, prostate, primary	81–100

NOS, not otherwise specified.

the pancreatic acinar cells and salivary glands. The amylases assist in the breakdown of complex carbohydrates. Immunohistochemical staining for amylase is useful in the identification of such cells, but it may also be observed in lungs, ovaries, and gastrointestinal tract (Table 2–35).

TABLE 2–35

Selected Neoplasms Demonstrating Immunoreactivity for Amylase

Diagnosis	Percentage of Cases Demonstrating Immunoreactivity
Cystadenocarcinoma, ovary	19–46
Carcinoma, acinar cell	11–47
Mesothelioma, NOS	4–32

NOS, not otherwise specified.

The amylase genes are found on chromosome 1p21[335] in 100-kb clusters consisting either of two pancreatic amylase genes and one salivary amylase gene or in 300-kb clusters containing four additional salivary amylase genes and two pseudogenes.[336, 337] A selective deficiency of pancreatic amylase has been described.[338]

Amylase shares with such enzymes as neuron-specific enolase an α/β barrel structure.[339] Because of the structural similarity to other α/β barrel proteins, similar conformational changes are expected during catalysis.

Epithelial Membrane Antigen and Milk Fat Globulin

Epithelial membrane antigen (EMA, episialin, polymorphic epithelial mucin, MUC1, PUM) is used in the immunohistochemical identification of both tumors demonstrating glandular differentiation and plasma cells (Table 2–36). Although there are at least seven genes encoding human mucins,[340] the majority of antibodies used in immunohistochemistry appear to be directed against the 400-kd product of a single gene, *MUC1*, which is localized to chromosome 1q21-24.[341] The product of this gene, human EMA (episialin, MUC1), consists largely of between 30 and 90 nearly identical 20-residue tandem repeats, which form the majority of the extracellular domain of the glycoprotein. The repeated structure is dominated by a hydrophilic domain of seven amino acids, extending into two flanking β turns.[342] The transmembrane and cytoplasmic domains are about 90% conserved between human and mouse.[343] Multiple forms of the gene product, generated by alternative splicing,[344] account for the large variation in the number of 20-residue tandem repeats observed in the molecule. After transcription, the protein is cleaved within the endoplasmic reticulum at a site that is upstream of the transmembrane domain[345]; the cleavage products remain associated with each other, allowing the amino-terminal mucin-like domain to remain anchored to the cell membrane through interaction with the carboxyl-terminal subunit. In contrast to CEA, which

TABLE 2–36

Immunoreactivity of Selected Neoplasms for Epithelial Membrane Antigen

Diagnosis	Percentage of Cases Demonstrating Immunoreactivity
Acinar cell carcinoma	29–71
Adenocarcinoma, breast	100
Adenocarcinoma, colorectal	80–95
Adenocarcinoma, endometrial	91–100
Adenocarcinoma, lung	97–100
Adenocarcinoma, prostate	8–44
Adenocarcinoma, stomach	64–100
Adrenal cortical carcinoma	0–7
Anaplastic carcinoma, thyroid	19–48
Anaplastic large cell lymphoma (P80+)	89–100
Anaplastic large cell lymphoma (P80-)	14–52
Angiosarcoma, epithelioid	0
Carcinoid, NOS	12–55
Carcinoma, thymus	37–73
Chondrosarcoma, extraskeletal, myxoid	10–36
Chordoma	91–99
Choriocarcinoma	38–71
Cystadenocarcinoma, ovary, NOS	100
Cystadenocarcinoma, ovary, serous	100
Cystadenoma, hepatobiliary	100
Dermatofibrosarcoma protuberans	0
Embryonal carcinoma	0–8
Endodermal sinus tumor	0–11
Epidermoid carcinoma, NOS	95–100
Epithelioid sarcoma, rhabdoid features	84–100
Follicular adenoma, thyroid	25–66
Granular cell tumor	0
Granulosa cell tumor	0
Hemangioblastoma, cerebellar	0–7
Hemangioendothelioma, epithelioid	0–11
Hemangiosarcoma	0
Hepatocellular carcinoma	24–43
Hodgkin's disease, lymphocyte predominance, nodular	48–69
Hodgkin's disease, lymphocyte predominance	39–80
Hodgkin's disease, mixed cellularity	9–18
Hodgkin's disease, nodular sclerosis	2–5
Hodgkin's disease, NOS	8–15
Inflammatory pseudotumor	0
Intra-abdominal desmoplastic small cell tumor	89–100
Ki-1 lymphoma	49–60
Leiomyoma, cellular	0
Leiomyosarcoma, NOS	0
Malignant fibrous histiocytoma	10–28
Malignant lymphoma, B-cell, NOS	2–6
Malignant lymphoma, large cell, diffuse	0
Malignant lymphoma, lymphoblastic, T-cell	2–14
Malignant lymphoma, T-cell, NOS	9–29
Malignant lymphoma, T-cell rich, B-cell	18–37
Melanocytic neuroectodermal tumor of infancy	16–56
Meningioma, fibrous	75–99
Meningioma, hemangioblastic	0–11
Meningioma, NOS	65–81
Meningioma, secretory	0
Merkel cell carcinoma	73–95
Mesothelial proliferation, NOS	4–9
Mesothelioma, epithelioid	78–96
Mesothelioma, NOS	66–73
Neuroblastoma, olfactory	0
Neurofibroma, NOS	0
Osteosarcoma, NOS	5–32
Osteosarcoma, extraskeletal	34–74
Paget's disease, breast	73–97
Papillary carcinoma, thyroid	73–92
Renal cell carcinoma	88–97
Seminoma, NOS	0–3
Small cell carcinoma, lung	82–96
Squamous cell carcinoma, basaloid	70–95
Synovial sarcoma, biphasic	100
Synovial sarcoma, monophasic	48–68
Thymoma, benign	39–75
Transitional cell carcinoma, NOS	85–100

NOS, not otherwise specified.

appears to be an adhesion molecule, high levels of cell-surface EMA inhibit cellular aggregation.[346]

In addition to antibodies identified as directed against EMA, the murine monoclonal antibodies E29, H23, HMFG-1, HMFG-2, MA5, MA6, and MA9 all react with the 20 residue repeat motif; all except MA-9 react with the carboxyl-terminal half.[347]

NEUROENDOCRINE MARKERS

S-100 Proteins

Antibodies directed against "S-100 proteins" have long proved useful in the identification of tumors believed to arise from the neural crest, such as malignant melanoma. The S-100 proteins were originally identified as a group of low-molecular-weight (10 to 12 kd) acidic proteins that were present predominantly in nervous tissue. S-100 derived from nerve actually contains two different subunits (α and β) with two different amino acid compositions. These subunits can form both homodimers and heterodimers in solution. Structurally similar S-100 proteins have been derived from many other tissues.[348] These proteins each contain two calcium-binding motifs, known as "EF hands." Each of these domains consists of a loop of 12 amino acids that is flanked on both sides by two nearly perpendicular α-helical domains. Although structurally similar, the various EF hands associated with S-100 proteins are not identical and may have significantly different calcium binding affinities. The amino-

and carboxyl-terminal regions of S-100 proteins are highly conserved hydrophobic domains.

The S-100 β subunit is responsible for the tissue-specific immunohistochemical reactivity (Table 2–37) of most anti–S-100 antibodies; it is also the best characterized of the S-100 proteins from a biochemical perspective; the protein has been crystallized, and a partial crystal structure is available.[349] The functions of the S-100 proteins have not been clearly elucidated, however. It is generally believed that S-100 proteins (Table 2–38), like other members of the calmodulin family, transduce calcium signals into a cellular response by modulating the activity of target proteins, rather than through a direct effect.[350] Although its function has been extensively studied, the actions of S-100 in vivo cannot be simply characterized. S-100β is expressed predominantly in the G_1 phase of the cell cycle, and predominantly in glial cells (within the central nervous system). S-100β stimulates intracellular calcium flux in both glial and neuronal cells, possibly by means of a phosphatidylinositol pathway. S-100β can stimulate neuritic outgrowth from both central and peripheral neurons,[351] alter microtubule dissociation and assembly,[352, 353] and bind p53.[354] The extracellular effects appear to require that S-100 be dimerized by means of a disulfide link.

Genetic analysis of S-100β indicates that it is highly conserved; the nucleic acid sequences of human and mouse are 85% homologous, and the protein products differ by only a single amino acid. This high degree of conservation implies a vital role for S-100 in maintaining normal life.[348]

Chromogranin

There are three distinct chromogranins (A, B, and C) that are found in neuroendocrine cells, such as those of the adrenal medulla. Chromogranin A is the most abundant and is the species against which most commercially available immunohistochemical reagents have been derived. Immunohistochemical identification of chromogranin suggests neuroendocrine differentiation (Table 2–39); because the intensity of staining is proportional to the number of neurosecretory granules present, tumors demonstrating only a few granules may not stain immunohistochemically. Tumors that typically exhibit chromogranin A immunoreactivity include pheochromocytoma, parathyroid adenoma, medullary carcinoma of the thyroid, carcinoid, oat-cell lung carcinoma of the lung, and pancreatic islet-cell tumors.

Chromogranin A is a protein that both stores and is released together with catecholamines in neurosecretory granules of neuroendocrine cells. It is coded by a highly conserved 11-kb gene[355] that localizes to 14q32,[356] near the immunoglobulin heavy-chain locus. Sequence analysis demonstrates that human chromogranin A contains 439 amino acid residues preceded by an 18-residue

TABLE 2–37

Immunoreactivity of Selected Neoplasms for S100

Diagnosis	Percentage of Cases Demonstrating Immunoreactivity
Adenocarcinoma, breast	30–58
Adenocarcinoma, colorectal	7–26
Adenocarcinoma, endometrium	62–86
Adenocarcinoma, lung	4–17
Adenocarcinoma, prostate	0
Adenocarcinoma, salivary glands	41–75
Anaplastic carcinoma, thyroid	18–51
Angiomyolipoma	8–42
Atypical fibroxanthoma	6–20
Basal cell carcinoma, NOS	0
Blue nevus, cellular	64–96
Blue nevus, NOS	100
Carcinoid, goblet cell	0
Carcinoid, insular	0
Carcinoid, mixed	0
Carcinoid, NOS	1–12
Carcinoma, thymus	0
Chondrosarcoma, extraskeletal myxoid	30–53
Chondrosarcoma, NOS	91–99
Chordoma	84–93
Choriocarcinoma, NOS	0
Clear cell sarcoma	54–86
Cystadenocarcinoma, ovary, NOS	65–80
Cystadenocarcinoma, serous, ovary	58–84
Cystadenocarcinoma, mucinous, ovary	0
Dermal nevus	100
Dermatofibroma	0
Dermatofibosarcoma protuberans	0–3
Endodermal sinus tumor	0–11
Embryonal carcinoma	0
Epidermoid carcinoma, NOS	0
Ewing's sarcoma	9–29
Fibrohistiocytic tumor, plexiform	0–15
Ganglioglioma	100
Glomus tumor	0–5
Granular cell tumor	94–100
Granulosa cell tumor	31–50
Hemangioblastoma, cerebellar	52–81
Hemangioendothelioma, epithelioid	0
Hemangiopericytoma	0–21
Hemangiosarcoma	0–12
Histiocytosis X	100
Inflammatory pseudotumor	0
Intra-abdominal desmoplastic small cell tumor	2–17
Large cell neuroendocrine carcinoma	0–21
Leiomyosarcoma	6–19
Malignant fibrous histiocytoma	0–5
Malignant lymphoma, NOS	0–10
Malignant melanoma, desmoplastic	92–100
Malignant melanoma, NOS	94–99
Medulloblastoma, NOS	0–15
Melanocytic neuroectodermal tumor of infancy	0–19
Meningioma, fibrous	34–69
Meningioma, hemangioblastic	0

Table 2–37 *Continued*

Diagnosis	Percentage of Cases Demonstrating Immunoreactivity
Meningioma, NOS	5–19
Meningioma, secretory	12–38
Merkel cell carcinoma	0
Mesothelioma, epithelioid	0
Mesothelioma, NOS	3–11
Myofibroblastoma	0
Myofibroma	0
Myxoma	20–42
Neurilemoma	100
Neuroblastoma	23–51
Neuroblastoma, olfactory	78–95
Neuroepithelioma, peripheral	46–74
Neurofibroma	65–85
Neurothecoma	0
Nevus, congenital	100
Nevus, dysplastic	49–82
Nodular fasciitis	0
Osteosarcoma	23–56
Paget's disease, breast	32–63
Paget's disease, extramammary	0
Peripheral nerve sheath tumor, NOS	48–94
Pleomorphic adenoma (mixed tumor), salivary glands	90–100
Primitive neuroectodermal tumor	34–66
Renal cell carcinoma	26–49
Rhabdomyosarcoma	0–13
Schwannoma, malignant, epithelioid	64–96
Schwannoma, malignant, NOS	48–83
Seminoma, NOS	0
Sinus histiocytosis with massive lymphadenopathy	88–100
Squamous cell carcinoma, basaloid	23–55
Synovial sarcoma, monophasic	0
Xanthogranuloma	0

NOS, not otherwise specified.

signal peptide.[357] Three regions are highly conserved—multiple paired basic residues that may serve as proteolytic processing signals, a region homologous to

TABLE 2–38

Tissue Localization of Various S-100 Subunits

Name	Tissue/Cell Type
S-100β	Glial and other neural crest cells
S-100α	Many cells, including kidney tubules and muscle cells
p11	Many cells, tyrosine kinase substrate
2A9	Fibroblasts
18A2	Fibroblasts, placenta
MRP8	Myeloid cells, serum of rheumatoid arthritis patients
MRP14	Myeloid cells, serum of rheumatoid arthritis patients
ICaBP	Intestinal cells (vitamin D–induced)

TABLE 2–39

Immunoreactivity of Selected Neoplasms for Chromogranin A

Diagnosis	Percentage of Cases Demonstrating Immunoreactivity
Acinar cell carcinoma	14–52
Adenocarcinoma, lung	0–10
Adenocarcinoma, pancreas	0
Adenocarcinoma, prostate	21–37
Adenoma, pituitary	100
Adrenal cortical carcinoma	0
Atypical carcinoid, lung	100
Carcinoid, NOS	85–93
Chordoma	0
Choriocarcinoma, NOS	0
Endodermal sinus tumor	0
Epidermoid carcinoma, NOS	0
Ganglioglioma	71–100
Glomus tumor	69–100
Granular cell tumor	0
Hemangioblastoma, cerebellar	0–13
Intra-abdominal desmoplastic small cell tumor	0–15
Intraductal carcinoma	0–19
Islet cell tumor	45–76
Large cell neuroendocine carcinoma	60–78
Medullary carcinoma, thyroid	90–100
Melanocytic neuroectodermal tumor of infancy	0–12
Meningioma, secretory	0
Merkel cell carcinoma	46–74
Neuroblastoma, NOS	60–82
Neuroblastoma, olfactory	41–66
Neuroepithelioma, peripheral	0
Pheochromocytoma	90–100
Renal cell carcinoma	0
Sclerosing hemangioma, lung	72–100
Seminoma	0
Small cell carcinoma, lung	28–39

NOS, not otherwise specified.

pancreastatin, and a short hydrophobic disulfide loop near the amino terminus.[358]

Chromogranin B (Table 2–40) is a 657 amino acid polypeptide that is preceded by a 20 residue signal peptide.[359] Chromogranin B is coded by a gene on chromosome 20pter-p12.[360] Chromogranin C is an 86-kd protein found in the pituitary and in the adrenal medulla.[361]

The precise function of the chromogranins is unknown, although chromogranin A is thought to participate in chromaffin granule calcium release.[362] Circular dichroism measurements from chromogranin A reveal a protein that is about 40% α helix. Chromogranin A binds calcium with low affinity; calcium causes a decrease in the α-helix content at intracellular pH.[363] Chromogranin A interacts with the inositol 1,4,5-triphosphate receptor on the intraluminal side of the secretory vesicle membrane at the intravesicular pH of 5.5 but dissociates at physiologic pH.[364]

TABLE 2–40

Immunoreactivity of Selected Neoplasms for Chromogranin B

Diagnosis	Percentage of Cases Demonstrating Immunoreactivity
Adenocarcinoma, prostate	34–69
Medullary carcinoma, thyroid	100
Merkel cell carcinoma	100
Mucinous carcinoma, breast	20–43
Pituitary adenoma	100

Synaptophysin

Synaptophysin, a 38-kd glycoprotein, is the major integral membrane protein of synaptic and neurosecretory vesicle membranes[365]; thus, it is a particularly useful immunohistochemical marker of neural and neuroendocrine differentiation (Table 2–41). Synaptophysin is coded by a 20-kb gene,[366–368] which maps to the locus Xp11.23-p11.22. The gene has been cloned and sequenced.[367, 368] The deduced amino acid suggests that the protein spans the synaptic vesicle membrane four times and that both amino and carboxyl termini face the cytoplasm. The structure of synaptophysin suggests that the protein may function as a channel in the synaptic vesicle membrane, with the carboxyl terminus serving as a binding site for cellular factors.[367] Synaptophysin binds calcium on the cytoplasmic side of the membrane and appears to form dimers and oligomers within the membrane.[365] This may allow it to form transmembrane channels.[367] Synaptophysin contains a novel tandem repeat motif that it shares with the proteins rhodopsin, synexin, RNA polymerase II, and gliadin. This motif allows ready interconversion of several conformations and suggests that the mechanism of action of these proteins may have common elements.[369]

TABLE 2–41

Immunoreactivity of Selected Neoplasms for Synaptophysin

Diagnosis	Percentage of Cases Demonstrating Immunoreactivity
Adrenal cortical carcinoma	72–99
Adenocarcinoma, lung	16–37
Adenocarcinoma, pancreas	0
Adenoma, pituitary	82–100
Astrocytoma	0
Carcinoid, atypical	100
Carcinoid, NOS	84–100
Chordoma	0–19
Ganglioglioma	100
Gastrointestinal stromal tumor	0
Glomus tumor	85–100
Intra-abdominal desmoplastic small cell tumor	10–39
Islet cell tumor	90–100
Large cell neuroendocrine carcinoma	28–53
Medulloblastoma	89–100
Melanocytic neuroectodemal tumor of infancy	45–83
Neuroblastoma	46–75
Neuroblastoma, olfactory	56–82
Neurocytoma, central	77–98
Neuroepithelioma, peripheral	58–89
Primitive neuroectodermal tumor, central	100
Primitive neuroectodermal tumor, peripheral	60–88
Renal cell carcinoma	0–10
Small cell carcinoma, cervix	33–77
Small cell carcinoma, lung	31–48
Squamous cell carcinoma, lung	3–19
Thymic carcinoma	14–45

NOS, not otherwise specified.

Neuron-Specific Enolase

Neuron-specific enolase (NSE) is useful in the identification of neural and neural crest cells. Like all enolases, NSE catalyzes the dehydration of 2-phosphoglycerate to phosphoenolpyruvate in the glycolytic pathway. The protein is coded by the 9-kb *ENO2* gene,[370] which localizes to chromosome 12pter-p11.[371] The enzyme consists of two subunits, each of which forms two distinctive domains. The larger domain is an eightfold β/α barrel, similar to that found in pyruvate kinase and several other glycolytic enzymes.[372] The β strand contains a hydrophobic patch that fits into a hydrophobic pocket on the α helix.[373]

Enolase requires two divalent metal (generally magnesium) ions per active site for activity. Binding of the first metal ion (conformational) results in a conformational change that allows substrate binding. The second metal ion (catalytic) binds only in the presence of a substrate or substrate analogue, is coordinated to an active site hydroxyl group,[374] and is important in the catalytic reaction.[375]

ALZHEIMER'S DISEASE MARKERS

Amyloid of Alzheimer's Disease

Amyloid is a cerebral protein that forms the plaque core in Alzheimer's disease and in older persons with Down syndrome. Immunohistochemical demonstration of amyloid is useful in the identification of Alzheimer's plaques. The cerebral amyloid proteins consist of aggregated 4.2-kd 29 amino acid polypeptides,[376, 377] which condense in the β-sheet conformation typical of all amyloid proteins. Several different isoforms of the protein are coded by alternative splicing of a complex gene[378] that localizes to 21q21.3-q22.11.[379] This gene appears to code for a 695 amino acid protease inhibitor, protease nexin-II[380]; the major protein subunit of cerebral amyloid is a cleavage product of this larger peptide.[380]

Although mutations in the amyloid gene account for early-onset Alzheimer's disease in some families,[381] the majority of such familial Alzheimer's disease cases are not associated with amyloid gene abnormalities.[382, 383]

Ubiquitin

Ubiquitin is a small (76 amino acid) protein that may be the most highly conserved protein in eukaryotes; the amino acid sequence is 95% conserved from yeast to humans (73 of 76 amino acids).[384] Ubiquitin functions in an extralysosomal protein degradation pathway,[384–386] which relies on conjugation of ubiquitin to proteolytic substrates as a signal for selective degradation of intracellular proteins. Apparently, binding of ubiquitin to the NH_2 groups of proteins signals the degradation pathway, whereas α-acetylation of cellular proteins blocks the ubiquitin-mediated degradation system.[387] Although ubiquitin is found in many tissues, it is valuable as an immunohistochemical target predominantly in the identification of neurofibrillary tangles, the demonstration of Lewy and Pick bodies, and the localization of Rosenthal fibers and axonal spheroids.

In humans, ubiquitin synthesis is directed by any of four different transcriptionally active genes; one of these genes *(UBC)* localizes to 12q24.3[134]; another *(UBB)* localizes to 17p11.1-17p12[388]; a third *(UBA52)* localizes to 19p13.1-p12.[389] Although the location of the fourth ubiquitin gene is not yet confirmed, chromosomal in situ hybridization results suggest that it may localize to chromosome 2q21.[134]

The conformation of ubiquitin has been studied by protein engineering and spectroscopic and crystallographic methods.[390–393] Although the protein engineering results suggest that ubiquitin must be conformationally mobile to trigger proteolysis,[390] crystallographic and nuclear magnetic resonance spectroscopic results demonstrate ubiquitin to be highly compact and tightly bonded to hydrogen; approximately 87% of the polypeptide chain is involved in a hydrogen-bonded secondary structure, which includes three and one-half turns of α helix, a short piece of 3(10) helix, a mixed five-strand β sheet, and seven reverse turns.[391–393]

Tau Protein

Tau proteins are microtubule-associated proteins (50 to 70 kd) that serve as immunohistochemical markers of Alzheimer's disease plaques but also may occasionally be observed in glial tumors. Although a single gene, localized to chromosome 17q21,[394] codes all tau proteins, alternative splicing with differential expression gives rise to both high- and low-molecular-weight forms,[395] which are expressed in brain but not other human tissues.[394]

Structural analysis shows that tau proteins are 2-nm diameter triple-stranded left-helical structures composed of three 1-nm strands. Each trimer is joined with other trimers to form long tau polymers.[396]

Tau protein plays a role in the extension and maintenance of neuronal processes through a direct association with microtubules.[397] The affinity of tau protein for microtubules is concentrated in a large region of the carboxyl terminus that contains 18 amino acid repeat sequences separated by flexible sequences of 13 to 14 amino acids.[397, 398]

Although the mechanism of tau action is unknown, it appears that both the initiation and the continued outgrowth of neurites are dependent on tau.[399] In Alzheimer's disease, the tau protein appears to be excessively phosphorylated[400]; phosphorylation may be mediated by a double-stranded DNA-stimulated protein kinase.[400, 401] There is evidence that proteins that phosphorylate tau are important in β-amyloid–mediated neuronal cell death.[402]

CELLULAR ADHESION MOLECULES

Integrins

The integrins are cell adhesion molecules that are involved in the interaction between cells and the extracellular matrix. Because cell-matrix interactions are believed to be important in tumor metastasis, immunohistochemical assessment of integrins has been investigated as a prognostic marker in cancer. In several tumors, including malignant melanoma,[403] renal cell carcinoma,[404] and others,[405] altered patterns of integrin expression have been correlated with tumor progression. In addition, integrin expression is of intense interest in understanding the basement membrane changes associated with renal glomerular disease.[406]

The integrins are a family of membrane glycoproteins that serve as cell-cell adhesion molecules and receptors for extracellular matrix. As such, they play important roles in inflammation, wound healing, tumor metastasis, and tissue migration during embryogenesis.[8] All integrins consist of two noncovalently linked peptides: α (120 to 180 kd) and β (90 to 110 kd). There are at least 14 different α and 8 different β subunits, and individual α subunits may associate with several different β subunits. The β subunits are highly conserved, showing 48 to 56 conserved cysteine residues arranged in four repeating units. The α subunits show less sequence homology but contain seven repeating domains. Both the α and β subunit span the membrane; the extracellular portion of the α subunit contains three magnesium-binding domain sites. Collectively, the integrins bind a wide variety of extracellular matrix proteins, including collagen, laminin, fibronectin, and fibrinogen, as well as the intercellular adhesion molecules; most integrins bind a specific sequence motif, Arg-Gly-Asp (the RGD sequence), on the extracellular or adhesion protein. Ligand binding requires both subunits and is cation dependent.

Deficiencies in one group of integrin proteins, CD18/CD11A, CD18/CD11B, and CD18/CD11C, all of which contain the β_2 subunit (ITGB2) of the leukocyte cell adhesion molecule, result in an autosomal recessive disorder of neutrophil function—leukocyte adhesion deficiency—characterized by recurrent bacterial infections. CD18 is coded by a 40-kb gene on chromosome 21q22.3[407, 408] and has been sequenced.[409]

Several of the integrins serve as laminin receptors. Integrin $\alpha_6\beta_4$ localizes to the basal surface of epithelial cells and is thought to be important in wound healing and metastasis. The α_6 gene is localized to chromosome 2, and β_4 is localized to chromosome 17q11-ter.[410] Both the α and β chains appear in various sizes, possibly as a result of post-translational cleavage.[8] Integrin $\alpha_7\beta_1$ is expressed in malignant melanoma and in muscle.

The secondary structure of the integrins has not been established experimentally, although inferences may be made from the nucleic acid sequence. Chemical studies demonstrate that binding of integrin receptor RGD sequences appears to be related both to the secondary structure of the matrix protein and to that of the integrin.[411–413]

Intercellular Adhesion Molecule-1

Immunohistochemical assessment of intercellular adhesion molecules, such as intracellular adhesion molecule-1 (ICAM-1, CD54), has been suggested as a prognostic marker in malignant disease.[414]

ICAM-1 is a member of the immunoglobulin superfamily and appears to be important in mediating inflammatory responses, particularly those that depend on cellular migration.[415] It is also the major receptor for rhinovirus.[416] ICAM-1 maps to chromosome 19p13.2[417]; the gene has been sequenced and is highly homologous to the neural cell adhesion molecule (NCAM).[418] Although fragments of the ICAM-1 molecule have been crystallized, the structures have not been determined to sufficient detail to allow determination of secondary structure.[419] ICAM-1 demonstrates an extracellular region composed of five immunoglobulin-like domains. It has a bent-rod shape, with the long arm (which contains all known ligand binding) positioned outward.[420]

ICAM-1 is expressed on monocytes, B and T lymphocytes, fibroblasts, and various epithelial cells.[8] It can be induced, or up-regulated, by several interferons and appears to mediate T-cell responses in several different ways.

Neural Cell Adhesion Molecule

Immunohistochemical assessment of the NCAM has been proposed as a prognostic marker in lung cancer; NCAM expression seems to reflect a poor prognosis.[421]

NCAM, another member of the immunoglobulin superfamily, is coded by a highly conserved gene at chromosome 11q23.1.[422] Although NCAMs are coded by a single gene, alternative splicing and post-translational modification give rise to NCAMs with molecular weights of 120, 140, and 180 kd.[8, 423] NCAM-140 and NCAM-180 are transmembrane proteins that differ in the size of their cytoplasmic domains; NCAM-120 is attached to the membrane by means of a glycosyl phosphatidylinositol link.

The NCAM appears on early embryonic cells and is thought to be important in the development of normal tissue architecture. In the adult it is found on neurons, astrocytes, Schwann cells, myoblasts, and NK lymphocytes, where it is assumed to mediate intercellular contact among neurons and between neurons and muscle.[424]

EXTRACELLULAR MATRIX PROTEINS

Collagen Type IV

Type IV collagen is found only in basement membranes, where it is the major structural protein. Each collagen molecule is composed of three α chains having molecular weights of 160 to 170 kd, each of which arises from one of six distinct genes.[6] The three-chain assembly contains a 350-nm triple-helical domain that includes about 20 interruptions that lend flexibility to the molecule. Extensive intermolecular disulfide bonding, together with noncovalent interactions, causes the molecules to self-assemble into a meshwork that interacts with other basement membrane components.[425]

Because of the multiple ways in which a type 4 collagen molecule can be assembled, there are many chemically distinct variants of type IV collagen. The most abundant form consists of two α_1 chains and a single α_2 chain. Complete sequences are available for collagen chains α_1, α_2, and α_5. The α_1 and α_2 genes, each of which is greater than 100 kb long, are transcribed from a common bidirectional promoter on chromosome 13q34. Similar head-to-head arrangements are found for the α_3 and α_4 genes, also found on chromosome 13q34, and for the α_5 and α_6 genes, found on chromosome Xq22.[6]

The secondary structure of collagen molecules has been investigated using a variety of spectroscopic techniques, theoretical analysis, and x-ray diffraction.[426–428] The triple-helical structure of the collagen molecule results from supercoiling of polyproline II.[426, 428] Each triple helix is extensively hydrated, with an extensive hydrogen bonding network between water molecules and peptide acceptor groups; the distribution of the water network is determined by the distribution of hydroxyproline residues.[426, 427]

The α_1 chain of type IV collagen contains integrin recognition sites.[429]

Laminin

Immunohistochemical assessment of laminin is used primarily as a tool to assess basement membrane integrity. The laminins are members of a large family of glycoproteins that are distributed throughout basement membranes. They appear to mediate both differentiation and cellular migration through their interactions with cell surface receptors and other basement membrane components. Each laminin is composed of one of two possible heavy chains (A or M) of molecular weight 30 to 40 kd, and two of three possible light chains (B1, B2, S). The three chains of the laminin heterotrimer are held together in an α-helical coiled-coil structure.[430] Each chain is coded by a separate gene.

The α-helical coiled-coil domain of the long arm is the only domain composed of multiple chains; cell attachment sites are found in the terminus of this arm. Additional cell attachment sites, demonstrating some homology to epidermal growth factor, are found in the short arms.[431]

The laminin A chain is encoded by a 9.5-kb gene localized to chromosome 18p11.3.[432, 433] This predicted amino acid sequence shows four globular regions, three cysteine-rich domains, and an α-helical region. The carboxyl-terminal globular domain contains five subdomains characterized by a conserved seven-amino acid (heptad) repeat within each subdomain.

The A chain is expressed in kidney, testis, and brain.[434] The laminin M chain is encoded by a 7-kb gene localized to chromosome 6q22-q23[434] and consists of 3088 amino acids preceded by a 22 residue signal peptide. M chain is expressed in many organs, including heart, pancreas, lung, spleen, kidney, adrenal gland, skin, testis, and brain, but not in liver, thymus, or bone.

The laminin B1 gene maps to chromosome 7q31-q32 and encodes a 21 amino acid signal sequence followed by a 1765 amino acid B1 chain.[435] The laminin B2 gene maps to chromosome 1q25-q31.[436] The B2 gene encodes a polypeptide containing a 33 residue signal peptide and a 1576 B2 chain. The B1 chain and the B2 chain are highly homologous and consist of distinct domains that contain helical structures, cysteine-rich repeats, and globular regions.[437, 438]

Study of laminin secondary structure is complicated by the complexity of the laminin assembly. Data suggest that the rod of the long arm of laminin contains several distinct α-helical segments; segments lacking α helix are also present.[439] The long arm also serves as the site for laminin/collagen IV interaction.[440] Formation of heterotrimers seems to depend on the presence of a heptad sequence repeat within the carboxyl-terminal α-helical region of the laminin long arm, resulting in interchain hydrophobic and charge-charge interactions.[441, 442] The heterotrimeric configuration appears to be essential to the adhesive function.[443]

Fibronectin

Fibronectin is a glycoprotein found in the extracellular matrix and in plasma; it serves as an adhesion protein and mediates cell-matrix interactions. Fibronectin is coded for by a single gene that is located on chromosome 2, either at 2p14-16 or 2q34-36.[6, 444] Nonidentical subunits, created by alternative splicing,[6, 445] are linked through disulfide bonds near the carboxyl terminus.[6]

Circular dichroism spectra of human plasma fibronectin suggest that the molecule contains approximately 79% β-sheet and 21% β-turn structures. These structures are arranged in a tandem array of seven-strand β sandwiches,[446, 447] from which the molecule obtains elastic properties. The "type III" domains may exist in either folded or stretched forms; the latter is sevenfold longer than the former.[446, 447] They may also mediate cell adhesion.[447]

MUSCLE PROTEINS

Identification of muscle differentiation is aided by immunohistochemical assessment of intermediate filaments (particularly desmin), together with proteins that are expressed exclusively or primarily in muscle. Although desmin has been in use for the longest period, it is less often identified than are the various isoforms of actin. For this reason, it is seldom employed alone. Myoglobin, although less often useful than desmin or actin, provides a third, often utilized, immunohistochemical target for determining muscle differentiation.

Myoglobin

Myoglobin is a 152 residue protein coded by a 10.5 kb gene that localizes to chromosome 22q11-q13.[448, 449] Myoglobin serves as an oxygen transport protein in muscle. Immunohistochemical demonstration of myoglobin is thus useful in the recognition of muscle differentiation.

Human myoglobin has been crystallized, and its structure has been determined both spectroscopically[450] and by x-ray diffraction.[451] Myoglobin consists of a single subunit protein, which holds a heme (oxygen-binding) group within a pocket near the protein surface. The protein portion of human myoglobin is predominantly (85%) α helix, together with 7% β sheet and 8% β turn.

Actin Proteins

Immunohistochemical staining for actin is used for the identification of muscle cells and for distinguishing smooth muscle and myoepithelial cells from those of skeletal and cardiac muscle. These distinctions are facilitated by the availability of reagents reacting relatively specifically with the smooth muscle isotype of actin or with both skeletal and smooth muscle isotypes.

Actins are microfilamentous proteins that participate in muscle contraction and in cellular locomotion. As such, they are ubiquitous proteins that are found in cells of many different histologic derivations. The six known actin proteins may be divided into two broad classes (muscle and cytoplasmic), which are coded by different genes.[452] The four muscle actins are in turn divided into α-skeletal and α-cardiac actins and into α and γ smooth muscle actins.[453] These actins are coded by between 6 and 20 different genes.[454]

Cardiac and skeletal muscle actin genes are coexpressed in both striated muscle types.[455, 456] The cardiac muscle actin[457] is coded by a gene localized to chromosome 15q11-ter, whereas a gene for skeletal muscle actin localizes to 1q42.1-42.3.[458] The γ smooth muscle actin is coded by a 27-kb gene localized to chromosome 2.[459]

The cytoskeletal actins are referred to as β and γ. The actin cytoskeletal β gene maps to 7p12-15,[460] whereas that for γ maps to 17p11-qter.[461] The β and γ cytoplasmic actins differ by only four amino acids at the amino terminus[461] and are coexpressed. The cytoplasmic actins self-assemble into linear polymers (microfilaments) that assist in cell mobility and organelle transport. Identification of these actins currently has no use in pathologic diagnosis, but cross-reactivity between supposedly "muscle specific" anti-actin antibodies with these nonmuscle actins may be observed with some reagents.

Actin exists intracellularly in two conformations—a monomeric globular form and the filamentous polymeric form. Actin monomers take on a conformation that is approximately 45% α helix and 27% β form.[462] It assembles into helical microfilament polymers, which interact with similar polymers of tropomyosin.[463] When viewed in an electron microscope, actin filaments display transverse bands whose 5.5-nm repeat and 15-degree pitch are consistent with the helical conformation.[464] Contraction depends on interaction of two actin filaments with protuberances (cross-bridges) from a myosin filament.[465] Each tropomyosin molecule winds along the filament in contact with seven consecutive actin monomers on the same strand of the two-stranded actin helix.[466]

STEROID RECEPTORS

Assessment of steroid receptors may be useful in predicting tumor prognosis. More importantly, however, identification of receptor expression allows an improved prediction of the response to hormonal manipulation in patients with breast and prostate cancer.

Estrogen Receptor

Immunohistochemical determination of estrogen receptor (ER) protein is used to predict prognosis and response to hormonal therapy in adenocarcinoma of the breast. The presence of estrogen receptor (Fig. 2–15) is associated with better overall survival[467]; about half of ER-positive patients respond to various hormonal manipulation.

ER, like the other steroid receptors, is a ligand-activated DNA-binding transcription factor. It is coded by a highly conserved 140-kb gene[468] that maps to 6q25.1.[469] A 66 amino acid segment of the DNA-binding domain determines the specificity of target gene recognition. A cDNA for ER has been sequenced.[470] Sequence analysis reveals that ER is a 595 amino acid protein.

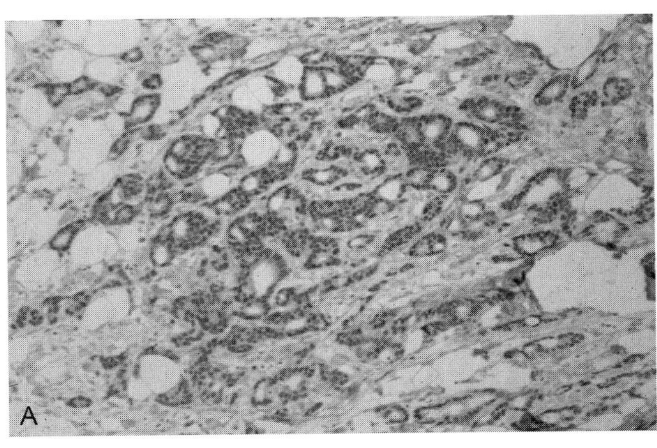

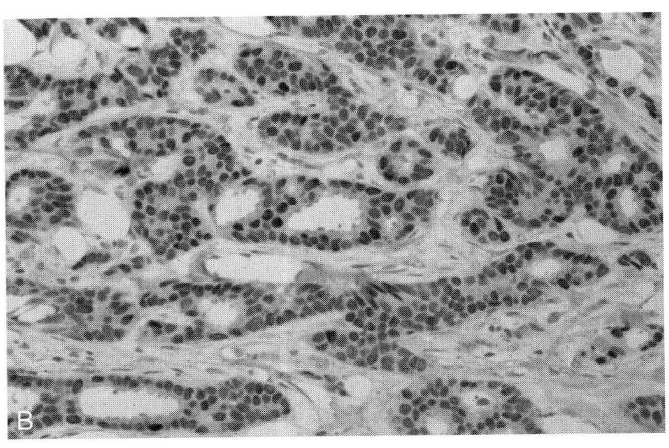

FIGURE 2–15
Section of tubular carcinoma of breast immunohistochemically stained for estrogen receptor protein, ×100 (*A*) and ×200 (*B*). (See also Color Fig. 2–15.)

ER acts by binding to an intranuclear receptor molecule that associates weakly with nuclear components in the absence of ligand, but strongly when steroid is bound. The secondary structure of the ER DNA binding domain, which is highly conserved among the steroid-binding proteins, includes two α helices in a structure similar to that seen in a variety of other nuclear hormone receptors.[471] These perpendicular α helices contain two zinc-binding sequence motifs, which loosely resemble "zinc-finger" DNA binding motifs.[472] On binding estradiol, ER undergoes a dramatic decrease in surface hydrophobicity; this conformational change is localized in the steroid binding domain[473] and is apparently required for ER to bind to DNA and activate transcription.[474] The changes in conformational alterations induced by estrogens are different than those induced by antiestrogens, such as tamoxifen.[475, 476] ER binds as a symmetrical dimer to a palindromic DNA binding site consisting of two 6-bp consensus half sites with three intervening base pairs; all steroid receptors recognize one or the other of these two consensus half-site sequences.[477] Binding of antiestrogens to the ER may disrupt dimer formation.[478] DNA binding further allosterically modulates the structure of the steroid binding domain of the ER[479]; this may be important for ER-binding to cause transcriptional activation of the target genes.

Estrogen receptor protein is localized immunohistochemically to the nucleus. Although it is somewhat useful in the identification of gynecologic neoplasms, thyroid and soft tissue tumors both occasionally show immunohistochemical reactions (Table 2–42).

TABLE 2–42

Immunoreactivity of Selected Neoplasms for Estrogen Receptor Protein

Diagnosis	Percentage of Cases Demonstrating Immunoreactivity
Adenocarcinoma, breast (primary)	61–73
Adenocarcinoma, breast (metastatic)	23–53
Adenocarcinoma, colon (primary)	0
Adenocarcinoma, colon (metastatic)	0–31
Adenocarcinoma, endocervix	12–39
Adenocarcinoma, endometrium	45–71
Adenocarcinoma, lung	0–3
Adenocarcinoma, pancreas	0
Adenocarcinoma, stomach	0
Cystadenocarcinoma, ovary	27–63
Hepatocellular carcinoma	0
Papillary carcinoma, thyroid	8–33
Poorly differentiated carcinoma, thyroid	28–65
Smooth muscle tumor, uncertain malignant potential	56–97

Progesterone Receptor

Immunohistochemical assessment of progesterone receptor (PR) protein (Table 2–43) is used as a prognostic indicator for adenocarcinoma of the breast; tumors positive for progesterone receptor (PR) have a better prognosis than those that are negative for the protein. Binding of monoclonal antibodies may depend on the conformational state of the PR[480]; whether this finding has significance for immunohistochemical assessments of PR is unknown.

PR is coded for by a gene that localizes to chromosome 11q22.1-q22.3.[481, 482] The amino acid sequence has been deduced from a cloned cDNA.[483] PR recognizes an imperfect palindrome, with the conserved half-sequence TGTYCY, whereas ER recognizes a palindrome with the half-sequence TGACC.[484] DNA recognition results from a PR structure that is similar to that of the estrogen receptor, and the conformational transitions occurring with steroid binding are also similar.[485] Binding of antiprogestins, such as RU486, to PR causes changes in the DNA-binding domain that are distinct from those induced by progestins.[486] This may reduce the formation of dimers, which are required for optimal binding of PR to its DNA-binding site.[487]

Androgen Receptor

The androgen receptor (AR) is a 919 amino acid transcriptional regulatory protein that mediates androgen-induced male sexual development and function. A single receptor protein binds both testosterone and dihydrotestosterone. AR is coded by a 90-kb gene[488, 489] that localizes to Xq11-q12.[490] The complete coding sequence for the gene has been established.[489] There are

TABLE 2–43

Immunoreactivity of Selected Neoplasms for Progesterone Receptor Protein

Diagnosis	Percentage of Cases Demonstrating Immunoreactivity
Adenocarcinoma, breast	2–30
Adenocarcinoma, breast, metastatic	84–100
Adenocarcinoma, endocervix	18–37
Adenocarcinoma, endometrium	42–67
Adenocarcinoma, lung	58–91
Capillary hemangioma	0
Endometrial hyperplasia	87–100
Meningioma, NOS	54–100
Meningioma, secretory	100
Paget's disease, breast	0–12

NOS, not otherwise specified.

four major binding domains. A central cysteine-rich DNA-binding domain, coded by exons 2 and 3, is flanked by the NH_2 terminal region and a hinge region. This, in turn, is flanked by a steroid binding domain. The NH_2 domain contains sequences involved in transcriptional activation and inhibition; most antibodies bind to this large amino-terminal domain. The androgen receptor is expressed in testes and prostate, where both 10- and 7-kb mRNA transcripts are found.[489, 491] AR is susceptible to proteolytic cleavage that results in multiple forms that retain high-affinity androgen binding.[492]

The structure of AR is similar to that of ER and PR, as are the mechanisms of action. Binding of androgen causes conformational changes in the receptor; different conformational changes occur on binding of antiandrogens. These changes may affect proteolytic degradation of the AR.[493] The conformational changes that occur on binding of antiandrogens are different than those that occur in ER and PR on binding of their antagonists. In ER and PR, antagonist binding results in conformational changes in the steroid binding domain. In contrast, binding of antagonists to AR causes no change in the steroid binding domain but rather alters the carboxyl-terminal domain of the receptor.[493, 494]

Mutations that consist of an increase in size of a polymorphic tandem CAG repeat in the first exon of AR (triplet repeat expansion) give rise to the disease known as X-linked spinal and bulbar muscular atrophy.[495, 496] Deletion or mutation in the steroid-binding domain of the AR gene may give rise to an androgen insensitivity syndrome.[497, 498] Mutations in the androgen receptor are also seen frequently in advanced prostate carcinoma.[499]

PROGNOSTIC MARKERS

A variety of different immunohistochemical assays have been proposed as indicators of prognosis for various tumors. Although none of these markers is universally accepted as having clinically useful prognostic value, they nonetheless have generated considerable interest in the medical literature.

Information on some of the more frequently cited immunohistochemical prognostic markers follows.

Epidermal Growth Factor Receptor

Immunohistochemical analysis of the epidermal growth factor receptor (EGFR) may be useful in predicting breast cancer prognosis. The gene for EGFR is approximately 110 kb[500] and localizes to chromosome 7; the precise site is uncertain.[501–503] The EGFR is a tyrosine protein kinase demonstrating three distinct domains: an extracellular EGF binding domain, a transmembrane domain, and a cytoplasmic domain. The intracellular domain contains the tyrosine kinase function (approximately 290 amino acids), as well as a COOH-terminal regulatory domain (approximately 230 amino acids) containing five phosphorylation sites.[504] The secondary structure has not been completely determined, but it is apparent that the dephosphorylated form of EGFR is more compact, suggesting that conformational changes may be involved in the mechanism of EGFR action.

ERBB2

Overexpression of the *ERBB2* oncogene *(HER2/neu)*, as assessed immunohistochemically, is a putative prognostic factor in cancers of the breast, ovaries, and other sites.[505] It may also prove useful in predicting response to treatment with cyclophosphamide, doxorubicin, and fluorouracil[506] and may be used to predict response to treatment with the monoclonal antibody Herceptin.[507, 508] Care must be taken, however, because various assays used to determine *ERBB2* gene overexpression do not always give equivalent results, either qualitatively or quantitatively.

ERBB2 encodes a tumor antigen that is similar to EGFR.[509] The gene maps to 17q12-q22[510]; the gene product is a 185-kd glycoprotein with tyrosine kinase activity.[511] Overexpression allows this gene, which is a normal growth factor, to behave as an oncogene.[512]

Few structural details are available for the ERBB2 protein. The protein can form both homodimers and heterodimers with related tyrosine kinases, such as EGFR[513]; such dimerization is apparently required for enzyme activity. A 45-kd protein that induces phosphorylation of ERBB2 has been identified and may be the natural ligand.[514]

p53

The *TP53* gene is altered in a wide variety of human cancers; immunohistochemical demonstration of the p53 tumor protein may be useful in predicting prognosis of several types of tumors. Immunohistochemical detection of p53 appears to reflect, in most cases, accumulation associated with binding of heat-shock proteins to mutant p53 molecules. Different antibody preparations demonstrate significantly different staining within the same tissue sections, complicating both interpretation of staining patterns as well as of the literature relating p53 staining to tumor prognosis.

TP53 is located at 17p13.105-p12[515]; the open reading frame is 393 amino acids long and contains a central DNA-binding domain, a carboxyl-terminal oligomerization domain, and an amino-terminal transcription activation domain.[516] *TP53* has at least two promoters: one is found 100 to 250 bp upstream of exon 1, and the second is within the first intron.[517]

The p53 molecule consists of a large β sandwich composed of two antiparallel β sheets containing 4 and 5 β strands, respectively, that act as scaffolding for three loops: the first loop binds to DNA within the major groove, the second loop binds to DNA within the minor groove, and the third loop stabilizes the second (Fig. 2–16).[518] Most cancer-related mutations are found near the protein/DNA interface in one of the DNA loops.[516]

The p53 protein appears to play a critical role in cell cycle regulation. p53 synthesis increases after mitogen stimulation. Induction of apoptosis by DNA damage depends on p53 function; p53 does not appear to directly activate apoptosis but either represses genes necessary for cell survival or assists in DNA repair. Normal p53 induces a gene, *WAF1 (CIP1)*,[519] whose product binds to cyclin complexes and inhibits the function of cyclin-dependent kinases.[520] The following picture emerges: DNA damage stimulates p53 expression. In turn, p53 binds to *WAF1* regulatory elements, activating synthesis of WAF1 protein. WAF1 protein prevents phosphorylation of cyclin-dependent kinase substrates, interrupting the cell cycle. Mutational inactivation of *TP53* would inactivate this pathway, permitting unregulated cycling.[519]

Alteration of the *TP53* gene is strongly associated with cancer[521] and appears to be responsible for the most common genetic mutations in cancer. Almost 98% of *TP53* mutations are found in exons 5 through 8, and there are at least three "hot spots"—residues 175, 248, and 273. In addition to mutational inactivation, it appears that p53 function can be altered by the presence of papillomavirus E6 protein. This may represent a pathway for the development of cervical cancer. Altogether, there are at least four possible mechanisms for p53 inactivation[516]: (1) deletion of one or both *TP53* alleles reduces expression of the growth inhibitory genes, (2) nonsense or splice site mutations may result in truncation of the protein, (3) missense mutations may result in conformationally altered p53 protein, and (4) expression of the human papillomavirus E6 gene, or overexpression of the *MDM2* gene, causes inactivation of p53 through binding and degradation.

Alterations of the *TP53* gene can occur as germline mutations in some cancer-prone families and gives rise to the Li-Fraumeni syndrome.[522–524]

Proliferation-Related Ki-67 Antigen

Ki-67 is a monoclonal antibody that reacts with a nuclear antigen expressed in proliferating cells; it appears to be useful in predicting prognosis of some tumors. Ki-67 expression occurs during late G_1, S, G_2, and M phases of the cell cycle; the antigen cannot be detected in G_0 phase cells[525]. The *MKI67* gene maps

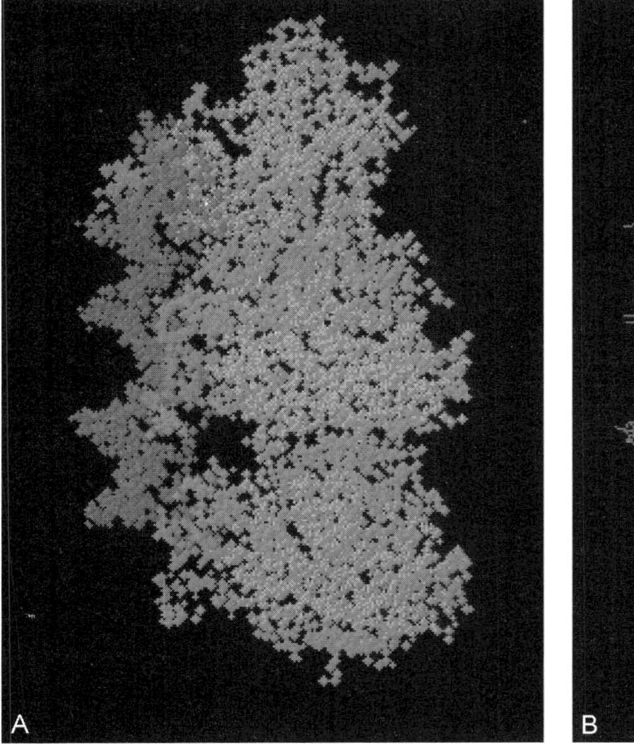

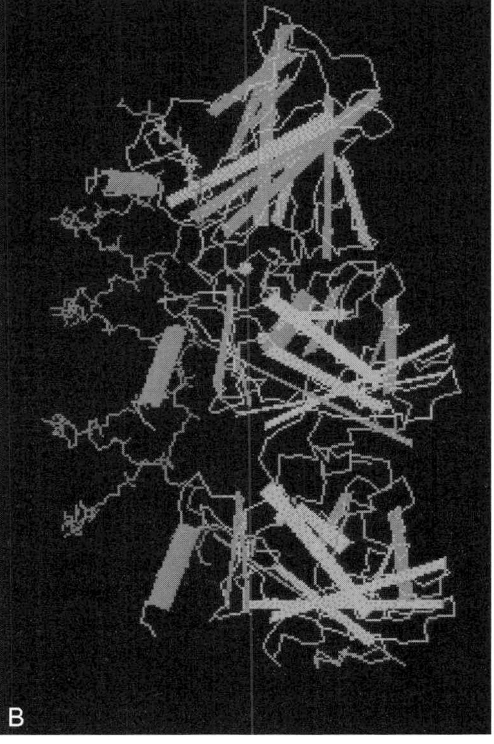

FIGURE 2–16
Space-filling (*A*) and secondary structure (*B*) models showing p53 bound to DNA. The models were generated using Cn3D and Brookhaven Protein Structure Data Base data. (See also Color Fig. 2–16.)

to 10q25-qter. Neither the sequence of the gene encoding Ki-67 nor the structure of the protein has been determined.

Proliferating Cell Nuclear Antigen

Proliferating cell nuclear antigen (PCNA, cyclin) has been utilized as an immunohistochemical prognostic marker in a variety of tissues. Several different commercial monoclonal antibodies are available; their reactivities differ somewhat as to the fixation conditions appropriate for optimal use.

PCNA is a 36-kd nuclear protein that is encoded by a gene localized to chromosome 20p12-13.[526] PCNA plays a key role in the initiation of cellular DNA synthesis and regulation of cell cycle progression.[527] The protein functions in replication as a processivity factor for DNA polymerase.[528] Gene expression is induced by a variety of stimuli, including platelet-derived growth factor and epidermal growth factor.[529] Synthesis of PCNA occurs predominantly in S phase; the synthesis rate appears to correlate well with proliferation in normal cultured cells and tissues but is less well correlated in neoplastic tissue.

BCL2

BCL2 is an oncogene that maps to chromosome 18q21 and encodes a 26-kd protein.[530, 531] Overexpression of *BCL2* blocks apoptotic cell death[532]; overexpression resulting from translocation of the *BCL2* gene to the immunoglobulin heavy-chain locus t(14;18) appears to be important in the pathogenesis of follicular lymphoma.[533] Immunohistochemical demonstration of BCL2 protein in the lymph node mantle zone is characteristic of normal and hyperplastic nodes, whereas expression in the germinal center is typical of follicular lymphoma.

Because of its role in blocking cell death, immunohistochemical assessment of *BCL2* expression has been suggested as a tumor prognostic marker. Most studies have not demonstrated independent prognostic utility, however.[534, 535]

The secondary structure of BCL2 has not been determined. It appears that *BCL2* can integrate into the cytoplasmic face of membranes and serves as an integral membrane protein.[536] The carboxyl-terminal hydrophobic region is essential for membrane integration.[532]

NM23

In 1988, Steeg and associates described a gene, NME1, that, when expressed at high levels, inhibited the metastatic potential of tumor cells.[537] The protein, which exhibits a nucleoside diphosphate (NDP) kinase activity,[538] consists of two chains, NM23-H1 and NM23-H2, the genes for which, *NME1* and *NME2*, have been mapped to chromosome 17q21.3-22.[539, 540] Allelic deletion of this region is associated with metastasis and shortened survival in colon carcinoma[539, 541]; decreased gene expression is associated with invasion in several types of cancer.[538, 542–545]

Although the structure of the NM23 gene products has not been determined, that of a related NDP kinase from *Dictyostelium discoideum* has been determined by x-ray diffraction. The enzyme is made of six identical subunits with a mononucleotide-binding fold. Each subunit contains an α/β domain with a four-stranded, antiparallel β sheet[546]; the structure of the *NME1* and *NME2* gene products are thought to be similar on the basis of sequence similarities.

Cathepsin D

Cathepsin D has been proposed as an immunohistochemical marker of prognosis in breast cancer. The studies that have appeared in the literature have yielded inconsistent results as to its clinical utility. Cathepsin D is a lysosomal proteinase that is coded by a gene localized at 11p15.[547] Cathepsin D is a 412 amino acid polypeptide that is synthesized as a pre-procathepsin having 476 amino acids. The final enzyme results from sequential cleavage of 20 and 44 amino acid units.[548] As an aspartic proteinase, cathepsin D falls in the same family as pepsin and chymosin; it shares with other members of this family the same catalytic apparatus and the ability to function in acid solutions.[549] It appears that the gene is estrogen inducible.[550]

Cathepsin D occurs either as a single 44-kd polypeptide chain or as a noncovalent complex consisting of a 14-kd peptide and a 30-kd peptide derived by cleavage of the 44-kd peptide.[551] The structure of cathepsin D and of a cathepsin-pepstatin complex have been determined by x-ray diffraction.[552] Cathepsin D is bilobed and contains one asparagine-linked oligosaccharide, as well as UDP-GlcNAc:lysosomal enzyme *N*-acetylglucosamine-1-phosphotransferase binding domains on each lobe.[553]

REFERENCES

1. Elias JM: Immunohistopathology: A Practical Approach to Diagnosis. Chicago, American Society of Clinical Pathology, 1990.
2. Taylor CR, Cote RJ: Immunomicroscopy: A Diagnostic Tool for the Surgical Pathologist, ed 2. Philadelphia, WB Saunders, 1994.
3. Colvin RB, Bhan AK, McClusky RT: Diagnostic Immunopathology, ed 2. New York, Raven Press, 1994.
4. Marchler-Bauer A, Addess KJ, Chappey C, et al: MMDB: Entrez's 3D structure database [In Process Citation]. Nucleic Acids Res 1999;27:240–243.
5. Hogue CW: Cn3D: A new generation of three-dimensional molecular structure viewer. Trends Biochem Sci 1997;22:314–316.

6. Ayad S, Boot-Handford RP, Humphries MJ, et al: The Extracellular Matrix FactsBook. San Diego, CA, Academic, 1994.
7. Barclay AN, Birkeland ML, Brown MH, et al: The Leukocyte Antigen FactsBook. San Diego, CA, Academic, 1993.
8. Pigott R, Power C: The Adhesion Molecule FactsBook. San Diego, CA, Academic, 1993.
9. Fuchs EV, Coppock SM, Green H, Cleveland DW: Two distinct classes of keratin genes and their evolutionary significance. Cell 1981;27(1 Pt 2):75–84.
10. Moll R, Franke WW, Schiller DL, et al: The catalog of human cytokeratins: Patterns of expression in normal epithelia, tumors and cultured cells. Cell 1982;31:11–24.
11. Lessin SR, Huebner K, Isobe M, et al: Chromosomal mapping of human keratin genes: Evidence of non-linkage. J Invest Dermatol 1988;91:572–578.
12. Rothnagel JA, Dominey AM, Dempsey LD, et al: Mutations in the rod domains of keratins 1 and 10 in epidermolytic hyperkeratosis. Science 1992;257:1128–1130.
13. Collin C, Moll R, Kubicka S, et al: Characterization of human cytokeratin 2, an epidermal cytoskeletal protein synthesized late during differentiation. Exp Cell Res 1992;202:132–141.
14. McLean WH, Morley SM, Lane EB, et al: Ichthyosis bullosa of Siemens—a disease involving keratin 2e. J Invest Dermatol 1994;103:277–281.
15. Schermer A, Galvin S, Sun TT: Differentiation-related expression of a major 64K corneal keratin in vivo and in culture suggests limbal location of corneal epithelial stem cells. J Cell Biol 1986;103:49–62.
16. Raimondi E, Moralli D, De Carli L, et al: Assignment of the human cytokeratin 3 gene *(KRT3)* to 12q12→q13 by FISH. Cytogenet Cell Genet 1994;66:162–163.
17. Barletta C, Batticane N, Ragusa RM, et al: Subchromosomal localization of two human cytokeratin genes (*KRT4* and *KRT15*) by in situ hybridization. Cytogenet Cell Genet 1990;54:148–150.
18. Lersch R, Fuchs E: Sequence and expression of a type II keratin, K5, in human epidermal cells. Mol Cell Biol 1988;8:486–493.
19. Bonifas JM, Bare JW, Lynch ED, et al: Regional assignment of the human keratin 5 *(KRT5)* gene to chromosome 12q near D12S14 by PCR analysis of somatic cell hybrids and multicolor in situ hybridization. Genomics 1992;13:452–454.
20. Lane EB, Rugg EL, Navsaria H, et al: A mutation in the conserved helix termination peptide of keratin 5 in hereditary skin blistering. Nature 1992;356:244–246.
21. Dong W, Ryynanen M, Uitto J: Identification of a leucine-to-proline mutation in the keratin 5 gene in a family with the generalized Kobner type of epidermolysis bullosa simplex. Hum Mutat 1993;2:94–102.
22. Rosenberg M, Fuchs E, Le Beau MM, et al: Three epidermal and one simple epithelial type II keratin genes map to human chromosome 12. Cytogenet Cell Genet 1991;57: 33–38.
23. Waseem A, Alexander CM, Steel JB, Lane EB: Embryonic simple epithelial keratins 8 and 18: Chromosomal location emphasizes difference from other keratin pairs. New Biol 1990;2:464–478.
24. Darmon MY, Semat A, Darmon MC, Vasseur M: Sequence of a cDNA encoding human keratin No 10 selected according to structural homologies of keratins and their tissue-specific expression. Mol Biol Rep. 1987;12:277–283.
25. Zhou XM, Idler WW, Steven AC, et al: The complete sequence of the human intermediate filament chain keratin 10: Subdomainal divisions and model for folding of end domain sequences. J Biol Chem 1988;263: 15584–15589.
26. Cheng J, Syder AJ, Yu QC, et al: The genetic basis of epidermolytic hyperkeratosis: A disorder of differentiation-specific epidermal keratin genes. Cell 1992;70: 811–819.
27. Chipev CC, Yang JM, DiGiovanna JJ, et al: Preferential sites in keratin 10 that are mutated in epidermolytic hyperkeratosis. Am J Hum Genet 1994;54:179–190.
28. Coulombe PA, Hutton ME, Letai A, et al: Point mutations in human keratin 14 genes of epidermolysis bullosa simplex patients: Genetic and functional analyses. Cell 1991;66:1301–1311.
29. Troyanovsky SM, Leube RE, Franke WW: Characterization of the human gene encoding cytokeratin 17 and its expression pattern. Eur J Cell Biol 1992;59:127–137.
30. Kulesh DA, Oshima RG: Complete structure of the gene for human keratin 18. Genomics 1989;4:339–347.
31. Heath P, Elvin P, Jenner D, et al: Localisation of a cDNA clone for human cytokeratin 18 to chromosome 17p11–p12 by in situ hybridisation. Hum Genet 1990; 85:669–670.
32. Bader BL, Magin TM, Hatzfeld M, Franke WW: Amino acid sequence and gene organization of cytokeratin no. 19, an exceptional tail-less intermediate filament protein. EMBO J 1986;5:1865–1875.
33. Stasiak PC, Lane EB: Sequence of cDNA coding for human keratin 19. Nucleic Acids Res 1987;15:10058.
34. Bader BL, Jahn L, Franke WW: Low level expression of cytokeratins 8, 18 and 19 in vascular smooth muscle cells of human umbilical cord and in cultured cells derived therefrom, with an analysis of the chromosomal locus containing the cytokeratin 19 gene. Eur J Cell Biol 1988;47:300–319.
35. Eng LF, Gerstl B, Vanderhaeghen JJ: A study of proteins in old multiple sclerosis plaques. Trans Am Soc Neurochem 1970;1:42.
36. Eng LF, Shiubra LA, Marangos PJ, et al (eds): Glial fibrillary acidic protein: A review of structure, function and clinical application. *In* Neuron and Glial Proteins: Structure, Function and Clinical Application. San Diego, CA, Academic, 1988.
37. Bongcam-Rudloff E, Nister M, Betsholtz C, et al: Human glial fibrillary acidic protein: Complementary DNA cloning, chromosome localization, and messenger RNA expression in human glioma cell lines of various phenotypes. Cancer Res 1991;51:1553–1560.
38. Brownell E, Lee AS, Pekar SK, et al: Glial fibrillary acid protein, an astrocytic-specific marker, maps to human chromosome 17. Genomics 1991;10:1087–1089.
39. Reeves SA, Helman LJ, Allison A, Israel MA: Molecular cloning and primary structure of human glial fibrillary acidic protein. Proc Natl Acad Sci USA 1989;86: 5178–5182.
40. Huston JS, Bignami A: Structural properties of the glial fibrillary acidic protein: Evidence for intermolecular disulfide bonds. Biochim Biophys Acta 1977;493:93–103.

41. Levy E, Liem RK, D'Eustachio P, Cowan NJ: Structure and evolutionary origin of the gene encoding mouse NF-M, the middle-molecular-mass neurofilament protein. Eur J Biochem 1987;166:71–77.
42. Lees JF, Shneidman PS, Skuntz SF, et al: The structure and organization of the human heavy neurofilament subunit (NF-H) and the gene encoding it. EMBO J 1988;7: 1947–1955.
43. Hurst J, Flavell D, Julien JP, et al: The human neurofilament gene *(NEFL)* is located on the short arm of chromosome 8. Cytogenet Cell Genet 1987;45:30–32.
44. Somerville MJ, McLachlan DR, Percy ME: Localization of the 68,000-Da human neurofilament gene *(NF68)* using a murine cDNA probe. Genome 1988;30: 499–500.
45. Julien JP, Grosveld F, Yazdanbaksh K, et al: The structure of a human neurofilament gene *(NF-L):* A unique exon-intron organization in the intermediate filament gene family. Biochim Biophys Acta 1987;909:10–20.
46. Mattei MG, Dautigny A, Pham-Dinh D, et al: The gene encoding the large human neurofilament subunit *(NF-H)* maps to the q121–q131 region on human chromosome 22. Hum Genet 1988;80:293–295.
47. Rouleau GA, Merel P, Lutchman M, et al: Alteration in a new gene encoding a putative membrane-organizing protein causes neuro-fibromatosis type 2 [see comments]. Nature 1993;363:515–521.
48. Clark EA, Lee VM: Dynamics of mammalian high-molecular-weight neurofilament subunit phosphorylation in cultured rat sympathetic neurons. J Neurosci Res 1991;30:116–123.
49. Hollosi M, Urge L, Perczel A, et al: Metal ion-induced conformational changes of phosphorylated fragments of human neurofilament (NF-M) protein. J Mol Biol 1992; 223:673–682.
50. Hollosi M, Shen ZM, Perczel A, Fasman GD: Stable intrachain and interchain complexes of neurofilament peptides: A putative link between Al3+ and Alzheimer disease. Proc Natl Acad Sci USA 1994;91:4902–4906.
51. Eagles PAM, Pant HC, Ganier H, et al (eds): Neurofilaments. *In* Cellular and Molecular Biology of Intermediate Filaments. New York, Plenum, 1990, pp 37–94.
52. Stromer MH, Bendayan M: Arrangement of desmin intermediate filaments in smooth muscle cells as shown by high-resolution immunocytochemistry. Cell Motil Cytoskeleton 1988;11:117–125.
53. Stromer MH, Bendayan M: Immunocytochemical identification of cytoskeletal linkages to smooth muscle cell nuclei and mitochondria. Cell Motil Cytoskeleton 1990;17:11–18.
54. Viegas-Pequignot E, Li ZL, Dutrillaux B, et al: Assignment of human desmin gene to band 2q35 by nonradioactive in situ hybridization. Hum Genet 1989;83: 33–36.
55. Edstrom L, Thornell LE, Eriksson A: A new type of hereditary distal myopathy with characteristic sarcoplasmic bodies and intermediate (skeletin) filaments. J Neurol Sci 1980;47:171–190.
56. Porte A, Stoeckel ME, Sacrez A, Batzenschlager A: Unusual familial cardiomyopathy with storage of intermediate filaments in the cardiac muscular cells. Virchows Arch [Pathol Anat] 1980;386:43–58.
57. Vajsar J, Becker LE, Freedom RM, Murphy EG: Familial desminopathy: Myopathy with accumulation of desmin-type intermediate filaments. J Neurol Neurosurg Psychiatry 1993;56:644–648.
58. Huiatt TW, Robson RM, Arakawa N, Stromer MH: Desmin from avian smooth muscle: Purification and partial characterization. J Biol Chem 1980;255:6981–6989.
59. Geisler N, Weber K: The amino acid sequence of chicken muscle desmin provides a common structural model for intermediate filament proteins. EMBO J 1982;1:1649–1656.
60. Quax W, Meera KP, Quax-Jeuken Y, Bloemendal H: The human desmin and vimentin genes are located on different chromosomes. Gene 1985;38:189–196.
61. Ferrari S, Cannizzaro LA, Battini R, et al: The gene encoding human vimentin is located on the short arm of chromosome 10. Am J Hum Genet 1987;41:616–626.
62. Perreau J, Lilienbaum A, Vasseur M, Paulin D: Nucleotide sequence of the human vimentin gene and regulation of its transcription in tissues and cultured cells. Gene 1988;62:7–16.
63. Traub P, Scherbarth A, Wiegers W, Shoeman RL: Salt-stable interaction of the amino-terminal head region of vimentin with the alpha-helical rod domain of cytoplasmic intermediate filament proteins and its relevance to protofilament structure and filament formation and stability. J Cell Sci 1992;101(Pt 2):363–381.
64. Raats JM, Henderik JB, Verdijk M, et al: Assembly of carboxy-terminally deleted desmin in vimentin-free cells. Eur J Cell Biol 1991;56:84–103.
65. Marshall CJ: Evolutionary relationships among the serpins. Philos Trans R Soc Lond B Biol Sci 1993;342: 101–119.
66. Billingsley GD, Walter MA, Hammond GL, Cox DW: Physical mapping of four serpin genes: Alpha 1-antitrypsin, alpha 1-antichymotrypsin, corticosteroid-binding globulin, and protein C inhibitor, within a 280-kb region on chromosome I4q32.1. Am J Hum Genet 1993;52:343–353.
67. Bao JJ, Sifers RN, Kidd VJ, et al: Molecular evolution of serpins: Homologous structure of the human alpha 1-antichymotrypsin and alpha 1-antitrypsin genes [published erratum appears in Biochemistry 1988;27:8508]. Biochemistry 1987;26:7755–7759.
68. Rubin H, Wang ZM, Nickbarg EB, et al: Cloning, expression, purification, and biological activity of recombinant native and variant human alpha 1-antichymotrypsins. J Biol Chem 1990;265:1199–1207.
69. Mast AE, Enghild JJ, Pizzo SV, Salvesen G: Analysis of the plasma elimination kinetics and conformational stabilities of native, proteinase-complexed, and reactive site cleaved serpins: Comparison of alpha 1-proteinase inhibitor, alpha 1-antichymotrypsin, antithrombin III, alpha 2-antiplasmin, angiotensinogen, and ovalbumin. Biochemistry 1991;30:1723–1730.
70. Perkins SJ, Smith KF, Nealis AS, et al: Secondary structure changes stabilize the reactive-centre cleaved form of SERPINs: A study by 1H nuclear magnetic resonance and Fourier transform infrared spectroscopy. J Mol Biol 1992;228:1235–1254.
71. Baumann U, Huber R, Bode W, et al: Crystal structure of cleaved human alpha-1-antichymotrypsin at 2.7 Å

resolution and its comparison with other serpins. J Mol Biol 1991;218:595–606.
72. Bruch M, Weiss V, Engel J: Plasma serine proteinase inhibitors (serpins) exhibit major conformational changes and a large increase in conformational stability upon cleavage at their reactive sites. J Biol Chem 1988;263: 16626–16630.
73. Taylor CR, Shi SR, Cote RJ: Antigen retrieval for immunohistochemistry: Status and need for greater standardization. Appl Immunohistochemistry 1996;4: 144–166.
74. Byth BC, Billingsley GD, Cox DW: Physical and genetic mapping of the serpin gene cluster at 14q32.1: Allelic association and a unique haplotype associated with alpha-1-antitrypsin deficiency. Am J Hum Genet 1994;55:126–133.
75. Long GL, Chandra T, Woo SL, et al: Complete sequence of the cDNA for human alpha-1-antitrypsin and the gene for the S variant. Biochemistry 1984;23:4828–4837.
76. Hafeez W, Ciliberto G, Perlmutter DH: Constitutive and modulated expression of the human alpha-1-antitrypsin gene: Different transcriptional initiation sites used in three different cell types. J Clin Invest 1992; 89:1214–1222.
77. Takahara H, Shibata S, Sinohara H: Conformational differences between mouse contrapsin and alpha-1-antitrypsin as studied by ultraviolet absorption and circular dichroism spectroscopy. Tohoku J Exp Med 1984;142: 261–273.
78. Song HK, Lee KN, Kwon KS, et al: Crystal structure of an uncleaved alpha-1-antitrypsin reveals the conformation of its inhibitory reactive loop. FEBS Lett 1995; 377:150–154.
79. Stein PE, Leslie AG, Finch JT, et al: Crystal structure of ovalbumin as a model for the reactive centre of serpins. Nature 1990;347:99–102.
80. Mega T, Lujan E, Yoshida A: Studies on the oligosaccharide chains of human alpha-1-protease inhibitor: II. Structure of oligosaccharides. J Biol Chem 1980;255: 4057–4061.
81. Harper ME, Barrera-Saldana HA, Saunders GF: Chromosomal localization of the human placental lactogen-growth hormone gene cluster to 17q22–24. Am J Hum Genet 1982;34:227–234.
82. Beattie WG, Dugaiczyk A: Structure and evolution of human alpha-fetoprotein deduced from partial sequence of cloned cDNA. Gene 1982;20:415–422.
83. Cooke NE, David EV: Serum vitamin D–binding protein is a third member of the albumin and alpha-fetoprotein gene family. J Clin Invest 1985;76:2420–2424.
84. Urano Y, Sakai M, Watanabe K, Tamaoki T: Tandem arrangement of the albumin and alpha-fetoprotein genes in the human genome. Gene 1984;32:255–261.
85. Sakai M, Morinaga T, Urano Y, et al: The human alpha-fetoprotein gene: Sequence organization and the 5′ flanking region. J Biol Chem 1985;260:5055–5060.
86. Gibbs PE, Zielinski R, Boyd C, Dugaiczyk A: Structure, polymorphism, and novel repeated DNA elements revealed by a complete sequence of the human alpha-fetoprotein gene. Biochemistry 1987;26:1332–1343.
87. Morinaga T, Sakai M, Wegmann TG, Tamaoki T: Primary structures of human alpha-fetoprotein and its mRNA. Proc Natl Acad Sci USA 1983;80:4604–4608.
88. Zizkovsky V, Strop P, Korcakova J, et al: Fluorescence spectroscopy, fluorescence polarization, and circular dichroism in studies on pH-dependent changes in the alpha-fetoprotein molecule. Ann NY Acad Sci 1983;417: 49–56.
89. Murray JC, Mills KA, Demopulos CM, et al: Linkage disequilibrium and evolutionary relationships of DNA variants (restriction enzyme fragment length polymorphisms) at the serum albumin locus. Proc Natl Acad Sci USA 1984;81:3486–3490.
90. Minghetti PP, Ruffner DE, Kuang WJ, et al: Molecular structure of the human albumin gene is revealed by nucleotide sequence within q11–22 of chromosome 4. J Biol Chem 6;261:6747–6757.
91. Gordon LM, Curtain CC, McCloyn V, et al: The amino-terminal peptide of HIV-1 gp41 interacts with human serum albumin. AIDS Res Hum Retroviruses 1993;9: 1145–1156.
92. Madison J, Arai K, Sakamoto Y, et al: Genetic variants of serum albumin in Americans and Japanese. Proc Natl Acad Sci USA 1991;88:9853–9857.
93. Madison J, Galliano M, Watkins S, et al: Genetic variants of human serum albumin in Italy: Point mutants and a carboxyl-terminal variant. Proc Natl Acad Sci USA 1994;91:6476–6480.
94. Ruiz M, Rajatanavin R, Young RA, et al: Familial dysalbuminemic hyperthyroxinemia: A syndrome that can be confused with thyrotoxicosis. N Engl J Med 1982;306: 635–639.
95. Chikishev AY, Lucassen GW, Koroteev NI, et al: Polarization-sensitive coherent anti-Stokes Raman scattering spectroscopy of the amide I band of proteins in solutions. Biophys J 1992;63:976–985.
96. Carter DC, He XM, Munson SH, et al: Three-dimensional structure of human serum albumin. Science 1989;244:1195–1198.
97. He XM, Carter DC: Atomic structure and chemistry of human serum albumin [published erratum appears in Nature 1993;364:362]. Nature 1992;358:209–215.
98. Watanabe S, Saito T: Conformational effects in the interaction of phenylbutazone with albumin studied by circular dichroism. Biochem Pharmacol 1992;43:931–935.
99. Le Gal JM, Manfait M: Conformational changes of human serum albumin in vivo induced by free fatty acids as studied by Fourier transform infrared spectroscopy. Biochim Biophys Acta 1990;1041:257–263.
100. Oda Y, Katsuda S, Nakanishi I: An autopsy case of hepatic sarcomatoid tumor: Immunohistochemical comparison with a sarcomatous component of hepatocellular carcinoma. Pathol Int 1994;44:230–236.
101. Deguchi S, Shimatani K, Tada T, et al: Solvent dependence of optical rotation of (S)-N- [1-(2-fluorophenyl)—3,4,6,7-tetrahydro-4-oxo-pyrrolo [3,2,1-jk] [1,4]benzodiazepine-3-yl]—1H-indole-2-carboxamide. J Pharm Sci 1993;82:734–736.
102. Slugen I, Horvathova J, Cernay P, et al: The importance of immunohistochemical examination of glomerulonephritis. Int Urol Nephrol 1988;20:679–683.

103. Hoeprich PDJ, Doolittle RF: Dimeric half-molecules of human fibrinogen are joined through disulfide bonds in an antiparallel orientation. Biochemistry 1983;22: 2049–2055.
104. Conway JF, Parry DA: Three-stranded alpha-fibrous proteins: The heptad repeat and its implications for structure. Int J Biol Macromol 1991;13:14–16.
105. Weisel JW, Stauffacher CV, Bullitt E, Cohen C: A model for fibrinogen: Domains and sequence. Science 1985;230:1388–1391.
106. Ohta N, Yotsuyanagi T: Alteration of fibrinogen secondary structure by *cis*-diaminedichloroplatinum(II) and calcium protection. Biol Pharm Bull 1993;16: 631–634.
107. Azpiazu I, Chapman D: Spectroscopic studies of fibrinogen and its plasmin-derived fragments. Biochim Biophys Acta 1992;1119:268–274.
108. Ugarova TP, Budzynski AZ, Shattil SJ, et al: Conformational changes in fibrinogen elicited by its interaction with platelet membrane glycoprotein GPIIb–IIIa. J Biol Chem 1993;268:21080–21087.
109. Apap-Bologna A, Webster A, Raitt F, Kemp G: The influence of calcium ions on fibrinogen conformation. Biochim Biophys Acta 1989;995:70–74.
110. Marino MW, Fuller GM, Elder FF: Chromosomal localization of human and rat A alpha, B beta, and gamma fibrinogen genes by in situ hybridization. Cytogenet Cell Genet 1986;42:36–41.
111. Kant JA, Fornace AJJ, Saxe D, et al: Evolution and organization of the fibrinogen locus on chromosome 4: Gene duplication accompanied by transposition and inversion. Proc Natl Acad Sci USA 1985;82:2344–2348.
112. Kant JA, Crabtree GR: The rat fibrinogen genes: Linkage of the A alpha and gamma chain genes. J Biol Chem 1983;258:4666–4667.
113. Fowlkes DM, Mullis NT, Comeau CM, Crabtree GR: Potential basis for regulation of the coordinately expressed fibrinogen genes: Homology in the 5′ flanking regions. Proc Natl Acad Sci USA 1984;81: 2313–2316.
114. Rixon MW, Chan WY, Davie EW, Chung DW: Characterization of a complementary deoxyribonucleic acid coding for the alpha chain of human fibrinogen. Biochemistry 1983;22:3237–3244.
115. Kant JA, Lord ST, Crabtree GR: Partial mRNA sequences for human A alpha, B beta, and gamma fibrinogen chains: Evolutionary and functional implications. Proc Natl Acad Sci USA 1983;80:3953–3957.
116. Chung DW, Chan WY, Davie EW: Characterization of a complementary deoxyribonucleic acid coding for the gamma chain of human fibrinogen. Biochemistry 1983; 22:3250–3256.
117. Chung DW, Que BG, Rixon MW, et al: Characterization of complementary deoxyribonucleic acid and genomic deoxyribonucleic acid for the beta chain of human fibrinogen. Biochemistry 1983;22:3244–3250.
118. Rixon MW, Chung DW, Davie EW: Nucleotide sequence of the gene for the gamma chain of human fibrinogen. Biochemistry 1985;24:2077–2086.
119. Crabtree GR, Kant JA: Coordinate accumulation of the mRNAs for the alpha, beta, and gamma chains of rat fibrinogen following defibrination. J Biol Chem 1982; 257:7277–7279.
120. Fornace AJJ, Cummings DE, Comeau CM, et al: Structure of the human gamma-fibrinogen gene: Alternate mRNA splicing near the 3′ end of the gene produces gamma A and gamma B forms of gamma-fibrinogen. J Biol Chem 1984;259:12826–12830.
121. Chung DW, Davie EW: Gamma and gamma′ chains of human fibrinogen are produced by alternative mRNA processing. Biochemistry 1984;23:4232–4236.
122. Donahue JP, Patel H, Anderson WF, Hawiger J: Three-dimensional structure of the platelet integrin recognition segment of the fibrinogen gamma chain obtained by carrier protein-driven crystallization. Proc Natl Acad Sci USA 1994;91:12178–12182.
123. Rupp C, Beck EA. Congenital dysfibrogenemia. *In* Beck EA, Furlan M (eds): Variants of Human Fibrinogen. Bern, Hans Huber, 1984, pp 65–130.
124. Collins CJ, Underdahl JP, Levene RB, et al: Molecular cloning of the human gene for von Willebrand factor and identification of the transcription initiation site. Proc Natl Acad Sci USA 1987;84:4393–4397.
125. Barrow LL, Simin K, Mohlke K, et al: Conserved linkage of neurotrophin-3 and von Willebrand factor on mouse chromosome 6. Mamm Genome 1993;4: 343–345.
126. Bonthron D, Orr EC, Mitsock LM, et al: Nucleotide sequence of pre-pro-von Willebrand factor cDNA. Nucleic Acids Res 1986;14:7125–7127.
127. Loscalzo J, Handin RI: Conformational domains and structural transitions of human von Willebrand protein. Biochemistry 1984;23:3880–3886.
128. Knott HM, Berndt MC, Kralicek AV, et al: Determination of the solution structure of a platelet-adhesion peptide of von Willebrand factor. Biochemistry 1992;31: 11152–11158.
129. Ohmori K, Fretto LJ, Harrison RL, et al: Electron microscopy of human factor VIII/von Willebrand glycoprotein: Effect of reducing reagents on structure and function. J Cell Biol 1982;95(2 Pt 1):632–640.
130. Shelton-Inloes BB, Chehab FF, Mannucci PM, et al: Gene deletions correlate with the development of alloantibodies in von Willebrand disease. J Clin Invest 1987;79:1459–1465.
131. Yamanishi K, Liew FM, Konishi K, et al: Molecular cloning of human epidermal transglutaminase cDNA from keratinocytes in culture. Biochem Biophys Res Commun 1991;175:906–913.
132. Rozenfeld MA, Vasileva MV: Mechanism of aggregation of fibrinogen molecules: The influence of fibrin-stabilising factor. Biomed Sci 1991;2:155–161.
133. Board PG, Chapple R, Coggan M: Haplotypes of the coagulation factor XIII A subunit locus in normal and deficient subjects. Am J Hum Genet 1988;42:712–717.
134. Board PG, Coggan M, Baker RT, et al: Localization of the human UBC polyubiquitin gene to chromosome band 12q24.3. Genomics 1992;12:639–642.
135. Takahashi N, Takahashi Y, Putnam FW: Primary structure of blood coagulation factor XIIIa (fibrinoligase, transglutaminase) from human placenta. Proc Natl Acad Sci USA 1986;83:8019–8023.

136. Board PG, Webb GC, McKee J, Ichinose A: Localization of the coagulation factor XIII A subunit gene (F13A) to chromosome bands 6p24–p25. Cytogenet Cell Genet 1988;48:25–27.
137. Yee VC, Pedersen LC, Le Trong I, et al: Three-dimensional structure of a transglutaminase: Human blood coagulation factor XIII. Proc Natl Acad Sci USA 1994;91:7296–7300.
138. Webb GC, Coggan M, Ichinose A, Board PG: Localization of the coagulation factor XIII B subunit gene *(F13B)* to chromosome bands 1q31–32.1 and restriction fragment length polymorphism at the locus. Hum Genet 1989;81:157–160.
139. Monig H, Ali IU, Oldfield EH, Schulte HM: Structure of the POMC promoter region in pituitary and extrapituitary ACTH producing tumors. Exp Clin Endocrinol 1993;101:36–38.
140. Feder J, Migone N, Chang AC, et al: A DNA polymorphism in close physical linkage with the proopiomelanocortin gene. Am J Hum Genet 1983;35:1090–1096.
141. Zabel BU, Naylor SL, Sakaguchi AY, et al: High-resolution chromosomal localization of human genes for amylase, proopiomelanocortin, somatostatin, and a DNA fragment *(D3S1)* by in situ hybridization. Proc Natl Acad Sci USA 1983;80:6932–6936.
142. Wallis M, Howell SL, Taylor KW: The Biochemistry of the Peptide Hormones. New York, John Wiley & Sons, 1985.
143. Stefaneanu L, Kovacs K, Horvath E, Lloyd RV: In situ hybridization study of pro-opiomelanocortin (POMC) gene expression in human pituitary corticotrophs and their adenomas. Virchows Arch A Pathol Anat Histopathol 1991;419:107–113.
144. Makarov AA, Esipova NG, Pankov IA, Lobachev VM: [left-helical conformation (type poly-L-proline II) of the polypeptide chain of adrenocorticotropic hormone in water]. Biofizika 1976;21:754–755.
145. Jeannotte L, Trifiro MA, Plante RK, et al: Tissue-specific activity of the pro-opiomelanocortin gene promoter. Mol Cell Biol 1987;7:4058–4064.
146. Konig W: Peptide and Protein Hormones: Structure, Regulation, Activity—a Reference Manual. Weinheim, Germany, VCH Publishers, 1992.
147. Spindel ER, Gibson BW, Reeve JRJ, Kelly M: Cloning of cDNAs encoding amphibian bombesin: Evidence for the relationship between bombesin and gastrin-releasing peptide. Proc Natl Acad Sci USA 1990;87:9813–9817.
148. Naylor SL, Sakaguchi AY, Spindel E, Chin WW: Human gastrin-releasing peptide gene is located on chromosome 18. Somat Cell Mol Genet 1987;13: 87–91.
149. Lebacq-Verheyden AM, Bertness V, Kirsch I, et al: Human gastrin-releasing peptide gene maps to chromosome band 18q21. Somat Cell Mol Genet 1987;13:81–86.
150. Spindel ER, Zilberberg MD, Chin WW: Analysis of the gene and multiple messenger ribonucleic acids (mRNAs) encoding human gastrin-releasing peptide: Alternate RNA splicing occurs in neural and endocrine tissue. Mol Endocrinol 1987;1:224–232.
151. Cavatorta P, Sartor G, Neyroz P, et al: Fluorescence and CD studies on the conformation of the gastrin releasing peptide in solution and in the presence of model membranes. Biopolymers 1991;31:653–661.
152. Hamid QA, Bishop AE, Springall DR, et al: Detection of human probombesin mRNA in neuroendocrine (small cell) carcinoma of the lung: In situ hybridization with cRNA probe. Cancer 1989;63:266–271.
153. Sunday ME, Wolfe HJ, Roos BA, et al: Gastrin-releasing peptide gene expression in developing, hyperplastic, and neoplastic human thyroid C-cells. Endocrinology 1988;122:1551–1558.
154. Hoppener JW, Steenbergh PH, Zandberg J, et al: Localization of the polymorphic human calcitonin gene on chromosome 11. Hum Genet 1984;66:309–312.
155. Hoovers JM, Redeker E, Speleman F, et al: High-resolution chromosomal localization of the human calcitonin/CGRP/IAPP gene family members. Genomics 1993;15:525–529.
156. Peleg S, Abruzzese RV, Cote GJ, Gagel RF: Transcription of the human calcitonin gene is mediated by a C cell–specific enhancer containing E-box–like elements. Mol Endocrinol 1990;4:1750–1757.
157. Brain SD, Williams TJ, Tippins JR, et al: Calcitonin gene–related peptide is a potent vasodilator. Nature 1985;313:54–56.
158. Amara SG, Jonas V, Rosenfeld MG, et al: Alternative RNA processing in calcitonin gene expression generates mRNAs encoding different polypeptide products. Nature 1982;298:240–244.
159. Nelkin BD, Rosenfeld KI, de Bustros A, et al: Structure and expression of a gene encoding human calcitonin and calcitonin gene–related peptide. Biochem Biophys Res Commun 1984;123:648–655.
160. Motta A, Morelli MA, Goud N, Temussi PA: Sequential 1H NMR assignment and secondary structure determination of salmon calcitonin in solution. Biochemistry 1989;28:7996–8002.
161. Meyer JP, Pelton JT, Hoflack J, Saudek V: Solution structure of salmon calcitonin. Biopolymers 1991;31: 233–241.
162. Meadows RP, Nikonowicz EP, Jones CR, et al: Two-dimensional NMR and structure determination of salmon calcitonin in methanol. Biochemistry 1991;30: 1247–1254.
163. Epand RM, Stahl GL, Orlowski RC: Conformational and biological properties of partial sequences of salmon calcitonin. Int J Pept Protein Res 1986;27: 501–507.
164. Epand RM, Epand RF, Orlowski RC, et al: Amphipathic helix and its relationship to the interaction of calcitonin with phospholipids. Biochemistry 1983;22:5074–5084.
165. Lund T, Geurts vKA, Haun S, Dixon JE: The genes for human gastrin and cholecystokinin are located on different chromosomes. Hum Genet 1986;73:77–80.
166. Loomis RE, Lee PC, Tseng CC: Conformational analysis of the cholecystokinin C-terminal octapeptide: A nuclear magnetic resonance and computer-simulation approach. Biochim Biophys Acta 1987;911:168–179.
167. Fournie-Zaluski MC, Durieux C, Lux B, et al: Conformational analysis of cholecystokinin fragments CCK4, CCK5, and CCK6 by 1H-NMR spectroscopy and fluorescence-transfer measurements. Biopolymers 1985;24: 1663–1681.

168. Bidart JM, Bellet D (eds): Immunohistochemical Approaches to the Study of Gonadotropins. New York, Raven, 1989, pp 21–33.
169. Sairam MR, Li CH: Gonadotropic hormones: Relationship between structure and function with emphasis on antagonists. *In* Hormonal Proteins and Peptides: Gonadotropic Hormones. New York, Academic, 1983, pp 1–79.
170. Dracopoli NC, Rettig WJ, Whitfield GK, et al: Assignment of the gene for the beta subunit of thyroid-stimulating hormone to the short arm of human chromosome 1. Proc Natl Acad Sci USA 1986;83:1822–1826.
171. Watkins PC, Eddy R, Beck AK, et al: DNA sequence and regional assignment of the human follicle-stimulating hormone beta-subunit gene to the short arm of human chromosome 11. DNA 1987;6:205–212.
172. Luderer U, Schwartz NB: An overview of FSH regulation and action. *In* Hunzicker-Dunn M, Schwartz NB (eds): Follicle Stimulating Hormone: Regulation of Secretion and Molecular Mechanisms of Action. New York, Springer Verlag, 1992.
173. Agris PF, Guenther RH, Sierzputowska-Gracz H, et al: Solution structure of a synthetic peptide corresponding to a receptor binding region of FSH (hFSH-beta 33–53). J Protein Chem 1992;11:495–507.
174. Roth KE, Liu C, Shepard BA, et al: The flanking amino acids of the human follitropin beta-subunit 33–53 region are involved in assembly of the follitropin heterodimer. Endocrinology 1993;132:2571–2577.
175. Debas HT: Gastrin. Clin Invest Med 1987;10:222–225.
176. Couch FJ, Abel KJ, Brody LC, et al: Localization of the gene for ATP citrate lyase *(ACLY)* distal to gastrin *(GAS)* and proximal to D17S856 on chromosome 17q12–q21. Genomics 1994;21:444–446.
177. Pincus MR, Murphy RB, Carty RP, et al: Conformational analysis of possible biologically active (receptor-bound) conformations of peptides derived from cholecystokinin, cerulein and little gastrin and the opiate peptide, met-enkephalin. Peptides 1988;9(Suppl 1):145–152.
178. Torda AE, Baldwin GS, Norton RS: High-resolution proton nuclear magnetic resonance studies of human gastrin. Biochemistry 1985;24:1720–1777.
179. Bell GI: The glucagon superfamily: Precursor structure and gene organization. Peptides 1986;7(Suppl 1):27–36.
180. Schroeder WT, Lopez LC, Harper ME, Saunders GF: Localization of the human glucagon gene *(GCG)* to chromosome segment 2q36–37. Cytogenet Cell Genet 1984;38:76–79.
181. White JW, Saunders GF: Structure of the human glucagon gene. Nucleic Acids Res 1986;14:4719–4730.
182. Drucker DJ, Philippe J, Jepeal L, Habener JF: Glucagon gene 5′-flanking sequences promote islet cell–specific gene transcription. J Biol Chem 1987;262: 15659–15665.
183. Drucker DJ, Mojsov S, Habener JF: Cell-specific post-translational processing of preproglucagon expressed from a metallothionein-glucagon fusion gene. J Biol Chem 1986;261:9637–9643.
184. Mojsov S, Weir GC, Habener JF: Insulinotropin: Glucagon-like peptide I (7–37) co-encoded in the glucagon gene is a potent stimulator of insulin release in the perfused rat pancreas. J Clin Invest 1987;79:616–619.
185. Unson CG, Gurzenda EM, Iwasa K, Merrifield RB: Glucagon antagonists: Contribution to binding and activity of the amino-terminal sequence 1–5, position 12, and the putative alpha-helical segment 19–27. J Biol Chem 1989;264:789–794.
186. Bodanszky M, Bodanszky A: Conformation of peptides of the secretin-VIP-glucagon family in solution. Peptides 1986;7(Suppl 1):43–48.
187. Murphy J, Zhang WJ, Macaulay W, et al: The relation of predicted structure to observed conformation and activity of glucagon analogs containing replacements at positions 19, 22, and 23. J Biol Chem 1987;262:17304–17312.
188. Sasaki K, Dockerill S, Adamiak DA, et al: X-ray analysis of glucagon and its relationship to receptor binding. Nature 1975;257:751–757.
189. Barsh GS, Seeburg PH, Gelinas RE: The human growth hormone gene family: Structure and evolution of the chromosomal locus. Nucleic Acids Res 1983;11: 3939–3958.
190. George DL, Phillips JA, Francke U, Seeburg PH: The genes for growth hormone and chorionic somatomammotropin are on the long arm of human chromosome 17 in region q21 to qter. Hum Genet 1981;57:138–141.
191. Abdel-Meguid SS, Shieh HS, Smith WW, et al: Three-dimensional structure of a genetically engineered variant of porcine growth hormone. Proc Natl Acad Sci USA 1987;84:6434–6437.
192. Ultsch M, de Vos AM, Kossiakoff AA: Crystals of the complex between human growth hormone and the extracellular domain of its receptor. J Mol Biol 1991; 222:865–868.
193. Aubert ML, Bewley TA, Grumbach MM, et al: Structure-function studies on human growth hormone: Evidence that tertiary structure is essential for biological activity. Int J Pept Protein Res 1986;28:45–57.
194. Julier C, Weil D, Couillin P, et al: The beta chorionic gonadotropin–beta luteinizing gene cluster maps to human chromosome 19. Hum Genet 1984;67:174–177.
195. Campain JA, Gutkin DW, Cox GS: Differential DNA methylation of the chorionic gonadotropin beta-subunit multigene family. Mol Endocrinol 1993;7:1331–1346.
196. Puett D, Birken S: Helix formation in reduced, S-carboxymethylated human choriogonadotropin beta subunit and tryptic peptides. J Protein Chem 1989;8: 779–794.
197. Willey KP, Leidenberger F: Functionally distinct agonist and receptor-binding regions in human chorionic gonadotropin: Development of a tertiary structure model. J Biol Chem 1989;264:19716–19729.
198. Keutmann HT, Charlesworth MC, Mason KA, et al: A receptor-binding region in human choriogonadotropin/lutropin beta subunit. Proc Natl Acad Sci USA 1987;84:2038–2042.
199. Gray CJ: Glycoprotein gonadotropins: Structure and synthesis. Acta Endocrinol Suppl (Copenh) 1988;288: 20–7.
200. Keutmann HT, Johnson L, Ryan RJ: Evidence for a conformational change in deglycosylated glycoprotein hormones. FEBS Lett 1985;185:333–338.
201. Lapthorn AJ, Harris DC, Littlejohn A, et al: Crystal structure of human chorionic gonadotropin [see comments]. Nature 1994;369:455–461.

202. Talwar GP, Singh O, Rao LV: An improved immunogen for anti–human chorionic gonadotropin vaccine eliciting antibodies reactive with a conformation native to the hormone without cross-reaction with human follicle-stimulating hormone and human thyroid-stimulating hormone. J Reprod Immunol 1988;14:203–212.
203. Gani M, Coley J, Porter P: Epitope masking and immunodominance—complications in the selection of monoclonal antibodies against HCG. Hybridoma 1987; 6:637–643.
204. Chandrasekharappa SC, Friedman L, King SE, et al: The gene for pancreatic polypeptide (PPY) and the anonymous marker D17S78 are within 45 kb of each other on chromosome 17q21. Genomics 1994;21: 458–460.
205. Takeuchi T, Gumucio DL, Yamada T, et al: Genes encoding pancreatic polypeptide and neuropeptide Y are on human chromosomes 17 and 7. J Clin Invest 1986;77:1038–1041.
206. Leiter AB, Montminy MR, Jamieson E, Goodman RH: Exons of the human pancreatic polypeptide gene define functional domains of the precursor. J Biol Chem 1985;260:13013–13017.
207. Glover ID, Moss DS, Tickle IJ, et al: Anisotropic thermal motion and polypeptide secondary structure studied by X-ray analysis at 0.98A resolution. Adv Biophys 1985; 20:1–12.
208. Taylor TC, Thompson DO, Ebner KE, et al: An immunochemical study of avian pancreatic polypeptide: The nature of the principal epitope. Mol Immunol 1988;25: 961–973.
209. Lemaigre FP, Peers B, Lafontaine DA, et al: Pituitary-specific factor binding to the human prolactin, growth hormone, and placental lactogen genes. DNA 1989;8: 149–159.
210. Berwaer M, Monget P, Peers B, et al: Multihormonal regulation of the human prolactin gene expression from 5000 bp of its upstream sequence. Mol Cell Endocrinol 1991;80:53–64.
211. Jacquemin P, Oury C, Peers B, et al: Characterization of a single strong tissue-specific enhancer downstream from the three human genes encoding placental lactogen. Mol Cell Biol 1994;14:93–103.
212. Shimomura K, Bremel RD: Characterization of bovine placental lactogen as a glycoprotein with N-linked and O-linked carbohydrate side chains. Mol Endocrinol 1988;2:845–853.
213. Lowman HB, Cunningham BC, Wells JA: Mutational analysis and protein engineering of receptor-binding determinants in human placental lactogen. J Biol Chem 1991;266:10982–10988.
214. Bell GI, Pictet RL, Rutter WJ, et al: Sequence of the human insulin gene. Nature 1980;284:26–32.
215. Bentley G, Dodson E, Dodson G, et al: Structure of 4-zinc insulin. Nature 1976;261:166–168.
216. Amodeo P, Naider F, Picone D, et al: Conformational sampling of bioactive conformers: A low-temperature NMR study of 15N-Leu-enkephalin. J Pept Sci 1998; 4:253–265.
217. Meirovitch E, Meirovitch H: New theoretical methodology for elucidating the solution structure of peptides from NMR data: II. Free energy of dominant microstates of Leu-enkephalin and population-weighted average nuclear Overhauser effects intensities. Biopolymers 1996;38:69–88.
218. Behnam BA, Deber CM: Evidence for a folded conformation of methionine—and leucine-enkephalin in a membrane environment. J Biol Chem 1984;259:14935–14940.
219. Mohrenweiser HW, Tynan KM, Branscomb EW, et al: Development of an integrated genetic, functional and physical map of human chromosome 19 [abstract]. Cytogenet Cell Genet 1991;58:2021.
220. Thompson J, Koumari R, Wagner K, et al: The human pregnancy-specific glycoprotein genes are tightly linked on the long arm of chromosome 19 and are coordinately expressed [published erratum appears in Biochem Biophys Res Commun 1990;168:1325]. Biochem Biophys Res Commun 1990;167:848–859.
221. Owerbach D, Rutter WJ, Cooke NE, et al: The prolactin gene is located on chromosome 6 in humans. Science 1981;212:815–816.
222. Evans AM, Petersen JW, Sekhon GS, DeMars R: Mapping of prolactin and tumor necrosis factor-beta genes on human chromosome 6p using lymphoblastoid cell deletion mutants. Somat Cell Mol Genet 1989;15: 203–213.
223. Bewley TA, Colosi P, Talamantes F: Conformational studies of secreted mouse pituitary prolactin. Biochemistry 1982;21:4238–4243.
224. Luck DN, Gout PW, Kelsay K, et al: Recombinant methionyl bovine prolactin: Loss of bioactivity after single amino acid deletions from putative helical regions. Mol Endocrinol 1990;4:1011–1016.
225. Watahiki M, Tanaka M, Masuda N, et al: Primary structure of chicken pituitary prolactin deduced from the cDNA sequence: Conserved and specific amino acid residues in the domains of the prolactins. J Biol Chem 1989;264:5535–5539.
226. Gotoh E, Yamagami T, Yamamoto H, Okamoto H: Chromosomal assignment of human VIP/PHM-27 gene to 6q26–q27 region by spot blot hybridization and in situ hybridization. Biochem Int 1988;17:555–562.
227. Yamagami T, Ohsawa K, Nishizawa M, et al: Complete nucleotide sequence of human vasoactive intestinal peptide/PHM-27 gene and its inducible promoter. Ann NY Acad Sci 1988;527:87–102.
228. Linder S, Barkhem T, Norberg A, et al: Structure and expression of the gene encoding the vasoactive intestinal peptide precursor. Proc Natl Acad Sci USA 1987;84: 605–609.
229. Fink JS, Verhave M, Kasper S, et al: The CGTCA sequence motif is essential for biological activity of the vasoactive intestinal peptide gene cAMP-regulated enhancer. Proc Natl Acad Sci USA 1988;85: 6662–6666.
230. Tsukada T, Horovitch SJ, Montminy MR, et al: Structure of the human vasoactive intestinal polypeptide gene. DNA 1985;4:293–300.
231. Fry DC, Madison VS, Bolin DR, et al: Solution structure of an analogue of vasoactive intestinal peptide as determined by two-dimensional NMR and circular dichroism spectroscopies and constrained molecular dynamics. Biochemistry 1989;28:2399–2409.

232. Musso GF, Patthi S, Ryskamp TC, et al: Development of helix-based vasoactive intestinal peptide analogues: Identification of residues required for receptor interaction. Biochemistry 1988;27:8174–8181.
233. Haghjoo K, Cash PW, Farid RS, et al: Solution structure of vasoactive intestinal polypeptide (11–28) NH2, a fragment with analgesic properties. Pept Res 1996;9: 327–331.
234. Calabi F, Bradbury A: The CD1 system. Tissue Antigens 1991;37:1–9.
235. Moingeon P, Chang HC, Sayre PH, et al: The structural biology of CD2. Immunol Rev 1989;111: 111–144.
236. Beyers AD, Barclay AN, Law DA, et al: Activation of T lymphocytes via monoclonal antibodies against rat cell surface antigens with particular reference to CD2 antigen. Immunol Rev 1989;111:59–77.
237. Lang G, Wotton D, Owen MJ, et al: The structure of the human CD2 gene and its expression in transgenic mice. EMBO J 1988;7:1675–1682.
238. Tunnacliffe A, Buluwela L, Rabbitts TH: Physical linkage of three CD3 genes on human chromosome 11. EMBO J 1987;6:2953–2957.
239. Tunnacliffe A, Sims JE, Rabbitts TH: T3 delta pre-mRNA is transcribed from a non-TATA promoter and is alternatively spliced in human T cells. EMBO J 1986;5:1245–1252.
240. Clevers HC, Dunlap S, Wileman TE, Terhorst C: Human CD3-epsilon gene contains three miniexons and is transcribed from a non-TATA promoter. Proc Natl Acad Sci USA 1988;85:8156–8160.
241. Wilson RK, Lai E, Concannon P, et al: Structure, organization and polymorphism of murine and human T-cell receptor alpha and beta chain gene families. Immunol Rev 1988;101:149–172.
242. Lefranc MP, Chuchana P, Dariavach P, et al: Molecular mapping of the human T cell receptor gamma (TRG) genes and linkage of the variable and constant regions. Eur J Immunol 1989;19:989–994.
243. Satyanarayana K, Hata S, Devlin P, et al: Genomic organization of the human T-cell antigen-receptor alpha/delta locus. Proc Natl Acad Sci USA 1988;85: 8166–8170.
244. Iwashima M, Green A, Davis MM, Chien YH: Variable region (V delta) gene segment most frequently utilized in adult thymocytes is 3′ of the constant (C delta) region. Proc Natl Acad Sci USA 1988;85:8161–8165.
245. Klausner RD, Samelson LE: T cell antigen receptor activation pathways: The tyrosine kinase connection. Cell 1991;64:875–878.
246. Matsui K, Boniface JJ, Reay PA, et al: Low affinity interaction of peptide-MHC complexes with T cell receptors. Science 1991;254:1788–1791.
247. Parnes JR: Molecular biology and function of CD4 and CD8. Adv Immunol 1989;44:265–311.
248. Shin J, Doyle C, Yang Z, et al: Structural features of the cytoplasmic region of CD4 required for internalization. EMBO J 1990;9:425–434.
249. Turner JM, Brodsky MH, Irving BA, et al: Interaction of the unique N-terminal region of tyrosine kinase p56lck with cytoplasmic domains of CD4 and CD8 is mediated by cysteine motifs. Cell 1990;60:755–765.
250. Wang JH, Yan YW, Garrett TP, et al: Atomic structure of a fragment of human CD4 containing two immunoglobulin-like domains [see comments]. Nature 1990; 348:411–418.
251. Maddon PJ, Molineaux SM, Maddon DE, et al: Structure and expression of the human and mouse T4 genes. Proc Natl Acad Sci USA 1987;84:9155–9159.
252. Schanberg LE, Fleenor DE, Kurtzberg J, et al: Isolation and characterization of the genomic human CD7 gene: Structural similarity with the murine Thy-1 gene. Proc Natl Acad Sci USA 1991;88:603–607.
253. D'Adamio L, Shipp MA, Masteller EL, Reinherz EL: Organization of the gene encoding common acute lymphoblastic leukemia antigen (neutral endopeptidase 24.11): Multiple miniexons and separate 5′ untranslated regions. Proc Natl Acad Sci USA 1989;86: 7103–7107.
254. LeBien TW, McCormack RT: The common acute lymphoblastic leukemia antigen (CD10)—emancipation from a functional enigma. Blood 1989;73:625–635.
255. Lee S, Zambas ED, Marsh WL, Redman CM: Molecular cloning and primary structure of Kell blood group protein. Proc Natl Acad Sci USA 1991;88:6353–6357.
256. Stocks SC, Albrechtsen M, Kerr MA: Expression of the CD15 differentiation antigen (3-fucosyl-N-acetyl-lactosamine, LeX) on putative neutrophil adhesion molecules CR3 and NCA-160. Biochem J 1990;268:275–280.
257. Zhou LJ, Ord DC, Hughes AL, Tedder TF: Structure and domain organization of the CD19 antigen of human, mouse, and guinea pig B lymphocytes: Conservation of the extensive cytoplasmic domain. J Immunol 1991;147:1424–1432.
258. Tedder TF, Isaacs CM: Isolation of cDNAs encoding the CD19 antigen of human and mouse B lymphocytes: A new member of the immunoglobulin superfamily. J Immunol 1989;143:712–717.
259. Kansas GS, Tedder TF: Transmembrane signals generated through MHC class II, CD19, CD20, CD39, and CD40 antigens induce LFA-1-dependent and independent adhesion in human B cells through a tyrosine kinase-dependent pathway. J Immunol 1991;147: 4094–4102.
260. Tedder TF, Disteche CM, Louie E, et al: The gene that encodes the human CD20 (B1) differentiation antigen is located on chromosome 11 near the t(11;14) (q13;q32) translocation site. J Immunol 1989;142: 2555–2559.
261. Tedder TF, Streuli M, Schlossman SF, Saito H: Isolation and structure of a cDNA encoding the B1 (CD20) cell-surface antigen of human B lymphocytes. Proc Natl Acad Sci USA 1988;85:208–212.
262. Bubien JK, Bell PD, Frizzell RA, Tedder TF: CD20 directly regulates transmembrane ion flux in B-lymphocytes. Leukocyte Typing 1989;IV:51—54.
263. Fujisaku A, Harley JB, Frank MB, et al: Genomic organization and polymorphisms of the human C3d/Epstein-Barr virus receptor. J Biol Chem 1989;264:2118–2125.
264. Ahearn JM, Fearon DT: Structure and function of the complement receptors, CR1 (CD35) and CR2 (CD21). Adv Immunol 1989;46:183–219.

265. Delcayre AX, Salas F, Mathur S, et al: Epstein Barr virus/complement C3d receptor is an interferon alpha receptor. EMBO J 1991;10:919–926.
266. Stamenkovic I, Seed B: The B-cell antigen CD22 mediates monocyte and erythrocyte adhesion. Nature 1990; 345:74–77.
267. Wilson GL, Fox CH, Fauci AS, Kehrl JH: cDNA cloning of the B cell membrane protein CD22: A mediator of B-B cell interactions. J Exp Med 1991;173:137–146.
268. Stamenkovic I, Sgroi D, Aruffo A, et al: The B lymphocyte adhesion molecule CD22 interacts with leukocyte common antigen CD45RO on T cells and alpha 2–6 sialyltransferase, CD75, on B cells [see comments]. Cell 1991;66:1133–1144.
269. Suter U, Bastos R, Hofstetter H: Molecular structure of the gene and the 5′-flanking region of the human lymphocyte immunoglobulin E receptor. Nucleic Acids Res 1987;15:7295–7308.
270. Schwab U, Stein H, Gerdes J, et al: Production of a monoclonal antibody specific for Hodgkin and Sternberg-Reed cells of Hodgkin's disease and a subset of normal lymphoid cells. Nature 1982;299:65–67.
271. Schwarting R, Gerdes J, Durkop H, et al: BER-H2: A new anti-Ki-1 (CD30) monoclonal antibody directed at a formol-resistant epitope. Blood 1989;74:1678–1689.
272. Durkop H, Latza U, Hummel M, et al: Molecular cloning and expression of a new member of the nerve growth factor receptor family that is characteristic for Hodgkin's disease. Cell 1992;68:421–427.
273. Shelley CS, Remold-O'Donnell E, Rosen FS, Whitehead AS: Structure of the human sialophorin (CD43) gene: Identification of features atypical of genes encoding integral membrane proteins. Biochem J 1990;270:569–576.
274. Rosenstein Y, Park JK, Hahn WC, et al: CD43, a molecule defective in Wiskott-Aldrich syndrome, binds ICAM-1. Nature 1991;354:233–235.
275. Fernandez-Luna JL, Matthews RJ, Brownstein BH, et al: Characterization and expression of the human leukocyte-common antigen (CD45) gene contained in yeast artificial chromosomes. Genomics 1991;10:756–764.
276. Streuli M, Hall LR, Saga Y, et al: Differential usage of three exons generates at least five different mRNAs encoding human leukocyte common antigens. J Exp Med 1987;166:1548–1566.
277. Strubin M, Berte C, Mach B: Alternative splicing and alternative initiation of translation explain the four forms of the Ia antigen-associated invariant chain. EMBO J 1986;5:3483–3488.
278. O'Sullivan DM, Larhammar D, Wilson MC, et al: Structure of the human Ia-associated invariant (gamma)-chain gene: Identification of 5′ sequences shared with major histocompatibility complex class II genes. Proc Natl Acad Sci USA 1986;83:4484–4488.
279. Kudo J, Chao LY, Narni F, Saunders GF: Structure of the human gene encoding the invariant gamma-chain of class II histocompatibility antigens. Nucleic Acids Res 1985;13:8827–8841.
280. Bast BJ, Zhou LJ, Freeman GJ, et al: The HB-6, CDw75, and CD76 differentiation antigens are unique cell-surface carbohydrate determinants generated by the beta-galactoside alpha 2,6-sialyltransferase. J Cell Biol 1992;116:423–435.
281. Stamenkovic I, Asheim HC, Deggerdal A, et al: The B cell antigen CD75 is a cell surface sialytransferase. J Exp Med 1990;172:641–643.
282. Prasad L, Waygood EB, Lee JS, Delbaere LT: The 2.5 Å resolution structure of the jel42 Fab fragment/HPr complex. J Mol Biol 1998;280:829–845.
283. Cox DW, Markovic VD, Teshima IE: Genes for immunoglobulin heavy chains and for alpha 1-antitrypsin are localized to specific regions of chromosome 14q. Nature 1982;297:428–430.
284. Matsuda F, Shin EK, Nagaoka H, et al: Structure and physical map of 64 variable segments in the 3′ 0.8-megabase region of the human immunoglobulin heavy-chain locus. Nat Genet 1993;3:88–94.
285. Tomlinson IM, Cook GP, Carter NP, et al: Human immunoglobulin VH and D segments on chromosomes 15q11.2 and 16p11.2. Hum Mol Genet 1994;3: 853–860.
286. Emanuel BS: Chromosomal in situ hybridization and the molecular cytogenetics of cancer. Surv Synth Pathol Res 1985;4:269–281.
287. Emanuel BS, Selden JR, Chaganti RS, et al: The 2p breakpoint of a 2;8 translocation in Burkitt lymphoma interrupts the V kappa locus. Proc Natl Acad Sci USA 1984;81:2444–2446.
288. Malcolm S, Barton P, Murphy C, et al: Localization of human immunoglobulin kappa light chain variable region genes to the short arm of chromosome 2 by in situ hybridization. Proc Natl Acad Sci USA 1982;79: 4957–4961.
289. Vasicek TJ, Leder P: Structure and expression of the human immunoglobulin lambda genes. J Exp Med 1990;172:609–620.
290. White MB, Shen AL, Word CJ, et al: Human immunoglobulin D: Genomic sequence of the delta heavy chain. Science 1985;228:733–737.
291. Nishida Y, Miki T, Hisajima H, Honjo T: Cloning of human immunoglobulin epsilon chain genes: Evidence for multiple C epsilon genes. Proc Natl Acad Sci USA 1982;79:3833–3837.
292. Koshland ME: The coming of age of the immunoglobulin J chain. Annu Rev Immunol 1985;3:425–453.
293. Peters CW, Kruse U, Pollwein R, et al: The human lysozyme gene: Sequence organization and chromosomal localization. Eur J Biochem 1989;182:507–516.
294. Yoshimura K, Toibana A, Nakahama K: Human lysozyme: Sequencing of a cDNA, and expression and secretion by *Saccharomyces cerevisiae*. Biochem Biophys Res Commun 1988;150:794–801.
295. Marx J, Jacquot J, Berjot M, et al: Characterization and conformational analysis by Raman spectroscopy of human airway lysozyme. Biochim Biophys Acta 1986; 870:488–494.
296. Artymiuk PJ, Blake CC, Grace DE, et al: Crystallographic studies of the dynamic properties of lysozyme. Nature 1979;280:563–568.
297. Blake CC, Pulford WC, Artymiuk PJ: X-ray studies of water in crystals of lysozyme. J Mol Biol 1983;167: 693–723.
298. Artymiuk PJ, Blake CC: Refinement of human lysozyme at 1.5 Å resolution analysis of non-bonded and

hydrogen-bond interactions. J Mol Biol 1981;152: 737–762.

299. Berthou J, Lifchitz A, Artymiuk P, Jolles P: An X-ray study of the physiological-temperature form of hen egg-white lysozyme at 2 Å resolution. Proc R Soc Lond B Biol Sci 1983;217:471–489.

300. Perkins SJ, Johnson LN, Machin PA, Phillips DC: Crystal structures of egg-white lysozyme of hen in acetate-free medium and of lysozyme complexes with *N*-acetylglucosamine and beta-methyl *N*-acetylglucosaminide. Biochem J 1978;173:607–616.

301. White A, Handler P, Smith EL: Principles of Biochemistry, ed 5. New York, McGraw-Hill, 1973.

302. Baas F, Bikker H, Geurts VK, et al: The human thyroglobulin gene: A polymorphic marker localized distal to C-*MYC* on chromosome 8 band q24. Hum Genet 1985; 69:138–143.

303. Berge-Lefranc JL, Cartouzou G, Mattei MG, et al: Localization of the thyroglobulin gene by in situ hybridization to human chromosomes. Hum Genet 1985;69: 28–31.

304. Baas F, van Ommen GJ, Bikker H, et al: The human thyroglobulin gene is over 300 kb long and contains introns of up to 64 kb. Nucleic Acids Res 1986;14: 5171–5186.

305. Malthiery Y, Lissitzky S: Primary structure of human thyroglobulin deduced from the sequence of its 8448-base complementary DNA. Eur J Biochem 1987;165: 491–498.

306. Malthiery Y, Marriq C, Berge-Lefranc JL, et al: Thyroglobulin structure and function: Recent advances. Biochimie 1989;71:195–209.

307. Hansen C, Javaux F, Juvenal G, et al: cAMP-dependent binding of a *trans*-acting factor to the thyroglobulin promoter. Biochem Biophys Res Commun 1989;160: 722–731.

308. Libert F, Vassart G, Christophe D: Methylation and expression of the human thyroglobulin gene. Biochem Biophys Res Commun 1986;134:1109–1113.

309. Formisano S, Moscatelli C, Zarrilli R, et al: Prediction of the secondary structure of the carboxy-terminal third of rat thyroglobulin. Biochem Biophys Res Commun 1985;133:766–772.

310. Formisano S, Di Jeso B, Acquaviva R, et al: Calcium-induced changes in thyroglobulin conformation. Arch Biochem Biophys 1983;227:351–357.

311. Acquaviva R, Consiglio E, Di Jeso B, et al: Calcium interaction with bovine thyroglobulin: Stoichiometry and structural consequences of calcium binding. Mol Cell Endocrinol 1991;82:175–181.

312. Kiso Y, Furmaniak J, Morteo C, Smith BR: Analysis of carbohydrate residues on human thyroid peroxidase (TPO) and thyroglobulin (Tg) and effects of deglycosylation, reduction and unfolding on autoantibody binding. Autoimmunity 1992;12:259–269.

313. Kohno Y, Tarutani O, Sakata S, Nakajima H: Monoclonal antibodies to thyroglobulin elucidate differences in protein structure of thyroglobulin in healthy individuals and those with papillary adenocarcinoma. J Clin Endocrinol Metab 1985;61:343–350.

314. Narkar AA, Shah DH, Yadav J, et al: Monoclonal antibodies to human thyroglobulin: Evaluation of immunoreactivity. Hybridoma 1992;11:803–813.

315. Schrewe H, Thompson J, Bona M, et al: Cloning of the complete gene for carcinoembryonic antigen: Analysis of its promoter indicates a region conveying cell type-specific expression. Mol Cell Biol 1990;10: 2738–2748.

316. Nuti M, Teramoto YA, Mariani-Costantini R, et al: A monoclonal antibody (B72.3) defines patterns of distribution of a novel tumor-associated antigen in human mammary carcinoma cell populations. Int J Cancer 1982;29:539–545.

317. Tavassoli FA, Jones MW, Majeste RM, et al: Immunohistochemical staining with monoclonal Ab B72.3 in benign and malignant breast disease. Am J Surg Pathol 1990;14:128–133.

318. Latza U, Niedobitek G, Schwarting R, et al: Ber-EP4: New monoclonal antibody which distinguishes epithelia from mesothelia. J Clin Pathol 1990;43:213–219.

319. Jensen ML, Johansen P: Immunocytochemical staining of smears and corresponding cell blocks from serous effusions: A follow-up and comparative investigation. Diagn Cytopathol 1996;15:33–36.

320. Frisman DM, McCarthy WF, Schleiff P, et al: Immunocytochemistry in the differential diagnosis of effusions: Use of logistic regression to select a panel of antibodies to distinguish adenocarcinomas from mesothelial proliferations. Mod Pathol 1993;6:179–184.

321. Diaz-Arias AA, Loy TS, Bickel JT, Chapman RK: Utility of BER-EP4 in the diagnosis of adenocarcinoma in effusions: An immunocytochemical study of 232 cases. Diagn Cytopathol 1993;9:516–521.

322. Gaffey MJ, Mills SE, Swanson PE, et al: Immunoreactivity for BER-EP4 in adenocarcinomas, adenomatoid tumors, and malignant mesotheliomas. Am J Surg Pathol 1992;16:593–599.

323. Sheibani K, Shin SS, Kezirian J, Weiss LM: Ber-EP4 antibody as a discriminant in the differential diagnosis of malignant mesothelioma versus adenocarcinoma. Am J Surg Pathol 1991;15:779–784.

324. Riegman PH, Vlietstra RJ, van der Korput JA, et al: Characterization of the prostate-specific antigen gene: A novel human kallikrein-like gene. Biochem Biophys Res Commun 1989;159:95–102.

325. Sutherland GR, Baker E, Hyland VJ, et al: Human prostate-specific antigen (APS) is a member of the glandular kallikrein gene family at 19q13. Cytogenet Cell Genet 1988;48:205–207.

326. Riegman PH, Vlietstra RJ, Suurmeijer L, et al: Characterization of the human kallikrein locus. Genomics 1992;14:6–11.

327. Lundwall A, Lilja H: Molecular cloning of human prostate specific antigen cDNA. FEBS Lett 1987;214:317–322.

328. Schulz P, Stucka R, Feldmann H, et al: Sequence of a cDNA clone encompassing the complete mature human prostate-specific antigen (PSA) and an unspliced leader sequence. Nucleic Acids Res 1988;16:6226.

329. Sharief FS, Li SS: Nucleotide sequence of human prostatic acid phosphatase ACPP gene, including seven Alu repeats. Biochem Mol Biol Int 1994;33:561–565.

330. Li SS, Sharief FS: The prostatic acid phosphatase (ACPP) gene is localized to human chromosome 3q21–q23. Genomics 1993;17:765–766.

331. Sharief FS, Lee H, Leuderman MM, et al: Human prostatic acid phosphatase: cDNA cloning, gene mapping and protein sequence homology with lysosomal acid phosphatase. Biochem Biophys Res Commun 1989; 160:79–86.
332. Ostrowski W, Bhargava AK, Dziembor E, et al: Acid phosphomonoesterase of human prostate: Carbohydrate content and optical properties. Biochim Biophys Acta 1976;453:262–269.
333. Schneider G, Lindqvist Y, Vihko P: Three-dimensional structure of rat acid phosphatase. EMBO J 1993;12: 2609–2615.
334. Lindqvist Y, Schneider G, Vihko P: Crystal structures of rat acid phosphatase complexed with the transition-state analogs vanadate and molybdate: Implications for the reaction mechanism. Eur J Biochem 1994;221:139–142.
335. Tricoli JV, Shows TB: Regional assignment of human amylase (AMY) to p22–p21 of chromosome 1. Somat Cell Mol Genet 1984;10:205–210.
336. Groot PC, Mager WH, Frants RR, et al: The human amylase-encoding genes *amy2* and *amy3* are identical to *AMY2A* and *AMY2B*. Gene 1989;85:567–568.
337. Groot PC, Mager WH, Frants RR: Interpretation of polymorphic DNA patterns in the human alpha-amylase multigene family. Genomics 1991;10:779–785.
338. Brock A, Mortensen PB, Mortensen BB, Roge HR: Familial occurrence of diminished pancreatic amylase in serum—a "silent" Amy-2 allelic variant? Clin Chem 1988;34:1516–1517.
339. Scheerlinck JP, Lasters I, Claessens M, et al: Recurrent alpha beta loop structures in TIM barrel motifs show a distinct pattern of conserved structural features. Proteins 1992;12:299–313.
340. Bobek LA, Tsai H, Biesbrock AR, Levine MJ: Molecular cloning, sequence, and specificity of expression of the gene encoding the low molecular weight human salivary mucin (MUC7). J Biol Chem 1993;268:20563–20569.
341. Swallow DM, Gendler S, Griffiths B, et al: The hypervariable gene locus PUM, which codes for the tumour associated epithelial mucins, is located on chromosome 1, within the region 1q21–24. Ann Hum Genet 1987; 51(Pt 4):289–294.
342. Price MR, Hudecz F, O'Sullivan C, et al: Immunological and structural features of the protein core of human polymorphic epithelial mucin. Mol Immunol 1990;27: 795–802.
343. Vos HL, de Vries Y, Hilkens J: The mouse episialin *(Muc1)* gene and its promoter: Rapid evolution of the repetitive domain in the protein. Biochem Biophys Res Commun 1991;181:121–130.
344. Williams CJ, Wreschner DH, Tanaka A, et al: Multiple protein forms of the human breast tumor–associated epithelial membrane antigen (EMA) are generated by alternative splicing and induced by hormonal stimulation. Biochem Biophys Res Commun 1990;170:1331–1338.
345. Ligtenberg MJ, Kruijshaar L, Buijs F, et al: Cell-associated episialin is a complex containing two proteins derived from a common precursor. J Biol Chem 1992; 267:6171–6177.
346. Ligtenberg MJ, Buijs F, Vos HL, Hilkens J: Suppression of cellular aggregation by high levels of episialin. Cancer Res 1992;52:2318–2324.
347. Dion AS, Smorodinsky NI, Williams CJ, et al: Recognition of peptidyl epitopes by polymorphic epithelial mucin (PEM)-specific monoclonal antibodies. Hybridoma 1991;10:595–610.
348. Kligman D, Hilt DC: The S100 protein family. Trends Biochem Sci 1988;13:437–443.
349. St Charles R, Kumar VD: Crystallization and preliminary X-ray analysis of apo-S100 beta and S100 beta with Ca^{2+}. J Mol Biol 1994;236:953–957.
350. Barger SW, Van Eldik LJ: S100 beta stimulates calcium fluxes in glial and neuronal cells. J Biol Chem 1992;267: 9689–9694.
351. Kligman D, Marshak DR: Purification and characterization of a neurite extension factor from bovine brain. Proc Natl Acad Sci USA 1985;82:7136–7139.
352. Baudier J, Briving C, Deinum J, et al: Effect of S-100 proteins and calmodulin on Ca^{2+}-induced disassembly of brain microtubule proteins in vitro. FEBS Lett 1982;147:165–168.
353. Endo T, Hidaka H: Effect of S-100 protein on microtubule assembly-disassembly. FEBS Lett 1983;161: 235–238.
354. Baudier J, Delphin C, Grunwald D, et al: Characterization of the tumor suppressor protein p53 as a protein kinase C substrate and a S100b-binding protein. Proc Natl Acad Sci USA 1992;89:11627–11631.
355. Wu HJ, Rozansky DJ, Parmer RJ, et al: Structure and function of the chromogranin A gene: Clues to evolution and tissue-specific expression. J Biol Chem 1991; 266:13130–13134.
356. Modi WS, Levine MA, Seuanez HN, et al: The human chromogranin A gene: Chromosome assignment and RFLP analysis. Am J Hum Genet 1989;45:814–818.
357. Konecki DS, Benedum UM, Gerdes HH, Huttner WB: The primary structure of human chromogranin A and pancreastatin. J Biol Chem 1987;262:17026–17030.
358. Parmer RJ, Koop AH, Handa MT, O'Connor DT: Molecular cloning of chromogranin A from rat pheochromocytoma cells. Hypertension 1989;14:435–444.
359. Benedum UM, Lamouroux A, Konecki DS, et al: The primary structure of human secretogranin I (chromogranin B): Comparison with chromogranin A reveals homologous terminal domains and a large intervening variable region. EMBO J 1987;6:1203–1211.
360. Craig SP, Lamouroux A, Mallet J, et al: Localization of the human gene for secretogranin 1 (chromogranin B) to chromosome 20 [abstract]. Cytogenet Cell Genet 1987; 46:600.
361. Rosa P, Zanini A: Purification of a sulfated secretory protein from the adenohypophysis: Immunochemical evidence that similar macromolecules are present in other glands. Eur J Cell Biol 1983;31:94–98.
362. Yoo SH, Albanesi JP: High capacity, low affinity Ca^{2+} binding of chromogranin A: Relationship between the pH-induced conformational change and Ca^{2+} binding property. J Biol Chem 1991;266:7740–7745.
363. Yoo SH, Albanesi JP: Ca^{2+}-induced conformational change and aggregation of chromogranin A. J Biol Chem 1990;265:14414–14421.
364. Yoo SH, Lewis MS: pH-dependent interaction of an intraluminal loop of inositol 1,4,5-trisphosphate receptor with chromogranin A. FEBS Lett 1994;341:28–32.

365. Rehm H, Wiedenmann B, Betz H: Molecular characterization of synaptophysin, a major calcium-binding protein of the synaptic vesicle membrane. EMBO J 1986; 5:535–541.
366. Ozcelik T, Lafreniere RG, Archer BT, et al: Synaptophysin: Structure of the human gene and assignment to the X chromosome in man and mouse. Am J Hum Genet 1990;47:551–561.
367. Sudhof TC, Lottspeich F, Greengard P, et al: A synaptic vesicle protein with a novel cytoplasmic domain and four transmembrane regions. Science 1987;238:1142–1144.
368. Sudhof TC, Lottspeich F, Greengard P, et al: The cDNA and derived amino acid sequences for rat and human synaptophysin. Nucleic Acids Res 1987;15: 9607.
369. Matsushima N, Creutz CE, Kretsinger RH: Polyproline, beta-turn helices: Novel secondary structures proposed for the tandem repeats within rhodopsin, synaptophysin, synexin, gliadin, RNA polymerase II, hordein, and gluten. Proteins 1990;7:125–155.
370. Oliva D, Cali L, Feo S, Giallongo A: Complete structure of the human gene encoding neuron-specific enolase. Genomics 1991;10:157–165.
371. Mattei JF, Baeteman MA, Mattei MG, et al: Regional assignments of CS and ENO2 on chromosome 12 [abstract]. Cytogenet Cell Genet 1982;32:297.
372. Lebioda L, Stec B: Crystal structure of enolase indicates that enolase and pyruvate kinase evolved from a common ancestor. Nature 1988;333:683–686.
373. Rice PA, Goldman A, Steitz TA: A helix-turn-strand structural motif common in alpha-beta proteins. Proteins 1990;8:334–340.
374. Lebioda L, Stec B: Mechanism of enolase: The crystal structure of enolase-$Mg^{2(+)}$-2-phosphoglycerate/phosphoenolpyruvate complex at 2.2—Å resolution. Biochemistry 1991;30:2817–2822.
375. Zhang E, Hatada M, Brewer JM, Lebioda L: Catalytic metal ion binding in enolase: The crystal structure of an enolase-Mn^{2+}-phosphonoacetohydroxamate complex at 2.4-Å resolution. Biochemistry 1994;33:6295–6300.
376. Glenner GG, Wong CW, Quaranta V, Eanes ED: The amyloid deposits in Alzheimer's disease: Their nature and pathogenesis. Appl Pathol 1984;2:357–369.
377. Masters CL, Simms G, Weinman NA, et al: Amyloid plaque core protein in Alzheimer disease and Down syndrome. Proc Natl Acad Sci USA 1985;82:4245–4249.
378. Yoshikai S, Sasaki H, Doh-ura K, et al: Genomic organization of the human amyloid beta-protein precursor gene [published erratum appears in Gene 1991;102: 291–292]. Gene 1990;87:257–263.
379. Blanquet V, Goldgaber D, Turleau C, et al: The beta amyloid protein (AD-AP) cDNA hybridizes in normal and Alzheimer individuals near the interface of 21q21 and q22.1. Ann Genet 1987;30:68–69.
380. Kang J, Lemaire HG, Unterbeck A, et al: The precursor of Alzheimer's disease amyloid A4 protein resembles a cell-surface receptor. Nature 1987;325:733–736.
381. Lawrence S, Keats BJ, Morton NE: The AD1 locus in familial Alzheimer disease. Ann Hum Genet 1992; 56(Pt 4):295–301.
382. Tanzi RE, Vaula G, Romano DM, et al: Assessment of amyloid beta-protein precursor gene mutations in a large set of familial and sporadic Alzheimer disease cases. Am J Hum Genet 1992;51:273–282.
383. Kamino K, Orr HT, Payami H, et al: Linkage and mutational analysis of familial Alzheimer disease kindreds for the APP gene region. Am J Hum Genet 1992;51:998–1014.
384. Ozkaynak E, Finley D, Varshavsky A: The yeast ubiquitin gene: Head-to-tail repeats encoding a polyubiquitin precursor protein. Nature 1984;312:663–666.
385. Orlowski M: The multicatalytic proteinase complex, a major extralysosomal proteolytic system. Biochemistry 1990;29:10289–10297.
386. Busch H: Ubiquitination of proteins. Methods Enzymol 1984;106:238–262.
387. Hershko A, Heller H, Eytan E, et al: Role of the alpha-amino group of protein in ubiquitin-mediated protein breakdown. Proc Natl Acad Sci USA 1984;81: 7021–7025.
388. Webb GC, Baker RT, Fagan K, Board PG: Localization of the human UbB polyubiquitin gene to chromosome band 17p11.1–17p12. Am J Hum Genet 1990;46: 308–315.
389. Webb GC, Baker RT, Coggan M, Board PG: Localization of the human UBA52 ubiquitin fusion gene to chromosome band 19p13.1–p12. Genomics 1994;19: 567–569.
390. Ecker DJ, Butt TR, Marsh J, et al: Ubiquitin function studied by disulfide engineering. J Biol Chem 1989; 264:1887–1893.
391. Weber PL, Brown SC, Mueller L: Sequential 1H NMR assignments and secondary structure identification of human ubiquitin. Biochemistry 1987;26:7282–7290.
392. Di Stefano DL, Wand AJ: Two-dimensional 1H NMR study of human ubiquitin: A main chain directed assignment and structure analysis. Biochemistry 1987;26: 7272–7281.
393. Vijay-Kumar S, Bugg CE, Cook WJ: Structure of ubiquitin refined at 1.8 Å resolution. J Mol Biol 1987; 194:531–544.
394. Neve RL, Harris P, Kosik KS, et al: Identification of cDNA clones for the human microtubule-associated protein tau and chromosomal localization of the genes for tau and microtubule-associated protein 2. Brain Res 1986;387:271–280.
395. Mavilia C, Couchie D, Mattei MG, et al: High and low molecular weight tau proteins are differentially expressed from a single gene. J Neurochem 1993;61: 1073–1081.
396. Ruben GC, Iqbal K, Grundke-Iqbal I, et al: The microtubule-associated protein tau forms a triple-stranded left-hand helical polymer [published erratum appears in J Biol Chem 1992;267:5013–5015]. J Biol Chem 1991;266:22019–22027.
397. Butner KA, Kirschner MW: Tau protein binds to microtubules through a flexible array of distributed weak sites. J Cell Biol 1991;115:717–730.
398. Goode BL, Feinstein SC: Identification of a novel microtubule binding and assembly domain in the developmentally regulated inter-repeat region of tau. J Cell Biol 1994;124:769–782.
399. Shea TB, Beermann ML, Nixon RA, Fischer I: Microtubule-associated protein tau is required for axonal neurite

elaboration by neuroblastoma cells. J Neurosci Res 1992;32:363–374.
400. Wu JM, Chen Y, An S, et al: Phosphorylation of protein tau by double-stranded DNA-dependent protein kinase. Biochem Biophys Res Commun 1993;193:13–18.
401. Roder HM, Ingram VM: Two novel kinases phosphorylate tau and the KSP site of heavy neurofilament subunits in high stoichiometric ratios. J Neurosci 1991;11:3325–3343.
402. Takashima A, Noguchi K, Sato K, et al: Tau protein kinase I is essential for amyloid beta-protein-induced neurotoxicity. Proc Natl Acad Sci USA 1993;90:7789–7793.
403. Schadendorf D, Gawlik C, Haney U, et al: Tumour progression and metastatic behaviour in vivo correlates with integrin expression on melanocytic tumours. J Pathol 1993;170:429–434.
404. Terpe HJ, Tajrobehkar K, Gunthert U, Altmannsberger M: Expression of cell adhesion molecules alpha-2, alpha-5 and alpha-6 integrin, E-cadherin, N-CAM, and CD-44 in renal cell carcinomas: An immunohistochemical study. Virchows Arch A Pathol Anat Histopathol 1993;422:219–224.
405. Bartolazzi A, Cerboni C, Nicotra MR, et al: Transformation and tumor progression are frequently associated with expression of the alpha 3/beta 1 heterodimer in solid tumors. Int J Cancer 1994;58:488–491.
406. Ogawa T, Yorioka N, Yamakido M: Immunohistochemical studies of vitronectin, C5b-9, and vitronectin receptor in membranous nephropathy. Nephron 1994;68:87–96.
407. Weitzman JB, Wells CE, Wright AH, et al: The gene organisation of the human beta 2 integrin subunit (CD18). FEBS Lett 1991;294:97–103.
408. Petersen MB, Slaugenhaupt SA, Lewis JG, et al: A genetic linkage map of 27 markers on human chromosome 21. Genomics 1991;9:407–419.
409. Kishimoto TK, Hollander N, Roberts TM, et al: Heterogeneous mutations in the beta subunit common to the LFA-1, Mac-1, and p150,95 glycoproteins cause leukocyte adhesion deficiency. Cell 1987;50:193–202.
410. Hogervorst F, Kuikman I, van Kessel AG, Sonnenberg A: Molecular cloning of the human alpha 6 integrin subunit: Alternative splicing of alpha 6 mRNA and chromosomal localization of the alpha 6 and beta 4 genes. Eur J Biochem 1991;199:425–433.
411. Pfaff M, Tangemann K, Muller B, et al: Selective recognition of cyclic RGD peptides of NMR defined conformation by alpha IIb beta 3, alpha V beta 3, and alpha 5 beta 1 integrins. J Biol Chem 1994;269:20233–20238.
412. Tuckwell DS, Ayad S, Grant ME, et al: Conformation dependence of integrin-type II collagen binding: Inability of collagen peptides to support alpha 2 beta 1 binding, and mediation of adhesion to denatured collagen by a novel alpha 5 beta 1-fibronectin bridge. J Cell Sci 1994;107(Pt 4):993–1005.
413. Tuckwell DS, Weston SA, Humphries MJ: Integrins: A review of their structure and mechanisms of ligand binding. Symp Soc Exp Biol 1993;47:107–136.
414. Kageshita T, Yoshii A, Kimura T, et al: Clinical relevance of ICAM-1 expression in primary lesions and serum of patients with malignant melanoma. Cancer Res 1993;53:4927–4932.
415. Sligh JEJ, Ballantyne CM, Rich SS, et al: Inflammatory and immune responses are impaired in mice deficient in intercellular adhesion molecule 1. Proc Natl Acad Sci USA 1993;90:8529–8533.
416. Greve JM, Davis G, Meyer AM, et al: The major human rhinovirus receptor is ICAM-1. Cell 1989;56:839–847.
417. Trask B, Fertitta A, Christensen M, et al: Fluorescence in situ hybridization mapping of human chromosome 19: Cytogenetic band location of 540 cosmids and 70 genes or DNA markers. Genomics 1993;15:133–145.
418. Simmons D, Makgoba MW, Seed B: ICAM, an adhesion ligand of LFA-1, is homologous to the neural cell adhesion molecule NCAM. Nature 1988;331:624–627.
419. Kolatkar PR, Oliveira MA, Rossmann MG, et al: Preliminary X-ray crystallographic analysis of intercellular adhesion molecule-1. J Mol Biol 1992;225:1127–1130.
420. Kirchhausen T, Staunton DE, Springer TA: Location of the domains of ICAM-1 by immunolabeling and single-molecule electron microscopy. J Leukoc Biol 1993;53:342–346.
421. Pujol JL, Simony J, Demoly P, et al: Neural cell adhesion molecule and prognosis of surgically resected lung cancer. Am Rev Respir Dis 1993;148(4 Pt 1):1071–1075.
422. Bello MJ, Salagnon N, Rey JA, et al: Precise in situ localization of NCAM, ETS1, and D11S29 on human meiotic chromosomes. Cytogenet Cell Genet 1989;52:7–10.
423. Cunningham BA, Hemperly JJ, Murray BA, et al: Neural cell adhesion molecule: Structure, immunoglobulin-like domains, cell surface modulation, and alternative RNA splicing. Science 1987;236:799–806.
424. Rutishauser U, Acheson A, Hall AK, et al: The neural cell adhesion molecule (NCAM) as a regulator of cell-cell interactions. Science 1988;240:53–57.
425. Yurchenco PD, Ruben GC: Basement membrane structure in situ: Evidence for lateral associations in the type IV collagen network. J Cell Biol 1987;105:2559–2568.
426. Bella J, Eaton M, Brodsky B, Berman HM: Crystal and molecular structure of a collagen-like peptide at 1.9-Å resolution [see comments]. Science 1994;266:75–81.
427. Lazarev YA, Grishkovsky BA, Khromova TB, et al: Bound water in the collagen-like triple-helical structure. Biopolymers 1992;32:189–195.
428. Bachinger HP, Davis JM: Sequence specific thermal stability of the collagen triple helix. Int J Biol Macromol 1991;13:152–156.
429. Eble JA, Golbik R, Mann K, Kuhn K: The alpha 1 beta 1 integrin recognition site of the basement membrane collagen molecule [alpha 1(IV)]2 alpha 2(IV). EMBO J 1993;12:4795–4802.
430. Nomizu M, Otaka A, Utani A, et al: Assembly of synthetic laminin peptides into a triple-stranded coiled-coil structure. J Biol Chem 1994;269:30386–30392.
431. Beck K, Hunter I, Engel J: Structure and function of laminin: Anatomy of a multidomain glycoprotein. FASEB J 1990;4:148–160.
432. Nagayoshi T, Mattei MG, Passage E, et al: Human laminin A chain (LAMA) gene: Chromosomal mapping to locus 18p11.3. Genomics 1989;5:932–935.

433. Haaparanta T, Uitto J, Ruoslahti E, Engvall E: Molecular cloning of the cDNA encoding human laminin A chain. Matrix 1991;11:151–160.
434. Vuolteenaho R, Nissinen M, Sainio K, et al: Human laminin M chain (merosin): Complete primary structure, chromosomal assignment, and expression of the M and A chain in human fetal tissues. J Cell Biol 1994;124: 381–394.
435. Pikkarainen T, Eddy R, Fukushima Y, et al: Human laminin B1 chain: A multidomain protein with gene *(LAMB1)* locus in the q22 region of chromosome 7. J Biol Chem 1987;262:10454–10462.
436. Fukushima Y, Pikkarainen T, Kallunki T, et al: Isolation of a human laminin B2 *(LAMB2)* cDNA clone and assignment of the gene to chromosome region 1q25–q31. Cytogenet Cell Genet 1988;48:137–141.
437. Pikkarainen T, Kallunki T, Tryggvason K: Human laminin B2 chain: Comparison of the complete amino acid sequence with the B1 chain reveals variability in sequence homology between different structural domains. J Biol Chem 1988;263:6751–6758.
438. Sasaki M, Yamada Y: The laminin B2 chain has a multidomain structure homologous to the B1 chain. J Biol Chem 1987;262:17111–17117.
439. Paulsson M, Deutzmann R, Timpl R, et al: Evidence for coiled-coil alpha-helical regions in the long arm of laminin. EMBO J 1985;4:309–316.
440. Charonis AS, Tsilibary EC, Saku T, Furthmayr H: Inhibition of laminin self-assembly and interaction with type IV collagen by antibodies to the terminal domain of the long arm. J Cell Biol 1986;103:1689–1697.
441. Utani A, Nomizu M, Timpl R, et al: Laminin chain assembly: Specific sequences at the C terminus of the long arm are required for the formation of specific double- and triple-stranded coiled-coil structures. J Biol Chem 1994;269:19167–19175.
442. Beck K, Dixon TW, Engel J, Parry DA: Ionic interactions in the coiled-coil domain of laminin determine the specificity of chain assembly. J Mol Biol 1993;231:311–323.
443. Lissitzky JC, Cantau P, Martin PM: Heterotrimeric configuration is essential to the adhesive function of laminin. J Cell Biochem 1992;48:141–149.
444. Jhanwar SC, Jensen JT, Kaelbling M, et al: In situ localization of human fibronectin (FN) genes to chromosome regions 2p14–p16, 2q34–q36, and 11q12.1–q13.5 in germ line cells, but to chromosome 2 sites only in somatic cells. Cytogenet Cell Genet 1986;41:47–53.
445. Schwarzbauer JE, Spencer CS, Wilson CL: Selective secretion of alternatively spliced fibronectin variants. J Cell Biol 1989;109(6 Pt 2):3445–3453.
446. Erickson HP: Reversible unfolding of fibronectin type III and immunoglobulin domains provides the structural basis for stretch and elasticity of titin and fibronectin. Proc Natl Acad Sci USA 1994;91:10114–10118.
447. Baron M, Main AL, Driscoll PC, et al: 1H NMR assignment and secondary structure of the cell adhesion type III module of fibronectin. Biochemistry 1992;31: 2068–2073.
448. Jeffreys AJ, Wilson V, Blanchetot A, et al: The human myoglobin gene: A third dispersed globin locus in the human genome. Nucleic Acids Res 1984;12:3235–3243.
449. Akaboshi E: Cloning of the human myoglobin gene. Gene 1985;33:241–249.
450. Dong A, Huang P, Caughey WS: Protein secondary structures in water from second-derivative amide I infrared spectra. Biochemistry 1990;29:3303–3308.
451. Hubbard SR, Hendrickson WA, Lambright DG, Boxer SG: X-ray crystal structure of a recombinant human myoglobin mutant at 2.8 Å resolution. J Mol Biol 1990;213:215–218.
452. Vandekerckhove J, Weber K: Mammalian cytoplasmic actins are the products of at least two genes and differ in primary structure in at least 25 identified positions from skeletal muscle actins. Proc Natl Acad Sci USA 1978;75:1106–1110.
453. Kedes L, Ng SY, Lin CS, et al: The human beta-actin multigene family. Trans Assoc Am Physicians 1985;98: 42–46.
454. Humphries SE, Whittall R, Minty A, et al: There are approximately 20 actin gene in the human genome. Nucleic Acids Res 1981;9:4895–4908.
455. Gunning P, Ponte P, Kedes L, et al: Chromosomal location of the co-expressed human skeletal and cardiac actin genes. Proc Natl Acad Sci USA 1984;81:1813–1817.
456. Buckingham M, Alonso S, Barton P, et al: Actin and myosin multigene families: Their expression during the formation and maturation of striated muscle. Am J Med Genet 1986;25:623–634.
457. Hamada H, Petrino MG, Kakunaga T: Molecular structure and evolutionary origin of human cardiac muscle actin gene. Proc Natl Acad Sci USA 1982; 79:5901–5905.
458. Akkari PA, Eyre HJ, Wilton SD, et al: Assignment of the human skeletal muscle alpha actin gene (ACTA1) to 1q42 by fluorescence in situ hybridisation. Cytogenet Cell Genet 1994;65:265–267.
459. Miwa T, Manabe Y, Kurokawa K, et al: Structure, chromosome location, and expression of the human smooth muscle (enteric type) gamma-actin gene: Evolution of six human actin genes. Mol Cell Biol 1991;11: 3296–3306.
460. Habets GG, van der Kammen RA, Willemsen V, et al: Sublocalization of an invasion-inducing locus and other genes on human chromosome 7. Cytogenet Cell Genet 1992;60:200–205.
461. Erba HP, Eddy R, Shows T, et al: Structure, chromosome location, and expression of the human gamma-actin gene: Differential evolution, location, and expression of the cytoskeletal beta- and gamma-actin genes. Mol Cell Biol 1988;8:1775–1789.
462. Wu CS, Yang JT: Reexamination of the conformation of muscle proteins by optical activity. Biochemistry 1976; 15:3007–3014.
463. Toyoshima C, Wakabayashi T: Three-dimensional image analysis of the complex of thin filaments and myosin molecules from skeletal muscle: I. Tilt angle of myosin subfragment-1 in the rigor complex. J Biochem (Tokyo) 1979;86:1887–1890.
464. Heuser JE, Cooke R: Actin-myosin interactions visualized by the quick-freeze, deep-etch replica technique. J Mol Biol 1983;169:97–122.
465. Holmes KC, Goody RS: The molecular basis of muscle contraction. Ciba Found Symp 1983;93:139–155.

466. Censullo R, Cheung HC: Tropomyosin length and two-stranded F-actin flexibility in the thin filament. J Mol Biol 1994;243:520–529.
467. Clark GM, McGuire WL: Steroid receptors and other prognostic factors in primary breast cancer. Semin Oncol 1988;15(2 Suppl 1):20–25.
468. Ponglikitmongkol M, Green S, Chambon P: Genomic organization of the human oestrogen receptor gene. EMBO J 1988;7:3385–3388.
469. Menasce LP, White GR, Harrison CJ, Boyle JM: Localization of the estrogen receptor locus (ESR) to chromosome 6q25.1 by FISH and a simple post-FISH banding technique. Genomics 1993;17:263–265.
470. Greene GL, Gilna P, Waterfield M, et al: Sequence and expression of human estrogen receptor complementary DNA. Science 1986;231:1150–1154.
471. Katahira M, Knegtel RM, Boelens R, et al: Homo- and heteronuclear NMR studies of the human retinoic acid receptor beta DNA-binding domain: Sequential assignments and identification of secondary structure elements. Biochemistry 1992;31:6474–6480.
472. Schwabe JW, Neuhaus D, Rhodes D: Solution structure of the DNA-binding domain of the oestrogen receptor. Nature 1990;348:458–461.
473. Fritsch M, Leary CM, Furlow JD, et al: A ligand-induced conformational change in the estrogen receptor is localized in the steroid binding domain. Biochemistry 1992;31:5303–5311.
474. Beekman JM, Allan GF, Tsai SY, et al: Transcriptional activation by the estrogen receptor requires a conformational change in the ligand binding domain. Mol Endocrinol 1993;7:1266–1274.
475. Sabbah M, Gouilleux F, Sola B, et al: Structural differences between the hormone and antihormone estrogen receptor complexes bound to the hormone response element. Proc Natl Acad Sci USA 1991;88:390–394.
476. Schwartz JA, Skafar DF: Ligand-mediated modulation of estrogen receptor conformation by estradiol analogs. Biochemistry 1993;32:10109–10115.
477. Schwabe JW, Chapman L, Finch JT, Rhodes D: The crystal structure of the estrogen receptor DNA-binding domain bound to DNA: How receptors discriminate between their response elements. Cell 1993;75:567–578.
478. Ruh MF, Turner JW, Paulson CM, Ruh TS: Differences in the form of the salt-transformed estrogen receptor when bound by estrogen versus antiestrogen. J Steroid Biochem 1990;36:509–516.
479. Fritsch M, Welch RD, Murdoch FE, et al: DNA allosterically modulates the steroid binding domain of the estrogen receptor. J Biol Chem 1992;267:1823–1828.
480. Traish AM, Netsuwan N: 7-Alpha-17-alpha-dimethyl-19-nortestosterone (mibolerone) induces conformational changes in progesterone receptors distinct from those induced by ORG 2058. Steroids 1994;59:362–370.
481. Mattei MG, Krust A, Stropp U, et al: Assignment of the human progesterone receptor to the q22 band of chromosome 11 using in situ hybridization [abstract]. Cytogenet Cell Genet 1987;46:658.
482. Mattei MG, Krust A, Stropp U, et al: Assignment of the human progesterone receptor to the q22 band of chromosome 11. Hum Genet 1988;78:96–97.
483. Misrahi M, Atger M, d'Auriol L, et al: Complete amino acid sequence of the human progesterone receptor deduced from cloned cDNA. Biochem Biophys Res Commun 1987;143:740–748.
484. Truss M, Chalepakis G, Slater EP, et al: Functional interaction of hybrid response elements with wild-type and mutant steroid hormone receptors. Mol Cell Biol 1991;11:3247–3258.
485. Allan GF, Tsai SY, Tsai MJ, O'Malley BW: Ligand-dependent conformational changes in the progesterone receptor are necessary for events that follow DNA binding. Proc Natl Acad Sci USA 1992;89:11750–11754.
486. Allan GF, Leng X, Tsai SY, et al: Hormone and antihormone induce distinct conformational changes which are central to steroid receptor activation. J Biol Chem 1992;267:19513–19520.
487. Skafar DF: Differential DNA binding by calf uterine estrogen and progesterone receptors results from differences in oligomeric states. Biochemistry 1991;30:6148–6154.
488. Chang CS, Kokontis J, Liao ST: Molecular cloning of human and rat complementary DNA encoding androgen receptors. Science 1988;240:324–326.
489. Lubahn DB, Joseph DR, Sullivan PM, et al: Cloning of human androgen receptor complementary DNA and localization to the X chromosome. Science 1988;240:327–330.
490. Brown CJ, Goss SJ, Lubahn DB, et al: Androgen receptor locus on the human X chromosome: Regional localization to Xq11–12 and description of a DNA polymorphism. Am J Hum Genet 1989;44:264–269.
491. Lubahn DB, Joseph DR, Sar M, et al: The human androgen receptor: Complementary deoxyribonucleic acid cloning, sequence analysis and gene expression in prostate. Mol Endocrinol 1988;2:1265–1275.
492. Zhou ZX, Wong CI, Sar M, Wilson EM: The androgen receptor: An overview. Recent Prog Horm Res 1994;49:249–274.
493. Kuil CW, Mulder E: Mechanism of antiandrogen action: Conformational changes of the receptor. Mol Cell Endocrinol 1994;102:R1–R5.
494. Kallio PJ, Janne OA, Palvimo JJ: Agonists, but not antagonists, alter the conformation of the hormone-binding domain of androgen receptor. Endocrinology 1994;134:998–1001.
495. La Spada AR, Wilson EM, Lubahn DB, et al: Androgen receptor gene mutations in X-linked spinal and bulbar muscular atrophy. Nature 1991;352:77–79.
496. La Spada AR, Paulson HL, Fischbeck KH: Trinucleotide repeat expansion in neurological disease. Ann Neurol 1994;36:814–822.
497. Brown TR, Lubahn DB, Wilson EM, et al: Deletion of the steroid-binding domain of the human androgen receptor gene in one family with complete androgen insensitivity syndrome: Evidence for further genetic heterogeneity in this syndrome. Proc Natl Acad Sci USA 1988;85:8151–8155.
498. Griffin JE: Androgen resistance—the clinical and molecular spectrum. N Engl J Med 1992;326:611–618.

499. Gaddipati JP, McLeod DG, Heidenberg HB, et al: Frequent detection of codon 877 mutation in the androgen receptor gene in advanced prostate cancers. Cancer Res 1994;54:2861–2864.
500. Haley J, Whittle N, Bennet P, et al: The human EGF receptor gene: Structure of the 110 kb locus and identification of sequences regulating its transcription. Oncogene Res 1987;1:375–396.
501. Shimizu N, Behzadian MA, Shimizu Y: Genetics of cell surface receptors for bioactive polypeptides: Binding of epidermal growth factor is associated with the presence of human chromosome 7 in human-mouse cell hybrids. Proc Natl Acad Sci USA 1980;77:3600–3604.
502. Carlin CR, Knowles BB: Identity of human epidermal growth factor (EGF) receptor with glycoprotein SA-7: Evidence for differential phosphorylation of the two components of the EGF receptor from A431 cells. Proc Natl Acad Sci USA 1982;79:5026–5030.
503. Kondo I, Shimizu N: Mapping of the human gene for epidermal growth factor receptor (EGFR) on the p13 leads to q22 region of chromosome 7. Cytogenet Cell Genet 1983;35:9–14.
504. Cadena DL, Chan CL, Gill GN: The intracellular tyrosine kinase domain of the epidermal growth factor receptor undergoes a conformational change upon autophosphorylation. J Biol Chem 1994;269: 260–265.
505. Slamon DJ, Godolphin W, Jones LA, et al: Studies of the HER-2/neu proto-oncogene in human breast and ovarian cancer. Science 1989;244:707–712.
506. Muss HB, Thor AD, Berry DA, et al: c-erbB-2 expression and response to adjuvant therapy in women with node-positive early breast cancer [see comments] [published erratum appears in N Engl J Med 1994;331: 211]. N Engl J Med 1994;330:1260–1266.
507. Pegram MD, Lipton A, Hayes DF, et al: Phase II study of receptor-enhanced chemosensitivity using recombinant humanized anti-p185HER2/neu monoclonal antibody plus cisplatin in patients with HER2/neu-overexpressing metastatic breast cancer refractory to chemotherapy treatment. J Clin Oncol 1998;16: 2659–2671.
508. Baselga J, Norton L, Albanell J, et al: Recombinant humanized anti-HER2 antibody (Herceptin) enhances the antitumor activity of paclitaxel and doxorubicin against HER2/neu overexpressing human breast cancer xenografts. Cancer Res 1998;58:2825–2831.
509. Coussens L, Yang-Feng TL, Liao YC, et al: Tyrosine kinase receptor with extensive homology to EGF receptor shares chromosomal location with neu oncogene. Science 1985;230:1132–1139.
510. Yang-Feng TL, Schechter AL, Weinberg RA, et al: Oncogene from rat neuro/glioblastomas (human gene symbol *NGL*) is located on the proximal long arm of human chromosome 17 and EGFR is confirmed at 17p13–q11.2 [abstract]. Cytogenet Cell Genet 1985;40:7084.
511. Akiyama T, Sudo C, Ogawara H, et al: The product of the human c-*erbB-2* gene: A 185-kilodalton glycoprotein with tyrosine kinase activity. Science 1986;232:1644–1646.
512. Di Fiore PP, Pierce JH, Kraus MH, et al: *erbB-2* is a potent oncogene when overexpressed in NIH/3T3 cells. Science 1987;237:178–182.
513. Qian X, LeVea CM, Freeman JK, et al: Heterodimerization of epidermal growth factor receptor and wild-type or kinase-deficient Neu: A mechanism of interreceptor kinase activation and transphosphorylation. Proc Natl Acad Sci USA 1994;91:1500–1504.
514. Holmes WE, Sliwkowski MX, Akita RW, et al: Identification of heregulin, a specific activator of p185erbB2. Science 1992;256:1205–1210.
515. van Tuinen P, Ledbetter DH: Construction and utilization of a detailed somatic cell hybrid mapping panel for human chromosome 17: Localization of an anonymous clone to the critical region of Miller-Dieker syndrome, deletion 17p13 [abstract]. Cytogenet Cell Genet 1987; 46:708–709.
516. Vogelstein B, Kinzler KW: p53 function and dysfunction. Cell 1992;70:523–526.
517. Reisman D, Greenberg M, Rotter V: Human p53 oncogene contains one promoter upstream of exon 1 and a second, stronger promoter within intron 1. Proc Natl Acad Sci USA 1988;85:5146–5150.
518. Cho Y, Gorina S, Jeffrey PD, Pavletich NP: Crystal structure of a p53 tumor suppressor-DNA complex: Understanding tumorigenic mutations [see comments]. Science 1994;265:346–355.
519. el-Deiry WS, Tokino T, Velculescu VE, et al: WAF1, a potential mediator of p53 tumor suppression. Cell 1993; 75:817–825.
520. Harper JW, Adami GR, Wei N, et al: The p21 Cdk-interacting protein Cip1 is a potent inhibitor of G1 cyclin-dependent kinases. Cell 1993;75:805–816.
521. Levine AJ, Momand J, Finlay CA: The p53 tumour suppressor gene. Nature 1991;351:453–456.
522. Malkin D, Li FP, Strong LC, et al: Germ line p53 mutations in a familial syndrome of breast cancer, sarcomas, and other neoplasms [see comments]. Science 1990;250: 1233–1238.
523. Malkin D, Friend SH, Li FP, Strong LC: Germ-line mutations of the p53 tumor-suppressor gene in children and young adults with second malignant neoplasms [letter]. N Engl J Med 1997;336:734.
524. Malkin D, Friend SH: Correction: A Li-Fraumeni syndrome p53 mutation [letter; comment]. Science 1993; 259:878.
525. Fonatsch C, Duchrow M, Rieder H, et al: Assignment of the human Ki-67 gene (MK167) to 10q25-qter. Genomics 1991;11:476–477.
526. Webb G, Parsons P, Chenevix-Trench G: Localization of the gene for human proliferating nuclear antigen/cyclin by in situ hybridization. Hum Genet 1990;86:84–86.
527. Rao VV, Schnittger S, Hansmann I: Chromosomal localization of the human proliferating cell nuclear antigen *(PCNA)* gene to or close to 20p12 by in situ hybridization. Cytogenet Cell Genet 1991;56:169–170.
528. Tinker RL, Kassavetis GA, Geiduschek EP: Detecting the ability of viral, bacterial and eukaryotic replication proteins to track along DNA. EMBO J 1994;13: 5330–5337.
529. Chang CD, Ottavio L, Travali S, et al: Transcriptional and posttranscriptional regulation of the proliferating cell nuclear antigen gene. Mol Cell Biol 1990;10: 3289–3296.

530. Tsujimoto Y, Finger LR, Yunis J, et al: Cloning of the chromosome breakpoint of neoplastic B cells with the t (14;18) chromosome translocation. Science 1984;*226*: 1097–1099.
531. Pegoraro L, Palumbo A, Erikson J, et al: A 14;18 and an 8;14 chromosome translocation in a cell line derived from an acute B-cell leukemia. Proc Natl Acad Sci USA 1984;81:7166–7170.
532. Nakai M, Takeda A, Cleary ML, Endo T: The bcl-2 protein is inserted into the outer membrane but not into the inner membrane of rat liver mitochondria in vitro. Biochem Biophys Res Commun 1993;196:233–239.
533. McDonnell TJ, Deane N, Platt FM, et al: bcl-2-immunoglobulin transgenic mice demonstrate extended B cell survival and follicular lymphoproliferation. Cell 1989; 57:79–88.
534. Silvestrini R, Veneroni S, Daidone MG, et al: The Bcl-2 protein: A prognostic indicator strongly related to p53 protein in lymph node-negative breast cancer patients. J Natl Cancer Inst 1994;86:499–504.
535. Pezzella F, Jones M, Ralfkiaer E, et al: Evaluation of bcl-2 protein expression and 14;18 translocation as prognostic markers in follicular lymphoma. Br J Cancer 1992; 65:87–89.
536. Chen-Levy Z, Cleary ML: Membrane topology of the Bcl-2 proto-oncogenic protein demonstrated in vitro. J Biol Chem 1990;265:4929–4933.
537. Steeg PS, Bevilacqua G, Kopper L, et al: Evidence for a novel gene associated with low tumor metastatic potential. J Natl Cancer Inst 1988;80:200–204.
538. Golden A, Benedict M, Shearn A, et al: Nucleoside diphosphate kinases, nm23, and tumor metastasis: Possible biochemical mechanisms. Cancer Treat Res 1992; 63:345–358.
539. Kelsell DP, Black DM, Solomon E, Spurr NK: Localization of a second NM23 gene, NME2, to chromosome 17q21–q22. Genomics 1993;17:522–524.
540. Backer JM, Mendola CE, Kovesdi I, et al: Chromosomal localization and nucleoside diphosphate kinase activity of human metastasis-suppressor genes *NM23-1* and *NM23-2*. Oncogene 1993;8:497–502.
541. Campo E, Miquel R, Jares P, et al: Prognostic significance of the loss of heterozygosity of *Nm23-H1* and *p53* genes in human colorectal carcinomas. Cancer 1994;73:2913–2921.
542. Bevilacqua G, Sobel ME, Liotta LA, Steeg PS: Association of low nm23 RNA levels in human primary infiltrating ductal breast carcinomas with lymph node involvement and other histopathological indicators of high metastatic potential. Cancer Res 1989;49: 5185–5190.
543. Lu C, Kerbel RS: Cytokines, growth factors and the loss of negative growth controls in the progression of human cutaneous malignant melanoma. Curr Opin Oncol 1994;6:212–220.
544. Porter-Jordan K, Lippman ME: Overview of the biologic markers of breast cancer. Hematol Oncol Clin North Am 1994;8:73–100.
545. Konishi N, Nakaoka S, Tsuzuki T, et al: Expression of nm23-H1 and nm23-H2 proteins in prostate carcinoma. Jpn J Cancer Res 1993;84:1050–1054.
546. Dumas C, Lascu I, Morera S, et al: X-ray structure of nucleoside diphosphate kinase. EMBO J 1992;11: 3203–3208.
547. Augereau P, Garcia M, Mattei MG, et al: Cloning and sequencing of the 52K cathepsin D complementary deoxyribonucleic acid of MCF7 breast cancer cells and mapping on chromosome 11. Mol Endocrinol 1988; 2:186–192.
548. Faust PL, Kornfeld S, Chirgwin JM: Cloning and sequence analysis of cDNA for human cathepsin D. Proc Natl Acad Sci USA 1985;82:4910–4914.
549. Tang J, Wong RN: Evolution in the structure and function of aspartic proteases. J Cell Biochem 1987;33: 53–63.
550. Westley BR, May FE: Oestrogen regulates cathepsin D mRNA levels in oestrogen responsive human breast cancer cells. Nucleic Acids Res 1987;15:3773–3786.
551. Pain RH, Lah T, Turk V: Conformation and processing of cathepsin D. Biosci Rep 1985;5:957–967.
552. Baldwin ET, Bhat TN, Gulnik S, et al: Crystal structures of native and inhibited forms of human cathepsin D: Implications for lysosomal targeting and drug design. Proc Natl Acad Sci USA 1993;90:6796–6800.
553. Cantor AB, Baranski TJ, Kornfeld S: Lysosomal enzyme phosphorylation: II. Protein recognition determinants in either lobe of procathepsin D are sufficient for phosphorylation of both the amino and carboxyl lobe oligosaccharides. J Biol Chem 1992;267:23349–23356.
554. Ultsch M, de Vos AM: Crystals of human growth hormone-receptor complexes: Extracellular domains of the growth hormone and prolactin receptors and a hormone mutant designed to prevent receptor dimerization. J Mol Biol 1993;231:1133–1136.
555. Mariuzza RA, Amit AG, Boulot G, et al: Crystallization of the fab fragments of monoclonal anti-*p*-azophenylarsonate antibodies and their complexes with haptens. J Biol Chem 1984;259:5954–5958.
556. Lascombe MB, Alzari PM, Boulot G, et al: Three-dimensional structure of Fab R19.9, a monoclonal murine antibody specific for the *p*-azobenzenearsonate group. Proc Natl Acad Sci USA 1989;86:607–611.

II

ADVANCED DIAGNOSTIC METHODS

Protocols

MARY B. KENNY-MOYNIHAN
ELIZABETH R. UNGER

3

Immunohistochemical and In Situ Hybridization Techniques

IMMUNOHISTOCHEMISTRY

Immunohistochemistry is the marriage of immunologic and histochemical techniques, allowing phenotypic markers to be detected and interpreted within a morphologic context. The birth of immunohistochemistry is attributable to Coons and colleagues,[1] who, in 1941, introduced fluorescent-labeled antibodies. The development of enzyme-labeled antibodies that were reactive in fixed, paraffin-embedded tissue, provided the basis for modern immunohistochemistry.[2–4] Subsequent modifications of techniques, including the peroxidase-antiperoxidase method[5] and avidin-biotin-peroxidase method,[6] as well as the development and commercial availability of a wide range of polyclonal and monoclonal antibodies, have combined to make immunohistochemistry an essential element of contemporary pathology practice.

The most widespread use of immunohistochemistry in pathology is to supplement morphologic criteria in determining the appropriate classification of an "undifferentiated" neoplasm. For this type of application the immunohistochemistry results are used to aid in the differential diagnosis suggested by the clinical setting and histology of the lesion. In the detection of infectious agents or identification of physiologic substances in aberrant locations, immunohistochemical assays more directly determine the diagnosis. In other applications, such as the detection of prognostic markers including hormone receptors, oncogene products, or proliferation markers, immunohistochemistry is used as an analytical assay. The addition of analytical assays has served to alert the pathology community to the need for more stringent controls in all aspects of immunohistochemistry.

Antigen-Antibody Reaction

Central to the immunohistochemical assay is the specific binding of an antibody to its corresponding antigen. The binding is dependent on noncovalent interactions between the molecules. The strength (avidity) and specificity of that binding are attributable to the multiplicative effect of numerous weak bonds, including electrostatic bonds, hydrophobic bonds, van der Waals forces, and hydrogen bonds. A detailed consideration of all aspects of the biology and biochemistry of these molecules is beyond the scope of this chapter, but a brief description emphasizing aspects important for development and use of immunohistochemical assays follows.

Antigens

Briefly, an antigen is any substance that evokes an antibody response. Antigens are composed of multiple molecular binding sites (epitopes), each of which may be a target for antibody. Epitopic determinants on an antigen are contiguous amino acids, nucleotides, or sugars that are in a linear sequence in the molecule or that join as a result of conformational arrangements.[7] One antigenic determinant stimulates production of multiple different clonal antibodies of varying degrees of affinity. The normal immune response in vivo involves the selection of high-affinity antibodies over low-affinity antibodies (affinity maturation) and is probably driven by competitive binding. Affinity of an antibody is a reflection of the quality of the fit between a single antigen-binding site with the antigen and is independent of the number of antigenic sites. Avidity of an antibody is the total binding strength of all its binding sites together. The nature of many common antigens is discussed in detail in Chapter 2.

Antibodies

An antibody is an immunoglobulin with a specific binding domain for its corresponding antigen. The majority of antibodies pertinent to immunohistochemistry are of the immunoglobulin G class, with a small percentage belonging to the immunoglobulin M class. The immunoglobulin molecule is composed of two heavy chains and two variable light chains. The latter form the antigen-binding sites (Fab) and have hypervariable domains, which account for the diversity and specificity of the immunoglobulin-antigen interaction. The other major functional component of the immunoglobulin molecule from the immunohistochemical perspective is the Fc binding domain. The Fc domain is itself antigenic. Depending on its class, it can also bind complement, protein A of *Staphylococcus* species, and cells including neutrophils, macrophages, and trophoblast cells. In some applications, the Fc portion of the immunoglobulin molecule is removed, leaving only Fab fragments to participate in the reaction.

Polyclonal Antibodies. Polyclonal antibodies are the product of a particular animal that has been challenged (immunized) with an antigen. Adjuvants, complex mixtures of lipids, emulsifying agents, and other compounds are often used to stimulate the antigenic response of the animal. In response to the antigenic challenge, the animal produces an idiosyncratic mixture of antibodies of varying specificity and affinity. One of the major limitations of polyclonal antibodies is the reliance on the individual animal's response to an antigen that contributes to significant lot-to-lot variability. Adjuvants may result in the production of an antibody mixture of low avidity and specificity.[7] The heterogeneous nature of the antibody response contributes to the potential for antibodies to be present that are directed against a contaminant in the immunogen or that cross-react with other antigens. Affinity-purification techniques may be used to fractionate polyclonal antibodies on the basis of antigenic recognition to eliminate such undesired reactivities. However, affinity-purification can result in an antiserum that contains predominantly low-avidity antibodies.[8] Polyclonal antibodies are relatively easy to prepare and have a broader tolerance to antigen fixation than monoclonal antibodies.[9(p54)] Because of the presence of a mixture of antibodies against different epitopes of the same antigen, polyclonal antibodies may result in a more intense signal than a corresponding monoclonal antibody.[9(p54)]

Monoclonal Antibodies. The polyclonal antibody response is the product of multiple clones of plasma cells, each secreting a unique immunoglobulin molecule. Isolation of a single clone of plasma cells would result in the production of a single immunoglobulin species, a monoclonal antibody (Fig. 3–1). This has been achieved through the use of cell fusion technology, referred to as hybridoma techniques. An animal is immunized, and immunoglobulin-producing lymphocytes are isolated. A lymphocyte producing the antibody of interest is fused with a nonsecreting myeloma cell to produce an immortalized hybrid cell line that can produce the desired antibody in cell culture or as a tumor in the body cavity of an animal. Monoclonal antibody from ascitic fluid of an animal may be contaminated by constitutive polyclonal antibodies. The use of cell culture supernatant avoids this difficulty.

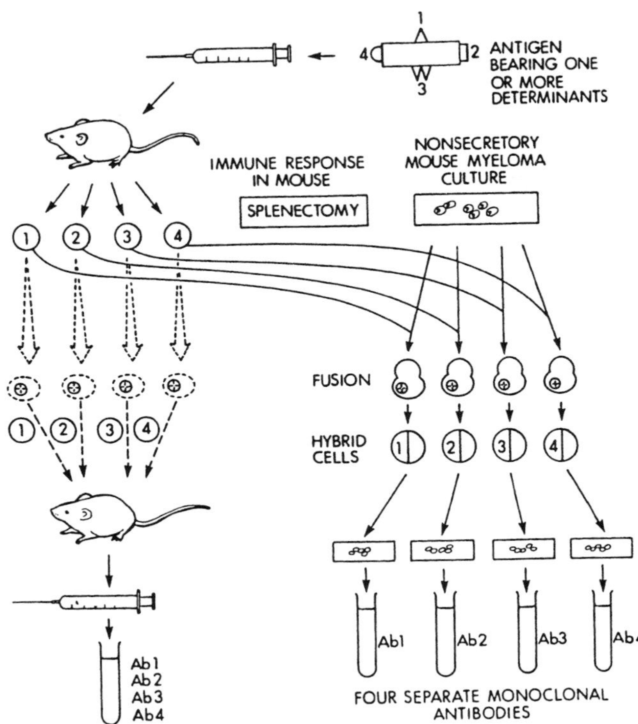

FIGURE 3–1
Production of hybridoma (monoclonal) antibody. A single antigen induces the formation of several different antibodies of differing specificity and affinity against various epitopes of the antigen. On the left, these antibodies are not separated, resulting in conventional mouse antiserum. On the right, separate antibody clones are isolated, resulting in the production of distinct monoclonal antibodies. (From Taylor CR: Principles of immunomicroscopy. *In* Taylor CR, Shi SR, Cote RJ [eds]: Immunomicroscopy: A Diagnostic Tool for the Surgical Pathologist, ed 2. Philadelphia, WB Saunders, 1994, p 18.)

Whichever production method is used, the result is the ability to indefinitely produce a unique well-characterized immunoglobulin.

Despite the cost of the technology to produce monoclonal antibodies, these purified reagents are increasingly used in immunohistochemistry because of greatly reduced background staining, absence of contaminating antibodies, consistency between production lots, and applicability as detection reagents in the form of secondary antibodies (see "Immunohistochemical Assay Formats"). However, these reagents do have limitations. Because the initial cells for fusion are isolated by affinity techniques, the selected clones may be of lowered affinity compared with the starting polyclonal response.[9(p35)] A mixture of monoclonal antibodies with specificities directed against different epitopes can result in sensitivity comparable to corresponding polyclonal antibodies.[10,11] An additional problem unique to monoclonal antibodies is that intrinsic cross-reactivity may occur because of shared epitopes between unrelated antigens. Because epitopic determinants are often short sequences of amino acids or carbohydrates, the chance that the same sequence may be shared by other cells or structures is significant.

This undesired cross-reaction cannot always be anticipated and may not be discovered until the antibody is in use.[12]

Conditions Affecting Antigen-Antibody Reaction

Time, temperature, and pH during the incubation of antigen and antibody will influence the binding of antibody to antigen. Increased temperature generally increases the rate of antigen-antibody complex formation. Within limits, the time of incubation may be shortened as the temperature of the incubation is raised. For polyclonal antibodies, which are composed of a mixture of antibodies with potentially different antigen-binding characteristics, long or repeated incubations should favor binding by the highest avidity antibodies, owing to displacement of low-avidity antibodies. However, these steps have little enhancing effect on the ultimate signal achieved with monoclonal antibodies. Although numerous permutations of incubation time and temperature have been utilized, the trend is away from 24- to 48-hour incubations at 4°C toward shorter incubations at room temperature, or 37°C, to facilitate the rapid turnaround time in demand in the current laboratory environment.

The buffer used as the antibody diluent controls the pH during the incubation. An alteration in the reaction pH can alter both the strength and specificity of the antigen-antibody interaction.[13(p160)] The majority of reactions between antigen and polyclonal antibody are tolerant of a pH range between 6.5 and 8.5. Monoclonal antibodies, however, are less tolerant of pH changes.[9(p42)] Most incubations utilize a pH between 7.2 and 7.6 maintained by phosphate-saline or TRIS-saline.

Antibody dilution is a critical factor in the antigen-antibody reaction. Antibody should be used at as high a dilution as possible without loss of detection of specific staining. This is economical, will diminish any prozone effect (false negative owing to high antigen content), and favors lower background staining. The highest dilution is selected during optimization of an antibody before implementing its use in the laboratory.

The cellular antigen must be accessible for the antigen-antibody reaction to occur optimally. For antigens located on the cell surface, this is usually not problematic. Intracellular antigens are made more accessible to antibody, which normally does not cross the cell membrane, by disrupting the cell membrane. This is partially accomplished by tissue fixation and sectioning. Antibody penetration is also enhanced by use of digestion techniques or by addition of detergent to the various reagents used in the immunohistochemical sequence. Addition of detergent, however, can occasionally result in antigen damage.[13(p155)] Lower-molecular-weight reagents will penetrate tissue sections more uniformly, hence enhancing reactivity with antigen. Because of this effect, in some settings Fab fragments of immunoglobulins may enhance the immunohistochemical result. Even penetration will occur only when antiserum uniformly covers the tissue section on the glass slide. Humidity is important to minimize dehydration of the tissue sections and reagents that can lead to a higher antibody concentration in solution than is desirable.

Immunohistochemical Assay Formats

DIRECT IMMUNOHISTOCHEMISTRY

The direct immunohistochemical method was originally developed by Coons and colleagues,[1] who conjugated a fluorescent molecule to antibody for use as a label (1941). For direct immunohistochemistry, the detection system (i.e., the enzyme or fluorochrome) is covalently linked (conjugated) directly to the primary antibody (Fig. 3–2). The primary antibody is applied to the specimen, followed by washing and direct detection by viewing or development with substrate. Because so few steps are involved, the direct technique is quite rapid. The principal utility of the direct method is in the immunofluorescent detection of immune complexes in skin and kidney biopsy specimens. The final sensitivity of the method is dependent on the chemistry of labeling the primary antibody. The chemical conjugation must be carefully controlled to ensure that the antigen-binding site is not damaged and that the reaction is nearly 100% efficient. Unlabeled primary antibody will efficiently compete with the labeled molecules for antigen binding and greatly reduce the signal. In practice, it is usually more efficient to use unlabeled primary antibody and devise alternative methods for detection.

INDIRECT IMMUNOHISTOCHEMISTRY

Indirect immunohistochemical methods exploit the natural capacity of immunoglobulin to act as antigen. In this approach, the primary antibody is raised in one species, for example, the rabbit, and is not conjugated.

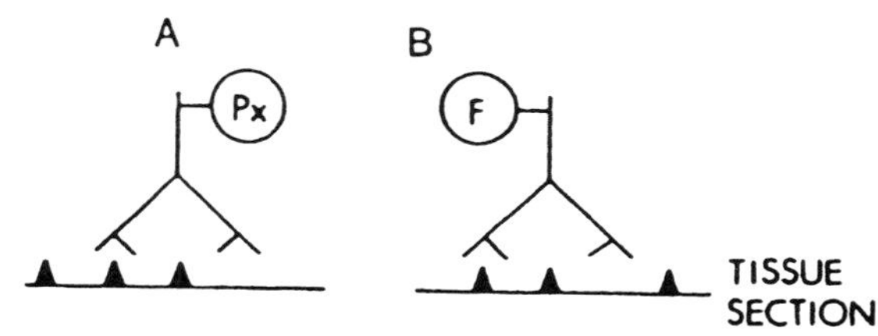

FIGURE 3–2
Direct immunohistochemistry. The label is attached directly to the antibody having specificity for the antigen under study. F, fluorescein; Px, peroxidase. (From Taylor CR: Principles of immunomicroscopy. *In* Taylor CR, Shi SR, Cote RJ [eds]: Immunomicroscopy: A Diagnostic Tool for the Surgical Pathologist, ed 2. Philadelphia, WB Saunders, 1994, p 10.)

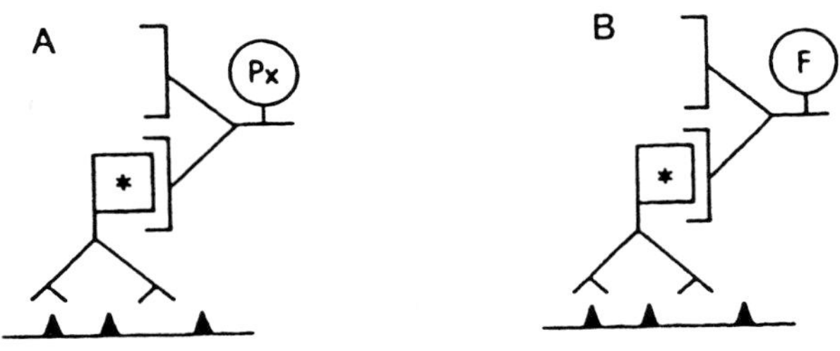

FIGURE 3–3
Indirect immunohistochemistry. The primary antibody is unlabeled. The method uses a labeled secondary antibody having specificity against the primary antibody. Boxed *asterisk* indicates antigen determinant on primary antibody. F, fluorescein; Px, peroxidase. (From Taylor CR: Principles of immunomicroscopy. *In* Taylor CR, Shi SR, Cote RJ [eds]: Immunomicroscopy: A Diagnostic Tool for the Surgical Pathologist, ed 2. Philadelphia, WB Saunders, 1994, p 11.)

Immunoglobulins from this species are then used as an immunogen in a second species, for example, the goat, resulting in antibodies recognizing immunoglobulin in the primary serum (in this example, goat anti-rabbit). Immunoglobulin from the secondary serum is then conjugated to a detection system as described earlier for the direct system (Fig. 3–3). The complete assay involves incubation with unlabeled primary antibody, washing, incubation with secondary antibody, followed by washing and detection.

The labeled secondary antibody can allow for signal amplification compared with the direct method, and this permits the primary antibody to be used at a higher dilution. Sensitivity is generally increased compared with direct detection. The labeled secondary antibody can be used to detect any primary antibody that has been raised in the species it recognizes. This versatility allows for commercial development and standardization of these detection reagents. Background staining associated with polyvalent secondary antibodies can be a problem with this technique.[7]

A recently developed variation of this technique uses a large dextran backbone to covalently link secondary antibody and enzyme molecules. The complex includes up to 100 enzyme molecules and 20 secondary antibody molecules. Improved sensitivity, attributed to increased localization of enzyme activity, has been reported.[14]

Antibody Bridge Techniques

The antibody bridge technique ("three-step method") is a further modification of the indirect method. In addition to the primary and secondary antibodies used in the indirect method, a tertiary labeled antibody is used in the antibody bridge technique. The primary and tertiary antibodies must be from the same or closely related species, and the secondary or bridge antibody is directed against that species, hence binding both primary and tertiary antibodies as a "bridge." (In this application the secondary antibody is unlabeled.)

In a variation on the same theme, the tertiary antibody can be an unlabeled antienzyme antibody. Addition of the enzyme (usually horseradish peroxidase) as the fourth step results in an immunologic reaction between enzyme (e.g., horseradish peroxidase) and antienzyme (anti-horseradish peroxidase) for detection. Preformed enzyme antienzyme complexes such as peroxidase antiperoxidase (PAP),[5] alkaline phosphatase anti-alkaline phosphatase (APAAP), and glucose oxidase anti-glucose oxidase (GAG), are available. This combination of tertiary antibody and enzyme into one complex that is linked to the primary antibody by an unlabeled bridge antibody reduces the four-step technique to a three-step technique (Fig. 3–4). Reproducibility and specificity are enhanced with use of PAP, which is a small, stable complex from the same or closely related species that shares antigenic determinants against which the bridge antibody is directed. The efficacy of these techniques depends on the development of high-affinity bridging antibodies, tertiary antibodies, and antienzyme antibodies.

Affinity Labeling Methods

Avidin-Biotin Methods. The extremely high affinity of avidin for biotin has been used as an alternative to relying on the antigenic nature of immunoglobulins to provide links between antigen localization and detection reagents. Avidin is a high-molecular-weight protein (mol. wt. 67,000) found in egg white that has very high affinity for biotin, a low-molecular-weight water-soluble vitamin. The avidin-biotin disassociation constant approaches the strength of a covalent bond ($K_d = 10^{-15}$), and the chemistry of utilizing these molecules as reagents for

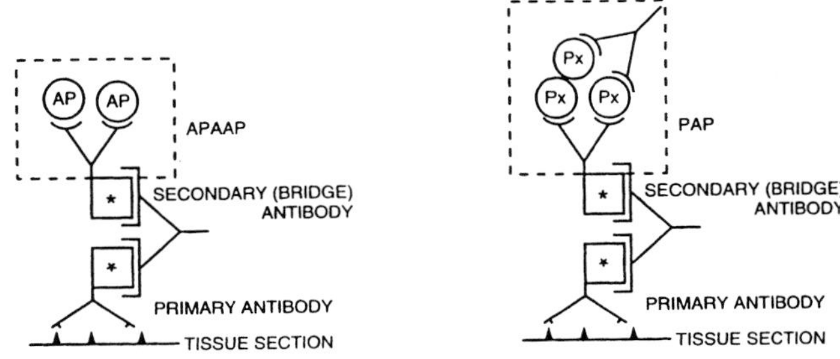

FIGURE 3–4
Antibody bridge techniques. The use of preformed enzyme-antienzyme complexes is illustrated. Primary and secondary antibodies are unlabeled. Primary antibody and antibody in preformed complex are from the same species. The secondary antibody forms a bridge between the two molecules by recognizing the same epitope. AP, alkaline phosphatase; APAAP, alkaline phosphatase anti-alkaline phosphatase, a stable soluble enzyme antibody complex; P, peroxidase; PAP, peroxidase anti-peroxidase, a stable soluble enzyme antibody complex; boxed *asterisk* indicates antigen determinant on primary antibody and PAP or APAAP complex. (From Taylor CR, Tandon A: Theoretical and practical aspects of the different immunoperoxidase techniques. *In* Taylor CR, Shi SR, Cote RJ [eds]: Immunomicroscopy: A Diagnostic Tool for the Surgical Pathologist, ed. 2. Philadelphia, WB Saunders, 1994, p 32.)

affinity purification has been well characterized.[15] One molecule covalently labeled with avidin will bind to another molecule covalently labeled with biotin, assuming labels are introduced in a fashion that does not sterically limit the interaction of the affinity labels. Because avidin molecules have four binding sites for biotin, the geometry and proportions may be arranged to allow for multi–molecular complex formation between avidin- and biotin-labeled reagents.

Although biotin can be attached to any component of the immunohistochemical reaction—primary, secondary, or histochemical enzyme—the use of a biotinylated secondary antibody is employed most frequently because of the great flexibility in the approach for detection. A simple layered approach may be used. After localization of the biotinylated secondary antibody, detection can be achieved with unlabeled avidin followed by biotinylated label as the fourth step, known as the bridged avidin-biotin method. The biotinylated label is most commonly a histochemical enzyme. The third and fourth steps of the bridged avidin-biotin method could be combined though complex formation between avidin and biotinylated enzyme, in the same way that the PAP complex eliminated one step. This was first described for biotinylated peroxidase[6] and is known as the avidin-biotin complex (ABC) method (Fig. 3–5). Because of the polyvalent biotin-binding capacity of avidin, mixing of the biotinylated enzyme and avidin can be done in a ratio that allows for multiple enzyme molecules to be complexed to avidin while the overall complex still retains the excess biotin-binding sites required for interaction with the biotinylated secondary antibody. The significant advantage of the three-step ABC is its great sensitivity, which has been attributed to the localization of several molecules of peroxidase at the antigenic site. The avidin-biotin peroxidase-antiperoxidase (ABPAP) complex involves

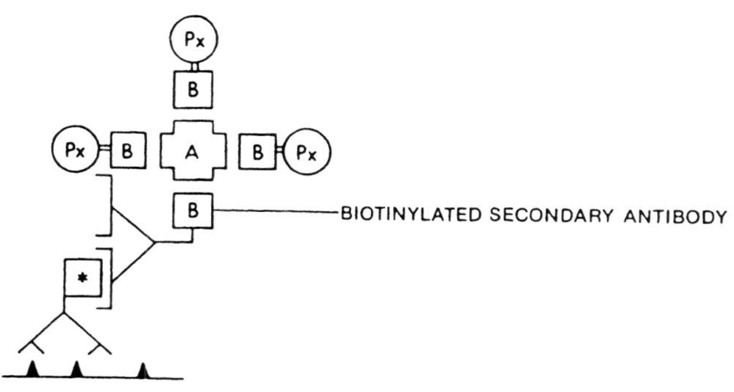

FIGURE 3–5
Avidin-biotin complex method (ABC). Primary antibody is unlabeled. Secondary antibody carries biotin tag, which is detected with a noncovalent complex of avidin (A)- and biotin (B)-labeled histochemical enzyme, in the case illustrated, peroxidase (Px). Boxed *asterisk* indicates antigen determinant on primary antibody. (From Taylor CR, Tandon A: Theoretical and practical aspects of the different immunoperoxidase techniques. *In* Taylor CR, Shi SR, Cote RJ [eds]: Immunomicroscopy: A Diagnostic Tool for the Surgical Pathologist, ed. 2 Philadelphia, WB Saunders, 1994, p 36.)

sequential use of the PAP and ABC techniques in an attempt to further increase the number of enzyme molecules at an antigen site. Signal amplification by these techniques reaches a limit because of steric effects. Binding of large complexes is less efficient, and enzymes buried within layers of other molecules may not be as accessible to substrates required to generate the colored products. Although first described for peroxidase, alkaline phosphatase can be biotinylated and complexed with avidin in a similar fashion.

Avidin reagents have been made by covalent reaction to a histochemical enzyme. For horseradish peroxidase, the resulting conjugate can include two or three enzymes bound to an avidin molecule. The use of conjugates is referred to as labeled avidin-biotin (LAB). The conjugates require no mixing before use, and the sensitivity of complex versus that of the conjugate is similar. Well-standardized commercial reagents are available for either approach.

Whereas the previous discussion has centered on avidin, a very similar protein, streptavidin, is available. It is produced by *Streptomyces avidinii* and has nearly identical biotin-binding characteristics. Unlike avidin, streptavidin has a neutral isoelectric charge because it lacks the carbohydrate side chains of avidin. In some applications, substituting streptavidin for avidin may contribute to lower background.

Protein A Methods. Protein A is a major cell wall component of most strains of *Staphylococcus aureus*. It has a very high affinity for the Fc component of immunoglobulin, particularly IgG. Its affinity for different subclasses of IgG and for other immunoglobulins varies from species to species.[16] It can be conjugated to various labels (e.g., fluorescein, gold, alkaline phosphatase, peroxidase) without impairment of its immunoglobulin-binding capacity,[11,17,18] allowing for shorter incubation times.[8,11,17] Lack of sensitivity limits widespread application in light microscopy; however, because of its low molecular weight, protein A is quite useful in immunoelectron microscopy.

Lectin Histochemistry. Lectins are proteins and glycoproteins of plant origin that bind in a noncovalent fashion to specific polysaccharides. In most applications, the lectin is substituted for a primary antibody to specifically localize a complex carbohydrate group. The bound lectin is then detected in a fashion similar to immunohistochemistry, for example, peroxidase with an appropriate label or a fluorescent or metallic label. Lectin histochemistry and diagnostic applications have been reviewed.[19,20]

Immunoelectron Microscopy

Immunoelectron microscopy serves to accurately localize antigen at the ultrastructural level. The technique is complex because of the need to balance antigen preservation and accessibility with adequate fixation for ultrastructural morphology. In pre-embedding techniques the antibody is applied to relatively thick sections of unfixed tissue. Subsequently, these sections are fixed and processed for electron microscopy. Although useful for very labile antigens susceptible to fixation, significant disadvantages include the need for fresh tissue and relatively poor ultrastructural preservation. Postembedding techniques, whereby the tissue is fixed, processed, and resin embedded before thin sectioning for immunoelectron microscopy, are much more practical. Morphology is improved, less tissue is needed, double staining is possible, and retrospective studies can be performed. Immunoelectron microscopy has been reviewed,[21] and a detailed discussion is beyond the scope of this chapter.

Detection Systems

As implied in the previous description of assay formats, antibody alone cannot be visualized. Each assay format uses a different technique for localizing a reporter molecule or detection system to specifically bound primary antibody. These detection systems include nonenzymatic systems as well as systems using enzyme to generate a signal.

NONENZYMATIC LABELS

Fluorescent labels, such as fluorescein isothiocyanate, were among the first labels used in immunohistochemistry and are most commonly used for detection of the abnormal deposition of physiologic substances in renal and skin biopsy specimens. Disadvantages associated with fluorescent labels include the need for a special light source, limited morphology because of poor counterstaining, fading of the signal on storage, and intrinsic tissue autofluorescence that is increased by fixation.

Heavy metals, such as silver, gold, ferritin, and mercuryl compounds may be used as labels, particularly at the ultrastructural level. Depending on particle size, metal labels may be visible with the light microscope. Immunogold techniques, involving conjugation of colloidal gold particles to antibody, protein A, or avidin, are increasingly being used at both the light and electron microscopic levels. The size of gold particles used ranges from 1 to 20 nm. Smaller particles improve signal resolution but may require silver enhancement for detection. Particles of 20 nm are readily visible at the light microscopic level but may be associated with steric hindrance[9(p29)] and produce a granular signal.[8,18]

HISTOCHEMICAL ENZYMES AND SUBSTRATES

Histochemical enzymes are enzymes that have been used as visualization tools for the localization of targets in tissues or cells. To be useful in such a capacity, the enzyme must have a substrate system that generates a product that can be visualized (i.e., a chromogen) and has minimal diffusion from the site of production. This latter characteristic is referred to as the substantivity of the chromogen. The final sensitivity of detection is determined by the combined efficiency of the enzyme-substrate system in generating signal. The enzyme-specific activity, substrate concentration and purity, time, and temperature of reaction will all impact results. In practice, these variables have been minimized because of the commercial availability of these key reagents. Table 3–1 summarizes the commonly used enzyme-substrate chromogens, color of product, and solubility of product in alcohol.

TABLE 3–1

Summary of Enzyme Substrate Systems

Enzyme	Chromogens	Color	Solubility in Alcohol
Horseradish peroxidase	Diaminobenzidine (DAB)	Brown	Insoluble
	Aminoethylcarbazole (AEC)	Red	Soluble
	Alpha-naphthol pyronin	Red	Soluble
	4-chloro-1-napthol	Blue	Soluble
	Paraphenylenediamine pyrocatechol	Blue	Insoluble
Alkaline phosphatase	Fast red TR	Red	Soluble
	Fast blue BB	Blue	Soluble
	BCIP/NBT	Blue/black	Insoluble*
Glucose oxidase	Tetrazolium blue	Blue	Insoluble
β-Galactosidase	BCI	Indigo	Insoluble

*Slight loss of intensity in alcohol.

BCI, 5-bromo-4-chloro-3-indolyl-β-D-galactopyranoside; BCIP/NBT, 5-bromo-4-chloro-3-indolyl phosphate/nitroblue tetrazolium.

Horseradish Peroxidase. Horseradish peroxidase is the most commonly used histochemical enzyme. It is a relatively small protein (mol. wt. 40,000) that uses peroxide as a substrate and is inactivated by substrate excess. The enzyme substrate reaction is rapid and enzyme activity is quenched within 15 to 30 minutes. Color development occurs using an electron donor as histochemically demonstrable material. There are several different histochemical systems for this enzyme. The two most commonly used are diaminobenzidine (DAB) and 3-amino-9-ethyl carbazole (AEC), either of which yields comparable results,[22] although less diffusion from site of liberation is noted for DAB. Peroxidase is most active at neutral pH and is reversibly inhibited by azide, cyanide, and sulfide.

DAB results in a mahogany brown reaction product that does not fade and is insoluble in organic solvents. The contrast with a light hematoxylin counterstain is good, and standard mounting media can be used. Intensification of the DAB reaction product, changing the color to black, can be accomplished by addition of heavy metals (e.g., nickel chloride, cobalt chloride, copper chloride, imidazole or osmium tetroxide).[9(p58)] DAB is a chemical carcinogen, and the powdered form must be handled in a hood using mask and gloves. Liquid forms, reducing the hazard of handling the reagent, are now commercially available.

AEC gives a red reaction product that is soluble in alcohol and can fade with long-term storage. The contrast with a light hematoxylin counterstain is good, but nonalcoholic forms (i.e., Mayer's hematoxylin) must be used to avoid removal of signal. Aqueous mounting media must be used. AEC was first introduced because of a reportedly lower carcinogenic potential than DAB. The reagent is not free of hazard and should still be handled with care for laboratory workers and the environment.

Other less frequently used chromogens include 4-chloro-1-naphthol, benzidine, alpha-naphthol pyronin, *p*-phenylenediamine pyrocatechol (Hanker-Yates reagent), and tetramethyl benzidine.[23] 4-Chloro-1-naphthol gives a blue end product, but it tends to diffuse from the site of precipitation. Successful use of the Hanker-Yates reagent for immunohistochemistry on renal biopsies is reported.[24]

Alkaline Phosphatase. Alkaline phosphatase is the other most commonly used histochemical enzyme. It is much larger than horseradish peroxidase (mol. wt. 140,000), and its size can influence geometry of complex formation and reagent penetration. The enzyme is most active at alkaline pH in the presence of magnesium and is inactivated by acid. There is no enzyme inactivation associated with the reaction with substrate, so color development can be extended to result in more signal (within limits). A variety of substrates are available. The resulting chromogens are variously colored; red, blue, or black products can be formed. The substrates are not carcinogenic. The final sensitivity depends on the substrate system. The chromogens are not stable in organic reagents and require protection from organic mounting medium or the use of aqueous based systems. Choice of counterstain is dictated by the color of the chromogen. Chromogens for use with alkaline phosphatase include fast dyes (Fast Red TR, Fast Blue BB) in conjunction with naphthol substrates or nitroblue tetrazolium 5-bromo-4 chloro-3 indolyl phosphate (NBT-BCIP).[25] The NBT-BCIP substrate results in a dark blue-black product that is very substantive and yields the highest sensitivity of any colorimetric detection system.

Glucose Oxidase. Glucose oxidase is most often employed with tetrazolium blue as the chromogen. Although this enzyme-substrate system is less sensitive than methods using peroxidase- and alkaline phosphatase–based colorimetric systems, it has the advantage that human tissues lack endogenous glucose oxidase activity. It is also useful in double immunohistochemical labeling techniques.

β-Galactosidase. β-Galactosidase is isolated from *Escherichia coli*. At the optimal pH for use (7.0 to 7.5), interference from mammalian β-galactosidase is not a problem. The substrate, 5-bromo-4-chloro-3-indolyl-β-D-galactopyranoside, results in an insoluble indigo-colored reaction product.

Double- or Multiple-Staining Techniques. This topic has been thoroughly reviewed by van der Loos and associates,[26] who provide practical suggestions on when and how to apply double-staining methods, including selection of the best methodologic combinations. Whereas immunohistochemistry for different antigens performed on adjacent serial sections usually suffices for routine purposes, occasionally the need arises to visualize more than one antigen in cells. Double or multiple staining procedures can be performed either sequentially or simultaneously and may involve use of more than one enzyme-chromogen combination, resulting in different colored reaction products. Many permutations are described.[27] A sequential procedure is used when both primary antibodies are raised in the same species. Elution of the first primary antibody or adequate development of the first reaction product before proceeding with the second reaction may be necessary.[9(p32)] When the two primary antibodies are raised in different species, a simultaneous procedure using different enzyme-chromogen combinations can be performed. The optimal end result in a case containing the antigens of interest will be two highly contrasting visually different signals. Combinations of immunogold-silver staining with horseradish peroxidase and alkaline phosphatase results in successful triple staining.[28]

Signal Amplification Techniques. A significant new approach to improving the sensitivity of histochemical detection involves the use of novel substrates that, rather than directly generating signal, generate additional affinity labels. The newly formed labels are subsequently detected with a second round of histochemical enzyme localization and conventional signal generating substrates.[29] The systems have been called varying names, including catalyzed reported deposition (CARD), tyramide signal amplification (TSA), and catalyzed signal amplification (CSA). The most common approach uses any of the conventional histochemistry methods to localize horseradish peroxidase. The horseradish peroxidase activity is used against a tyramide substrate covalently linked to an affinity label. Horseradish peroxidase acts on the phenolic part of the affinity-labeled tyramide to produce a highly reactive short-lived intermediate that forms a covalent link with adjacent protein molecules. The newly deposited affinity labels are subsequently detected with another round of histochemical detection (either horseradish peroxidase or alkaline phosphatase, with standard colorimetric substrates) or fluorescence. Alternatively, additional rounds of signal amplification with the tyramide reagent may be used to generate still more targets. Tyramide conjugates have been made with biotin or fluorescein affinity tags. This approach has been reported to result in greatly improved sensitivity.[30,31] Because the reactive affinity–labeled intermediates have an extremely short half-life, signal localization remains good, although some loss of precision occurs with additional rounds of amplification. Care must be taken to optimize the system because any background in the initial histochemical localization is amplified in the subsequent reactions. Signal amplification applies equally to detection of in situ hybridization reactions and is an attractive alternative to in situ PCR reactions for detection of low copies of target.

Optimization of Test Material

A crucial requirement for a valid immunohistochemical assay is to have adequate test material that will yield valid results. Although this component of the assay is often taken for granted, it is clear that no refinement of immunohistochemical technique can compensate for inadequate starting material. Adequate test material means that the sample must be representative of the lesion and be prepared to allow for preservation of morphologic detail and antigenicity. Some method of fixation is undertaken to arrest autolysis and to preserve morphologic detail. Unfortunately, from the perspective of the immunohistochemist, fixation may result in variable target antigen loss or may render the antigen target inaccessible.

Under ideal situations, the tissue specimen would be rapidly submitted to the pathologist in the fresh state and equally rapidly examined and processed. The pathologist would then control the nature and duration of fixation. A representative sample of all tumors could be snap frozen and maintained in a tumor bank, in case a particular target antigen is susceptible to fixation and to allow for validation of results or extension of results by current or future molecular assays. Although this idealized strategy is unlikely to be implemented, some improvement on the widely used practice of immersing a whole specimen in fixative for an unspecified period of time before sending it to the pathologist needs to be considered.

The biochemical and ultrastructural alterations known as autolysis occur immediately after tissue is removed from the body, or after the body dies. Just as tissues do not autolyze at a standard rate, so tissue antigens and nucleic acids autolyze at variable rates. Minor changes are inevitable, and even extensively autolyzed tissue may still be useful for immunohistochemistry.[32] Knowledge about the effect of autolysis on any particular antigen is necessary for reliable interpretation. The goal of each method of tissue fixation and processing is to obtain reproducible preservation of morphology and biochemical macromolecules.

Methods of Tissue Fixation

Freezing. Rapidly frozen tissue is of use for immunohistochemistry because of superior preservation of antigens, in particular cell membrane surface antigens. The pattern of immunoreactivity in frozen sections remains the gold standard against which all other assays are judged. If antigen is detected in frozen sections but not in paraffin sections of formalin-fixed tissue, then the fixation and processing sequence has resulted in antigen loss, change, or masking, rendering it unavailable. Frozen tissue is used to demonstrate the optimal pattern of reactivity of an antibody. A wider range of antibodies is applicable to frozen tissues, and generally frozen tissues have been promptly handled and are well preserved.

Snap freezing tissue for immunohistochemical analysis is not routine, so frozen material will not always be available. The frozen sample must be protected from freeze-thaw cycles and from dehydration during storage. The morphology of the cryostat section is not as good as can be obtained with paraffin sections, and adherence of frozen tissue to the glass slide can be difficult. In addition, unfixed antigens may diffuse or be dislocated to other areas during sectioning. Rapid fixation of cryostat sections in acetone or periodate lysine paraformaldehyde or by microwave irradiation is used to minimize the problem of antigen dislocation and to improve morphology. Variations in duration of fixation and nature of the fixative will influence antigen preservation and the eventual staining intensity and patterns.[9(p3)] In current diagnostic practice, the use of frozen section immunohistochemistry is largely confined to hematopathology[33] and the diagnosis of renal and dermatologic diseases. The availability of antibodies reactive in fixed tissues[34–37] and the use of plastic embedding media[38,39] and enhanced antigen retrieval systems[34,35,40] have reduced the need for frozen tissue studies.

Freeze-drying or freeze-substitution of tissue as a means of fixation can be used for either electron or light microscopic study. In combination with both liquid- and vapor-phase fixatives and resin-embedding, excellent preservation of small antigens, such as intracellular enzymes, is achieved. Intracellular location of antigen within specific organelles can also be demonstrated morphologically by such means.[41,42]

Cross-linking Fixatives. Formaldehyde at 37% (wt/wt) or 40% (wt/vol) in aqueous solution is diluted 1 in 10 and buffered to pH 7.0 to make a working solution that is known as 10% buffered formalin or 4% formaldehyde. Formalin is inexpensive, readily available, widely used, and probably the closest approach to a universal fixative. Morphologic preservation and antigen immobilization is superior when compared with coagulant fixatives.[43] Although formaldehyde penetrates tissues rapidly, fixation occurs slowly. It acts to form covalent cross-links between adjacent reactive groups on macromolecules. The highest reactivity is with amino groups such as lysine, and thiols such as cysteine, but amides will also react with the aldehyde.[44] This cross-linking process can result in direct loss of epitopes that include these reactive groups or indirect loss of antigenicity through cross-linking of adjacent molecules resulting in steric hindrance.

Tissue fixation is dependent on reagent penetration and on the rate of reaction. For the chemical reaction to be even, the tissues must be thinly cut, 0.2 cm ideally, and no larger than 1.5 cm in diameter. The rate of chemical reaction is temperature dependent, and times range from 16 hours at 37°C to 24 hours at room temperature for the chemical reaction to reach equilibrium. Prolonged fixation time, 72 or 96 hours, has no deleterious effect on morphology; however, increased cross-linkage limits antigen accessibility. For this reason the fixation time should be minimized. The response of each antigen to fixation is somewhat different, making broad generalizations about optimal fixation times difficult. A minimum of 12 hours and a maximum of 24 hours formalin fixation have been advocated.[45] The use of freshly made 10% buffered formalin, rather than commercial preparations that may contain methanol or other contaminants, may also enhance target preservation. With shorter fixation times in formalin, the periphery of the specimen is formalin fixed, but fixation of the central portion is accomplished by the dehydrating alcohols of the tissue processor, resulting in uneven immunohistochemical signal limited to either the central portion or the edge of the tissue.[45] At the other extreme, formalin fixation for prolonged periods of time can result in potentially irretrievable antigen loss. Antigens such as vimentin filaments are particularly susceptible to formalin fixation. Tissues fixed in formalin for more than 72 hours show marked decrease or complete loss of vimentin immunoreactivity.[46] The use of such ubiquitous targets as internal controls of fixation is useful in the interpretation of immunohistochemical panels wherein results seem erratic or aberrant.

Addition of other substances to formalin may enhance morphologic detail and antigenicity. However, the improved antigen preservation with any of these modified formalin fixatives may be more related to control of the duration of fixation than to the chemical reaction of the fixative with the tissue.[8] Mercuric chloride, picric acid, acetic acid, and periodate lysine paraformaldehyde (PLP) are the most common additives. Mercuric chloride–containing fixatives such as B5 (formalin/mercuric chloride/sodium acetate mixture) and Zenker's fluid result in improved nuclear morphology. Enhancement of intracellular immunoglobulin staining is reported.[47] The mercury results in a precipitate that must be removed from the tissue and adds to cost for appropriate disposal of an environmental toxin. Fixatives containing picric acid, such as Bouin's fluid or Zamboni's fluid, have been shown to enhance cytoplasmic immunoglobulin signal, obviating the need for predigestion of tissue sections.[48] Picric acid reacts with histones and basic proteins, with the formation of crystalline picrates.[8] PLP fixation permits the use of monoclonal antibodies directed against some lymphocyte surface antigens in paraffin-fixed tissue and is useful for immunofluorescent techniques because it does not induce tissue autofluorescence.[49,50] PLP requires fresh preparation for each specimen.

Glutaraldehyde is another cross-linking aldehyde fixative that differs from formaldehyde in that it penetrates tissues slowly but cross-links tissue rapidly. It is the preferred fixative for small pieces of tissue intended for electron microscopic study or for light microscopic immunohistochemistry of low-molecular-weight substances.[43] However, its potent cross-linking ability can result in antigen masking. Strong background fluorescence after fixation in glutaraldehyde renders it an unsuitable fixative for immunofluorescence studies.

Coagulant Fixatives. Coagulant fixatives fix tissues by precipitating proteins without introducing covalent bonds. The primary protein structure may be relatively unaffected by these methods. Absolute ethanol is probably the most commonly used coagulant fixative; and in comparison with formalin, it appears to afford greater preservation of immunoreactivity of filament proteins.[51] Another advantage of non–cross-linking fixatives is that a predigestion step can often be avoided.[52]

Coagulant fixatives are not without disadvantages. Low-molecular-weight antigens are susceptible to loss (extraction) during fixation and processing. Dislocation artifacts occur; for example, instead of the usual cytoplasmic distribution of myeloperoxidase, ethanol-fixed neutrophils demonstrate perinuclear myeloperoxidase immunohistochemical signal.[43] Tissue shrinkage and distortion can also be a problem. Enzymes responsible for autolysis may not be completely inactivated by ethanol fixation; and if a lengthy incubation step is necessary subsequent to fixation, focal tissue autolysis may occur. Proprietary alcohol-based fixatives are available and reportedly result in less tissue shrinkage than ethanol. Other coagulant fixatives include Carnoy's fluid, methacarn, acetone, and methanol.[53] Carnoy's fluid and methacarn reportedly penetrate tissue more rapidly than ethanol.

Microwave Irradiation Fixation. The physics of microwave technology in histochemistry has been reviewed in detail.[54] The predominant physical effect of microwaving is to increase the temperature, resulting in acceleration of reagent permeation and chemical reactions. Microwave-assisted fixation in dilute aldehydes is reported to give superior morphology and eliminate the need for a predigestion step.[55] This approach may result in rapid fixation of the outer zone of tissue with subsequent decrease in diffusion of fixative into the tissue. The central portion of the tissue would be stabilized secondary to heat coagulation of proteins rather than by cross-linking.[56]

In another variation, microwave stabilization of tissue in buffered salt solution such as normal saline can result in good preservation of morphology and enhanced immunoreactivity against common antigens compared with conventional formalin fixation.[57] Additional advantages include speed of fixation and use of normal saline rather than chemical fixatives; however, preservation of fine ultrastructural detail may be suboptimal.

All microwave methods are highly temperature dependent. The size, shape, and volume of the material to be microwaved, dilution and ionic strength of the medium, position in the microwave oven, and presence of other loads in the oven may all significantly affect temperature. In addition, the size and power of the microwave oven and age of the magnetron may affect the temperature achieved. Some control of these variables can be achieved by using the same oven for defined periods of time in a standardized fashion.[54,58] Horobin and Flemming[56] have summarized artifacts and hazards associated with microwave use and provided examples of useful flow charts for pinpointing specific problems.[46]

Tissue Processing and Embedding Media

In the majority of histology laboratories, tissue is dehydrated and infiltrated with paraffin on automated tissue processors with or without vacuum. It is then subsequently embedded in paraffin wax at its melting point. In most instances all tissues cut throughout the day are processed together in group fashion to allow for the processing to be complete for embedding the following morning. Because the process is automated and "routine," the impact of tissue processing on immunohistochemical and molecular preservation tends to be overlooked. As part of tissue processing, fixation is completed. For optimal results, reagents on the tissue processors must be changed at appropriate intervals, depending on the number of cases processed. Times and temperatures at each step of the processor should be controlled. As commonly used, the processor includes one or two additional changes of formalin before initiation of the alcohol-based dehydration steps. These are added to ensure adequate fixation, but significant variation in fixation occurs depending on the size of the tissues and time of fixation before the tissue is placed on the processor. Weekend processing introduces further variation because of the common practice of holding tissue blocks in the formalin step from Friday through Sunday. Separate processing of smaller tissues (biopsy specimens) with appropriate adjustment of times has been used by some laboratories to minimize variation. Weekend holding stations may be modified to avoid prolonged exposure to formalin.

At the completion of the dehydration steps, tissue is infiltrated with paraffin at its melting temperature in preparation for manual embedding. The melting temperature of the paraffin embedding medium varies depending on the commercial preparation and additives but varies between 50°C and 60°C. Prolonged exposure of tissue to this elevated temperature may result in antigen loss or denaturation.[59]

Alternative tissue processing procedures can be developed to attempt to introduce more standardization. One, known as the AMeX procedure, involves initial fixation in acetone and clearing in methylbenzoate and xylene before paraffin embedding, has been reported to result in improved antigen detection using antibodies usually only reactive in frozen sections.[60]

Numerous alternative embedding media in combination with various fixatives have been used on various tissues for "routine" light microscopy immunohistochemistry and for immunoelectron microscopy. Briefly, the main alternatives are acrylic resins, of which the best known are methyl methacrylate or glycol methacrylate, epoxy resins, and, more recently, LR resins and lowicryl. Advantages of plastic embedding media include ability to embed tissue at low temperature, minimal tissue shrinkage, ability to cut 1- to 2-μm sections (of use for serial sections of the same cell), improved preservation of hematolymphoid antigens, and obviation of the need for decalcification.[39] Disadvantages include expense, need for additional equipment and expertise, difficulty with antigen preservation, and need for removal of embedding medium before immunohistochemistry. There are reports of simplified methods and documented success with immunohistochemistry on plastic embedded tissues.[39,41,42,61–64] Plastic embedded blocks may require special storage conditions either at low temperatures or in conditions of low humidity. Epoxy resins are most commonly used for electron microscopy because of their sturdiness. Removal of epoxy resins requires a harsh chemical procedure that may result in antigen loss. Combinations of freeze-drying or freeze-substitution fixation and resin embedding are used for immunoelectron microscopy.[42] Most antigens and intracellular enzymes are preserved well with this technique.

Digestion and Antigen Retrieval

Recognizing that tissue fixation is often a poorly controlled part of the immunohistochemistry sequence and that tissue antigens may undergo deleterious yet reversible alteration as a result of excessive or harsh fixation, both enzymatic and nonenzymatic methods have been used in attempts to retrieve or "unmask" target antigen. Such techniques may lead to unanticipated or aberrant cross-reactivity and should be introduced with appropriate controls to exclude that possibility.

Enzyme Digestion. Enzymes such as trypsin, pepsin, pronase, or DNase, either singly or in combination or sequence, have been used to digest tissue sections before incubation with antibody. The digestion may function to reduce steric hindrance of antibody and detection reagents. Variables to be considered during optimization and standardization of the digestion include enzyme concentration, time and temperature of digestion, nature of the tissue, and duration of fixation as well as thickness of tissue section. Time of digestion needed for maximum target antigen unmasking varies inversely with the duration of fixation.[52] For formalin-fixed tissues, no significant advantage of any one protease over another has been identified. Optimal conditions for enzyme digestion vary considerably between antibodies, and a decrease or abolition of immunoreactivity with certain antibodies is reported after enzyme digestion.[65] The digestion conditions must be optimized whenever a new antibody is introduced[8] and must be closely monitored to ensure that maximum antigen unmasking is not achieved at the cost of suboptimal tissue morphology. Because lot-to-lot variability can occur, the activity of a new lot of enzyme used for digestion must be compared with the previous lot before it is put into use. Similarly, the enzyme must be stored under appropriate conditions to minimize loss of activity.

Antigen Retrieval. Nonenzymatic methods of antigen retrieval are becoming more popular. Refixation of the tissue block in zinc formalin[66] or immersion of tissue sections in strong alkaline solution[67,68] is reported to improve immunohistochemical staining. "Antigen retrieval solutions" of proprietary composition are available commercially, and enhanced immunoreactivity has been reported.[69,70]

Microwave-assisted antigen retrieval has been reviewed.[71,72] Reversal of formalin-induced protein cross-linkage at high temperature was noted originally in the 1940s,[73,74] and this is thought to be a partial basis for microwave irradiation enhancement of immunohistochemical signal. Various solutions (ranging from heavy metal solutions or salt solutions to distilled water) have been used.[75–78] Similar enhancement of signal is observed after simple boiling of tissue sections in a domestic pressure cooker,[79] whereas heating of tissue sections in a conventional oven has proved less successful. Various factors intrinsic to microwave ovens as discussed in the previous section on microwave fixation need to be at least partially standardized for the procedure to be reproducible. Different conditions result in optimal antigen retrieval depending on the target and its cellular location.[78–80] Enhancement of detection is reported for most antigens tested, although some examples of reduced or abolished signal are demonstrated.[75,78] It is not yet clear which antigenic characteristics can predict whether enhancement or abolition of signal will occur after antigen retrieval.

There are several advantages associated with microwave antigen retrieval. There is potential for reduction in incubation time with primary antibody resulting in cost savings. Positive immunohistochemical signal can be identified after microwave antigen retrieval in tissues that have been formalin fixed for extended periods of time or in tissues that are usually unreactive for that particular antibody after formalin fixation. Improved signal-to-noise ratio is usually demonstrated. A disadvantage is that in tissues prone to high background, antigen retrieval can lead to exacerbation of background staining.[78] Use of microwave antigen retrieval in determining the differentiation of neoplasms does not appear to result in aberrant staining patterns. The enhanced sensitivity of microwave antigen retrieval in the immunohistochemical detection of potentially prognostically significant antigens such as cellular proliferation markers or overexpression or mutation of oncogenes is more problematic. Correlation with results of molecular assays will be required to establish the appropriate cutoff for a true positive result.

Testing Samples of Minimal Size

Previously Stained Slides. In some instances, such as in the examination of consultation material, immunohistochemistry is required but additional material may not be available. In such a situation, hematoxylin-and-eosin–stained tissue sections can successfully be submitted for immunostaining after de-staining,[81] or without de-staining because multiple washes during immunostaining will lighten the stain.[82,83] Gentle treatment of slides is necessary to ensure that tissue remains adherent to the slides. If only one slide with multiple tissue levels is available, two different approaches can be used so that more than one immunostain and control can be performed. Tissue can be removed and placed on other slides using the "peel and stick" method,[84] or the slide can be divided into "wells" for different antibodies using a diamond pen.[83] When removing the coverslip from previously stained slides, immersion time in xylene should be minimized to avoid false-negative results or increased background staining.[82] Higher antibody concentration may be needed to achieve a positive result in previously stained tissues.[9(p58)]

Cytology Specimens. Immunohistochemistry can also be a valuable adjunct to cytopathology. Cytology cell blocks that are processed as "tissue" are the preferred material for immunohistochemistry. Some special considerations apply to other cytology specimens. Filter preparations are not suitable for immunohistochemistry because the filter adsorbs immunologic reagents, resulting in very high background staining. Smears, cytospins, or imprints that are briefly fixed (1–20 minutes) in formalin or alcohol are all suitable substrates for immunohistochemistry.[83,85] Cellular loss can be minimized by the use of coated slides during preparation of smears, cytospins, or imprints. If detection of surface antigen is sought, the cytospins, smears, or imprints are best air-dried and subsequently briefly fixed. Cytologic material is particularly useful for detection of surface antigens because these are more easily demonstrated in cytologic material and because loss of intracellular antigen in cytologic material predisposes to false-negative results for those targets.[85] Cytology preparations for estrogen and progesterone receptor study must be kept frozen unfixed, because these antigens are labile at room temperature and sensitive to fixation. Interpretative pitfalls in immunohistochemistry of cytologic preparations include nonspecific positive signal in three-dimensional cell clusters or in cells that contain phagocytic materials such as neutrophils within their cytoplasm.[83,86]

Decalcified Specimens. Immunohistochemistry can be successfully performed on sections of fixed decalcified bone. Individual antigens vary in their resistance to decalcification procedures, however; immunoglobulins are particularly sensitive.[87,88] Successful immunohistochemistry is reported on glycol methacrylate–embedded bone marrow biopsy specimens in which the decalcification step is avoided altogether.[62]

Previously Frozen Tissue. Immunohistochemistry performed on a tissue block that has been frozen for intraoperative diagnosis, with subsequent slow thawing, fixation, and processing, can give aberrant or suboptimal results, possibly associated with antigen diffusion or destruction. This is an important consideration in intraoperative evaluation of tumors by frozen section. If at all feasible, some tissue should be routinely fixed or rapidly frozen in anticipation of the need for immunohistochemistry or molecular studies.

QUALITY CONTROL FOR IMMUNOHISTOCHEMISTRY

Titration and Optimization of Reagents

As discussed briefly in the description of the antibody antigen reaction, optimal results are obtained with the primary antibody diluted to the point at which background is minimized and signal is maximized. This optimal dilution is determined empirically for a given set of working conditions, that is, time and temperature of incubation as well as detection conditions. The tissue used for titration should be processed in a manner as close as possible to that used for test tissues.

In practice, most primary antibodies are obtained commercially and laboratories rely on the manufacturer to extensively validate the reactivity of the primary antiserum. Commercial preparations include recommendations for optimal working dilutions as well as for storage of the reagent. Some antibodies are sold as working solutions. Such "pre-diluted" solutions are intended to be used without alteration by the consumer. Although the quality of commercial reagents can in general be trusted, good laboratory practice requires verification of results with several dilutions on either side of the manufacturer's recommendation. As an additional component of this titration process, the reactivity of the primary antibody may be evaluated using one or more tissue or reagent controls described in the next section.

Detection reagents also require empirical optimization. Commercial reagents are generally sold in sets with each component adjusted to give optimal results. In general, components from one detection system should not be mixed with those from another if reproducible results are to be expected. Even different lots from one manufacturer may yield slightly different results.

Reagent Quality Control

Once the reactivity of the primary antibody has been characterized, appropriate storage conditions are required to ensure that there is no deterioration. The manufacturer's instructions on commercial kits should be followed strictly. Repeated freezing and thawing can lead to antibody degradation or precipitation. Overgrowth of microorganisms in antiserum can be prevented by storage of antiserum aliquots at −20°C. Storage at 4°C of working dilutions prevents repeated freezing and thawing of the antiserum. Addition of sodium azide 0.1% suppresses microorganism growth.[11,65] Addition of proteins such as bovine serum albumin stabilizes the working dilutions stored at 4°C.[89] A possible explanation for loss of antibody activity in working dilutions in the absence of albumin additives is that immunoglobulin may adsorb to the walls of the glass or plastic containers used for storage.[90] Deterioration in the working dilutions or in the stock antiserum will lead to inconsistencies in the final results.

Although the primary antibody is central to the immunohistochemistry assay, it is clear that accurate reproducible results will be obtained only when all reagents used throughout the assay are prepared and stored under controlled conditions. Dewaxing agents, buffers, protease, detection reagents, and substrates all will impact on the quality of the final product. Changes in buffers and dewaxing agents should be noted in case variable results are seen, but testing before introducing new lots is not required. Change in all other reagents requires comparison of new and old lot results to ensure reproducibility.

Assay Controls

Because so many variables exist in the immunohistochemistry staining sequence, controls are of paramount importance to monitor each assay for validity. The purpose of controls is to provide assurance that tissues without signal are devoid of the antigen and that tissues with signal contain the antigen. Controls also allow problems in any assay to be detected so that appropriate corrective measures can be instituted. Routine controls for immunohistochemistry are briefly summarized in Table 3–2. Controls can be divided into tissue controls and reagent controls.

Tissue Controls. Positive tissue controls contain a known quantity of the antigen of interest and have been fixed and processed identically to the patient material to be tested. In practice, antigen quantitation is seldom achieved in tissues. It is recognized that neoplasms may not express antigen in the same density as normal tissues, so a positive result in the control tissue and negative result in the tumor may reflect differences in antigen density rather than true absence of antigen.[9(p54)] In some instances, the patient material may include an internal positive control, such as normal nerve that is S-100 protein positive. This can be helpful in monitoring loss of antigenicity because of problems with fixation and processing. The most commonly used positive control is tissue known to contain the antigen of interest in either normal or abnormal cells. When feasible, use of a "low-positive" control, that is, a control in which the target antigen is present in small quantities, will establish the limits of sensitivity of the procedure. This concept is of particular importance with respect to hormone receptor, oncogene, and proliferation assays, in which the clinical importance of a strong versus weak positive result may be as yet unknown.

Some authors advocate the use of multi-tissue blocks as control tissues. This allows confirmation of reactivity with appropriate antigens and evaluation of any unexpected spurious reaction.[91,92] The tissue control, whether multi-tissue or single tissue, can be sectioned and placed on the same slide as the patient's section, allowing fewer slides to be manipulated during the assay and providing exact monitoring of reagents used for the patient material. This facilitates interpretation and retrospective review of immunostains, in addition to removing variables in the staining steps, because the tissues are stained simultaneously[92]; however, valuable control blocks can be rapidly depleted with this approach.

The main purpose of the negative control is to confirm that any positive signal in patient tissue represents specific rather than nonspecific reaction. The simplest approach to the negative tissue control is to study the patient tissue section, to ensure that unexpected staining patterns are not detected (e.g., antibodies directed against keratin demonstrating positive signal in segments of peripheral nerve). Alternatively, a tissue section known to lack the antigen of interest can be used in parallel with the patient's

TABLE 3–2

Controls for Immunohistochemistry

Control	Requirement	Purpose
Positive control tissue (handle as additional tissue sample)	Processed in manner identical to test tissue Known to contain antigen that binds to the primary antibody	Positive results verify reaction of antibody and detection reagents
Negative control tissue (handle as additional tissue sample; may be a component of test tissue)	Processed in manner identical to test tissue Known to lack the antigen that binds to the primary antibody	Negative results monitor specificity of primary antibody and detection reagents
Negative antibody control (reagent control, use on each tissue)	Omission of primary antibody; nonimmune serum or buffer diluent for antibody is substituted for primary antibody	Negative results monitor specificity of detection reagents

tissue to confirm absence of staining. The remainder of the issues that pertain to negative control tissues are best discussed under reagent control.

Reagent Controls. Reagent controls serve to determine that any positive signal detected is not caused by spurious reaction associated with each individual step in the immunohistochemical staining procedure. Therefore, under ideal conditions, the immunohistochemical staining procedure would be repeated multiple times, each time omitting one particular step. This is particularly important when multistep procedures involving more than one antibody are performed.[93] The more commonly used negative reagent control represents substitution of preimmune or hyperimmune serum from the same species as the primary antibody for the primary antibody in the incubation step. Preimmune serum is generally not available for commercial marketed antibodies.[93] In practice, substitution of diluent or of an antibody of irrelevant specificity from the same species as the primary antibody, in place of the primary antibody at the incubation step, is the recommended negative control for nonspecific staining and should be performed on the patient's tissue.[94]

Another approach to the negative control is to use adsorbed antiserum. Incubation of antibody with excess purified antigen should result in abolition of signal. The specificity of this method relies on the purity of the antigen used for adsorption. Any extraneous contaminating material in the adsorption antigen would allow removal of cross-reacting antibodies as well as those directed against the truly pure antigen. This problem can be minimized by rigorous purification and the use of different preparations for immunization and adsorption. The lack of signal adsorption should raise questions about the validity of the reaction, but there are situations in which the reacting epitopes, usually part of the secondary structure, are modified in the adsorbing antigen. Similarly, lack of adsorption may reflect inability of the antigen-antibody complex to precipitate. Although this approach has these difficulties, is expensive, and is difficult to employ for most commercial antibodies, it is a useful control for those laboratories preparing their own serum and when a poorly characterized antibody is being introduced into the laboratory.

Independent Validation of Results. Independent validation of the results of immunohistochemistry assays with assay using different technology is an ideal approach. For example, when introducing hormone receptor immunohistochemical assays, samples could be also tested by the biochemical method for comparison. Similarly, for an infectious agent, aliquots could be tested by a molecular assay or by culture. Although complete concordance between methods can never be expected, this approach will allow the laboratory to demonstrate sensitivity and specificity of immunohistochemistry relative to another currently used method. This approach is essential for those immunohistochemical assays that are designed to be analytical (i.e., those for hormone receptors, oncogene prognostic markers, and proliferation markers). Participation in interlaboratory comparison programs is recommended to allow the laboratory to see how its results compare with other laboratories using the same starting material. This program will allow for significant technical problems to be discovered but will not test for difficulties in "routine" specimen fixation and processing that could impair reliability of immunohistochemical analysis.

Troubleshooting

Appropriate controls will allow the laboratory to recognize that a problem exists. Recognition that there is a problem is a key first step. Troubleshooting can be thought of as the subsequent steps to specifically identifying and correcting the problem.

SIGNAL IN NEGATIVE CONTROLS OR ABERRANT LOCATIONS

Endogenous Enzyme Activity. When the signal is generated by histochemical enzymes, any enzyme activity remaining in the tissues will contribute to the signal. Endogenous peroxidase or pseudo-peroxidase (catalase and cytochrome oxidase) is present in granulocytes, hepatocytes, and erythrocytes and can survive freezing or fixation and paraffin-embedding. Difficulty in interpretation of immunostains performed on tissues naturally rich in these cells may occur. An extra step can be undertaken to quench endogenous peroxidase, and numerous methods have been reported. Taylor has used 80% methanol containing 0.6% hydrogen peroxide for 15 minutes without detectable loss of antigenicity.[95] A need for quenching endogenous peroxidase may not be present in all situations. When a quenching step is used, the appearance of signal should suggest preparation of fresh quenching solution, because peroxide is labile.

Endogenous alkaline phosphatase activity is present in intestinal mucosa, placenta, renal tubular cells, osteoblasts, lymphoid cells, and some mesenchymal cells. Although quite problematic in frozen sections, formalin fixation and embedding inactivates the majority of such activity. Endogenous alkaline phosphatase activity is most efficiently removed by quenching with acid. Alkaline phosphatase as an enzyme marker may be particularly useful in tissues that possess much intrinsic peroxidase activity such as bone marrow. It is also useful in dual staining when combined with the peroxidase-antiperoxidase technique. Glucose oxidase, which is not present in human tissues, can also be used as an enzyme marker.

Cellular Pigment. Cells containing abundant pigment such as melanin or hemosiderin may cause difficulty in interpretation of signal when diaminobenzidine is used as chromogen. The pigment may be the reason why the negative control section appears positive. Switching to a substrate producing a different colored product, such as AEC, or changing the histochemical enzyme system may allow the problem to be verified as caused by endogenous pigment. By careful comparison with the negative control tissues, signals in the test tissues can be "read around" the endogenous pigment.

Avidin-Biotin Interactions. Nonspecific binding of detection reagents, resulting in spurious signal, can occur as the result of interaction between cellular components and the highly charged avidin molecules in solution. Similarly, human tissue may contain endogenous biotin that will bind to avidin. Both undesired reactions can be partially ameliorated by incubating in nonfat dry milk or by preincubation with free avidin or biotin, but this approach will also block specific avidin binding. A useful alternative is simply to "read around" the unwanted background or to substitute an alternative detection system that does not rely on avidin-biotin interactions.

Endogenous Fc Receptors. Fc receptors on mononuclear cells do not survive tissue fixation and processing. In frozen tissue subject only to brief fixation, Fc receptors on lymphoid and monocytic cells can result in unwanted binding of primary antiserum. The Fc portion of antibody can also bind to basic groups present in collagen fibers. Substitution of Fab fragments for primary antibody, bridge antibody, and antiperoxidase complex eliminates the problem.

Antigen Dislocation. Diffusion of antigen from its primary location and subsequent attachment to or permeation of other cells can result in "aberrant" signal. Antigen dislocation reflects events that occurred during fixation and processing and cannot be corrected. Thyroglobulin and immunoglobulin can be particularly problematic and may result in thyroglobulin signal in thyroid endothelial cells or immunoglobulin signal in Reed-Sternberg cells of Hodgkin's disease. Recognition of such a signal as aberrant with respect to the cellular morphology will aid the pathologist in avoiding a pitfall of interpretation.

Edge Artifact. Other spurious reactions such as the positive tissue "edge artifact" in which the only signal is identified at the edge of the tissue section, plague the unsuspecting pathologist who must interpret the stain. A possible explanation for edge artifact is that tissue may curl slightly at the edge, allowing nonspecific trapping of antibody and subsequent spurious positive signal. Alternatively, the edge of the tissue may be the only part that is adequately fixed and may represent the only true detection of signal in the tissue.

LACK OF SIGNAL IN POSITIVE CONTROL

Error in Assay. Probably the simplest and most frustrating possibility is omission of one step or use of incorrect reagents in one step. This type of error is reduced with experience and may be almost eliminated with the introduction of automated methods. In most instances the problem will affect more than one assay in the run.

Change in Reagents. When an assay that has been working at an acceptable level suddenly no longer works, or works with reduced signal, the first area to investigate is the key reagents of antibody and detection. Out-of-date reagents cannot be used reliably. Changes of lots can result in different results. Careful introduction of new lots of any reagent by comparison with old lots will allow the laboratory to pinpoint the problem before introduction of the faulty reagent. This not only eliminates errors on patient material but also provides cogent evidence to the manufacturer when the problem occurs with commercial reagents.

If loss of signal is only observed in a test that requires protease digestion, a change in that reagent's activity could be suspected. Similarly, microwave unmasking reagents and conditions should be investigated. Other reagents, such as buffers and dewaxing agents, are less likely sources of error but should not be overlooked.

Fixation Problems. These problems are difficult to detect with routine controls and may be restricted to a specific tissue. Once they occur, there is no way to correct for them, although microwave antigen retrieval techniques can be tried to overcome overfixation. Problems with fixation can be suspected when there is difficulty identifying good normal controls processed in the laboratory. Similarly, difficulty with antigens known to be susceptible to fixation, such as vimentin, also suggest that fixation and processing should be investigated. Finally, a laboratory that gets better results with the interlaboratory comparison programs than it does with its own tissues should seriously review protocols to improve standardization of fixation and processing.

OTHER PROBLEMS

Loss of Tissue from Slides. Some method of enhancement of tissue adherence to glass slides is usually necessary, owing to extensive manipulations of the tissue on the glass slides during the immunohistochemical staining procedure. Clean glass slides must be used. A number of different products such as poly-L-lysine, albumin, and Elmer's glue can be used to coat the slides. Description of six different methods is available.[11,38] Use of electrostatically charged glass slides can also enhance tissue adherence. Gentle handling during the various steps of the staining procedure is necessary. Excessive use of digestion techniques or microwave antigen retrieval methods can also result in loss of tissue from the slides, and particular care is necessary when using these methods.

Excess Chromogen on Glass Surrounding Tissue. The presence of chromogen on the glass slides on completion of the immunohistochemical procedure indicates an imbalance between primary and secondary antibodies or between primary antibody and detection reagents.

IN SITU HYBRIDIZATION

Principles of Hybridization Assay

The basis for any hybridization assay is the specificity of the interaction of a probe with target nucleic acid. This interaction shares some similarities to the antibody-antigen reaction that forms the basis for immunohistochemistry. In both instances the remarkable specificity of the interaction is caused by many weak noncovalent interactions that will be influenced by assay conditions. However, it is nucleic acid chemistry rather than protein chemistry that dictates the nature of the noncovalent interactions and the optimal conditions for these interactions. Nucleic acid chemistry and principles of hybridization assays have been reviewed elsewhere,[96–100] and readers not familiar with nucleic acids may benefit from additional reading.

Briefly, in an aqueous environment, the thermodynamically stable conformation of nucleic acid is a double-stranded helix. The negatively charged sugar-phosphate backbone is exposed, and the hydrophobic bases are shielded from the aqueous phase. The bases are flat and stack centrally, interacting between strands through hydrogen bonds. Chemistry and geometry dictate that only certain base pairs fit into this stable configuration; adenine pairs with thymine (or uracil) and cytosine with guanine. Bases that "fit together" are termed *complementary*, as are two strands of nucleic acid that will combine to form a stable double-stranded helix. Clearly, the sequence of bases in one strand will determine the sequence of bases in its complementary strand.

A double-stranded molecule may be separated or denatured into two single strands by conditions that disrupt the stabilizing hydrogen bonds between bases. This process is referred to as *melting* because the change is from order to disorder often through the application of heat. Formamide, which breaks hydrogen bonds, is another commonly used denaturant. The melting process is reversible, and complementary strands will re-form a helix when denaturants are removed (Fig. 3–6). When complementary strands from two different sources are mixed, some of the duplex structures will be composed of one strand from each source, molecules known as "hybrids." In a hybridization assay, the two sources are the target (sample) and the probe nucleic acids. A probe is simply a known fragment of nucleic acid with a label that can be detected in some fashion. A probe will form a hybrid molecule with a sample that contains nucleic acids complementary to its sequence. The process of searching a sample for specific nucleic acid sequences is termed a *hybridization reaction*. Both DNA and RNA may participate in the hybridization process, and duplex structures

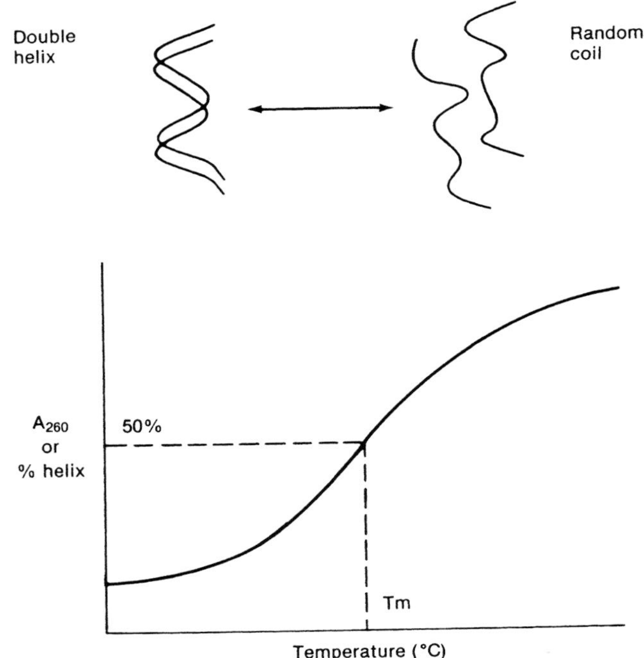

FIGURE 3–6
DNA melting curve. A double-stranded DNA molecule will dissociate into single strands with the application of heat. The change from "order" to "disorder" is referred to as "melting" and can be followed by the increased absorption of single-stranded DNA (A_{260}). The process is reversible; when temperature is reduced, the double-stranded structure will re-form. The ability of DNA to denature and re-form specific duplex structures based on complementary base sequence forms the basis of hybridization assays. (From Piper MA, Unger ER: Nucleic Acid Probes: A Primer for Pathologists. Chicago, ASCP, 1989, p 20.)

may be composed of DNA:DNA, DNA:RNA, or RNA:RNA, in order of increasing stability. Depending on the conditions, some degree of base-pair mismatching will be tolerated in a duplex structure. Conditions that require exact or nearly exact base-pair matching are called "stringent."

All hybridization assays share some similarities. They require the probe and sample nucleic acid to be mixed under conditions allowing complementary base-pairing as well as a method to detect that hybridization has occurred. Although there is a bewildering array of techniques published for in situ hybridization, all share the same basic steps. These steps are shown in Figure 3–7 and are in turn compared with the basic steps for an immunohistochemical assay. In situ hybridization is a specialized form of a solid support assay in which sample nucleic acid is affixed to a solid matrix and interacts with a probe in solution. The microscopic slide is the solid support, and the affixed tissue with preserved morphology is the sample. It is the nature of the sample that makes the in situ hybridization unique. The goal of in situ hybridization is to allow the assay to occur and to be interpreted within a morphologic context. The requirement for morphologic preservation means that the sample nucleic acid must remain at least partially

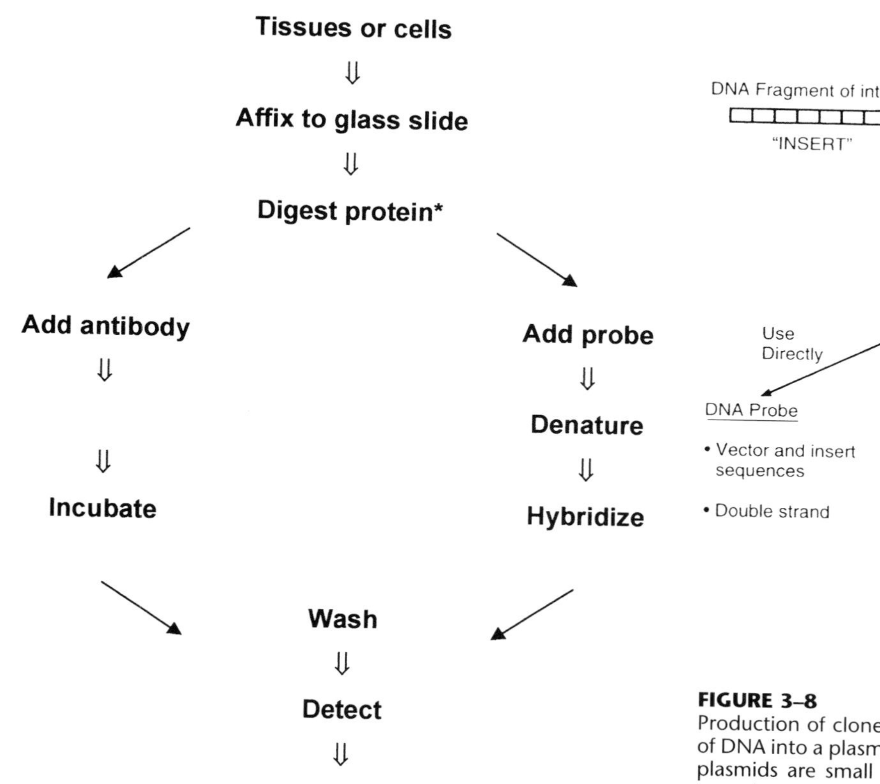

FIGURE 3–7
Generalized steps of in situ hybridization/immunohistochemical assay. The schematic for in situ hybridization is shown on the right; that for immunohistochemistry is on the left.

*Pretreatment for immunohistochemistry may not require enzyme digestion or may include antigen retrieval techniques.

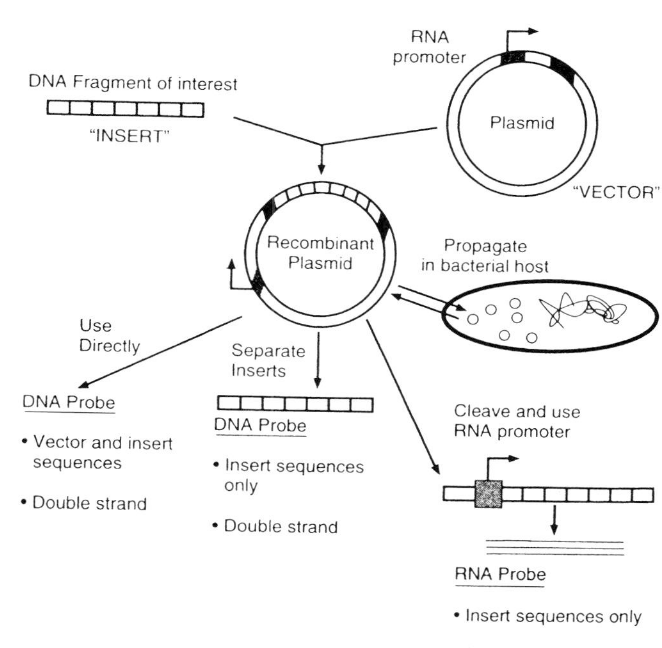

FIGURE 3–8
Production of cloned probes. Insertion of a known foreign segment of DNA into a plasmid vector results in a recombinant plasmid. These plasmids are small circular pieces of DNA that are propagated by growth in a bacterial host. The plasmid DNA is easily separated from the bacterial chromosomal DNA on the basis of size. Either DNA or RNA probes may be produced, depending on the nature of the plasmid. Purified recombinant plasmid may be used as the probe. This produces a double-stranded DNA probe with both insert and vector sequences; alternatively insert sequences may be purified from the vector sequences and used as a probe. If the plasmid contains an RNA promoter region, then RNA probes may be produced using RNA polymerase to transcribe the insert sequences. Because only one strand is transcribed, the resulting RNA probes are single stranded. (From Unger ER: In situ hybridization: Principles and practice. Clin Immunol Newslett 1990;10[8]:121.)

associated with membranes, proteins, and other cellular components forming the framework recognized as cell and tissue structure by light microscopy. This places a restraint on the availability of the target nucleic acids for interaction with probe. The final conditions therefore represent a compromise between morphologic integrity and sample availability.

Probes

PROBE TYPES

Genomic probes are composed of purified genomic material from a particular organism. Before the advent of recombinant nucleic acid technology, these were the only probes available. For example, to get a probe for a virus, the virus was grown in tissue culture and then the virions were isolated and nucleic acid was extracted. The chemical nature of the probe (i.e., DNA or RNA, double- or single-stranded) depended on the isolated organism's genomic structure. Genomic probes are still used in some circumstances, but the vast majority of probes are now produced either by recombinant nucleic acid technology or through chemical synthesis.

Cloned probes consist of a known segment of DNA inserted into a plasmid vector that is propagated by growth in bacterium (Fig. 3–8). The small circular plasmids are easily separated from the bacterial genome on the basis of their size difference. Many different plasmid vectors are now available; pBR322 was one of the first in common use. The probe may consist of the entire plasmid (insert plus vector sequences), or the insert may be purified from the vector sequence. The latter method is obviously more cumbersome, but may result in reduced background in some cases. As prepared by either of these two methods, the resulting probe is a double-stranded DNA probe. Such cloned DNA probes were the first type available and made much of the progress in molecular biology possible. They continue to have wide use and application. Because both complementary strands are included in the probe, it must be denatured before use and solution-phase self-hybridization will limit the extent of hybridization with the immobilized target.

New vectors contain RNA promoter regions adjacent to the inserted DNA sequence that permit generation of

RNA transcripts from the DNA insert. Because only one strand is copied during the RNA synthesis, single-strand RNA probes are generated. Controlling the orientation of the insert in relation to the promoter region allows the production of transcripts in the "sense" (i.e., same as messenger RNA [mRNA]) or "antisense" (i.e., complementary to mRNA) direction. These probes have several advantages. No self-hybridization is possible, favoring maximal interaction with target sequences. RNA probes oriented in the "sense" direction provide excellent negative controls for "antisense" probes. Nonspecifically bound RNA probe can be removed through RNase digestion that will degrade single strands but spare hybrids. The disadvantages of these probes are related to the requirement for placing the insert in a vector with one or two RNA promoters and the relative instability of RNA. RNA probes require careful handling and storage to prevent degradation. RNA is much more labile than DNA, and enzymes that digest RNA (known as RNase) are virtually everywhere. The use of RNA probes therefore dictates use of sterile technique and preparation of reagents and glassware to remove RNase.

Oligonucleotide probes are short segments (15 to 45 bases) of DNA that are chemically synthesized to a specified base sequence. Automated accurate methods of synthesis[101] continue to lower the price of production. Sequence information is increasingly available in data banks.[102] The probes can be generated to be "sense" or "antisense." These features combine to make chemical synthesis very competitive. However, selection of sequences and hybridization conditions to optimize specificity is somewhat empirical. The limited amount of genetic information in these short probes results in lower sensitivity than that achieved with recombinant DNA or RNA probes, which contain several kilobases of information. The result of increasing the genetic complexity of probe is that more of the total target sequence will hybridize with the probe. Thus, for equal numbers of targets, probes with highest representation of target sequence will result in highest signal. This problem has been addressed through the use of multiple oligonucleotide probes to increase the representation of the target sequence in the probe. This approach is somewhat reminiscent of combining monoclonal antibodies to increase the number of recognized epitopes.

A variation of the synthetic approach to probe production is the use of the PCR to produce amplified segments of DNA. In this application the PCR is used not to identify the presence of a target sequence but rather to produce copies of the sequence that can be used as probes. The resultant probe is double-stranded DNA, although asymmetric synthesis can be used to produce single-stranded probes. If the primers are designed to incorporate an RNA promoter, RNA probes can be produced with a subsequent reaction using RNA polymerase.

PROBE SIZE

The physical size of the probe (as opposed to complexity or amount of genetic information) is a crucial consideration for in situ hybridization. Most investigators have found that relatively short probes (fewer than 500 bases) favor increased signal and decreased background. This observation is attributable to penetrance of probe into morphologically constrained target. Oligonucleotide probes are short by nature of their construction; however, genetically complex recombinant probes have the potential for being too large for optimal hybridization. DNA probes can be reduced in size by treatment with DNase I, an endonuclease, whereas RNA probes are subjected to controlled alkaline hydrolysis. Often this reduction in size is achieved through the methods of label incorporation.

PROBE LABELING: ISOTOPIC LABELS

A wide variety of radioactive and nonradioactive labels have been described. Nucleic acid technology was founded with the use of isotopic labeling and detection. Radioactive labels are still favored in many research settings because of the unsurpassed sensitivity achieved with probes of high specific activity. Thus, in situ hybridization with radioactive probes and autoradiographic detection is generally accepted as the standard to which all other methods are compared. Tritium and sulfur 35 (^{35}S) are the two radioisotopes most commonly employed. Higher-energy isotopes, such as phosphorus 32 (^{32}P) and iodine 125, do not permit adequate localization of signal. Tritium has a very long half-life, so the probes are stable for years. This is in contrast to ^{35}S probes, which have a short half-life (80 to 90 days). Exposure times with ^{35}S are shorter than those with tritium because of its higher emission, with some loss of signal localization. Isotopic labeling is achieved through enzymatic incorporation of radioactive nucleotides.

The principles of enzymatic incorporation of label are exemplified by the nick translation reaction,[103] which was the first widely used method of labeling double-stranded DNA probes. As shown in Figure 3–9, single-stranded nicks are randomly introduced into the probe DNA by an enzyme, DNase I. The 3′-hydroxy groups generated form priming sites for the initiation of DNA synthesis by another enzyme, DNA polymerase, which incorporates labeled triphosphate nucleotides in the 5′ to 3′ direction using the opposite strand as template and removing unlabeled strand with its 5′ exonuclease activity. The single-stranded nicks are introduced randomly throughout the probe, the number of nicks being dependent on the amount of DNase I activity. The net result of the action of these two enzymes is to reduce the size of the probe and to incorporate label into both strands of the probe. Fragments will be of random size, but the size range can be controlled by the ratio of the two enzymes in the reaction mixture. The activity of both

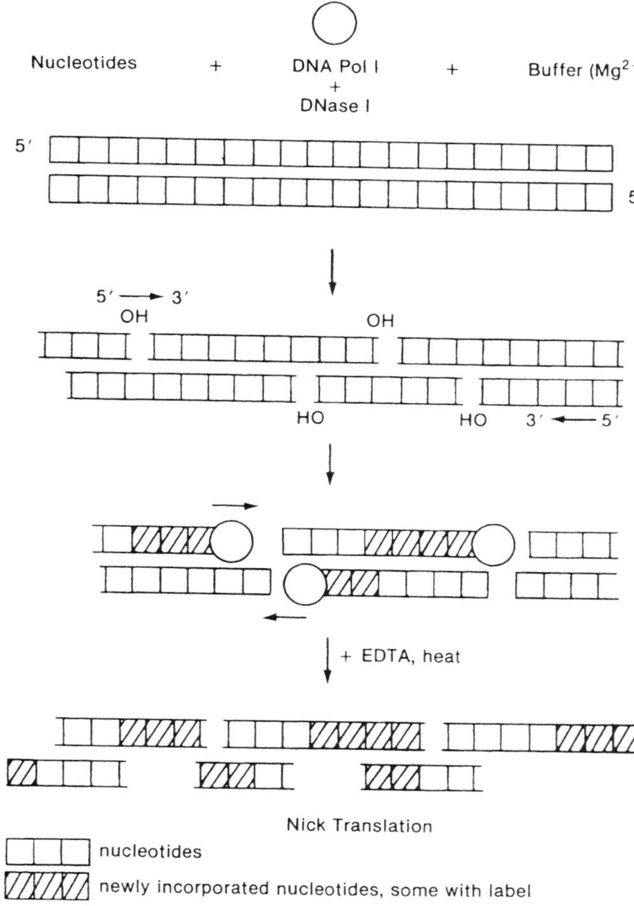

FIGURE 3–9
Nick translation reaction. The principle of in vitro enzymatic incorporation of label into probe is illustrated with the nick translation reaction. The starting material for the reaction includes double-stranded DNA, a mixture of all four nucleotides (at least one nucleotide is labeled), DNase I, and DNA polymerase I, all in a buffer containing magnesium. DNase I is an endonuclease that introduces single-strand nicks. DNA polymerase I uses the 3′OH groups at the nick sites to initiate DNA synthesis in the 5′ to 3′ direction using the opposite strand as template and incorporating nucleotides in the reaction mixture. Unlabeled DNA in the path of the polymerase is removed with the 5′ exonuclease activity of DNA polymerase I. The reaction is terminated by inactivation of both enzymes with heat and EDTA. The result is that label is incorporated into both strands to the DNA probe and the final size of the labeled probe is reduced. (From Unger ER, Piper MA: Nucleic acid biochemistry and diagnostic applications. *In* Burtis CA, Ashwood ER [eds]: Tietz Textbook of Clinical Chemistry, ed 2. Philadelphia, WB Saunders, 1994, p 603.)

enzymes is stopped with heat or by treating the sample with ethylenediaminetetraacetic acid (EDTA). The probe must be separated from unincorporated nucleotides by precipitation or gel filtration.

A newer method of labeling double-stranded DNA probes is referred to as *random-priming*.[104,105] The probe is denatured and allowed to anneal with short hexanucleotides (oligos) of random sequence. The 3′-hydroxy end of an annealed oligo forms the initiation site for the DNA polymerase enzyme, which will incorporate labeled nucleotides using single-stranded regions of the DNA as the template. This reaction also generates short random-sized fragments with both strands of plasmid template labeled. Depending on the reaction conditions, net synthesis of probe may occur and higher specific activity may result.

The generation of RNA probes with use of a transcription vector containing a promoter for RNA polymerase enzyme has been illustrated schematically in Figure 3–8. The transcription vector is linearized by digestion with a restriction endonuclease and then serves as a template for the RNA polymerase as directed by the promoter. The first such vector contained a promoter for SP6 polymerase.[106] When labeled ribonucleotides are present in the reaction mixture, the RNA polymerase will incorporate them using the DNA strand as template. Some vectors contain promoters for two different polymerases permitting generation of sense or anti-sense probes with the same plasmid depending on the choice of RNA polymerase. If conditions are optimized, the RNA polymerase will generate full-length single-stranded RNA transcripts, all the same length as the insert.

Different enzymatic reactions are useful for oligonucleotide probes. T4 polynucleotide kinase may be used to label the 5′ end with ^{32}P, but because that isotope is not generally useful for in situ work, an alternative labeling technique is more common. Terminal deoxynucleotidyl transferase (TdT) will add nucleotides onto the 3′ end in a "tailing" reaction. No template is required, and the number and type of nucleotide can be controlled by the reaction conditions. This will result in a slightly longer probe than the original oligonucleotide with additional "noncoding" labeled bases at the 3′-hydroxy end.

PROBE LABELING: NONRADIOACTIVE

The first practical example of nonisotopic labeling of a probe was achieved through production of a biotin-labeled analogue of deoxyuridine triphosphate,[107] shown in Figure 3–10. The biotin side chain is quite bulky, but despite the altered steric configuration, this nucleotide will be incorporated by DNA polymerase with only slightly lower efficiency than isotopic analogues. Biotin itself cannot generate signal. Polynucleotides with biotin incorporated into their structure are detected indirectly through high-affinity interaction with avidin or streptavidin chemically linked or complexed to a colorimetric enzyme or fluorescent tag. (Antibodies against biotin may be used in place of avidin.) Other functional groups such as bromodeoxyuridine or digoxigenin may be used as affinity labels for DNA and RNA probes. In each case the functional group is chemically linked to a nucleotide (e.g., digoxigenin-dUTP) with subsequent incorporation of the nucleotide analogue by polymerase enzymes. High-affinity antibodies specifically directed against the functional group hapten are produced. The incorporated label is then detected with this antibody linked with a colorimetric

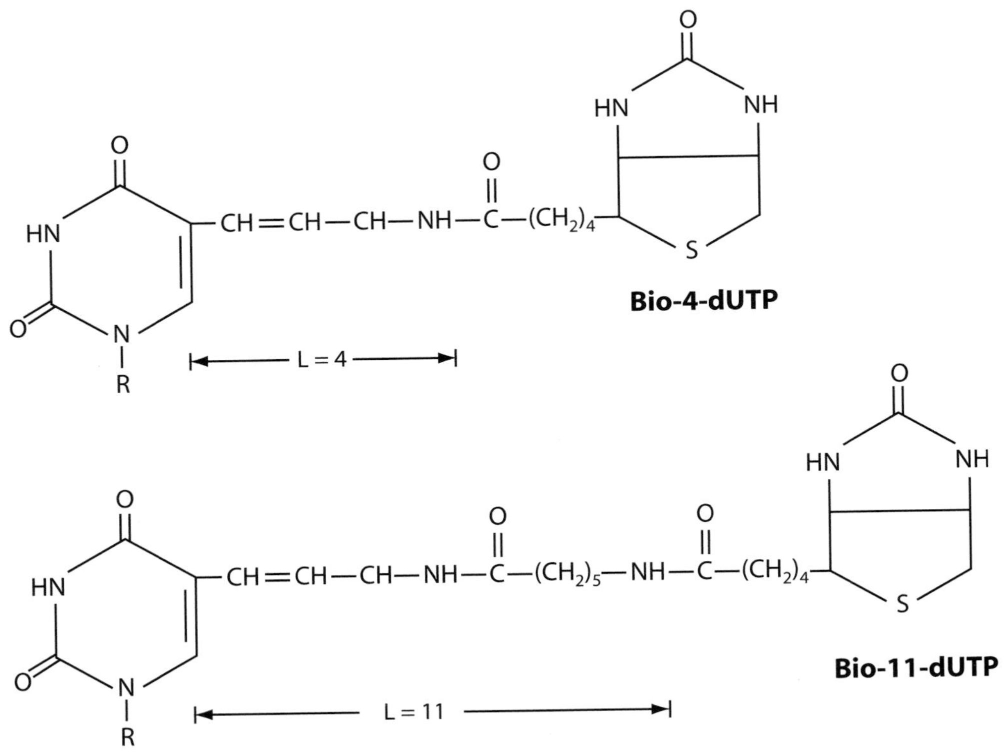

FIGURE 3–10
Biotin analogues of deoxyuridine triphosphate. The length of the carbon side-chain spacer may be varied; Bio-11-dUTP is the most commonly used analogue.

enzyme or fluorescent tag. Although either the nick translation or random priming method may be used to incorporate affinity labels, nick translation is more frequently used. The higher incorporation achieved with random priming is not advantageous for these indirectly detected labels. Final size of labeled product is more easily controlled with nick translation.

Incorporation of affinity-labeled ribonucleotides by RNA polymerases to generate nonradioactive RNA probes can be problematic. RNA polymerases have difficulty with efficient incorporation of these analogues, and short, poorly labeled transcripts may result. As an alternative, analogues with an activated amino group have been synthesized that are more efficiently utilized by the RNA polymerase.[108] Once incorporated, the active amino group can be affinity-labeled in a second direct chemical reaction.

Oligonucleotide probes can be affinity-labeled by several different methods. One of the most efficient is through incorporation of affinity-labeled nucleotide probes at the 3′ end with terminal transferase ("tailing reaction"). Affinity-labeled nucleotides may be incorporated during the synthetic reaction, resulting in label in the hybridizing portion of the probe. Affinity labels may also be added to the 5′ end of the molecule by beginning the synthesis with noncoding nucleotides with active amino groups that are subsequently derivatized. Labels at either the 5′ or the 3′ end have been found to be most efficient.[109]

Nonenzymatic methods of affinity-labeling probes have been described. These include activated analogues of biotin that chemically link to DNA, RNA, or protein when exposed to the light (photo-biotin). Probes can be modified through sulfonation or addition of other large groups (e.g., AAIF) that are subsequently detected with antibodies. Enzymes and fluorescent groups have also been directly chemically linked to probes. These methods have potential because of their simplicity; however, none has been optimized to compete with enzymatic methods of affinity labeling in terms of sensitivity and reproducibility.

COMMERCIAL PROBES

Although numerous well-characterized primary antibodies are readily available through commercial sources, nucleic acid probes are only beginning to be developed. For most clinical laboratories, the lack of commercial reagents is one of the most significant factors limiting diagnostic application.

Assay Conditions

The sensitivity and specificity of the hybridization reaction is greatly influenced by the physical-chemical environment during the reaction and subsequent detection of the hybrid molecules.

DENATURATION

Almost all assays utilize heat to denature probe and/or target nucleic acids. Efficient denaturation is especially important when both species are double-stranded. The time and temperature of denaturation are empirically determined; formalin-fixed cross-linked material requires higher temperatures than nucleic acid in solution.

HYBRIDIZATION COCKTAIL

The hybridization cocktail is the medium used to control the chemical environment during the hybridization reaction. Empirically designed, it is composed of a mixture of reagents selected to favor interaction of nucleic acids through sequence-specific hydrogen bonds rather than charge. The components vary widely but include buffers, salts, denaturants such as formamide, high-molecular-weight polymers, carrier DNA or RNA, various components added to reduce background (e.g., detergents, bovine serum albumin, and Ficoll) and, of course, the probe. The ionic strength of both the hybridization cocktail and the subsequent washes is most often modulated by the concentration of a saline sodium citrate (SSC) buffer composed of 0.15 mol/L sodium chloride and 0.015 mol/L trisodium citrate with a pH of 7.0. The shorthand notation for these conditions refers to the strength of the SSC (i.e., 0.1X SSC). The final stringency of the hybridization reaction is controlled by the formamide and salt concentration of the hybridization cocktail, the temperature of the hybridization reaction, and the temperature and salt concentration of the washing steps.

The concentration of the probe in the hybridization cocktail is another important variable. Unlike antibody, serial dilutions or titrations are not used to determine optimal concentrations. Within limits, kinetics of the solid liquid hybridization rate are influenced by the probe concentration. If probe is double-stranded, solution phase self-hybridization is favored at higher concentration and with increased time, limiting the final sensitivity of probe target interaction. High probe concentration also contributes to high background, that is, interaction with tissues through charge or other mechanisms not involving specific base-pairing. Isotopically labeled probes are especially prone to this problem and are generally used at much lower concentrations than affinity-labeled probes. Similar to the situation with immunohistochemical assays, the time of the hybridization reaction can be reduced with increased probe concentration.

DETECTION

After hybridization, excess probe is removed with buffer washes. The salt concentration and temperature during the washes control the final stringency of the hybridization reaction. Even exactly matched hybrids may be destabilized and removed with improper washing. Detection methods are, of course, dictated by the type of label on the probe.

Detection of radiolabeled probes is achieved with autoradiography. Slides are dipped in a silver emulsion while protected from light and, after time of exposure, developed to demonstrate deposition of silver grains over the areas of localized isotope. The time of exposure and degree of signal localization depend on the isotope. After an optimal hybridization assay, the specific activity of the radiolabeled probe is the major determinant of sensitivity. Within limits, increasing the time of exposure can increase the sensitivity of detection. Longer times will increase background, and background eventually limits resolution of signal. Low-energy isotopes such as tritium require long exposure (month) and provide highest resolution of signal.

Detection of affinity-labeled probes is achieved with methods identical to those previously discussed for immunohistochemistry. Colorimetric detection is guided by the same considerations as those in immunohistochemistry, except that final sensitivity is an even more important consideration for in situ hybridization. In most applications the amount of antigen greatly exceeds the amount of nucleic acid target in tissues. Low background is essential for optimal results and is greatly influenced by the colorimetric detection reagents. The histochemical enzyme/substrate combination also needs to be selected with final sensitivity in mind. Alkaline phosphatase systems with NBT-BCIP substrate are reported to yield the best results,[110,111] although there are many options.

Optimization of Test Material

FIXATION AND PROCESSING

These topics have been considered in detail in the section on immunohistochemistry, and the same considerations apply for in situ hybridization. Optimal results will be achieved only with carefully fixed and processed tissue samples. Although snap freezing and coagulant fixatives have been used with success in research settings, formalin-fixed paraffin-embedded material remains the best choice in a diagnostic setting. Cross-linking fixatives result in improved morphology and increased retention of small nucleic acids. At the same time, cross-linking limits permeation of probe into the tissue, so final probe size, denaturation conditions, and protein digestion must be adjusted to maximize target accessibility.

The concerns with the adequacy of "routine" histopathology practice for adequate preservation of antigens are magnified for preservation of nucleic acids, especially RNA. The extreme lability of RNA requires tissues to be rapidly cut thin enough to allow for even penetration of fixative. DNA is much more stable than RNA and will tolerate more variation in fixation and processing conditions. Because the nucleic acids are bound to tissue, more degradation of target is tolerated for an in situ hybridization assay than for extraction-based hybridization assays such as Northern or Southern hybridization. Nonetheless, there is a point at which the molecular information becomes inadequate for analysis. Clearly variations in fixation and processing that may go unnoticed by hematoxylin-and-eosin staining will result in significant alterations in nucleic acid preservation and cross-linking and will influence the results of molecular analysis.

Protease Pretreatment

Protease treatment is required for all cross-linked samples. Digestion removes proteins and makes the target more accessible to the probe. Acid conditions also contribute to tissue permeabilization and protein removal. Conditions depend on the type of sample and degree of cross-linking. Because of variations in tissue fixation and processing, optimal digestion conditions must be established for each tissue using hybridization to an endogenous target as a guide (see "Controls"). Proteinase K, pronase, and pepsin, as well as other proteases have all been used successfully.

Controls

The same basic considerations discussed for controls and quality assurance in immunohistochemistry apply to in situ hybridization so need not be repeated in detail. With so many facets of the in situ hybridization assay being empirically determined, it is clear that laboratories must carefully control and monitor the results of each test. Interpretation of a precipitated product as evidence of an identified segment of nucleic acid requires that all other explanations be eliminated. Ideally, the specificity of the probe should be established through the use of other hybridization assay formats, such as Southern or Northern blot. Although there are many different kinds of controls that can be included, the three essential controls are listed in Table 3–3. The College of American Pathologists (CAP) Laboratory Checklist for molecular pathology requires these three as a minimum.

With each assay, a sample known to contain the target must be run to demonstrate that all components of the assay are working. This positive control tissue should be fixed and processed identically to test tissues and should be run as an additional sample in each assay. It is often helpful to use a sample with a low level of target to verify the lower limit of assay sensitivity. This allows for small variations between runs to be noticed and corrected.

Because of unavoidable variations in tissue fixation and processing, the use of an endogenous positive control probe on each sample is absolutely essential. This probe is selected to be positive on all tissues if the target nucleic acid has been adequately preserved and made available. This probe should be labeled and used at the same concentration as the test probe. If the positive control probe does not give positive results on a tissue, a negative result for the test probe cannot be interpreted. Adjustment of digestion conditions will often allow positive results to be obtained, but, at times, preservation is poor or tissues are so overfixed that the assay must be termed unsatisfactory.

TABLE 3–3
Controls for In Situ Hybridization

Control	Requirement	Purpose
Positive control tissue (handle as additional tissue sample)	Processed in manner identical to test tissue Known to contain target that hybridizes to test probe	Positive results verify reaction of probe and detection reagents
Positive control probe (use on each tissue)	Hybridizes with a target present in all tissues Labeled in similar manner to test probe and used at similar concentration	Positive result verifies preservation of nucleic acid and availability to probe
Negative control probe (use on each tissue)	Probe of similar base-pair composition to test probe, that should not hybridize to test and control tissues Labeled in similar manner to test probe and used at similar concentration	Negative results monitor specificity of hybridization and detection

The negative control probe is selected to evaluate the specificity of probe target interaction. It should be of similar size and base-pair composition as the test probe but should not hybridize in the absence of the specific target. For recombinant DNA probes, unmodified plasmid sequences are commonly used as the negative control. The negative control probe is labeled and used at the same concentration as the test probe. A negative result with the negative control probe does not prove specificity of the test probe interaction but is at least a guide to monitoring that specificity. The negative control also monitors nonspecific interaction of detection reagents and tissue. If the negative control probe yields positive results, use of a cocktail-only reaction (no probe) will demonstrate if the problem is attributable to detection reagents.

Troubleshooting

Again, because of the similarities between the techniques of in situ hybridization and immunohistochemistry, the approach to many troubleshooting problems in the in situ hybridization assay will be similar to that for immunohistochemistry and will not be repeated.

Tissue Loss

Because the conditions for hybridization assays are more harsh than those used for immunohistochemistry, tissue loss is a bigger problem. The use of silanized glass is almost required. The tissue will form a covalent bond to the glass. This will occur immediately as the tissue is picked up from a protein-free tap water bath. If the glass is properly treated, the tissue will not be able to be "refloated" or moved around on the slide once it has been lifted from the surface of the water. Difficulties with the procedure can be attributed to poorly treated glass, dirty glass, or protein in the water bath.

Overdigestion of tissues will cause poor morphology and result in increased tissue loss. Digestion conditions should be adjusted to the minimum required for probe penetrance.

No Signal with Endogenous Positive Control Probe

Assuming the positive control probe has been properly prepared and stored, this problem reflects either inadequate preservation of target or inadequate pretreatment to make target available. Obviously, if target is degraded, nothing can be done. Increasing concentration of protease, time, and temperature of digestion may all be attempted to improve detection. Conditions of denaturation should also be verified because no hybridization will occur if the target is not denatured. Increasing the time and temperature of denaturation can be attempted.

Signal with Negative Control Probe

This problem could result from endogenous histochemical enzyme, nonspecific binding of detection reagent, or nonspecific binding of probe. The first two possibilities are discussed earlier in the immunohistochemistry section. Nonspecific binding of probe in most instances reflects low-stringency conditions in hybridization and/or wash. The probe may be used at a concentration that is too high or when the time of hybridization is too long. Drying of tissue during the hybridization reaction will result in very high nonspecific sticking of a probe.

REFERENCES

1. Coons AH, Creech HJ, Jones RN: Immunological properties of an antibody containing a fluorescent group. Proc Soc Exp Biol Med 1941;47:200–202.
2. DiStefano HS, Marucci AA, Dougherty RM: Immunohistochemical demonstration of avian leukosis virus antigen in paraffin embedded tissue. Proc Soc Exp Biol Med 1973;142:1111–1115.
3. Nakane PK, Pierce GBJ: Enzyme-labeled antibodies for the light and electron microscopic localization of tissue antigens. J Cell Biol 1967;33:308.
4. Taylor CR, Burns J: The demonstration of plasma cells and other immunoglobulin-containing cells in formalin-fixed, paraffin-embedded tissues using peroxidase-labeled antibody. J Clin Pathol 1974;27:14–20.
5. Sternberger LA, Hardy PHJ, Cuculis JJ, Meyer HG: The unlabeled antibody enzyme method of immunohistochemistry: Preparation and properties of soluble antigen-antibody complex (horseradish peroxidase/anti-horseradish peroxidase) and its use in identification of spirochetes. J Histochem Cytochem 1970;18:315–333.
6. Hsu SM, Raine L, Fanger H: Use of avidin-biotin-peroxidase complex (ABC) in immunoperoxidase techniques: A comparison between ABC and unlabeled antibody (PAP) procedures. J Histochem Cytochem 1981;29:577–580.
7. Swanson PE: Foundations of immunohistochemistry: A practical review. Am J Clin Pathol 1988;90:333–339.
8. Taylor CR, Shi SR, Cote RJ (eds): Immunomicroscopy: A Diagnostic Tool for the Surgical Pathologist, ed 2. Philadelphia, WB Saunders, 1994, pp 42–70.
9. Elias JM: Immunohistopathology: A Practical Approach to Diagnosis. Chicago, ASCP, 1990.
10. Battifora H: p53 immunohistochemistry: A word of caution. Hum Pathol 1994;25:435–437.
11. True LD: Atlas of Diagnostic Immunohistopathology. New York, JB Lippincott, 1990, p 1.
12. Hickey WF, Lee V, Trojanowski JQ, et al: Immunohistochemical application of monoclonal antibodies

against myelin basic protein and neurofilament triple protein subunits: Advantages over antisera and technical limitations. J Histochem Cytochem 1983;31:1126–1135.
13. Larsson L: Immunohistochemistry: Theory and Practice. Boca Raton, FL, CRC, 1988.
14. Sabattini E, Bisgaard K, Poggi S, et al: The Envision system: A new immunohistochemical method for diagnosis and research: Critical comparison with the APAAP, ChemMate, LABC and SABC techniques. J Clin Pathol 1998;51:506–511.
15. Bayer EA, Wilchek M: The use of the avidin-biotin complex as a tool in molecular biology. Methods Biochem Anal 1980;26:1–45.
16. Goding JW: Use of staphylococcal protein A as an immunological reagent. J Immunol Methods 1978;20:241–253.
17. Charalambous C, Singh N, Isaacson PG: Immunohistochemical analysis of Hodgkin's disease using microwave heating. J Clin Pathol 1993;46:1085–1088.
18. Roth J, Heitz PU: Immunolabeling with the protein A-gold technique: An overview. Ultrastruct Pathol 1989; 13:467–484.
19. Damjanov I: Lectin cytochemistry and histochemistry. Lab Invest 1987;57:5–20.
20. Walker RA: The use of lectins in histopathology. Pathol Res Pract 1989;185:826–835.
21. Herrera GA: Ultrastructural immunolabeling: A general overview of techniques and applications. Ultrastruct Pathol 1992;16:37–45.
22. Tubbs RR, Velasco ME, Benjamin SP: Immunocytochemical identification of human chorionic gonadotropin: Comparative study of diaminobenzidine and 3-amino, 9-ethylcarbazole, a nonhazardous chromogen. Arch Pathol Lab Med 1979;103:534–536.
23. Trojanowski JQ, Obrocka MA, Lee VM: A comparison of eight different chromogen protocols for the demonstration of immunoreactive neurofilaments or glial filaments in rat cerebellum using the peroxidase-antiperoxidase method and monoclonal antibodies. J Histochem Cytochem 1983;31:1217–1223.
24. Sheibani K, Tubbs RR, Gephardt GN, et al: Comparison of alternative chromogens for renal immunohistochemistry. Hum Pathol 1981;12:349–354.
25. McGadey J: A tetrazolium method for non-specific alkaline phosphatase. Histochemie 1970;23:180–184.
26. van der Loos CM, Becker AE, van den Oord JJ: Practical suggestions for successful immunoenzyme double-staining experiments. Histochem J 1993;25:1–13.
27. Van Rooijen N: Six methods for separate detection of two different antigens in the same tissue section. J Histochem Cytochem 1980;28:716.
28. Krenacs T, Laszik Z, Dobo E: Application of immunogold-silver staining and immunoenzymatic methods in multiple labeling of human pancreatic Langerhans islet cells. Acta Histochem 1989;85:79–85.
29. Bobrow MN, Shaughnessy KJ, Litt GJ: Catalyzed reported deposition, a novel method of signal amplification: II. Application to membrane immunoassays. J Immunol Methods 1991;137:101–112.
30. Adams JC: Biotin amplification of biotin and horseradish peroxidase signals in histochemical stains. J Histochem Cytochem 1992;40:1457–1463.
31. Kerstens HMJ, Poddighe PJ, Hanselaar AGJM: A novel in situ hybridization signal amplification method based on the deposition of biotinylated tyramine. J Histochem Cytochem 1995;43:347–352.
32. Pelstring RJ, Allred DC, Esther RJ, et al: Differential antigen preservation during tissue autolysis. Hum Pathol 1991;22:237–241.
33. Hsu SM: The use of monoclonal antibodies and immunohistochemical techniques in lymphomas: Review and outlook. Hematol Pathol 1988;2:183–197.
34. Norton AJ, Isaacson PG: Lymphoma phenotyping in formalin-fixed and paraffin wax-embedded tissues: I. Range of antibodies and staining patterns. Histopathology 1989; 14:437–446.
35. Norton AJ, Isaacson PG: Lymphoma phenotyping in formalin-fixed and paraffin wax-embedded tissues: II. Profiles of reactivity in the various tumour types. Histopathology 1989;14:557–579.
36. Perkins SL, Kjeldsberg CR: Immunophenotyping of lymphomas and leukemias in paraffin-embedded tissues. Am J Clin Pathol 1993;99:362–373.
37. Pileri S, Falini B, Sabattini E, et al: Immunohistochemistry of malignant lymphomas: Advantages and limitations of the new monoclonal antibodies working in paraffin sections. Haematologica 1991;76:226–234.
38. Casey TT, Cousar JB, Collins RD: A simplified plastic embedding and immunohistologic technique for immunophenotypic analysis of human hematopoietic and lymphoid tissues. Am J Pathol 1988;131:183–189.
39. Casey TT, Olson SJ, Cousar JB, Collins RD: Plastic section immunohistochemistry in the diagnosis of hematopoietic and lymphoid neoplasms. Clin Lab Med 1990;10:199–213.
40. Merz H, Rickers O, Schrimel S, et al: Constant detection of surface and cytoplasmic immunoglobulin heavy and light chain expression in formalin-fixed and paraffin-embedded material. J Pathol 1993;170: 257–264.
41. Grube D, Kusumoto Y: Serial semithin sections in immunohistochemistry: Techniques and applications. Arch Histol Jpn 1986;49:391–410.
42. Murray GI: Enzyme histochemistry and immunohistochemistry with freeze-dried or freeze-substituted resin-embedded tissue. Histochem J 1992;24:399–408.
43. Larsson L: Tissue preparation methods for light microscopic immunohistochemistry. Appl Immunohistochemistry 1993;1:2–16.
44. Fox CH, Johnson FB, Whiting J, Roller PP: Formaldehyde fixation. J Histochem Cytochem 1985;33: 845–853.
45. Elias JM, Gown AM, Nakamura RM, et al: Quality control in immunohistochemistry: Report of a workshop sponsored by the Biological Stain Commission. Am J Clin Pathol 1989;92:836–843.
46. Battifora H: Assessment of antigen damage in immunohistochemistry. Am J Clin Pathol 1991;96:669–671.
47. Curran RC, Gregory J: Effects of fixation and processing on immunohistochemical demonstration of immunoglobulin in paraffin sections of tonsil and bone marrow. J Clin Pathol 1980;33:1047–1057.
48. Mepham BL: Influence of fixatives on the immunoreactivity of paraffin sections. Histochem J 1982;14: 731–737.

49. McLean IW, Nakane PK: Periodate-lysine-paraformaldehyde fixative: A new fixation for immunoelectron microscopy. J Histochem Cytochem 1974;22:1077–1083.
50. Brenes F, Harris S, Paz MO, et al: PLP fixation for combined routine histology and immunocytochemistry of liver biopsies. J Clin Pathol 1986;39:459–463.
51. Azumi N, Battifora H: The distribution of vimentin and keratin in epithelial and nonepithelial neoplasms: A comprehensive immunohistochemical study on formalin- and alcohol-fixed tumors. Am J Clin Pathol 1987; 88: 286–296.
52. Battifora H, Kopinski M: The influence of protease digestion and duration of fixation on the immunostaining of keratins: A comparison of formalin and ethanol fixation. J Histochem Cytochem 1986;34: 1095–1100.
53. Mitchell D, Ibrahim S, Gusterson BA: Improved immunohistochemical localization of tissue antigens using modified methacarn fixation. J Histochem Cytochem 1985;33:491–495.
54. Kok LP, Boon ME: Physics of microwave technology in histochemistry. Histochem J 1990;22:381–388.
55. Login GR, Schnitt SJ, Dvorak AM: Rapid microwave fixation of human tissues for light microscopic immunoperoxidase identification of diagnostically useful antigens. Lab Invest 1987;57:585–591.
56. Horobin RW, Flemming L: "Trouble-shooting" microwave accelerated procedures in histology and histochemistry: Understanding and dealing with artefacts, errors and hazards. Histochem J 1990;22:371–376.
57. Leong AS, Milios J, Duncis CG: Antigen preservation in microwave-irradiated tissues: A comparison with formaldehyde fixation. J Pathol 1988;156:275–282.
58. Suurmeijer AJ, Boon ME, Kok LP: Notes on the application of microwaves in histopathology. Histochem J 1990;22:341–346.
59. Rickert RR, Maliniak RM: Intralaboratory quality assurance of immunohistochemical procedures: Recommended practices for daily application. Arch Pathol Lab Med 1989; 113:673–679.
60. Sato Y, Mukai K, Watanabe S, et al: The AMeX method: A simplified technique of tissue processing and paraffin embedding with improved preservation of antigens for immunostaining. Am J Pathol 1986;125: 431–435.
61. Beckstead JH, Halverson PS, Ries CA, Bainton DF: Enzyme histochemistry and immunohistochemistry on biopsy specimens of pathologic human bone marrow. Blood 1981;57:1088–1098.
62. Islam A, Archimbaud E, Henderson ES, Han T: Glycol methacrylate (GMA) embedding for light microscopy: II. Immunohistochemical analysis of semithin sections of undecalcified marrow cores. J Clin Pathol 1988;41: 892–896.
63. Larsson L: Immunohistochemistry: Theory and Practice. Boca Raton, FL, CRC Press, 1988, p 61.
64. Lazzaro B, Munger R, Lumb G: Antigen localization in immunoperoxidase-stained plastic-embedded soft tissues. Hum Pathol 1988;19:902–909.
65. Andrade RE, Hagen KA, Swanson PE, Wick MR: The use of proteolysis with ficin, for immunostaining of paraffin sections: A study of lymphoid, mesenchymal, and epithelial determinants in human tissues. Am J Clin Pathol 1988;90:33–39.
66. Abbondanzo SL, Allred DC, Lampkin S, Banks PM: Enhancement of immunoreactivity among lymphoid malignant neoplasms in paraffin-embedded tissues by refixation in zinc sulfate-formalin. Arch Pathol Lab Med 1991;115:31–33.
67. Shi SR, Cote C, Kalra KL, et al: A technique for retrieving antigens in formalin-fixed, routinely acid-decalcified, celloidin-embedded human temporal bone sections for immunohistochemistry. J Histochem Cytochem 1992;40:787–792.
68. Shi SR, Tandon AK, Haussmann RR, et al: Immunohistochemical study of intermediate filament proteins on routinely processed, celloidin-embedded human temporal bone sections by using a new technique for antigen retrieval. Acta Otolaryngol (Stockh) 1993;113: 48–54.
69. Greenwell A, Foley JF, Maronpot RR: An enhancement method for immunohistochemical staining of proliferating cell nuclear antigen in archival rodent tissues. Cancer Lett 1991;59:251–256.
70. van den Berg FM, Baas IO, Polak MM, Offerhaus GJ: Detection of p53 overexpression in routinely paraffin-embedded tissue of human carcinomas using a novel target unmasking fluid. Am J Pathol 1993; 142:381–385.
71. Suurmeijer AJ, Boon ME: Notes on the application of microwaves for antigen retrieval in paraffin and plastic tissue sections. Eur J Morphol 1993;31:144–150.
72. Swanson PE: Microwave antigen retrieval in citrate buffer. Lab Med 1994;25:520–522.
73. Fraenkel-Conrat H, Brandon BA, Olcott HS: The reaction of formaldehyde with proteins: IV. Participation of indole groups: Gramicidin. J Biol Chem 1947;168: 99–117.
74. Fraenkel-Conrat H, Olcott HS: Reaction of formaldehyde with proteins: VI. Cross-linking of amino groups with phenol, imidazole, or indole groups. J Biol Chem 1948; 174:837–843.
75. Cattoretti G, Pileri S, Parravicini C, et al: Antigen unmasking on formalin-fixed, paraffin-embedded tissue sections. J Pathol 1993;171:83–98.
76. Gown AM, DeWever N, Battifora H: Microwave-based antigenic unmasking. Appl Immunohistochemistry 1993; 1:256–266.
77. Leong AS: Microwave techniques for diagnostic laboratories. Scanning 1993;15:88–98.
78. Shi SR, Key ME, Kalra KL: Antigen retrieval in formalin-fixed, paraffin-embedded tissues: An enhancement method for immunohistochemical staining based on microwave oven heating of tissue sections. J Histochem Cytochem 1991;39:741–748.
79. Norton AJ: Microwave oven heating for antigen unmasking in routinely processed tissue sections. J Pathol 1993;171:79–80.
80. Shi SR, Chaiwun B, Young L, et al: Antigen retrieval technique utilizing citrate buffer or urea solution for immunohistochemical demonstration of androgen receptor in formalin-fixed paraffin sections. J Histochem Cytochem 1993;41:1599–1604.

81. Milios J, Leong AS: The application of the avidin-biotin technique to previously stained histological sections. Stain Technol 1987;62:411–416.
82. Myers JD: Development and application of immunocytochemical staining techniques: A review. Diagn Cytopathol 1989;5:318–330.
83. Nadji M, Ganjei P, Morales AR: Immunocytochemistry in contemporary cytology: Technique and its application. Lab Med 1994;25:502–508.
84. Mehta P, Battifora H: How to do multiple immunostains when only one tissue slide is available. Appl Immunohistochemistry 1993;1:297–298.
85. Nadji M, Ganjei P: Special report: Immunocytochemistry in diagnostic cytology: A 12-year perspective. Am J Clin Pathol 1990;94:470–475.
86. Miller RT: Immunohistochemistry in the community practice of pathology: Part I. General considerations, technical factors and quality assurance. Lab Med 1991; 22:457–464.
87. Matthews JB, Mason GI: Influence of decalcifying agents on immunoreactivity of formalin-fixed, paraffin-embeded tissue. Histochem J 1984;16:771–787.
88. Mullink H, Hezen-Logmans SC, Tadema TM, et al: Influence of fixation and decalcification on the immunohistochemical staining of cell-specific markers in paraffin-embedded human bone biopsies. J Histochem Cytochem 1985;33:1103–1109.
89. Ciocca DR, Adams DJ, Bjercke RJ, et al: Monoclonal antibody storage conditions and concentration effects on immunohistochemical specificity. J Histochem Cytochem 1983;31:691–696.
90. Larsson L: Immunohistochemistry: Theory and Practice. Boca Raton, FL, CRC, 1988, p 158.
91. Battifora H: The multitumor (sausage) tissue block: Novel method for immunohistochemical antibody testing. Lab Invest 1986;55:244–248.
92. Miller RT, Groothuis CL: Multitumor "sausage" blocks in immunohistochemistry: Simplified method of preparation, practical uses, and roles in quality assurance. Am J Clin Pathol 1991;96:228–232.
93. Taylor CR, Tandon AK: Theoretical and practical aspects of the different immunoperoxidase techniques. *In* Taylor CR, Shi SR, Cote RJ (eds): Immunomicroscopy: A Diagnostic Tool for the Surgical Pathologist, ed 2. Philadelphia, WB Saunders, 1994, pp 21–41.
94. Taylor CR: Report of the Immunohistochemistry Steering Committee of the Biological Stain Commission: "Proposed format: package insert for immunohistochemistry products." Biotech Histochem 1992;67: 323–338.
95. Taylor CR, Shi SR: Fixation processing, special applications. *In* Taylor CR, Shi SR, Cote RJ (eds): Immunomicroscopy: A Diagnostic Tool for the Surgical Pathologist, ed 2. Philadelphia, WB Saunders, 1994, pp 42–70.
96. Fenoglio-Preiser CM, Willman CL: Molecular Diagnostics in Pathology. Baltimore, Williams & Wilkins, 1991.
97. Herrington CS, McGee JO: Diagnostic Molecular Pathology: A Practical Approach. Oxford, Oxford University Press, 1992.
98. Piper MA, Unger ER: Nucleic Acid Probes: A Primer for Pathologists. Chicago, ASCP, 1989.
99. Tenover FC, Unger ER: Use of nucleic acid probes for detection and identification of infectious agents. *In* Persing DH, Smith TF, Tenover FC (eds): Diagnostic Molecular Microbiology. Washington, DC, American Society of Microbiology, 1993, pp 3–25.
100. Unger ER, Piper MA, Burtis CA, Ashwood ER (eds): Tietz Textbook of Clinical Chemistry. Philadelphia, WB Saunders, 1993, pp 594–624.
101. Caruthers MH: Gene synthesis machines: DNA chemistry and its uses. Science 1985;230:281–285.
102. Mapping and Sequencing the Human Genome. Washington, DC, National Academy of Sciences Press, 1988.
103. Rigby PW, Dieckmann M, Rhodes C, Berg P: Labeling deoxyribonucleic acid to high specific activity in vitro by nick translation with DNA polymerase I. J Mol Biol 1977;113:237–251.
104. Feinberg AP, Vogelstein B: A technique for radiolabeling DNA restriction endonuclease fragments to high specificactivity: Addendum. Anal Biochem 1984;137: 266–267.
105. Feinberg AP, Vogelstein B: A technique for radiolabeling DNA restriction endonuclease fragments to high specific activity. Anal Biochem 1983;132:6–13.
106. Melton DA, Krieg PA, Rebagliati MR, et al: Efficient in vitro synthesis of biologically active RNA and RNA hybridization probes from plasmids containing a bacteriophage SP6 promoter. Nucleic Acids Res 1984;12:7035–7056.
107. Langer PR, Waldrop AA, Ward DC: Enzymatic synthesis of biotin-labeled polynucleotides: Novel nucleic acid affinity probes. Proc Natl Acad Sci U S A 1981;78: 6633–6637.
108. Folsom V, Hunkeler MJ, Haces A, Harding JD: Detection of DNA targets with biotinylated and fluoresceinated RNA probes: Effects of the extent of derivatization on detection sensitivity. Anal Biochem 1989;182:309–314.
109. Cook AF, Vuocolo E, Brakel CL: Synthesis and hybridization of a series of biotinylated oligonucleotides. Nucleic Acids Res 1988;16:4077–4095.
110. Unger ER, Hammer ML, Chenggis ML: Comparison of 35S and biotin as labels for in situ hybridization: Use of an HPV model system. J Histochem Cytochem 1991; 39:145–150.
111. Waller HA, Savage AK: Analysis of gene transcription in situ: Methodological considerations and applications in pathology. J Histotechnol 1994;17:203–218.

CHAPTER 3 APPENDIX

SOP 3.1*

ANTIGEN DETECTION IN TISSUE BY ABC IMMUNOHISTOCHEMISTRY

PRINCIPLE

The presence of a certain antigen is demonstrated using the avidin-biotin-peroxidase complex (ABC) method of immunohistochemistry. Tissue samples are submitted on appropriate slides.

SPECIMEN

Specimens are 4- to 6-μm sections of formalin-fixed, paraffin-embedded tissue that has been placed on coated glass microscope slides. Two slides are required at a minimum.

MATERIALS AND SOLUTIONS

Oven set at 60°C
Water bath set at 35°C to 40°C
Magnetic stir plate, stir bars
Gloves
Pipettes
Xylene
100% ethanol
0.05% protease VIII (Sigma, St. Louis) in 0.1 mol/L sodium phosphate buffer, pH 7.8
100% methanol with 3% hydrogen peroxide (H_2O_2)
0.01 mol/L sodium phosphate, pH 7.40, 0.15 mol/L NaCl (PBS)
Normal serum (specific for secondary antibody species)
Primary antibody
Biotinylated secondary antibody
Avidin-biotin complex (ABC) reagent
0.016% diaminobenzidine tetrahydrochloride (DAB), 0.24% H_2O_2 in PBS
Gill's hematoxylin
2% concentrated ammonia in deionized water
Permount (Fisher Scientific)

* SOP 3.1 by Gary L. Bratthauer, BA, MT, Department of Gynecologic and Breast Pathology, Armed Forces Institute of Pathology, Washington, DC.

CONTROL

POSITIVE CONTROL SLIDE. This is a slide known to demonstrate the antigen of interest; it should be weakly or moderately (not strongly) positive. A positive control is run with every patient specimen. This control ensures that the reagent system is functioning properly.

NEGATIVE CONTROL SLIDE. This is a patient slide with PBS substituting for the primary antibody, to control for nonspecitic binding of the detection system. Section should not give a signal.

PROCEDURE

1. Paraffin sections mounted on pretreated slides are heated in an oven for 30 minutes.
2. Deparaffinize sections using four changes of xylene for 5 minutes each, followed by four changes of 100% for 3 minutes each. For sections that do not require digestion, go directly to step 6.
3. For sections requiring digestion, rinse in deionized water for 3 minutes.
4. Incubate sections in buffered protease VIII at 37°C for 1 to 30 minutes. The standard time for digestion is 3 minutes.
5. Rinse sections in two changes of deionized water for 2 minutes each, then three changes of 100% ethanol for 3 minutes each.
6. Block endogenous peroxidase activity with 3% H_2O_2 methanol for 30 minutes.
7. Rinse sections three times with deionized water.
8. Reduce nonimmunologic binding of antiserum by placing sections in 10% normal serum-PBS derived from the same species as the biotinylated (secondary) antibody (e.g., if biotinylated antibody is goat anti-rabbit antiserum, use normal goat serum) at 4°C overnight.
9. Shake off excess normal serum and place slides in leveled staining trays. Distribute the slides according to the primary antiserum that is to be applied, Care should be taken so that the sections do not touch during incubation with primary antisera. The need to separate the slides into groups to preclude any chance of contaminating a section with the wrong antibody cannot be overemphasized. Cover section with primary antiserum (e.g., rabbit antiserum) specific for desired antigen for 30 minutes at room temperature. Make sure the chamber lid is on to prevent air-drying during the incubation.
10. Wash sections with PBS three times.
11. Flood sections twice with 10% normal serum for 10 minutes each, and then rinse in PBS.

12. Shake off excess buffer and cover sections with biotinylated secondary antibody. Incubate for 30 minutes at room temperature, making sure the chamber lid is on to prevent air-drying of sections.
13. Wash sections three times with PBS.
14. Shake off excess buffer and cover sections with ABC reagent, prepared according to the recommendations of the manufacturer, for 30 minutes at room temperature, making sure the chamber lid is on to prevent air-drying of the sections.
15. Wash sections three times with PBS. Place sections in staining racks for a final 10-minute soak in PBS.
16. Develop in 0.016% DAB and 0.24% H_2O_2 in PBS solution for 10 to 25 minutes at room temperature. The usual time for optimal development of DAB is 15 minutes, but this may vary with the lot of DAB being used.
17. Wash sections 1 or 2 minutes three times with deionized water.
18. Counterstain with Gill's hematoxylin.
19. "Blue" sections with ammonia water.
20. Wash in deionized water for 5 minutes.
21. Dehydrate and mount sections with Permount.

REPORTING RESULTS

Positive antibody-antigen reaction is brown, with nuclei blue. The assay is indeterminate if the assay is negative and the positive control section shows no reactivity. The negative control should be carefully examined to control for nonspecific staining.

PROCEDURE NOTES

Throughout the procedure, keep drying of the sections to a minimum to prevent destroying epitopes on the cell membrane. Drying also causes nonspecific background staining.

In step 2, it is important to complete deparaffinization because paraffin can mask epitopes from the primary antibody.

In step 16, special precautions should be taken when handling DAB because of its possible carcinogenic properties.

REFERENCES

Bratthauer GL, Adams LR: Immunohistochemistry: Antigen detection in tissue. In Mikel UV (ed): Advanced Laboratory Methods in Histology and Pathology. American Registry of Pathology, 1994, pp 1–40.

Hsu SM, Raine L, Fanger H: Use of avidin-biotin-peroxidase complex (ABC) in immunoperoxidase techniques: A comparison between ABC and unlabeled antibody (PAP) procedures. J Histochem Cytochem 1981;29:577–580.

CYNTHIA F. WRIGHT
ANN H. REID

4

Hybridization and Blotting Techniques

Investigational methods of molecular biology are rapidly transforming our understanding of the pathogenesis and diagnosis of many diseases. It is now possible to detect changes in the structure or expression of target genes within the entire context of the human genome. Finding one target in an array of targets is made possible by *hybridization*, the ability of nucleic acid molecules to find their complementary sequences in biologic specimens. The presence of one labeled, hybridized molecule, called a *probe*, can be detected by a variety of techniques. Hybridization forms the basis of nearly all of the techniques used in molecular pathology today, including polymerase chain reaction (PCR) (see Chapter 5) and Southern and Northern blotting techniques.

In addition to discussing PCR and blots, in this chapter we also describe techniques for extracting tissue DNA, RNA, proteins, and the subsequent manipulations that allow mixtures of molecules to be separated by size, transferred to solid supports, and detected by probes. Particular attention is given to applying these methods to formalin-fixed paraffin-embedded tissues.

EXTRACTION OF NUCLEIC ACIDS

Extraction of DNA

DNA that is suitable for filter hybridization can be obtained using a variety of techniques. The usual protocol is to lyse cells by incubation in a buffer containing protease and detergent, followed by phenol extraction, and then ethanol precipitation or dialysis of the nucleic acid. RNA is eliminated by including pancreatic ribonuclease (RNAse) in the extraction buffer. Choosing a protocol from the variety that is available depends on the molecular weight of the resulting DNA that is desired. By specifically modifying the extraction procedure, DNA can be isolated from blood, minced fresh tissue, or pulverized frozen tissue. Many commercial suppliers offer kits for isolating DNA from blood, tissue, or cells. Commercially prepared kits allow the option of isolating DNA using organic extraction (i.e., by phenol-chloroform removal of protein), nonorganic extraction (i.e., using high salt solutions to precipitate proteins), or column-based methods in which samples are run through a nucleic-acid binding resin from which DNA and RNA are later eluted.

DNA suitable for Southern blot analysis (described later) can sometimes be recovered from formalin-fixed, paraffin-embedded tissue.[1–4] In the protocol used by Goettz and co-workers,[3] for example, as much tissue as possible is cut away from paraffin and finely minced before proteinase K treatment and DNA extraction. Relatively intact DNA can be obtained if the sample was originally processed in a buffered fixative and if long periods of protease digestion in ionic detergents are used. The length of time the sample spends in fixative has influenced the results in some studies[2, 4] but not in others.[3] In the method of Dubeau and colleagues,[1, 2] the formalin-fixed, paraffin-embedded tissue is first cut with a microtome, then packed into a centrifuge tube, and finally deparaffinized with xylene before proteinase K treatment. Because the method emphasizes the use of high-molecular-weight DNA, the cell suspensions are centrifuged after 12 hours of proteinase K digestion to eliminate degraded DNA that remains in the supernatant. Only DNA that can be spooled with a glass rod from the final ethanol precipitate is used for subsequent blotting experiments. The ability to recover DNA from paraffin blocks permits the investigation of archived material in a variety of studies. Unfortunately, only 30% to 75% of paraffin blocks yield DNA that is intact enough for blotting. The preparation time for these samples is long, lasting many days, and most, if not all, of the tissue in a block must be used for the extraction procedure. Of course, any DNA suitable for Southern blot analysis also can be used for dot-blot testing (described later).

The PCR technique allows the DNA in archived tissue to be studied much more easily because the template

DNA does not have to be purified extensively or be of high molecular weight. We have found that the amount of DNA in a single 6-μm section (of 50 to 200 mm^2) of formalin-fixed, paraffin-embedded material can yield enough template for hundreds of PCR reactions. Even though the lysate contains both DNA and RNA, if no reverse transcriptase step is performed, this method is specific for amplification of DNA. Using a method adapted from Shibata and associates,[5] we routinely cut two 6-μm sections from a block, then deparaffinize the sections with xylene and ethanol, and resuspend the resulting tissue pellet in a buffer solution containing nonionic detergents and proteinase K (for details, see SOP 4.1). The amount of the resulting lysate used in subsequent PCR reactions depends on the starting amount of tissue. Generally, 1 to 2 μL of lysate will generate enough product to yield a visible signal on gel electrophoresis with ethidium bromide staining, provided that the expected product is in the range of 100 to 200 base pairs (bp). The signal can be amplified by performing a Southern blot (discussed later). If no signal is visible after PCR, diluting the lysate in serial dilutions is sometimes useful. Often, 1 μL of a 10-fold dilution will work when 1 μL of a stock lysate solution does not. This procedure may seem contradictory, but we believe that this may dilute inhibitors of PCR while retaining enough DNA to serve as a template. The fixative used to preserve the tissue before embedding has a profound effect on the subsequent ability to amplify the DNA. In our experience, formalin-fixed tissue will work 90% to 95% of the time, whereas tissue fixed in B5 has never worked in our laboratory. It may be possible, however, to remove inhibitors present in the tissue or in the fixative by modifying the lysate preparation procedure.

Isolating specific regions of a tissue block for amplification and subsequent analysis also is possible. In this case, an unstained tissue section on a glass slide can be deparaffinized by dipping the slide in xylene and ethanol, air-drying the tissue, and then comparing it with an adjacent section stained with hematoxylin and eosin. The region of interest can be removed from the slide using a scalpel or needle and placed in a separate tube. In this way, it is possible to compare the results obtained from normal cells, preneoplastic lesions, and overtly neoplastic areas from the same tissue section.

Techniques to examine small populations of cells from a tissue section have become even more refined with the recently described technique called *laser capture microdissection*.[6] In this technique, a plastic film is placed on a tissue section, the section is placed under a microscope, and the plastic is activated to adhere to the cells of interest by a laser pulse. The desired cells bound to the plastic can then be selectively removed and analyzed for DNA, RNA, or protein content. Techniques such as this are making it possible to analyze gene content and expression in sharply defined cell populations.

Extraction of RNA

RNA suitable for blotting also can be isolated from a variety of sources, and many different protocols have been published.[7–9] To isolate RNA from tissues rich in ribonuclease, for example, Chirgwin and co-workers[7] homogenize cells in the presence of guanidinium thiocyanate and a reducing agent. The RNA is separated from contaminating protein by ethanol precipitation or sedimentation through a cesium chloride "cushion." In a variation of this method, RNA can be isolated by a single extraction with an acid guanidinium thiocyanate/phenol/chloroform mixture.[8] These techniques and variations have been exploited commercially to manufacture kits that aid in RNA isolation. These kits are total RNA isolation systems that allow rapid purification of RNA from tissues, cells, or biologic fluids. Commercially, kits also are available for isolating mRNA from total RNA, based on oligo-dT cellulose technologies or on isolating mRNA directly from tissue or cultured cells using magnetic separation technology.

To obtain RNA of sufficient quality for dot-blot hybridization does not require extensive purification of the RNA or a large number of sample cells. In one method used for cytoplasmic dot hybridization, cells are lysed in nonionic detergent, the nuclei are pelleted, and the supernatant is denatured with formaldehyde and spotted onto nitrocellulose.[10] Alternatively,[11] cells are solubilized in guanidine hydrochloride, the viscous lysate is passed through a syringe, and the RNA is precipitated with ethanol, dissolved in formaldehyde, and applied to nitrocellulose.

It has been known for many years that intact RNA exists in formalin-fixed, paraffin-embedded tissue. The first application was to extract RNA for Northern and dot-blot analysis.[12] In that extraction application, minced tissue from paraffin blocks was homogenized in a Waring blender, digested in a sodium dodecyl sulfate (SDS)/proteinase K solution, phenol-extracted, and precipitated with lithium chloride and, finally, residual paraffin was removed. Subsequently, RNA has successfully been isolated from formalin-fixed, paraffin-embedded tissue for PCR analysis.[13–16] RNA present in fixed tissues also has been detected using in situ hybridization[17] and even in situ PCR.[18] We also have had success in performing reverse transcriptase PCR to analyze formalin-fixed paraffin-embedded tissues for the presence of influenza viruses, morbilliviruses, and hepatitis C virus.[19] We have obtained amplifiable RNA from paraffin blocks dating back to 1918.[20] We deparaffinize sections in xylene and ethanol, digest the tissue in a buffer containing SDS and proteinase K, extract in phenol-chloroform, and then precipitate the nucleic acids in ethanol. The precipitates are resuspended in distilled diethyl pyrocarbonate (DEPC)–treated water, and an aliquot is reverse-transcribed with Moloney murine leukemia virus (MMLV) reverse transcriptase. If a single gene product is sought, the reverse-transcription reaction can be performed with a specific downstream primer. The other specific primer is then added, along with Taq polymerase, and the sample is cycled in a thermal cycler. If the lysate is to be used to amplify many different viral targets, random hexamers can be used for reverse transcription to ensure that complementary DNA (cDNA) is made from all the RNA in the sample.

Quality Control

DNA and RNA isolated for subsequent PCR applications must be handled under conditions that prevent contamination from extraneous samples. We cut formalin-fixed, paraffin-embedded tissues with disposable microtome blades, using a different blade for each sample. Lysates from these tissues are prepared in a PCR-setup room that is physically separate from the rooms used to analyze the amplified product. Reagents and aliquots are prepared in this room, with pipettes that are used solely for applications performed without template DNA. Also, pipette tips containing plugs are used to help prevent contaminating pipettes with aerosolized samples. Additionally, empty tubes and sections cut from paraffin blocks in which no tissue has been embedded are carried through the lysate preparation procedure to serve as controls for the introduction of contamination during preparation (see SOP 4.1).

BLOTTING TECHNIQUES

Blotting techniques are used to separate biologic molecules by size and then to transfer them to a solid support that can be probed for the molecule of interest. (The blotting of DNA is called *Southern* blotting after its inventor, E. M. Southern.[21] RNA blots are called *Northern*, and protein blots are called *Western*, in deference to Southern's initial innovation.) The idea behind each of these techniques is the same: A complex mixture is separated by molecular mass by loading a sample into a semisolid gel and passing an electric current through the gel. Smaller molecules travel through the gel more quickly so that the mixture is spread out through the gel in order of molecular size. The separated molecules are then transferred out of the gel onto a solid support, such as a nitrocellulose or nylon membrane. The membrane can then be incubated in a solution containing a labeled probe, or *detector* molecule, which binds to the molecule of interest. When the excess, unbound probe is washed off, a signal will be visible wherever the molecule of interest has become bound to the membrane. The results of blotting can yield information about the presence or absence of a molecule, its size, its amount relative to other species, and, if appropriate standards are used, its absolute amount.

Southern Blotting

Southern blotting can be used to characterize any mixture of DNA, including high-molecular-weight genomic DNA extracted from tissue, plasmids grown in bacteria, and fragments generated in a PCR reaction. The type of DNA to be analyzed will affect the type and percentage of agarose used in the gel. Generally, the larger the DNA fragments to be analyzed, the lower the percentage of agarose used to make the gel. Genomic DNA, for example, is run on gels containing 0.5% to 1.5% agarose. Plasmid digests, which generally contain fragments between 0.2 and 5.0 kilobases (kb), usually are run in 1.2% to 1.5% agarose. PCR products, which generally range from 0.1 to 1.0 kb, are run in 2% to 4% gels. There also are different types of agarose that vary with respect to melting point, strength, and clarity. A standard molecular biology grade of agarose, however, is adequate for most purposes. Low-melting-point agaroses are useful for the high-percentage gels used to separate and blot small DNA fragments (<500 bp) generated by PCR.

Agarose powder is melted in buffer (usually TRIS-borate ethylenediaminetetraacetic acid [EDTA], but sometimes, especially for genomic DNA, Tris-acetate-EDTA) and poured into a mold. Wells are formed by inserting a well-forming comb into the molten agarose. Solutions of DNA mixed with loading buffer, which contains tracking dyes, are loaded into the wells after the solidified gel is submerged in buffer. Ethidium bromide, a chemical that intercalates with DNA and fluoresces under ultraviolet light, can be included in the gel or the buffer, or both, to visualize the DNA after the gel is run. A current is applied to the gel so that the DNA, which migrates toward the anode, travels through the length of the gel. When the DNA has migrated far enough (amount of migration depends on the size of the DNA target, the percentage of agarose, and the current applied), the gel can be placed on an ultraviolet transilluminator and examined. The DNA will be visible as bright orange lines (plasmid digests or PCR products) or as a blur extending the length of the lane (genomic DNA). One or more lanes are usually reserved for mixtures of DNA of known lengths; these markers allow determination of the size of the target DNA.

Many scientific supply companies sell horizontal "submarine" gel devices for running agarose gels, ranging in size from 8×10 cm to 15×20 cm. A gel device, a power supply, and a heat source for melting the agarose are the only major pieces of equipment necessary for running an agarose DNA gel.

For plasmid digests and PCR products, visualization of the ethidium-bromide–stained gel can be sufficient to identify the target DNA, and a Southern blot is unnecessary. For complex mixtures of DNA, or when the target DNA is present in very small amounts, the gel must be blotted and probed. In blotting, the DNA is forced out of the gel onto a membrane. Once it has become bound to the membrane, the DNA can be probed with a labeled fragment of DNA complementary to the DNA of interest.

Classic Southern blotting is a passive process in which buffer diffuses up through the gel and then through a membrane. As the buffer flows through the gel, the DNA is carried out of the gel and binds to the membrane. Nitrocellulose was the membrane originally used and is still favored by some researchers because it gives exceptionally low background signals. Nitrocellulose must be baked for 2 hours to bind the DNA and consequently is quite fragile; and, as a result, stripping and reprobing nitrocellulose blots is difficult. There are now a variety of nylon membranes available for Southern blotting. Each manufacturer recommends slightly different conditions for optimal blotting, so package directions should be carefully followed.

Whether using nitrocellulose or nylon membrane, the "upward" technique of Southern blotting is similar. The gel is first soaked in a mildly basic solution to denature the DNA. When very large DNA fragments are to be blotted, it is useful to first soak the gel in a solution that depurinates the DNA. Depurinated strands will break on denaturation, and smaller fragments will blot more efficiently. Depurination is not necessary and may be harmful for DNA fragments smaller than 15kb.[23] After denaturation, the gel is soaked in a neutralizing buffer.

Finally, the gel is placed on a platform in a tray of high-salt buffer (usually 20×SSC [standard sodium citrate]). The platform is covered with a piece of heavy filter paper that hangs down into the buffer and acts as a wick to draw buffer upward through the gel. The gel is placed directly on top of this filter-paper wick and is covered with the nitrocellulose or nylon membrane, which has been wetted with transfer buffer. On top of the membrane are placed several thicknesses of filter paper and a stack of paper towels, which soak up the buffer as it is drawn through the gel and membrane. A weight is placed on top of the entire stack to ensure close contact among the various layers. Transfer of small (<500 bp) fragments of DNA is complete in a few hours. Genomic blots usually are allowed to transfer overnight.

DNA also can be blotted "downward" out of a gel. In this modification of the Southern protocol, the stack of paper towels is placed on the laboratory bench and a piece of filter paper is placed on top. The nitrocellulose or nylon membrane, prewetted in denaturing solution, is placed on the filter paper. The gel is placed on top of the membrane, covered with plastic wrap, and then covered by a glass plate. Finally, a medium weight (such as a liter bottle filled with liquid or a heavy catalog) is placed on the plate. The weight presses the liquid out of the gel, downward through the membrane, and into the paper towels below. As with classic Southern blotting, the DNA is carried out of the gel with the buffer and binds to the membrane.

The downward method is easier to set up than the classic upward method and, in our laboratory, has provided satisfactory results for the transfer of PCR products. The transfer efficiency of large fragments (>1 kb) has not been extensively evaluated and may be much lower than in the classic method.

DNA also can be transferred out of agarose gels using a vacuum method. The gel is placed on top of the membrane on a vacuum manifold; when a vacuum is applied, buffer is pulled through the gel, depositing the DNA on the membrane. Several companies sell vacuum devices. Generally, however, the vacuum sources are strong enough only for low-percentage gels, with an upper limit of approximately 1.5%; therefore, the vacuum extraction method is unsuitable for the 2.5% to 4% gels used for the resolution of small PCR fragments. Comprehensive systems are available in which gels can be poured, run, washed, and blotted in place, but only relatively low-percentage gels can be transferred.

Devices that electrophoretically transfer DNA out of agarose gels also are available. Given the ease and efficiency of the passive and vacuum techniques already described, however, the electrophoretic transfer techniques are more commonly used for transfer of DNA or proteins out of polyacrylamide gels. A detailed protocol for Southern blotting using a radioactive probe is given in SOP 4.2.

Southern blotting is now a staple for many molecular pathology laboratories, especially in its application to testing lymphoproliferative disorders for clonal B- or T-cell gene rearrangements. The College of American Pathologists began proficiency testing for the B- and T-cell gene rearrangement test in 1992, and laboratories may subscribe to this survey. The reader is referred to the text of Farkas[22] for a detailed protocol of this test and an in-depth discussion of quality control procedures.

Northern Blotting

RNA also can be electrophoretically fractionated by size through gels and transferred to membranes in a manner similar to Southern blotting. (When the species transferred is RNA, the blots are called Northerns.) Some of the basic characteristics of RNA make Northern blot procedures more complicated than Southern blots. First, RNA is vulnerable to the action of RNAse, which is a common and hardy laboratory contaminant. The apparatus used for Northern blots should be reserved for that procedure, and gloves should be worn while performing preparations involving RNA. Second, RNA, because it is single stranded, can assume complicated secondary structures that do not travel through the gel at a rate proportional to their lengths; therefore, RNA must first be thoroughly denatured and then run through a gel containing strong denaturants, most commonly formaldehyde or glyoxal (the reader is referred to laboratory manuals[9, 23] that provide detailed protocols for running Northern blots). Because RNA is vulnerable to degradation, the likelihood of isolating enough full-length mRNA from paraffin-embedded tissues to run a successful Northern blot is very low. Techniques for the analysis of RNA from fixed tissue are therefore limited to dot-blot and PCR-based methods (as described earlier under RNA isolation).

Dot and Slot Blots

Both Southern and Northern blotting use electrophoresis to separate nucleic acids by size, before analysis. Separation by size is useful for confirming that binding of a specific probe has occurred, that the correct species is being analyzed, for providing evidence of mutation or rearrangement when the pattern of bands changes, and for allowing the analysis of more than one species at a time if the targets and the probes are well characterized. Both Southern and Northern blots, however, require relatively large quantities of high-quality starting material and can take several days to complete. Dot and slot blotting bypass the step of electrophoresis of the sample nucleic acid and are therefore quicker and depend less on the quality of the starting material.

In its simplest form, dot blotting can be performed by literally dotting samples of denatured DNA or RNA onto nitrocellulose or nylon membrane. To make quantitation possible, however, most researchers use a vacuum apparatus into which the membrane is inserted. The samples are loaded into uniformly sized wells (in the shape of dots or slots) and are then pulled onto the membrane by vacuum. If the samples are loaded as serial dilutions and appropriate controls are included, dot and slot blots can provide accurate information about the presence and quantity of a specific nucleic acid.

Western Blotting

Just as DNA and RNA can be analyzed by Southern and Northern blotting, proteins also can be extracted, separated electrophoretically, and detected on blots. Often, to prepare proteins for Western blotting, cells or tissue samples are simply resuspended in gel-loading buffer[24] that contains SDS and a reducing agent and will immediately lyse the cells. The viscosity of these solutions, which is caused by the release of high-molecular-weight DNA, can be reduced by sonicating the lysate or by passing it through a hypodermic needle. The resulting solution usually is then run on an SDS-polyacrylamide gel in a discontinuous buffer system.[25, 26] In this system, the proteins all become complexed to SDS and assume a net negative charge, causing them to separate by size alone in the gel. After electrophoresis, the proteins are transferred to a solid support, traditionally nitrocellulose, using an electric current in devices especially manufactured for this purpose. Other commonly used membranes are those based on polyvinylidene difluoride (PVDF). Originally described by Towbin and associates,[27] the electrophoretic transfer procedure was performed in a buffer consisting of TRIS, glycine, and methanol. Adding a low percentage of SDS to the transfer buffer can assist in transferring some proteins.[28] After transfer to the membrane, additional binding sites in the membrane are blocked with excess protein, often by incubating the membrane in a solution of nonfat dry milk.[23] After incubation, the membrane is ready for the probe.

Probes for Western blots usually are antibodies that are specific for epitopes on the target protein. The membrane is incubated in a solution containing this primary antibody—the appropriate dilution must be determined empirically. The binding sites of the primary antibody are then determined by using either of two techniques: by incubation with a second antibody raised against the first and enzymatically labeled, or labeled with biotin; or by incubation with radiolabeled or enzymatically labeled protein A. For example, we routinely incubate the blot containing the bound primary antibody along with a secondary antibody directly conjugated to horseradish peroxidase; then the blot is subjected to colorimetric or chemiluminescent detection of the enzyme. This two-step probe process avoids the necessity of labeling the individual primary antibodies. Labeled protein A and secondary antibodies are readily available commercially. For a detailed description of the Western technique, see the text by Sambrook and colleagues.[9] It should be mentioned that this technique is not applicable to formalin-fixed tissue. The proteins in such tissues are cross-linked in high-molecular-weight complexes and thus cannot easily be electrophoretically separated.

NUCLEIC ACID PROBES

Almost any nucleic acid can be labeled and used as the detector molecule, or probe, for Southern and Northern blots. Theoretically, the probe will hybridize or form a duplex structure only with a target molecule that is complementary to it. The degree of specificity required between the two can be changed by manipulating the experimental conditions so that the probe must find its exact complement (*high stringency*) or so that mismatches will be tolerated in the hybrid structure (*low stringency*). Discussions of hybridization theory and detailed experimental protocols for hybridizing and washing blots have been provided by Hames and associates.[29]

Recombinant DNA technology allows practically any DNA sequence to be subcloned into a bacterial vector and produced in large quantities. These vectors, or fragments from them, can be uniformly labeled by either nick translation or random primer labeling. Details of these protocols can be found in many references.[30, 31] These procedures can be performed either in the presence of radioactive nucleotides, to create radiolabeled probes, or in the presence of biotinylated or fluorescein-conjugated precursors, to create nonradiolabeled probes. Double-stranded DNA also can be radioactively end-labeled at the 5′ or 3′ end using enzymes such as T4 polynucleotide kinase (5′ end), by the Klenow fragment of *Escherichia coli* DNA polymerase I (3′ end), or using terminal deoxynucleotidyl transferase (3′ end). More detailed discussion of these protocols can be found in other references.[30, 31]

Probes also can be labeled with chemiluminescent markers. In these systems, a dideoxy nucleotide bearing a substrate such as digoxigenin or biotin is attached to the specific probe by terminal transferase. An antibody to the substrate, bound to an enzyme such as horseradish peroxidase, is incubated with the blot and binds to the labeled probe. A chemiluminescent substrate that emits light when cleaved by the probe-bound enzyme is then added. The advantages of chemiluminescent detection systems over radioactive labeling are that signals are visible in minutes rather than hours and that the safety and regulatory issues involved in the use of radioactivity are avoided. The blots require more incubation and washing steps, however, so the chemoluminescent procedure involves more hands-on time than does radioactive probing.

The presence of radioactively labeled probes is detected by autoradiography (see SOP 4.2). Additionally, many companies sell machines that facilitate the detection of radioisotopes on blots, detecting radioactivity either directly or by a phosphor screen that generates a latent image, which is scanned by a laser. Whatever detection method is used, automated imaging of the labeled filter can greatly facilitate quantitation of the results. Biotin-labeled probes usually are detected by incubating them with a streptavidin/alkaline phosphatase or horseradish peroxidase conjugate, followed by adding substrates that detect these enzymes colorimetrically or, more popularly today, by chemiluminescence. Similarly, if the probes are labeled with fluorescein-conjugated nucleotides, they are detected by incubation with an antifluorescein antibody conjugated to alkaline phosphatase or horseradish peroxidase. A substrate is then added which is converted to a stable, colored precipitate or emits light when acted on by the probe-bound enzyme. The colorimetric reactions are detected by the deposition of a colored precipitate on the filter; chemiluminescent detection is performed with film. Alternatively, the phosphor screen imaging system of at least one company is capable of using filters that have been processed for chemiluminescent detection (Typhoon System, Moleculer Dynamics, Sunnyvale, CA). Radioactive probes have been the method of choice because of their sensitivity; however, chemiluminescent detection now approaches the sensitivity of radioactivity.[32–35]

The advent of machines that can synthesize short pieces of single-stranded DNA (called *oligonucleotides*, usually 20 to 50 bases long) allows the user to design probes for any sequence of interest. Oligonucleotides can be radioactively labeled at the 5′ end with T4 polynucleotide kinase, substituted with biotin during synthesis, or directly conjugated to enzymes such as alkaline phosphatase. A detailed protocol for radioactive 5′-end labeling with kinase can be found in SOP 4.3.

RNA also can be used as a probe for blots or solution hybridization studies. In this case, DNA encoding the RNA of interest is cloned into one of a variety of commercially available plasmids that contain bacteriophage RNA polymerase promoter sequences. The DNA can then be transcribed in vitro, using the appropriate RNA polymerase in the presence of radioactive or non-radioactive nucleotide precursors. This process results in uniformly labeled RNA of highly specific activity. Like oligonucleotide probes, RNA probes are single stranded and thus cannot reassociate during hybridization, making them nearly 10 times more efficient at detecting target sequences[36] than are double-stranded probes.

REFERENCES

1. Dubeau L, Chandler LA, Gralow JR, et al: Southern blot analysis of DNA extracted from formalin-fixed pathology specimens. Cancer Res 1986;46:2964–2969.
2. Dubeau L, Weinberg K, Jones PA, et al: Studies on immunoglobulin gene rearrangement in formalin-fixed, paraffin-embedded pathology specimens. Am J Pathol 1988;130:588–594.
3. Goeltz SE, Hamilton SR, Vogelstein B: Purification of DNA from formaldehyde fixed and paraffin embedded human tissue. Biochem Biophys Res Commun 1985; 130:118–126.
4. Warford A, Pringle JH, Hay J, et al: Southern blot analysis of DNA extracted from formal-saline fixed and paraffin wax embedded tissue. J Pathol 1988;154:313–320.
5. Shibata DK, Arnheim N, Martin WJ: Detection of human papilloma virus in paraffin-embedded tissue using the polymerase chain reaction. J Exp Med 1988; 167:225–230.
6. Emmert-Buck MR, Bonner RF, Smith PD, et al: Laser capture microdissection. Science 1996;274:998–1001.
7. Chirgwin JM, Przybyla AE, MacDonald RJ, et al: Isolation of biologically active ribonucleic acid from sources enriched in ribonuclease. Biochemistry 1979;18:5294–9.
8. Chomczynski P, Sacchi N: Single-step method of RNA isolation by acid guanidinium thiocyanate-phenol-chloroform extraction. Anal Biochem 1987;162:156–159.
9. Sambrook J, Fritsch EF, Maniatis T: Molecular Cloning: A Laboratory Manual. Cold Spring Harbor, NY, Cold Spring Harbor Laboratory, 1989.
10. White BA, Bancroft FC: Cytoplasmic dot hybridization: Simple analysis of relative mRNA levels in multiple

small cell or tissue samples. J Biol Chem 1982;257: 8569–8572.

11. Cheley S, Anderson R: A reproducible microanalytical method for the detection of specific RNA sequences by dot-blot hybridization. Anal Biochem 1984;137:15–19.
12. Rupp GM, Locker J: Purification and analysis of RNA from paraffin-embedded tissues. Biotechniques 1988;6: 56–60.
13. Finke J, Fritzen R, Ternes P, et al: An improved strategy and a useful housekeeping gene for RNA analysis from formalin-fixed, paraffin-embedded tissues by PCR. Biotechniques 1993;14:448–453.
14. Jackson DP, Quirke P, Lewis F, et al: Detection of measles virus RNA in paraffin-embedded tissue [letter]. Lancet 1989;1:1391.
15. Stanta G, Schneider C: RNA extracted from paraffin-embedded human tissues is amenable to analysis by PCR amplification. Biotechniques 1991;11:304, 306, 308.
16. von Weizsacker F, Labeit S, Koch HK, et al: A simple and rapid method for the detection of RNA in formalin-fixed, paraffin-embedded tissues by PCR amplification. Biochem Biophys Res Commun 1991;174:176–180.
17. Tanaka Y, Enomoto N, Kojima S, et al: Detection of hepatitis C virus RNA in the liver by in situ hybridization. Liver 1993;13:203–208.
18. Nuovo GJ, Lidonnici K, MacConnell P, et al: Intracellular localization of polymerase chain reaction (PCR)-amplified hepatitis C cDNA. Am J Surg Pathol 1993; 17:683–690.
19. Krafft AE, Duncan BW, Bijwaard KE, et al: Optimization of the isolation and amplification of RNA from formalin-fixed, paraffin-embedded tissue: The Armed Forces Institute of Pathology experience and literature review. Mol Diagn 1997;2:217–230.
20. Taubenberger JK, Reid AH, Krafft AE, et al: Initial genetic characterization of the 1918 "Spanish" influenza virus [see comments]. Science 1997;275:1793–1796.
21. Southern EM: Detection of specific sequences among DNA fragments separated by gel electrophoresis. J Mol Biol 1975;98:503–517.
22. Farkas DH. Molecular Biology and Pathology: A Guidebook for Quality Control. San Diego, Academic, 1993.
23. Ausubel FM, Brent R, Kingston RE, et al: Current Protocols in Molecular Biology Inc., New York, NY, John Wiley & Sons, 1988.
24. Laemmli UK: Cleavage of structural proteins during the assembly of the head of bacteriophage T4. Nature 1970; 227:680–685.
25. Davis BJ: Disc electrophoresis: II. Method and application to human serum proteins. Ann NY Acad Sci 1964; 121:404–412.
26. Ornstein L: Disc electrophoresis: I. Background and theory. Ann NY Acad Sci 1964;121:321–328.
27. Towbin H, Staehelin T, Gordon J: Electrophoretic transfer of proteins from polyacrylamide gels to nitrocellulose sheets: Procedure and some applications. Proc Natl Acad Sci USA 1979;76:4350–4354.
28. Aebersold RH, Leavitt J, Saavedra RA, et al: Internal amino acid sequence analysis of proteins separated by one- or two-dimensional gel electrophoresis after in situ protease digestion on nitrocellulose. Proc Natl Acad Sci USA 1987;84:6970–6974.
29. Hames BD, Higgens SJ, Hames BD, et al (eds): Nucleic Acid Hybridization: A Practical Approach. Oxford, IRL, 1999.
30. Amersham Corporation: Nucleic Acid Labeling. Arlington Heights, IL, Amersham Corporation 1999.
31. Symons RH (ed): Nucleic Acid Probes. Boca Raton, FL, CRC, 1989.
32. Barlet V, Cohard M, Thelu MA, et al: Quantitative detection of hepatitis B virus DNA in serum using chemiluminescence: Comparison with radioactive solution hybridization assay. J Virol Methods 1994;49:141–151.
33. Geiger CP, Caselmann WH: Non-radioactive hybridization with hepatitis C virus-specific probes created during polymerase chain reaction: A fast and simple procedure to verify hepatitis C virus infection. J Hepatol 1992;15: 387–390.
34. Zachar V, Mayer V, Aboagye-Mathiesen G, et al: Enhanced chemiluminescence-based hybridization analysis for PCR-mediated HIV-1 DNA detection offers an alternative to ^{32}P-labelled probes. J Virol Methods 1991;33:391–395.
35. Shaap AP, Sandison MD, Handley RS: Chemical and enzymatic triggering of 1,2 dioxetanes: III. Alkaline phosphatase-catalyzed chemiluminescence from an aryl phosphate-substituted dioxetane. Tetrahedron Letters 1987; 8:1159–1162.
36. Krieg PA, Melton DA: In vitro RNA synthesis with SP6 RNA polymerase. Methods Enzymol 1987;155:397–415.

CHAPTER 4 APPENDIX

SOP 4.1*

EXTRACTION OF DNA FROM FORMALIN-FIXED, PARAFFIN-EMBEDDED TISSUE

PRINCIPLE

In the polymerase chain reaction (PCR) technique, DNA polymerase makes repeated copies of a specific sequence of DNA. For the DNA contained within a formalin-fixed, paraffin-embedded tissue sample to be made available in a PCR reaction, the tissue must be deparaffinized and digested with protease. Once the DNA has been released into the lysis buffer, cellular debris can be centrifuged out, and the lysate is suitable for use in a PCR reaction to amplify any DNA target sequence.

MATERIALS AND SOLUTIONS

Gloves
2 small beakers
1.5-mL microcentrifuge tubes
Microtome
Extra microtome blades
Pipetaid
One or two 1-mL pipettes
Microcentrifuge
Sterile cotton swabs or 5-μL microcapillary pipettes
Water bath set at 55°C
Water bath or heat block set at 95°C
Xylene
Absolute ethanol
Proteinase K (2.5 mg/mL in water, store at −20°C)
1 mol/L KCl (100 mL):
  KCl 7.46 g
  H_2O to 100 mL final volume
0.5 mol/L TRIS, pH 8.3 (100 mL):
  TRIS-base 3.52 g
  TRIS-HCl 3.31 g
  H_2O to 100 mL final volume
1 mol/L $MgCl_2$ (100 mL):
  $MgCl_2$ 9.52 g
  H_2O to 100 mL final volume
Extraction buffer (store in 1-mL aliquots at (−20°C):

	Stock Concentration	Final Concentration	Amount to Add
KCl	1.0 mol/L	50 mmol/L	0.5 mL
Tris, pH 8.3	0.5 mol/L	10 mmol/L	0.2 mL
$MgCl_2$	1.0 mol/L	2.5 mmol/L	25 μL
Tween 20	100%	0.45%	45 μL
Nonidet P-40	100%	0.45%	45 μL
H_2O			9.2 mL

PROCEDURE

1. Wear gloves.
2. Change the microtome blade between blocks. The microtome itself and any tools that may have touched the specimen also must be wiped off with xylene.
3. Place two 6-μm sections into each of two sterile 1.5-mL microcentrifuge tubes.
4. Cut an additional section that will be mounted and stained with hematoxylin and eosin. This section will be used to verify the presence of the feature that is of pathologic interest.
5. Pour approximately 1 mL per sample of xylene into one beaker and approximately 2 mL per sample of ethanol into another beaker. Do not pipette directly from stock bottles.
6. Thaw 1 mL of extraction buffer for every nine samples. Add 25 μL of 2.5 mg/mL proteinase K. Keep on ice until ready to use.
7. Include an empty tube with each set of samples. Label this tube "paraffin negative control." Treat this empty tube exactly the same as a sample tube.
8. Add 800 μL of xylene to each sample, and vortex at full speed for 5 seconds.
9. Add 400 μL of ethanol, and vortex at full speed for 5 seconds; then centrifuge at full speed for 5 minutes.
10. CAREFULLY decant the liquid. Resuspend the tissue in 800 μL of 100% ethanol, and vortex at full speed for 5 seconds.
11. Centrifuge at full speed for 5 minutes.
12. Remove the ethanol by decanting or pipetting, and remove residual ethanol with a microcapillary pipette or cotton swab.
13. Resuspend the pellet in a solution of 100-μL extraction buffer and proteinase K. Incubate in a water bath at 55°C for 1 hour.

* SOP 4.1, 4.2, 4.3 by Ann H. Reid, MA, Research Biologist, Department of Cellular Pathology, Armed Forces Institute of Pathology, Rockville, Maryland, and Cynthia F. Wright, PhD, Associate Professor, Department of Pathology and Laboratory Medicine, Medical University of South Carolina, Charleston, South Carolina

14. Place in a water bath or heat block at 95°C for 10 minutes to inactivate the proteinase K.
15. Centrifuge at full speed for 5 minutes to pellet debris. The supernatant now contains the DNA from the lysed cells and is called the lysate sample. The sample can be stored with the pelleted debris in place and is usually resistant to multiple freeze-thaw cycles. Label the tube and store at −20°C.

Reporting Results

Lysate is suitable for use as template DNA in a standard PCR reaction. Each set of cases has an internal negative control—the paraffin-negative control—used to demonstrate that no contamination was introduced during the extraction process.

Procedure Notes

1. The specimen may consist of any formalin-fixed, paraffin-embedded tissue. Specimens that have been fixed in B-5 or other mercury-based fixatives are unsuitable for PCR analysis.
2. The most common problem in this protocol is loss of sample because the pellet does not stick to the microcentrifuge tube after step 4.
   - If you experience difficulty because none of your samples stick to the tube after centrifugation, try different brands of microcentrifuge tubes until you find one to which most samples stick.
   - If an occasional sample floats off after centrifugation, try either removing most of the xylene-ethanol mixture by pipetting before adding pure ethanol, or, if the problem is severe, add more ethanol to the xylene-ethanol mixture and repeat the centrifuge step.
3. If, after PCR, the paraffin-negative control gives a positive signal, discard all reagents used for that set of samples and repeat the extraction using decontaminated pipetmen and disposable plasticware.
4. Removal of ethanol after step 6 is important. If too much ethanol is left in the tube, the PCR reaction may be inhibited. The goal is to leave no more than 1 or 2 μL in the tube. If a large proportion of samples (more than 20%) fail to amplify the positive control gene, it would be appropriate to make sure that virtually all the alcohol is removed at this step.

SOP 4.2

SOUTHERN BLOTTING, HYBRIDIZATION, AND AUTORADIOGRAPHY

PRINCIPLE

Ultraviolet-light visualization of ethidium-bromide–stained PCR product often is not sufficiently sensitive to detect all positive signals. Much greater sensitivity can be obtained by probing the PCR product with a radioactively labeled probe that is complementary to a sequence between the two primers. The DNA is transferred from the agarose gel to a specialized membrane to which the DNA binds irreversibly. The membrane, or *blot*, is then placed in a plastic bag with the labeled probe in a hybridization solution. After allowing time for hybridization of the probe to its complementary sequence (called *annealing*), the unbound probe is washed off and the blot is exposed to x-ray film. When the film (now called an *autoradiogram*) is developed, a band will be visible wherever the probe has become bound to DNA on the blot.

MATERIALS AND SOLUTIONS

Gloves
Plastic or glass tray (slightly larger than gel and at least 1 inch deep)
Rocker apparatus
Paper towels
Whatman 3-mm paper
Nylon membrane (e.g., Nytran, Hybond-c, or Sureblot)
Plastic wrap
Glass plate (slightly larger than the gel)
2- to 4-lb weight (e.g., a large book, or a 1-L bottle filled with liquid)
Forceps
15-mL tubes
Heat-sealable plastic bags, approximately 6×8 inches
Heat sealer for bags
Water bath set at 55°C
X-ray film cassette
Intensifying screen
Kodak XAR film or equivalent
−70°C freezer
1×membrane blocking solution (diluted from 2.5×Oncor stock)
Hybrisol III (Oncor)
Phosphorus 32 (^{32}P)-labeled probe (see Hybridization section later)
Denaturing solution (0.5 mol/L NaOH, 0.6 mol/L NaCl):
  NaOH 20 g
  NaCl 35 g
  H_2O to bring up to 1000 mL
Washing solution (0.16 × standard sodium citrate [SSC], 0.1% SDS)
  20×SSC (8 mL, available from many suppliers as a 20× stock)
  20% SDS (5 mL, available from many suppliers as a 20% stock)
H_2O to bring up to 1000 mL

PROCEDURE

Blotting (Downward Method)

1. Put on gloves.
2. Place the gel in a plastic box and cover it with denaturing solution.
3. Place the plastic box on a rocker and rock it gently for 20 minutes. During this time, the DNA in the gel will become denatured (single-stranded). In its single-stranded form it will be able to migrate out of the gel, bind to the nylon membrane, and bind to the labeled probe.
4. Cut a piece of Whatman 3-mm paper slightly larger than the gel.
5. Cut a piece of nylon membrane exactly the same size as the gel.
6. Place a 3-inch stack of paper towels (towels must be larger than gel) on a laboratory bench where they will not be disturbed.
7. Place the Whatman paper on top of the paper towels.
8. Gently ease the nylon membrane into the denaturing solution so that it wets evenly (this can be done on the surface of the denaturing solution in which the gel is soaking). Lift the wet membrane out by its edges and lay it on top of the Whatman paper. Be careful not to

introduce bubbles between the paper and the membrane. If necessary, a 10-mL pipette can be rolled over the membrane to push out any bubbles.

9. Lift the gel out of the denaturing solution and lay it precisely on top of the membrane. Starting in the middle and working outward toward the edges, gently press the gel to eliminate any bubbles between the gel and the membrane. Again, a 10-mL pipette can be gently rolled over the surface of the gel to remove any bubbles. If any bubbles remain, the DNA will not transfer properly.
10. Place plastic wrap over the whole stack.
11. Place the glass plate on top of the plastic wrap and place the weight on top of the glass plate.
12. Leave the stack undisturbed overnight. During this time, moisture from the gel will be absorbed through the membrane into the stack of paper towels, carrying the DNA with it. The DNA will bind to the membrane.

Hybridization

1. Dismantle the stack carefully, gently pulling the membrane away from the gel with forceps. The gel should be less than $\frac{1}{8}$-inch thick. Mark the location of the first well by cutting off that corner of the membrane. Use a pencil or ballpoint pen to label and date the membrane in another corner.
2. Place the membrane in a plastic box and cover it with approximately 50 mL of 1× membrane blocking solution. Rock the plastic box on the rocker for 20 minutes.
3. Remove the membrane from the membrane blocking solution and place it in a plastic heat-sealable bag, which has been sealed on three sides. The bag should be approximately 1 cm larger than the membrane on three sides and approximately 5 cm larger than the membrane on the open side. Roll a pipette over the bag to squeeze out any excess membrane blocking solution.
4. ALL SUBSEQUENT STEPS INVOLVE THE USE OF RADIOACTIVE REAGENTS. WEAR APPROPRIATE PROTECTIVE CLOTHING (COAT, GLOVES), AND A DOSIMETRY DEVICE, AS REQUIRED BY WORKPLACE REGULATIONS. WORK BEHIND A SHIELD AS MUCH AS POSSIBLE.
5. In a 15-mL tube, place 5 mL (for blots 50 to 150 cm2) or 10 mL (for blots 150 to 300 cm^2) of Hybrisol III. Add 1 μL of labeled probe for each milliliter of Hybrisol IIII. Cap and vortex gently.
6. Pour the probe mixture into the plastic bag containing the membrane. Seal the edge of the open side, trying not to leave too much air in the bag—do not be concerned about small bubbles.
7. Use a pipette to roll any small bubbles up to the last sealed edge. Seal the bag again between the membrane and the bubbles, trapping the bubbles between the two seals. This double-seal technique allows elimination of bubbles with minimal leakage of the highly radioactive probe mixture. Roll the pipette firmly over the bag to ensure that there are no leaks.
8. Place the sealed bag in the 55°C water bath and leave it to hybridize for at least 4 hours or overnight.

NOTE: Hybridization ovens, in which the blots and probe mixtures are gently rotated in glass tubes, are available.

Washing

1. Cut a corner of the hybridization bag and squeeze the probe mixture into a 15-mL tube. The probe mixture can be stored in a −20°C freezer and used again several times.
2. Cut the bag open and gently remove the membrane using forceps. Place the membrane in a plastic box and cover it with washing solution. Rock the plastic box for 5 minutes.
3. Discard the washing solution by pouring it out into radioactive waste. Cover the membrane with fresh washing solution and rock it for 5 minutes.
4. Repeat step 3, EXCEPT, instead of rocking the plastic box for 5 minutes, cover it and place it in the 55°C water bath for 5 minutes.
5. Remove the membrane and place it on a piece of paper towel. Allow the membrane to air dry for 5 to 10 minutes. There should be no visibly wet patches on the membrane.
6. Transfer the membrane from the paper towel to a flat piece of plastic wrap. Cover the membrane with another piece of plastic wrap, avoiding wrinkles as much as possible.
7. In the darkroom, place the plastic-wrapped membrane into an x-ray film cassette. Cover it with a sheet of XAR film and an intensifying screen. Expose at −70°C in a freezer for 2 hours to overnight.

Reporting Results

Developed film will reveal bands wherever the probe became bound to amplified DNA, indicating that those samples contained the target DNA of interest (see Principle under SOP 4.3).

Procedure Notes

1. The most common errors in this procedure are failing to denature the gel and failing to remove all bubbles from between the gel and the nylon membrane. If care is taken in these steps, this blotting technique yields very consistent results.
2. When the gel/membrane/paper towel stack is dismantled, check to make sure that the gel thickness has been markedly reduced. If it has not, something has prevented the absorption of moisture from the gel through the membrane and into the paper towels. In this case, very little of the DNA is likely to have been transferred to the membrane. Check the organization of the stack for errors and re-blot.
3. It is important to remove bubbles from the hybridization bag because bubbles can prevent the labeled probe from reaching all parts of the blot.
4. Interpreting autoradiograms:

a. The autoradiogram is completely blank, even though labeled markers were used:
   (1) The gel was not markedly thinner after blotting, then the gel stack was improperly constructed. Check the blotting stack for errors and re-blot (see note 3 above).
   (2) The gel was markedly thinner after blotting, then
      (a) The stack was assembled improperly so that moisture from the blot did not flow through the nylon membrane (e.g., if the membrane was placed above the blot instead of below it). Run the gel again and re-blot.
      (b) The gel was not properly denatured. Run the gel again and denature it for 20 minutes before blotting.

b. The autoradiogram is completely black:
   (1) The film was exposed to light before development. Allow the film cassette to thaw completely and load with a fresh piece of film to reprint the exposure.

c. The lanes with positive signals have more than one band:
   (1) When blotting PCR products, occasionally a band will appear slightly below the band of interest; this band is thought to be single-stranded DNA from the target sequence that migrates at a different rate from double-stranded DNA; the appearance of this band is caused by one primer of the pair binding to the target more efficiently than the other; as long as this band is always accompanied by a band of the expected size, it should not be a concern.

d. A band that was visible by ethidium bromide is not visible on the autoradiogram:
   (1) The ethidium bromide band represents nonspecific PCR product, which is unable to bind to the target-specific probe.
   (2) A bubble in the blotting stack prevented the PCR product from binding to the nylon membrane.

e. The autoradiogram is obscured by black blotches and spider web–like lines:
   (1) The nylon membrane was not sufficiently dry when wrapped in plastic and exposed to the film (see step 5 under WASHING); remove the membrane from the plastic wrap, place it in the washing solution and incubate it at 55°C for 3 to 5 minutes; remove it from the solution and let it air dry until no visible moisture remains; wrap it in plastic wrap, as described in step 6 under WASHING, and re-expose it to a fresh sheet of film.

SOP 4.3

END-LABELING OF OLIGONUCLEOTIDE PROBES

PRINCIPLE

When the probe is annealed to a target sequence, immobilized on a blot, and exposed to x-ray film, the radioactivity exposes the film so that a black band is seen when the film is developed. The labeling of an oligonucleotide is a simple reaction that can be carried out in any laboratory equipped and approved for the use of ^{32}P. In the labeling reaction, T4 polynucleotide kinase transfers the ^{32}P-labeled terminal phosphate from commercially labeled adenosine triphosphate (ATP) to the 5′ end of the oligonucleotide.

The probe itself should be a 30- to 40-base length of DNA. When choosing the sequence, look for an area without internal complementarity, that is, a sequence that will not be able to fold on itself. There are vendors who custom synthesize oligonucleotides or sell oligonucleotides already designed for certain applications.

MATERIALS AND SOLUTIONS

1.5-mL microcentrifuge tubes
Microcentrifuge tube rack
Microcentrifuge floater (rack to hold tubes in a water bath)
Water bath set at 37°C
Water bath set at 65°C
Pipetman (1 to 20 μL)
Microcentrifuge
Vortex
Oligonucleotide probe at 2.5 μmol/L (2.5 pmol/mL [pmol = 10^{-12} mol/L])
Adenosine 5′-(γ-^{32}P) triphosphate, triethylammonium salt-3000 Ci/mmol (γ-^{32}P-ATP)
5′ End-labeling kit (available from many suppliers); OR, instead of using a kit, the following reagents can be made; check pH and adjust with concentrated HCl:

1 mol/L $MgCl_2$ (see SOP 4.1)
1.5 mol/L TRIS, pH 9.5

TRIS base	18.16 g
H_2O	to bring solution up to 100 mL

10× kinase buffer (0.5 mol/L TRIS [pH 9.5], 0.1 mol/L $MgCl_2$, 50% glycerol)

	Stock Concentration	Final Concentration	Amount to Add
Tris base (pH 9.5)	1.5 mol/L	0.5 mol/L	333 μL
$MgCl_2$	1.0 mol/L	0.1 mol/L	100 μL
Glycerol	100%	50%	500 μL
H_2O			67 μL

100 mmol/L dithiothreitol (1.54 g DTT in 100 mL); store frozen in 1-mL aliquots
T4 polynucleotide kinase (available from many suppliers)

PROCEDURE

1. Place the following reagents in a 1.5-mL microcentrifuge tube
   4 μL oligonucleotide probe (10 pmol)
   2 μL 10× kinase buffer
   1 μL 100 mm DTT
   3 μL γ-32P-ATP
   1 μL T4 polynucleotide kinase (10 U/μL)
   9 μL water
2. Vortex and spin down the solution.
3. Place the solution in a 37°C water bath for 45 minutes.
4. Place in 65°C water bath for 10 minutes (to inactivate the kinase).
5. Spin down briefly and store in −20°C freezer until used.

ALAN E. HUBBS

5

Amplification Methods

Increasingly, medical diagnosis demands that more information be extracted from less sample material. Sample size for molecular testing is often limited by the choice of biopsy techniques, such as fine-needle aspiration, and by the need to reserve material for light microscopy. Less invasive tests, which have lower risks and costs associated with greater diagnostic benefits, are favored for economic reasons. Finally, the expanding base of knowledge about genetics and disease is increasing the number of potential prognostic and diagnostic targets to detect. As a result, smaller portions of a patient's biopsy sample are available for any single test. Sample size limitations are even more acute when performing studies on archived material. The amount of an archived sample decreases with each round of analysis, and its quality may degrade with time.

To meet the growing demand for information, tests with greater sensitivity and less sample destruction must be developed. Nucleic acid amplification technologies represent a means to this end. It has been demonstrated that not only can genetic tests be made highly sensitive,[1–4] but immunoassays[5–8] and tests for small analytes[9] also can be brought to the theoretical limits of detection by coupling them to a nucleic acid amplification method. A discussion of the use of these techniques as a general amplification tool is outside the scope of this chapter, but the reader should be aware that nucleic acid amplification pervades all areas of diagnostics. It is therefore critical that those in the field of medicine understand the basis for this technology.

At the molecular level, all nucleic acid amplifications start with a hybridization reaction between a nucleic acid probe and a target sequence; and they all result in the target-dependent enzymatic production of a nucleic acid product. More important than these similarities, however, are the differences between the methods. The differences address the suitability of the method to the task at hand. Understanding these differences requires a rudimentary understanding of molecular biology, including double-stranded DNA (dsDNA) structure, hybridization, and enzymatic specificity. A review of background material is recommended if these concepts are foreign to the reader.

This chapter provides pathologists with an understanding of the nucleic acid amplification methods required to match sample handling and analysis methods with the diagnostic goals. These goals might include the discovery of previously unidentified gene sequences, the determination of the presence of known hereditary or somatic genetic defects, the detection of gene expression, the detection of infectious agents, or the production of large amounts of known targets for further study at the research level. Genetic counselors also may benefit from a molecular-level understanding of amplification-based tests, so that they may interpret the results of these tests in their proper context.

GENERAL FEATURES

All nucleic acid diagnostic methods are based on hybridization. This is the process by which complementary bases on two nucleic acid strands bond noncovalently to form the double-stranded helical structure generally attributed to DNA—a reaction that represents detection at the molecular level. It is the molecular recognition of a target sequence by a complementary nucleic acid probe. The specificity of hybridization is the degree to which only precise complementary sequences are recognized. When nucleic acid amplification techniques are applied as diagnostic tests, absolute control of specificity is required. It is the sequence specificity of the hybridization steps that determines whether a valid result will be obtained from an amplification. As a practical matter, this specificity is primarily controlled by adjusting the hybridization temperature.

The nature of hybridization is the same in amplification as in the traditional Southern or Northern blotting techniques (see Chapter 4).[2, 10–12] Once a probe is hybridized to its specific target, however, recognition of the probe-target hybrid is distinct between filter-based hybridization and amplification reactions. Traditional methods call for the target to be immobilized on a membrane (or other solid support), then probed by hybridization. After the hybridization phase is completed, unhybridized probe is washed away and the immobilized *probe-target hybrids* are then detected. The hybridized probe and unhybridized probe are distinguished by virtue of the mechanical removal of the probe from solution, on hybridization to the target. In contrast, in an amplification reaction, it is enzymatic specificity that distinguishes unhybridized probes from probe-target hybrids. Once formed, the probe-target hybrid becomes a substrate for the enzyme used in the amplification.

A variety of enzymatic activities, including polymerases,[13–16] ligases,[17, 18] and restriction endonucleases,[19, 20] are now used in the different amplification methods.[1–4, 21–25] It is the substrate specificity of these enzymes that translates the sequence-specific probe hybridization into a meaningful and detectable result. As such, the enzymes, substrates, and conditions required for activity are a matched set for a given assay, and they can only be altered in concert. Fortunately, the reaction conditions for a great number of applications have already been worked out in detail, so the pathologist need understand only which strategy to apply for a particular set of circumstances.

Assay design may depend on direct, indirect, or signal-sequence-amplification strategies. These designs differ in the arrangement of the initial target recognition and its subsequent amplification. The *direct amplification* strategy uses a single set of probes that are responsible for both target recognition and amplification. The resulting amplification product contains nucleic acids identical to the original target. In contrast, the *indirect amplification* strategy first generates an amplifiable pseudotarget and then amplifies the pseudotarget. The original target is either destroyed or it becomes irrelevant to the amplification. The products are representations of the original target sequence but are not necessarily identical to the original target. The *signal-sequence–amplification* strategy uses either a direct or an indirect method as a means of increasing assay sensitivity, but does not necessarily generate copies of the original nucleic acid target. Signal-sequence amplification often places a routine amplification in series with a traditional hybridization.

METHODS

Polymerase Chain Reaction

The polymerase chain reaction (PCR) was the first technique invented specifically for the purpose of amplifying diagnostic targets.[26–28] It is the most widely applied nucleic acid amplification technique, and many of the techniques that have followed are variations and combinations of the PCR. This section first will explain in detail the polymerase chain reaction, and then variations and techniques. This is not to imply that PCR is the best method for all applications; the particular strengths of each method will be explicitly pointed out.

The PCR is very flexible in the type, quality, and size of the target that can be amplified.[28, 29] As a result, it has become a valuable tool for genetic research, clinical diagnosis, and forensics. It has been applied in gene discovery,[30, 31] in prenatal detection of fetal DNA sequences,[32] in early detection of viral or mycobacterial infection,[33–35] and in mutation detection from archived tissue,[36, 37] to name only a few examples. Despite numerous other available methods of nucleic acid amplification, PCR remains the gold standard and starting point in building a modern clinical nucleic acid diagnostic. The latest advances in PCR are not in the technique itself but in its coupling to high-throughput screening and homogeneous detection systems,[22] as discussed later in this chapter.

PCR targets may be single- or double-stranded DNA, but minor modifications allow for the detection of RNA. The PCR reaction yields an exponential replication of the target sequence, using a direct-amplification strategy that relies on temperature cycling. The reaction mixture contains a thermostable DNA polymerase, free deoxynucleotide triphosphates (dNTPs), and two oligonucleotide primers that act as the sequence-specific probes. Primers generally are 15 to 40 nucleotides in length, are designed to be complementary to the opposite strands of the target, and are located such that they flank the target sequence. The reaction solution maintains a magnesium concentration and pH that are optimized to allow DNA annealing and enzymatic nucleotide incorporation. Thermal cycling provides the mechanism for releasing product DNA strands from the target. The copies of the target are referred to as *amplicons*, and they double in amount with each temperature cycle.

The cycling scheme is shown in Fig. 5–1. Typically, the temperature cycling is performed as a three-temperature sequence. First, the temperature is brought to above the melting point of DNA, or approximately 95°C. This temperature will render a target single-stranded and thereby accessible by the primers. The temperature is then lowered so that the primers can hybridize to the complementary portion of the target sequence. A temperature that is approximately 5°C below the predicted annealing temperature of the primer sequences (usually 50°C to 65°C) is satisfactory. Because the primers are present in excess, they effectively compete for all of the available target sites in the sample, and each primer anneals to the opposite DNA strand. The temperature required for DNA strand dissociation would destroy most enzymes, but the *Thermus aquaticus* (*Taq*) DNA polymerase used in this technique is resistant to such temperatures.[38, 39]

Once formed, the primer–target hybrids and the free dNTPs act as substrates for the DNA polymerase.

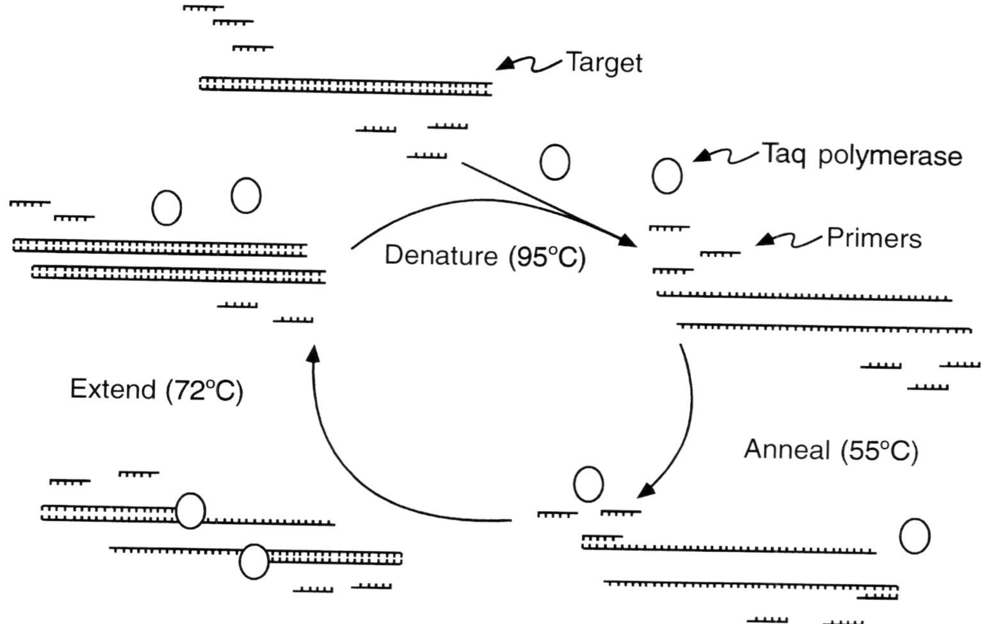

FIGURE 5–1
The polymerase chain reaction (PCR) relies on temperature cycling to render a single-stranded target and to release newly formed product into solution. The product is formed by a process of adding nucleotides to two target-directed primers. The primers are complementary to opposite strands of the target and bracket the target sequence. The incorporation reaction is catalyzed by a thermostable polymerase. Continued thermal cycling results in the exponential production of target copies.

The polymerase begins extending the primers by processively adding nucleotides that are complementary to the target sequence. Primer extension begins as soon as the hybrids are formed, but the temperature is brought to 72° C, which is the optimal temperature of the Taq polymerase and ensures rapid completion of the extension reaction. Each of these temperatures needs to be maintained for less than 1 minute, depending on the application. Target sequences of 1000 or more nucleotides, for example, may require longer primer extension times.[40, 41] These are generally useful guidelines, but, as with all nucleic acid hybridizations and enzymatic reactions, the precise conditions must be tailored to the application.

Selection of primer sequences and annealing temperature are the most critical aspects of a successful PCR-reaction design.[42–45] The primers are responsible for target recognition. Only proper hybridization of the primers to the target can discriminate between target and nontarget DNA. The primers must reside at opposite ends of the sequence to be amplified, and they must anneal to opposite strands of the target. In addition, they must be positioned such that their 3′ ends are aimed inward, toward the sequence to be amplified. If any of these conditions are not met, amplification will not take place. PCR primers should be designed in pairs, and their design depends on the particular application. Computer-aided primer-design software is available to deal with most of the complexities, but it cannot substitute for common sense.

The annealing temperature must match the characteristics of the primers.[44, 45] Placing the reaction at an annealing temperature that is too low can cause the primers to partially anneal to nontarget sequence and may result in the generation of nontarget amplicons. Ideally, paired primers should anneal to their targets at the same temperature, within 2° C. This temperature should be only a few degrees higher than the lowest temperature used in the thermocycling routine, to ensure specificity. It is also important that the primers do not anneal to themselves or to each other at any temperature near the annealing temperature. Such interactions result in the production of very short products, generally referred to as *primer-dimers*,[43, 46, 47] a side reaction that can often deplete the supply of primer available for target amplification and render the reaction useless. Moreover, if primer-dimers are formed during the first cycle of the PCR reaction, they will likely be produced in greater quantity than the desired target. This can often complicate the analysis of the PCR products in such applications as sequencing or real-time product detection.

Mispriming at temperatures well below those required for sequence specificity will be a problem, if measures are not taken to prevent it. To avoid mispriming, polymerase enzymatic activity can be blocked until after the initial melting of the double-stranded target. Physical separation of the enzyme from the rest of the polymerization mixture effectively restricts enzymatic activity until after the first heat-denaturation step, and a commercially available wax can be used for this purpose.[48, 49] As soon as the reaction is heated to greater than 90° C, the wax melts and allows the enzyme to enter the reaction mixture. Alternatively, polymerase enzymes have been developed that remain inactive until they are heated to 95° C.[50–52]

Carryover contamination also can interfere with test accuracy by generating false-positive results.[53, 54] Carryover of amplicons, for example, can be minimized by conducting the PCR setup with barrier tips in a laboratory area that is separate from the area used for post-PCR analysis.[55] The most desirable analysis methods are those that do not require reaction tubes to be opened.

Additional methods of ensuring against false-positive results include the use of uracil-DNA glycosylase (UNG) kits, which use deoxyuridine-triphosphate (dUTP) in place of deoxythymidine-triphosphate (dTTP).[56–58] At the start of the reaction, UNG degrades previously formed amplicons that contain uracil residues, but natural targets that contain dTTP are unaffected. The high-temperature step, required for activating the polymerase, inactivates UNG before the start of the amplification. Despite inactivation, residual UNG may interfere with electrophoretic analysis.[59] Signature primers can be used to detect carryover amplicons from prior PCR reactions.[60] False-positives also may be generated from contamination resulting from the DNA that remains on equipment, even after sterilization.[61] Meticulous attention should be given to decontamination procedures and proper controls in all assays.

Inhibitors of PCR are widely reported and may be inherent in the tissue being analyzed,[62–64] or they may be inadvertently introduced during sample processing[65–67] or patient treatment.[68, 69] For example, guanine analogues such as acyclovir triphosphate, used to treat immunocompromised patients, can inhibit Taq polymerase, which makes negative PCR results difficult to interpret in these patients.[68] Heparin, heme, and heme-containing proteins also inhibit some polymerases and transcriptases. Thus, blood[70, 71] and muscle tissue[63] samples may yield false-negative results in some circumstances. Even materials routinely used in PCR-related procedures have been found to be sources of inhibitory actions.[65, 66] Solutions to these problems include alternative methods of sample preparation[69, 72, 73] or the use of an alternative polymerase.[74] Recent systematic examinations of these phenomena are well worth consulting.[67, 75] In all cases, proper positive and negative controls should be designed to detect possible inhibitors inherent in the sample.[75]

In some cases, the analysis of point mutations can be obscured by a high background of wild-type sequences that coamplify with the genetic feature of interest. Microdissection can be used to selectively analyze different tissue elements.[76] Cell enrichment is a valuable aid in developing correlates between genotypic changes and clinical outcome.[36, 37, 77, 78] The identification of genetic changes associated with particular histologic subtypes also can be addressed.[37] Analysis with respect to invasive margins, different tumor cell populations within a given tumor (as evident by microscopy), and relative enrichment of tumor-to-nontumor ratio sampling can be reliably performed with this methodology. Thus, microdissection in conjunction with PCR is generally useful in the study of tumor progression.[79, 80]

Typically, one or more 5-mm sections of formalin-fixed, paraffin-embedded (FFPE) tissue are microdissected with a sterile scalpel blade or injection needle, and the material recovered from different areas of the tissue is subjected to further analysis.[81, 82] Stained slides are used as maps of the tissue being dissected, and unstained slides are used for the microdissection procedure. The unstained slide can be stained after the dissection if a demonstration of the accuracy of the procedure is needed. The tissues can be deparaffinized after the dissection or directly on the glass slide, before the dissection.[82] An alternative method is to place the entire section, recut from a block, directly into a microfuge tube, wherein the tissue can be deparaffinized—a useful method in the investigation of genes that normally would not be present in the subject (e.g., viruses). Similarly, microdissection has been applied to the analysis of fine-needle aspirates and cytology smears.[83, 84]

Reverse Transcription PCR

Reverse transcription PCR (RT-PCR) represents an extension of the PCR technique in which an RNA target sequence can be detected.[85] The amplification is indirect: an amplifiable DNA replica of the target RNA is produced first, then the DNA is amplified. Thus, the amplicons represent the target sequence but are not copies of the original target. The initial step of copying the RNA target into DNA form is catalyzed with a reverse transcriptase. This enzyme catalyzes DNA primer extension by RNA-template–directed deoxynucleotide incorporation. Once the complementary DNA (cDNA) has been created, it can serve as a single-stranded DNA target for the PCR reaction.

Most reverse transcriptase enzymes are not heat stable; however, because RNA is primarily single-stranded, heat denaturation is not necessarily required for the primer to access its hybridization site on the RNA molecule. The initial preparation of a cDNA template is conducted at approximately 42°C, a temperature suitable for the RT enzyme. In some cases, this temperature may result in the production of undesirable, nonspecific products. Reverse transcription at 55°C improves the specificity of cDNA synthesis and is compatible with the avian myeloblastosis virus (AMV) RT.[86] Alternatively, a thermostable RT can be used. The *Thermus thermophilus* DNA polymerase catalyzes both cDNA generation and DNA amplification in a single reaction, thereby increasing throughput and reducing the chance of contamination.[13]

RT-PCR is used for the detection of infectious agents in general[87] but also is particularly useful for those agents that have an RNA genome.[88, 89] In formalin-fixed tissue, RT-PCR can detect viral RNA despite severe degradation of the nucleic acids.[90] In fresh sample material, T-PCR can determine the presence of RNA viruses faster and with increased sensitivity than the viral culture method.[91] The relationship between gene expression and disease can be examined at the transcriptional level,[92] and gene expression can be correlated with protein expression by immunologic detection of the gene products. [93–95] A variety of experimental designs can be used to obtain quantitative data from RT-PCR reactions.[104–105] The RT-PCR is more complex than ordinary PCR, and therefore carries more potential points of failure. Direct inhibitors of the RT enzyme, as well as inhibitors of the DNA polymerase, can cause the RT-PCR reaction to give false-negative results.[71, 72] Moreover, there are reports that using too much RT enzyme can inhibit the reaction.[46, 102] The RNA substrate presents its own unique challenges. RNA may be degraded by endogenous ribonuclease (RNase) activity acting before the tissue is fixed, or from RNases introduced during the lysate preparation procedure. Rapid sample processing, reduced temperatures, and the use of RNase inhibitors should all be used to optimize RNA target recovery.[103] The loss of amplifiable RNA targets can also result from chemical modification of the nucleic acid strands by tissue fixatives. The unpaired nucleotide-bases of RNA are more reactive than the paired nucleotide-bases found in DNA. In order to confidently interpret negative results from an RT-PCR, internal control reactions should be run in parallel with diagnostic samples. An example of an RT-PCR control reaction that detects β_2-microglobulin RNA as the *internal control* is shown in SOP 5.1. The RT-PCR analysis has been successfully applied for detecting translocations and for monitoring the expression of fusion transcripts.[96–99] Recently, RT-PCR has been used in conjunction with sentinel lymph node mapping to detect micrometastases.[100] Many of the cited references use multiplex assay formats, with up to nine targets being detected in a single reaction.[87, 101] RNA also can be specifically detected in the presence of contaminating genomic DNA by choosing a target region that covers more than one exon.[92] In some cases, the DNA may still serve as a template during amplification, but the distance between exons is great enough that the DNA target is not efficiently amplified.

In Situ PCR

In situ PCR is performed by conducting RT-PCR directly on slide-mounted tissue sections, and it can be combined with in situ hybridization (ISH) techniques. This technique is an alternative to microdissection, but because the skeletal architecture of both the cells and tissue remains intact, there is the potential for increased resolution. In situ PCR can be used to determine which cells in a tissue are expressing a gene[106, 107] or to pinpoint the cellular location of infectious agents.[108, 109] It can also be used in conjunction with fluorescent antibody-cell sorting, but the characteristics of the individual antibodies used must be considered.[110] In situ PCR is considered more sensitive than ISH.[111, 112]

Commercial thermal-cyclers have been designed to accommodate the slide format. The technical complexity associated with in situ PCR, however, has restricted the use of thermocyclers primarily to the research laboratory, and, particularly, to situations in which there is no other way to get the desired information. Consistent results require proper tissue fixation and permeabilization.[106, 111, 113] Improperly fixed tissue will yield different results depending on the proximity of the cells to the outer edge of the tissue block.[114] As with ordinary RT-PCR, timely fixation also is critical. Poorly fixed cells will suffer from marked RNA degradation, and no results will be obtained. Insufficiently permeabilized cells will not allow the infusion of reagents into the subcellular site of the transcripts of interest. The permeabilization must allow macromolecules such as primers and enzymes to reach the site of the transcript because that is where the amplification will take place. Also, properly permeabilized tissues do not allow the targets or the amplicons to diffuse from their original cellular location to other sites in the tissue.[106]

The analysis of archived samples is affected by the fixative, fixation time, and the ex vivo prefixation period.[114–116] Samples fixed in mercury-based fixatives (e.g., B5), for example, are not as readily amplifiable as those fixed with neutral buffered formalin.[117] Short- and intermediate-length DNA targets can be routinely amplified by PCR from FFPE samples.[115, 117–119] The recovery of amplifiable RNA targets from FFPE material is generally less efficient and will yield less product than a similar amplification from fresh tissue.[116, 120] RNA is particularly prone to degradation resulting from suboptimal sample handling. The loss of amplifiability may result from nucleic acid strand breaks, or *adducts* (chemical modifications). When designing a retrospective study, multiple potential target sequences should be tested from representative samples, and it is best to select as short a target as possible.[121] This is the best way to compensate for fixation parameters that are not under the investigator's control. Proper target selection and RNA preparation methods can yield amplifiable RNA even from archived tissue blocks that are decades old.[90, 116]

Prospective studies offer the opportunity to ensure success by requesting specific sample handling procedures. Arranging for the immediate fixation of the tissues will ensure that the gene expression profile represents the state of the cell in its native environment. In contrast, if a tissue is removed from its natural environment without immediate fixation, the messenger RNA (mRNA) pool within the cell may not reflect a native state.[103] Some RNA targets will be lost due to degradation by endogenous RNase activity,[122–125] while new RNA will continue to be synthesized and will shift the gene expression profile.

This continuous adjustment of expression is a natural process that does not come to a halt on the surgical separation of the tissue from the body. In addition to immediate fixation, the choice of fixative may also be specified to best suit the diagnostic procedures that will be used to analyze the tissue.

Ligase Chain Reaction

The ligase chain reaction (LCR) is a direct-amplification method that relies on oligonucleotide probes and a single enzymatic activity combined in a temperature-cycling format. Unlike PCR, however, LCR uses four oligonucleotides that together make up both strands of the complete target sequence, and the enzyme is a heat-stable DNA ligase[126, 127] instead of a polymerase. Because the complete target sequence must be known in order to design an LCR reaction, it is not an appropriate method for gene discovery. This reaction is best suited for the detection of known sequences and for its ability to distinguish between sequences that differ by a single nucleotide base (Fig. 5–2).

As with PCR, the temperature is first elevated to render a single-stranded target, and then the temperature is lowered to allow for the formation of target-probe hybrids. Both strands form these hybrids, which act as the substrates for the DNA ligase. Each hybrid consists of two oligonucleotide probes annealed to adjacent portions of a strand of the target. Thus, the original double-stranded target is completely re-formed except that a single phosphodiester linkage is now missing between neighboring nucleotides on the adjacent probes. This missing bond is known as a "nick." Once formed, this nick can be enzymatically repaired by the ligase, which generates a phosphodiester linkage at that site, to complete the cycle. The newly formed copies act as targets in the subsequent cycles. The ligase chain reaction can be thought of as a target-dependent assemblage of amplicons from half targets that were supplied at the start of the reaction.

The four probes used in LCR are typically longer than the average PCR primer. Naturally, each of the probes can hybridize to its complementary probe at the annealing temperature; however, the ligase will only join probes that are annealed to adjacent bases on the target. In the original LCR design, blunt-ended ligation would take place and cause some background noise. Because of the four olignucleotide probes that make up the complete sequence, this artifact actually produces a small amount of product that is indistinguishable from the real product. This limited the resolution of the technique to detecting one target copy in a background of 10^4 wild-type sequences.[128] Modifications made since to the LCR, known as gap-LCR and asymmetric gap-LCR, reduce background noise and allow for the detection of RNA.[129]

In its simplest form, the LCR method can determine the presence or absence of a target sequence in a sample; however, it can also be used to query the identity of the base at a particular nucleotide position on a target.[130, 131] Competing probes are designed with the base in question represented at the ligation site, on the 3′-side of the nick.[17] When these probes are placed in the same reaction with the target, they will likely bind equally well to the target, but only the probes that are fully hybridized at the ligation site will be joined. This strategy forms the basis of a simple and accurate test for

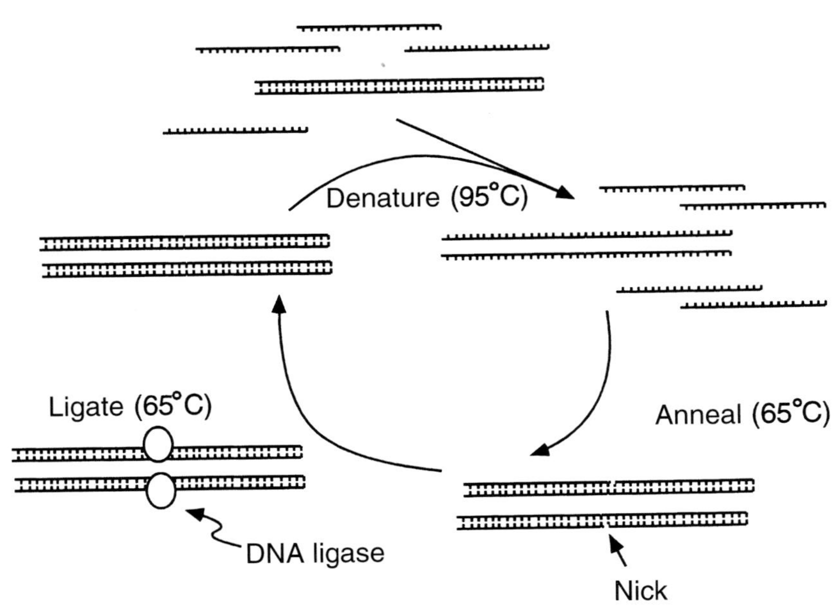

FIGURE 5–2
The ligase chain reaction relies on temperature cycling to render a single-stranded target and to release newly formed product into solution. Product is formed by joining adjacently annealed probes. Four probes are used, and together they represent the entire target sequence. A thermostable ligase catalyzes the reaction.

the detection of previously characterized single-nucleotide polymorphisms or mutations in the target. The LCR method has been used to distinguish between closely related species, such as *Mycobacterium tuberculosis*, *Chlamydia trachomatis*, and *Neisseria gonorrhoeae* (commercial LCR assay kits also are available [e.g., Abbott]).[132–137] In some cases, however, it has been suggested that the sensitivity of LCR is significantly improved when used in series with PCR.[138]

Ligase chain reaction and PCR achieve their exponential target amplification by using both strands of the target as templates. In a variation of the LCR technique, a single strand of the target may be used as a template but only a linear increase in the number of copies will occur. This procedure is known as *ligase detection reaction* (LDR) because it is generally used to couple a detection system to the PCR reaction. The PCR portion of the assay provides the exponential target amplification whereas the LDR creates a detectable signal, proportional to the amplicon concentration.

A key advantage of LDR is the simplicity with which such a reaction can be "multiplexed" or coupled to a detection method. Multiplex capabilities are critical when analyzing genetic disorders that arise from a variety of single nucleotide polymorphisms, such as cystic fibrosis. Fluorescently labeled probes have been used to detect 30 possible mutations in the cystic fibrosis gene using the PCR-LDR method.[139] In another study, all 19 of the currently identified single-base mutations in exons 12, 13, and 61 of *KRAS* were detected in a single reaction.[140] Ligation-dependent fluorescence also can be used to make these assays compatible with real-time detection systems for high-throughput screening.[141]

Strand Displacement Amplification

Strand displacement amplification (SDA) is an indirect-amplification method used specifically for the detection of short DNA sequences. It is a conceptually complex method, but in practice it is currently supported by a user-friendly platform developed by Becton-Dickinson for the identification of microorganisms.[142] The amplification reaction is an isothermal process, but a brief period at elevated temperatures in the presence of the nucleic acid probes is required at the start of the reaction. This method requires four primers, a modified DNA polymerase, a restriction endonuclease, and nucleotide triphosphates. One of the four nucleotide triphosphates must have a sulfur substituted for the alpha phosphate to make it uncleavable by the restriction enzyme. Thermostability of the enzymes is not required.[19, 143]

The primers are designed as a pair of "bumper" primers, which flank the target, and a pair of amplification primers that nest between the bumper primers on the target sequence. The amplification primers contain a sequence for target recognition, but they also carry a sequence at the 5′-tail end, which contains a restriction-endonuclease recognition sequence. This *restriction site* is not usually present in the original target. The bumper primers are important for the initial generation of an amplifiable copy of the target, but they do not participate in the amplification. At the start of the reaction, the target DNA and primers are heated to denaturing temperature in the absence of the enzymes and are then cooled to a temperature compatible with primer annealing and enzymatic activity. This allows all four primers to anneal.

The isothermal process begins as soon as the enzymes are added to the reaction, and the process continues until one of the reagents is used up, or until the reaction is stopped. An exonuclease-deficient Klenow fragment derived from the *Escherichia coli* DNA polymerase I is used for the primer extention reaction. This enzyme displaces DNA strands that are in its path as it extends the primer. This *strand displacement* mechanism allows the amplification to operate at a single temperature by releasing product DNA strands from the template without the need for thermal denaturation. Initially, all four primers are extended. Extension of the amplification primers creates the amplifiable copy of the target, and simultaneously the extension of the bumper primers displaces this amplifiable copy from the original target DNA. Once these reactions occur, the bumper primers and the original target are no longer relevant to the amplification, because they remain double-stranded, but the amplification primers continue to participate in the reaction.

Two critical features distinguish the amplifiable copy of the target from the original target DNA. First, a restriction site has been introduced at both ends of the newly formed amplifiable copy, by the 5′ end of the primer. Second, modified nucleotides have been introduced into the DNA as it was extended by the polymerase. As a result, each end of the amplifiable copy has a restriction site composed of modified (sulfur-containing) nucleotides on one strand but unmodified nucleotides on its complementary sequence. The restriction enzyme is capable of binding to its recognition sequence despite the presence of modified nucleotides, but only the strand containing the unmodified nucleotides can act as a substrate for the enzyme. Thus, the restriction enzyme creates a single stranded cut, or *nick*, at the restriction site on the strand containing the unmodified nucleotides. The DNA polymerase can recognize the nicked site and extend from that site while displacing the previous extension product into solution. The continuous regeneration of the nick by the restriction enzyme allows the process to be repeated spontaneously. Additional subtleties of this method are not relevant to understanding its applicability and, therefore, are not covered here. Only a select set of restriction endonucleases is capable of performing the described nicking activity, which is referred to as *hemirestriction*.

The strand displacement amplification reaction is complex, but it remains relevant for clinical diagnoses because Becton-Dickinson has developed a user-friendly, closed-amplification system in which the reactions are monitored in real time, using fluorescent probes.[144] *M. tuberculosis*, *C. trachomatis*, and *N. gonorrhoeae* detection have each been demonstrated using this system (available as BDProbeTecET).[142, 144, 145] In addition, multiplex SDA and reverse transcription SDA have been demonstrated.[146, 147]

Nucleic Acid Sequence–Based Amplification

Nucleic acid sequence–based amplification (NASBA) is an indirect method that will amplify specifically an RNA target, even in the presence of dsDNA of an identical sequence. The enzymatic activities of an RT, an RNase, and an RNA polymerase are combined into a single, self-sustained isothermal reaction. Two oligonucleotide primers are also required, and one of them must carry a promoter sequence that is specifically recognizable by the RNA polymerase. The amplification can be directed toward DNA by the addition of a denaturation step at the start of the reaction. The principle end product is single-stranded RNA, but low levels of RNA-DNA hybrids and dsDNA remain at the end of the reaction.[23, 148]

The chain of events begins when the primer hybridizes to the target RNA, and the hybrid acts as a substrate for the reverse transcriptase. Avian myeloblastosis virus RT can extend a DNA primer that is annealed to either RNA or DNA. A cDNA of the original target RNA is created to form an RNA-DNA hybrid. The RNA strand of this hybrid is then degraded by RNase, while the cDNA strand is left intact.[15, 149, 150] This allows the second primer to access the cDNA, and the reverse transcriptase can extend this primer to form a double-stranded cDNA. This dsDNA carries a complete RNA-polymerase promoter sequence at one end, which was introduced by the primer. The RNA polymerase recognizes this sequence as the starting point for RNA synthesis, and 10 to 1000 new RNA copies are produced per cDNA. Because these new RNA copies are released directly into solution, they are immediately available as targets. Thus, the reaction repeats itself until some substrate is depleted or the reaction is stopped.

NASBA is a generally applicable technique that can be used as an alternative to RT-PCR. It has been applied to the detection of tumor necrosis factor (TNF)-α mRNA[151] and *BCR-ABL* mRNA[152] and has been multiplexed to detect two separate mRNAs.[153] It can be used for the detection of viral or bacterial pathogens[154–158] or known human genetic defects.[159] As with the PCR and RT-PCR methods, NASBA does not require full knowledge of the sequence of the target, which makes it suitable for gene discovery; and the products of a NASBA reaction can be directly sequenced.[160] Furthermore, detecting mRNA in a dsDNA background with this technique requires no special design changes, which is most useful when the amplification of a region of the RNA that crosses an intron-exon boundary is not possible, as in the case for an intronless gene.[161] Kits for NASBA-based detection of human immunodeficiency virus (HIV) and hepatitis C virus (HCV) are available and have compared favorably to other commercial kits.[162, 163] Transcription-mediated amplification is conceptually similar to NASBA and is also commercially available in kit form for some clinical assays.[164]

Ligation-Dependent PCR

Ligation-dependent PCR (LD-PCR) is a signal-sequence-amplification method. LD-PCR uses a PCR reaction that occurs only if ligation takes place between two probe sequences. The design includes two hemiprobes that carry both a target-hybridization sequence and a primer binding site. Both probes recognize the same strand of the target. Once hybridized to the target, the hemiprobes are located adjacent to each other, separated only by a nick, as in the LCR technique. If both probes hybridize to the target, then a ligase can effectively repair the nick and assemble an amplifiable signal sequence.

Typically, the assay is conducted in several steps. First, a hybridization reaction is conducted in a mixture that includes both hemiprobes and one or two capture probes. Whereas the hemiprobes are designed to bind to the target sequence, the capture probes bind nearby (Fig. 5–3). The capture probes allow the target-probe hybrids to be rapidly purified from solution. Often, biotin is attached to the probe for this purpose and beads coated with immobilized streptavidin are used to pull the biotin-labeled nucleic acid from solution. These beads are washed free of unbound nucleic acid with a series of wash steps—residual, unbound probe will generate background noise if care is not taken at this step. These wash steps will also remove inhibitory substances before the amplification reaction. Once washed, the beads containing the captured target-probe hybrids are placed into a reaction mixture containing a DNA ligase. It is in this reaction that the ligase joins the two hemiprobes to form a single, complete probe that can be amplified in a subsequent PCR reaction. The target itself is not amplified at all, but amplification of the probe is proportional to the amount of target present because probe capture was mediated by the target.

The requirements for separate hybridization, wash, ligation, and PCR steps make this a more complex technique than those discussed earlier. Consistent results have been demonstrated, however, and the labor-intensive

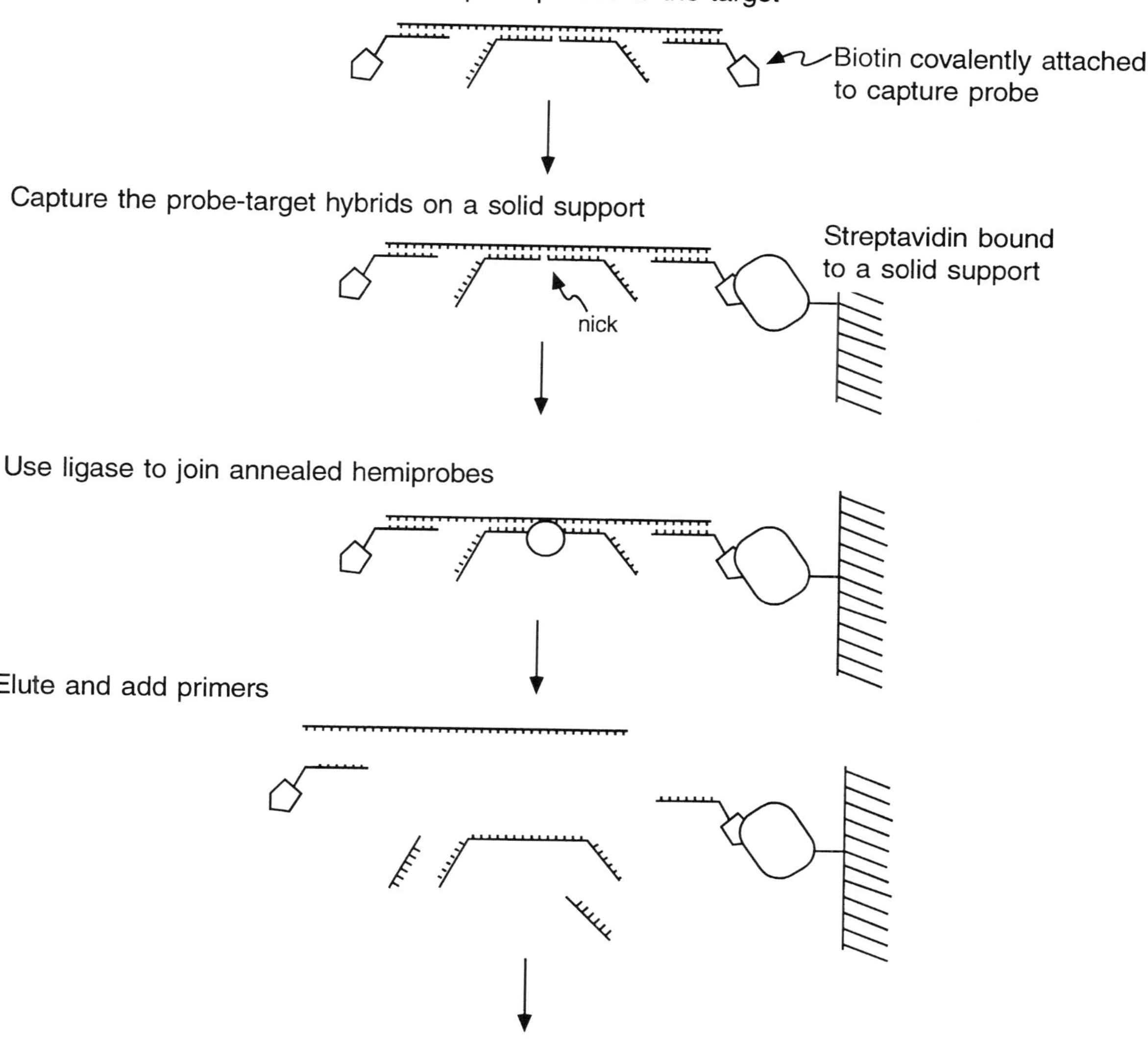

FIGURE 5–3
Ligation-dependent PCR (LD-PCR) represents a complex assay in which the target recognition and amplification steps take place in separate reactions. First, specific probes are hybridized to the target; then the probe-target hybrids are recovered from solution, and hybridized probes are ligated together to form an amplifiable reporter sequence. The resulting ligation product is then placed in a PCR reaction and amplified.

nature of the method can be overcome by using automated instruments. The complexity can be justified by the advantage gained from conducting the hybridization separately from the amplification. In this assay, hybridization can be conducted under optimal conditions that can be adjusted on sample-to-sample and target-to-target bases without affecting the efficiency of the amplification reaction—in contrast to PCR conditions, which are compromised to allow both hybridization and enzymatic activity to proceed in the same reaction.

The analysis of FFPE tissue, which often contains nucleic acid strands that have cross links, adducts, or areas of depurination, also can benefit from the LD-PCR method. Because processive incorporation of nucleotides along the target DNA strand is not involved, there is no chance that modifications to the target will interfere with the amplification step. Hybridization is not affected as dramatically by nucleic acid modifications, and selection of appropriate hybridization targets and conditions can allow recognition of the sequence of interest despite these alterations. Additionally, target recognition by both a capture probe and an amplification probe can potentially increase assay specificity. Finally, the use of more than one capture probe ensures that if one hybridization capture site is blocked, the target will still be captured, provided that the alternate capture site is not blocked.

The LD-PCR has been used to detect human papillomavirus, and hepatitis C and Epstein-Barr viruses.[165–167] In each of these studies, successful detection was demonstrated using FFPE tissues. Recently, a modified LD-PCR method using "circularizable" probes has been developed. This improvement results in "superexponential" amplification by combining the PCR reaction with a rolling-circle form of replication.[168]

Q-Beta Replicase

The Q-beta replicase (QBR) technique is a signal-sequence–amplification system that relies on a specialized RNA replicase originally derived from the QB-bacteriophage. The natural substrate for this enzyme is the midivariant RNA 1 (MDV-1) from the same phage. MDV-1 RNA is replicated by the QB-replicase without the need for primers. By embedding a target-directed probe sequence within the sequence of the MDV-1 RNA, a combined probe capable of target recognition and amplification is formed.[4, 169] First, a hybridization reaction is used to anneal the probe to the target. Capture probes are included in the hybridization reaction and are used to recover the target from solution, as discussed earlier for the LD-PCR method. The recovered material is extensively washed to remove traces of nonspecifically bound probe. Then the remaining probe, which is specifically bound to the target, is amplified.

Amplification of the probe by the QBR enzyme proceeds isothermally at 37°C, and the product is naturally displaced into solution. The method has the added convenience of not requiring primers, which eliminates one of the rate-limiting steps in the amplification. A single molecule can be replicated to produce 1×10^{12} copies in less than 10 minutes. Typical reactions are conducted for up to 30 minutes and can be quantified through 11 orders of magnitude by measuring the rate of production of the MDV-1 RNA.[16] The advantages and disadvantages are similar to those of the LD-PCR method when a ligation-dependent pair of MDV-1 hemiprobes is used.[170] If a single-hybridization probe design is used, sufficient carryover of nonspecifically bound probe will generate a false-positive signal. It is worth noting that the QBR technique randomly synthesizes nucleic acid strands in the absence of a template, but this activity is nominal and therefore can be ignored when designing diagnostic assays.[171] Laboratory instruments have been designed that adequately handle the necessary washing steps and combine the amplification with a real-time detection system. The QBR technique has been applied to the detection of *M. tuberculosis* and compares favorably with diagnostic cell culture method.[172]

BRANCHED DNA SIGNAL AMPLIFICATION

The branched DNA (b-DNA) signal amplification system has gained acceptance in clinical laboratory settings; several commercial kits that use this method are widely used clinically. This technique uses only traditional hybridization methods, but they are arranged in a unique format that provides signal amplification but not nucleic acid amplification.

First, sample RNA or DNA is hybridized with probes that have both target and capture sequences. The hybrids can bind to a solid support through the hybridization of some of the capture sequences. Additional capture sequences are available for further hybridization that incorporate an amplifier probe. The amplifier is a highly branched structure that provides numerous hybridization sites for a final round of hybridization. The final hybridization incorporates nucleic acids that are linked

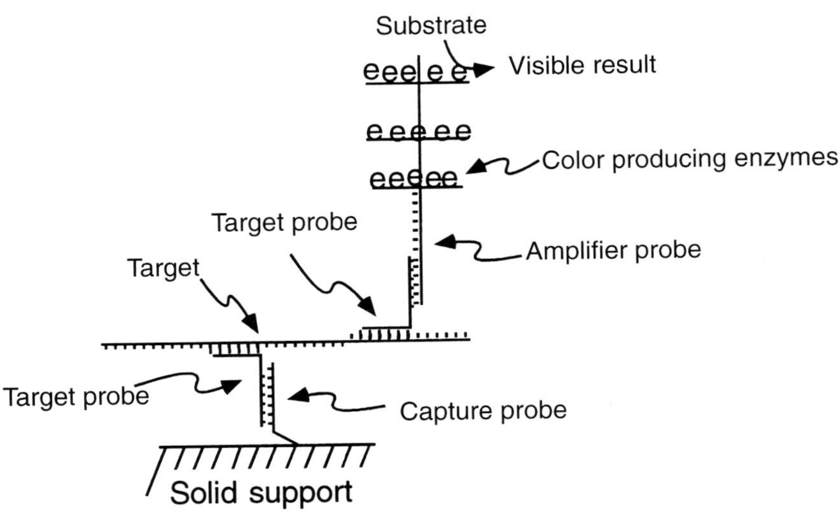

FIGURE 5–4
Branched DNA (b-DNA) signal amplification does not rely on amplification of nucleic acids for its sensitivity. Instead, a series of hybridizations are used to create a highly branched structure with many detectable sites; then a probe that carries a signal-producing enzyme is hybridized to this structure. In the final step, substrate is added, and the enzyme produces a detectable signal.

to a signal-producing enzyme. A schematic of this strategy is shown in Fig. 5–4, but it does not do justice to the well-designed commercial kits, which are based on carefully derived sets of target-directed probes.

Simply stated, the signal amplification in this method is generated by stepwise increases in the number of hybridization sites, followed by attachment of enzymes to those sites. Enzymatic signal production can then be measured to indicate the amount of target in the sample. The sensitivity of this method has been compared favorably with PCR and NASBA for monitoring HIV-1 viral load.[162] An advantage of b-DNA signal amplification is that it is not subject to inhibition by the inhibitors found in a variety of biologic samples.[173] This technique is well presented, along with its applications for detecting hepatitis B, C, and G; HIV-1; cytomegalovirus, and *Trypanosoma brucei*, in a single review.[174]

DETECTION OF AMPLIFICATION PRODUCTS

Regardless of the amplification method used, a method of detection must be used to determine the results. In the simplest case, the DNA can be separated by electrophoresis and visualized on an ethidium bromide–stained agarose gel to determine if an amplification product of the expected length has been generated. This method is simple and effective and is still applied during the development of an assay. Agarose gel electrophoresis is the preferred separation method to use in conjunction with filter hybridization analysis, such as a Southern or Northern blot. The size separation, primer specificity, and subsequent high stringency hybridization create an effective combination of independent verifications of the target identity. Quantitation can be accomplished by simultaneously amplifying an internal control sequence, which ideally should use the same primers.[104, 147, 153, 156]

Automated sequencing methods have proven to be cost-effective and labor conservative, while generating full sequence information not obtainable by blotting. This is useful in cases in which obtaining sequence information is more important than absolute quantitation. In some cases, PCR amplification products can be sequenced directly without extensive preprocessing steps. Generally, a portion of the PCR reaction can be placed directly into a sequencing reaction, provided that the reaction yields a single product and uses up all of the primer. If excess primer from the PCR step is present, then a simple filtration step will prepare the product for sequencing. In cases in which more than one product is amplified, the bands can be purified from an agarose gel and then sequenced.[175] Microdissection followed by PCR and sequencing is a powerful combination when applied to a retrospective analysis.

Large-scale screening methods based in part on sequencing can be applied to the analysis of gene expression. Serial analysis of gene expression (SAGE) provides sequence information sufficient for the identification of 15 to 30 expressed transcripts per sequencing reaction. A unique cloning process is used to concatenate multiple sequence tags into a single plasmid insert.[176] A library of these tags is then produced in bacteria and analyzed by sequencing. Direct PCR from the bacterial clones can be used to avoid the plasmid purification step. When SAGE is used to compare identical cells in a diseased or healthy state, the profiles of expressed genes can reveal disease-specific changes.[177, 178] A recently described modification of the method even offers to extract similar information from small samples, such as biopsy samples.[31]

Modern detection methods now allow for the real-time quantitation of amplicon production during the amplification process, which offers multiple advantages: most obvious is the ability to obtain reproducible quantitative data from a sample. For an end-point quantitiation to be accurate, all the reactions being compared must be stopped at the same time, and they must not be limited by any reagents in the reaction. Real-time systems simplify this problem by collecting data throughout the course of the reaction and then use data collected during the exponential phase of the reaction for quantitative analysis.[16, 179, 180]

Real-time detection systems are based primarily on the detection of a fluorescence signal from reporter moieties attached to nucleic acid probes. Because most researchers rely on commercially available fluorescent tags to design their assays, the physics related to the production of a fluorescent signal are ignored here; instead, the focus of the discussion is on an explanation of relevant assay design strategies. Only the techniques that couple to the PCR reaction are addressed, but similar methods have been worked out for the other amplification techniques. The material provided here gives a sufficient basis for the more detailed study of other strategies.

There are a variety of sequence-specific and non–sequence-specific strategies for coupling signal production to amplicon production. Some probes rely on a quenched fluorescent signal on unhybridized probes, which is then unquenched on hybridization. Other probes assemble a functional fluorogenic entity at the hybridization site through the closely proximal hybridization of labeled probes. Alternatively, fluorescence may remain quenched on hybridization and then be unquenched on preferential degradation of the hybridized probe. Finally, dyes are available that fluoresce on intercalation between the bases of double-stranded nucleic acids. The most popular intercalating dye for real-time detection is SYBR Green, because its absorption and emission characteristics are consistent with commercial instruments currently on the market,[181–184] but the use of propidium iodide also has been demonstrated.[16] Such dyes can be used to monitor the continuous production of amplicons without the specificity provided by linking the signal to a nucleic acid probe. This is most advantageous in the development of new assays. Other strategies used to date are largely variations on these models.

Probes that undergo a fluorogenic conformational change on hybridization have been dubbed "molecular beacons."[185] These probes are designed with a target-recognition sequence surrounded by a self-hybridization sequence. When they are not hybridized to their target, the ends of the probe self-hybridize to take on the conformation of a stem and loop. The fluorogenic tags are chemically bonded to the self-hybridizing region of the probe. At one end is a fluorophore that will emit detectable light on excitation from a laser light source. At the other end is a quencher that is capable of absorbing the light emitted by the excitable fluorophore. When the probe is self-hybridized, the fluorophore and the quencher are in close proximity and any fluorescence emitted is absorbed by the quencher. When the probe is annealed to its target, the hybridization to the target recognition sequence causes the probe to take on a linear conformation that moves the fluorogenic components of the probe to their farthest distance apart. In this conformation, emission from the fluorophore is detectable. Thus, detectable fluorescence depends on target hybridization.

Typically, there is a 100-fold increase in the fluorescence of a molecular beacon on hybridization. The self-annealing region of the probe may be 5 or more nucleotides in length, whereas the loop is generally 15 or more nucleotides in length. Thermodynamic studies have demonstrated that stem-and-loop probes such as molecular beacons show enhanced sequence specificity compared with linear probes of similar sequences.[186] Enhanced specificity is advantageous when distinguishing sequences that differ by a single base. The full potential and relative importance of molecular beacons compared with other specific probe systems has yet to be determined. A similar stem-and-loop quenched-probe design has been used in conjunction with SDA, but the unquenching of the probe is accomplished by endonucleolytic cleavage of the probe.[144]

Probes that hybridize to form a detectable fluorogen at the target site have been referred to as *fluorescence resonance energy transfer* (FRET) probes. These probes may be designed as adjacent hybridization probes[187, 188] or as probe-primer pairs.[189] Adjacent probes anneal to the same strand of the target in a tandem configuration. As a result, the Cy-5 label at the back end of the first probe is brought in close proximity to the fluorescein label at the front of the second probe. When excited by laser light, the combined action of the fluorescein and Cy-5 produces a detectable emission. FRET probe-primer pairs work by bringing the fluorescein label of the probe into the proximity of a Cy-5 label, carried on the PCR primers. The probe is hybridized to the DNA strand generated from the labeled primer, and, while it is hybridized, fluorescence occurs.

When designing adjacent FRET probes, the probes should be 23 to 30 nucleotides in length and should have nearly equal melting temperatures. The melting temperature should be 5°C to 10°C above that of the PCR primers. The probes should also be blocked at their 3′ ends so that they do not become extended by the polymerase. Placement of the fluorescein at the 3′ end of the one probe will block it from being extended, but the Cy-5–labeled probe should be blocked at the 3′ end by phosphorylation. It is best that the hybridization site be located as far from the extending primer as possible to allow time for hybridization and hybrid detection, before the probe is displaced by the strand being newly synthesized. When designing a FRET primer-probe pair, the same rules apply for the probe that will carry the fluorescein label. The primer, however, must be selected to have a thymidine residue 3 to 6 bases from its 3′ end. This residue will be modified during its synthesis to carry the Cy-5 label on a "linker" arm. Optimal fluorescence intensity will be achieved if, on hybridization, the fluorescein and Cy-5 labels are separated by four or five nucleotides.

Single-target–directed probes that contain both a fluorescent reporter and a fluorescent quencher dye on the same molecule can be designed so that their fluorescence intensity increases on degradation.[190] Typically, the reporter dye is attached to the 5′ end of the probe and a quencher is placed at the opposite end. The probe is designed so that it anneals next to the extending primer. As the primer is extended during the PCR reaction, the 5′ to 3′ exonuclease activity of the Taq polymerase degrades the probe, releasing the reporter dye that is no longer quenched. Thus, detectable fluorescence accumulates in proportion to amplicon production, and quantity can be reverse-calculated based on the PCR cycle, at which signal intensity surpasses some threshold.[179, 180]

Because nuclease-based assays depend on the nucleolytic activity of the *Taq* polymerase as it extends the primer, it is critical that the detection probe be hybridized to its target before primer extension begins.[191] Therefore, the hybridization probe must have an annealing temperature at least 10°C higher than the primers. The primers should be designed with melting temperatures of 58°C to 60°C. The efficiency of probe hydrolysis also may depend on its close proximity to the extending primer. In addition, amplicon size should be restricted to less than 150 nucleotides to ensure an efficient PCR reaction. Guanidine residues should not be located at the 5′ end of the hydrolysis probe.

Real-time fluorescence applications for multiplex detection have been demonstrated for each of the popular probe formats.[187, 192–195] Each of these detection modes are well suited to genotyping and allelic discrimination assays.[188, 189, 193, 196–198] Real-time in situ DNA detection has been demonstrated using 5′-nuclease probes.[199] When detection alone is important, an end-point determination may be useful; but real-time methods allow very precise relative or absolute quantitation of gene amplification or transcript expression across a broader linear range than do end-point determinations.[179, 200, 201]

SUMMARY

The PCR is the most flexible and powerful nucleic acid amplification technique for research and diagnostic purposes. It can be applied to DNA or RNA and is therefore the ideal platform for the early development of any amplification assay. Ligase chain reaction (LCR), when combined with PCR, couples an amplification reaction to a detection reaction and has great potential for multiplex analysis of single nucleotide sites. Nucleic acid sequence-based amplification (NASBA) is particularly useful when the detection of RNA in the presence of a similar DNA sequence is required. Ligation-dependent PCR (LD-PCR) and Q-Beta replicase (QBR) are signal-sequence amplification technologies that separately detect the target, then amplify a nontarget sequence to indicate the presence of the original target. As such, they offer the greatest chance for detecting damaged nucleic acids, situations that are commonly encountered in the analysis of archived formalin-fixed paraffin-embedded samples.

The complexity of amplification methods is becoming less relevant to both the clinical and research laboratory. New generations of laboratory instruments are automating the sample handling and processing steps and combining amplification methods with real-time detection methods. Thus, there are few technical barriers that specifically exclude a technique from success in the clinical setting. Nucleic acid amplification techniques will continue to pervade the clinical setting. They will be applied to the detection of genetic differences and gene expression, as they have since their inception. Interestingly, however, most of these techniques can be coupled to tests that detect proteins and small analytes. It is therefore most important that students of the medical sciences be well versed about the molecular basis of the different nucleic acid amplification methods and their potential strengths and weaknesses.

Acknowledgment

I would like to acknowledge the entire staff of the Molecular Pathology Division of the Armed Forces Institute of Pathology for their support in putting together this chapter. I would especially like to thank Ron Przygodzki and Karen Bijwaard for input, and Ying Liu for carrying extra work while I was involved in this effort.

REFERENCES

1. Landegren U: Molecular mechanics of nucleic acid sequence amplification. Trends Genet 1993;9:199–204.
2. Wolcott MJ: Advances in nucleic acid-based detection methods. Clin Microbiol Rev 1992;5:370–386.
3. Birkenmeyer LG, Mushahwar IK: DNA probe amplification methods. J Virol Methods 1991;35:117–126.
4. Lizardi PM, Kramer FR: Exponential amplification of nucleic acids: New diagnostics using DNA polymerases and RNA replicases. Trends Biotechnol 1991;9:53–58.
5. Monteiro L, Cabrita J, Megraud F: Evaluation of performances of three DNA enzyme immunoassays for detection of *Helicobacter pylori* PCR products from biopsy specimens. J Clin Microbiol 1997;35:2931–2936.
6. Sano T, Smith CL, Cantor CR: Immuno-PCR: Very sensitive antigen detection by means of specific antibody-DNA conjugates. Science 1992;258:120–122.
7. Saito K, Kobayashi D, Sasaki M, et al: Detection of human serum tumor necrosis factor-alpha in healthy donors, using a highly sensitive immuno-PCR assay. Clin Chem 1999;45:665–669.
8. Case MC, Burt AD, Hughes J, et al: Enhanced ultrasensitive detection of structurally diverse antigens using a single immuno-PCR assay protocol [erratum appears in J Immunol Methods 1999;226:189–190]. J Immunol Methods 1999; 223:93–106.
9. Joerger RD, Truby TM, Hendrickson ER, et al: Analyte detection with DNA-labeled antibodies and polymerase chain reaction. Clin Chem 1995;41:1371–1377.
10. Sealey PG, Whittaker PA, Southern EM: Removal of repeated sequences from hybridisation probes. Nucleic Acids Res 1985;13:1905–1922.
11. Southern EM: Detection of specific sequences among DNA fragments separated by gel electrophoresis. J Mol Biol 1975;98:503–517.
12. Thomas PS: Hybridization of denatured RNA and small DNA fragments transferred to nitrocellulose. Proc Natl Acad U S A 1980;77:5201–5205.
13. Myers TW, Gelfand DH: Reverse transcription and DNA amplification by a *Thermus thermophilus* DNA polymerase. Biochemistry 1991;30:7661–7666.
14. Lawyer FC, Stoffel S, Saiki RK, et al: High-level expression, purification, and enzymatic characterization of full-length *Thermus aquaticus* DNA polymerase and a truncated form deficient in 5′ to 3′ exonuclease activity. PCR Methods Appl 1993;2:275–287.
15. Watson KF, Schendel PL, Rosok MJ, et al: Model RNA-directed DNA synthesis by avian myeloblastosis virus DNA polymerase and its associated RNase H. Biochemistry 1979;18:3210–3219.
16. Burg JL, Cahill PB, Kutter M, et al: Real-time fluorescence detection of RNA amplified by Q beta replicase. Anal Biochem 1995;230:263–272.
17. Luo J, Bergstrom DE, Barany F: Improving the fidelity of *Thermus thermophilus* DNA ligase. Nucleic Acids Res 1996;24:3071–3078.

18. Tong J, Cao W, Barany F: Biochemical properties of a high fidelity DNA ligase from *Thermus* species AK16D. Nucleic Acids Res 1999;27:788–794.
19. Walker GT, Fraiser MS, Schram JL, et al: Strand displacement amplification: An isothermal, in vitro DNA amplification technique. Nucleic Acids Res 1992; 20:1691–1696.
20. Spargo CA, Fraiser MS, Van Cleve M, et al: Detection of *M. tuberculosis* DNA using thermophilic strand displacement amplification. Mol Cell Probes 1996;10:247–256.
21. Rogers BB: Nucleic acid amplification and infectious disease. Hum Pathol 1994;25:590–593.
22. Whitcombe D, Newton CR, Little S: Advances in approaches to DNA-based diagnostics. Curr Opin Biotechnol 1998;9:602–608.
23. Compton J: Nucleic acid sequence-based amplification. Nature 1991;350:91–92.
24. Fox RI, Dotan I, Compton T, et al: Use of DNA amplification methods for clinical diagnosis in autoimmune diseases. J Clin Lab Anal 1989;3:378–387.
25. Malek L, Sooknanan R, Compton J: Nucleic acid sequence-based amplification (NASBA). Methods Mol Biol 1994;28:253–260.
26. Saiki RK, Gelfand DH, Stoffel S, et al: Primer-directed enzymatic amplification of DNA with a thermostable DNA polymerase. Science 1988;239:487–491.
27. Saiki RK, Scharf S, Faloona F, et al: Enzymatic amplification of beta-globin genomic sequences and restriction site analysis for diagnosis of sickle cell anemia. Science 1985;230:1350–1354.
28. Gibbs RA: DNA amplification by the polymerase chain reaction. Anal Chem 1990;62:1202–1214.
29. Bell J: The polymerase chain reaction. Immunol Today 1989;10:351–355.
30. Velculescu VE, Zhang L, Vogelstein B, et al: Serial analysis of gene expression [see comments]. Science 995; 270:484–487.
31. Datson NA, van der Perk-de Jong J, van den Berg MP, et al: MicroSAGE: A modified procedure for serial analysis of gene expression in limited amounts of tissue. Nucleic Acids Res 1999;27:1300–1307.
32. Artlett CM, Smith JB, Jimenez SA: Identification of fetal DNA and cells in skin lesions from women with systemic sclerosis. N Engl J Med 1998; 338:1186–1191.
33. Collandre H, Aubin JT, Agut H, et al: Detection of HHV-6 by the polymerase chain reaction. J Virol Methods 1991;31:171–179.
34. Buchbinder A, Josephs SF, Ablashi D, et al: Polymerase chain reaction amplification and in situ hybridization for the detection of human B-lymphotropic virus. J Virol Methods 1988;21:191–197.
35. Keller GH, Huang DP, Shih JW, et al: Detection of hepatitis B virus DNA in serum by polymerase chain reaction amplification and microtiter sandwich hybridization. J Clin Microbiol 1990;28:1411–1416.
36. Ernst SI, Hubbs AE, Przygodzki RM, et al: KIT mutation portends poor prognosis in gastrointestinal stromal/-smooth muscle tumors. Lab Invest 1998;78:1633–1636.
37. Przygodzki RM, Finkelstein SD, Langer JC, et al: Analysis of p53, K-ras-2, and C-raf-1 in pulmonary neuroendocrine tumors: Correlation with histological subtype and clinical outcome. Am J Pathol 1996;148:1531–1534.
38. Kaledin AS, Sliusarenko AG, Gorodetskii SI, et al: [Isolation and properties of DNA polymerase from extreme thermophylic bacteria Thermus aquaticus YT-1]. Biokhimiia 1980;45:644–651.
39. Saiki RK, Gelfand DH, Stoffel S, et al: Primer-directed enzymatic amplification of DNA with a thermostable DNA polymerase. Science 1988;239:487–491.
40. Cheng S, Chang SY, Gravitt P, et al: Long PCR. Nature 1994;369:684–685.
41. Cheng S, Fockler C, Barnes WM, et al: Effective amplification of long targets from cloned inserts and human genomic DNA. Proc Natl Acad U S A 1994;91:5695–5699.
42. Rychlik W: Priming efficiency in PCR. Biotechniques 1995;18:84–90.
43. Rychlik W: Selection of primers for polymerase chain reaction. Mol Biotechnol 1995;3:129–134.
44. Mitsuhashi M: Technical report: Part 1. Basic requirements for designing optimal oligonucleotide probe sequences. J Clin Lab Anal 1996;10:277–284.
45. Mitsuhashi M: Technical report: Part 2. Basic requirements for designing optimal PCR primers. J Clin Lab Anal 1996;10:285–293.
46. Chumakov KM: Reverse transcriptase can inhibit PCR and stimulate primer-dimer formation. PCR Methods Appl 1994;4:62–64.
47. Brownie J, Shawcross S, Theaker J, et al: The elimination of primer-dimer accumulation in PCR. Nucleic Acids Res 1997;25:3235–3241.
48. Chou Q, Russell M, Birch DE, et al: Prevention of pre-PCR mis-priming and primer dimerization improves low-copy-number amplifications. Nucleic Acids Res 1992;20:1717–1723.
49. De la Viuda M, Fille M, Ruiz J, et al: Use of AmpliWax to optimize amplicon sterilization by isopsoralen. J Clin Microbiol 1996;34:3115–3119.
50. Birch DE: Simplified hot start PCR. Nature 1996; 381:445–446.
51. Moretti T, Koons B, Budowle B: Enhancement of PCR amplification yield and specificity using AmpliTaq Gold DNA polymerase. Biotechniques 1998;25:716–722.
52. Sharkey DJ, Scalice ER, Christy KGJ, et al: Antibodies as thermolabile switches: High temperature triggering for the polymerase chain reaction. Biotechnology 1994; 12:506–509.
53. Hartley JL, Rashtchian A: Dealing with contamination: enzymatic control of carryover contamination in PCR. PCR Methods Appl 1993;3:S10–S14.
54. Thornton CG, Hartley JL, Rashtchian A: Utilizing uracil DNA glycosylase to control carryover contamination in PCR: Characterization of residual UDG activity following thermal cycling. Biotechniques 1992;13:180–184.
55. Reid AH: Polymerase chain reaction. *In* Mikel UV (ed): advanced laboratory methods in histology and pathology. Washington, DC, American Registry of Pathology, 1994, pp 77–106.
56. Pang J, Modlin J, Yolken R: Use of modified nucleotides and uracil-DNA glycosylase (UNG) for the control of contamination in the PCR-based amplification of RNA. Mol Cell Probes 1992;6:251–256.
57. Niederhauser C, Hofelein C, Wegmuller B, et al: Reliability of PCR decontamination systems. PCR Methods Appl 1994; 4:117–123.

58. Rys PN, Persing DH: Preventing false-positives: Quantitative evaluation of three protocols for inactivation of polymerase chain reaction amplification products. J Clin Microbiol 1993;31:2356–2360.
59. Ritzler M, Perschil I, Altwegg M: Influence of residual uracil-DNA glycosylase activity on the electrophoretic migration of dUTP-containing PCR products. J Microbiol Methods 1999;35:73–76.
60. Abbott LZ, Spicer T, Bryz-Gornia V, et al: Design and use of signature primers to detect carry-over of amplified material. J Virol Methods 1994;46:51–59.
61. Kaul K, Luke S, McGurn C, et al: Amplification of residual DNA sequences in sterile bronchoscopes leading to false-positive PCR results. J Clin Microbiol 1996;34: 1949–1951.
62. Wiedbrauk DL, Werner JC, Drevon AM: Inhibition of PCR by aqueous and vitreous fluids. J Clin Microbiol 1995;33:2643–2646.
63. Belec L, Authier J, Eliezer-Vanerot MC, et al: Myoglobin as a polymerase chain reaction (PCR) inhibitor: A limitation for PCR from skeletal muscle tissue avoided by the use of *Thermus thermophilus* polymerase. Muscle Nerve 1998;21:1064–1067.
64. Deneer HG, Knight I: Inhibition of the polymerase chain reaction by mucolytic agents. Clin Chem 1994;40:171–172.
65. Gilgen M, Hofelein C, Luthy J, et al: Hydroxyquinoline overcomes PCR inhibition by UV-damaged mineral oil. Nucleic Acids Res 1995;23(19):4001–4002.
66. de Lomas JG, Sunzeri FJ, Busch MP: False-negative results by polymerase chain reaction due to contamination by glove powder. Transfusion 1992;32(1):83–85.
67. Farnert A, Arez AP, Correia AT, et al: Sampling and storage of blood and the detection of malaria parasites by polymerase chain reaction. Trans R Soc Trop Med Hyg 1999;93:50–53.
68. Yedidag EN, Koffron AJ, Mueller KH, et al: Acyclovir triphosphate inhibits the diagnostic polymerase chain reaction for cytomegalovirus. Transplantation 1996;62: 238–242.
69. Taylor AC: Titration of heparinase for removal of the PCR-inhibitory effect of heparin in DNA samples. Mol Ecol 1997;6:383–385.
70. Imai H, Yamada O, Morita S, et al: Detection of HIV-1 RNA in heparinized plasma of HIV-1 seropositive individuals. J Virol Methods 1992;36:181–184.
71. Jung R, Lubcke C, Wagener C, et al: Reversal of RT-PCR inhibition observed in heparinized clinical specimens. Biotechniques 1997;23:24, 26, 28.
72. Witt DJ, Kemper M: Techniques for the evaluation of nucleic acid amplification technology performance with specimens containing interfering substances: Efficacy of boom methodology for extraction of HIV-1 RNA. J Virol Methods 1999;79:97–111.
73. Bourke MT, Scherczinger CA, Ladd C, et al: NaOH treatment to neutralize inhibitors of Taq Polymerase [in process citation]. J Forensic Sci 1999;44:1046–1050.
74. Abu A, Radstrom P: Capacity of nine thermostable DNA polymerases to mediate DNA amplification in the presence of PCR-inhibiting samples. Appl Environ Microbiol 1998;64:3748–3753.
75. Miyachi H, Masukawa A, Ohshima T, et al: Monitoring of inhibitors of enzymatic amplification in polymerase chain reaction and evaluation of efficacy of RNA extraction for the detection of hepatitis C virus using the internal control. Clin Chem Lab Med 1998;36:571–575.
76. Vortmeyer AO, Devouassoux-Shisheboran M, Li G, et al: Microdissection-based analysis of mature ovarian teratoma. Am J Pathol 1999;154:987–991.
77. Przygodzki RM, Finkelstein SD, Keohavong P, et al: Sporadic and Thorotrast-induced angiosarcomas of the liver manifest frequent and multiple point mutations in K-ras-2. Lab Invest 1997;76:153–159.
78. Przygodzki RM, Koss MN, Moran CA, et al: Pleomorphic (giant and spindle cell) carcinoma is genetically distinct from adenocarcinoma and squamous cell carcinoma by K-*ras*-2 and p53 analysis. Am J Clin Pathol 1996;106:487–492.
79. Zhuang Z, Bertheau P, Emmert-Buck MR, et al: A microdissection technique for archival DNA analysis of specific cell populations in lesions <1 mm in size. Am J Pathol 1995;146:620–625.
80. Zhuang Z, Emmert-Buck MR, Roth MJ, et al: von Hippel-Lindau disease gene deletion detected in microdissected sporadic human colon carcinoma specimens. Hum Pathol 1996;27:152–156.
81. Berger DH, Chang H, Wood M, et al: Mutational activation of K-ras in nonneoplastic exocrine pancreatic lesions in relation to cigarette smoking status. Cancer 1999;85:326–332.
82. Przygodzki RM, Moran CA, Suster S, et al: Primary mediastinal and testicular seminomas: A comparison of K-*ras*-2 gene sequence and p53 immunoperoxidase analysis of 26 cases. Hum Pathol 1996;27:975–979.
83. Abati A, Sanjuan X, Wilder A, et al: Utilization of microdissection and the polymerase chain reaction for the diagnosis of adrenal cortical carcinoma in fine-needle aspiration cytology. Cancer 1999;87:231–237.
84. Przygodzki RM, Goodman ZD, Rabin L, et al.: Hemochromatosis (HFE) gene sequence analysis of formalin-fixed, paraffin-embedded liver biopsy specimens. Mol Diagn. 2001;6:227–32.
85. Hagen-Mann K, Mann W: RT-PCR and alternative methods to PCR for in vitro amplification of nucleic acids. Exp Clin Endocrinol Diabetes 1995;103:150–155.
86. Freeman WM, Vrana SL, Vrana KE: Use of elevated reverse transcription reaction temperatures in RT-PCR. Biotechniques 1996;20:782–783.
87. Grondahl B, Puppe W, Hoppe A, et al: Rapid identification of nine microorganisms causing acute respiratory tract infections by single-tube multiplex reverse transcription-PCR: Feasibility study. J Clin Microbiol 1999;37:1–7.
88. Adeyefa CA, Quayle K, McCauley JW: A rapid method for the analysis of influenza virus genes: Application to the reassortment of equine influenza virus genes. Virus Res 1994;32:391–399.
89. Osiowy C: Direct detection of respiratory syncytial virus, parainfluenza virus, and adenovirus in clinical respiratory specimens by a multiplex reverse transcription-PCR assay. J Clin Microbiol 1998;36:3149–3154.

90. Taubenberger JK, Reid AH, Krafft AE, et al: Initial genetic characterization of the 1918 "Spanish" influenza virus [see comments]. Science 1997;275:1793–1796.
91. Pena MJ, Bolanos M, Perez MC, et al: The importance of polymerase chain reaction in the diagnosis of enterovirus infections of the central nervous system in children Clinico-epidemiologic characteristics. Enferm Infecc Microbiol Clin 1999;17:227–230.
92. Wingo ST, Ringel MD, Anderson JS, et al: Quantitative reverse transcription-PCR measurement of thyroglobulin mRNA in peripheral blood of healthy subjects. Clin Chem 1999;45(6 Pt 1):785–789.
93. Saegusa M, Okayasu I: DCC expression is related to mucinous differentiation but not changes in expression of p21(WAF1/Cip1) and p27Kip1, apoptosis, cell proliferation and human papillomavirus infection in uterine cervical adenocarcinomas. Br J Cancer 1999;80:51–58.
94. Vonlanthen S, Heighway J, Tschan MP, et al: Expression of p16INK4a/p16alpha and p19ARF/p16beta is frequently altered in non-small cell lung cancer and correlates with p53 overexpression. Oncogene 1998;17: 2779–2785.
95. Shields DJ, Byrd JC, Abbondanzo SL, et al: Detection of Epstein-Barr virus in transformations of low-grade B-cell lymphomas after fludarabine treatment. Mod Pathol 1997;10:1151–1159.
96. Nogva HK, Evensen SA, Madshus IH: One-tube multiplex RT-PCR of BCR-ABL transcripts in analysis of patients with chronic myeloid leukaemia and acute lymphoblastic leukaemia. Scand J Clin Lab Invest 1998;58: 647–654.
97. Downing JR, Khandekar A, Shurtleff SA, et al: Multiplex RT-PCR assay for the differential diagnosis of alveolar rhabdomyosarcoma and Ewing's sarcoma. Am J Pathol 1995;146:626–634.
98. Scurto P, Hsu RM, Kane JR, et al: A multiplex RT-PCR assay for the detection of chimeric transcripts encoded by the risk-stratifying translocations of pediatric acute lymphoblastic leukemia. Leukemia 1998;12:1994–2005.
99. Preudhomme C, Chams-Eddine L, Roumier C, et al: Detection of BCR-ABL transcripts in chronic myeloid leukemia (CML) using an in situ RT-PCR assay. Leukemia 1999;13:818–823.
100. Blaheta HJ, Schittek B, Breuninger H, et al: Detection of melanoma micrometastasis in sentinel nodes by reverse transcription-polymerase chain reaction correlates with tumor thickness and is predictive of micrometastatic disease in the lymph node basin. Am J Surg Pathol 1999;23:822–828.
101. Pallisgaard N, Hokland P, Riishoj DC, et al: Multiplex reverse transcription-polymerase chain reaction for simultaneous screening of 29 translocations and chromosomal aberrations in acute leukemia. Blood 1998; 92:574–588.
102. Chandler DP, Wagnon CA, Bolton HJ: Reverse transcriptase (RT) inhibition of PCR at low concentrations of template and its implications for quantitative RT-PCR. Appl Environ Microbiol 1998;64:669–677.
103. O'Leary TJ: Reducing the impact of endogenous ribonucleases on reverse transcription-PCR assay systems [editorial; comment]. Clin Chem 1999;45(4):449–450.
104. Haberhausen G, Pinsl J, Kuhn CC, et al: Comparative study of different standardization concepts in quantitative competitive reverse transcription-PCR assays. J Clin Microbiol 1998;36:628–633.
105. Dostal DE, Rothblum KN, Baker KM: An improved method for absolute quantification of mRNA using multiplex polymerase chain reaction: determination of renin and angiotensinogen mRNA levels in various tissues. Anal Biochem 1994;223:239–250.
106. Uhlmann V, Rolfs A, Mix E, et al: A novel, rapid in-cell RNA amplification technique for the detection of low-copy mRNA transcripts. Mol Pathol 1998;51:160–163.
107. Gey A, Hamdi S, Vielh P, et al: Development of a direct in situ RT-PCR method using labeled primers to detect cytokine mRNA inside cells. J Immunol Methods 1999; 227:149–160.
108. O'Leary JJ, Landers RJ, Silva I, et al: Molecular analysis of ras oncogenes in CIN III and in stage I and II invasive squamous cell carcinoma of the uterine cervix. J Clin Pathol 1998;51:576–582.
109. Shieh B, Lee SE, Tsai YC, et al: Detection of hepatitis B virus genome in hepatocellular carcinoma tissues with PCR-in situ hybridization. J Virol Methods 1999;80: 157–167.
110. Mutty CE, Timm EAJ, Stewart CC: Effects of thermal exposure on immunophenotyping combined with in situ PCR, measured by flow cytometry. Cytometry 1999;36:303–311.
111. Li VR, Bianchi UA, Carosi G, et al: Successful application of indirect in-situ polymerase chain reaction to tissues fixed in Bouin's solution. Histopathology 1999;35: 134–143.
112. Liu HJ, Liao MH, Chang CD, et al: Comparison of two molecular techniques for the detection of avian reoviruses in formalin-fixed, paraffin-embedded chicken tissues [in process citation]. J Virol Methods 1999;80: 197–201.
113. Uhlmann V, Silva I, Luttich K, et al: In-cell amplification. Mol Pathol 1998;51:119–130.
114. Tbakhi A, Totos G, Hauser-Kronberger C, Pettay J, et al: Fixation conditions for DNA and RNA in situ hybridization: A reassessment of molecular morphology dogma. Am J Pathol 1998;152:35–41.
115. Tbakhi A, Totos G, Pettay JD, et al: The effect of fixation on detection of B-cell clonality by polymerase chain reaction. Mod Pathol 1999;12:272–278.
116. Mizuno T, Nagamura H, Iwamoto KS, et al: RNA from decades-old archival tissue blocks for retrospective studies. Diagn Mol Pathol 1998;7:202–208.
117. Crisan D, Mattson JC: Amplification of intermediate-size DNA sequences from formalin and B-5 fixed tissue by polymerase chain reaction. Clin Biochem 1992;25:99–103.
118. Crisan D, Mattson JC: Retrospective DNA analysis using fixed tissue specimens. DNA Cell Biol 1993;12: 455–464.
119. Koopmans M, Monroe SS, Coffield LM, et al: Optimization of extraction and PCR amplification of RNA extracts from paraffin-embedded tissue in different fixatives. J Virol Methods 1993;43:189–204.
120. Goldsworthy SM, Stockton PS, Trempus CS, et al: Effects of fixation on RNA extraction and amplification

from laser capture microdissected tissue. Mol Carcinog 1999;25:86–91.

121. Krafft AE, Duncan BW, Bijwaard KE, et al: Optimization of the isolation and amplification of RNA from formalin-fixed, paraffin-embedded tissue: The Armed Forces Institute of Pathology experience and literature review. Mol Diagn 1997;2:217–230.
122. Hamalainen MM, Eskola JU, Hellman J, et al: Major interference from leukocytes in reverse transcription-PCR identified as neurotoxin ribonuclease from eosinophils: Detection of residual chronic myelogenous leukemia from cell lysates by use of an eosinophil-depleted cell preparation. Clin Chem 1999;45:465–471.
123. Rosenberg HF, Dyer KD: Human ribonuclease 4 (RNase 4): Coding sequence, chromosomal localization and identification of two distinct transcripts in human somatic tissues. Nucleic Acids Res 1995;23:4290–4295.
124. Rosenberg HF, Dyer KD: Molecular cloning and characterization of a novel human ribonuclease (RNase k6): Increasing diversity in the enlarging ribonuclease gene family. Nucleic Acids Res 1996;24(18):3507–3513.
125. Futami J, Tsushima Y, Murato Y, et al: Tissue-specific expression of pancreatic-type RNases and RNase inhibitor in humans. DNA Cell Biol 1997;16:413–419.
126. Barany F: Genetic disease detection and DNA amplification using cloned thermostable ligase. Proc Natl Acad U S A 1991;88:189–193.
127. Barany F: The ligase chain reaction in a PCR world [erratum appears in PCR Methods Appl 1991 Nov; 1(2):149]. PCR Methods Appl 1991;1:5–16.
128. Kalin I, Shephard S, Candrian U: Evaluation of the ligase chain reaction (LCR) for the detection of point mutations. Mutat Res 1992;283:119–123.
129. Marshall RL, Laffler TG, Cerney MB, et al: Detection of HCV RNA by the asymmetric gap ligase chain reaction. PCR Methods Appl 1994;4:80–84.
130. Batt CA, Wagner P, Wiedmann M, et al: Detection of bovine leukocyte adhesion deficiency by nonisotopic ligase chain reaction. Anim Genet 1994;25:95–98.
131. Wiedmann M, Wilson WJ, Czajka J, et al: Ligase chain reaction (LCR): Overview and applications. PCR Methods Appl 1994;3(Suppl 4):51–64.
132. Pfeffer M, Meyer H, Wiedmann M: A ligase chain reaction targeting two adjacent nucleotides allows the differentiation of cowpox virus from other Orthopoxvirus species. J Virol Methods 1994;49:353–360.
133. Palacios JJ, Ferro J, Ruiz PN, et al: Comparison of the ligase chain reaction with solid and liquid culture media for routine detection of *Mycobacterium tuberculosis* in nonrespiratory specimens. Eur J Clin Microbiol Infect Dis 1998;17:767–772.
134. Jouveshomme S, Cambau E, Trystram D, et al: Clinical utility of an amplification test based on ligase chain reaction in pulmonary tuberculosis. Am J Respir Crit Care Med 1998;158:1096–1101.
135. Tortoli E, Tronci M, Tosi CP, et al: Multicenter evaluation of two commercial amplification kits (Amplicor, Roche and LCx, Abbott) for direct detection of *Mycobacterium tuberculosis* in pulmonary and extrapulmonary specimens. Diagn Microbiol Infect Dis 1999;33: 173–179.
136. Doing KM, Curtis K, Long JW, et al: Prospective comparison of the Gen-probe PACE 2 assay and the Abbott ligase chain reaction for the direct detection of *Chlamydia trachomatis* in a low prevalence population. J Med Microbiol 1999;48:507–510.
137. Xu K, Glanton V, Johnson SR, et al: Detection of *Neisseria gonorrhoeae* infection by ligase chain reaction testing of urine among adolescent women with and without *Chlamydia trachomatis* infection. Sex Transm Dis 1998;25:533–538.
138. Minamitani S, Nishiguchi S, Kuroki T, et al: Detection by ligase chain reaction of precore mutant of hepatitis B virus. Hepatology 1997;25:216–222.
139. Eggerding FA, Iovannisci DM, Brinson E, et al: Fluorescence-based oligonucleotide ligation assay for analysis of cystic fibrosis transmembrane conductance regulator gene mutations. Hum Mutat 1995;5:153–165.
140. Khanna M, Park P, Zirvi M, et al: Multiplex PCR/LDR for detection of K-ras mutations in primary colon tumors. Oncogene 1999;18:27–38.
141. Chen X, Livak KJ, Kwok PY: A homogeneous, ligase-mediated DNA diagnostic test. Genome Res 1998;8: 549–556.
142. Pfyffer GE, Funke-Kissling P, Rundler E, et al: Performance characteristics of the BDProbeTec system for direct detection of *Mycobacterium tuberculosis* complex in respiratory specimens. J Clin Microbiol 1999;37:137–140.
143. Walker GT, Little MC, Nadeau JG, et al: Isothermal in vitro amplification of DNA by a restriction enzyme/DNA polymerase system. Proc Natl Acad USA 1992;89:392–396.
144. Little MC, Andrews J, Moore R, et al: Strand displacement amplification and homogeneous real-time detection incorporated in a second-generation DNA probe system, BDProbeTecET. Clin Chem 1999;45(6 Pt 1): 777–784.
145. Bergmann JS, Woods GL: Clinical evaluation of the BDProbeTec strand displacement amplification assay for rapid diagnosis of tuberculosis. J Clin Microbiol 1998;36:2766–2768.
146. Badak FZ, Kiska DL, O'Connell M, et al: Confirmation of the presence of *Mycobacterium tuberculosis* and other mycobacteria in mycobacterial growth indicator tubes (MGIT) by multiplex strand displacement amplification. J Clin Microbiol 1997;35:1239–1243.
147. Nycz CM, Dean CH, Haaland PD, et al: Quantitative reverse transcription strand displacement amplification: quantitation of nucleic acids using an isothermal amplification technique. Anal Biochem 1998;259:226–234.
148. Kievits T, van Gemen B, van Strijp D, et al: NASBA isothermal enzymatic in vitro nucleic acid amplification optimized for the diagnosis of HIV-1 infection. J Virol Methods 1991;35:273–286.
149. Olsen JC, Watson KF: RNase H-mediated release of the retrovirus RNA polyadenylate tail during reverse transcription. J Virol 1985;53:324–329.
150. Oyama F, Kikuchi R, Crouch RJ, et al: Intrinsic properties of reverse transcriptase in reverse transcription: Associated RNase H is essentially regarded as an endonuclease. J Biol Chem 1989;264:18808–18817.

151. Darke BM, Jackson SK, Hanna SM, et al: Detection of human TNF-alpha mRNA by NASBA. J Immunol Methods 1998;212:19–28.
152. Sooknanan R, Malek L, Wang XH, et al: Detection and direct sequence identification of BCR-ABL mRNA in Ph+ chronic myeloid leukemia. Exp Hematol 1993;21: 1719–1724.
153. van Deursen PB, Gunther AW, van Riel CC, et al: A novel quantitative multiplex NASBA method: Application to measuring tissue factor and CD14 mRNA levels in human monocytes. Nucleic Acids Res 1999; 27:e15.
154. Romano JW, van Gemen B, Kievits T: NASBA: A novel, isothermal detection technology for qualitative and quantitative HIV-1 RNA measurements. Clin Lab Med 1996;16:89–103.
155. Parekh B, Phillips S, Granade TC, et al: Impact of HIV type 1 subtype variation on viral RNA quantitation. AIDS Res Hum Retroviruses 1999;15:133–142.
156. van Gemen B, Kievits T, Nara P, et al: Qualitative and quantitative detection of HIV-1 RNA by nucleic acid sequence-based amplification. AIDS 1993;7(Suppl 2): 107–110.
157. Uyttendaele M, Schukkink R, van Gemen B, et al: Development of NASBA, a nucleic acid amplification system, for identification of *Listeria monocytogenes* and comparison to ELISA and a modified FDA method. Int J Food Microbiol 1995;27:77–89.
158. van der Vliet GM, Schukkink RA, van Gemen B, et al: Nucleic acid sequence-based amplification (NASBA) for the identification of mycobacteria. J Gen Microbiol 1993;139(pt 10):2423–2429.
159. Reitsma PH, van der Velden PA, Vogels E, et al: Use of the direct RNA amplification technique NASBA to detect factor V Leiden, a point mutation associated with APC resistance. Blood Coagul Fibrinolysis 1996;7:659–663.
160. Chadwick N, Wakefield AJ, Pounder RE, et al: Comparison of three RNA amplification methods as sources of DNA for sequencing. Biotechniques 1998;25:818–820, 822.
161. Heim A, Grumbach IM, Zeuke S, et al: Highly sensitive detection of gene expression of an intronless gene: Amplification of mRNA, but not genomic DNA by nucleic acid sequence based amplification (NASBA). Nucleic Acids Res 1998;26:2250–2251.
162. Prud'homme IT, Kim JE, Pilon RG, et al: Amplicor HIV monitor, NASBA HIV-1 RNA QT and quantiplex HIV RNA version 2.0 viral load assays: A Canadian evaluation. J Clin Virol 1998;11:189–202.
163. Saldanha J, Lelie N, Heath A: Establishment of the first international standard for nucleic acid amplification technology (NAT) assays for HCV RNA. World Health Organization Collaborative Study Group. Vox Sang 1999;76:149–158.
164. Pasternack R, Vuorinen P, Miettinen A: Comparison of a transcription-mediated amplification assay and polymerase chain reaction for detection of *Chlamydia trachomatis* in first-void urine. Eur J Clin Microbiol Infect Dis 1999;18:142–144.
165. Punwaney R, Brandwein MS, Zhang DY, et al: Human papillomavirus may be common within nasopharyngeal carcinoma of caucasian Americans: Investigation of Epstein-Barr virus and human papillomavirus in eastern and western nasopharyngeal carcinoma using ligation-dependent polymerase chain reaction. Head Neck 1999; 21:21–29.
166. Park YN, Abe K, Li H, et al: Detection of hepatitis C virus RNA using ligation-dependent polymerase chain reaction in formalin-fixed, paraffin-embedded liver tissues. Am J Pathol 1996;149:1485–1491.
167. Miyauchi I, Moriyama M, Zhang DY, et al: Further study of hepatitis C virus RNA detection in formalin-fixed, paraffin-embedded liver tissues by ligation-dependent polymerase chain reaction. Pathol Int 1998;48: 428–432.
168. Zhang DY, Brandwein M, Hsuih TC, et al: Amplification of target-specific, ligation-dependent circular probe. Gene 1998;211:277–285.
169. Nishihara T, Mills DR, Kramer FR: Localization of the Q beta replicase recognition site in MDV-1 RNA. J Biochem (Tokyo) 1983;93:669–674.
170. Tyagi S, Landegren U, Tazi M, et al: Extremely sensitive, background-free gene detection using binary probes and beta replicase. Proc Natl Acad USA 1996;93: 5395–5400.
171. Biebricher CK, Eigen M, Luce R: Template-free RNA synthesis by Q beta replicase. Nature 1986;321:89–91.
172. Shah JS, Liu J, Buxton D, et al: Detection of *Mycobacterium tuberculosis* directly from spiked human sputum by Q-beta replicase-amplified assay. J Clin Microbiol 1995;33:322–328.
173. Nolte FS, Boysza J, Thurmond C, et al: Clinical comparison of an enhanced-sensitivity branched-DNA assay and reverse transcription-PCR for quantitation of human immunodeficiency virus type 1 RNA in plasma. J Clin Microbiol 1998;36:716–720.
174. Nolte FS: Branched DNA signal amplification for direct quantitation of nucleic acid sequences in clinical specimens. Adv Clin Chem 1998;33:201–235.
175. Marshall VM, Lew AM: Direct automated DNA sequencing of ds and ss PCR products. *In* Griffin HG, Griffin AM (eds): PCR Technology: Current Innovations. Boca Raton, FL, CRC, 1994, pp 85–100.
176. Velculescu VE, Zhang L, Vogelstein B, et al: Serial analysis of gene expression. Science 1995;270:484–487.
177. Zhang L, Zhou W, Velculescu VE, et al: Gene expression profiles in normal and cancer cells. Science 1997; 276:1268–1272.
178. Zhou W, Sokoll LJ, Bruzek DJ, et al: Identifying markers for pancreatic cancer by gene expression analysis. Cancer Epidemiol Biomarkers Prev 1998;7:109–112.
179. Gibson UE, Heid CA, Williams PM: A novel method for real-time quantitative RT-PCR. Genome Res 1996;6:995–1001.
180. Heid CA, Stevens J, Livak KJ, et al: Real-time quantitative PCR. Genome Res 1996;6:986–994.
181. Bohling SD, King TC, Wittwer CT, et al: Rapid simultaneous amplification and detection of the MBR/JH chromosomal translocation by fluorescence melting curve analysis. Am J Pathol 1999;154: 97–103.
182. Bohling SD, Wittwer CT, King TC, et al: Fluorescence melting curve analysis for the detection of the bcl-1/JH translocation in mantle cell lymphoma. Lab Invest 1999;79:337–345.

183. Woo TH, Patel BK, Smythe LD, et al: Identification of *Leptospira inadai* by continuous monitoring of fluorescence during rapid cycle PCR. Syst Appl Microbiol 1998;21:89–96.
184. Morrison TB, Weis JJ, Wittwer CT: Quantification of low-copy transcripts by continuous SYBR Green I monitoring during amplification. Biotechniques 1998;24: 954–958, 960, 962.
185. Tyagi S, Kramer FR: Molecular beacons: Probes that fluoresce upon hybridization. Nat Biotechnol 1996;14: 303–308.
186. Bonnet G, Tyagi S, Libchaber A, et al: Thermodynamic basis of the enhanced specificity of structured DNA probes. Proc Natl Acad USA 1999;96:6171–6176.
187. Bernard PS, Ajioka RS, Kushner JP, et al: Homogeneous multiplex genotyping of hemochromatosis mutations with fluorescent hybridization probes. Am J Pathol 1998;153:1055–1061.
188. Bernard PS, Lay MJ, Wittwer CT: Integrated amplification and detection of the C677T point mutation in the methylenetetrahydrofolate reductase gene by fluorescence resonance energy transfer and probe melting curves. Anal Biochem 1998;255:101–107.
189. Lay MJ, Wittwer CT: Real-time fluorescence genotyping of factor V Leiden during rapid-cycle PCR. Clin Chem 1997;43:2262–2267.
190. Holland PM, Abramson RD, Watson R, et al: Detection of specific polymerase chain reaction product by utilizing the 5′–3′ exonuclease activity of *Thermus aquaticus* DNA polymerase. Proc Natl Acad USA 1991;88: 7276–7280.
191. Livak KJ, Flood SJ, Marmaro J, et al: Oligonucleotides with fluorescent dyes at opposite ends provide a quenched probe system useful for detecting PCR product and nucleic acid hybridization. PCR Methods Appl 1995;4:357–362.
192. Vet JA, Majithia AR, Marras SA, et al: Multiplex detection of four pathogenic retroviruses using molecular beacons. Proc Natl Acad U S A 1999;96:6394–9639.
193. Marras SA, Kramer FR, Tyagi S: Multiplex detection of single-nucleotide variations using molecular beacons. Genet Anal 1999;14:151–156.
194. Bernard PS, Pritham GH, Wittwer CT: Color multiplexing hybridization probes using the apolipoprotein E locus as a model system for genotyping. Anal Biochem 1999;273:221–228.
195. Lee LG, Livak KJ, Mullah B, et al: Seven-color, homogeneous detection of six PCR products. Biotechniques 1999;27:342–349.
196. Nauck MS, Gierens H, Nauck MA, et al: Rapid genotyping of human platelet antigen 1 (HPA-1) with fluorophore-labelled hybridization probes on the LightCycler. Br J Haematol 1999;105:803–810.
197. Livak KJ: Allelic discrimination using fluorogenic probes and the 5′ nuclease assay. Genet Anal 1999;14:143–149.
198. Happich D, Schwaab R, Hanfland P, et al: Allelic discrimination of factor V Leiden using a 5′ nuclease assay. Thromb Haemost 1999;82:1294–1296.
199. Patterson BK, Jiyamapa D, Mayrand E, et al: Detection of HIV-1 DNA in cells and tissue by fluorescent in situ 5′-nuclease assay (FISNA). Nucleic Acids Res 1996;24: 3656–3658.
200. Kreuzer KA, Lass U, Bohn A, et al: LightCycler technology for the quantitation of bcr/abl fusion transcripts. Cancer Res 1999;59:3171–3174.
201. Ortiz E, Estrada G, Lizardi PM: PNA molecular beacons for rapid detection of PCR amplicons. Mol Cell Probes 1998;12:219–226.

CHAPTER 5 APPENDIX

SOP 5.1*

RT-PCR PROCEDURE FOR β_2-MICROGLOBULIN (HUMAN RNA CONTROL)

PRINCIPLE

RT-PCR is performed on a control gene to assess the integrity of the sample RNA (an internal control). The β_2-microglobulin primers span intron 2 of the gene, which is highly expressed in almost all nucleated cells. The 158 base pair product is separated by agarose gel electrophoresis, Southern blotted, and probed with a specific ^{32}P labeled oligonucleotide. Lysates derived from a cell line are analyzed for β_2-microglobulin, in parallel with patient samples, to assess the assay variability (an external positive control). Negative controls which are devoid of RNA are used to monitor potential points of cross-contamination.

ABBREVIATIONS AND CONVENTIONS

The usual source of a reagent is abbreviated in BRACKETS [ ]. An asterisk [*] is used when the source varies, Fisher [F1], Advanced Biosystems Incorporated [ABI], promega [PR], Invitrogen [IVG], PGC Scientific [PGC], Integrated DNA Technologies Incoporated [IDT], Molecular Bioproducts Incorporated [MBP], American type culture collection [ATCC], in-house reagents [MDL].

Other abberviation and definitions used in ths SOP include: Moloney murine leukemia virus (M-MLV), reverse transcriptase (RT), *Taq* polymerase *Taq*, polymerase chain reaction (PCR), agarose gel electrophoresis (AGE), formalin-fixed paraffin-embedded (FFPE), Dithithreitol (DTT), aerosol-resistant pipette tips (ARTs), Advanced Biosystems Incorporated Model 9600 or model 9700 Thermal Cycler (TC 9600), ethylene-diamine-tetraacetic acid (EDTA), Tris-borate-EDTA solution (TBE, 10× contains 0.9 M boric acid and 0.01 M EDTA in 1 M Tris-Base at pH8.3), sodium dodecyl sulfate (SDS), saline sodium citrate buffer (SSC, 20× contains 3 M NaCl in 0.3 M sodium citrate at pH 7), deoxynucleotide triphosphate mixture containing 10 mM each of dATP, dTTP, dCTP, and dGTP (dNTP) reaction (rxn), master mix (MM), nucleotide base pairs (bp), microliters (µL), milliliters (mL), arbitrary units of enzymatic activity as defined by the manufacture (U).

* This procedure has been generalized from a procedure developed in the Molecular Diagnostics Laboratory at the Department of Cellular Pathology and Genetics, Armed Forces Institute of Pathology, Washington, DC. Typical sources of reagents and supplies are indicated here for the purpose of illustration only.

MATERIALS

Specimens (see SOP 1 in Appendix at end of book)

Patient RNA samples—[derived by RNA extraction (SOP 5 in Appendix at end of book) of recut archival FFPE blocks (SOP 3 in Appendix at end of book) OR other patient sample material.]

RNA Positive Control—[derived by RNA extraction (SOP 5 in Appendix at end of book) of K562 cells.

Storage and Handling

The primers and probes for β_2-microglobulin were selected from published sequences. Primers are stored in the −20°C RNA-freezer in a working dilution of 15 µmol/L. RT, Taq, and PCR primers and all RT-PCR reagents, except $MgCl_2$, are stored according to manufacturer's instructions in areas specially designated for RNA-related work. RNA extracts may be kept at −20°C for up to one week. For long term storage of RNA, extracts and positive controls are stored at −70°C. Probes for β_2-microglobulin are kept at −20°C in the post-PCR room. Aliquots of reagents and standards are stored in microcentrifuge tubes (1.5 and 0.5 mL). **Do not put unused aliquots back in tubes or containers. Throw them away. Always wear gloves when handling reagents and samples and follow procedures for avoiding contamination of PCR reaction (See SOP 2 in Appendix at end of book)!!**

Primers and Probes [IDT]

Reverse Transcriptase primer (working stock = 15 µmol/L)
BM3 5′-CCT CCA TGA TGC TGC TTA CAT GTC (1023–1046);

PCR primer (working stock = 15 µmol/L)
BM5 5′-CTT GTC TTT CAG CAA GGA CTG G (274–295);

β_2-microglobulin Probe (working stock = 15 µmol/L)
BMP1 5′-AGT ATG CCT GCC GTG TGA ACC ATG (345–368)

Reagents

HPLC-grade water	[FI]
First-strand buffer (5×)	[IVG]
DTT (0.1 M)	[IVG]
PCR buffer II (10×)	[ABI]
dNTPs (10 mM)	[PR]
M-MLV RT (200 U/L)	[IVG]
Taq polymerase (5 Units/L)	[ABI]
$MgCl_2$ (25 mM)	[ABI]

Master Mixes

Master mixes are prepared from the primary reagents exclusive of enzymes and nucleic acid primers or probes (see SOP 13 in Appendix at end of book). Aliquots of the MMs are stored at $-70°$C and are thawed on the day of use. Enzymes and primers are added immediately before use, and tubes must be maintained strictly on ice after enzyme addition. Note that the reverse-transcriptase and PCR-RNA master mix used for β_2-microglobulin is the same as that used for *bcr-abl*, actin, and t(2;5) assays.

REVERSE TRANSCRIPTASE MASTER MIX

The volumes given are per 20 μL reaction with 5-μL of RNA sample will be used, and final concentrations are indicated in parentheses.

4.0 μL	5× first strand buffer
2.0 μL	100 mmol/L DTT (0.01 M)
1.6 μL	10 mmol/L dNTPs (200 μM @ RT rxn)
6.1 μL	water
13.7 μL	total volume per sample before primer or enzyme addition

Immediately before use make the following additions:

1.0 μL	15 μmol/L RT-primer BM3 (300 nmol/L)
0.3 μL	M-MLV RT (1.2 U/reaction)

PCR-RNA MASTER MIX

The volumes given are per 50.0 μL final reaction volume where 30 μL of PCR-RNA master mix will be added to 20 μL of the RT-PCR reaction, and final concentrations are indicated in parentheses.

3.0 μL	10 × PCR buffer II
2.0 μL	25 mM $MgCl_2$ (2.2 mM)
23.7 μL	water
28.7 μL	total volume per sample

Immediately before use make the following additons:

1.0 μL	15 μmol/L PCR-primer BM5 primer
0.3 μL	5 U/μl Taq polymerase (1.25 U/50 μL rxn)

Supplies

Microcentrifuge tubes (1.5 mL and 0.5 mL)	[PGC]
Microcentrifuge tube rack	[PGC]
ART tips	[MBP]
Disposable latex or vinyl gloves	[FI]
Extra fine tip permanent markers	[FI]

Equipment

Note: All equipment used in the preparation and setup for RNA analysis should be reserved solely for that purpose.

Pipetters	[FI]
Microcentrifuge	[FI]
TC9600 Thermal Cycler	[ABI]
Vortexer	[FI]

Materials Described in Other SOPs Included in this Text

Agarose gel electrophoresis	SOP 6
Southern blotting of PCR products	SOP 9
End-labeling oligonucleotide probes	SOP 7
Hybridization and washing Southern blots	SOP 10
Exposing and developing film	SOP 11

QUALITY CONTROL PROCEDURES (see SOP 13 for more details)

Positive Assay Controls

β_2-microglobulin serves as a control gene for the assessment of RNA integrity. The amplified β_2-microglobulin product is 158 base pairs.

Amplification Control. RNA lysate of cell line K562 [ATCC].

Southern Blotting and Hybridization Control. A separate previously tested 158 bp product may be optionally included in a separate lane of the AGE and blotting procedures.

Negative Assay Controls

These control for the possible introduction of human RNA or DNA from external sources such as sample cross-contamination or the introduction of skin cells from persons setting up the assay. Separate controls monitor the reagents, lysate preparation and RT-PCR setup steps.

Reagent Control. An RT-PCR reaction mix containing water as the sample tested is set up *before* patient sample lysates are opened. The purpose is to assess the purity of the reagents.

Lysate Preparation Control. A tube containing no patient sample is processed in parallel with patient samples throughout the lysate preparation procedure to generate a *false lysate*. The false lysate is then tested as a control for cross contamination at steps prior to RT-PCR setup.

PCR Setup Control. An RT-PCR reaction mix containing water as the sample tested is set up *after* patient sample reactions setup is completed. The purpose is to assess the purity of the reagents.

Standard Format for Controls

Positive control and negative controls are always run in parallel with patient samples.

Positive controls are tested at two concentrations (1 μL and 5 μL of the 1:100 dilution of a K562 lysate, with the difference in volume made up by adding water).

Negative controls and patient samples are tested at one concentration (5 μL of the undiluted extract).

All master mix batch lots (containing all reaction components except RNA, enzymes, and primers) are tested in advance with positive and negative controls, to validate lot-specific preparation variables.

PROCEDURE

Lysate Preparation

Refer to the preparation procedure that applies for the samples being tested. If archival FFPE samples are being tested refer to cutting blocks (see SOP 3). Extract RNA from recut samples (See SOP 5)

RT-Polymerase Chain Reaction (RT-PCR).

1. Determine the number of samples to be assayed (include one dilution of each patient extract, plus two dilutions of positive amplification control, and one dilution of each negative control per run). Take this number and increase it by 10% and round up to the next whole number to get the value "N" for subsequent calculations.

   Example: six patient samples, plus two positive controls, plus three negative controls gives eleven samples. Adding 10% gives 12.1 samples. Rounding up makes a total of 13 samples. This allows for pipetting inaccuracies.

2. Thaw all necessary frozen materials on ice (include MM aliquots, enzymes, primers). Record the MM lot numbers on the standardized assay worksheet.

   NOTE: The RT master mix aliquots are stored as multiples of 13.7 μl per sample; the PCR-RNA master mix aliquots are stored as multiples of 28.7 μl per sample. Calculate the amount of RT master mix needed by multiplying "N" × 13.7 μL. Calculate the amount of PCR-RNA master mix by multiplying "N" × 28.7 μL.
3. Label all microfuge tubes consecutively starting with "1." This is the "assay-tube number." Use an extra-fine marker and label only the sides of the tube. Immediately after labeling, record the assay-tube number and the actual identity of the sample on the standard worksheet. Place all tubes in consecutive order in a PCR tray and leave one space between each tube. Lock the tubes in place and ensure that the tubes are oriented in the tray with sample number 1 in position A1 (numbering should proceed horizontally on a row-by-row basis).
4. Add the enzymes and primers to the master mixes and store on ice until use.
   - Add [("N" × 0.3 μl of M-MLV RT), **AND** ("N" × 1.0 μL of BM3 RT-primer) **TO** ("N" × 13.7 μl of the RT master mix)], **THEN** tap the tube gently to mix.
   - Add [("N" × 0.3 μl of Taq polymerase), **AND** ("N" × 1.0 μl of MB5 PCR-primer) **TO** ("N" × 28.1 μl of the PCR-master mix)] **THEN** tap the tube gently to mix.
5. Add 15 μL of RT-Master mix to each reaction tube, then cap the tubes.
6. Prepare the negative reagent-control and negative lysate-preparation controls.
   - Add 5.0 μL of water to the reagent-control tube.
   - Add 5.0 μL of the false lysate to the lysate-preparation control tube.
   - Recap the tubes
7. Adjust the volume for the diluted positive amplification control by adding 4 μL of water to the diluted amplification-control tube, then recap the tube.
8. Add patient sample to each tube (5.0 μL of the undiluted extract). The final volume of the RT reaction is 20.0 μL. Recap the tubes.
9. *After* all the patient sample tubes have been capped, add positive amplification control lysate to appropriate tubes.
   - Add 1.0 μL of the K562 RNA (1:100 dilution) lysate to the dilute positive control.
   - Add 5.0 μL of the K562 RNA (1:100 dilution) lysate to the neat positive control.
   - Recap the positive control tubes.
10. Add 5.0 μL of water to the PCR-setup control and cap the tube.
11. Place the tray of tubes in a TC9600 thermal cycler and incubate at 37°C for 1 hour.
12. Remove the tray from the TC9600 and place it on ice.
13. Add 30.0 μL of PCR-RNA master mix to each reaction tube. Recap the tubes.
14. Place the tray back into a TC9600 thermal cycler and apply the following preprogrammed thermal cycling protocol. (m = minutes, @ = at):
    one cycle (5 m @ 94°C);
    40 cycles (1 m @ 94°C, 1 m @ 55°C, 1 m @ 72°C);
    one cycle (5 m @ 72°C); rapid ramp down to 4°C and hold indefinitely
15. Remove the rack from the TC9600 and refrigerate in the post-PCR room for analysis by agarose gel electrophoresis.

Agarose Gel Electrophoresis (See SOP 6)

All reagents are in the post-PCR room. The 158-bp product is resolved on 2.5% agarose (2% low melting point agarose, 0.5% agarose) in 1X TBE.

Southern Blotting of PCR Products (See SOP 9)

End-Labeling Oligonucleotide Probes (See SOP 7)

Hybridization and Washing Southern Blots (See SOP 10)

Add 100 μL of ^{32}P-labeled probe to 5 ml of pre-warmed hybrisol I.
Hybridize blot with probe for 4 hr at 42°C.
Wash three times for 5 minutes per wash at 42°C in 0.1X SSC and 0.1% SDS.

Exposing and Developing film (See SOP 11)

If there is a negative signal for the acting gene, the viral assay is reported as *indeterminate*.

REPORTING RESULTS

A *positive* result for β_2-microglobulin is reported if a positive signal is seen with the specific probe and the patient sample, provided all the appropriate controls are working. If not, repeat the assay.

PROCEDURE NOTES

Avoid repeated freeze-thaw cycles of patient sample material, enzymes, and reagents. The lysates may be heated to 90°C and then placed on ice immediately prior to the RT reaction, but not after addition of the RT master mix. This will enhance target-sequence exposure by denaturing the target.

REFERENCES

Gussow, D., Rein, R., Ginjaar, I., et al: The human B_2-microglobulin gene. J Immunol 1987;139:3132–3138.

III

ADVANCED DIAGNOSTIC METHODS

Practice

TIMOTHY J. O'LEARY

6

Infectious Diseases

Diagnosis of infectious diseases from tissue specimens is one of the most common, most important, and most difficult tasks in diagnostic pathology. For most organisms, culture of freshly obtained tissue specimens remains the gold standard. In some cases, such as infection with *Mycobacterium tuberculosis*, unambiguous identification can be obtained in tissue sections using classic histochemical stains. For many organisms, however, histochemical staining is insufficient, either because the organism is inapparent on morphologic examination or because its morphologic characteristics are sometimes ambiguous. In these cases, and in some cases of previously unidentified microorganisms, characterization using either immunohistochemical (IHC) or molecular biologic techniques may enable diagnosis even in formalin-fixed, paraffin-embedded tissue. The differing biology of the various infectious diseases makes reliance on a single approach inadvisable. For some diseases, presenting in certain types of tissue specimens, polymerase chain reaction (PCR) tests may actually prove to be less sensitive than morphologic examination! Great care must be taken, therefore, to match the clinical situation and the testing strategy.

In spite of this caveat, IHC methods and PCR are usually the diagnostic approaches of choice when an organism cannot be identified by morphologic examination of histochemically stained sections. When an antibody is available that demonstrates an organism in formalin-fixed, paraffin-embedded tissue, the sensitivity of the IHC assay generally is competitive with that of in situ hybridization (ISH) methods, with fewer "technical complications." On the other hand, when an assay needs to be brought online quickly, PCR and reverse transcriptase/PCR (RT-PCR) assays are most quickly designed and implemented; these assays can often be validated in less than a week. As a result, there are very few organisms for which we employ ISH assays for routine diagnosis.

The focus in this chapter is on the identification of infectious agents in tissues other than blood and urine. For this reason, the discussion of methods excludes some powerful molecular approaches that are commonly used in these fluids, such as ligase chain reaction[1, 2] and branched-chain amplification (bDNA),[3] and focuses instead on PCR, ISH, and IHC approaches. Little attention is given to use of molecular methods to provide prognostic information regarding the probable clinical course, although this may be very valuable, particularly in the case of human immunodeficiency virus (HIV) infection. The previously cited references provide a useful introduction to these topics. Finally, a few classes of infectious agent that are frequently included in the differential diagnosis in tissue specimens are discussed.

VIRAL DISEASES

Although some disorders, such as cytomegalovirus (CMV) disease, may occasionally be identified on the basis of characteristic viral inclusions, there is no viral disease for which morphology of classically stained histologic sections provides the sensitivity required to allow confidence in a "negative" diagnosis. For this reason, immunocytochemical and molecular biologic approaches provide powerful tools useful in the diagnosis of all viral diseases.

The Adenoviruses

The adenoviruses are common causes of upper respiratory tract infections, bronchitis, interstitial pneumonia, and otitis media. The "classic" histologic appearance is that of the "smudge cell"—a cell with a darkly basophilic, somewhat indistinct nucleus that appears to be undergoing necrosis. Unfortunately, this appearance is not sufficiently specific to allow a specific etiologic diagnosis, nor is it invariably seen in cases of proven adenoviral infection.

Adenovirus may readily be identified in formalin-fixed, paraffin-embedded sections by IHC (Fig. 6–1)[4] or ISH.[5] Although ISH offers, in principle, an opportunity for subtyping, the existence of more than 40 different adenovirus

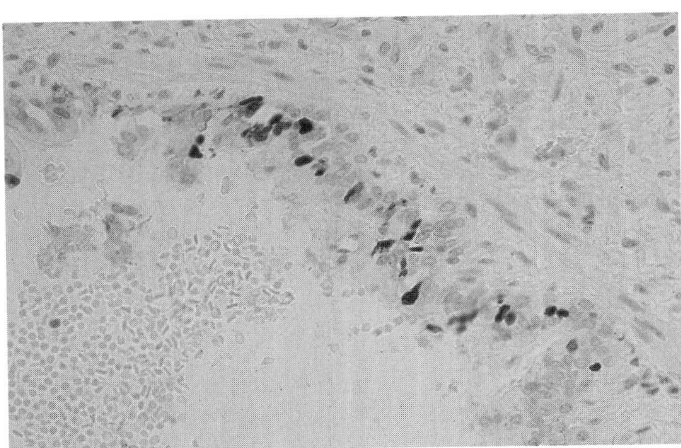

FIGURE 6–1
Immunohistochemical demonstration of adenovirus species in airway tissue (×200). (See also Color Fig. 6–1.)

types strongly limits its practical utility. PCR assays for formalin-fixed, paraffin-embedded tissue specimens are also available and have demonstrated considerably higher sensitivity than ISH.[6, 7]

The Coronaviruses

Coronavirus infection is often associated with clinical presentation as a "common cold."[8] Although coronavirus is rarely suspected, much less diagnosed, on tissue specimens, it may be detected in formalin-fixed, paraffin-embedded tissues by IHC[4] or by ISH.[9] PCR assays have been published but have not been adapted to formalin-fixed, paraffin-embedded tissues, and the relative sensitivity and specificity of the three approaches have not been determined.

The Hantaviruses

The hantaviruses cause a wide variety of disorders, including hantavirus pulmonary syndrome (such as that caused by the Sin Nombre virus in the southwestern United States)[10] and hemorrhagic fevers giving rise to renal insufficiency (as with Hantaan virus).[11–13] Although the general nature of the pathologic process is usually sufficient to raise hantavirus infection as a diagnostic possibility, the "tissue clues" are insufficient to establish the diagnosis of "hantavirus infection," much less precise etiologic agent, with certainty.

Sensitive IHC assays for the hantaviruses have been developed, are applicable to archival tissue, and correlate highly with serologic and molecular biologic tests.[14–16] Although at least some of these assays demonstrate cross-reactivity with a number of hantaviruses, a positive finding, together with clinical and epidemiologic information, is sufficient to establish a precise diagnosis in many cases.

Even early in the course of disease, most patients have viral RNA not only in affected tissues but also in peripheral blood mononuclear cells. Thus, tissue biopsies or blood both can be used for diagnosis. RT-PCR assays may be used to identify hantaviruses and differentiate among them,[11, 17, 18] but, in general, a large number of assays is required for complete molecular characterization. For this reason, serologic tests are often more useful in clinical practice. There are similarities in the hantaviruses that can be exploited to simplify diagnosis, however. A single pair of consensus primers can be used to amplify a conserved region of the small genome segment that is common to several hantavirus genera and viruses differentiated by differences in the molecular weight distributions of fragments generated by digestion with restriction enzymes.[19] Because the amplification products are 280 to 320 base pairs (bp), adaptation of this method to formalin-fixed, paraffin-embedded tissue may be challenging, but use in peripheral mononuclear cells or fresh tissue should be straightfoward.

Hepatitis Viruses

Although the hepatitis viruses belong to several distinct families, all must be simultaneously considered in the differential diagnosis of hepatitis. Hepatic architecture and clinical course provide excellent clues as to etiologic agent. The orcein stain, now infrequently used, is capable of identifying some cases of hepatitis B infection, and CMV inclusions also yield unequivocal diagnoses, but, in general, precise etiologic diagnosis of viral hepatitis requires the use of IHC or molecular biologic techniques. Although methods are available for identifying most hepatitis viruses in tissue, most laboratories find it unnecessary to implement assays for hepatitis viruses other than those causing hepatitis B and hepatitis C.

HEPATITIS A

Hepatitis A is a mild, self-limited infection characterized by food-borne transmission, particularly from seafood or infected food service workers. It is rarely diagnosed on the basis of histologic examination; clinical characteristics, together with serologic testing and stool isolation, are generally sufficient to make the diagnosis. Although an IHC assay is available that works in formalin-fixed, paraffin-embedded tissue,[20] it has not been characterized in the literature, nor is there a an ISH assay. PCR assays have been used to detect the virus in food,[21] water,[22] and stool[23]; these should be readily adaptable to formalin-fixed, paraffin-embedded tissues as well as fresh clinical samples of all types.

HEPATITIS B

Hepatitis B is a serious infection, transmitted through blood or sexual contact, that may lead to liver failure or hepatocellular carcinoma. IHC assays for hepatitis B core and surface antigens have been available for many years[24] and in most cases can establish the diagnosis unequivocally (Fig. 6–2). ISH assays for hepatitis B are also available and may demonstrate replicating virus even in the absence of detectable IHC staining.[25–27] Nevertheless, we generally find immunohistochemistry to be sufficient to make a diagnosis.

PCR-based assays, not surprisingly, are more sensitive than either IHC or ISH for the detection of hepatitis B[28–32] and may detect viral sequences even in patients who do not have viral antigens or nucleic acids detectable by IHC or ISH.

HEPATITIS C

Hepatitis C is a chronic, blood-borne infection that has become the most common cause of end-stage liver disease. Antiviral therapy is available and sometimes effective; thus, an accurate diagnosis carries significant therapeutic implications. Viral antigens may be immunohistochemically detected in formalin-fixed, paraffin-embedded tissues.[33, 34] Some commercially available antibodies may cross-react with non–hepatitis C epitopes, however.[35]

Both ISH[36, 37] and RT-PCR assays are available for detecting hepatitis C. The sensitivity of the PCR assay is higher than that of ISH, and both the sensitivity and specificity are higher than IHC.[35] We have found the RT-PCR assay described in SOP 6.1 to be highly reliable and to give results in the vast majority of archival specimens submitted for analysis.

There is evidence that nucleic acid sequence analysis (genotyping) may have both prognostic and therapeutic implications in patients with hepatitis C infection, but the literature does not yet yield a consensus on this matter.[38] Quantitation of serum hepatitis C virus is also important in establishing prognosis and response and may be accomplished using either quantitative PCR or bDNA assays.[39]

HEPATITIS DELTA

Hepatitis delta is an uncommon defective virus that requires co-infection with hepatitis B to replicate; it is often associated with other hepatitis viruses. The diagnosis is usually made serologically,[40] but the virus may be detected in tissue by IHC,[41] ISH,[42] or RT-PCR.[43, 44]

HEPATITIS E

The diagnosis of hepatitis E, a relatively uncommon hepatitis virus, is usually made serologically,[45] but IHC assays for the virus have been reported.[45–47] In addition, RT-PCR assays have been reported for use on stool samples[48, 49]; these should be adaptable to tissue.

The Herpesviruses

Rapid and correct identification of herpesviruses is important because effective antiviral therapy is

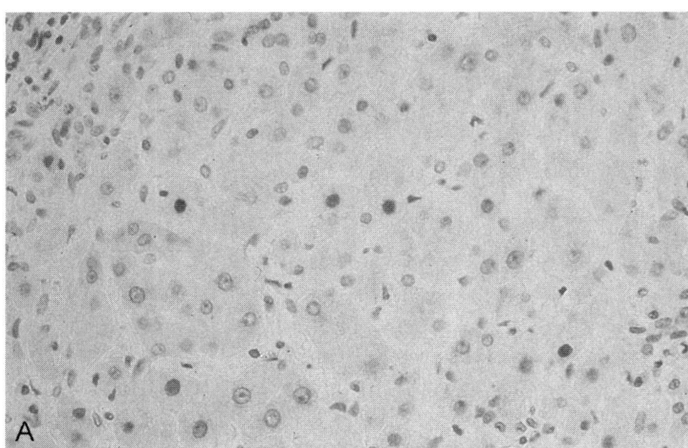

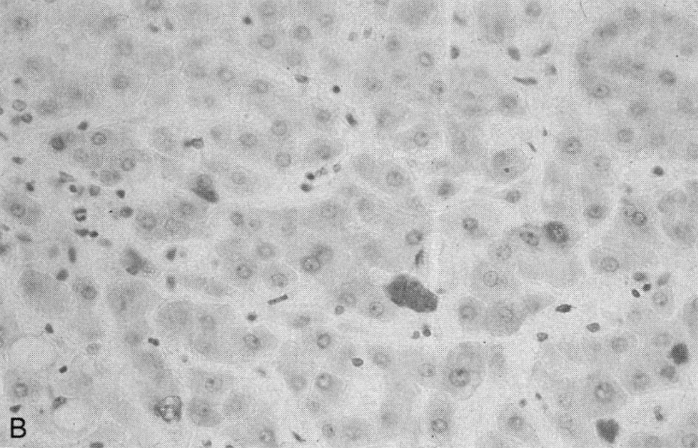

FIGURE 6–2
Immunohistochemical demonstration of *(A)* hepatitis B core antigen (×200) and *(B)* hepatitis B surface antigen (×400) in liver tissue. (See also Color Fig. 6–2.)

available and because some of the herpesvirus diseases, such as herpes encephalitis, rapidly progress to irreversible damage and/or death if not successfully treated in a timely manner. In some sites, such as cerebrospinal fluid, molecular diagnosis by PCR or other amplification method is the preferred diagnostic method, both for sensitivity and speed of diagnosis, but in other sites the use of more than one diagnostic strategy may be required.

HERPES SIMPLEX VIRUSES TYPES 1 AND 2

The herpes simplex viruses (HSV) may be successfully treated with antiviral agents. Particularly when disease is present in the central nervous system, rapid diagnosis is vital. In these cases, PCR-based assays are clearly the diagnostic method of choice, because they provide very rapid, highly accurate, and highly specific results.[50–58] Both HSV type 1 and type 2 can be amplified using the same reaction, even from formalin-fixed, paraffin-embedded tissue, and differentiated by type-specific oligonucleotide hybridization of the PCR products[59, 60] A PCR assay for HSV, which works in both cerebrospinal fluid and in formalin-fixed, paraffin-embedded sections, is shown in SOP 6.2.

Localization of HSV in tissue section can be accomplished using either IHC or ISH assays. ISH assays, although more technically challenging than the IHC methods, allow differentiation of types 1 and 2 through the use of type-specific probes.[5, 61, 62] They are, however, more likely to "fail" in the laboratory as a result of tissue "wash-off." IHC assays are about as sensitive as the ISH methods, are less likely to result in tissue wash-off, and are able to reliably distinguish HSV infections from varicella-zoster virus (VZV) infections.[63, 64] They cannot, however, distinguish between HSV types 1 and 2. IHC assays can also be used on cytologic preparations and seem to be about as sensitive as culture for the detection of virus in the uterine cervix.[65]

VARICELLA-ZOSTER VIRUS

Although VZV gives rise to intranuclear inclusions, these inclusions cannot be reliably distinguished from those of HSV in routinely stained sections. IHC, ISH, and PCR may all be used to make this distinction or to detect viral infections that have not produced characteristic inclusions.

Both monoclonal and polyclonal antibodies are available for the detection of VZV infection and can be used alone, or in combination with ISH, to diagnose this infection.[66–69] Viral genomes can be detected late in the course of infection, when immunocytochemical evidence of the virus has disappeared,[68] and may appear earlier in the course of infection than do viral proteins.[69]

PCR assays are more sensitive and specific for VZV DNA than are ISH assays.[70] Assays are applicable to both fresh and formalin-fixed, paraffin-embedded tissue.[59, 70] We prefer PCR methods to both ISH assay and immunocytochemistry for the diagnosis of VZV infection, because it is more straightforward to maintain readily available control tissue for PCR assay than for immunocytochemistry and because both PCR and immunocytochemistry are less technically challenging and more likely to give definitive results on the first try than is ISH. The assay that we use for VZV appears as SOP 6.3.

CYTOMEGALOVIRUS

When characteristic nuclear and cytoplasmic inclusions (often best demonstrated with periodic acid–Schiff stain) are present, the diagnosis of CMV is not challenging. Early in disease, however, CMV inclusions may not be present; and in small biopsy specimens, characteristic inclusions may not be observed even when disease is well established and widespread. IHC[64, 71–75] (Fig. 6–3*A*), ISH[64, 71–75] (see Fig. 6–3*B*),

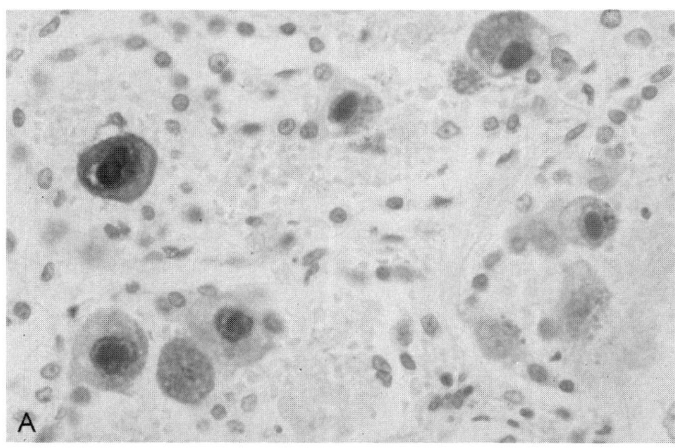

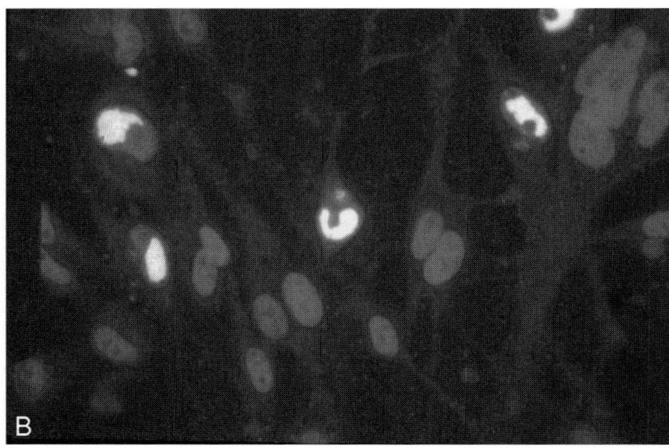

FIGURE 6–3
A, Immunohistochemical demonstration of cytomegalovirus in lung tissue (×400). *B*, Demonstration of fluorescent in situ hybridization of a cytomegalovirus genome in cultured fibroblasts (×400). (See also Color Fig. 6–3.)

and PCR-based assays[76, 77] are all capable of identifying the virus.

In most cases, the PCR-based assays are most sensitive, even in formalin-fixed, paraffin-embedded tissue.[78] Even when only rare cells are infected, the tissue preparation procedure ensures that viral genomes will be distributed throughout the initial lysate and present in the amplification mix. Quantitative PCR CMV assays are also available and are useful in viral load quantitation, particularly in patients who have been immunosuppressed after transplantation.[79–83]

The sensitivity of PCR is rarely required for diagnosis, however, and may occasionally result in confusion (particularly in fresh or frozen specimens—rarely in paraffin-embedded tissue), because rare copies of quiescent CMV are frequently found in individuals who do not demonstrate clinical evidence of infection.[84] ISH assays for CMV do not suffer from these limitations. When used for early confirmation of CMV infection in viral culture, these assays are more sensitive than IHC methods (although less sensitive than PCR). They are probably also more sensitive for fresh tissue, but, in my experience and that of others, are no more sensitive than IHC assays for CMV in formalin-fixed, paraffin-embedded tissues.[64] The nuclear antigens may appear and be detected by immunocytochemistry within several hours of infection; enzymatic pretreatment or antigen-retrieval techniques significantly enhance the sensitivity of this assay. Because in most hands IHC assays are technically easier and less expensive than ISH assays, they are probably preferable in most cases.[64]

Although in situ PCR assays for CMV have been published,[85] these assays are generally too complex and offer too little improvement in sensitivity to be useful for routine diagnostic work.

EPSTEIN-BARR VIRUS

Detection, quantitation, and characterization of Epstein-Barr virus (EBV) are important in the diagnosis of EBV-associated tumors, the monitoring of immunosuppressed patients, and the diagnosis of EBV disease. Unlike cytomegalovirus, HSV, and herpes zoster, EBV seldom gives rise to viral inclusions. Hence, the diagnosis rests in all cases on identification by culture, IHC, or molecular biologic methods. IHC assays that work in frozen or paraffin-embedded tissue are available. Most laboratories that deal with paraffin-embedded tissue use an antibody directed against the EBV latent membrane protein 1 (LMP1) or EBV nuclear protein 1 (EBNA1), although assays intended to detect the *BZLF1* gene product have also been published.[86–89] ISH assays may detect EBV genome in a small percentage of cases in which these antigens cannot be detected immunohistochemically,[89] and PCR assays will detect genome in cases in which ISH is negative.[90] The approach to PCR for EBV that we use is shown in SOP 6.4.[91]

EBV may persist in a latent state and be present at low copy number but not be involved in the pathogenesis of disease. Both ISH and PCR assays are sufficiently sensitive to detect these nonreplicating viruses. Viral replication can be identified by utilizing assays that detect viral RNA[92, 93]

Viral load quantitation may be useful in distinguishing latent virus from active infection and also for identifying patients at risk for post-transplant immunoproliferative disorders.[94] Several approaches to viral load quantitation are available, including a PCR/enzyme-linked immunosorbent assay method,[95] competitive PCR,[96] and limiting dilution methods.[93]

HUMAN HERPESVIRUS TYPE 6

Human herpesvirus type 6 causes exanthem subitum and has been linked with a variety of other diseases, particularly respiratory tract infections. This virus may be demonstrated in formalin-fixed, paraffin-embedded tissue by IHC assay[97, 98] and by PCR.[99]

HUMAN HERPESVIRUS TYPE 7

Human herpesvirus type 7 is closely related to human herpesvirus type 6,[100] is responsible for a febrile exanthem that resembles exanthem subitum, and is frequently associated with febrile convulsions.[101] An IHC assay has been demonstrated in formalin-fixed, paraffin-embedded tissue.[102] The virus can also be demonstrated by PCR, either alone or using an assay that simultaneously detects and discriminates between human herpesvirus types 6 and 7.[103, 104]

HUMAN HERPESVIRUS TYPE 8

Human herpesvirus type 8 has been associated with Kaposi's sarcoma, multicentric Castleman's disease, and body cavity–based lymphoma.[105] Although routinely stained sections may occasionally show cells with eosinophilic intranuclear inclusions, they are generally inconspicuous or inapparent. IHC assays are not available for routine diagnosis; both DNA and RNA ISH assays have been published, however.[106–108] Human herpesvirus type 8 is also readily identified from fresh or archival specimens by PCR.[109, 110]

HUMAN IMMUNODEFICIENCY VIRUS

HIV-1 and HIV-2 cause the acquired immunedeficiency syndrome, a blood-borne and sexually transmitted disease that eventually kills approximately 98% of those infected. The diagnosis is rarely made on the basis of tissue biopsy but is sometimes suspected when a lymph node biopsy demonstrates hyperplasia in the absence of another cause. A variety of antibodies are available to detect HIV in both frozen and formalin-fixed, paraffin-embedded tissue.[111–114] Monoclonal antibodies directed against the p24, gp41, and gp120 are all effective in detecting the virus; none is quite as sensitive as carefully conducted ISH assays.[113, 115, 116] PCR assays are more sensitive yet.

Although HIV is frequently detectable in brain or hyperplastic lymph nodes by IHC or ISH, this is usually not possible by the time lymph nodes are depleted. PCR assays are still useful at this point, and complementary DNA from the virus can usually be easily detected using PCR.[117–120] The PCR assay that we use for formalin-fixed, paraffin-embedded tissues is shown as SOP 6.5.

Viral load quantitation may be carried out using either PCR[121] or the bDNA[122] method with commercially available kits. Measurement of blood (serum) viral load has become a cornerstone of management of patients with HIV disease and is an excellent indicator of both response to therapy and prognosis.[123–125]

Influenza Viruses

Like the adenoviruses, influenza viruses infect the upper respiratory tract and lungs. Viral replication only occurs for 1 to 2 days, during which time cells resembling the "smudge cells" of adenovirus infection may occasionally be observed. Two major (A and B) and one minor (C) type infect humans. Influenza A, responsible for most infections, undergoes continuous evolution based on mutation and reassortment of both hemagglutinin and neuraminidase antigens. Although the use of IHC methods for detecting influenza in formalin-fixed, paraffin-embedded tissue specimens has been reported,[20] there are no details in the literature. An assay intended for use on swine would likely work also in humans, however.[126] RT-PCR assays are available for identification and typing of influenza viruses,[127, 128] and RT-PCR methods have been used for sequence determination in formalin-fixed, paraffin-embedded tissue.[129]

Morbillivirus

The only significant morbillivirus disease in humans is measles. Although this is generally a self-limited disease that does not give rise to a need for tissue diagnosis, histologic specimens will occasionally present in which a diagnosis of measles encephalitis or measles pneumonia is suspected either clinically or histologically. Viral antigens may be identified immunohistochemically[130] or by RT-PCR[131] in formalin-fixed, paraffin-embedded tissues.

An assay that has been used to identify and speciate animal morbilliviruses[132] is also applicable to the detection of measles virus. Surprisingly, this assay works well even in highly degraded tissue and appears to be more robust and sensitive than the IHC assay under most circumstances.

Papillomaviruses

There are over 80 human papillomaviruses (HPVs), which together are responsible for a variety of benign and malignant growths ranging from the plantar wart to cervical carcinoma. For the most part, the various papillomavirus types responsible for these growths have been well characterized and there is little diagnostic benefit to identifying or typing the papillomaviruses within. The uterine cervix may be an exception, however. Many cases of HPV infection are transient and do not give rise to malignancy.[133] However, cervical carcinoma almost never arises without prolonged persistence of demonstrable HPV infection with one of the "high-risk" HPV types (HPV 16, 18, 31, 33, 35, 39, 45, 51, 52, 56, 68, and others); progression to a high-grade squamous intraepithelial lesion (SIL) is rare in women who are HPV negative at the time of cytologic screening.[134] This may enable one to use HPV testing to improve the treatment of women whose Papanicolaou smears are given a diagnosis of "atypical squamous cells of undetermined significance (ASCUS)." If women with a diagnosis of ASCUS are referred to colposcopy only if high-risk HPV is identified, far fewer women are unnecessarily subjected to this procedure, and few cases of high-grade SIL will be missed.[135, 136] HPV testing may also be useful in interpretation of cellular atypia in postmenopausal women; the rate of HPV infection in biopsy-proven SIL is as high as for younger women, although few cases of cytologic atypia are associated with SIL.[137]

Although available IHC assays can detect many HPV types, they often fail to demonstrate virus even in the presence of a high viral load. ISH allows visualization of HPV-infected cells, but the conditions necessary for the assay are harsh and multiple samples are often required. The most commonly used approaches for diagnosis and typing are the MY09/MY11 L1 consensus primer PCR-based test and the hybrid capture method.[138, 139] These tests do not give equivalent results. The PCR test is clearly more sensitive and detects a greater range of HPV types. The sensitivity of the hybrid capture method is significantly higher for women with concurrent SILs than for women with normal cytologic findings.[138] Although the hybrid-capture assay is slightly less expensive and challenging technically, neither is difficult for the routine molecular diagnostic laboratory.

Although PCR assay for HPV can be used in formalin-fixed, paraffin-embedded tissue, the simpler hybrid capture assay cannot. In our laboratory, we use a combined assay that uses hybrid capture to detect the presence of

HPV and characterize the amplimers as reflecting the presence of high- or low-risk HPV types.

Parvoviruses

Parvovirus infections give rise to a wide spectrum of clinical disease. Intrauterine parvovirus B19 infection is a frequent cause of hydrops fetalis and fetal death. Infection of the bone marrow of immune-deficient patients with parvovirus can cause severe anemia; patients with other anemias may develop aplastic crises after infection. The virus can also cause a fulminant hepatitis, particularly in children. Characteristic viral inclusions, when present in one of these settings, enable the diagnosis to be made reliably on conventionally stained material but are occasionally not observed. In these cases, parvovirus infection may be diagnosed immunohistochemically[140–142] or by ISH.[141, 143, 144] Although some studies have found ISH to be more sensitive,[141] this may depend on the specific characteristics of the ISH and IHC assays compared. Some IHC assays appear to offer comparable sensitivity.[142] The reliability of histologic examination is sufficiently high that PCR-based assays generally add little useful information.[145]

Fetal loss caused by parvovirus infection may occur in the third trimester without the presence of demonstrable antigen or nucleic acid in the fetus. Maternal serology may help to establish the diagnosis in these cases.[140]

Picornaviruses

The picornaviruses, in particular coxsackieviruses, are most frequently encountered in diagnostic anatomic pathology as suspected etiologic agents in myocarditis/dilated cardiomyopathy (see Chapter 7). Surprisingly, IHC methods have not been routinely employed, although an IHC assay that works in formalin-fixed, paraffin-embedded tissue sections has been developed using a polyclonal rabbit antibody raised against coxsackievirus types B1 through B6.[146] Immunofluorescent antibody staining is also useful for identification of coxsackieviruses and other enteroviruses,[147–149] but specimens must be stained before fixation to avoid difficulties in interpretation arising from formaldehyde-induced autofluorescence. ISH has been employed in formalin-fixed, paraffin-embedded tissue,[150] but it may be limited to studying early stages of infection. RT-PCR assays are also appropriate for detecting picornavirus in formalin-fixed archival specimens[151–153] and are probably the most robust approach to diagnosis of picornavirus infection in routinely processed tissue. Even so, results must be interpreted with caution, because picornavirus infection may persist without causing disease[154] and because, in many patients, virus does not persist throughout the course of disease.

Polyomaviruses

Infection with the JC virus causes progressive multifocal leukoencephalopathy (PML), frequently observed in patients with immune deficiencies; BK virus infection of the urinary tract is frequently seen in immunosuppressed patients and occasionally in healthy individuals. The histologic appearances of PML and BK virus infections are both generally distinctive, and immunohistologic or molecular biologic confirmation is rarely required, except in cases in which only tiny biopsy specimens or cytologic material is available. Commercially available monoclonal antibodies can be used in IHC assays to detect either virus.[155, 156] ISH assays (Fig. 6–4) are unquestionably more sensitive for detection of JC virus, however.[155] An example of an ISH assay for JC virus is given in SOP 6.6.

PCR assays for JC virus are also available, and PCR of the cerebrospinal fluid is nearly as sensitive as brain biopsy for confirmation of a diagnosis of PML.[157–159] Quantitation of cerebrospinal fluid viral load may be useful in monitoring therapy.[160] The diagnosis of PML may also be confirmed by tissue PCR,[161] but a positive PCR for JC virus in brain tissue must not be automatically equated with a clinical diagnosis of

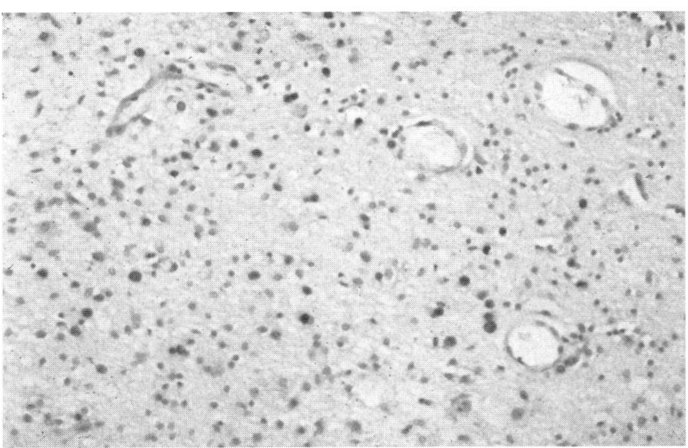

FIGURE 6–4
Demonstration of a JC virus genome by in situ hybridization in brain tissue from a patient with progressive multifocal leukoencephalopathy (×100). (See also Color Fig. 6–4.)

PML, because viral sequences are frequently detected in normal brain.[159, 162] JC virus is not normally shed into the cerebrospinal fluid, and the identification of JC virus sequences by PCR of the cerebrospinal fluid is a reliable diagnostic tool.

BK virus infection in tissue, urine, and bladder washings can usually be diagnosed on cytomorphologic characteristics alone, but IHC[155, 156] and ISH assays are available as diagnostic adjuncts.[163] PCR assays are probably "overkill" in most cases, but they may prove useful in monitoring the urine of immunosuppressed patients.[164]

Respiratory Syncytial Virus

Respiratory syncytial virus (RSV) causes an acute pulmonary infection that may be responsible for some cases of sudden infant death syndrome (SIDS). Although the diagnosis of RSV infection may be made reliably when characteristic histologic changes accompany a typical clinical picture, ancillary diagnostic approaches may be useful in cases in which the presentation is atypical or only small amounts of tissue are available for examination. Virus may be identified in formalin-fixed, paraffin-embedded tissue either immunohistochemically,[165, 166] by ISH,[167, 168] or by RT-PCR.[168] Although it seems likely that IHC methods are adequate in most cases, comparative studies of the sensitivity and specificity of these methods have not been performed.

Chlamydia

The three *Chlamydia* species that commonly cause disease in humans are *C. trachomatis*, *C. pneumoniae*, and *C. psittaci*. Of these, only *C. trachomatis* is routinely diagnosed in the clinical laboratory; *C. pneumoniae* is under active investigation as an etiologic agent in atherosclerosis. The discussion of laboratory methods for diagnosing *Chlamydia* infections in tissue is restricted here to these two agents.

CHLAMYDIA TRACHOMATIS

Chlamydia trachomatis, a major cause of pelvic inflammatory disease, can be demonstrated in formalin-fixed, paraffin-embedded tissue either immunohistochemically or by ISH.[169–174] Unfortunately, neither technique detects about half the cases in which the organism is successfully cultured.[170] Immunoperoxidase is more sensitive than ISH, and the combination of both is more sensitive yet.[171] PCR is far more sensitive than either technique for the detection of *C. trachomatis* in formalin-fixed, paraffin-embedded tissues.[175]

C. trachomatis can be detected sensitively and inexpensively by PCR or the ligase chain reaction, not only in cervical swabs but also in the urine of infected women. There is considerable evidence that the screening and treatment of young asymptomatic women by amplification methods is a cost-effective intervention for the prevention of pelvic inflammatory disease.[176–178]

CHLAMYDIA PNEUMONIAE

Chlamydia pneumoniae is a common respiratory pathogen that has been implicated in the pathogenesis of coronary artery disease. Diagnosis in surgical pathology material is usually required by research, rather than clinical, needs. It may be demonstrated by IHC,[179, 180] by ISH,[179, 180] or by PCR.[179]

BACTERIAL AND MYCOPLASMAL DISEASES

Adjunct diagnostic methods are less often used for the tissue diagnosis of bacterial diseases than for the tissue diagnosis of viral diseases. Bacterial disease can often be cultured or sufficiently identified with special stains such as the Braun-Bren, Braun-Hoppes, Warthin-Starry, and acid-fast stains. Although these stains assist greatly in visualizing and characterizing bacteria, they often do not permit unambiguous identification. Hence, when culture is not possible, unambiguous identification of bacteria may require IHC or molecular biologic methods.

Several species-specific approaches are available for the identification of bacteria in tissue sections. IHC identification is relatively inexpensive and can often be accomplished with the same antibodies used for assisting in the identification of cultured microorganisms in the clinical laboratory. PCR-based identification, on the other hand, is relatively expensive and often requires many, many reactions. The work may sometimes be reduced by using for identification assays that depend on the analysis of PCR products from 16S RNA, but such assays must be implemented in the laboratory with great care, because some commercial Taq polymerase contain a great deal of Taq 16S RNA. Identification of microorganisms by this approach is beyond the scope of this chapter.

References to IHC and molecular biologic assays for a number of bacterial diseases are shown in Table 6–1. Here, the discussion is limited to the diagnosis of *Mycobacteria*, *Helicobacter*, and *Mycoplasma* infections.

Helicobacter pylori

Helicobacter pylori can be visualized by modified Giemsa or silver stains in most cases.[181, 182] Although the modified Giemsa stain has the highest sensitivity

TABLE 6–1

Selected Bacteria for Which Immunohistochemical or Molecular Biologic Methods Allow Identification in Formalin-Fixed, Paraffin-Embedded Tissues

Organism	References	
	Immunocyto-chemical Method	Molecular Method
Borrelia burgdorferi	4209	209–211
Campylobacter species	20	
Escherichia coli	212	
Helicobacter pylori	182, 183	213
Klebsiella	20	
Legionella pneumophila	214, 215	
Mycobacterium species	185	191–197
Pseudomonas aeruginosa	20	
Salmonella	20	
Shigella	20	
Staphylococcus	20	
Streptococcus	216	
Treponema pallidum	217, 218	219, 220
Yersinia	20	221

for diagnosis, the specificity and interobserver reproducibility is low.[182] IHC methods offer a sensitivity comparable to that of modified Giemsa staining, but with a much higher specificity.[182, 183] ISH is a sensitive and specific alternative, but it is technically more complicated than IHC.[184] PCR assays are available but are no more sensitive, and may be less sensitive, than IHC.

We have frequently observed that PCR is often not sensitive for the detection of bacteria, such as *H. pylori*, in formalin-fixed, paraffin-embedded tissue. With careful examination, a single organism can often be identified by classic stains or IHC methods within a tissue section. In contrast, lysate amounting to less than a single tissue section is often used to obtain amplification in formalin-fixed, paraffin-embedded tissues; unless multiple organisms are present in the original tissue sections, their genomes may not appear in the lysate to be amplified! This is seldom an issue for fresh or frozen tissue, however, and in our experience PCR is usually more sensitive than visual examination for the identification of bacteria in unfixed tissue.

Mycobacteria

The identification *of Mycobacterium tuberculosis, M. avium-intracellulare*, or *M. leprae* in formalin-fixed, paraffin-embedded tissue is accomplished with highest sensitivity and specificity by a trained observer using Ziehl-Nielsen or modified acid-fast stained tissue. In some cases, IHC staining for mycobacterial antigens can assist in the visualization of these organisms.[185–187] Occasionally, when classic techniques are unable to demonstrate and/or speciate mycobacteria, PCR analysis can provide a solution.[188–197] Nevertheless, I have observed several cases in which expert examination of acid-fast stained specimens has been able to identify organisms not detectable by PCR.

Mycoplasma

The diagnosis of *Mycoplasma* infection is only rarely made on the basis of cytologic or biopsy material. Although the histologic appearance of an interstitial pneumonia may suggest the possibility of *Mycoplasma* infection, organisms cannot be identified in routinely stained sections. Mycoplasmas can occasionally be demonstrated immunohistochemically,[20] but the sensitivity of IHC assay is generally quite low. *M. fermentans*

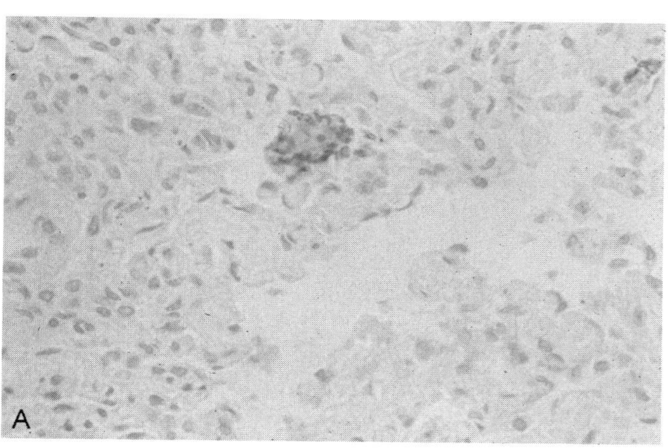

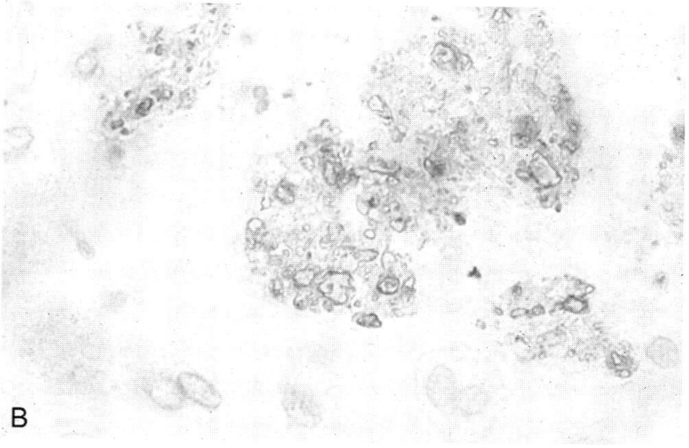

FIGURE 6–5
Immunohistochemical demonstration of *Pneumocystis carinii* in the "foamy exudate" of lung tissue, seen at ×100 *(A)* and at ×400 *(B)*. (See also Color Fig. 6–5.)

TABLE 6–2

Selected Fungi, Protozoa, and Parasites for Which Immunohistochemical or Molecular Biologic Methods Allow Identification in Formalin-Fixed, Paraffin-Embedded Tissues or Cytologic Specimens

	References	
Organism	**Immunocyto-chemical Method**	**Molecular Method**
Aspergillus sp.	222-224	
Blastomyces sp.	20	
Candida sp.	223-226	227
Cryptococcus neoformans	223-225	228, 229
Cryptosporidium sp.		230
Entamoeba histolytica	231, 232	233
Fasciola hepatica	20	
Fusarium anthophilum	223, 224	234
Giardia lamblia	235, 236	
Histoplasma capsulatum	20, 237	238
Leishmania sp.	239	240, 241
Pneumocystis carinii	200, 201	242
Sporothrix schenckii	223, 225	
Toxoplasma gondii	207, 243	208, 244
Trichomonas sp.	20	245–247
Trichophyton sp.	20	
Trichosporon beigelii	223, 248, 249	
Trypanosoma cruzi	250	251

has been demonstrated in tissue both immunohistochemically and by PCR,[198] a technique by which, using consensus primers, a large variety of mycoplasmas can be identified and speciated.[199]

PROTOZOANS, FUNGI, AND HELMINTHS

For the most part, these organisms are readily suspected or identified on the basis of hematoxylin-and-eosin–stained sections. Identification and speciation of fungi is further assisted by the use of periodic acid–Schiff or methenamine silver stains, and protozoa and helminths may sometimes be recognized more easily with May-Grünwald or Wolbach's stain. Masson's trichrome stain may assist in recognition of *Entamoeba* trophozoites. It is rare that the molecular biologic or IHC methods provide significant assistance in the identification of these organisms; as a result, the focus here is on only two of them, relegating references on IHC and molecular biologic diagnostic methods for the remainder to Table 6–2.

PNEUMOCYSTIS CARINII

Pnemocystis carinii is readily suspected on the basis of the characteristic foamy exudate in hematoxylin-and-eosin–stained sections. The diagnosis is readily confirmed, or rare organisms found, using methenamine silver–stained sections. Although IHC assays *for P. carinii* are available (Fig. 6–5), they generally offer no perceptible advantage over silver staining.[200, 201] IHC staining is occasionally helpful when atypical morphology makes differentiation between *P. carinii* and yeast forms uncertain.

I have not found molecular biologic methods to improve diagnosis of *Pneumocystis* in formalin-fixed, paraffin-embedded tissue. PCR assays can be used to detect the organism with high sensitivity in blood and oral secretions, however, sometimes eliminating the need for bronchoscopy and/or peripheral lung biopsy.[202–205] The sensitivity of PCR exceeds that of histologic examination when fresh tissue is available, however, and also exceeds that of cytologic examination, with or without histochemical/IHC stains, in the detection of *Pneumocystis* in sputum or bronchioloalveolar lavage specimens.

TOXOPLASMA GONDII

Toxoplasma gondii can often be identified in hematoxylin-and eosin– or methenamine silver–stained sections, but it is often difficult to be certain of the diagnosis when a few organisms are present in the midst of abundant necrotic debris. In these cases, IHC assays

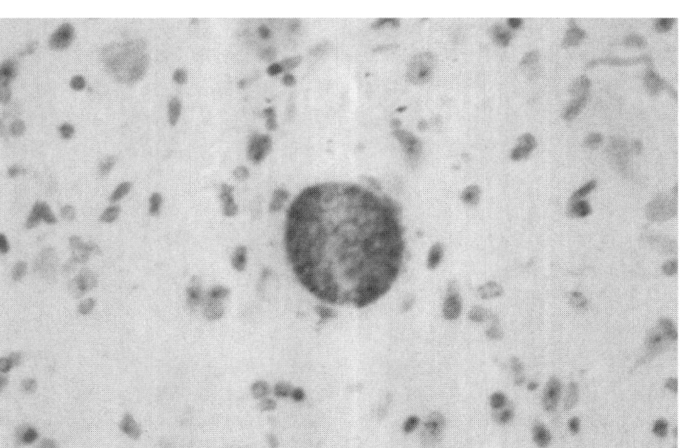

FIGURE 6–6
Immunohistochemical demonstration of a *Toxoplasma gondii* cyst in brain tissue of a patient with acquired immunodeficiency syndrome (×400). (See also Color Fig. 6–6.)

(Fig. 6–6) may facilitate diagnosis.[206, 207] PCR is somewhat more sensitive than either of these techniques, even in formalin-fixed, paraffin-embedded tissue.[208] Unfortunately, PCR of the cerebrospinal fluid is not a reliable way to confirm the diagnosis of cerebral toxoplasmosis[157]; brain biopsy is still required.

REFERENCES

1. LeBar WD: Keeping up with new technology: New approaches to diagnosis of *Chlamydia* infection. Clin Chem 1996;42:809–812.
2. Birkenmeyer LG, Mushahwar IK: DNA probe amplification methods. J Virol Methods 1991;35:117–126.
3. Urdea MS, Wuestehube LJ, Laurenson PM, Wilber JC: Hepatitis C—diagnosis and monitoring. Clin Chem 1997;43:1507–1511.
4. Cartun RW, Van Kruiningen HJ, Pedersen CA, Berman MM: An immunocytochemical search for infectious agents in Crohn's disease. Mod Pathol 1993;6:212–219.
5. Brigati DJ, Myerson D, Leary JJ, et al: Detection of viral genomes in cultured cells and paraffin-embedded tissue sections using biotin-labeled hybridization probes. Virology 1983;126:32–50.
6. Matsuse T, Matsui H, Shu CY, et al: Adenovirus pulmonary infections identified by PCR and in situ hybridisation in bone marrow transplant recipients. J Clin Pathol 1994; 47:973–977.
7. Turner PC, Bailey AS, Cooper RJ, Morris DJ: The polymerase chain reaction for detecting adenovirus DNA in formalin-fixed, paraffin-embedded tissue obtained post mortem. J Infect 1993;27:43–46.
8. Makela MJ, Puhakka T, Ruuskanen O, et al: Viruses and bacteria in the etiology of the common cold. J Clin Microbiol 1998;36:539–542.
9. Murray RS, Brown B, Brian D, Cabirac GF: Detection of coronavirus RNA and antigen in multiple sclerosis brain. Ann Neurol 1992;31:525–533.
10. Nichol ST, Spiropoulou CF, Morzunov S, et al: Genetic identification of a hantavirus associated with an outbreak of acute respiratory illness. Science 1993;262:914–917.
11. Kim EC, Kim IS, Choi Y, et al: Rapid differentiation between Hantaan and Seoul viruses by polymerase chain reaction and restriction enzyme analysis. J Med Virol 1994;43:245–248.
12. Hjelle B, Goade D, Torrez-Martinez N, et al: Hantavirus pulmonary syndrome, renal insufficiency, and myositis associated with infection by Bayou hantavirus. Clin Infect Dis 1996;23:495–500.
13. Lundkvist A, Hukic M, Horling J, et al: Puumala and Dobrava viruses cause hemorrhagic fever with renal syndrome in Bosnia-Herzegovina: Evidence of highly cross-neutralizing antibody responses in early patient sera. J Med Virol 1997;53:51–59.
14. Khan AS, Khabbaz RF, Armstrong LR, et al: Hantavirus pulmonary syndrome: The first 100 US cases. J Infect Dis 1996;173:1297–1303.
15. Ksiazek TG, Peters CJ, Rollin PE, et al: Identification of a new North American hantavirus that causes acute pulmonary insufficiency. Am J Trop Med Hyg 1995;52:117–123.
16. Zaki SR, Khan AS, Goodman RA, et al: Retrospective diagnosis of hantavirus pulmonary syndrome, 1978–1993: Implications for emerging infectious diseases. Arch Pathol Lab Med 1996;120:134–139.
17. Mertz G, Chapman L: Hantavirus infections in the United States: Diagnosis and treatment. Adv Exp Med Biol 1996;394:153–162.
18. Schwarz TF, Zaki SR, Morzunov S, et al: Detection and sequence confirmation of Sin Nombre virus RNA in paraffin-embedded human tissues using one-step RT-PCR. J Virol Methods 1995;51:349–356.
19. Arthur RR, Lofts RS, Gomez J, et al: Grouping of hantaviruses by small (S) genome segment polymerase chain reaction and amplification of viral RNA from wild-caught rats [published erratum appears in Am J Trop Med Hyg 1993; 48(3):v]. Am J Trop Med Hyg 1992;47:210–224.
20. Cartun RW, Taylor CR, Cote RJ (eds): Immunomicroscopy: A Diagnostic Tool for the Surgical Pathologist, 2nd ed. Philadelphia, WB Saunders, 1994, pp 401–415.
21. Atmar RL, Neill FH, Romalde JL, et al: Detection of Norwalk virus and hepatitis A virus in shellfish tissues with the PCR. Appl Environ Microbiol 1995;61:3014–3018.
22. Tsai YL, Tran B, Sangermano LR, Palmer CJ: Detection of poliovirus, hepatitis A virus, and rotavirus from sewage and ocean water by triplex reverse transcriptase PCR. Appl Environ Microbiol 1994;60:2400–2407.
23. Apaire-Marchais V, Ferre-Aubineau V, Colonna F, et al: Development of RT-semi-nested PCR for detection of hepatitis A virus in stool in epidemic conditions. Mol Cell Probes 1994;8:117–124.
24. Huang SN: Immunohistochemical demonstration of hepatitis B core and surface antigens in paraffin sections. Lab Invest 1975;33:88–95.
25. Brambilla C, Tackney C, Hirschman SZ, et al: Varying nuclear staining intensity of hepatitis B virus DNA in human hepatocellular carcinoma. Lab Invest 1986;55: 475–481.
26. Infantolino D, Pinarello A, Ceccato R, Barbazza R: HBV-DNA by in situ hybridization: A method to improve sensitivity on formalin-fixed, paraffin-embedded liver biopsies. Liver 1989;9:360–366.
27. Lau JY, Naoumov NV, Alexander GJ, Williams R: Rapid detection of hepatitis B virus DNA in liver tissue by in situ hybridisation and its combination with immunohistochemistry for simultaneous detection of HBV antigens. J Clin Pathol 1991;44:905–908.
28. De Lamballerie, Chapel F, Vignoli C, Zandotti C: Improved current methods for amplification of DNA from routinely processed liver tissue by PCR. J Clin Pathol 1994; 47:466–467.
29. Diamantis ID, McGandy C, Pult I, et al: Polymerase chain reaction detects hepatitis B virus DNA in paraffin-embedded liver tissue from patients sero- and histo-negative for active hepatitis B. Virchows Arch A Pathol Anat Histopathol 1992;420:11–15.
30. Lampertico P, Malter JS, Colombo M, Gerber MA: Detection of hepatitis B virus DNA in formalin-fixed, paraffin-embedded liver tissue by the polymerase chain reaction. Am J Pathol 1990;137:253–258.
31. Lo YM, Mehal WZ, Fleming KA: In vitro amplification of hepatitis B virus sequences from liver tumour DNA and from paraffin wax embedded tissues using the polymerase chain reaction. J Clin Pathol 1989;42:840–846.

32. Nainan OV, Cromeans TL, Margolis HS: Sequence-specific, single-primer amplification and detection of PCR products for identification of hepatitis viruses. J Virol Methods 1996;61:127–134.
33. Chamlian A, Benkoel L, Sahel J, et al: Immunohistochemical detection of hepatitis C virus related C100–3 and core antigens in formalin-fixed liver tissue. Cell Mol Biol 1996;42:557–566.
34. Nouri-Aria KT, Sallie R, Mizokami M, et al: Intrahepatic expression of hepatitis C virus antigens in chronic liver disease. J Pathol 1995;175:77–83.
35. Komminoth P, Adams V, Long AA, et al: Evaluation of methods for hepatitis C virus detection in archival liver biopsies: Comparison of histology, immunohistochemistry, in situ hybridization, reverse transcriptase polymerase chain reaction (RT-PCR) and in situ RT-PCR. Pathol Res Pract 1994;190:1017–1025.
36. Endo H, Yamada G, Nakane PK, Tsuji T: Localization of hepatitis C virus RNA in human liver biopsies by in situ hybridization using thymine-thymine dimerized oligo DNA probes: Improved method. Acta Med Okayama 1992; 46:355–364.
37. Felgar RE, Montone KT, Furth EE: A rapid method for the detection of hepatitis C virus RNA by in situ hybridization. Mod Pathol 1996;9:696–702.
38. Craxi A, Magrin S, Fabiano C, et al: Host and viral features in chronic HCV infection: Relevance to interferon responsiveness. Res Virol 1995;146:273–278.
39. Cribier B, Rey D, Uhl G, et al: Quantification of hepatitis C virus RNA in peripheral blood mononuclear cells: A comparison between patients chronically infected by HCV and patients co-infected by HIV. Res Virol 1996;147:325–332.
40. Greer S, Alexander GJ: Viral serology and detection. Baillieres Clin Gastroenterol 1995;9:689–721.
41. Hytiroglou P, Dash S, Haruna Y, et al: Detection of hepatitis B and hepatitis C viral sequences in fulminant hepatic failure of unknown etiology. Am J Clin Pathol 1995;104:588–593.
42. Pacchioni D, Negro F, Chiaberge E, et al: Detection of hepatitis delta virus RNA by a nonradioactive in situ hybridization procedure. Hum Pathol 1992;23:557–561.
43. Huang YH, Wu JC, Sheng WY, et al: Diagnostic value of anti-hepatitis D virus (HDV) antibodies revisited: A study of total and IgM anti-HDV compared with detection of HDV-RNA by polymerase chain reaction. J Gastroenterol Hepatol 1998;13:57–61.
44. Edamato Y, Tani M, Kurata T, Abe K: Hepatitis C and B virus infections in hepatocellular carcinoma: Analysis of direct detection of viral genome in paraffin embedded tissues. Cancer 1996;77:1787–1791.
45. Lok AS, Soldevila-Pico C: Epidemiology and serologic diagnosis of hepatitis E. J Hepatol 1994;20:567–569.
46. Purdy MA, Carson D, McCaustland KA, et al: Viral specificity of hepatitis E virus antigens identified by fluorescent antibody assay using recombinant HEV proteins. J Med Virol 1994;44:212–214.
47. Lau JY, Sallie R, Fang JW, et al: Detection of hepatitis E virus genome and gene products in two patients with fulminant hepatitis E. J Hepatol 1995;22:605–610.
48. Zhao SY, Zhou LY, Zhou WY, et al: A comparative study of detection of hepatitis E virus RNA by RT-PCR and digoxin probe techniques. Kansenshogaku Zasshi 1996; 70:485–489.
49. Turkoglu S, Lazizi Y, Meng H, et al: Detection of hepatitis E virus RNA in stools and serum by reverse transcription-PCR. J Clin Microbiol 1996;34:1568–1571.
50. Anderson NE, Powell KF, Croxson MC: A polymerase chain reaction assay of cerebrospinal fluid in patients with suspected herpes simplex encephalitis. J Neurol Neurosurg Psychiatry 1993;56:520–525.
51. Ando Y, Kimura H, Miwata H, et al: Quantitative analysis of herpes simplex virus DNA in cerebrospinal fluid of children with herpes simplex encephalitis. J Med Virol 1993;41:170–173.
52. Aslanzadeh J, Osmon DR, Wilhelm MP, et al: A prospective study of the polymerase chain reaction for detection of herpes simplex virus in cerebrospinal fluid submitted to the clinical virology laboratory. Mol Cell Probes 1992;6: 367–373.
53. Aslanzadeh J, Garner JG, Feder HM, Ryan RW: Use of polymerase chain reaction for laboratory diagnosis of herpes simplex virus encephalitis. Ann Clin Lab Sci 1993;23: 196–202.
54. Guffond T, Dewilde A, Lobert PE, et al: Significance and clinical relevance of the detection of herpes simplex virus DNA by the polymerase chain reaction in cerebrospinal fluid from patients with presumed encephalitis. Clin Infect Dis 1994;18:744–749.
55. Puchhammer-Stockl E, Popow-Kraupp T, Heinz F, et al: Establishment of PCR for the early diagnosis of herpes simplex encephalitis. J Med Virol 1990;32:77–82.
56. Ratnamohan VM, Cunningham AL, Rawlinson WD: Removal of inhibitors of CSF-PCR to improve diagnosis of herpesviral encephalitis. J Virol Methods 1998; 72:59–65.
57. Sakrauski A, Weber B, Kessler HH, et al: Comparison of two hybridization assays for the rapid detection of PCR amplified HSV genome sequences from cerebrospinal fluid. J Virol Methods 1994;50:175–184.
58. Uren EC, Johnson PD, Montanaro J, Gilbert GL: Herpes simplex virus encephalitis in pediatrics: Diagnosis by detection of antibodies and DNA in cerebrospinal fluid. Pediatr Infect Dis J 1993;12:1001–1006.
59. Nicoll JA, Maitland NJ, Love S: Use of the polymerase chain reaction to detect herpes simplex virus DNA in paraffin sections of human brain at necropsy. J Neurol Neurosurg Psychiatry 1991;54:167–168.
60. Vago L, Nebuloni M, Sala E, et al: Coinfection of the central nervous system by cytomegalovirus and herpes simplex virus type 1 or 2 in AIDS patients: Autopsy study on 82 cases by immunohistochemistry and polymerase chain reaction. Acta Neuropathol (Berl) 1996;92:404–408.
61. Bruner JM: Oligonucleotide probe for herpes virus: Use in paraffin sections. Mod Pathol 1990;3:635–638.
62. Nicoll JA, Love S, Burton PA, Berry PJ: Autopsy findings in two cases of neonatal herpes simplex virus infection: Detection of virus by immunohistochemistry, in situ hybridization and the polymerase chain reaction. Histopathology 1994;24:257–264.
63. Nikkels AF, Debrus S, Sadzot-Delvaux C, et al: Comparative immunohistochemical study of herpes simplex and varicella-zoster infections. Virchows Arch A Pathol Anat Histopathol 1993;422:121–126.
64. Strickler JG, Manivel JC, Copenhaver CM, Kubic VL: Comparison of in situ hybridization and immunohistochemistry for detection of cytomegalovirus and herpes simplex virus. Hum Pathol 1990;21:443–448.

65. Marsella RC, Buckner SB, Bratthauer GL, et al: Identification of genital herpes simplex virus infection by immunoperoxidase staining: Comparison with culture results and cytology. Appl Immunohistochem 1995;3:184–189.
66. Nikkels AF, Delvenne P, Sadzot-Delvaux C, et al: Distribution of varicella zoster virus and herpes simplex virus in disseminated fatal infections. J Clin Pathol 1996;49: 243–248.
67. Schmidbauer M, Budka H, Pilz P, et al: Presence, distribution and spread of productive varicella zoster virus infection in nervous tissues. Brain 1992;115(pt 2): 383–398.
68. Wenkel H, Rummelt V, Fleckenstein B, Naumann GO: Detection of varicella zoster virus DNA and viral antigen in human eyes after herpes zoster ophthalmicus. Ophthalmology 1998;105:1323–1330.
69. Mendez JC, Procop GW, Espy MJ, et al: Detection and semiquantitative analysis of human herpesvirus 8 DNA in specimens from patients with Kaposi's sarcoma. J Clin Microbiol 1998;36:2220–2222.
70. Annunziato P, Lungu O, Gershon A, et al: In situ hybridization detection of varicella zoster virus in paraffin-embedded skin biopsy samples. Clin Diagn Virol 1996;7: 69–76.
71. Mullink H, Walboomers JM, Tadema TM, et al: Combined immuno- and non-radioactive hybridocytochemistry on cells and tissue sections: Influence of fixation, enzyme pretreatment, and choice of chromogen on detection of antigen and DNA sequences. J Histochem Cytochem 1989;37: 603–609.
72. Porter HJ, Heryet A, Quantrill AM, Fleming KA: Combined non-isotopic in situ hybridisation and immunohistochemistry on routine paraffin wax embedded tissue: Identification of cell type infected by human parvovirus and demonstration of cytomegalovirus DNA and antigen in renal infection. J Clin Pathol 1990;43:129–132.
73. Rimsza LM, Vela EE, Frutiger YM, et al: Rapid automated combined in situ hybridization and immunohistochemistry for sensitive detection of cytomegalovirus in paraffin-embedded tissue biopsies. Am J Clin Pathol 1996;106:544–548.
74. Unger ER, Budgeon LR, Myerson D, Brigati DJ: Viral diagnosis by in situ hybridization: Description of a rapid simplified colorimetric method. Am J Surg Pathol 1986;10:1–8.
75. Wolber RA, Lloyd RV: Cytomegalovirus detection by nonisotopic in situ DNA hybridization and viral antigen immunostaining using a two-color technique. Hum Pathol 1988;19:736–741.
76. Chen YT, Mercer GO, Cheigh JS, Mouradian JA: Cytomegalovirus infection of renal allografts: Detection by polymerase chain reaction. Transplantation 1992;53:99–102.
77. Rogers BB, Alpert LC, Hine EA, Buffone GJ: Analysis of DNA in fresh and fixed tissue by the polymerase chain reaction. Am J Pathol 1990;136:541–548.
78. Persons DL, Moore JA, Fishback JL: Comparison of polymerase chain reaction, DNA hybridization, and histology with viral culture to detect cytomegalovirus in immunosuppressed patients. Mod Pathol 1991;4:149–153.
79. Kuhn JE, Wendland T, Eggers HJ, et al: Quantitation of human cytomegalovirus genomes in the brain of AIDS patients. J Med Virol 1995;47:70–82.
80. Boeckh M, Boivin G: Quantitation of cytomegalovirus: Methodologic aspects and clinical applications. Clin Microbiol Rev 1998;11:533–554.
81. Boivin G, Gilbert C, Morissette M, et al: A case of ganciclovir-resistant cytomegalovirus (CMV) retinitis in a patient with AIDS: Longitudinal molecular analysis of the CMV viral load and viral mutations in blood compartments. AIDS 1997;11:867–673.
82. Cope AV, Sweny P, Sabin C, et al: Quantity of cytomegalovirus viruria is a major risk factor for cytomegalovirus disease after renal transplantation. J Med Virol 1997; 52:200–205.
83. Mendez J, Espy M, Smith TF, et al: Clinical significance of viral load in the diagnosis of cytomegalovirus disease after liver transplantation. Transplantation 1998;65: 1477–1481.
84. Brainard JA, Greenson JK, Vesy CJ, et al: Detection of cytomegalovirus in liver transplant biopsies: A comparison of light microscopy, immunohistochemistry, duplex PCR and nested PCR. Transplantation 1994;57:1753–1757.
85. Zhaori G, Shen K, Jiang Z, et al: Detection of cytomegalovirus DNA in paraffin-embedded lung tissue specimens using in situ polymerase chain reaction. Chin Med J (Engl) 1996;109:361–365.
86. Grasser FA, Murray PG, Kremmer E, et al: Monoclonal antibodies directed against the Epstein-Barr virus–encoded nuclear antigen 1 (EBNA1): Immunohistologic detection of EBNA1 in the malignant cells of Hodgkin's disease. Blood 1994;84:3792–3798.
87. Kanavaros P, Sakalidou A, Tzardi M, et al: Frequent detection of Epstein-Barr virus (EBV), EBER transcripts and latent membrane protein-1 (LMP-1) in tumor cells in Hodgkin's disease arising in childhood. Pathol Res Pract 1994;190:1026–1030.
88. Ogutcen-Toller M: Detection of Epstein-Barr virus early replicative phase using monoclonal antibody BZ-1 in oral hairy leukoplakia and other hyperkeratotic oral mucosal lesions: A retrospective study. J Nihon Univ Sch Dent 1996;38:37–48.
89. Vera-Sempere FJ, Burgos JS, Botella MS, et al: Immunohistochemical expression of Epstein-Barr virus–encoded latent membrane protein (LMP-1) in paraffin sections of EBV-associated nasopharyngeal carcinoma in Spanish patients. Eur J Cancer B Oral Oncol 1996; 32B:163–168.
90. Ohshima K, Kikuchi M, Eguchi F, et al: Analysis of Epstein-Barr viral genomes in lymphoid malignancy using Southern blotting, polymerase chain reaction and in situ hybridization. Virchows Arch B Cell Pathol Incl Mol Pathol 1990;59:383–390.
91. Wright CF, Reid AH, Tsai MM, et al: Detection of Epstein-Barr virus sequences in Hodgkin's disease by the polymerase chain reaction. Am J Pathol 1991;139: 393–398.
92. Ohshima K, Kikuchi M, Kobari S, et al: Demonstration of Epstein-Barr virus genomes, using polymerase chain reaction in situ hybridization in paraffin-embedded lymphoid tissues. Pathol Res Pract 1995;191:139–147.
93. Orentas RJ: Determination of Epstein-Barr virus (EBV) load by RT-PCR and cellular dilution. Mol Cell Probes 1998;12:427–430.

94. Lucas KG, Burton RL, Zimmerman SE, et al: Semiquantitative Epstein-Barr virus (EBV) polymerase chain reaction for the determination of patients at risk for EBV-induced lymphoproliferative disease after stem cell transplantation. Blood 1998;91:3654–3661.
95. Bazzichi A, Guidi FV, Rindi L, et al: PCR ELISA for the quantitative detection of Epstein-Barr virus genome. J Virol Methods 1998;74:15–20.
96. Rowe DT, Qu L, Reyes J, et al: Use of quantitative competitive PCR to measure Epstein-Barr virus genome load in the peripheral blood of pediatric transplant patients with lymphoproliferative disorders. J Clin Microbiol 1997;35:1612–1615.
97. Hammerling JA, Lambrecht RS, Kehl KS, Carrigan DR: Prevalence of human herpesvirus 6 in lung tissue from children with pneumonitis. J Clin Pathol 1996;49: 802–804.
98. Pitalia AK, Liu-Yin JA, Freemont AJ, et al: Immunohistological detection of human herpes virus 6 in formalin-fixed, paraffin-embedded lung tissues. J Med Virol 1993; 41:103–107.
99. Luppi M, Marasca R, Barozzi P, et al: Frequent detection of human herpesvirus-6 sequences by polymerase chain reaction in paraffin-embedded lymph nodes from patients with angioimmunoblastic lymphadenopathy and angioimmunoblastic lymphadenopathy-like lymphoma. Leuk Res 1993;17:1003–1011.
100. Nicholas J: Determination and analysis of the complete nucleotide sequence of human herpesvirus. J Virol 1996; 70:5975–5989.
101. Clark DA, Kidd IM, Collingham KE, et al: Diagnosis of primary human herpesvirus 6 and 7 infections in febrile infants by polymerase chain reaction. Arch Dis Child 1997;77:42–45.
102. Yadav M, Nambiar S, Khoo SP, Yaacob HB: Detection of human herpesvirus 7 in salivary glands. Arch Oral Biol 1997;42:559–567.
103. Kidd IM, Clark DA, Bremner JA, et al: A multiplex PCR assay for the simultaneous detection of human herpesvirus 6 and human herpesvirus 7, with typing of HHV-6 by enzyme cleavage of PCR products. J Virol Methods 1998;70:29–36.
104. Osiowy C, Prud'homme I, Monette M, Zou S: Detection of human herpesvirus 6 DNA in serum by a microplate PCR-hybridization assay. J Clin Microbiol 1998;36: 68–72.
105. Orenstein JM, Alkan S, Blauvelt A, et al: Visualization of human herpesvirus type 8 in Kaposi's sarcoma by light and transmission electron microscopy. AIDS 1997;11: F35–F45.
106. Sturzl M, Blasig C, Schreier A, et al: Expression of HHV-8 latency-associated T0.7 RNA in spindle cells and endothelial cells of AIDS-associated, classical and African Kaposi's sarcoma. Int J Cancer 1997;72:68–71.
107. Blasig C, Zietz C, Haar B, et al: Monocytes in Kaposi's sarcoma lesions are productively infected by human herpesvirus 8. J Virol 1997;71:7963–7968.
108. Reed JA, Nador RG, Spaulding D, et al: Demonstration of Kaposi's sarcoma–associated herpes virus cyclin D homolog in cutaneous Kaposi's sarcoma by colorimetric in situ hybridization using a catalyzed signal amplification system. Blood 1998;91:3825–3832.
109. Cathomas G, McGandy CE, Terracciano LM, et al: Detection of herpesvirus-like DNA by nested PCR on archival skin biopsy specimens of various forms of Kaposi sarcoma. J Clin Pathol 1996;49:631–633.
110. Li N, Anderson WK, Bhawan J: Further confirmation of the association of human herpesvirus 8 with Kaposi's sarcoma. J Cutan Pathol 1998;25:413–419.
111. Ward JM, O'Leary TJ, Baskin GB, et al: Immunohistochemical localization of human and simian immunodeficiency viral antigens in fixed tissue sections. Am J Pathol 1987;127:199–205.
112. Morrison HL, Neal JW, Parkes AB, Jasani B: Immunohistochemical retrieval of the principal HIV antigens p24, gp41, and gp120 in formalin fixed tissue: An investigation using HIV infected lymphoblasts and postmortem brain tissue from AIDS cases. Mol Pathol 1998;51:227–231.
113. Shapshak P, Yoshioka M, Sun NC, et al: HIV-1 in postmortem brain tissue from patients with AIDS: A comparison of different detection techniques. AIDS 1992;6: 915–923.
114. Strappe PM, Wang TH, McKenzie CA, et al: Enhancement of immunohistochemical detection of HIV-1 p24 antigen in brain by tyramide signal amplification. J Virol Methods 1997;67:103–112.
115. Daugharty H, Long EG, Swisher BL, et al: Comparative study with in situ hybridization and immunocytochemistry in detection of HIV-1 in formalin-fixed paraffin-embedded cell cultures. J Clin Lab Anal 1990;4:283–288.
116. Unger ER, Chandler FW, Chenggis ML, et al: Demonstration of human immunodeficiency virus by colorimetric in situ hybridization: A rapid technique for formalin-fixed paraffin-embedded material. Mod Pathol 1989;2:200–204.
117. An SF, Ciardi A, Scaravilli F: PCR detection of HIV proviral DNA (gag) in the brains of patients with AIDS: Comparison between results using fresh frozen and paraffin wax embedded specimens. J Clin Pathol 1994;47:990–994.
118. Embretson J, Zupancic M, Beneke J, et al: Analysis of human immunodeficiency virus–infected tissues by amplification and in situ hybridization reveals latent and permissive infections at single-cell resolution. Proc Natl Acad Sci U S A 1993;90:357–361.
119. Kimmel PL, Ferreira-Centeno A, Farkas-Szallasi T, et al: Viral DNA in microdissected renal biopsy tissue from HIV infected patients with nephrotic syndrome. Kidney Int 1993;43:1347–1352.
120. Slavik T, Wolfaardt M, van Zyl H, Simson IW: Retrospective determination of HIV-1 status by a PCR method on paraffin wax embedded sections. J Clin Pathol 1995;48: 733–736.
121. Triques K, Coste J, Perret JL, et al: Efficiencies of four versions of the AMPLICOR HIV-1 MONITOR test for quantification of different subtypes of human immunodeficiency virus type 1 [in process citation]. J Clin Microbiol 1999;37:110–116.
122. Urdea MS, Wilber JC, Yeghiazarian T, et al: Direct and quantitative detection of HIV-1 RNA in human plasma with a branched DNA signal amplification assay. AIDS 1993;7(Suppl 2):S11–S14.
123. Vidal C, Garcia F, Gatell JM, et al: Predictive factors influencing peak viral load drop in response to nucleoside reverse transcriptase inhibitors in antiretroviral-naive

HIV-1-infected patients. J Acquir Immune Defic Syndr Hum Retrovirol 1998;19:55–60.
124. Trauger RJ, Giermakowska WK, Ferre F, et al: Cell-mediated immunity to HIV-1 in Walter Reed stages 1–6 individuals: Correlation with virus burden. Immunology 1993;78:611–615.
125. Rubio A, Leal M, Rey C, et al: Short-term evolution of HIV-1 viraemia and $CD4^+$ cell counts in patients who have a primary mutation to zidovudine. AIDS 1998; 12:395–398.
126. Haines DM, Waters EH, Clark EG: Immunohistochemical detection of swine influenza A virus in formalin-fixed and paraffin-embedded tissues. Can J Vet Res 1993;57:33–36.
127. Claas EC, Sprenger MJ, Kleter GE, et al: Type-specific identification of influenza viruses A, B and C by the polymerase chain reaction. J Virol Methods 1992;39:1–13.
128. Wright KE, Wilson GA, Novosad D, et al: Typing and subtyping of influenza viruses in clinical samples by PCR. J Clin Microbiol 1995;33:1180–1184.
129. Taubenberger JK, Reid AH, Krafft AE, et al: Initial genetic characterization of the 1918 "Spanish" influenza virus [see comments]. Science 1997;275:1793–1796.
130. Kumanishi T, In S: SSPE: Immunohistochemical demonstration of measles virus antigen(s) in paraffin sections. Acta Neuropathol (Berl) 1979;48:161–163.
131. Godec MS, Asher DM, Swoveland PT, et al: Detection of measles virus genomic sequences in SSPE brain tissue by the polymerase chain reaction. J Med Virol 1990;30: 237–244.
132. Krafft A, Lichy JH, Lipscomb TP, et al: Postmortem diagnosis of morbillivirus infection in bottlenose dolphins *(Tursiops truncatus)* in the Atlantic and Gulf of Mexico epizootics by polymerase chain reaction–based assay. J Wildl Dis 1995;31:410–415.
133. Ho GY, Bierman R, Beardsley L, et al: Natural history of cervicovaginal papillomavirus infection in young women. N Engl J Med 1998;338:423–428.
134. Rozendaal L, Walboomers JM, van der Linden JC, et al: PCR-based high-risk HPV test in cervical cancer screening gives objective risk assessment of women with cytomorphologically normal cervical smears. Int J Cancer 1996;68:766–769.
135. Cox JT, Lorincz AT, Schiffman MH, et al: Human papillomavirus testing by hybrid capture appears to be useful in triaging women with a cytologic diagnosis of atypical squamous cells of undetermined significance. Am J Obstet Gynecol 1995;172:946–954.
136. Cox JT, Schiffman MH, Winzelberg AJ, Patterson JM: An evaluation of human papillomavirus testing as part of referral to colposcopy clinics. Obstet Gynecol 1992;80: 389–395.
137. Symmans F, Mechanic L, MacConnell P, et al: Correlation of cervical cytology and human papillomavirus DNA detection in postmenopausal women. Int J Gynecol Pathol 1992;11:204–209.
138. Cope JU, Hildesheim A, Schiffman MH, et al: Comparison of the hybrid capture tube test and PCR for detection of human papillomavirus DNA in cervical specimens. J Clin Microbiol 1997;35:2262–2265.
139. Shah KV, Solomon L, Daniel R, et al: Comparison of PCR and hybrid capture methods for detection of human papillomavirus in injection drug–using women at high risk of human immunodeficiency virus infection. J Clin Microbiol 1997;35:517–519.
140. Essary LR, Vnencak-Jones CL, Manning SS, et al: Frequency of parvovirus B19 infection in nonimmune hydrops fetalis and utility of three diagnostic methods. Hum Pathol 1998;29:696–701.
141. Liu W, Ittmann M, Liu J, et al: Human parvovirus B19 in bone marrows from adults with acquired immunodeficiency syndrome: A comparative study using in situ hybridization and immunohistochemistry. Hum Pathol 1997;28:760–766.
142. Morey AL, O'Neill HJ, Coyle PV, Fleming KA: Immunohistological detection of human parvovirus B19 in formalin-fixed, paraffin-embedded tissues. J Pathol 1992; 166:105–108.
143. Hassam S, Briner J, Tratschin JD, et al: In situ hybridization for the detection of human parvovirus B19 nucleic acid sequences in paraffin-embedded specimens. Virchows Arch B Cell Pathol Incl Mol Pathol 1990; 59:257–261.
144. Walters C, Powe DG, Padfield CJ, Fagan DG: Detection of parvovirus B19 in macerated fetal tissue using in situ hybridisation [see comments]. J Clin Pathol 1997; 50:749–754.
145. Mark Y, Rogers BB, Oyer CE: Diagnosis and incidence of fetal parvovirus infection in an autopsy series: II. DNA amplification. Pediatr Pathol 1993;13:381–386.
146. Kamei S, Hersch SM, Kurata T, Takei Y: Coxsackie B antigen in the central nervous system of a patient with fatal acute encephalitis: Immunohistochemical studies of formalin-fixed paraffin-embedded tissue. Acta Neuropathol (Berl) 1990;80:216–221.
147. Burch GE, Sun SC, Colcolough HL, et al: Coxsackie B viral myocarditis and valvulitis identified in routine autopsy specimens by immunofluorescent techniques. Am Heart J 1967;74:13–23.
148. Burch GE, Sun SC, Chu KC, et al: Interstitial and coxsackievirus B myocarditis in infants and children: A comparative histologic and immunofluorescent study of 50 autopsied hearts. JAMA 1968;203:1–8.
149. Burch GE, Harb JM, Hiramoto Y: Coxsackie viral infection of human myocardium. Hum Pathol 1975;6: 120–125.
150. Hilton DA, Variend S, Pringle JH: Demonstration of Coxsackie virus RNA in formalin-fixed tissue sections from childhood myocarditis cases by in situ hybridization and the polymerase chain reaction. J Pathol 1993; 170:45–51.
151. Arola A, Kalimo H, Ruuskanen O, Hyypia T: Experimental myocarditis induced by two different coxsackievirus B3 variants: Aspects of pathogenesis and comparison of diagnostic ethods. J Med Virol 1995;47:251–259.
152. Nicholson F, Ajetunmobi JF, Li M, et al: Molecular detection and serotypic analysis of enterovirus RNA in archival specimens from patients with acute myocarditis. Br Heart J 1995;74:522–527.
153. Woodall CJ, Watt NJ, Clements GB: Simple technique for detecting RNA viruses by PCR in single sections of wax embedded tissue. J Clin Pathol 1993;46:276–277.
154. Ueno H, Yokota Y, Shiotani H, et al: Significance of detection of enterovirus RNA in myocardial tissues by reverse

transcription-polymerase chain reaction. Int J Cardiol 1995;51:157–164.
155. Aksamit AJ, Sever JL, Major EO: Progressive multifocal leukoencephalopathy: JC virus detection by in situ hybridization compared with immunohistochemistry. Neurology 1986;36:499–504.
156. Greenlee JE, Keeney PM: Immunoenzymatic labelling of JC papovavirus T antigen in brains of patients with progressive multifocal leukoencephalopathy. Acta Neuropathol (Berl) 1986;71:150–153.
157. d'Arminio MA, Cinque P, Vago L, et al: A comparison of brain biopsy and CSF-PCR in the diagnosis of CNS lesions in AIDS patients. J Neurol 1997;244:35–39.
158. Hammarin AL, Bogdanovic G, Svedhem V, et al: Analysis of PCR as a tool for detection of JC virus DNA in cerebrospinal fluid for diagnosis of progressive multifocal leukoencephalopathy. J Clin Microbiol 1996; 34:2929–2932.
159. Vago L, Cinque P, Sala E, et al: JCV-DNA and BKV-DNA in the CNS tissue and CSF of AIDS patients and normal subjects: Study of 41 cases and review of the literature. J Acquir Immune Defic Syndr Hum Retrovirol 1996;12:139–146.
160. Koralnik IJ, Boden D, Mai V, et al: JC virus DNA load in patients with and without progressive multifocal leukoencephalopathy. Neurology 1999;52:253–260.
161. Telenti A, Aksamit AJJ, Proper J, Smith TF: Detection of JC virus DNA by polymerase chain reaction in patients with progressive multifocal leukoencephalopathy. J Infect Dis 1990;162:858–861.
162. Ferrante P, Caldarelli-Stefano R, Omodeo-Zorini E, et al: PCR detection of JC virus DNA in brain tissue from patients with and without progressive multifocal leukoencephalopathy. J Med Virol 1995;47:219–225.
163. Hukkanen V, Haarala M, Nurmi M, et al: Viruses and interstitial cystitis: Adenovirus genomes cannot be demonstrated in urinary bladder biopsies. Urol Res 1996;24:235–238.
164. Arthur RR, Beckmann AM, Li CC, et al: Direct detection of the human papovavirus BK in urine of bone marrow transplant recipients: Comparison of DNA hybridization with ELISA. J Med Virol 1985;16:29–36.
165. Wright C, Oliver KC, Fenwick FI, et al: A monoclonal antibody pool for routine immunohistochemical detection of human respiratory syncytial virus antigens in formalin-fixed, paraffin-embedded tissue. J Pathol 1997; 182:238–244.
166. Neilson KA, Yunis EJ: Demonstration of respiratory syncytial virus in an autopsy series. Pediatr Pathol 1990;10:491–502.
167. An SF, Gould S, Keeling JW, Fleming KA: Role of respiratory viral infection in SIDS: Detection of viral nucleic acid by in situ hybridization. J Pathol 1993;171: 271–278.
168. Cubie HA, Duncan LA, Marshall LA, Smith NM: Detection of respiratory syncytial virus nucleic acid in archival postmortem tissue from infants. Pediatr Pathol Lab Med 1997;17:927–938.
169. Gencay M, Puolakkainen M, Wahlstrom T, et al: *Chlamydia trachomatis* detected in human placenta. J Clin Pathol 1997;50:852–855.
170. Meddens MJ, Quint WG, van der Willigen H, et al: Detection of *Chlamydia trachomatis* in culture and urogenital smears by in situ DNA hybridization using a biotinylated DNA probe. Mol Cell Probes 1988;2:261–269.
171. Patton DL, Askienazy-Elbhar M, Henry-Suchet J, et al: Detection of *Chlamydia trachomatis* in fallopian tube tissue in women with postinfectious tubal infertility. Am J Obstet Gynecol 1994;171:95–101.
172. Shurbaji MS, Dumler JS, Gage WR, et al: Immunohistochemical detection of chlamydial antigens in association with cystitis. Am J Clin Pathol 1990;93: 363–366.
173. Edwards JM, Campbell AR, Tait A, Lusher M: Demonstration of *Chlamydia trachomatis* in colposcopic cervical biopsy specimens by an immunoperoxidase method. J Clin Pathol 1991;44:1027–1029.
174. Shurbaji MS, Gupta PK, Myers J: Immunohistochemical demonstration of chlamydial antigens in association with prostatitis. Mod Pathol 1988;1:348–351.
175. Stern RA, Svoboda-Newman SM, Frank TS: Analysis of chronic endometritis for *Chlamydia trachomatis* by polymerase chain reaction. Hum Pathol 1996;27: 1085–1088.
176. Gaydos CA, Howell MR, Pare B, et al: *Chlamydia trachomatis* infections in female military recruits. N Engl J Med 1998;339:739–744.
177. Howell MR, Quinn TC, Brathwaite W, Gaydos CA: Screening women for *Chlamydia trachomatis* in family planning clinics: The cost-effectiveness of DNA amplification assays. Sex Transm Dis 1998;25:108–117.
178. Howell MR, Quinn TC, Gaydos CA: Screening for *Chlamydia trachomatis* in asymptomatic women attending family planning clinics: A cost-effectiveness analysis of three strategies. Ann Intern Med 1998;128: 277–284.
179. Grayston JT, Kuo CC, Coulson AS, et al: *Chlamydia pneumoniae* (TWAR) in atherosclerosis of the carotid artery. Circulation 1995;92:3397–3400.
180. Pai J, Knoop FC, Hunter WJ, Agrawal DK: *Chlamydia pneumoniae* and occlusive vascular disease: Identification and characterization. J Pharmacol Toxicol Methods 1998;39:51–61.
181. Doglioni C, Turrin M, Macri E, et al: HpSS: A new silver staining method for *Helicobacter pylori*. J Clin Pathol 1997;50:461–464.
182. Jonkers D, Stobberingh E, de Bruine A, et al: Evaluation of immunohistochemistry for the detection of *Helicobacter pylori* in gastric mucosal biopsies. J Infect 1997;35: 149–154.
183. Faraker CA: Diagnosis of *Helicobacter pylori* in gastric brush and biopsy specimens stained by Romanowsky and immunocytochemical methods: Comparison with the CLOtest. Cytopathology. 1996;7:108–119.
184. Barrett DM, Faigel DO, Metz DC, et al: In situ hybridization for *Helicobacter pylori* in gastric mucosal biopsy specimens: Quantitative evaluation of test performance in comparison with the CLOtest and thiazine stain. J Clin Lab Anal 1997;11:374–379.
185. Ang SC, Moscovic EA: Cross-reactive and species-specific *Mycobacterium tuberculosis* antigens in the immunoprofile of Schaumann bodies: A major clue to the etiology of sarcoidosis. Histol Histopathol 1996;11: 125–134.
186. Natrajan M, Katoch K, Katoch VM, Bharadwaj VP: Enhancement in the histological diagnosis of indetermi-

nate leprosy by demonstration of mycobacterial antigens. Acta Leprol 1995;9:201–207.

187. Radhakrishnan VV, Mathai A, Radhakrishnan NS, et al: Immunohistochemical demonstration of mycobacterial antigens in intracranial tuberculoma. Indian J Exp Biol 1991;29:641–644.

188. Alcantara-Payawal DE, Matsumura M, Shiratori Y, et al: Direct detection of *Mycobacterium tuberculosis* using polymerase chain reaction assay among patients with hepatic granuloma. J Hepatol 1997;27:620–627.

189. Ghossein RA, Ross DG, Salomon RN, Rabson AR: Rapid detection and species identification of mycobacteria in paraffin-embedded tissues by polymerase chain reaction. Diagn Mol Pathol 1992;1:185–191.

190. Moatter T, Mirza S, Siddiqui MS, Soomro IN: Detection of *Mycobacterium tuberculosis* in paraffin embedded intestinal tissue specimens by polymerase chain reaction: Characterization of IS6110 element negative strains. JPMA J Pak Med Assoc 1998;48:174–178.

191. Frank TS, Cook SM: Analysis of paraffin sections of Crohn's disease for *Mycobacterium paratuberculosis* using polymerase chain reaction. Mod Pathol 1996; 9:32–35.

192. Hardman WJ, Benian GM, Howard T, et al: Rapid detection of mycobacteria in inflammatory necrotizing granulomas from formalin-fixed, paraffin-embedded tissue by PCR in clinically high-risk patients with acid-fast stain and culture-negative tissue biopsies. Am J Clin Pathol 1996;106:384–389.

193. Komiyama K, Horie N, Yoshimura M, et al: Rapid diagnosis of oral tuberculosis by amplification of *Mycobacterium* DNA from paraffin embedded specimens. J Oral Sci 1998;40:31–36.

194. Marchetti G, Gori A, Catozzi L, et al: Evaluation of PCR in detection of *Mycobacterium tuberculosis* from formalin-fixed, paraffin-embedded tissues: Comparison of four amplification assays. J Clin Microbiol 1998;36:1512–1517.

195. Nishimura M, Kwon KS, Shibuta K, et al: Methods in pathology: An improved method for DNA diagnosis of leprosy using formaldehyde-fixed, paraffin-embedded skin biopsies. Mod Pathol 1994;7:253–256.

196. Ozkara HA, Kocagoz T, Ozcelik U, et al: Comparison of three different primer pairs for the detection of *Mycobacterium tuberculosis* by polymerase chain reaction in paraffin-embedded tissues. Int J Tuberc Lung Dis 1998;2:451–455.

197. Perosio PM, Frank TS: Detection and species identification of mycobacteria in paraffin sections of lung biopsy specimens by the polymerase chain reaction. Am J Clin Pathol 1993;100:643–647.

198. Macon WR, Lo SC, Poiesz BJ, et al: Acquired immunodeficiency syndrome-like illness associated with systemic *Mycoplasma fermentans* infection in a human immunodeficiency virus–negative homosexual man. Hum Pathol 1993;24:554–558.

199. Chan PJ, Seraj IM, Kalugdan TH, King A: Prevalence of mycoplasma conserved DNA in malignant ovarian cancer detected using sensitive PCR-ELISA. Gynecol Oncol 1996;63:258–260.

200. Amin MB, Mezger E, Zarbo RJ: Detection of *Pneumocystis carinii:* Comparative study of monoclonal antibody and silver staining. Am J Clin Pathol 1992;98:13–18.

201. Travis WD, Pittaluga S, Lipschik GY, et al: Atypical pathologic manifestations of *Pneumocystis carinii* pneumonia in the acquired immune deficiency syndrome: Review of 123 lung biopsies from 76 patients with emphasis on cysts, vascular invasion, vasculitis, and granulomas. Am J Surg Pathol 1990;14:615–625.

202. Atzori C, Agostoni F, Angeli E, et al: *P. carinii* DNA detected by ITSs nested PCR in serum and PBMC of AIDS patients with PCP. J Eukaryot Microbiol 1996;43:42S.

203. Atzori C, Agostoni F, Angeli E, et al: Combined use of blood and oropharyngeal samples for noninvasive diagnosis of *Pneumocystis carinii* pneumonia using the polymerase chain reaction. Eur J Clin Microbiol Infect Dis 1998;17:241–246.

204. Lipschik GY, Gill VJ, Lundgren JD, et al: Improved diagnosis of *Pneumocystis carinii* infection by polymerase chain reaction on induced sputum and blood. Lancet 1992;340:203–206.

205. Wagner D, Koniger J, Kern WV, Kern P: Serum PCR of *Pneumocystis carinii* DNA in immunocompromised patients. Scand J Infect Dis 1997;29:159–164.

206. Conley FK, Jenkins KA, Remington JS: *Toxoplasma gondii* infection of the central nervous system: Use of the peroxidase-antiperoxidase method to demonstrate *Toxoplasma* in formalin-fixed, paraffin-embedded tissue sections. Hum Pathol 1981;12:690–698.

207. Ito M, Hara K, Saga S, et al: Two cases of acquired toxoplasmic lymphadenitis: Light and electron microscopic and immunohistochemical studies. Acta Pathol Jpn 1988;38:1565–1573.

208. Tsai MM, O'Leary TJ: Identification of *Toxoplasma gondii* in formalin-fixed, paraffin-embedded tissue by polymerase chain reaction. Mod Pathol 1993;6:185–188.

209. Lebech AM, Clemmensen O, Hansen K: Comparison of in vitro culture, immunohistochemical staining, and PCR for detection of *Borrelia burgdorferi* in tissue from experimentally infected animals. J Clin Microbiol 1995; 33:2328–2333.

210. Brettschneider S, Bruckbauer H, Klugbauer N, Hofmann H: Diagnostic value of PCR for detection of *Borrelia burgdorferi* in skin biopsy and urine samples from patients with skin borreliosis. J Clin Microbiol 1998;36:2658–2665.

211. Wienecke R, Neubert U, Volkenandt M: Molecular detection of *Borrelia burgdorferi* in formalin-fixed, paraffin-embedded lesions of Lyme disease. J Cutan Pathol 1993;20:385–388.

212. Hori S, Tsutsumi Y: Histological differentiation between chlamydial and bacterial epididymitis: Nondestructive and proliferative versus destructive and abscess forming immunohistochemical and clinicopathological findings. Hum Pathol 1995;26:402–407.

213. Scholte GH, van Doorn LJ, Quint WG, Lindeman J: Polymerase chain reaction for the detection of *Helicobacter pylori* in formaldehyde-sublimate fixed, paraffin-embedded gastric biopsies. Diagn Mol Pathol 1997; 6:238–243.

214. Suffin SC, Kaufmann AF, Whitaker B, et al: *Legionella pneumophila:* Identification in tissue sections by a new immunoenzymatic procedure. Arch Pathol Lab Med 1980;104:283–286.

215. Theaker JM, Tobin JO, Jones SE, et al: Immunohistological detection of *Legionella pneumophila* in lung sections. J Clin Pathol 1987;40:143–146.
216. Feldman RG, Law SM, Salisbury JR: Detection of group B streptococcal antigen in necropsy specimens using monoclonal antibody and immunoperoxidase staining. J Clin Pathol 1986;39:223–226.
217. Lee WS, Lee MG, Chung KY, Lee JB: Detection of *Treponema pallidum* in tissue: A comparative study of the avidin-biotin-peroxidase complex, indirect immunoperoxidase, FTA-ABS complement techniques and the darkfield method. Yonsei Med J 1991;32:335–341.
218. Beckett JH, Bigbee JW: Immunoperoxidase localization of *Treponema pallidum:* Its use in formaldehyde-fixed and paraffin-embedded tissue sections. Arch Pathol Lab Med 1979;103:135–138.
219. Genest DR, Choi-Hong SR, Tate JE, et al: Diagnosis of congenital syphilis from placental examination: Comparison of histopathology, Steiner stain, and polymerase chain reaction for *Treponema pallidum* DNA. Hum Pathol 1996;27:366–372.
220. Burstain JM, Grimprel E, Lukehart SA, et al: Sensitive detection of *Treponema pallidum* by using the polymerase chain reaction. J Clin Microbiol 1991;29: 62–69.
221. Odinot PT, Meis JF, Hoogkamp-Korstanje JA, Melchers WJ: In situ localisation of *Yersinia enterocolitica* by catalysed reported deposition signal amplification. J Clin Pathol 1998;51:444–449.
222. Verweij PE, Smedts F, Poot T, et al: Immunoperoxidase staining for identification of *Aspergillus* species in routinely processed tissue sections. J Clin Pathol 1996;49: 798–801.
223. Fukuzawa M, Inaba H, Hayama M, et al: Improved detection of medically important fungi by immunoperoxidase staining with polyclonal antibodies. Virchows Arch 1995;427:407–414.
224. Kobayashi K, Hayama M, Hotchi M: The application of immunoperoxidase staining for the detection of causative fungi in tissue specimens of mycosis: I. Mycopathologia 1988;102:107–113.
225. Reed JA, Hemann BA, Alexander JL, Brigati DJ: Immunomycology: Rapid and specific immunocytochemical identification of fungi in formalin-fixed, paraffin-embedded material. J Histochem Cytochem 1993;41: 1217–1221.
226. Monteagudo C, Marcilla A, Mormeneo S, et al: Specific immunohistochemical identification of *Candida albicans* in paraffin-embedded tissue with a new monoclonal antibody (1B12). Am J Clin Pathol 1995;103:130–135.
227. Makimura K, Murayama SY, Yamaguchi H: Detection of a wide range of medically important fungi by the polymerase chain reaction. J Med Microbiol 1994;40: 358–364.
228. Rappelli P, Are R, Casu G, et al: Development of a nested PCR for detection of *Cryptococcus neoformans* in cerebrospinal fluid. J Clin Microbiol 1998;36: 3438–3440.
229. Tanaka K, Miyazaki T, Maesaki S, et al: Detection of *Cryptococcus neoformans* gene in patients with pulmonary cryptococcosis. J Clin Microbiol 1996;34: 2826–2828.
230. Laxer MA, D'Nicuola ME, Patel RJ: Detection of *Cryptosporidium parvum* DNA in fixed, paraffin-embedded tissue by the polymerase chain reaction. Am J Trop Med Hyg 1992;47:450–455.
231. Hoffman EO, Miller MJ: Immunofluorescent staining of amebae in routine paraffin-embedded tissues. J Parasitol 1975;61:1104–1105.
232. Tsutsumi Y, Kawai K, Nagakura K: Use of patients' sera for immunoperoxidase demonstration of infectious agents in paraffin sections. Acta Pathol Jpn 1991;41: 673–679.
233. Ohnishi K, Murata M, Kojima H, et al: Brain abscess due to infection with *Entamoeba histolytica.* Am J Trop Med Hyg 1994;51:180–182.
234. Alexandrakis G, Sears M, Gloor P: Postmortem diagnosis of *Fusarium panophthalmitis* by the polymerase chain reaction. Am J Ophthalmol 1996;121:221–223.
235. Fleck SL, Hames SE, Warhurst DC: Detection of *Giardia* in human jejunum by the immunoperoxidase method: Specific and non-specific results. Trans R Soc Trop Med Hyg 1985;79:110–113.
236. Sydler T, Pospischil A, Gottstein B, Eckert J: Immunohistochemical labeling of *Giardia* trophozoites spp. in formalin fixed paraffin embedded tissues. Zentralbl Veterinarmed [B] 1991;38:135–141.
237. Kaufman L: Immunohistologic diagnosis of systemic mycoses: An update. Eur J Epidemiol 1992;8:377–382.
238. Collins MH, Jiang B, Croffie JM, et al: Hepatic granulomas in children: A clinicopathologic analysis of 23 cases including polymerase chain reaction for *Histoplasma.* Am J Surg Pathol 1996;20:332–338.
239. Esterre P, Guerret S, Ravisse P, et al: Immunohistochemical analysis of the mucosal lesion in mucocutaneous leishmaniasis. Parasite 1994;1:305–309.
240. Laskay T, Miko TL, Negesse Y, et al: Detection of cutaneous *Leishmania* infection in paraffin-embedded skin biopsies using the polymerase chain reaction. Trans R Soc Trop Med Hyg 1995;89:273–275.
241. Schubach A, Haddad F, Oliveira-Neto MP, et al: Detection of *Leishmania* DNA by polymerase chain reaction in scars of treated human patients. J Infect Dis 1998; 178:911–914.
242. Sattler F, Nichols L, Hirano L, et al: Nonspecific interstitial pneumonitis mimicking *Pneumocystis carinii* pneumonia. Am J Respir Crit Care Med 1997;156: 912–917.
243. Chen BX, Szabolcs MJ, Matsushima AY, Erlanger BF: A strategy for immunohistochemical signal enhancement by end-product amplification. J Histochem Cytochem 1996;44:819–824.
244. Brezin AP, Egwuagu CE, Burnier MJ, et al: Identification of *Toxoplasma gondii* in paraffin-embedded sections by the polymerase chain reaction. Am J Ophthalmol 1990;110:599–604.
245. Lin PR, Shaio MF, Liu JY: One-tube, nested-PCR assay for the detection of *Trichomonas vaginalis* in vaginal discharges. Ann Trop Med Parasitol 1997;91: 61–65.
246. Madico G, Quinn TC, Rompalo A, et al: Diagnosis of *Trichomonas vaginalis* infection by PCR using vaginal swab samples. J Clin Microbiol 1998;36: 3205–3210.

247. Shaio MF, Lin PR, Liu JY: Colorimetric one-tube nested PCR for detection of *Trichomonas vaginalis* in vaginal discharge. J Clin Microbiol 1997;35:132–138.
248. Takeuchi T, Kobayashi M, Moriki T, Miyoshi I: Application of a monoclonal antibody for the detection of *Trichosporon beigelii* in paraffin-embedded tissue sections. J Pathol 1988;156:23–27.
249. Kobayashi M, Kotani S, Fujishita M, et al: Immunohistochemical identification of *Trichosporon beigelii* in histologic section by immunoperoxidase method. Am J Clin Pathol 1988;89:100–105.
250. Chandler FW, Watts JC: Immunofluorescence as an adjunct to the histopathologic diagnosis of Chagas' disease. J Clin Microbiol 1988;26:567–569.
251. Jones EM, Colley DG, Tostes S, et al: Amplification of a *Trypanosoma cruzi* DNA sequence from inflammatory lesions in human chagasic cardiomyopathy. Am J Trop Med Hyg 1993;48:348–357.

CHAPTER 6 APPENDIX

SOP 6.1*

RT PCR-HEPATITIS C VIRUS (HCV) PCR/SOUTHERN BLOT PROCEDURE

PRINCIPLE

Hepatitis C, an RNA virus, must be identified after reverse transcriptase/polymerase chain reaction (RT-PCR) amplification because of the low viral load often present. To amplify the viral genomic sequences, viral RNA must first be converted to complementary DNA (cDNA) through an RT step. The subsequent cDNA may then be amplified in a standard PCR assay.

SPECIMEN (see SOP 1)

REAGENTS, SUPPLIES, AND EQUIPMENT

ALWAYS WEAR GLOVES WHEN HANDLING REAGENTS. FOLLOW PROCEDURES FOR AVOIDING CONTAMINATION OF PCR REACTIONS!! (See SOP 2)

The primers and a probe for the HCV genome were selected from published sequences (see Reference). HCV reverse transcriptase and PCR primers and all RT-PCR reagents, except $MgCl_2$, are stored in the RNA freezer in the PCR setup room. $MgCl_2$ is stored in the RNA refrigerator in the PCR setup area. RNA extracts and an HCV-positive control are kept in the −70°C freezer in the hall for long-term storage (more than 1 week). Extracts are kept in the RNA freezer for up to 1 week. Probes for HCV are kept in the freezer in the post-PCR room. Aliquots of reagents and standards are stored in microcentrifuge tubes (1.5 and 0.5 mL). Do not put unused aliquots back in tubes or containers. Throw them away.

The usual source of a reagent is indicated in brackets [ ]: Fisher [FI], PerkinElmer [PE], Promega [PR], etc. Homemade reagents are abbreviated [MDL] and have been quality control tested before use. An asterisk [*] is used when the source varies.

Cutting Blocks (see SOP 3)

RNA Extraction (see SOP 5)

RT-Polymerase Chain Reaction (RT-PCR)

Reagents

*SOPs 6.1, 6.2, 6.3, and 6.4, and 6.5 were written by Amy E. Krafft, Ph D, Department of Cellular Pathology and Genetics, Armed Forces Institute of Pathology. SOP 6.6 was written by Robert E. Cunningham, M S.

HPLC-grade water [FI]
First strand buffer (5X) [BRL]
DTT (0.1 mol/L) [BRL]
PCR buffer II (10X) [PE]
dNTP-2.5 mmol/L each [PR] [MDL]

1. To prepare, first make a 10-mmol/L solution from a 100-mmol/L stock (1:10 dilution) of each dNTP (dATP, dCTP, dGTP, and dTTP) as follows. To four microcentrifuge tubes, add 900 μL of water, then add 100 μL of dNTP (100 mmol/L). Mix well.
2. Next, mix equal volumes of each 10-mmol/L solution to make each dNTP 2.5 mmol/L in the final mix.
3. Aliquot and label tubes. Store in DNA freezer.

MMLV reverse transcriptase (200 U/μL) [BRL]
Taq polymerase (5 U/μL) [PE]
$MgCl_2$ (25 mmol/L) [PE]

Primers [MDL] [Research Genetics]

Primers are stored in the RNA freezer in a working dilution of 15 mol/L.

HCV RT PRIMER
5′-CCC AAC ACT ACT CGG CTA-3′

HCV PRIMER 1
5′-AGT CTT GCG GCC GCA CGC CCA AAT C-3′

HCV PRIMER 19
5′-GCC ATG GCG TTA GTA TGA GTG TCG TGC-3′

Master Mixes

Master mixes are used for this assay. Refer to SOP 13 for additional information on master mixes and their setup. The RT and PCR-RNA master mix used for HCV is different from that used for *BCR-ABL*, actin, DMV, and t(2;5) assays.

These master mixes do not contain primers or enzymes.

REVERSE TRANSCRIPTASE MASTER MIX

The volumes per 20-μL reaction with 5-μL sample are as follows:

4 μL 5X first strand buffer
2 μL DTT (0.01 mol/L)
1.6 μL dNTPs (200 mol/L final concentration in RT)
5.1 μL water

12.7 μL total volume per sample

One microliter of the HCV RT primer (15 mol/L working dilution, final concentration = 300 nmol/L) and 0.3 μL of MMLV-RT (1.2 U/reaction) is added to the RT master mix before use.

PCR-RNA MASTER MIX (UPPER MIX)

The volumes to prepare 30 μL of reaction mix are as follows:

3 μL 10X PCR buffer II
4.8 μL Mg^{2+} (3.6 mmol/L final concentration)
19.9 μL water

27.7 μL total volume per sample

One microliter of HCV primer 1 (15 mol/L), 1 μL of HCV primer 19 (15 mol/L), and 0.3 μL Taq polymerase (1.25 U/reaction) is added to the PCR-RNA master mix before use.

Supplies and Equipment
- Microcentrifuge tubes (1.5 and 0.5 mL)
- Aerosol-resistant pipette tips (ART tips)
- Disposable gloves
- Extra-fine-tip permanent marker and racks
- Pipetters
- Microcentrifuge (reserved for pre-PCR use only)
- PerkinElmer Thermal Cycler Model 9600
- Vortexer

Agarose Gel Electrophoresis (see SOP 6)

All reagents are in the post-PCR room. Use 2.5% agarose.

Southern Blotting of PCR Products (see SOP 9)

End-Labeling Oligonucleotide Probes (see SOP 6)

Oligo probes are stored in the post-PCR room freezer in a working dilution of 15 mol/L.

HCV OLIGO PROBE

5′-CCA TAG TGG TCT GCG GAA CCG GTG AGT ACA

Hybridization and Washing Southern Blots (see SOP 10)

Exposing and Developing Film (see SOP 11)

QUALITY CONTROL

Positive Assay Control

The positive control lysate is RNA prepared from a paraffin-embedded sample of HCV-infected tissue as described in SOP 5. Alternately, HCV RNA can be isolated from HCV-positive serum using the RNAzol method. The amplified HCV product is 169 bp.

Negative Assay Controls

WATER CONTROL. An RT-PCR reaction mix containing water as the sample tested is set up first in the RT-PCR run, before patient samples, to assess the purity of the reagents.

LYSATE CONTROL. A lysate (no RNA template) prepared in parallel to patient samples should give no detectable band, indicating that the tube was not contaminated with patient RNA during extraction.

CONTAMINATION CONTROL. A negative control PCR reaction containing water as the sample tested is also set up last in the PCR run, after the positive control. This reaction assesses the overall quality of the assay setup procedure in avoiding carryover contamination from a positive to an adjacent negative sample.

Assay Controls

Run positive control and negative controls along with patient samples.

Positive controls are tested at two concentrations: 1 μL of the 1:100 diluted extract and 5 μL of the 1:100 diluted extract.

A water control (5 μL water), 5 μL of lysate control (an empty tube that was treated with the same reagents used during the preparation of the patient RNA extracts), and a contamination control (5 μL water) at the end of each run serve as negative controls.

Patient samples are tested at one concentration: 5 μL of the undiluted extract.

The current master mix lot, containing all reaction components except RNA, enzymes, and HCV-specific primers, is prepared and tested in advance with positive and negative controls.

Amplification Control

A control gene must be tested to assess RNA integrity. β_2 microglobulin is used as the control gene to assess RNA integrity. The amplified product is 158 bp. See SOP 13.

PROCEDURE

FOLLOW PROCEDURES FOR AVOIDING CONTAMINATION OF PCR REACTIONS!! (See SOP 2)

Cutting Blocks (see SOP 3)

RNA Extraction (see SOP 5)

RT-Polymerase Chain Reaction (RT-PCR)

Use PerkinElmer Thermal Cycler Model 9600.

1. Determine the number of samples to be assayed (one dilution of each patient extract, a water control, at least one lysate control, and two positive controls). Prepare enough reagents for 2 additional assays; two plus the number of samples and controls = N. Remove the appropriate number of master mix aliquots for the setup. Aliquots of master mix are sufficient for 12 assays. Record the master mix lot numbers on the worksheet. The RT master mix is aliquotted with 13.7 μL per sample; the PCR-RNA master mix is aliquotted with 27.7 μL per sample. Calculate the amount of RT master mix needed by multiplying N × 13.7 μL. Calculate the amount of PCR-RNA master mix by multiplying N × 27.7 μL.
2. Number the side of each MicroAmp tube, consecutively, with an extra-fine-point permanent marker. Record assay number and identity of sample (MDL#, control) on worksheet.
3. Add 0.3 μL × N MMLV and 1 μL × N HCV RT primer to N × 13.7 μL of the RT master mix (0.3 μL + 1 μL + 13.7 μL = 15 μL). Tap tube gently to mix. Store on ice until use.
4. Add 0.3 μL × N Taq polymerase, 1 μL × N HCV primer 1, 1 μL × N of HCV primer 19 to N × 27.7 μL of the PCR master mix (0.3 μL + 1 μL + 1 μL + 27.7 μL = 30 μL). Tap tube gently to mix. Store the master mixes on ice until use.
5. Add 15 μL of RT master mix to each reaction tube. Cap tubes.

6. Add 5 μL of water to water control and 4 μL of water to the positive control that will contain 1 μL of extract.
7. Add 5 μL of the negative control lysate to the negative lysate control.
8. Add sample to each tube (5 μL of the undiluted extract). The final volume of the RT reaction is 20 μL.
9. After all samples have been added, add controls to appropriate tube. For the positive controls, add 1 μL and 5 μL of the 1:100 dilution of the HCV RNA lysate.
10. Add 5 μL of water to the contamination control.
11. Place in PerkinElmer Thermal Cycler Model 9600 and incubate at 37°C for 1 hour.
12. Remove tubes from thermal cycler and place in racks with at least one space between each tube.
13. Add 30 μL PCR-RNA master mix to each reaction tube. Cap tubes.
14. Place in PerkinElmer Thermal Cycler Model 9600 and cycle with times and temperatures below.

Initial step:	5 min 94°C
40 cycles of:	1 min 94°C
	1 min 55°C
	1 min 72°C
Final step:	5 min 72°C

15. Remove tube from thermal cycler and place in refrigerator in post-PCR room for analysis by gel electrophoresis.

Agarose Gel Electrophoresis (see SOP 6)

All reagents are in the post-PCR room. The 169-bp product is resolved on 2.5% agarose (2% LMP, 0.5% agarose) in 1X TBE.

Southern Blotting of PCR Products (see SOP 9)

End-Labeling Oligonucleotide Probes (see SOP 6)

Hybridization and Washing Southern Blots (see SOP 10)

1. Add 100 μL of ^{32}P-labeled probe to 5 mL of pre-warmed Hybrisol I.
2. Hybridize blot with probe for 4 hours at 42°C.
3. Wash 3× for 5 minutes at 42°C in 0.1X SSC and 0.1% SDS.

Exposing and Developing Film (see SOP 11)

REPORTING RESULTS

A positive result for HCV is repor ed if a positive signal is seen with the patient sample, provided all the appropriate controls are working. If not, repeat the assay.

If there is a positive signal for the actin gene and a negative signal for HCV, the HCV assay is reported as negative.

If there is a negative signal for the actin gene and a negative signal for HCV, the HCV assay is reported as indeterminate.

PROCEDURE NOTES

Avoid freeze/thawing the sample too often. The sample may be heated to 90°C before RT reaction.

REFERENCE

Bresters D, Cuypers HTM, Reesink HW, et al: Detection of hepatitis C viral RNA sequences in fresh and paraffin-embedded liver biopsy specimens of non-A, non-B, hepatitis patients. J Hepatol 1992;15:391–395.

SOP 6.2

PCR PROCEDURE: HERPES SIMPLEX VIRUS (HSV)

PRINCIPLE

A 118-bp segment of the thymidine kinase gene of HSV can be identified using the PCR and Southern blot hybridization with a ^{32}P-labeled HSV-1– or HSV-2– specific oligonucleotide probe.

SPECIMEN (see SOP 1)

REAGENTS, SUPPLIES, AND EQUIPMENT

ALWAYS WEAR GLOVES WHEN HANDLING REAGENTS. FOLLOW PROCEDURES FOR AVOIDING CONTAMINATION OF PCR REACTIONS!! (See SOP 2)

HSV primers and the HSV positive control are kept in the DNA freezer in the PCR setup room. HSV probes are in the post-PCR freezer. Aliquots of reagents and standards are stored in microcentrifuge tubes (1.5 and 0.5 mL). Do not put unused aliquots back in tubes or containers. Throw them away.

The usual source of a reagent is indicated in brackets [ ]: Fisher [FI], PerkinElmer [PE], Promega [PR], etc. Homemade reagents are abbreviated [MDL], and the lot number in use has been quality control tested. An asterisk [*] is used when the source varies.

Cutting Blocks (see SOP 3)

Preparation of DNA Lysates (see SOP 4)

Polymerase Chain Reaction (PCR)

Reagents

HPLC-grade water [FI]
PCR buffer II (10X) [PE]
dNTP 2.5 mmol/L each [PR] [MDL]

1. To prepare, first make a 10-mmol/L solution from a 100-mmol/L stock (1:10 dilution) of each dNTP (dATP, dCTP, dGTP, and dTTP) as follows. To prepare 1 mL of a 10-mmol/L solution of each dNTP, add 900 μL of water to four microcentrifuge tubes, then add 100 μL of each dNTP (100 mmol/L). Mix well.
2. Next, mix equal volumes of each 10-mmol/L solution to make each dNTP 2.5 mmol/L in the final mix.
3. Aliquot and label tubes. Store in DNA freezer.

Taq polymerase (5 U/μL) [PE]
$MgCl_2$ (25 mmol/L) [PE]

Primers

Primers are stored in the post-PCR room freezer in a working dilution of 5 mol/L.

HSV5 PRIMER

5′-TAC CCG AGC CGA TGA CTT AC-3′

HSV3 PRIMER

5′-GCG CTT GTC ATT ACC ACC GC-3′

Master Mix

Use a master mix. Refer to SOP 13 for additional information on master mixes and their setup. The same master mix is used for HSV, EBV, HIV, and *ERBB2* assays.

The volumes per 50-μL reaction with 5-μL sample are as follows:

5.0 μL	10X PCR buffer II
4.0 μL	dNTP Mix I (200 mol/L final concentration)
3.4 μL	25 mmol/L $MgCl_2$ (2.5 mmol/L final concentration)
30.3 μL	HPLC water
42.7 μL	total volume/sample

Add 0.3 μL × N Taq polymerase and 1 μL × N each of HSV 5 and HSV 3 immediately before use.

Supplies and Equipment

- Microcentrifuge tubes (1.5 and 0.5 mL)
- Aerosol-resistant pipette tips (ART tips)
- Disposable gloves
- Extra-fine-tip permanent marker and racks
- Pipetters
- Microcentrifuge (reserved for pre-PCR use only)
- PerkinElmer Thermal Cycler Model 9600
- Vortexer

Agarose Gel Electrophoresis (see SOP 6)

All reagents are in the post-PCR room. Use 2.5% agarose.

Southern Blotting of PCR Products (see SOP 9)

End-Labeling Oligonucleotide Probes (see SOP 6)

Oligo probes are stored in the post-PCR room freezer in a working dilution of 15 M (15 pmol/μL).

HSV-1 OLIGO PROBE

5′-CGA GAC AAT CGC GAA CAT CT-3′

HSV-2 OLIGO PROBE

5′-CGA GAC CCT GAC GAA CAT CT-3′

Hybridization and Washing Southern Blots (see SOP 10)

Exposing and Developing Film (see SOP 11)

QUALITY CONTROL

Several types of positive and negative controls are run with each assay as controls for test performance. The placement of the controls within an assay is crucial to the detection of contamination at each step in the test system.

Positive Assay Control

The HSV positive control is a lysate from a paraffin-embedded patient sample of herpes keratitis. The amplified HSV product is 118 bp. The amount of HSV template added per assay is at a level near the lower detection ability of the assay and at a level low enough so as not to serve as a source of crossover contamination.

Negative Assay Controls

A negative control is used to control for each step in the test system: lysate preparation, reagent mix preparation, and carryover contamination from sample to sample in the assay setup procedure.

WATER CONTROL. A PCR reaction mix containing water as the sample tested is set up as first in the PCR run, before patient samples, to assess the purity of the assay reagents.

LYSATE CONTROL. A lysate (no DNA template) prepared in parallel with patient samples should give no detectable band, indicating that the tube was not contaminated with DNA during lysate preparation.

CONTAMINATION CONTROL. A negative control PCR reaction containing water as the sample tested is also set up last in the PCR run, after the positive control. This reaction assesses the overall quality of the assay setup procedure in avoiding carryover contamination from a positive to an adjacent negative sample.

Assay Controls

Run positive control and negative controls along with patient samples. The positive control is tested at one concentration: 1 μL of the undiluted positive lysate.

A water control (5 μL of water) and 1 μL of lysate controls (an empty tube that was treated with the same reagents used during the preparation of the patient DNA lysates) serve as negative controls.

Patient samples are tested at three concentrations: 1 μL of a 1:5 dilution (1:5) of tissue lysate,1 μL of the undiluted lysate (1X), and 5 μL of the undiluted lysate (5X).

Amplification Control

Paraffin-embedded tissues may contain inhibitors of PCR or fixatives that severely compromise nucleic acid integrity. A control gene must be tested for each sample to assess whether amplifiable nucleic acid is present in the sample. If a gene rearrangement assay such as TCR or immunoglobulin heavy chain is not performed, an *ERBB2* assay must be set up. See SOP 13A. The *ERBB2* product is 241 bp.

The current master mix lot, containing all reaction components except DNA, Taq polymerase, and HSV-specific primers, is prepared and tested in advance with positive and negative controls.

PROCEDURE

FOLLOW PROCEDURES FOR AVOIDING CONTAMINATION OF PCR REACTIONS!! (See SOP 2)

Cutting Blocks (see SOP 3)

Preparation of DNA Lysates (see SOP 4)

Polymerase Chain Reaction (PCR)

Use PerkinElmer DNA Thermal Cycler Model 9600.

1. Determine the number of samples to be assayed (three dilutions of each patient lysate, a water control, one lysate control, one positive control, and one contamination control). Prepare enough reagents for 2 additional assays; two plus the number of samples and controls = N. Remove the appropriate number of master mix aliquots for the setup. Aliquots of master mix are sufficient for 12 assays. Record the master mix lot numbers on the worksheet. The master mix is aliquotted with 42.7 μL per reaction.
2. Number the top of each 0.5-mL microcentrifuge reaction tube, consecutively, with an extra-fine-point permanent marker. Record assay number and identity of sample (MDL#, control) on worksheet.
3. Add 42.7 μL × N of the master mix to a labeled 1.5-mL tube. Use a larger tube for total volumes of 1.5 mL. Add 0.3 μL × N Taq polymerase, 1 μL × N of HSV, and 1 μL × N of HSV to the master mix (0.3 μL + 1 μL + 1 μL + 42.7 μL = 45 μL). For total volumes less than 0.5 mL, tap tube gently to mix. For total volumes greater than 0.5 mL, invert tube. Store on ice until use.
4. Add master mix to each reaction tube (45 μL). Cap tubes.
5. Add 5 μL of water to water control, 4 μL of water to 1:5 tubes and 1X tubes, to give a combined volume of water and patient sample equal to 5 μL.
6. Add 1 μL of the negative control lysate (without DNA template) to the negative lysate control tube.
7. Make dilutions of patient samples and add 1 μL of a 1:5 dilution to the 1:5 tube. Add 1 μL of the undiluted lysate to the 1X tube. Add 5 μL of the undiluted lysate to the 5X tube.
8. Add positive control lysate to appropriate tubes after all samples have been prepared: 1 μL of an undiluted positive lysate. The setup order is (a) water, (b) lysate control, (c) patient samples, (d) positive controls, and (e) contamination control.
9. Add 5 μL of water to the contamination control.
10. Place in PerkinElmer Thermal Model 9600 and cycle with times and temperatures below:

Initial step:	5 min 94°C
40 cycles of:	1 min 94°C
	1 min 55°C
	1 min 72°C
Final step:	7 min 72°C

11. Remove sample tray from thermal cycler and place tubes in rack in refrigerator in post-PCR room for analysis by gel electrophoresis.

Agarose Gel Electrophoresis (see SOP 6)

The 118-bp product is resolved on 2.5% agarose (2% low melting point (LMP), 0.5% agarose) in 1X TBE.

Southern Blotting (see SOP 9)

End-Labeling Oligonucleotide Probes (see SOP 6)

Hybridization and Washing Southern Blots (see SOP 10)

1. Add 100 μL of ^{32}P-labeled probe to 5 mL of pre-warmed Hybrisol I.
2. Hybridize blot with probe for 4 hours at 42°C.
3. Wash 3× for 5 minutes at 42°C with room temperature-equilibrated 0.1X SSC and 0.1% SDS.

Exposing and Developing Film (see SOP 11)

REPORTING RESULTS

A positive result for HSV is reported if a positive signal is seen in at least two of three dilutions.

If there is a positive signal in only one of three dilutions, repeat the assay. A negative result for the HSV is reported if no signal is seen in at least two of three dilutions of the repeated assay.

The assay for HSV is indeterminate if the HSV assay is negative and the *ERBB2* gene is nonamplifiable.

REFERENCE

Cockerham GC, Krafft AE, McLean IW: Herpes simplex virus in primary graft failure. Arch Ophthalmol 1997;115:586–589. Reprinted in Wilson RP (ed): The Year Book of Ophthalmology. St. Louis, CV Mosby, 1998.

SOP 6.3

PCR PROCEDURE: VARICELLA ZOSTER VIRUS (VZV)

PRINCIPLE

A conserved region of the varicella-zoster genome is amplified. The 230-bp product is detected by Southern blot hybridization with a ^{32}P-labeled probe.

SPECIMEN (see SOP 1)

REAGENTS, SUPPLIES, AND EQUIPMENT

ALWAYS WEAR GLOVES WHEN HANDLING REAGENTS. FOLLOW PROCEDURES FOR AVOIDING CONTAMINATION OF PCR REACTIONS!! (See SOP 2)

VZV primers and the VZV positive control are kept in the DNA freezer in the pre-PCR room. VZV probes are in the post-PCR −20°C freezer. Aliquots of reagents and standards are stored in Eppendorf tubes (1.5 and 0.5 mL). Do not put unused aliquots back in tubes or containers. Throw them away.

The usual source of a reagent is indicated in brackets [ ]: Fisher [FI], PerkinElmer [PE], Promega [PR], etc. Homemade reagents are abbreviated [MDL] and have been quality control tested before use. An [*] is used when the source varies.

Cutting Blocks (see SOP 3)

Preparation of DNA Lysotes (see SOP 4)

Polymerase Chain Reaction (PCR)

Extracts and most PCR reagents are stored at −20°C in the pre-PCR DNA freezer. Mg^{2+} is stored at 4°C in the pre-PCR RNA refrigerator.

Reagents

HPLC-grade water [FI]

PCR buffer II (10X) [PE]

dNTP (Mix I) 2.5 mmol/L each [PR]

1. First, make a 10-mmol/L solution from a 100-mmol/L stock of each dNTP (dATP, dCTP, dGTP, and dTTP). Add 900 μL of water and 100 μL of dNTP (100 mmol/L) to an Eppendorf tube and mix well.
2. Next, mix equal volumes of each 10-mmol/L solution to make each dNTP 2.5 mmol/L in the final mix.

Taq polymerase (5 U/μL) [PE]

Do not add Taq to master mix and freeze. Add Taq to master mix immediately before use.

$MgCl_2$ (25 mmol/L) [PE]

Primers

Primers are stored at $-20°C$ in a stock concentration of 5 mol/L.

PRIMER 1

5′-CGT CAC ATA TTA TGC AAA CAT G-3′

PRIMER 2

5′-GT TTT TAA TAT TAC AAA TCC CGC-3′

Master Mix

N = the number of samples and controls plus two.

Multiply each volume by (N) to determine the volume of each reagent.

The volumes per 50-μL reaction with 5-μL sample are as follows:

5.0 μL	10× PCR buffer II [PE]
4.0 μL	dNTP mix I (200 μmol/L final concentration) [PR]
5.4 μL	25 mmol/L $MgCl_2$ (2.7 mmol/L final concentration) [PE]
1.0 μL	primer 1 (5 mol/L)
1.0 μL	primer 2 (5 mol/L)
28.3 μL	HPLC water [FI]
44.7 μL	total volume/sample

For sample volumes other than 5 μL, adjust the volume of water accordingly.

Add 0.3 μL × N Taq polymerase immediately before use.

Master mixes are prepared in batches and stored at $-20°C$. Stored batches are quality control tested before use.

Supplies and Equipment

Microcentrifuge tubes (1.5 and 0.5 mL)

Aerosol-resistant pipette tips (ART tips)

Disposable gloves

Permanent marker and racks

Pipetters

Microcentrifuge (reserved for pre-PCR use only)

PerkinElmer Thermal Cycler Model 9600

Agarose Gel Electrophoresis

All reagents are in the post-PCR room. The 230-bp product is resolved on 2.5% agarose (2% LMP, 0.5% agarose) in 1X TBE.

Southern Blotting (see SOP 9)

End-Labeling Oligonucleotide Probes (see SOP 6)

Oligos for probes are stored in the post-PCR room $-20°C$ freezer in a stock concentration of 15 mol/L.

VZV OLIGO PROBE

5′-CTT CTG CGC ACA ATC CCA CAG AGG CTT CGG CTT CAG TTT-3′

Hybridization and Washing Southern Blots (see SOP 10)

1. Hybridize blot with probe for 4 hours at 42°C.
2. Wash 3× for 5 minutes at room temperature in 0.1X SSC and 0.1 SDS.

Exposing and Developing Film (see SOP 11)

QUALITY CONTROL

Preparation of Controls

Prepare 100 μL of a VZV positive control lysate from a paraffin-embedded tissue sample of VZV-infected cells as described in SOP 4.

The amplified VZV product is 230 bp.

Negative Controls

A mock PCR reaction mix containing all reagents except the template (water control) is run with each batch of patient samples to assess the purity of the reagents. A lysate (no DNA template) prepared alongside patient samples should give no detectable band, indicating that the tube was not contaminated with patient DNA during extraction.

ERBB2 is used as a control to assess DNA integrity. The amplified *ERBB2* product is 241 bp.

Assay Controls

Run positive control and negative controls along with patient samples.

Patient samples are loaded at three concentrations: 1μL of a 1:5 dilution, 1 μL of the undiluted extract (1X), and 5 μL of the undiluted extract (5X).

A tube with all reagents and 1 μL of lysate controls (an empty tube that was treated with the same reagents used during the preparation of the patient DNA extracts) serve as negative controls.

Stored master mixes, containing all reaction components except DNA and Taq polymerase, are prepared and tested in advance with positive and negative controls. Taq polymerase should not be frozen; thus, it is added fresh before each assay. Unused portions of master mix aliquots are discarded.

PROCEDURE

FOLLOW PROCEDURES FOR AVOIDING CONTAMINATION OF PCR REACTIONS!! (See SOP 2)

Cutting Blocks (see SOP 3)

DNA Extraction (see SOP 4)

Polymerase Chain Reaction (PCR)

Use PerkinElmer Thermal Cycler Model 9600.

1. Determine the number (N) of samples to be assayed (three dilutions of each patient extract, a water control, at least one lysate control, and a positive control). To ensure an adequate volume of master mix for the batch, add enough reagents for two additional assays (N + 2).
2. Number the sides of each MicroAmp tube, consecutively, with an extra-fine-point permanent marker. Record assay number and identity of sample (e.g., MDL#, control) on worksheet.
3. Add water to tubes to give a combined volume of water + sample equal to 5 μL
4. Add 0.3 μL Taq polymerase to 44.7 μL master mix. Tap tube gently to mix.
5. Add master mix to each reaction tube (45 μL). Cap tubes.
6. Add sample to each tube (1 μL of a 1:5 dilution, 1 μL of the undiluted extract (1X), and 5 μL of the undiluted extract (5X).
7. Add controls to appropriate tube. For the positive controls, add 1 μL and 5 μL of the VZV DNA lysate. For the negative controls, add 5 μL of water to water control and 1 μL of the lysate without DNA template and 4 μL water to the lysate control.
8. Place in PerkinElmer Thermal Cycler Model 9600 and cycle with times and temperatures below.

Initial step:	5 min 94°C
40 cycles of:	1 min 94°C
	1 min 55°C
	1 min 72°C
Final step:	7 min 72°C

9. Remove tube from thermal cycler and place in refrigerator in post-PCR room for analysis by gel electrophoresis.

Agarose Gel Electrophoresis (see SOP 6)

All reagents are in the post-PCR room. The 230-bp product is resolved on 2.5% low-melting point agarose in 1X TBE.

Southern Blotting (see SOP 9)

End-Labeling Oligonucleotide Probes (see SOP 6)

Hybridization and Washing Southern Blots (see SOP 10)

1. Add 100 μL of ^{32}P-labeled probe to 5 mL of pre-warmed Hybrisol I.
2. Hybridize blot with probe for 4 hours at 42°C.
3. Wash 3× for 5 minutes at room temperature in 0.1X SSC and 0.1 SDS.

Exposing and Developing Film (see SOP 11)

REPORTING RESULTS

A positive result for the VZV is reported if a positive signal is seen in at least two of three dilutions. If there is a positive signal in only one of three dilutions, repeat the assay.

A negative result for the VZV is reported if no signal is seen in at least two of three dilutions of the repeated assay.

The assay for VZV is indeterminate if the VZV assay is negative and the *HER2* gene is nonamplifiable.

Rarely, the assay for VZV is positive whereas the *ERBB2* assay is negative. If the *ERBB2* assay controls worked appropriately, the VZV assay is reported as positive.

REFERENCE

Kido S, Ozaki T, Asada H, et al: Detection of varicella-zoster virus (VZV) DNA in clinical samples from patients with VZV by the polymerase chain reaction. J Clin Microbiol 1991; 29:76–79.

SOP 6.4

PCR PROCEDURE: EPSTEIN-BARR VIRUS (EBV)

PRINCIPLE

A 240-bp segment of the IR3 region of EBV can be identified using the PCR and Southern blot hybridization with a ^{32}P-labeled EBV-specific oligonucleotide probe.

SPECIMEN (see SOP 1)

REAGENTS, SUPPLIES, AND EQUIPMENT

ALWAYS WEAR GLOVES WHEN HANDLING REAGENTS. FOLLOW PROCEDURES FOR AVOIDING CONTAMINATION OF PCR REACTIONS!! (See SOP 2)

EBV primers and the EBV positive control are kept in the DNA freezer in the PCR setup room. EBV probes are in the post-PCR freezer. Aliquots of reagents and standards are stored in microcentrifuge tubes (1.5 and 0.5 mL). Do not put unused aliquots back in tubes or containers. Throw them away.

The usual source of a reagent is indicated in brackets [ ]: Fisher [FI], PerkinElmer [PE], Promega [PR], etc. Homemade reagents are abbreviated [MDL], and the lot number in use has been quality control tested. An asterisk [*] is used when the source varies.

Cutting Blocks (see SOP 3)

Preparation of DNA Lysates (see SOP 4)

Polymerase Chain Reaction (PCR)

Reagents

HPLC-grade water [FI]

PCR buffer II (10X) [PE]

dNTP 2.5 mmol/L each [PR] [MDL]

1. To prepare, first make a 10-mmol/L solution from a 100-mmol/L stock (1:10 dilution) of each dNTP (dATP, dCTP, dGTP, and dTTP) as follows. To prepare 1 mL of a 10-mmol/L solution of each dNTP, add 900 μL of water to four microcentrifuge tubes, then add 100 μL of each dNTP (100 mmol/L). Mix well.

2. Next, mix equal volumes of each 10-mmol/L solution to make each dNTP 2.5 mmol/L in the final mix.
3. Aliquot and label tubes. Store in DNA freezer.

Taq polymerase (5 U/μL) [PE]
$MgCl_2$ (25 mmol/L) [PE]

Primers

Primers are stored in the post-PCR room freezer in a working dilution of 5 mol/L.

EBV-1 SENSE PRIMER 1
5′-GAC GAG GGG CCA GGT ACA GG-3′

EBV-2 ANTISENSE PRIMER 2
5′-CA GCC AAT GCT TCT TGG ACG TTT TTG G-3′

Master Mix

Use a master mix. Refer to SOP 13 for additional information on master mixes and their setup. The same master mix is used for EBV, HIV, and HER2 assays.

The volumes per 50-μL reaction with 5-μL sample are as follows:

5.0 μL	10X PCR buffer II
4.0 μL	dNTP mix I (200 mol/L final concentration)
3.4 μL	25 mmol/L $MgCl_2$ (2.5 mmol/L final concentration)
30.3 μL	N HPLC water
42.7 μL	total volume/sample

Add 0.3 μL × N Taq polymerase and 1 μL × N each of EBV 1 and EBV 2 immediately before use.

Supplies and Equipment

Microcentrifuge tubes (1.5 and 0.5 mL)
Aerosol-resistant pipette tips (ART tips)
Disposable gloves
Extra-fine-tip permanent marker and racks
Pipetters
Microcentrifuge (reserved for pre-PCR use only)
PerkinElmer Thermal Cycler Model 9600
Vortexer

Agarose Gel Electrophoresis (see SOP 6)

All reagents are in the post-PCR room. Use 2.5% agarose.

Southern Blotting of PCR Products (see SOP 9)

End-Labeling Oligonucleotide Probes (see SOP 6)

Oligo probes are stored in the post-PCR room freezer in a working dilution of 15 mol/L (15 pmol/μL).

EBV OLIGO PROBE
5′-CGT CCT CGT CCT CTT CCC CGT CCA CGT CCA TGG TTA TCA CC-3′

Hybridization and Washing Southern Blots (see SOP 10)

Exposing and Developing Film (see SOP 11)

QUALITY CONTROL

Several types of positive and negative controls are run with each assay as controls for test performance. The placement of the controls within an assay is crucial to the detection of contamination at each step in the test system.

Positive Assay Control

The EBV positive control is a lysate from a paraffin-embedded sample of an EBV-containing Burkitt's lymphoma cell line (Raji).

The amplified EBV product is 240 bp. The amount of EBV template added per assay is at a level near the lower detection ability of the assay and at a level low enough so as not to serve as a source of cross-over contamination.

Negative Assay Controls

A negative control is used to control for each step in the test system: lysate preparation, reagent mix preparation, and carryover contamination from sample to sample in the assay setup procedure.

WATER CONTROL. A PCR reaction mix containing water as the sample tested is set up as first in the PCR run, before patient samples, to assess the purity of the assay reagents.

LYSATE CONTROL. A lysate (no DNA template) prepared in parallel with patient samples should give no detectable band, indicating that the tube was not contaminated with DNA during lysate preparation.

CONTAMINATION CONTROL. A negative control PCR reaction containing water as the sample tested is also set up last in the PCR run, after the positive control. This reaction assesses the overall quality of the assay setup procedure in avoiding carryover contamination from a positive to an adjacent negative sample.

Assay Controls

Run positive control and negative controls along with patient samples.

The positive control is tested at one concentration: 1 μL of the undiluted Raji cell lysate.

A water control (5 μL water) and 1 μL of lysate controls (an empty tube that was treated with the same reagents used during the preparation of the patient DNA lysates) serve as negative controls.

Patient samples are tested at three concentrations: 1 μL of a 1:5 dilution (1:5) of tissue lysate,1 μL of the undiluted lysate (1X), and 5 μL of the undiluted lysate (5X).

Amplification Control

Paraffin-embedded tissues may contain inhibitors of PCR or fixatives that severely compromise nucleic acid integrity. A control gene must be tested for each sample to assess whether amplifiable nucleic acid is present in the sample. If a gene rearrangement assay such as TCR or heavy chain is not performed, a *ERBB2* assay must be set up. See SOP 13. The *ERBB2* product is 241 bp.

The current master mix lot, containing all reaction components except DNA, Taq polymerase, and EBV-specific primers, is prepared and tested in advance with positive and negative controls.

PROCEDURE

FOLLOW PROCEDURES FOR AVOIDING CONTAMINATION OF PCR REACTIONS!! (See SOP 2)

Cutting Blocks (see SOP 3)

Preparation of DNA Lysates (see SOP 4)

Polymerase Chain Reaction (PCR)

Use PerkinElmer DNA Thermal Cycler Model 9600.

1. Determine the number of samples to be assayed (three dilutions of each patient lysate, a water control, one lysate control, one positive control, and one contamination control). Prepare enough reagents for 2 additional assays; two plus the number of samples and controls = N. Remove the appropriate number of master mix aliquots for the setup. Aliquots of master mix are sufficient for 12 assays. Record the master mix lot numbers on the worksheet. The master mix is aliquotted with 42.7 μL/reaction.
2. Number the top of each 0.5-mL microcentrifuge reaction tube, consecutively, with an extra-fine-point permanent marker. Record assay number and identity of sample (MDL#, control) on worksheet.
3. Add 42.7 μL × N of the master mix to a labeled 1.5-mL tube. Use a larger tube for total volumes greater than 1.5 mL. Add 0.3 μL × N Taq polymerase, 1 μL × N of EBV-1, and 1 μL × N of EBV-2 to the master mix (0.3 μL + 1 μL + 1 μL + 42.7 μL = 45 μL). For total volumes less than 0.5 mL, tap tube gently to mix. For total volumes greater than 0.5 mL, invert. Store on ice until use.
4. Add master mix to each reaction tube (45 μL). Cap tubes.
5. Add 5 μL of water to water control, 4 μL of water to 1:5 tubes and 1X tubes to give a combined volume of water and patient sample equal to 5 μL.
6. Add 1 μL of the negative control lysate (without DNA template) to the negative lysate control tube.
7. Make dilutions of patient samples and add 1 μL of a 1:5 dilution to the 1:5 tube. Add 1 μL of the undiluted lysate to the 1× tube. Add 5 μL of the undiluted lysate to the 5X tube.
8. Add positive control lysate to appropriate tubes after all samples have been prepared: 1 μL of an undiluted Raji cell lysate. The setup order is (a) water, (b) lysate control, (c) patient samples, (d) positive controls, and (e) contamination control.
9. Add 5 μL water to the contamination control.
10. Place in PerkinElmer Thermal Cycler Model 9600 and cycle with times and temperatures below:

Initial step:	5 min 94°C
40 cycles of:	1 min 94°C
	1 min 55°C
	1 min 72°C
Final step:	7 min 72°C

11. Remove sample tray from thermal cycler and place tubes in rack in refrigerator in post-PCR room for analysis by gel electrophoresis.

Agarose Gel Electrophoresis (see SOP 6)

The 240-bp product is resolved on 2.5% agarose (2% LMP, 0.5% agarose) in 1X TBE.

Southern Blotting (see SOP 9)

End-Labeling Oligonucleotide Probes (see SOP 6)

Hybridization and Washing Southern Blots (see SOP 10)

1. Add 100 μL of ^{32}P-labeled probe to 5 mL of pre-warmed Hybrisol I.
2. Hybridize blot with probe for 4 hours at 42°C.
3. Wash 3× for 5 minutes at 42°C with room temperature-equilibrated 0.1X SSC and 0.1% SDS.

Exposing and Developing Film (see SOP 11)

REPORTING RESULTS

A positive result for EBV is reported if a positive signal is seen in at least two of three dilutions. If there is a positive signal in only one of three dilutions, repeat the assay.

A negative result for EBV is reported if no signal is seen in at least two of three dilutions of the repeated assay.

The assay for EBV is indeterminate if the EBV assay is negative and the *ERBB2* gene is nonamplifiable.

REFERENCE

Wright CF, Reid AH, Tsai MM, et al: Detection of Epstein-Barr virus sequences in Hodgkin's disease by the polymerase chain reaction. Am J Pathol 1991;139:393–397.

SOP 6.5

PCR PROCEDURE: HUMAN IMMUNO DEFICIENCY VIRUS (HIV)

PRINCIPLE

PCR is used to amplify the *gag* region of the HIV-1 genome with primer pair SK 38 and SK 39. The 114-bp product is detected by Southern blot hybridization with a ^{32}P-labeled probe (SK 19).

SPECIMEN (see SOP 1)

REAGENTS, SUPPLIES, AND EQUIPMENT

ALWAYS WEAR GLOVES WHEN HANDLING REAGENTS. FOLLOW PROCEDURES FOR AVOIDING CONTAMINATION OF PCR REACTIONS!! (See SOP 2)

The primers for the *gag* region of HIV-1 are kept in the DNA freezer in the pre-PCR room. The HIV-1 probe is in the post-PCR −20°C freezer. Aliquots of reagents and standards are stored in Eppendorf tubes (1.5 and 0.5 mL). Do not put unused aliquots back in tubes or containers. Throw them away.

The usual source of a reagent is indicated in brackets [ ]: Fisher [FI], PerkinElmer [PE], Promega [PR], etc. Homemade reagents are abbreviated [MDL] and have been quality control tested before use. An [*] is used when the source varies.

Cutting Blocks (see SOP 3)

DNA Extraction (see SOP 4)

Polymerase Chain Reaction (PCR)

Extracts and most PCR reagents are stored at −20°C in the pre-PCR DNA freezer. Mg^{2+} is stored at 4°C in the pre-PCR RNA refrigerator.

Reagents

HPLC-grade water [FI]
PCR buffer II (10X) [PE]
dNTP (Mix I) 2.5 mmol/L each [PR]

1. First, make a 10-mmol/L solution from a 100-mmol/L stock of each dNTP (dATP, dCTP, dGTP, and dTTP). Add 900 μL of water and 100 μL of dNTP (100 mmol/L) to an Eppendorf tube and mix well.
2. Next, mix equal volumes of each 10 mmol/L solution to make each dNTP 2.5 mmol/L in the final mix.

Taq polymerase (5 U/μL) [PE]

Do not add Taq to master mix and freeze. Add Taq to master mix immediately before use.

$MgCl_2$ (25 mmol/L) [PE]

HIV Primers

Primers are stored at −20°C in a stock concentration of 5 mol/L.

SK 38-*gag* 1551–1578

5′ATA ATC CAC CTA TCC CAG TAG GAG AAA T-3′

SK 39-*gag* 1638–1665

5′TTT GGT CCT TGT CTT ATG TCC AGA ATG C-3′

Master Mix

NOTE: The same master mix is used for HIV, EBV, and *ERBB2* assays.

N = the number of samples and controls plus two.

Multiply each volume by N to determine the volume of each reagent.

The volumes per 5-μL reaction with 5-μL sample are as follows:

5.0 μL × N	10X PCR buffer (PE II)
4.0 μL × N	dNTP Mix I (200 mol/L final concentration) [PR]
3.4 μL × N	25 mmol/L $MgCl_2$ (2.5 mmol/L final concentration) [PE]
30.3 μL × N	HPLC water [FI]
42.7 μL	total volume/sample

For sample volumes other than 5 μL, adjust the volume of water accordingly.

Add 0.3 μL × N Taq polymerase and 1 μL each of SK 38 and SK 39 immediately before use.

Master mixes are prepared in batches and stored at −20°C. Stored batches are quality control tested before use.

Supplies and Equipment

Microcentrifuge tubes (1.5 and 0.5 mL)
Aerosol-resistant pipette tips (ART tips)
Disposable gloves
Permanent marker and racks
Pipetters
Microcentrifuge (reserved for pre-PCR use only)
PerkinElmer Thermal Cycler Model 9600

Agarose Gel Electrophoresis

All reagents are in the post-PCR room. The 114-bp product is resolved on 2.5% agarose (2% LMP, 0.5% agarose) in 1X TBE.

Southern Blotting (see SOP 9)

End-Labeling Oligonucleotide Probes (see SOP 6)

Oligos for probes are stored in the post-PCR room −20°C freezer in a stock concentration of 15 mol/L.

HIV PROBE: SK 19 *gag* 1595–1635

5′-ATC CTG GGA TTA AAT AAA ATA GTA AGA ATG TAT AGC CCT AC-3′

Hybridization and Washing Southern Blots (see SOP 10)

1. Hybridize blot with probe for 4 hours at 42°C.
2. Wash 3× for 5 minutes at room temperature in 0.1X SSC and 0.1 SDS.

Exposing and Developing Film (see SOP 11)

QUALITY CONTROL

Preparation of Controls

Prepare a 100-μL DNA lysate of an HIV positive control cell line 8E5 as described in SOP 4.

The amplified HIV product is 114 bp.

Negative Controls

A mock PCR reaction mix containing all reagents except the template (water control) is run with each batch of patient samples to assess the purity of the reagents. A lysate (no DNA template) prepared alongside patient samples should give no detectable band, indicating that the tube was not contaminated with patient DNA during extraction.

ERBB2 is used as a control to assess DNA integrity. The amplified *ERBB2* product is 241 bp.

Assay Controls

Run positive control and negative controls along with patient samples.

Patient samples are loaded at three concentrations: 1 μL of a 1:5 dilution, 1 μL of the undiluted extract (1X), and 5 μL of the undiluted extract (5X).

A tube with all reagents and 1 μL of lysate controls (an empty tube that was treated with the same reagents used during the preparation of the patient DNA extracts) serves as a negative control.

Stored master mixes, containing all reaction components except DNA, Taq polymerase, and HIV-specific primers, are prepared and tested in advance with positive and negative controls. Taq polymerase should not be frozen; thus, it is added fresh before each assay. Unused portion of master mix aliquots are discarded.

PROCEDURE

FOLLOW PROCEDURES FOR AVOIDING CONTAMINATION OF PCR REACTIONS!! (See SOP 2)

Cutting Blocks (see SOP 3)

DNA Extraction (see SOP 4)

Polymerase Chain Reaction (PCR)

Use PerkinElmer Thermal Cycler Model 9600.

1. Determine the number (N) of samples to be assayed (three dilutions of each patient extract, a water control, at least one lysate control, and a positive control). To ensure an adequate volume of master mix for the batch, add enough reagents for 2 additional assays (N + 2).
2. Number the side of each MicroAmp tube, consecutively, with an extra-fine-point permanent marker. Record assay number and identity of sample (e.g., MDL#, control) on worksheet.
3. Add water to tubes to give a combined volume of water + sample equal to 5 μL.
4. Add 0.3 μL Taq polymerase, 1 μL of SK 38 primer, and 1 μL of SK 39 primer to 42.7 μL master mix. Tap tube gently to mix.
5. Add master mix to each reaction tube (45 μL). Cap tubes.
6. Add sample to each tube (1 μL of a 1:5 dilution, 1 μL of the undiluted extract [1X], and 5 μL of the undiluted extract [5X]).
7. Add controls to appropriate tube. For the positive controls, add 1 μL of a 1:100 dilution (1X) and 5 μL of the 1:100 dilution (5X) of the 8E5 cell line lysate. For the negative controls add 5 μL of water to water control and 1 μL of the lysate without DNA template and 4 μL water to the lysate control.
8. Place in PerkinElmer Thermal Cycler Model 9600 and cycle with times and temperatures below:

Initial step:	5 min 94°C
40 cycles of:	1 min 94°C
	1 min 55°C
	1 min 72°C
Final step:	7 min 72°C

9. Remove tube from thermal cycler and place in refrigerator in post-PCR room for analysis by gel electrophoresis.

Agarose Gel Electrophoresis (see SOP 6)

All reagents are in the post-PCR room. The 114-bp product is resolved on 2.5% agarose (2% low-melting point, 0.5% agarose) in 1X TBE.

Southern Blotting (see SOP 9)

End-Labeling Oligonucleotide Probes (see SOP 6)

Hybridization and Washing Southern Blots (see SOP 10)

1. Add 100 μL of ^{32}P-labeled probe to 5 mL of pre-warmed Hybrisol I.
2. Hybridize blot with probe for 4 hours at 42°C.
3. Wash 3× for 5 minutes at room temperature in 0.1X SSC and 0.1 SDS.

Exposing and Developing Film (see SOP 11)

REPORTING RESULTS

A positive result for HIV is reported if a positive signal is seen in at least two of three dilutions.

If there is a positive signal in only one of three dilutions, repeat the assay. A negative result for HIV is reported if no signal is seen in at least two of three dilutions of the repeated assay.

The assay for HIV is indeterminate if the HIV assay is negative and the *ERBB2* gene is nonamplifiable.

Rarely, the assay for HIV is positive whereas the *ERBB2* assay is negative. If the *ERBB2* assay controls worked appropriately, the HIV assay is reported as positive.

REFERENCES

Folks TM, Powell D, et al: Biological and biochemical characterization of a cloned LEU-3-cell surviving infection with the acquired immune deficiency syndrome retrovirus. J Exp Med 1986;164:280–290.

Ou CY, Kwok S, et al: DNA amplification for direct detection of HIV-1 in DNA of peripheral blood mononuclear cells. Science 1988;239:295–297.

SOP 6.6

IN SITU HYBRIDIZATION PROCEDURE FOR JC VIRUS

PRINCIPLE

In situ hybridization of viral DNA is used to identify JC virus genome within tissue sections. DNA within the tissue is denatured by incubation at a high temperature, then biotinylated probe that is specific for the JC virus is allowed to hybridize. Probe that is not bound to the tissue section is washed off; bound probe is detected by a modified ABC method.

SPECIMEN

Specimens are 4- to 6-μm sections of formalin-fixed, paraffin-embedded tissue that have been placed on coated glass microscope slides. Two slides are required at a minimum.

REAGENTS, SUPPLIES, AND EQUIPMENT

ALWAYS WEAR GLOVES WHEN HANDLING REAGENTS.

Xylene, reagent grade
Absolute ethanol, nondenatured, reagent grade
95% Ethanol (in distilled, deionized water)

Proteinase K, 0.25 mg/mL in PBSE (see SOP 15)
0.3% Hydrogen peroxide in PBSE (see SOP 16)
PBSE, pH 7.4 (see SOP 14)
Coverslips
Diluted HRP-SA complex (see SOP 19)
Detection complex (see SOP 19)
1X SSC (see SOP 14)
2X SSC (see SOP 14)
0.2X SSC (see SOP 14)
Mayer's hematoxylin

JC VIRUS POSITIVE PROBE

From a 4-kb fragment of JC virus DNA cloned into the Eco R1 site of pBR322

Enzo Diagnostics No. BP-847

Concentration: 20 μg/mL

Quantity: 1.6 μg

Fragment size: 200 to 2000 bp, as estimated by gel electrophoresis

pBR322 NEGATIVE PROBE

Grown in *Escherichia coli* HB101, extracted by standard molecular procedures, and purified by isopyknic banding in CsCl gradient.

Enzo Diagnostics No. BP-841

Concentration: 25 μg/mL

Quantity: 2.5 μg

Fragment size: 200 to 2000 bp, as estimated by gel electrophoresis

CARRIER DNA

Salmon sperm DNA supplied at 10 mg/mL

Enzo Diagnostics

One vial is supplied with each vial of DNA probe

Used in ISH as a blocking agent. Remove desired amount from freezer and boil for 10 minutes, quickly cool, and add to DNA probe mixture at 100 μg/mL of hybridization solution.

DEXTRAN SULFATE 50% SOLUTION (W/V)

Sigma No. D-7140 mol. wt. 500,000

Diluted in quality water with long mixing and possibly sonication to drive it into solution. The 50% solution is very heavy, with a "syrupy" texture and light brown color.

DEIONIZED FORMAMIDE

Sigma No. F-7503

Concentrations of 40% to 50% are used in ISH. Each 1% formamide lowers the TM (melting temperature of DNA) by 0.7%.

Commercial preparations of this chemical usually contain salt impurities as well as hydrolysis products, ammonium formate, NH^{+}_{4}, and formic acid. The formamide should have a conductivity below 40 μS, and a 50% solution of it should have a pH below 7.5. The formamide can be cleaned by stirring 1 L with 10 g of Norite A (Fisher Sci) and 50 g of mixed bed resin (AG501-X8(d), 20 to 50 mesh, Biorad) at 4°C for 2 hours. Filter twice through Whatman #1 filter paper. Store aliquots at −70°C.

PREPARATION OF HYBRIDIZATION MIXTURE

Deionized formamide pH 6.8 to 7.2	50 μL
50% Dextran sulfate	20 μL
20× SSC	10 μL
JC virus probe	20 μL
Carrier DNA	4 μL

This mixture is stable for 12+ months at 4°C. This is enough for 5 samples of 20 × 20 mm.

CONTROLS

Positive Control Slide

This is a slide from a patient who has a known JC virus infection and generally represents a section from brain in which JC virus has been previously detected with this assay. A positive control is run with every patient specimen. This control ensures that the reagent system is functioning properly.

Negative Control Slide

Patient slide is run with pBR322 probe (instead of JC virus probe) to control for nonspecific binding of the probe. Sections should not give a signal with this probe.

PROCEDURE

1. Hydrate sections by first removing paraffin by dewaxing in two changes of xylene for 2 minutes each and then twice immersing sections in 100% ethanol for 2 minutes, 95% ethanol for 2 minutes, 50% ethanol for 2 minutes, and finally into PBSE (phosphate-buffered saline, pH 7.4, with 5 mmol/L EDTA) for 5 minutes.
2. Wash in deionized water and air dry at 37°C.
3. Digest sections in 0.125 mg of proteinase K/mL PBSE for 10 minutes at 37°C.
4. Block endogenous peroxidase by immersing sections in 3% hydrogen peroxide in PBSE for 10 minutes at 37°C.
5. Wash slides in three changes of PBSE, 2 minutes each; then wash in deionized water.
6. Dehydrate sections through graded alcohols (50%, 95%, and 100%) for 2 minutes each.
7. Add probe at 10 μL per 20 × 20-mm tissue area.
8. Add small amount (pipette dipped in vial) of glass beads to the probe, and add a coverslip large enough to cover the tissue.
9. Denature both probe and genomic DNA by heating the slides to 90°C on the hot plate for 10 minutes.
10. Remove slides from hot plate and place in the slide warmer to hybridize at 37°C for 1 hour.
11. Remove coverslip by immersing each slide in 2X SSC.
12. Wash slides in 2X SSC with 0.1% sodium dodecyl sulfate (SDS) 5 minutes.
13. Wash slides in 0.2X SSC with 0.1% SDS 5 minutes.
14. Wash slides in PBSE 5 minutes.
15. Add approximately 0.5 mL of detection complex (HRP-SA) to each slide 37°C for 15 minutes (see SOP 19).
16. Wash slides in three changes of PBSE, 2 minutes each.
17. Wash slides in deionized water.
18. Add approximately 5 drops of chromagen complex (AEC) to each slide at 37°C for 15 minutes (see SOP 20).
19. Wash in three changes of deionized water 2 minutes each.
20. Counterstain with Mayer's hematoxylin for 15 to 30 seconds.
21. Wash in tap water for 20 minutes.
22. Lightly dry slides and add Crystalmount to cover the sections.
23. Dry slides first at 25°C for 10 minutes; then completely dry sections by heating at 80°C for 10 minutes.
24. (Optional) Add 3 drops of Permount and coverslip.
25. Observe under a light microscope at 100× to 400× magnification.

REPORTING RESULTS

A positive result for JC virus is reported if a positive signal is seen in one or more nuclei within the tissue section. Positive results are reported as "JC virus–related sequences are identified within the tissue section."

The assay for JC is indeterminate if the assay is negative and the control section shows positive signal within one or more nuclei. Results are reported as "JC virus–related sequences are not identified within the tissue section." If the positive control slide is not stained, the procedure requires troubleshooting before reporting of a patient result.

REFERENCES

Brigati DJ, Myerson D, Leary JJ, et al: Detection of viral genomes in cultured cells and paraffin-embedded tissue sections using biotin-labeled hybridization probes. Virology 1983;126: 32–50.

Jones KW, Robertson FW: Localization of reiterated nucleotide sequences in *Drosophila* and mouse by in situ hybridization of complementary RNA. Chromosoma 1970;31:331–345.

Padget BL, Walker DL, Zu Rhein GM, et al: JC papovavirus in progressive multifocal leukoencephalopathy. J Infect Dis 1976;133:686–690.

TIMOTHY J. O'LEARY

7

Cardiovascular System

Cardiovascular disease is the single most important health problem in Western nations. With the recognition that about half the variability of major risk factors for cardiovascular disease is genetic, the importance of molecular diagnosis to the practice of cardiology has been rapidly increasing. The identification of numerous polymorphisms associated with hypertension, serum lipoprotein abnormalities, and hereditary cardiomyopathies has significantly increased our understanding of "ordinary" cardiovascular disease, as well as enabling specific diagnoses for many individuals with less common disorders. The result is an increased use of immunohistochemical and molecular biologic techniques not only in the research setting but also in the routine diagnostic laboratory.

Lipid and lipoprotein disorders account for much of the individual and familial predisposition to coronary artery disease. The genes responsible for the majority of proteins involved in lipid and lipoprotein metabolism have been identified and sequenced, and regulatory elements have been characterized. In addition, genes responsible for some developmental anomalies, hereditary arrhythmias, and thrombotic disorders have been discovered. This basic information enables the physician in some cases to provide molecular explanations for diseases that have become manifest in the patient, to provide risk assessment and counseling for the patient and his or her relatives, and sometimes to offer early intervention.

In this chapter we focus on the molecular biology of disorders for which the use of immunohistochemical and molecular biologic techniques is well understood and well established, as well as on some important disorders for which the diagnostic approach is less obvious. By so doing, we hope to provide an understanding not only of current applications of these tools but also insight into areas in which the use of molecular methods for disease characterization may be expected to play an important role in the near future.

CONGENITAL MALFORMATIONS

Relatively little is known about the molecular genetics of congenital heart disease. Deletions of chromosome 22q11 are found in approximately 50% of patients with an interrupted aortic arch, 35% of patients with truncus arteriosus, 33% of patients with ventricular septal defect, and 16% of patients with tetralogy of Fallot. The deletion appears never to be associated with transposition of the great vessels.[1] In patients with DiGeorge syndrome, the frequency of 22q11 deletion rises to approximately 90%.[2] Deletions of 22q11 are also associated with pulmonary artery anomalies.[3,4] There is as yet, however, little predictive value in molecular analysis of the 22q11 site.

Cardiovascular malformations are frequently seen in association with complex congenital malformation syndromes. For example, about one third of affected persons with the Marfan syndrome have, in addition to the characteristic skeletal and lens abnormalities, mitral valve prolapse, aortic root enlargement, or both. The disease results from mutations in the fibrillin-1 gene, which has a 9.3-kb coding sequence. Because the mutations are family specific,[5] molecular diagnosis of potentially affected family members is generally accomplished by segregation analysis of polymorphic markers.[6] Although some mutations have been associated with major cardiovascular system involvement[7] and others with a lack of cardiac abnormalities,[8] there is as yet no generally useful molecular basis on which to predict the likelihood of cardiovascular involvement.[9] However, identification of family-specific mutations is useful in identifying potentially affected family members and in genetic counseling.

Patients with Down syndrome (trisomy 21) are also frequently affected by cardiovascular malformations. It appears likely that the defects are localized to one or more loci on chromosome 21q22.2-q22.3.[10–12] Similarly, supravalvular aortic stenosis and pulmonary artery stenoses frequently accompany Williams syndrome, a phenotypically hypervariable developmental disorder associated with microdeletions at 7q11.23[13, 14] involving the elastin gene locus.[15–17] Mutations within the elastin gene are also responsible for many cases of familial supravalvular aortic stenosis that are not associated with the Williams syndrome.[18, 19] It appears that loss of elastin expression causes thickening of the arterial musculature and stenosis.[20]

HEREDITARY ARRHYTHMIAS

Long QT syndrome is a group of disorders characterized by prolonged ventricular repolarization, resulting in recurrent syncopal attacks, ventricular tachycardia, and sudden death. Mutations in at least four different genes, *KCNQ1*, *KCNH2*, *KCNE1*, or *SCN5A*, can result in this clinical spectrum.[21–24] These genes code for peptides forming the cardiac potassium and sodium ion channels.

The inheritance of long QT syndrome may be either autosomal dominant (Romano-Ward syndrome) or autosomal recessive (Jervell and Lange-Nielsen syndromes) depending on the gene and site of mutation. Most of the mutations are "private" or "family specific." Thus, molecular evaluation of affected kindreds must begin with complete sequencing of the coding regions of four genes. Once a specific mutation has been identified in the proband, remaining family members need only be screened for the family-specific mutation.

HEREDITARY DILATED CARDIOMYOPATHY

Although most cases of dilated cardiomyopathy appear to arise as a result of viral infections,[25] 20% to 30% of cases appear to be familial.[26] Diagnosis of a hereditary form generally requires both a positive family history and an exclusion of infectious etiology. Familial dilated cardiomyopathy frequently follows an autosomal dominant pattern; linkage studies have mapped genes to chromosomes 1q32,[26] 9q13,[27] and 10q21-23.[25] Specific genes or mutations have yet to be identified, however. X-linked dilated cardiomyopathies have been reported in both teenage boys and middle-aged women, and due to mutations in the dystrophin gene.[28–33] Mutations in the 5′ portion of this gene can apparently cause cardiac muscle abnormalities without the corresponding skeletal muscle changes seen in Duchenne or Becker muscular dystrophy.[28, 31] Dystrophin mutations are seldom[28] associated with sporadic dilated cardiomyopathy, however; and although cardiomyopathy is commonly seen in Duchenne/Becker muscular dystrophy, it rarely dominates the clinical presentation.[34] Mutations in the tafazzin gene (the site of the Barth syndrome mutation) at Xq28 result in an aggressive, X-linked, infantile dilated cardiomyopathy.[35, 36] Molecular assessment is useful in distinguishing this hereditary cardiomyopathy from viral disease, because the clinical presentation may be quite similar in spite of radically different implications for subsequent offspring.

The mutation rate of mitochondrial DNA is high, and mitochondrial DNA mutations associated with dilated cardiomyopathy have been reported.[37–41] Unlike mitochondrial DNA mutations associated with hypertrophic cardiomyopathy, these mutations are apparently a consequence of aging or increased oxidative stress in the failing heart rather than an etiologic factor in the pathogenesis of idiopathic cardiomyopathy.

HYPERTROPHIC CARDIOMYOPATHY

Hypertrophic cardiomyopathy (also known as asymmetrical septal hypertrophy or muscular subaortic stenosis), although only about a fourth as common as dilated cardiomyopathy, is nevertheless one of the most common causes of cardiac death in young athletes. The earliest clinical signs of this condition are a presystolic gallop and electrocardiographic changes, but the disorder frequently remains undetected until either congestive heart failure or sudden cardiac death intervenes. Although several types have been distinguished on morphologic grounds, the resulting categorization does not appear to correlate with molecular alterations that have been described. Both familial and sporadic cases occur.

Kindred studies most commonly suggest autosomal dominant inheritance,[42–44] although maternal[45] inheritance patterns have also been reported. The autosomal dominant forms have been most frequently associated with mutations in either the cardiac β-myosin heavy-chain gene (chromosome 1q3),[46–49] the α-tropomyosin gene (chromosome 15q2),[45, 51–53] or the troponin gene (Table 7–1).[44, 50, 52–59]

At least 20 different missense mutations in the β-myosin heavy-chain gene have been observed, scattered in 10 different exons.[50] Mutations in the cardiac β-myosin heavy-chain gene have been observed in patients without hypertrophic cardiomyopathy or in whom the diagnosis is questionable[46]; this has led some authors to suggest a limited role for molecular biologic analysis in patients with this disease. Nevertheless, some mutations (Arg719Trp, Arg403Gln) are associated with early onset of disease (often in childhood), complete penetrance, and early sudden cardiac death,[60–64] whereas patients with other mutations (Leu908Val, Arg403Trp) demonstrate late-onset disease with low penetrance.[43, 46, 48, 62, 63, 65, 66] The extent of left ventricular hypertrophy correlates strongly with the precise mutations observed.[60]

Abnormalities in the cardiac troponin T gene are associated with varying penetrance, a wide range of hypertrophy, and a varying incidence of sudden cardiac death, depending on the site of mutation.[44, 50, 52, 54–57, 59] The spectrum of clinical findings associated with mutations in the α-tropomyosin gene has not yet been

TABLE 7–1
Representative Mutations in Hypertrophic Cardiomyopathy and Their Clinical Impact

Gene	Mutation	Clinical Impact	Reference
β-Myosin heavy chain	Arg719Trp	48% risk of premature death	60
β-Myosin heavy chain	Glu930Lys+	19% risk of premature death	60
β-Myosin heavy chain	Val606Met	9% risk of premature death	60
β-Myosin heavy chain	Phe513Cys	Near-normal life expectancy	61
β-Myosin heavy chain	Gly716Arg	Increased risk of congestive failure	61
β-Myosin heavy chain	Leu908Val	Late onset, low penetrance, low risk of premature death	62
β-Myosin heavy chain	Arg403Gln	Early onset, completed penetrance, high risk of premature death	62
β-Myosin heavy chain	Arg453Cys	Complete penetrance, high risk of death	64
Troponin T	Arg102Leu	Complete pentrance, low risk of early death	54
Troponin T	Ala104Val	High risk of early cardiac death	44
Tropomyosin	Ala63Val	Unknown	52
Tropomyosin	Asp175Asn	Unknown	52

well defined.[44, 50–52] Myosin light-chain mutations have also been observed.[67] Families have been identified in which linkage to chromosomes 1, 11, 14, and 15 can be excluded, suggesting that additional, as yet unidentified, loci are associated with the development of hypertrophic cardiomyopathy in some families. Ethnic factors are important in determining whether a particular person or family is likely to harbor mutations in the β-myosin heavy-chain gene or in another gene. For example, although the cardiac β-myosin heavy-chain gene has been most frequently associated with this disease in United States, mutation of the β- and α-tropomyosin genes is significantly more frequent in the Finnish population.[51]

Hypertrophic cardiomyopathy may be associated with mitochondrial genome mutation. Patients have been reported in which skeletal muscle demonstrates typical "ragged red" fibers, in association with mitochondrial transfer RNA mutations.[40, 68–74] The mitochondrial form of hypertrophic cardiomyopathy is transmitted by a strictly maternal route.

Mutations in the cardiac β-myosin heavy-chain gene are associated with the presence of central core disease in the skeletal muscle, a predominance of type 1 "slow" fibers, and absence of mitochondria in the center of many of the type 1 fibers.[43] The calcium-activated force of contraction developed by myocytes with mutations in either troponin T or the cardiac β-myosin heavy chain is lower than that of myocytes with wild-type proteins. Diminished output force may therefore be a stimulus for cardiac hypertrophy.[59] Progressing hypertrophy is associated with increased expression of transforming growth factor-β_1 and insulin-like growth factor-1.[75] Hypertrophy of cardiac muscle can give rise to compression of the coronary arteries, with subsequent myocardial ischemia. In addition, septal hypertrophy can block both aortic and pulmonic outflow tracts. As heart failure ensues, down-regulation of α-myosin heavy-chain gene occurs.[76] The complications of hypertrophic cardiomyopathy have been dealt with by both medical and surgical means. However, the diverse clinical features make it difficult to define precise guidelines for management.

Polymorphism of the angiotensinogen gene, particularly the T235 variant, is a predisposing factor for hypertrophic cardiomyopathy, carrying an approximately twofold increase in risk.[77, 78] Angiotensin-converting enzyme genotype also affects the phenotypic expression of hypertrophic cardiomyopathy. The frequency of allele *DD* is substantially higher in hypertrophic cardiomyopathy families with a high incidence of sudden cardiac death than in those with a low incidence of sudden cardiac death.[79–81]

Both normal mutant β-cardiac myosin heavy-chain genes are transcribed in normal circulating lymphocytes.[49] As a result, deletions, abnormal splicing, and missense mutations may be identified through reverse transcriptase/polymerase chain reaction (RT-PCR) analysis of circulating cells. This enables preclinical diagnosis of familial hypertrophic cardiomyopathy in those cases in which the cardiac myosin chains are involved. Molecular testing of children, however, is controversial. Although there is little evidence that the long-term debilitation due to congestive heart failure can be prevented through early intervention, it is possible that the early sudden cardiac death associated with the "malignant" mutations could be prevented by an implanted defibrillator.

AMYLOIDOSIS

Although hereditary amyloidosis usually presents as peripheral neuropathy,[82] it is renal, cardiac, or autonomic

TABLE 7–2
Transthyretin Mutations

Mutation	Clinical Presentation	Reference
Gly6Ser	No disease	240
Gly6Ser	Increased thyroxine binding	241
Val20Ile	Late-onset cardiac amyloidosis	242
Val30Leu	Neuropathy	243
Val30Met	Peripheral nervous system only	244
Val30Met	Only homozygotes became symptomatic	245
Val30Met	Leptomeningeal amyloidosis	246
Val30Met	Heart failure before the onset of neurologic symptoms	247
Phe33Leu	Ascites	248
Phe44Ser	Headache and hearing loss	249
Ala45Thr	Prominent cardiomyopathy without peripheral neuropathy	250
Thr59Lys	Autosomal dominant systemic amyloidosis	251
Ala97Gly	Somatic sensory and motor neuropathy	252
Ile107Val	Carpal tunnel syndrome	253
Ile107Val	Cardiac and neurologic involvement	254
Thr119Met	Increased thyroxine binding	255
Val122Ile	Isolated cardiac amyloidosis	256

nervous system disease that leads to greatest disability and death[83]; approximately half of affected patients die of arrhythmia or cardiac failure.[82] Patients present in their mid 60s, with about a third demonstrating cardiomyopathy at the time of initial diagnosis. The median survival is just less than 6 years—significantly longer than the survival of patients with secondary amyloidosis.[82] Although the acquired amyloidoses most often result from accumulation of immunoglobulins, most cases of hereditary amyloidosis result from the accumulation of a 127 amino acid thyroxin-binding prealbumin, transthyretin.[83, 84] Mutations in this gene give rise to a wide variety of clinical presentations (Table 7–2); inheritance may be either autosomal dominant or autosomal recessive, depending on the particular mutation and family. More than 40 different mutations have been described.

Isolated cardiac amyloidosis is four times as common in blacks as in whites in the United States.[85] The reasons for this difference are unclear, although a high prevalence of the Val122Ile mutation in the general population (allele frequency 0.02)[86] has been suggested as one possibility.[85] Although some mutations have been specifically associated with the "cardiac" form of hereditary amyloidosis, Table 7–2 demonstrates the heterogeneity of disease presentation that may be seen in different individuals or families with identical transthyretin mutations.[85, 87] As a result, the various mutation identification and screening strategies that have been described,[88–97] although useful in identifying family members who carry a specific mutation, provide no information about likely clinical manifestations beyond that provided by the family history. Furthermore, the largely private and family-specific nature of the mutations that have been described necessitates that families suspected of the disease first undergo complete sequencing of the patient's transthyretin coding sequence, and then this gene sequence information is used to design the least laborious subsequent screening strategy.

VIRAL MYOCARDITIS AND DILATED CARDIOMYOPATHY

Viral myocarditis is thought to account for approximately 80% of cases of dilated cardiomyopathy. Although enteroviruses (most commonly coxsackievirus B) are most frequently implicated, myocarditis and dilated cardiomyopathy are frequently associated with human immunodeficiency virus (HIV) infection,[98, 99] hepatitis C virus infection,[100–102] adenovirus infection,[103] or infection with one of the herpesviruses.[103–105]

A number of studies have considered identification by PCR of enteroviruses in endomyocardial biopsy specimens of patients with myocarditis or dilated myopathy. The results have varied from 0%[106] to 72%[107] positive for virus; most studies have demonstrated virus by PCR in one third to one half of the cases examined.[108–113] These results suggest that many cases of dilated cardiomyopathy ultimately result from an enteroviral infection, possibly acting in a "hit and run" manner.[114]

The "gold standard" for the diagnosis of enteroviral infection is isolation and culture of the virus, followed by neutralization assay for serotype identification.[115] Unfortunately, this is a complex procedure requiring material fresher than may usually be obtained in the diagnostic setting. Immunofluorescent antibody staining, also useful for identification of coxsackieviruses and other enteroviruses,[116–118] has been employed on autopsy specimens; specimens must be stained before fixation to avoid difficulties in interpretation arising from formaldehyde-induced autofluorescence, however. Immunohistochemical[119] and in situ hybridization methods[120] have been employed in formalin-fixed, paraffin-embedded tissue, but they may be limited to studying early stages of infection when the viral load is high. RT-PCR assay for enterovirus has been carried out from formalin-fixed archival specimens,[119, 121, 122] and it is probably the most robust approach to diagnosis of enterovirus infection in the routinely obtained endomyocardial biopsy, or autopsy heart. Even so, results must be interpreted with caution, because enterovirus infection may persist without causing disease[123] and because in many patients virus does not persist throughout the course of disease.

Although enterovirus is most frequently implicated in the pathogenesis of myocarditis, hepatitis C virus has been identified in a significant proportion of patients; and there is evidence that the virus replicates in the myocardium of some of these patients.[100, 101] In our experience, this virus is reliably identified by RT-PCR in formalin-fixed, paraffin-embedded tissue. HIV infection is also associated with myocarditis and dilated cardiomyopathy.

Adenovirus has been implicated as a cause of myocarditis and is identified about twice as often as enteroviruses in patients with childhood myocarditis.[103] Parvovirus B19, Epstein-Barr virus, cytomegalovirus, and herpes simplex virus have all been implicated as causes of myocarditis, particularly in children.[103, 104, 125] Although PCR-based assays may be used to identify these agents, immunohistochemical assays that work well in formalin-fixed paraffin-embedded material are available and provide a suitable alternative.

Because they are RNA viruses, the enteroviruses, HIV, and hepatitis C all present special diagnostic difficulty. Unless meticulous care is taken, exogenous ribonucleases may be introduced during specimen processing, rapidly degrading viral RNA. Furthermore, the inflammatory cell infiltrate associated with myocarditis is an abundant source of potent ribonucleases.[126–132] As a result, viral RNA is extremely labile in these specimens and may be completely degraded by the time it has been removed from the patient. Hence, even with the best possible RNA extraction methods, identification of virus may be impossible in some of these patients.

HYPERTENSION

The regulation of blood pressure results from a complex interaction of autonomic nervous system, renal, and cardiovascular factors. It has been generally believed that multiple genes and multiple environmental factors contribute to the regulation of blood pressure and, hence, to the development of hypertension in some individuals.

The renin-angiotensin system is one of the mechanisms by which blood pressure is regulated in humans. When blood pressure drops, renin is secreted by the kidney. In the blood, renin enzymatically cleaves angiotensinogen, a protein secreted primarily by the liver, to form a 10 amino acid peptide, angiotensin I. Angiotensin-converting enzyme (ACE) then cleaves two additional amino acids from this peptide, leaving the octapeptide angiotensin II. Angiotensin II is an extremely potent vasoconstrictor and a major determinant of salt and water homeostasis. There is abundant evidence that abnormalities in the renin-angiotensin system contribute to the development of essential hypertension.[133–136]

A number of polymorphisms have been described in both angiotensinogen and ACE. Among the more common angiotensinogen polymorphisms is a variant in which a methionine at position 235 on the angiotensinogen polypeptide is replaced by a threonine (usually referred to as angiotensinogen Met235Thr). Approximately one third of whites have at least one copy of the angiotensinogen Met235Thr gene, and there is some evidence that individuals homozygous for this variant are at increased risk for hypertension, myocardial infarction, and stroke.[137–140]

The most extensively investigated polymorphism in the ACE gene is a 287 base-pair (bp) insertion (I)/deletion (D) polymorphism in intron 16. Patients demonstrating a *DD* genotype appear to have an increased risk of hypertension and associated disease; the effects of this polymorphism are synergistic with those of the angiotensinogen polymorphism.[133, 138, 139, 141, 142] There is some evidence that persons with ACE *DD* may have a greater response to ACE inhibitors such as captopril.[142] Nevertheless, the utility of molecular assessment of these gene polymorphisms remains unclear.

ATHEROSCLEROTIC CARDIOVASCULAR DISEASE

Atherosclerotic cardiovascular disease is arguably the most important health problem in the developed world. Many factors, including lifestyle (diet, smoking, and level of physical activity), blood pressure, serum lipid profiles, coagulation factor activities, and others contribute to the pathogenesis of arterial plaques and interact with each other in complex and as yet incompletely defined ways. Diseases such as diabetes predispose to its development. In addition, infective agents such as herpesviruses and *Chlamydia* have been postulated to contribute to the pathogenesis of atherosclerotic plaques.

In most cases, there is no single genetic abnormality that can be identified as the predominant contributor to the development of coronary artery disease.

Nevertheless, there are a variety of monogenic abnormalities that have been shown to contribute to the pathogenesis of disease in some patients and several infectious agents that have been postulated to play a role. In particular, plasma lipoprotein abnormalities, coagulation factors, and *Chlamydia pneumoniae* have all been postulated to contribute. In this chapter, we will consider each of these classes of agent in turn.

Lipoprotein Abnormalities

LIPOPROTEIN LIPASE DEFICIENCY

This relatively uncommon lipid disorder is characterized by massive chylomicronemia accompanied by reduced high-density and low-density lipoprotein levels when the patient is on a normal diet. If the patient undertakes a fat-free diet, the lipid profile returns to nearly normal.

Lipoprotein lipase is an enzyme found on capillary endothelial surfaces in fat and muscle; it is responsible for the hydrolysis of diglycerides and triglycerides in chylomicrons and very-low-density lipoproteins. Patients with lipoprotein lipase deficiency cannot metabolize these lipids properly. They are frequently afflicted with recurrent abdominal pain, pancreatitis, and vascular disease. Deficiency results from any of numerous mutations in the lipoproteins lipase gene. Unfortunately, most of the mutations are either private or familial.

Although one can employ single-strand conformational polymorphism, chemical mismatch screening, or protein truncation test assays to screen for a wide spectrum of mutations, these approaches miss a lot of mutations. Hence, a widely applicable molecular screening test is not possible. Approximately 25% of patients of European extraction with lipoprotein lipase deficiency have a 2-kb direct tandem duplication within the lipoprotein lipase gene,[143] and approximately 72% of mutant alleles in French-Canadian patients share a Pro207Leu mutation, with approximately 24.3% of mutant alleles caused by a Gly188Glu mutation.[144, 145] Within certain population groups, therefore, accurate molecular biologic screening may be possible.

APOLIPOPROTEIN C-II DEFICIENCY

Apolipoprotein C-II (apo C-II) is a 79 amino acid protein that serves as a necessary cofactor for lipoprotein lipase activation. Mutations in apo C-II cause a form of hypertriglyceridemia that is usually less severe than that seen in lipoprotein lipase deficiency but that can still result in pancreatitis in some patients. A variety of mutations have been identified in the apo C-II gene.[146–148] Most are private or familial; none of these mutations represents a high proportion of those found in any demographic group.

FAMILIAL HYPERCHOLESTEROLEMIA (HYPERLIPOPROTEINEMIA TYPE IIA)

Familial hypercholesterolemia is characterized clinically by an increase in low-density lipoprotein-cholesterol. Homozygous individuals often have xanthomas appearing at infancy, and both heterozygotes and homozygotes develop early coronary artery disease, often by the fourth decade. The disease results from mutations in the low-density lipoprotein receptor.[149–153] Normally, low-density lipoprotein is bound to the cell membrane, taken into the cell, and degraded in lysosomes. Cholesterol taken up in this way inhibits the enzyme 3-hydroxy-3-methylglutaryl coenzyme A (HMG-CoA) reductase, which is the rate-limiting enzyme in cholesterol synthesis. Mutation giving way to an internalization defect results in the clinical manifestations.

The frequency of heterozygosity for familial hypercholesterolemia is approximately 1 in 500 in populations of European descent but is as high as 1 in 100[154] in the Transvaal province of South Africa and 1 in 154[155] among French Canadians. Over 350 different mutations have been described.[156] A 10-kb deletion mutation is found in 63% of Canadians with heterozygous familial hypercholesterolemia,[157] but in specific demographic groups a much smaller number of mutations may account for most of the disease. For example, in South Africa, three mutations account for approximately three fourths of the cases.[154, 158]

FAMILIAL HYPOBETALIPOPROTEINEMIA

Apolipoprotein B, the main apolipoprotein of chylomicrons and low density lipoproteins, occurs in the plasma in two main forms, apo B-48 (synthesized in the intestines) and apo B-100 (synthesized by the liver). The two forms represent differential splicing of transcripts from the same gene. Persons who are homozygous for mutant apo B have unusually low levels of cholesterol and may demonstrate fat malabsorption and its complications. Disease usually results from mutations that cause the appearance of STOP codons, giving rise to truncated forms of the protein.[159–165]

Splice site mutations have also been reported[164, 166]; these may apparently give rise to inefficient transcription and low levels of the lipoprotein.

APOLIPOPROTEIN E POLYMORPHISM

Apolipoprotein E (apo E) is one of the major protein constituents of chylomicrons, very-low-density lipoproteins, and high-density lipoproteins. More than 30 allelic variants have been described; about half have been linked to various familial dyslipoproteinemias, but three major isoforms—E2 (allele frequency 0.11), E3 (allele frequency 0.72), and E4 (allele frequency 0.17) predominate in populations of European descent.[167] The three isoforms differ from each other at two amino acids; E2 contains cysteine at both positions 112 and 158, whereas E4 contains arginine at both of these positions. E3 contains cysteine at position 112 and arginine at position 158.

Apo E binds to a specific receptor on hepatic cells, enabling their endocytosis and catabolism. Whereas the E3 and E4 isoforms bind well, the E2 isoform binds poorly to these receptors. Nevertheless, only about 5% of patients who are homozygous for E2 demonstrate hyperlipidemia (although virtually all persons with type III hyperlipoproteinemia are E2 homozygotes). Such factors as obesity, diabetes, and exercise clearly play an important role in determining which E2 homozygous persons will become hyperlipidemic. There appears to be an association between the E2 allele and preeclampsia,[168] but the association with cardiovascular disease is not striking. In spite of the fact that it is the E2 isoform that is associated with hyperlipidemia, it is the E4 isoform that appears to predispose most strongly to both silent myocardial ischemia and myocardial infarction.[169, 170]

There are a variety of approaches that have been proposed for apo E genotyping.[171–189] For routine use, however, products from a PCR amplification that includes both the 112 and 158 positions are digested with the *Hha*I restriction enzyme, separated on an agarose gel, and visualized with ethidium bromide staining[179, 180] (see SOP 7.1). *Hha*I cleaves at GCGC encoding 112Arg (E4) and 158Arg (E3, E4) but does not cut at GTGC encoding 112Cys (E2, E3) and 158Cys (E2). Each isoform thus gives a different band pattern. Although occasionally rare isoforms may be mischaracterized by this assay,[188] variants of this method are both rapid and applicable to a wide variety of samples, ranging from buccal swabs[190] to formalin-fixed, paraffin-embedded tissue.[173]

Homocysteinemia

Homocysteinemia is found in about 10% of families in which coronary artery disease presents clinically before the sixth decade[191] and is also associated with cerebrovascular disease.[192] Elevated plasma homocysteine appears to be a risk factor for both arterial[193] and venous thrombosis[194, 195] and may increase susceptibility to endothelial injury.

Homocysteinemia is most often associated with folate deficiency or deficiency of cystathione β-synthetase deficiency.[196, 197] Vitamin deficiency probably accounts for more cases, particularly in the elderly,[198] and the vascular effects of homocysteinemia caused by vitamin deficiency can be corrected by folic acid supplementation.[198] Younger patients are more likely to have cystathione β-synthetase gene mutations. These mutations are largely familial or private, necessitating complete sequencing for initial identification.[199]

Fibrinogen Abnormalities

Polymorphisms of the β-fibrinogen gene affect plasma fibrinogen levels,[200–203] the risk of peripheral arterial disease,[204–206] and the risk and extent of coronary artery disease[207–209]; more than 10 such polymorphisms have been identified. The most extensively investigated polymorphism is a G→A transition 455 bases upstream of the transcription start site, but other polymorphisms may be identified throughout the gene. The effects of the polymorphisms are quite substantial, with an effect on fibrinogen levels similar to that of age, smoking, and body mass index,[210, 211] and represent an independent predictor of the risk of myocardial infarction.[212] Nevertheless, the specific relative risk associated with many of the reported polymorphisms has yet to be established, because only a small number of cases demonstrating these polymorphisms have been reported.

Although the clinical utility of identifying these polymorphisms has not yet been established, it seems likely that their analysis will find its way into clinical practice. Current methods for identification include single-strand conformational polymorphism analysis[208] and PCR followed by restriction digestion.[210] Each of these techniques is capable of identifying only a limited subset of possible polymorphisms, however, so direct sequencing is probably the most appropriate method by which to identify patients bearing polymorphisms that predispose to the development of vascular disease.

Platelet Glycoprotein IIIA

The platelet membrane glycoprotein IIb/IIIa binds fibrinogen, cross-links platelets, and initiates thrombus formation.[213] A Leu/Pro polymorphism at position 33 occurs in about one fourth of the population and has been associated with coronary artery stenosis[202, 214] and with myocardial infarction.[213] The polymorphism has also been related to the risk of restenosis after coronary stent placement.[215] Other authors have failed to demonstrate clinical implications of polymorphism at this site, however,[216–221] and there are no persuasive data that genotyping of patients should impact therapy.

Chlamydia pneumoniae

A number of publications have suggested on the basis of serologic studies of patient serum and immunohistochemical and PCR-based studies of arterial tissue that there is a causal link between *Chlamydia pneumoniae* infection and atherosclerotic cardiovascular disease.[222–233] *Chlamydia* can multiply in human endothelial cells,[234] as well as smooth muscle and macrophages[235]; rabbits infected with *C. pneumoniae* develop changes typically of early atherosclerotic lesions in humans.[236, 237] These latter

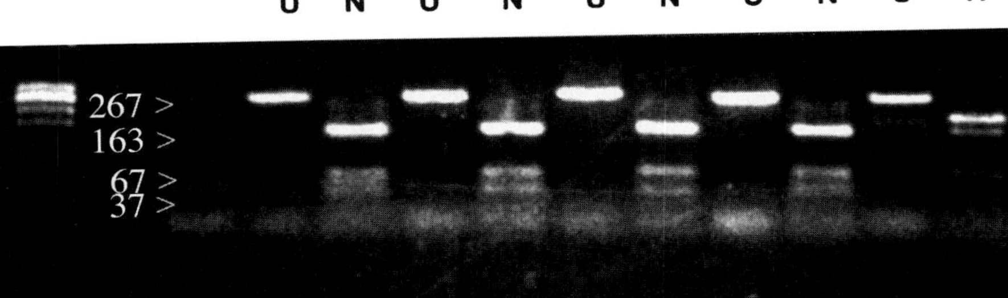

FIGURE 7–1
Ethidium-bromide–stained agarose gel showing results of a polymerase chain reaction (PCR)/restriction fragment length polymorphism (PCR-RFLP) assay for factor V Leiden. Undigested PCR products have been run in bands labeled U and demonstrate the characteristic 267-bp band. Products found in lanes marked N demonstrate fragments with sizes of 37, 67, and 163 bp, typical of patients demonstrating wild-type factor V. The product found in the lane marked H demonstrates a band of 200 pb. This indicates a factor V Leiden mutation in one of the two alleles, accompanied by one wild-type allele.

observations suggest that the presence of *C. pneumoniae* within arterial lesions is indicative of a pathogenetic role and that chronic treatment with macrolide antibiotics, such as erythromycin, could dramatically reduce the incidence of coronary artery disease.

Several investigators have failed to confirm the findings of organisms in atherosclerotic lesions, using highly sensitive techniques such as nested PCR,[238, 239] raising the possibility that the relationship between *Chlamydia* and atherosclerosis may vary from population to population, as well as raising issues of whether positive laboratory reports reflect either cross-reactions with other organisms/cellular constituents or laboratory contamination. In the absence of information that suggests possible treatment benefits for patients with *Chlamydia* infection, however, routine testing is probably not warranted.

VENOUS THROMBOSIS

The most common cause of familial venous thrombosis is a defect in the gene for factor V, a 286-kd glycoprotein. An Arg506Gln mutation gives rise to a variant of this protein known as factor V Leiden, leading to a hypercoagulable state; up to 90% of patients with venous thrombosis carry either one or two copies of this gene, which is seen in approximately 7% of the normal population. Both homozygous and heterozygous states are associated with increased risk. Individuals who are heterozygous for factor V Leiden have a risk of deep venous thrombosis approximately 7-fold higher than that of the general population. For homozygous individuals, this risk rises to approximately 70-fold greater than that of unaffected individuals.

The ease of molecular testing for factor V Leiden has made the PCR test one of the most frequently performed in the molecular diagnostic laboratory. After PCR, the amplified product is digested with the restriction enzyme *MnlI*. Because the factor V Leiden mutation destroys an *MnlI* restriction site, patients homozygous for this mutant demonstrate a different band pattern from individuals who do not have the mutation, as well as from individuals who are heterozygotes (Fig. 7–1). SOP 7.2 shows a method for simultaneously identifying both factor V Leiden and a common prothombin gene mutation (Gly20210Ala) that also predisposes to hypercoagulability.

REFERENCES

1. Goldmuntz E, Clark BJ, Mitchell LE, et al: Frequency of 22q11 deletions in patients with conotruncal defects. J Am Coll Cardiol 1998;32:492–498.
2. Momma K, Kondo C, Matsuoka R, Takao A: Cardiac anomalies associated with a chromosome 22q11 deletion in patients with conotruncal anomaly face syndrome. Am J Cardiol 1996;78:591–594.
3. Seaver LH, Pierpont JW, Erickson RP, et al: Pulmonary atresia associated with maternal 22q11.2 deletion: Possible parent of origin effect in the conotruncal anomaly face syndrome. J Med Genet 1994;31:830–834.
4. Hofbeck M, Rauch A, Buheitel G, et al: Monosomy 22q11 in patients with pulmonary atresia, ventricular septal defect, and major aortopulmonary collateral arteries. Heart 1998;79:180–185.
5. Tynan K, Comeau K, Pearson M, et al: Mutation screening of complete fibrillin-1 coding sequence: Report of five new mutations, including two in 8-cysteine domains. Hum Mol Genet 1993;2:1813–1821.
6. Rantamaki T, Lonnqvist L, Karttunen L, et al: DNA diagnostics of the Marfan syndrome: Application of amplifiable polymorphic markers. Eur J Hum Genet 1994;2:66–75.
7. Pepe G, Giusti B, Attanasio M, et al: A major involvement of the cardiovascular system in patients affected by Marfan syndrome: Novel mutations in fibrillin 1 gene. J Mol Cell Cardiol 1997;29:1877–1884.
8. Milewicz DM, Grossfield J, Cao SN, et al: A mutation in *FBN1* disrupts profibrillin processing and results in isolated skeletal features of the Marfan syndrome. J Clin Invest 1995;95:2373–2378.
9. Pereira L, Levran O, Ramirez F, et al: A molecular approach to the stratification of cardiovascular risk in

families with Marfan's syndrome. N Engl J Med 1994;331: 148–153.

10. Hubert RS, Mitchell S, Chen XN, et al: BAC and PAC contigs covering 3.5 Mb of the Down syndrome congenital heart disease region between D21S55 and MX1 on chromosome 21. Genomics 1997;41:218–226.
11. Korenberg JR, Bradley C, Disteche CM: Down syndrome: Molecular mapping of the congenital heart disease and duodenal stenosis. Am J Hum Genet 1992; 50:294–302.
12. Nadal M, Mila M, Pritchard M, et al: YAC and cosmid FISH mapping of an unbalanced chromosomal translocation causing partial trisomy 21 and Down syndrome. Hum Genet 1996;98:460–466.
13. del Rio T, Urban Z, Csiszar K, Boyd CD: A gene-dosage PCR method for the detection of elastin gene deletions in patients with Williams syndrome. Clin Genet 1998;54:129–135.
14. Urban Z, Kiss E, Kadar K, et al: Genetic diagnosis of Williams syndrome. Orv Hetil 1997;138:1749–1752.
15. Robinson WP, Waslynka J, Bernasconi F, et al: Delineation of 7q11.2 deletions associated with Williams-Beuren syndrome and mapping of a repetitive sequence to within and to either side of the common deletion. Genomics 1996;34:17–23.
16. Mari A, Amati F, Mingarelli R, et al: Analysis of the elastin gene in 60 patients with clinical diagnosis of Williams syndrome. Hum Genet 1995;96:444–448.
17. Nickerson E, Greenberg F, Keating MT, et al: Deletions of the elastin gene at 7q11.23 occur in approximately 90% of patients with Williams syndrome. Am J Hum Genet 1995;56:1156–1161.
18. Ewart AK, Jin W, Atkinson D, et al: Supravalvular aortic stenosis associated with a deletion disrupting the elastin gene. J Clin Invest 1994;93:1071–1077.
19. Olson TM, Michels VV, Lindor NM, et al: Autosomal dominant supravalvular aortic stenosis: Localization to chromosome 7. Hum Mol Genet 1993;2:869–873.
20. Li DY, Faury G, Taylor DG, et al: Novel arterial pathology in mice and humans hemizygous for elastin. J Clin Invest 1999;102:1783–1787.
21. Russell MW, Dick M, Collins FS, Brody LC: *KVLQT1* mutations in three families with familial or sporadic long QT syndrome. Hum Mol Genet 1996;5:1319–1324.
22. Curran M, Atkinson D, Timothy K, et al: Locus heterogeneity of autosomal dominant long QT syndrome. J Clin Invest 1993;92:799–803.
23. Keating M: Linkage analysis and long QT syndrome: Using genetics to study cardiovascular disease. Circulation 1992;85:1973–1986.
24. Wattanasirichaigoon D, Beggs AH: Molecular genetics of long-QT syndrome. Curr Opin Pediatr 1998;10: 628–634.
25. Bowles KR, Gajarski RJ, Porter P, et al: Gene mapping of familial autosomal dominant dilated cardiomyopathy to chromosome 10q21-23. J Clin Invest 1996;98: 1355–1360.
26. Durand JB, Bachinski LL, Bieling LC, et al: Localization of a gene responsible for familial dilated cardiomyopathy to chromosome 1q32. Circulation 1995;92:3387–3389.
27. Krajinovic M, Pinamonti B, Sinagra G, et al: Linkage of familial dilated cardiomyopathy to chromosome 9. Am J Hum Genet 1995;57:846–852.
28. Bies RD, Maeda M, Roberds SL, et al: A 5′ dystrophin duplication mutation causes membrane deficiency of alpha-dystroglycan in a family with X-linked cardiomyopathy. J Mol Cell Cardiol 1997;29:3175–3188.
29. Franz WM, Cremer M, Herrmann R, et al: X-linked dilated cardiomyopathy: Novel mutation of the dystrophin gene. Ann N Y Acad Sci 1995;752:470–491.
30. Mestroni L, Krajinovic M, Severini GM, et al: Molecular genetics of dilated cardiomyopathy. Herz 1994;19: 97–104.
31. Muntoni F, Wilson L, Marrosu G, et al: A mutation in the dystrophin gene selectively affecting dystrophin expression in the heart. J Clin Invest 1995;96:693–699.
32. Ortiz-Lopez R, Li H, Su J, et al: Evidence for a dystrophin missense mutation as a cause of X-linked dilated cardiomyopathy. Circulation 1997;95:2434–2440.
33. Towbin JA, Hejtmancik JF, Brink P, et al: X-linked dilated cardiomyopathy: Molecular genetic evidence of linkage to the Duchenne muscular dystrophy (dystrophin) gene at the Xp21 locus. Circulation 1993;87:1854–1865.
34. Michels VV, Pastores GM, Moll PP, et al: Dystrophin analysis in idiopathic dilated cardiomyopathy. J Med Genet 1993;30:955–957.
35. D'Adamo P, Fassone L, Gedeon A, et al: The X-linked gene G4.5 is responsible for different infantile dilated cardiomyopathies. Am J Hum Genet 1997;61:862–867.
36. Gedeon AK, Wilson M, Colley AC, et al: X linked fatal infantile cardiomyopathy maps to Xq28 and is possibly allelic to Barth syndrome. J Med Genet 1995;32:383–388.
37. Li YY, Hengstenberg C, Maisch B: Whole mitochondrial genome amplification reveals basal level multiple deletions in mtDNA of patients with dilated cardiomyopathy. Biochem Biophys Res Commun 1995;210:211–218.
38. Li YY, Maisch B, Rose ML, Hengstenberg C: Point mutations in mitochondrial DNA of patients with dilated cardiomyopathy. J Mol Cell Cardiol 1997;29:2699–2709.
39. Marin-Garcia J, Goldenthal MJ, Ananthakrishnan R, et al: Specific mitochondrial DNA deletions in idiopathic dilated cardiomyopathy. Cardiovasc Res 1996; 31:306–313.
40. Ozawa T, Tanaka M, Sugiyama S, et al: Multiple mitochondrial DNA deletions exist in cardiomyocytes of patients with hypertrophic or dilated cardiomyopathy. Biochem Biophys Res Commun 1990;170:830–836.
41. Remes AM, Hassinen IE, Ikaheimo MJ, et al: Mitochondrial DNA deletions in dilated cardiomyopathy: A clinical study employing endomyocardial sampling. J Am Coll Cardiol 1994;23:935–942.
42. Arai S, Matsuoka R, Hirayama K, et al: Missense mutation of the beta-cardiac myosin heavy-chain gene in hypertrophic cardiomyopathy. Am J Med Genet 1995;58: 267–276.
43. Fananapazir L, Dalakas MC, Cyran F, et al: Missense mutations in the beta-myosin heavy-chain gene cause central core disease in hypertrophic cardiomyopathy. Proc Natl Acad Sci U S A 1993;90:3993–3997.
44. Nakajima-Taniguchi C, Matsui H, Fujio Y, et al: Novel missense mutation in cardiac troponin T gene found

in Japanese patient with hypertrophic cardiomyopathy. J Mol Cell Cardiol 1997;29:839–843.

45. Merante F, Tein I, Benson L, Robinson BH: Maternally inherited hypertrophic cardiomyopathy due to a novel T-to-C transition at nucleotide 9997 in the mitochondrial tRNA(glycine) gene. Am J Hum Genet 1994;55: 437–446.
46. al-Mahdawi S, Chamberlain S, Chojnowska L, et al: The electrocardiogram is a more sensitive indicator than echocardiography of hypertrophic cardiomyopathy in families with a mutation in the *MYH7* gene. Br Heart J 1994;72: 105–111.
47. Nishi H, Kimura A, Harada H, et al: Possible gene dose effect of a mutant cardiac beta-myosin heavy chain gene on the clinical expression of familial hypertrophic cardiomyopathy. Biochem Biophys Res Commun 1994; 200:549–556.
48. Posen BM, Moolman JC, Corfield VA, Brink PA: Clinical and prognostic evaluation of familial hypertrophic cardiomyopathy in two South African families with different cardiac beta myosin heavy chain gene mutations. Br Heart J 1995;74:40–46.
49. Rosenzweig A, Watkins H, Hwang DS, et al: Preclinical diagnosis of familial hypertrophic cardiomyopathy by genetic analysis of blood lymphocytes. N Engl J Med 1991;325:1753–1760.
50. Hwang DS, Chen YT, Su JS, et al: Evidence of genetic heterogeneity of hypertrophic cardiomyopathy in eight Chinese patients. Chung Hua I Hsueh Tsa Chih (Taipei) 1996;57:315–321.
51. Jaaskelainen P, Soranta M, Miettinen R, et al: The cardiac beta-myosin heavy chain gene is not the predominant gene for hypertrophic cardiomyopathy in the Finnish population. J Am Coll Cardiol 1998;32:1709–1716.
52. Nakajima-Taniguchi C, Matsui H, Nagata S, et al: Novel missense mutation in alpha-tropomyosin gene found in Japanese patients with hypertrophic cardiomyopathy. J Mol Cell Cardiol 1995;27:2053–2058.
53. Anderson PA, Greig A, Mark TM, et al: Molecular basis of human cardiac troponin T isoforms expressed in the developing, adult, and failing heart. Circ Res 1995;76:681–686.
54. Forissier JF, Carrier L, Farza H, et al: Codon 102 of the cardiac troponin T gene is a putative hot spot for mutations in familial hypertrophic cardiomyopathy. Circulation 1996;94:3069–3073.
55. Gerull B, Osterziel KJ, Witt C, et al: A rapid protocol for cardiac troponin T gene mutation detection in familial hypertrophic cardiomyopathy. Hum Mutat 1998;11: 179–182.
56. Kai H, Muraishi A, Sugiu Y, et al: Expression of proto-oncogenes and gene mutation of sarcomeric proteins in patients with hypertrophic cardiomyopathy. Circ Res 1998;83:594–601.
57. Morimoto S, Yanaga F, Minakami R, Ohtsuki I: Ca^{2+}-sensitizing effects of the mutations at Ile79 and Arg92 of troponin T in hypertrophic cardiomyopathy. Am J Physiol 1998;275(1 Pt 1):C200–C207.
58. Oberst L, Zhao G, Park JT, et al: Dominant-negative effect of a mutant cardiac troponin T on cardiac structure and function in transgenic mice. J Clin Invest 1998;102: 1498–1505.
59. Watkins H, Seidman CE, Seidman JG, et al: Expression and functional assessment of a truncated cardiac troponin T that causes hypertrophic cardiomyopathy: Evidence for a dominant negative action. J Clin Invest 1996;98: 2456–2461.
60. Abchee A, Marian AJ: Prognostic significance of beta-myosin heavy chain mutations is reflective of their hypertrophic expressivity in patients with hypertrophic cardiomyopathy. J Investig Med 1997;45:191–196.
61. Anan R, Greve G, Thierfelder L, et al: Prognostic implications of novel beta cardiac myosin heavy chain gene mutations that cause familial hypertrophic cardiomyopathy. J Clin Invest 1994;93:280–285.
62. Epstein ND, Cohn GM, Cyran F, Fananapazir L: Differences in clinical expression of hypertrophic cardiomyopathy associated with two distinct mutations in the beta-myosin heavy chain gene: A 908Leu-Val mutation and a 403Arg-Gln mutation. Circulation 1992;86: 345–352.
63. Fananapazir L, Epstein ND: Genotype-phenotype correlations in hypertrophic cardiomyopathy: Insights provided by comparisons of kindreds with distinct and identical beta-myosin heavy chain gene mutations. Circulation 1994;89:22–32.
64. Ko YL, Chen JJ, Tang TK, et al: Malignant familial hypertrophic cardiomyopathy in a family with a 453Arg→Cys mutation in the beta-myosin heavy chain gene: Coexistence of sudden death and end-stage heart failure. Hum Genet 1996;97:585–590.
65. Marian AJ, Mares AJ, Kelly DP, et al: Sudden cardiac death in hypertrophic cardiomyopathy: Variability in phenotypic expression of beta-myosin heavy chain mutations. Eur Heart J 1995;16:368–376.
66. al-Mahdawi S, Chamberlain S, Cleland J, et al: Identification of a mutation in the beta cardiac myosin heavy chain gene in a family with hypertrophic cardiomyopathy. Br Heart J 1993;69:136–141.
67. Poetter K, Jiang H, Hassanzadeh S, et al: Mutations in either the essential or regulatory light chains of myosin are associated with a rare myopathy in human heart and skeletal muscle. Nat Genet 1996;13:63–69.
68. Bobba A, Giannattasio S, Pucci A, et al: Characterization of mitochondrial DNA in primary cardiomyopathies. Clin Chim Acta 1995;243:181–189.
69. Hiruta Y, Chin K, Shitomi K, et al: Mitochondrial encephalomyopathy with A to G transition of mitochondrial transfer RNA(Leu(UUR)) 3,243 presenting hypertrophic cardiomyopathy. Intern Med 1995;34:670–673.
70. Ito T, Hattori K, Obayashi T, et al: Mitochondrial DNA mutations in cardiomyopathy. Jpn Circ J 1992;56: 1045–1053.
71. Merante F, Myint T, Tein I, et al: An additional mitochondrial tRNA(Ile) point mutation (A-to-G at nucleotide 4295) causing hypertrophic cardiomyopathy. Hum Mutat 1996;8:216–222.
72. Obayashi T, Hattori K, Sugiyama S, et al: Point mutations in mitochondrial DNA in patients with hypertrophic cardiomyopathy. Am Heart J 1992;124:1263–1269.
73. Takeda N: Cardiomyopathies and mitochondrial DNA mutations. Mol Cell Biochem 1997;176:287–290.
74. Yoshida R, Ishida Y, Abo K, et al: Hypertrophic cardiomyopathy in patients with diabetes mellitus associated

with mitochondrial tRNA(Leu)(UUR) gene mutation. Intern Med 1995;34:953–958.
75. Li RK, Li G, Mickle DA, et al: Overexpression of transforming growth factor-beta1 and insulin-like growth factor-I in patients with idiopathic hypertrophic cardiomyopathy. Circulation 1997;96:874–881.
76. Lowes BD, Minobe W, Abraham WT, et al: Changes in gene expression in the intact human heart: Down-regulation of alpha-myosin heavy chain in hypertrophied, failing ventricular myocardium. J Clin Invest 1997;100: 2315–2324.
77. Brugada R, Kelsey W, Lechin M, et al: Role of candidate modifier genes on the phenotypic expression of hypertrophy in patients with hypertrophic cardiomyopathy. J Investig Med 1997;45:542–551.
78. Ishanov A, Okamoto H, Yoneya K, et al: Angiotensinogen gene polymorphism in Japanese patients with hypertrophic cardiomyopathy. Am Heart J 1997;133:184–189.
79. Lechin M, Quinones MA, Omran A, et al: Angiotensin-I converting enzyme genotypes and left ventricular hypertrophy in patients with hypertrophic cardiomyopathy. Circulation 1995;92:1808–1812.
80. Marian AJ, Yu QT, Workman R, et al: Angiotensin-converting enzyme polymorphism in hypertrophic cardiomyopathy and sudden cardiac death. Lancet 1993;342: 1085–1086.
81. Yoneya K, Okamoto H, Machida M, et al: Angiotensin-converting enzyme gene polymorphism in Japanese patients with hypertrophic cardiomyopathy. Am Heart J 1995;130:1089–1093.
82. Gertz MA, Kyle RA, Thibodeau SN: Familial amyloidosis: A study of 52 North American-born patients examined during a 30-year period. Mayo Clin Proc 1992;67: 428–440.
83. Benson MD, Wallace MR: Genetic amyloidosis: Recent advances. Adv Nephrol Necker Hosp 1989;18:129–137.
84. Gorevic PD, Prelli FC, Wright J, et al: Systemic senile amyloidosis: Identification of a new prealbumin (transthyretin) variant in cardiac tissue: Immunologic and biochemical similarity to one form of familial amyloidotic polyneuropathy. J Clin Invest 1989;83:836–843.
85. Jacobson DR, Pastore RD, Yaghoubian R, et al: Variant-sequence transthyretin (isoleucine 122) in late-onset cardiac amyloidosis in black Americans. N Engl J Med 1997;336:466–473.
86. Jacobson DR, Pastore R, Pool S, et al: Revised transthyretin Ile122 allele frequency in African-Americans. Hum Genet 1996;98:236–238.
87. Sakaki Y, Sasaki H, Yoshioka K, Furuya H: Genetic analysis of familial amyloidotic polyneuropathy, an autosomal dominant disease. Clin Chim Acta 1989;185: 291–297.
88. Ii S, Minnerath S, Ii K, et al: Two-tiered DNA-based diagnosis of transthyretin amyloidosis reveals two novel point mutations. Neurology 1991;41:893–898.
89. Jacobson DR: A specific test for transthyretin 122 (Val-Ile), based on PCR-primer–introduced restriction analysis (PCR-PIRA): Confirmation of the gene frequency in blacks. Am J Hum Genet 1992;50:195–198.
90. Lucotte G, Berriche S, David F, et al: Prenatal diagnosis of hereditary amyloidosis in a Portuguese family living in France. Genet Couns 1993;4:285–287.
91. Nichols WC, Padilla LM, Benson MD: Prenatal detection of a gene for hereditary amyloidosis. Am J Med Genet 1989;34:520–524.
92. Nichols WC, Benson MD: Hereditary amyloidosis: Detection of variant prealbumin genes by restriction enzyme analysis of amplified genomic DNA sequences. Clin Genet 1990;37:44–53.
93. Almeida MR, Alves IL, Sakaki Y, et al: Prenatal diagnosis of familial amyloidotic polyneuropathy: Evidence for an early expression of the associated transthyretin methionine 30. Hum Genet 1990;85:623–626.
94. Nichols WC, Liepnieks JJ, McKusick VA, Benson MD: Direct sequencing of the gene for Maryland/German familial amyloidotic polyneuropathy type II and genotyping by allele-specific enzymatic amplification. Genomics 1989;5:535–540.
95. Saeki Y, Ueno S, Yorifuji S, et al: New mutant gene (transthyretin Arg 58) in cases with hereditary polyneuropathy detected by non-isotope method of single-strand conformation polymorphism analysis. Biochem Biophys Res Commun 1991;180:380–385.
96. Saeki Y, Ueno S, Takahashi N, et al: A novel mutant (transthyretin Ile-50) related to amyloid polyneuropathy: Single-strand conformation polymorphism as a new genetic marker. FEBS Lett 1992;308:35–37.
97. Sheffield VC, Beck JS, Nichols B, et al: Detection of multiallele polymorphisms within gene sequences by GC-clamped denaturing gradient gel electrophoresis. Am J Hum Genet 1992;50:567–575.
98. Anderson DW, Virmani R, Reilly JM, et al: Prevalent myocarditis at necropsy in the acquired immunodeficiency syndrome. J Am Coll Cardiol 1988;11:792–799.
99. Reilly JM, Cunnion RE, Anderson DW, et al: Frequency of myocarditis, left ventricular dysfunction and ventricular tachycardia in the acquired immune deficiency syndrome. Am J Cardiol 1988;62:789–793.
100. Matsumori A, Matoba Y, Sasayama S: Dilated cardiomyopathy associated with hepatitis C virus infection. Circulation 1995;92:2519–2525.
101. Matsumori A, Sasayama S: Newer aspects of pathogenesis of heart failure: Hepatitis C virus infection in myocarditis and cardiomyopathy. J Card Fail 1996;2(4 Suppl): S187–S194.
102. Okabe M, Fukuda K, Arakawa K, Kikuchi M: Chronic variant of myocarditis associated with hepatitis C virus infection. Circulation 1997;96:22–24.
103. Martin AB, Webber S, Fricker FJ, et al: Acute myocarditis: Rapid diagnosis by PCR in children. Circulation 1994;90:330–339.
104. Hebert MM, Yu C, Towbin JA, Rogers BB: Fatal Epstein-Barr virus myocarditis in a child with repetitive myocarditis. Pediatr Pathol Lab Med 1995;15:805–812.
105. Schonian U, Crombach M, Maser S, Maisch B: Cytomegalovirus-associated heart muscle disease. Eur Heart J 1995;16(Suppl O):46–49.
106. Liljeqvist JA, Bergstrom T, Holmstrom S, et al: Failure to demonstrate enterovirus aetiology in Swedish patients with dilated cardiomyopathy. J Med Virol 1993;39:6–10.
107. Andreoletti L, Wattre P, Decoene C, et al: Detection of enterovirus-specific RNA sequences in explanted myocardium biopsy specimens from patients with dilated or

ischemic cardiomyopathy. Clin Infect Dis 1995;21:1315–1317.

108. Satoh M, Tamura G, Segawa I, et al: Expression of cytokine genes and presence of enteroviral genomic RNA in endomyocardial biopsy tissues of myocarditis and dilated cardiomyopathy. Virchows Arch 1996;427: 503–509.
109. Satoh M, Tamura G, Segawa I: Enteroviral RNA in endomyocardial biopsy tissues of myocarditis and dilated cardiomyopathy. Pathol Int 1994;44:345–351.
110. Satoh M, Tamura G, Segawa I, et al: Enteroviral RNA in dilated cardiomyopathy. Eur Heart J 1994;15:934–939.
111. Schwaiger A, Umlauft F, Weyrer K, et al: Detection of enteroviral ribonucleic acid in myocardial biopsies from patients with idiopathic dilated cardiomyopathy by polymerase chain reaction. Am Heart J 1993;126:406–410.
112. Andreoletti L, Hober D, Decoene C, et al: Detection of enteroviral RNA by polymerase chain reaction in endomyocardial tissue of patients with chronic cardiac diseases. J Med Virol 1996;48:53–59.
113. Archard LC, Khan MA, Soteriou BA, et al: Characterization of Coxsackie B virus RNA in myocardium from patients with dilated cardiomyopathy by nucleotide sequencing of reverse transcription-nested polymerase chain reaction products. Hum Pathol 1998;29:578–584.
114. Baboonian C, Treasure T: Meta-analysis of the association of enteroviruses with human heart disease. Heart 1997;78:539–543.
115. Rigonan AS, Mann L, Chonmaitree T: Use of monoclonal antibodies to identify serotypes of enterovirus isolates. J Clin Microbiol 1998;36:1877–1881.
116. Burch GE, Sun SC, Colcolough HL, et al: Coxsackie B viral myocarditis and valvulitis identified in routine autopsy specimens by immunofluorescent techniques. Am Heart J 1967;74:13–23.
117. Burch GE, Sun SC, Chu KC, et al: Interstitial and coxsackievirus B myocarditis in infants and children: A comparative histologic and immunofluorescent study of 50 autopsied hearts. JAMA 1968;203:1–8.
118. Burch GE, Harb JM, Hiramoto Y: Coxsackie viral infection of human myocardium. Hum Pathol 1975;6: 120–125.
119. Arola A, Kalimo H, Ruuskanen O, Hyypia T: Experimental myocarditis induced by two different coxsackievirus B3 variants: Aspects of pathogenesis and comparison of diagnostic methods. J Med Virol 1995;47:251–259.
120. Hilton DA, Variend S, Pringle JH: Demonstration of Coxsackievirus RNA in formalin-fixed tissue sections from childhood myocarditis cases by in situ hybridization and the polymerase chain reaction. J Pathol 1993;170: 45–51.
121. Nicholson F, Ajetunmobi JF, Li M, et al: Molecular detection and serotypic analysis of enterovirus RNA in archival specimens from patients with acute myocarditis. Br Heart J 1995;74:522–527.
122. Woodall CJ, Watt NJ, Clements GB: Simple technique for detecting RNA viruses by PCR in single sections of wax embedded tissue. J Clin Pathol 1993;46:276–277.
123. Ueno H, Yokota Y, Shiotani H, et al: Significance of detection of enterovirus RNA in myocardial tissues by reverse transcription-polymerase chain reaction. Int J Cardiol 1995;51:157–164.
124. Hyypia T: Etiological diagnosis of viral heart disease. Scand J Infect Dis Suppl 1993;88:25–31.
125. Schowengerdt KO, Ni J, Denfield SW, et al: Association of parvovirus B19 genome in children with myocarditis and cardiac allograft rejection: Diagnosis using the polymerase chain reaction. Circulation 1997;96:3549–3554.
126. Domachowske JB, Dyer KD, Adams AG, et al: Eosinophil cationic protein/RNase 3 is another RNase A-family ribonuclease with direct antiviral activity. Nucleic Acids Res 1998;26:3358–3363.
127. Domachowske JB, Dyer KD, Bonville CA, Rosenberg HF: Recombinant human eosinophil-derived neurotoxin/RNase 2 functions as an effective antiviral agent against respiratory syncytial virus. J Infect Dis 1998; 177:1458–1464.
128. Egesten A, Dyer KD, Batten D, et al: Ribonucleases and host defense: Identification, localization and gene expression in adherent monocytes in vitro. Biochim Biophys Acta 1997;1358:255–260.
129. Hamalainen MM, Eskola JU, Hellman J, Pulkki K: Major interference from leukocytes in RT-PCR identified as neurotoxin ribonuclease from eosinophils: Detection of residual CML directly from cell lysates by use of an eosinophil-depleted cell preparation. Clin Chem 1999;45: 465–471.
130. Rosenberg HF, Dyer KD: Molecular cloning and characterization of a novel human ribonuclease (RNase k6): Increasing diversity in the enlarging ribonuclease gene family. Nucleic Acids Res 1996;24:3507–3513.
131. Saxena SK, Rybak SM, Davey RT Jr, et al: Angiogenin is a cytotoxic, tRNA-specific ribonuclease in the RNase A superfamily. J Biol Chem 1992;267:21982–21986.
132. Molina HA, Kierszenbaum F: Immunohistochemical detection of deposits of eosinophil-derived neurotoxin and eosinophil peroxidase in the myocardium of patients with Chagas' disease. Immunology 1988;64:725–731.
133. Vasku A, Soucek M, Znojil V, et al: Angiotensin I-converting enzyme and angiotensinogen gene interaction and prediction of essential hypertension. Kidney Int 1998;53:1479–1482.
134. Mondorf UF, Russ A, Wiesemann A, et al: Contribution of angiotensin I converting enzyme gene polymorphism and angiotensinogen gene polymorphism to blood pressure regulation in essential hypertension. Am J Hypertens 1998;11:174–183.
135. Kiema TR, Kauma H, Rantala AO, et al: Variation at the angiotensin-converting enzyme gene and angiotensinogen gene loci in relation to blood pressure. Hypertension 1996;28:1070–1075.
136. Caulfield M, Lavender P, Farrall M, et al: Linkage of the angiotensinogen gene to essential hypertension. N Engl J Med 1994;330:1629–1633.
137. Ishigami T, Umemura S, Iwamoto T, et al: Molecular variant of angiotensinogen gene is associated with coronary atherosclerosis. Circulation 1995;91:951–954.
138. Tiret L, Blanc H, Ruidavets JB, et al: Gene polymorphisms of the renin-angiotensin system in relation to hypertension and parental history of myocardial infarction and stroke: The PEGASE study. Projet d' Étude des Genes de l'Hypertension Arterielle Severe a Moderée Essentielle. J Hypertens 1998;16:37–44.

139. Ludwig EH, Borecki IB, Ellison RC, et al: Associations between candidate loci angiotensin-converting enzyme and angiotensinogen with coronary heart disease and myocardial infarction: The NHLBI Family Heart Study. Ann Epidemiol 1997;7:3–12.
140. Jeunemaitre X, Ledru F, Battaglia S, et al: Genetic polymorphisms of the renin-angiotensin system and angiographic extent and severity of coronary artery disease: The CORGENE study. Hum Genet 1997;99:66–73.
141. Kamitani A, Rakugi H, Higaki J, et al: Enhanced predictability of myocardial infarction in Japanese by combined genotype analysis. Hypertension 1995;25:950–953.
142. Riegger GA: Role of the renin-angiotensin system as a risk factor for control of morbidity and mortality in coronary artery disease. Cardiovasc Drugs Ther 1996;(10 Suppl 2):613–615.
143. Devlin RH, Deeb S, Brunzell J, Hayden MR: Partial gene duplication involving exon-Alu interchange results in lipoprotein lipase deficiency. Am J Hum Genet 1990;46: 112–119.
144. Normand T, Bergeron J, Fernandez-Margallo T, et al: Geographic distribution and genealogy of mutation 207 of the lipoprotein lipase gene in the French Canadian population of Quebec. Hum Genet 1992;89:671–675.
145. Ma Y, Henderson HE, Murthy V, et al: A mutation in the human lipoprotein lipase gene as the most common cause of familial chylomicronemia in French Canadians. N Engl J Med 1991;324:1761–1766.
146. Parrott CL, Alsayed N, Rebourcet R, Santamarina-Fojo S: ApoC-IIParis2: A premature termination mutation in the signal peptide of apoC-II resulting in the familial chylomicronemia syndrome. J Lipid Res 1992;33:361–367.
147. Reina M, Brunzell JD, Deeb SS: Molecular basis of familial chylomicronemia: Mutations in the lipoprotein lipase and apolipoprotein C-II genes. J Lipid Res 1992;33: 1823–1832.
148. Zanelli T, Catapano AL, Averna MR, et al: A new case of apo C-II deficiency with a nonsense mutation in the apo C-II gene. Clin Chim Acta 1994;224:111–118.
149. Brown MS, Goldstein JL: Expression of the familial hypercholesterolemia gene in heterozygotes: Mechanism for a dominant disorder in man. Science 1974;185:61–63.
150. Brown MS, Dana SE, Goldstein JL: Regulation of 3-hydroxy-3-methylglutaryl coenzyme A reductase activity in human fibroblasts by lipoproteins. Proc Natl Acad Sci USA 1973;70:2162–2166.
151. Brown MS, Goldstein JL: Receptor-mediated control of cholesterol metabolism. Science 1976;191:150–154.
152. Goldstein JL, Dana SE, Brunschede GY, Brown MS: Genetic heterogeneity in familial hypercholesterolemia: Evidence for two different mutations affecting functions of low-density lipoprotein receptor. Proc Natl Acad Sci USA 1975;72:1092–1096.
153. Goldstein JL, Brown MS: Familial hypercholesterolemia: A genetic regulatory defect in cholesterol metabolism. Am J Med 1975;58:147–150.
154. Seftel HC, Baker SG, Sandler MP, et al: A host of hypercholesterolaemic homozygotes in South Africa. BMJ 1980;281:633–636.
155. Vohl MC, Couture P, Moorjani S, et al: Rapid restriction fragment analysis for screening four point mutations of the low-density lipoprotein receptor gene in French Canadians. Hum Mutat 1995;6:243–246.
156. Varret M, Rabes JP, Thiart R, et al: LDLR Database (second edition): New additions to the database and the software, and results of the first molecular analysis. Nucleic Acids Res 1998;26:248–252.
157. Hobbs HH, Brown MS, Russell DW, et al: Deletion in the gene for the low-density-lipoprotein receptor in a majority of French Canadians with familial hypercholesterolemia. N Engl J Med 1987;317:734–737.
158. Jenkins T, Nicholls E, Gordon E, et al: Familial hypercholesterolaemia—a common genetic disorder in the Afrikaans population. S Afr Med J 1980;57:943–947.
159. Ohashi K, Ishibashi S, Yamamoto M, et al: A truncated species of apolipoprotein B (B-38.7) in a patient with homozygous hypobetalipoproteinemia associated with diabetes mellitus. Arterioscler Thromb Vasc Biol 1998; 18:1330–1334.
160. Ruotolo G, Zanelli T, Tettamanti C, et al: Hypobetalipoproteinemia associated with apo B-48.4, a truncated protein only 14 amino acids longer than apo B-48. Atherosclerosis 1998;137:125–131.
161. Gabelli C, Bilato C, Martini S, et al: Homozygous familial hypobetalipoproteinemia: Increased LDL catabolism in hypobetalipoproteinemia due to a truncated apolipoprotein B species, apo B-87Padova. Arterioscler Thromb Vasc Biol 1996;16:1189–1196.
162. Welty FK, Ordovas J, Schaefer EJ, et al: Identification and molecular analysis of two apoB gene mutations causing low plasma cholesterol levels. Circulation 1995;92: 2036–2040.
163. Farese RVJ, Garg A, Pierotti VR, et al: A truncated species of apolipoprotein B, B-83, associated with hypobetalipoproteinemia. J Lipid Res 1992;33:569–577.
164. Huang LS, Kayden H, Sokol RJ, Breslow JL. ApoB gene nonsense and splicing mutations in a compound heterozygote for familial hypobetalipoproteinemia. J Lipid Res 1991;32:1341–1348.
165. Ross RS, Hoeg JM, Higuchi K, et al: Homozygous hypobetalipoproteinemia: Transcriptional regulation and 5′-flanking sequence analysis in an apolipoprotein B deficiency state. Biochim Biophys Acta 1989;1004:29–35.
166. Pulai JI, Zakeri H, Kwok PY, et al: Donor splice mutation (665 + 1 G_T) in familial hypobetalipoproteinemia with no detectable apoB truncation [in process citation]. Am J Med Genet 1998;80:218–220.
167. Zannis VI, Just PW, Breslow JL: Human apolipoprotein E isoprotein subclasses are genetically determined. Am J Hum Genet 1981;33:11–24.
168. Nagy B, Rigo JJ, Fintor L, et al: Apolipoprotein E alleles in women with severe pre-eclampsia. J Clin Pathol 1998; 51:324–325.
169. Nakai K, Fusazaki T, Zhang T, et al: Polymorphism of the apolipoprotein E and angiotensin I converting enzyme genes in Japanese patients with myocardial infarction. Coron Artery Dis 1998;9:329–334.
170. Nakata Y, Katsuya T, Rakugi H, et al: Polymorphism of the apolipoprotein E and angiotensin-converting enzyme genes in Japanese subjects with silent myocardial ischemia. Hypertension 1996;27:1205–1209.
171. Srinivasan JR, Kachman MT, Killeen AA, et al: Genotyping of apolipoprotein E by matrix-assisted laser de-

sorption/ionization time-of-flight mass spectrometry. Rapid Commun Mass Spectrom 1998;12:1045–1050.

172. Kohler T, Rost AK, Purschwitz K, et al: Genotyping of human apolipoprotein E alleles by the new qualitative, microplate-based CASSI-detection assay. Biotechniques 1998;25:80–85.

173. Ghebremedhin E, Braak H, Braak E, Sahm J: Improved method facilitates reliable APOE genotyping of genomic DNA extracted from formaldehyde-fixed pathology specimens. J Neurosci Methods 1998;79:229–231.

174. Baron H, Fung S, Aydin A, et al: Oligonucleotide ligation assay for detection of apolipoprotein E polymorphisms. Clin Chem 1997;43:1984–1986.

175. Zivelin A, Rosenberg N, Peretz H, et al: Improved method for genotyping apolipoprotein E polymorphisms by a PCR-based assay simultaneously utilizing two distinct restriction enzymes. Clin Chem 1997;43:1657–1659.

176. Little DP, Braun A, Darnhofer-Demar B, Koster H: Identification of apolipoprotein E polymorphisms using temperature cycled primer oligo base extension and mass spectrometry. Eur J Clin Chem Clin Biochem 1997;35:545–548.

177. Bolla MK, Haddad L, Humphries SE, et al: High-throughput method for determination of apolipoprotein E genotypes with use of restriction digestion analysis by microplate array diagonal gel electrophoresis. Clin Chem 1995;41:1599–1604.

178. Reymer PW, Groenemeyer BE, van de Burg R, Kastelein JJ: Apolipoprotein E genotyping on agarose gels. Clin Chem 1995;41:1046–1047.

179. Dallinga-Thie GM, van Linde-Sibenius T, Kock LA, De Bruin TW: Apolipoprotein E2/E3/E4 genotyping with agarose gels. Clin Chem 1995;41:73–75.

180. Crook R, Hardy J, Duff K: Single-day apolipoprotein E genotyping. J Neurosci Methods 1994;53:125–127.

181. Hansen PS, Gerdes LU, Klausen IC, et al: Genotyping compared with protein phenotyping of the common apolipoprotein E polymorphism. Clin Chim Acta 1994;224:131–137.

182. Tsai MY, Suess P, Schwichtenberg K, et al: Determination of apolipoprotein E genotypes by single-strand conformational polymorphism. Clin Chem 1993;39:2121–2124.

183. Stavljenic-Rukavina A, Sertic J, Salzer B, et al: Apolipoprotein E phenotypes and genotypes as determined by polymerase chain reaction using allele-specific oligonucleotide probes and the amplification refractory mutation system in children with insulin-dependent diabetes mellitus. Clin Chim Acta 1993;216:191–198.

184. Guo C, Marynen P, Cassiman JJ: A rapid, semiautomated method for apolipoprotein E genotyping. PCR Methods Appl 1993;2:348–350.

185. Green EK, Bain SC, Day PJ, et al: Detection of human apolipoprotein E3, E2, and E4 genotypes by an allele-specific oligonucleotide-primed polymerase chain reaction assay: Development and validation. Clin Chem 1991;37:1263–1268.

186. Wenham PR, Price WH, Blandell G: Apolipoprotein E genotyping by one-stage PCR [letter]. Lancet 1991;337:1158–1159.

187. Main BF, Jones PJ, MacGillivray RT, Banfield DK: Apolipoprotein E genotyping using the polymerase chain reaction and allele-specific oligonucleotide primers. J Lipid Res 1991;32:183–187.

188. Kontula K, Aalto-Setala K, Kuusi T, et al: Apolipoprotein E polymorphism determined by restriction enzyme analysis of DNA amplified by polymerase chain reaction: Convenient alternative to phenotyping by isoelectric focusing. Clin Chem 1990;36:2087–2092.

189. Hixson JE, Vernier DT: Restriction isotyping of human apolipoprotein E by gene amplification and cleavage with HhaI. J Lipid Res 1990;31:545–548.

190. Ilveskoski E, Lehtimaki T, Erkinjuntti T, et al: Rapid apolipoprotein E genotyping from mailed buccal swabs. J Neurosci Methods 1998;79:5–8.

191. Boers GH: Carriership for homocystinuria in juvenile vascular disease. Haemostasis 1989;19(Suppl 1):29–34.

192. Brattstrom LE, Hardebo JE, Hultberg BL: Moderate homocysteinemia—a possible risk factor for arteriosclerotic cerebrovascular disease. Stroke 1984;15:1012–1016.

193. Bienvenu T, Ankri A, Chadefaux B, et al: Elevated total plasma homocysteine, a risk factor for thrombosis: Relation to coagulation and fibrinolytic parameters. Thromb Res 1993;70:123–129.

194. Florell SR, Rodgers GM: Inherited thrombotic disorders: An update. Am J Hematol 1997;54:53–60.

195. Simioni P, Prandoni P, Burlina A, et al: Hyperhomocysteinemia and deep-vein thrombosis: A case-control study. Thromb Haemost 1996;76:883–886.

196. Brattstrom L, Israelsson B, Norrving B, et al: Impaired homocysteine metabolism in early-onset cerebral and peripheral occlusive arterial disease: Effects of pyridoxine and folic acid treatment. Atherosclerosis 1990;81:51–60.

197. Dudman NP, Wilcken DE, Wang J, et al: Disordered methionine/homocysteine metabolism in premature vascular disease: Its occurrence, cofactor therapy, and enzymology. Arterioscler Thromb 1993;13:1253–1260.

198. Selhub J, Jacques PF, Wilson PW, et al: Vitamin status and intake as primary determinants of homocysteinemia in an elderly population. JAMA 1993;270:2693–2698.

199. Kraus JP: Biochemistry and molecular genetics of cystathionine beta-synthase deficiency. Eur J Pediatr 1998;157(Suppl 2):S50–S53.

200. De Backer G, De Henauw S, Sans S, et al: A comparison of lifestyle, genetic, bioclinical and biochemical variables of offspring with and without family histories of premature coronary heart disease: The experience of the European Atherosclerosis Research Studies [in process citation]. J Cardiovasc Risk 1999;6:183–188.

201. Carter AM, Mansfield MW, Stickland MH, Grant PJ: Beta-fibrinogen gene-455 G/A polymorphism and fibrinogen levels: Risk factors for coronary artery disease in subjects with NIDDM. Diabetes Care 1996;19:1265–1268.

202. Carter AM, Ossei-Gerning N, Wilson IJ, Grant PJ: Association of the platelet Pl(A) polymorphism of glycoprotein IIb/IIIa and the fibrinogen Bbeta 448 polymorphism with myocardial infarction and extent of coronary artery disease. Circulation 1997;96:1424–1431.

203. Gensini GF, Comeglio M, Colella A: Classical risk factors and emerging elements in the risk profile for coronary artery disease. Eur Heart J 1998;19(Suppl A):A53–A61.

204. Nishiuma S, Kario K, Yakushijin K, et al: Genetic variation in the promoter region of the beta-fibrinogen gene is

associated with ischemic stroke in a Japanese population. Blood Coagul Fibrinolysis 1998;9:373–379.

205. Schmidt H, Schmidt R, Niederkorn K, et al: Beta-fibrinogen gene polymorphism (C148→T) is associated with carotid atherosclerosis: Results of the Austrian Stroke Prevention Study. Arterioscler Thromb Vasc Biol 1998;18: 487–492.

206. Kessler C, Spitzer C, Stauske D, et al: The apolipoprotein E and beta-fibrinogen G/A-455 gene polymorphisms are associated with ischemic stroke involving large-vessel disease. Arterioscler Thromb Vasc Biol 1997;17:2880–2884.

207. de Maat MP, Kastelein JJ, Jukema JW, et al: −455G/A polymorphism of the beta-fibrinogen gene is associated with the progression of coronary atherosclerosis in symptomatic men: Proposed role for an acute-phase reaction pattern of fibrinogen. REGRESS group. Arterioscler Thromb Vasc Biol 1998;18:265–271.

208. Behague I, Poirier O, Nicaud V, et al: Beta fibrinogen gene polymorphisms are associated with plasma fibrinogen and coronary artery disease in patients with myocardial infarction. The ECTIM Study: Étude Cas-Temoins sur l'Infarctus du Myocarde. Circulation 1996; 93:440–449.

209. Wang XL, Wang J, McCredie RM, Wilcken DE: Polymorphisms of factor V, factor VII, and fibrinogen genes: Relevance to severity of coronary artery disease. Arterioscler Thromb Vasc Biol 1997;17:246–251.

210. Heinrich J, Funke H, Rust S, et al: Impact of polymorphisms in the alpha- and beta-fibrinogen gene on plasma fibrinogen concentrations of coronary heart disease patients. Thromb Res 1995;77:209–215.

211. Margaglione M, Cappucci G, Colaizzo D, et al: Fibrinogen plasma levels in an apparently healthy general population-relation to environmental and genetic determinants. Thromb Haemost 1998;80:805–810.

212. Yu Q, Safavi F, Roberts R, Marian AJ: A variant of beta fibrinogen is a genetic risk factor for coronary artery disease and myocardial infarction. J Investig Med 1996;44: 154–159.

213. Anderson JL, King GJ, Bair TL, et al: Associations between a polymorphism in the gene encoding glycoprotein IIIa and myocardial infarction or coronary artery disease. J Am Coll Cardiol 1999;33:727–733.

214. Garcia-Ribes M, Gonzalez-Lamuno D, Hernandez-Estefania R, et al: Polymorphism of the platelet glycoprotein IIIa gene in patients with coronary stenosis. Thromb Haemost 1998;79:1126–1129.

215. Kastrati A, Schomig A, Seyfarth M, et al: PlA polymorphism of platelet glycoprotein IIIa and risk of restenosis after coronary stent placement. Circulation 1999;99: 1005–1010.

216. Durante-Mangoni E, Davies GJ, Ahmed N, et al: Coronary thrombosis and the platelet glycoprotein IIIA gene *PLA2* polymorphism. Thromb Haemost 1998;80: 218–219.

217. Herrmann SM, Poirier O, Marques-Vidal P, et al: The Leu33/Pro polymorphism (PlA1/PlA2) of the glycoprotein IIIa (GPIIIa) receptor is not related to myocardial infarction in the ECTIM Study. Étude Cas-Temoins de l'Infarctus du Myocarde. Thromb Haemost 1997;77: 1179–1181.

218. Kekomaki S, Hamalainen L, Kauppinen-Makelin R, et al: Genetic polymorphism of platelet glycoprotein IIIa in patients with acute myocardial infarction and acute ischaemic stroke. J Cardiovasc Risk 1999;6:13–17.

219. Laule M, Cascorbi I, Stangl V, et al: A1/A2 polymorphism of glycoprotein IIIa and association with excess procedural risk for coronary catheter interventions: A case-controlled study. Lancet 1999;353:708–712.

220. Mamotte CD, van Bockxmeer FM, Taylor RR: PIa1/a2 polymorphism of glycoprotein IIIa and risk of coronary artery disease and restenosis following coronary angioplasty. Am J Cardiol 1998;82:13–6.

221. Ridker PM, Hennekens CH, Schmitz C, et al: PIA1/A2 polymorphism of platelet glycoprotein IIIa and risks of myocardial infarction, stroke, and venous thrombosis. Lancet 1997;349:385–388.

222. Campbell LA, Kuo CC, Grayston JT: *Chlamydia pneumoniae* and cardiovascular disease [in process citation]. Emerg Infect Dis 1998;4:571–579.

223. Yamashita K, Ouchi K, Shirai M, et al: Distribution of *Chlamydia pneumoniae* infection in the atherosclerotic carotid artery. Stroke 1998;29:773–778.

224. Ossewaarde JM, Feskens EJ, De Vries A, et al: *Chlamydia pneumoniae* is a risk factor for coronary heart disease in symptom-free elderly men, but *Helicobacter pylori* and cytomegalovirus are not. Epidemiol Infect 1998;120:93–99.

225. Kuo CC, Coulson AS, Campbell LA, et al: Detection of *Chlamydia pneumoniae* in atherosclerotic plaques in the walls of arteries of lower extremities from patients undergoing bypass operation for arterial obstruction. J Vasc Surg 1997;26:29–31.

226. Wimmer ML, Sandmann-Strupp R, Saikku P, Haberl RL: Association of chlamydial infection with cerebrovascular disease. Stroke 1996;27:2207–2210.

227. Juvonen J, Juvonen T, Laurila A, et al: Immunohistochemical detection of *Chlamydia pneumoniae* in abdominal aortic aneurysms. Ann N Y Acad Sci 1996;800:236–238.

228. Blasi F, Denti F, Erba M, et al: Detection of *Chlamydia pneumoniae* but not *Helicobacter pylori* in atherosclerotic plaques of aortic aneurysms. J Clin Microbiol 1996;34: 2766–2769.

229. Ong G, Thomas BJ, Mansfield AO, et al: Detection and widespread distribution of *Chlamydia pneumoniae* in the vascular system and its possible implications. J Clin Pathol 1996;49:102–106.

230. Kuo CC, Grayston JT, Campbell LA, et al: *Chlamydia pneumoniae* (TWAR) in coronary arteries of young adults (15–34 years old). Proc Natl Acad Sci U S A 1995;92*(15)*: 6911–6914.

231. Melnick SL, Shahar E, Folsom AR, et al: Past infection by *Chlamydia pneumoniae* strain TWAR and asymptomatic carotid atherosclerosis. Atherosclerosis Risk in Communities (ARIC) Study Investigators. Am J Med 1993;95: 499–504.

232. Kuo CC, Gown AM, Benditt EP, Grayston JT: Detection of *Chlamydia pneumoniae* in aortic lesions of atherosclerosis by immunocytochemical stain. Arterioscler Thromb 1993;13:1501–1504.

233. Valtonen VV: Infection as a risk factor for infarction and atherosclerosis. Ann Med 1991;23:539–543.

234. Kaukoranta-Tolvanen SS, Laitinen K, Saikku P, Leinonen M: *Chlamydia pneumoniae* multiplies in human endothelial cells in vitro. Microb Pathog 1994;16:313–319.
235. Godzik KL, O'Brien ER, Wang SK, Kuo CC: In vitro susceptibility of human vascular wall cells to infection with *Chlamydia pneumoniae.* J Clin Microbiol 1995;33: 2411–2414.
236. Fong IW, Chiu B, Viira E, et al: Rabbit model for *Chlamydia pneumoniae* infection. J Clin Microbiol 1997;35: 48–52.
237. Laitinen K, Laurila A, Pyhala L, et al: *Chlamydia pneumoniae* infection induces inflammatory changes in the aortas of rabbits. Infect Immun 1997;65:4832–4835.
238. Paterson DL, Hall J, Rasmussen SJ, Timms P: Failure to detect *Chlamydia pneumoniae* in atherosclerotic plaques of Australian patients. Pathology 1998;30:169–172.
239. Lindholt JS, Ostergard L, Henneberg EW, et al: Failure to demonstrate *Chlamydia pneumoniae* in symptomatic abdominal aortic aneurysms by a nested polymerase chain reaction (PCR). Eur J Vasc Endovasc Surg 1998; 15:161–164.
240. Jacobson DR, Alves IL, Saraiva MJ, et al: Transthyretin Ser 6 gene frequency in individuals without amyloidosis. Hum Genet 1995;95:308–312.
241. Fitch NJ, Akbari MT, Ramsden DB: An inherited nonamyloidogenic transthyretin variant, [Ser6]-TTR, with increased thyroxine-binding affinity, characterized by DNA sequencing. J Endocrinol 1991;129:309–313.
242. Jacobson DR, Pan T, Kyle RA, Buxbaum JN: Transthyretin ILE20, a new variant associated with late-onset cardiac amyloidosis. Hum Mutat 1997;9:83–85.
243. Utsugisawa K, Tohgi H, Nagane Y, et al: Familial amyloid polyneuropathy related to transthyretin mutation Val30 to Leu in a Japanese family. Muscle Nerve 1998;21: 1783–1785.
244. Grateau G, Adams D, Malapert D, et al: Late-onset familial amyloid polyneuropathy with the TTR Met 30 mutation in France. Clin Genet 1993;43:143–145.
245. Skare J, Yazici H, Erken E, et al: Homozygosity for the met30 transthyretin gene in a Turkish kindred with familial amyloidotic polyneuropathy. Hum Genet 1990;86:89–90.
246. Herrick MK, DeBruyne K, Horoupian DS, et al: Massive leptomeningeal amyloidosis associated with a Val30Met transthyretin gene. Neurology 1996;47:988–992.
247. Aoki K, Koike R, Yuasa T, et al: [A sporadic case of late onset familial amyloidotic polyneuropathy preceded by cardiac involvement]. Rinsho Shinkeigaku 1993;33: 905–908.
248. Myers TJ, Kyle RA, Jacobson DR: Familial amyloid with a transthyretin leucine 33 mutation presenting with ascites. Am J Hematol 1998;59:249–251.
249. Klein CJ, Nakumura M, Jacobson DR, et al: Transthyretin amyloidosis (serine 44) with headache, hearing loss, and peripheral neuropathy. Neurology 1998;51: 1462–1464.
250. Saraiva MJ, Almeida MD, Sherman W, et al: A new transthyretin mutation associated with amyloid cardiomyopathy. Am J Hum Genet 1992;50:1027–1030.
251. Booth DR, Tan SY, Hawkins PN, et al: A novel variant of transthyretin, 59Thr→Lys, associated with autosomal dominant cardiac amyloidosis in an Italian family. Circulation 1995;91:962–967.
252. Yasuda T, Sobue G, Doyu M, et al: Familial amyloidotic polyneuropathy with late-onset and well-preserved autonomic function: A Japanese kindred with novel mutant transthyretin (Ala97 to Gly). J Neurol Sci 1994;121: 97–102.
253. Uemichi T, Gertz MA, Benson MD: Amyloid polyneuropathy in two German-American families: A new transthyretin variant (Val 107). J Med Genet 1994;31:416–417.
254. Jacobson DR, Gertz MA, Buxbaum JN: Transthyretin VAL107, a new variant associated with familial cardiac and neuropathic amyloidosis. Hum Mutat 1994;3: 399–401.
255. Scrimshaw BJ, Fellowes AP, Palmer BN, et al: A novel variant of transthyretin (prealbumin), Thr119 to Met, associated with increased thyroxine binding. Thyroid 1992;2:21–26.
256. Jacobson DR, Pastore RD, Yaghoubian R, et al: Variant-sequence transthyretin (isoleucine 122) in late-onset cardiac amyloidosis in black Americans. N Engl J Med 1997;336:466–473.

CHAPTER 7 APPENDIX

SOP 7.1*

APOLIPOPROTEIN E GENOTYPING

PRINCIPLE

Apolipoprotein (apo) E serves as a ligand for low-density lipoprotein receptor uptake (the apo B/E receptor) and mediates the binding of chylomicron remnants to the apo E receptor. The apo E gene is located on chromosome 19 and spans 3.7 kilobases, including four exons. The three major genotypes are the wild-type apo E3, as well as the isoforms apo E2 (frequency 10%) and apo E4 (frequency 15%). These proteins differ by amino acid substitution at one or both of the 112 and 158 positions. Apo E4 is associated with increased low-density lipoprotein cholesterol, coronary artery disease, and Alzheimer's disease. Many patients with type III hyperlipoproteinemia are either homozygous or heterozygous for apo E2.

SPECIMEN (SEE SOP 1)

Specimen: blood
Recommended volume: 5 mL in sodium citrate or EDTA anticoagulant
Minimum amount: 300 μL (0.3 mL)
Storage: up to 5 days at 4°C before initial processing

REAGENTS, SUPPLIES, AND EQUIPMENT

ALWAYS WEAR GLOVES WHEN HANDLING REAGENTS. FOLLOW PROCEDURES FOR AVOIDING CONTAMINATION OF PCR REACTIONS!! (See SOP 2)

The usual source of a reagent is indicated in brackets [ ]: Fisher [FI], PerkinElmer [PE], Promega [PR], Sigma [S], New England Biomedical [NEB], GibcoBRL [BRL], etc. Homemade reagents are abbreviated [MDL], and the lot number in use has been quality control tested. An asterisk [*] is used when the source varies.

* SOP 7.1 by Sherman A. McCall, MO, Department of Cellular Pathology and Genetics, Armed Forces Institute of Pathology, Washington, DC.

Preparation of DNA Lysates (see SOP 4)

Polymerase Chain Reaction (PCR)

REAGENTS

Water molecular grade [S]
PCR buffer II, 10X [PE]
dNTP 2.5 mmol/L each [PR] [MDL]

1. To prepare, first make a 10-mmol/L solution from a 100-mmol/L (1:10 dilution) stock dilution of each dNTP (dATP, dCTP, dGTP, and dTTP) as follows. To prepare 1 mL of a 10-mmol/L solution of each dNTP, add 900 μL of water to four microcentrifuge tubes; then add 100 μL of each dNTP (100 mmol/L) and mix well.
2. Next, mix equal volumes of each 10-mmol/L solution to make each dNTP 2.5 mmol/L in the final mix.
3. Aliquot and label tubes. Store in DNA freezer.

Ampli Taq Gold (5 U/mL) [PE]
$MgCl_2$ (25 mmol/L) [PE]

PRIMERS

Primers are stored in the post-PCR freezer in a dilution of 20 μmol/L.
PRIMER SM12 (3′ primer, 20-mer), APO E GENE EXON 4
5′-AAC AAC TGA CCC CGG TGG CG-3′
PRIMER SM13 (5′ primer, 20-mer), APO E GENE EXON 4
5′-ATG GCG CTG AGG CCG CGC TC-3′

PCR Mix	μL per Sample	Final Concentration	Aliquots	Total
10× Buff	5	1×	6	30
25 mmol/L MgCl2	3	1.5 mmol/L	6	18
10 mmol/L dNTPs	1	0.2 mmol/L	6	6
20 mmol/L SM12	1	0.4 μmol/L	6	6
20 mmol/L SM13	1	100 μmol/L	6	6
DMSO	5	100 mL/L	6	30
Ampli Tag Gold	0.25	1.25 U	6	1.5
Sample	2		6	12
dH_2O	31.75		6	190.5
Total	50			300

MASTER MIX

Use a master mix. Refer to SOP 13 for additional information on master mixes and their setup. The volume per 50-μL reaction (including 5-μL sample) is as follows. Add Taq polymerase and sample immediately before use.

SUPPLIES AND EQUIPMENT

Microcentrifuge tubes (1.5 and 0.5 mL)
Aerosol-resistant pipette tips (ART tips)
Disposable gloves
Extra-fine-tip permanent marker and racks
Pipetters
Microcentrifuge (reserved for pre-PCR use only)
PerkinElmer DNA Thermal Cycler Model 9600
Vortexer

Enzyme Digestion

Reagents

*Hha*I restriction enzyme, 20 U/μL

Supplier: New England Biolabs (NEB)
Storage: $-20°C$, Products Lab

10X NE (New England) Buffer #4 (1X = 10 mmol/L TRIS-HCl, 10 mmol/L $MgCl_2$, 50 mmol/L NaCl, 1 mmol/L DTT, pH = 7.9)

Supplier: NEB (supplied with enzyme)
Storage: $-20°C$, Products Lab

100X bovine serum albumin (BSA), 100 μg/mL

Supplier: NEB (supplied with enzyme)
Storage: $-20°C$, Products Lab
TEMED [Sigma]

QUALITY CONTROL

Several types of positive and negative controls are run with each assay. Placement of the controls within an assay is crucial to the detection of contamination at each step in the test system.

Positive Assay Control

Apo E2 or E4 heterozygotes will be identified as positive controls as clinical testing is performed.

Negative Assay Control

A negative control is placed at each step in the test system: lysate preparation, reagent mix preparation, and carryover contamination from sample to sample in the assay setup procedure.

WATER CONTROL. A PCR reaction mix containing water as the sample tested is set up first in the PCR run, before patient samples, to assess purity of the assay reagents.

LYSATE CONTROL. A lysate (no DNA template) prepared in parallel with patient samples should give no detectable band, indicating that the tube was not contaminated with DNA during lysate preparation.

CONTAMINATION CONTROL. A negative control PCR reaction containing water as the sample tested is set up last in the PCR run, after the positive control. This reaction assesses the quality of the setup procedure in avoiding carryover contamination from a positive to an adjacent negative sample.

Assay Controls

Run positive control and wild-type controls along with patient samples.

PROCEDURE

FOLLOW PROCEDURES FOR AVOIDING CONTAMINATION OF PCR REACTIONS!! (See SOP 2)

Preparation of DNA Lysates (see SOP 4)

Polymerase Chain Reaction (PCR)

Use PerkinElmer Thermal Cycler Model 9600.

1. Determine the number of reactions (one per sample, plus one water control, one lysate control, one positive control, and one contamination control). Prepare enough reagent for two additional assays (two plus the number of samples and controls = N). The master mix is aliquoted with 45 μL per reaction.
2. Number each 0.5-mL microcentrifuge tube consecutively with an extra-fine-point permanent marker. Record assay number and identity of sample (MDL#, control) on worksheet.
3. Mix the components of master mix to a total volume of 45 μL × N in a labeled 1.5-mL tube (or a larger tube for volumes greater than 1.5 mL). Add Ampli Taq Gold last and tap tube gently to mix. Store on ice until use.
4. Add 45 mL of master mix to each reaction tube and cap tubes.
5. Add 5 mL of water to water control.
6. Add 5 mL of the negative control lysate (without DNA template) to the lysate control tube.
7. Add positive control lysate (5 μL of a factor V heterozygote) to appropriate tubes after all samples have been prepared. The setup order is as follows:
   - Water
   - Lysate control
   - Patient samples
   - Positive controls
   - Contamination control
8. Add 5 μL of water to the contamination control.
9. Place in PerkinElmer Thermal Cycler Model 9600 and cycle with times and temperatures below:

Denaturation:	12 min 94°C
Initial PCR (5 cycles):	1 min 95°C
	3 min 72°C
PCR (40 cycles):	1 min 94°C
	1 min 65°C
	1 min 72°C
Extension:	7 min 72°C

10. Remove sample tray from thermal cycler, and place tubes in a rack in a refrigerator in post-PCR room for analysis by gel electrophoresis.
11. Save isolated DNA and remaining buffy coats at $-70°C$.

Restriction Enzyme Digestion

1. Make digestion buffer with 9 μL of 100X bovine serum albumin (BSA) [NEB] in 91 μL of *Hha*I buffer. Store buffer mix at $-20°C$ and reuse.
2. At time of digestion, add *Hha*I enzyme to buffer mix. Use 3 μL of buffer and 1 μL of enzyme (20 U/μL) for each reaction. Buffer/enzyme mix cannot be stored.
3. Pipette 4 μL of buffer/enzyme mix for each reaction, and add 26 μL of sample PCR product. Incubate at 37°C for at least 3 hours.
4. When digestion is complete, add 5 μL of agarose loading dye to the digested PCR products.

Polyacrylamide Gel Electrophoresis

The products are resolved on 10% nondenaturing polyacrylamide tall minigel run in 1X Tris, Boric acid, EDTA (TBE) at 100 V. Assemble the gel unit using the thin 0.75-mm spacers, and pour hot 1% agarose down the sides of the plate to seal the bottom. Make the gel with 15 mL of 40% 19:1 acrylamide/bis solution, to which add 50 μL 25% APS and 5 μL TEMED. Fill the rig and place the comb.

Ideally there should be a wild type, a heterozygote control, and size markers. Develop the gel in ethidium bromide, and photograph for documentation. The lower indicator, bromophenol blue, run between 20 and 30 bp. To visualize the smallest 35-bp fragment and the lower rungs of the ladder, stop the dye front just short of the end of the gel. The very small and closely spaced fragments are best interpreted if a 10-bp ladder is used [BRL]. To compensate for irregularities in the dye front it is useful to put the ladder last in both the first and last lanes.

REPORTING RESULTS

Interpretation

Undigested PCR product: 292 bp
Normal (E3): 91, 61, 48, 35 bp
E4: 72, 61, 48, 35 bp
E2: 91, 83, 61 bp
Water control: none

These bands are for homozygotes of these alleles. Heterozygotes share the bands of each allele. A hint in interpretation: with a single exception, a four-band pattern is a normal E3 homozygote. The exception is an E4 homozygote who is missing the normal 91-bp band and has an unexpected band at 72 bp. All other combinations express either three bands or more than four.

Limitations and Interference

Over 30 apo E variants have been described, 14 of which are associated with familial dysbetalipoproteinemia, a genetic lipid disorder characterized by elevated plasma cholesterol and triglyceride levels and risk of atherosclerosis. Seven apo E variants are associated with other forms of hyperlipoproteinemia.

PROCEDURE NOTES (ALTERNATIVE METHODS)

Phenotyping

The original classification of isoforms is based on global charge determined by isoelectric focusing (IFE). The wild type (E3) has zero charge, E4 has 1+, and E2 is −1. Minor variants may overlap in phenotype, however. Other methods include hybridization or sequencing.

REFERENCES

Contois J, Anamani D, Tsongalis G: The underlying molecular mechanism of apolipoprotein E polymorphism relationships to lipid disorders, cardiovascular disease, and Alzheimer's disease. Clin Lab Med 1996;16: 105–123.

Pascale R, Thomas G, de Zulueta M, et al: Common and rare genotypes of human apolipoprotein E determined by specific restriction profiles of polymerase chain reaction-amplified DNA. Clin Chem 1994;40:24–29.

SOP 7.2*

FACTOR V LEIDEN (PROTHROMBIN MUTATION MULTIPLEX)

PRINCIPLE

Factor V gene mutation analysis is useful for identifying the cause of activated protein C (APC) resistance identified by functional coagulation testing. It is also used to establish the diagnosis of APC resistance when functional coagulation testing is not feasible (e.g., with patients on anticoagulant therapy or possessing lupus anticoagulants). Assay for factor V genotype detects a novel polymorphism (Glu1691Arg) in exon 10 of the factor V gene that substitutes the arginine at amino acid 506 with glutamine. This mutation is associated with a sevenfold increased risk of venous thrombosis (representing up to 20% of cases).

A second common disorder is the Gly20210Ala mutation in the 3′ untranslated region of the prothrombin gene. It appears to increase prothrombin levels and is associated with an odds ratio of 2.8 for deep venous thrombosis.

Because it cannot be known a priori which defect a given hypercoagulation patient has, this is a multiplex assay for both defects. Mutagenic primers are used to create a *Taq*I endonuclease site in wild-type patients yielding digestion products 20 bp shorter than each of the original amplification products. When the mutation is present, no cleavage takes place.

SPECIMEN (see SOP 1)

Specimen: blood
Recommended volume: 5 mL in sodium citrate or EDTA anticoagulant
Minimum amount: 300 μL (0.3 mL)
Storage: up to 5 days at 4°C before initial processing

REAGENTS, SUPPLIES, AND EQUIPMENT

ALWAYS WEAR GLOVES WHEN HANDLING REAGENTS. FOLLOW PROCEDURES FOR AVOIDING CONTAMINATION OF PCR REACTIONS!! (See SOP 2).

Denaturation	**94 °C—12′**	
Initial PCR	95 °C—1′	
	72 °C—3′	5 cycles
PCR	94 °C—1′	
	65 °C—1′	
	72 °C—1′	40 cycles
Extension	72 °C—7′	

The usual source of a reagent is indicated in brackets [ ]: Fisher [FI], PerkinElmer [PE], Promega [PR], Sigma [S], New England Biomedical [NEB], etc. Homemade reagents are abbreviated [MDL], and the lot number in use has been quality control tested. An asterisk [*] is used when the source varies.

* SOP 7.2 by Karen E. Bijuaard, MS; Jack H. Lichy, MD, PhD; Sherman A. McCall, MD, all at the Department of Cellular Pathology and Genetics, Armed Forces Institute of Pathology, Washington, DC.

Preparation of DNA Lysates (see SOP 4)

Polymerase Chain Reaction (PCR)

REAGENTS

Water molecular grade [S]
PCR buffer II, 10× [PE]
dNTP 2.5 mmol/L each [PR] [MDL]

1. To prepare, first make a 10-mmol/L solution from a 100-mmol/L (1:10 dilution) stock dilution of each dNTP (dATP, dCTP, dGTP, and dTTP) as follows. To prepare 1 mL of a 10-mmol/L solution of each dNTP, add 900 μL of water to four microcentrifuge tubes, then add 100 μL of each dNTP (100 mmol/L) and mix well.
2. Next, mix equal volumes of each 10-mmol/L solution to make each dNTP 2.5 mmol/L in the final mix.
3. Aliquot and label tubes. Store in DNA freezer.

Ampli Taq Gold (5 U/μL) [PE]
$MgCl_2$ (25 mmol/L) [PE]

PRIMERS

Primers are stored in the post-PCR freezer in a dilution of 20 μM.

PRIMER SM2 (3′ primer, 20-mer); nt: 127 to 146 in intron 10 of factor V
5′-TGT TAT CAC ACT GGT GCT AA-3′

PRIMER SM9 (5′ primer, 18-mer); nt: 1673–1690 of factor V
5′-GCA GAT CCC TGG ACA GTC-3′

PRIMER SM10 (5′ primer, 20-mer)
5′-CAA TAA AAG TGA CTC TCA TC-3′ (20190–20209)

PRIMER SM11 (3′ primer, 20-mer)
5′-AGG TGG TGG ATT CTT AAG TC-3′ (20307–20288)

MASTER MIX

Use a master mix. Refer to SOP 13 for additional information on master mixes and their setup. The volume per 50-μL reaction (including 5-μL sample) is as follows. Add Taq polymerase and sample immediately before use.

SUPPLIES AND EQUIPMENT

Microcentrifuge tubes (1.5 and 0.5 mL)
Aerosol-resistant pipette tips (ART tips)
Disposable gloves
Extra-fine-tip permanent marker and racks
Pipetters
Microcentrifuge (reserved for pre-PCR use only)
PerkinElmer Thermal Cycler Model 9600
Vortexer

Enzyme Digestion

REAGENTS

Enzymes

TaqI restriction enzyme, 20 U/μL

Supplier: New England Biolabs (NEB)
Storage: −20°C, Products Lab

10X NE (New England) Buffer *Taq*I, (1X = 10 mmol/L TRIS HCl, 10 mmol/L $MgCl_2$, 50 mmol/L NaCl, 1 mmol/L DTT, pH = 7.9)

Supplier: NEB (supplied with enzyme)
Storage: −20°C, Products Lab

100X bovine serum albumin (BSA), 100 μg/mL

Supplier: NEB (supplied with enzyme)
Storage: −20°C, Products Lab

Agarose Gel Electrophoresis (see SOP 6)

All reagents are in the post-PCR room. Use 2.5% agarose.

QUALITY CONTROL

Several types of positive and negative controls are run with each assay. Placement of the controls within an assay is crucial to the detection of contamination at each step in the test system.

Positive Assay Control

The factor V positive control is a lysate from blood of a factor V Leiden heterozygote. The prothrombin control is a heterozygote.

Negative Assay Controls

A negative control is placed at each step in the test system: lysate preparation, reagent mix preparation, and carryover contamination from sample to sample in the assay setup procedure.

WATER CONTROL. A PCR reaction mix containing water as the sample tested is set up first in the PCR run, before patient samples, to assess purity of the assay reagents.

LYSATE CONTROL. A lysate (no DNA template) prepared in parallel with patient samples should give no detectable band, indicating that the tube was not contaminated with DNA during lysate preparation.

CONTAMINATION CONTROL. A negative control PCR reaction containing water as the sample tested is set up last in the PCR run, after the positive control. This reaction assesses the quality of the setup procedure in avoiding carryover contamination from a positive to an adjacent negative sample.

Assay Controls

Run positive control and wild-type controls along with patient samples.

PROCEDURE

FOLLOW PROCEDURES FOR AVOIDING CONTAMINATION OF PCR REACTIONS!! (See SOP 1 in Appendix at back of book)

Preparation of DNA Lysates (see SOP 4 in Appendix at back of book)

Polymerase Chain Reaction (PCR)

Use PerkinElmer Thermal Cycler Model 9600.

1. Determine the number of reactions (one per sample, plus one water control, one lysate control, one positive control, and one contamination control). Prepare enough reagent for two additional assays (two plus the number of samples and controls = N). The master mix is aliquoted with 45 μL per reaction.
2. Number each 0.5-mL microcentrifuge reaction tube, consecutively, with an extra-fine-point permanent marker. Record assay number and identity of sample (laboratory accession number, control) on worksheet.
3. Mix the components of master mix to a total volume of 45 μL × N in a labeled 1.5-mL tube (or a larger tube for volumes greater than 1.5 mL). Add Ampli Taq Gold last and tap tube gently to mix. Store on ice until use.
4. Add 45 μL of master mix to each reaction tube and cap tubes.
5. Add 5 μL of water to water control.
6. Add 5 μL of the negative control lysate (without DNA template) to the lysate control tube.
7. Add 2 μL of sample and 3 μL of water to each sample tube.

PCR Mix	μL per Sample	Final Concentration
10× Buff	5	1×
25 mmol/L $MgCl_2$	3	1.5 mmol/L
10 mmol/L dNTPs	1	0.2 mmol/L
20 mmol/L SM2	1.5	0.6 μmol/L
20 mmol/L SM9	1.5	0.6 μmol/L
20 mmol/L SM10	1.5	0.6 μmol/L
20 mmol/L SM11	1.5	0.6 μmol/L
Ampli Taq Gold	0.25	1.25 U
Sample	5	
dH_2O	29.75	
Total	50	

8. Add positive control lysate (5 μL of a factor V heterozygote) to appropriate tubes after all samples have been prepared. The setup order is (a) water, (b) lysate control, (c) patient samples, (d) positive controls, and (e) contamination control.
9. Add 5 μL of water to the contamination control.
10. Place in PerkinElmer Thermal Cycler Model 9600 and cycle with times and temperatures below:

Initial step:	10 min 94°C
40 cycles of:	1 min 94°C
	1 min 55°C
	1 min 72°C
Final step:	7 min 72°C

11. Remove sample tray from thermal cycler and place tubes in rack in refrigerator in post-PCR room for analysis by gel electrophoresis.

Restriction Enzyme Digestion

1. Make digestion buffer with 9 μL of 100X bovine serum albumin (BSA) [NEB] in 91 μL of *Taq*I buffer. Store buffer mix at −20°C and reuse.
2. At time of digestion, add *Taq*I enzyme to buffer mix. Use 3 μL of buffer and 1 μL of enzyme (5 U/μL) for each reaction. Buffer-enzyme mix cannot be stored.
3. Pipette 4 μL of buffer-enzyme mix for each reaction and add 26 μL of sample PCR product. Incubate at 65°C for at least 1 hour.

4. When digestion is complete, add 5 μL of agarose loading dye to the digested PCR products.
5. Add 3 μL of 5X agarose loading dye to 12 μL of the undigested PCR products. All samples are ready to be loaded on gel.

Agarose Gel Electrophoresis (see SOP 6)

The products are resolved on 2.5% agarose (2% LMP, 0.5% agarose) in 1X TBE at 120 V. Run undigested and digested products from each sample in adjacent wells. There should be a wild-type and heterozygote control and size markers for each row of samples. Photograph the gel for documentation. To better visualize the closely opposed bands, run the lower (bromphenol blue) indicator to the end of the gel. Interpretation is easiest if a 50-bp molecular-weight ladder is used, although a 100-bp ladder is also useful to identify the 98-bp fragment.

REPORTING RESULTS

Interpretation

Undigested product: factor V 175 bp, prothrombin 118 bp
Normal control: factor V 155 bp, prothrombin 98 bp
Heterozygote: factor V 175 and 155 bp, prothrombin 118 and 98 bp
Homozygote: factor V 175 bp, prothrombin 118 bp
Water control: none
Save isolated DNA and remaining buffy coats at −70°C.

Limitations and Interference

The factor V genotype should be interpreted in the context of the entire clinical picture. Genotype merely predisposes the individual toward a given clinical outcome and is not diagnostic alone.

Known PCR inhibitors may interfere with the amplification: sodium acetate >0.5 mmol/L or ethanol >1.25%. Hemoglobin, heparin, polyethylene glycol, dimethyl sulfoxide, and formamide variably interfere with the PCR reaction. Conditions must be determined empirically.

PROCEDURE NOTES (Alternative Methods)

Phenotyping by Functional APC Resistance Testing

Activated protein C resistance test (APC-R) is an activated partial prothrombin time (APTT)-based screening test. This assay is performed in the coagulation laboratory using sodium citrate plasma.

Genotyping (for Factor V)

Other laboratories are available to perform the analysis.

REFERENCE

Ripoll L, Paulin D, Thomas S, Drouet L: Multiplex PCR-mediated site-directed mutagenesis for one-step determination of Factor V Leiden and G20210A transition of the prothrombin gene. Thromb Haemost 1997;78:960–961.

RONALD M. PRZYGODZKI
MICHAEL N. KOSS

8

Pulmonary System

The application of molecular biologic and immunohistochemical (IHC) techniques has revealed to the pathologist and clinician the genetic events that lead to carcinogenesis, invasion, and metastasis of malignant neoplastic diseases. This statement is also true for genetic or heritable diseases, susceptibility to carcinoma, and issues relevant in nonmalignant neoplastic disease.[1–13] Molecular markers may also some day be used to monitor response to therapy, predict metastatic potential, and determine prognosis. Translational research using molecular methodologies deemed esoteric are in the forefront of clinical research, and they make a substantial contribution to analysis of disease.[14, 15] It is no wonder that major textbooks of physiology, pathophysiology, and pathology are adding information on molecular biology and molecular pathology.

Rather than merely classifying lung diseases by whether mutations or antigens are present, we will organize them into non-neoplastic and neoplastic diseases. Among the non-neoplastic diseases, many can be linked to a single gene alteration; therefore, the disease entity will be discussed with its pertinent genetic alteration(s). In contrast, the neoplastic diseases have combinations of gene alterations that are shared among many different malignant tumors. Therefore, when we turn to neoplastic disease, the gene alterations themselves will be discussed, followed by the tumor entities and the types of gene alteration(s) that they may harbor.

NON-NEOPLASTIC DISEASE

Congenital and Developmental Diseases

LARYNGEAL WEB

The usual cause of laryngeal web is failure to canalize the larynx during the 6th to 10th weeks of fetal life, leaving a membranous web localized at the level of the vocal cords. Although laryngeal webs can occur at any age, they are usually discovered in infancy, owing to respiratory stridor. Fokstuen and associates[16] described a 22q11.2 microdeletion in type III laryngeal atresia (glottic web) in three patients. One of the patients had clinical overlap with DiGeorge syndrome and velocardiofacial syndrome, whereas the other patients had heart defects and minor anomalies. The chromosome 22q11 deletion has been found in two additional children.[17] The finding of laryngeal atresia should prompt investigation for the 22q11.2 microdeletion, especially when congenital heart defects are also present, in particular, tetralogy of Fallot with pulmonary atresia or absent pulmonary valve.

Other studies have linked laryngeal web with an autosomal dominant variant trait. For example, three generations of a family have been found with laryngeal web occurring in their lineage.[18] The Schinzel (ulnar-mammary) syndrome[19] also shows laryngeal stenosis and web formation, in addition to ulnar ray defects, anal atresia, hand malformations, and pyloric stenosis. The Pallister-Hall syndrome (hypothalamic hamartoblastoma, hypopituitarism, imperforate anus, and postaxial polydactyly)[20, 21] can also show a cleft upper larynx and a posterior web in the subglottic area. All of these diseases are inherited as autosomal dominant disorders. Aside from cytogenetic analysis, there are no known molecular and histochemical techniques available to predict occurrence of laryngeal web.

TRACHEOESOPHAGEAL FISTULA

Tracheoesophageal fistulas are seen most often in conjunction with esophageal atresia. Five to eight subtypes have been described; the most common is esophageal atresia with tracheoesophageal fistula of the distal esophageal segment.[22] Tracheoesophageal fistulas are most commonly associated with the VATER (vertebral defect, anal atresia, tracheoesophageal fistula and esophageal atresia, radial dysplasia), VACTER (cardiac malformations), and VACTERL (limb defects) syndromes.[23, 24] In one study,[25, 26] two unrelated male subjects with hydrocephalus, bilateral radial aplasia, and absent thumbs underwent chromosomal analysis for Fanconi's anemia. The authors raise the possibility of an X-linked genetic trait in these cases.

BRONCHOGENIC CYST

Bronchogenic cysts are lined by ciliated respiratory epithelium and contain cartilage in their wall, which may or may not have bronchial glands and smooth muscle. They are usually single and found in the subhilar region or middle mediastinum or within the lung parenchyma. In one study, two male infants were described who had typical VACTERL syndrome branchial arch defects,[27] including bronchogenic cyst. An X-linked inheritance was suggested.

CONGENITAL LOBAR EMPHYSEMA

This autosomal dominant disease presents in very young children as sudden, progressive respiratory distress. It usually affects the upper or right middle lobes, and it produces overdistention of the airways and extrabronchial vascular compression. These patients typically have bronchial cartilage hypoplasia. There are two reports of the disease in siblings[28, 29] and a third describing it in both a mother and a daughter.[30]

CONGENITAL CYSTIC ADENOMATOID MALFORMATION

Congenital cystic adenomatoid malformation is primarily seen in neonates, but it occasionally presents in older children. It consists of one or more epithelial-lined cysts in the lung, and it is classified based on the size and histologic appearance of the cysts. The cysts are believed to arise from arrested development at different levels of the airway.[31, 32] This disorder appears to show a slight predilection for males.[33] A study of one child noted a polymorphism on chromosome 19; an identical alteration was found in the father of the patient.[34]

CYSTIC FIBROSIS

Cystic fibrosis (CF, mucoviscidosis) is an autosomal recessive disorder with an incidence of approximately 1 in 2000 Caucasian births and a carrier rate of 1 in 25 to 30. The disease results from mutations on chromosome 7q31.2. The salient finding of increased concentration of sweat chloride has long served as the diagnostic marker for the disorder. The current understanding of the disturbance in electrolyte transport is linked to the CF gene product, known as the cystic fibrosis transmembrane conductance regulator (CFTR).[35–41] Numerous genetic alterations have been noted, and continue to be discovered, in patients with CF. Currently, there are over 800 characterized variants.[9, 42] Some of the more common variants are listed in Table 8–1. A valuable source of the ever-expanding mutation types is available from the website run by L. Tsui in the Department of Genetics at the Hospital for Sick Children in Toronto, Ontario, Canada (http://www.genet.sickkids.on.ca/cftr/). The most common genetic alteration by far is the ΔF508 deletion. Several other mutations are also evident and are discussed below.

Mapping of the *CFTR* gene was a long journey. Quinton[43] and Knowles and colleagues[44] suggested the primary defect in CF might be in chloride transport. Widdicombe and co-workers[45] found a cyclic adenosine monophosphate (AMP)–dependent transepithelial chloride current in normal, but not CF, epithelia. The gene was found to have linkage to a polymorphic locus that controls the activity of the serum aryl esterase paraoxanase (PON) enzyme.[46] PON was subsequently localized to chromosome 7q[47]; the DNA probe pJ3.11 assigned it more specifically to 7cen-q22.[48] Finally, the *MET* oncogene was shown to be tightly linked with the CF gene locus, that is, the midportion of the 7q chromosome.[49] This finding is important in that the *MET* oncogene is a tyrosine kinase that could be involved in cyclic AMP signal transduction pathways and possibly the regulation of ion transport.[50] Further investigations lead to a 250-kb gene, and the presence of a 3-base pair (bp) deletion affecting phenylalanine at position 508 of the coding region of this gene (ΔF508), which was present only in CF patients.[36, 51] The ΔF508 deletion affects about 75% of CF patients; differences in population genetics change this value and are discussed

TABLE 8–1

Common Mutations of the *CFTR* Gene

ΔF508	G542X	G551D	N1303K	W1282X
R553X	621 + 1G→T	1717 − 1G→A	R117H	R1162X
R347P	3849 + 10kbC→T	Δ1507	394delTT	G85E
R560T	A455E	1078delT	2879 + 5G→A	3659delC
R334W	1989 + 1G→T	711 + 1G→T	2183AA→G	3905insT
S549N	2184delA	Q359K/T360K	M1101K	Y122X
1989 + 5G→T	3120 + 1G→A	I148T		

Data from Tsui LC: The cystic fibrosis transmembrane conductance regulator gene. Am J Respir Crit Care Med 1995;151(3 pt 2): S47–S53.

later. The ΔF508 deletion interferes with adenosine triphosphate (ATP) binding.

The *CFTR* gene contains 27 exons and spans over 250 kb of DNA. CFTR consists of 1480 amino acids. It has two amino acid sequence domains resembling consensus nucleotide ATP binding folds and two repeat sequence motifs, which suggest structures characteristic of membrane proteins. A putative regulatory element for the gene has been found.[52] The protein, in part, resembles the multidrug resistance factor P-glycoprotein, which functions as a pump removing toxins or drugs from the cells[53]; it contains hydrophobic transmembrane domains and nucleotide binding folds for ATP attachment. Studies on the effects of mutations in *CFTR* on ion channel selectivity show that it is a cyclic AMP–regulated chloride channel in which lysine, at position 95 and position 335, determines the ion selectivity.[54, 55]

Several possible reasons for the existence of CF have been postulated. They generally fall under the category of defense mechanisms against certain infectious diseases. One hypothesis is that *CFTR* mutation is a host defense mechanism that acts by preventing the bacterium *Pseudomonas aeruginosa* from adhering to respiratory epithelium.[56] Another study postulates that heterozygotes for ΔF508 show increased resistance to the uptake of *Salmonella typhi*, thereby making them more resistant to typhoid fever.[57] A third study in mice with an inserted stop codon in exon 10 of the *CFTR* gene showed that the mutation prevented secretion or loss of fluid in response to cholera toxin.[58] Other studies have reported that heterozygotes or homozygotes for CF are less likely to have secretory diarrhea.[59, 60]

Four haplotypes of CF have been postulated: A, B, C, D. Familial studies done of different ethnic origins show different chromosomal cross-over of the B haplotype, as seen by restriction fragment length polymorphism (RFLP) with subsequent reassociation by cross-over with A, C or D haplotypes in these subjects.[61] Because of the ethnic origins of the genetic mutation, different populations have different carrier frequencies of CF. This is especially true of the northern European population, in which the gene frequency reaches 1 in 20 to 25.[62] The European Working Group on CF Genetics found that approximately 88% of the Danish population and 30% of the Turkish population were afflicted with ΔF508.[63] In the United States, this mutation rate is found in about 70% of CF cases. Several ethnic groups have much lower mutation frequencies, notably African Americans (37%) and Ashkenazi Jews (35%).[51, 64] However, among the Ashkenazi Jewish population, the frequency of CF is 1:3300, which is relatively high and almost similar to that of the European white population. Among the Spanish and Italian populations, the ΔF508 mutation frequency is 46%.[65]

There is a 99% link between homozygous deletion of the ΔF508 mutation and the finding of pancreatic insufficiency, a 72% link in patients heterozygous for the deletion, and only a 36% link in all other types of mutation.[66] However, the ΔF508 mutation is not highly linked to pulmonary disease.[9, 67, 68] Alteration in the function of the CFTR chloride ion pump occurs in all types of *CFTR* mutations, but to a lesser or greater degree. These functional differences are likely caused by the varying consequences of mutations on the CFTR protein. Mutations are known to block processing of the protein (ΔF508, N1303K), block regulation (G551D), alter conductance (R117H, R347P), reduce synthesis of the protein (A455E, 3849 + 10kbC → T), or totally eliminate synthesis of it (G542X, 394delTT, 1717 − 1G → A).[9] Mutations that eliminate apical function (ΔF508) appear more detrimental than those (R344W, R347P, R177H) that allow partial function.[69] These findings have been supported by a number of investigations of "mild" pulmonary disease in patients with *CTFR* mutations.[70–72] Gan and associates[73] investigated 33 Dutch patients who were compound heterozygotes for the common ΔF508 mutation and A455E alleles. Compound heterozygotes can therefore modulate the expression of CFTR.[74] These patients had milder lung disease as well as pancreatic dysfunction; the onset of disease also occurred at a later age. Patients with a mutation alteration in intron 19(849 + 10kbC → T) have abnormal chest radiographs but an unremarkable sweat test; levels of transcripts are markedly reduced in these individuals.[75]

To reliably identify *CFTR* mutations, one needs to study the alterations that are found within a given ethnic group. This is imperative, because the population frequencies of mutations vary among the groups; prevalent markers specific for one ethnic group may not be frequent in another. An excellent source for marker variability is the reference by Tsui[9] and the website http://www.genet.sickkids.on.ca/cftr/. Among more recent and novel mutation sites is an unusual 3120 + 1G → A insertion mutation occurring in 12% of the black CF population.[76] This mutation is also found in Arab populations; the only European population that has a similar alteration is the Greek population.[77] El-Harith and associates[78] found six mutations that enable identification of 70% of Saudi *CFTR* mutations. Kerem and co-workers[79] identified 12 mutations unique to 91% of Israeli Jewish CF patients. Seven novel mutations among Spanish CF patients determine 90% of all *CFTR* mutations in this group.[80] One must also realize that double heterozygotes do exist, and they need to be taken into consideration when analyzing CF cases.[74] Therefore, DNA-based tests require evaluation not only for ΔF508 mutations but also for a limited number of other mutations that should be selected on the basis of their known prevalence in the population being tested.

Screening tests for CF include detection of high immunoreactive trypsin levels in serum as well as sweat chloride tests.[81, 82] Polymerase chain reaction (PCR) identification of mutations, in particular ΔF508, appears to be rather simple and cost effective. Homozygous

ΔF508 deletion will determine CF in an individual. However, a person with a heterozygote ΔF508 status either can be a carrier or can have other mutations that need to be sought. Herein lies the difficulty: how extensive must the investigation be in a given case to determine CF status?

PCR can be easily used to initially detect ΔF508 mutations.[83] The PCR product from a wild-type sequence is 95 bp long, whereas mutated product is 92 bp long. These products can be run on a gel; determination of the migration pattern determines the genotype. A single band that migrates where the 95-bp fragments normally are found eliminates from consideration the ΔF508 mutation, whereas migration to the 92-bp site determines homozygous ΔF508 mutation. Two bands, one at 95 and the other at 92, determine a heterozygous state. Additional heteroduplexes of wild-type and mutated DNA strands may be seen using this methodology; they can be identified as larger fragments migrating a shorter distance than either of the 92- or 95-bp fragments.

Mutations can also be detected by direct sequencing, a laborious and expensive task, given the fact that mutations can occur anywhere from exon 3 up to 24, not sparing intron segments. Rapid and inexpensive techniques include ligase chain reaction and reverse dot hybridization. Ligase chain reaction uses two oligonucleotides. One 3′ oligonucleotide end is wild type, and the second oligonucleotide end has the mutation codon in question. A common downstream wild-type oligonucleotide is used with both discriminating oligonucleotides. Heating and annealing of the oligonucleotides, with subsequent joining by DNA ligase, confirms the specific sequence in question.[84] This methodology does not require sequence analysis; however, at least two if not more oligonucleotide pairs need to be used to confirm or refute a given mutation site. Reverse dot hybridization has been successfully employed in human leukocyte haplotyping and has been extended for other mutant allele analyses. The methodology involves setting up an array of known oligonucleotide probes, both mutated and wild-type, on a nitrocellulose membrane or other commercially available membrane strip/chromogen technologies. On this membrane, amplified PCR product of the given gene sequence is hybridized. One of the oligonucleotides used for amplification of the product may be biotinylated or chemiluminated for detection.[85–89] Hybridization reveals whether a given case is wild type or a heterozygous or homozygous mutant. This methodologic approach can be carried out on a certain set of known mutations. Finally, allele-specific oligonucleotide PCR (ASO-PCR) is somewhat similar to ligase chain reaction in that two different oligonucleotide probes are used as the basis for determination of the base call. A second oligonucleotide primer several bases away from the 3′ determining primers is used. PCR amplification with stringent conditions determines the genotype. In a different twist to this approach, one corporation has added a fluorescent dye to the common oligonucleotide probe on the 3′ end and altered the lengths of the 5′ ends of the determining probes. Several base sites can be investigated simultaneously, determining the base calls on each site by the site of migration of the determining probe/common probe product.

As mentioned earlier, one problem with these tests is that the number of alleles to be evaluated is controversial. In general, screening should be performed only when at least 95% of the mutations in carriers can be detected. Some of the common mutations for which screening may be done are seen in Table 8–1. The American College of Medical Genetics recommends a panel of 25 alleles.[90] Determination of the presence or lack of alteration is most commonly determined by denaturing gradient gel electrophoresis determining heteroduplexes; this methodology is seen as the artifact in the Rommen approach to identify the ΔF508 mutation.[83] Other common approaches include reverse dot hybridization, membrane strip/chromogen techniques, and restriction digest analysis.[90, 91, 93, 94] In one test study, 91% of the laboratories performing *CFTR* mutation analysis correctly typed the alteration in a given sample but 35% incorrectly typed one or more alleles from a total of 12 alleles.[90] Although standardization is difficult, some form of it needs to be obtained and is an ongoing challenge.

ASTHMA

Allergic asthma is an acute, usually reversible, spasmodic and diffuse airway narrowing that affects 3% to 8% of the population.[95] Historically, it has been classified as extrinsic when an exogenous cause is known and intrinsic when no known cause is found. Although etiologic difference may exist, mediators of the allergic, or atopic, reaction are similar in both. They therefore are discussed together.

Asthma is more a syndrome than a distinct disease entity. Most asthmatics between the ages of 5 and 40 are atopic,[96] whereas older asthmatics usually are recognized as having "intrinsic" asthma, or asthma of unknown etiology. Histologically, one of the key features is bronchial inflammation, characterized by influx of eosinophils, as well as lymphocytes and plasma cells. This inflammation is mediated through a complex array of molecular and cellular mechanisms that only are partially understood. The central feature of the atopic response is the prolonged and augmented production of immunoglobulin E (IgE) directed against specific allergen, which is triggered by interleukin 4 (IL-4) and T and B lymphocyte interactions.[97] Allergen-specific IgE, bound to mast cells and located in the bronchial epithelium, reacts with the allergen, which results in degranulation of the mast cell. This results in the release of numerous intermediate inflammatory mediators, including histamine, leukotrienes, and prostaglandins, among others. The late bronchial inflammatory response is associated with influx of CD4+ T lymphocytes and eosinophils. The influx of cells may also be caused by the release of IL-4 from activated mast cells. The eosinophils release four basic proteins: cationic protein, eosinophil-derived neurotoxin, peroxidase, and major basic protein. They also release a plethora of other mediators, including platelet-activating factor, prostaglandins, and leukotrienes, all which contribute to the inflammatory response.

Initially, one approach to evaluating the "atopic" state of a given individual was to measure the total serum IgE by solid-phase immunoassay. However, the methodology was flawed because age and smoking could change the results. Furthermore, one could not evaluate whether the atopy was intrinsic or extrinsic.

The genetic techniques developed in the 1980s brought a partial solution to the problem. Eiberg and colleagues[98] found a strong suggestion of linkage between esterase D and IgE regulation on chromosome 13. Cookson and associates[99] suggested that an atopic person may produce a prolonged and exuberant IgE response in response to a small amount of allergen and that the general state of enhanced IgE responsiveness can cause an increase in antigen-specific IgE antibody levels, with or without a high total IgE serum level. In linkage studies, they found linkage to a hypervariable minisatellite probe, which has been assigned to 11q12-q13, and they further reconfirmed this result with the marker D11S97. Other studies, however, could not determine an association between the D11S97 marker with either atopy or bronchial hyperreactivity to methacholine.[100] However, a different study shows significant linkage of a highly polymorphic microsatellite marker in the fifth intron of the *MS4A2* gene to a diagnosis of asthma.[101] A study by De Sanctis and associates[102] noted significant linkage to two loci on the mouse chromosomes 2, 15, and 17: Bhr1, Bhr2, and Bhr3, respectively. These loci, collectively, account for approximately 25% of the genetic variants found in airway responsiveness of A/J and C57BL/6J mice. Human counterparts of the candidate genes include IL-1β; receptor for IL-2B and the B chain of platelet-derived growth factor (PDGF); and tumor necrosis factor-α (TNF-α), respectively.

A recent reanalysis of hyperresponsiveness and atopy has led to a linkage between serum IgE levels and chromosome 5q31-33, including D5S436.[103] The results were interpreted as indicating that a gene governing bronchial hyperresponsiveness is located near a major locus that regulates IgE levels on chromosome 5q. Other studies have shown a correlation between cytokines and asthma[104] and an increase in intercellular adhesion molecule (ICAM), vascular cell adhesion molecule (VCAM), and E-selectin immunohistochemistry (IHC) staining and in situ hybridization messenger RNA (mRNA) expression in the endothelial lining of asthmatic patients.[105, 106] There also appears to be a lack of association between asthma and nonasthmatic patients and tumor growth factor-β_1 (TGF-β_1) expression,[107] but there may be a link between increased nitric oxide and asthma.[108] There is no association between vasoactive intestinal polypeptide and substance P expression and asthma.[109]

Clearly, there are still no definitive genetic alterations linked to asthma or the atopic state, nor are there specific tests to predict either of them. There are, however, promising developments. One study notes a strong association between the finding of intrinsic asthma and the presence of the HLA-w6 locus.[110] Another study[111] found that G protein–linked receptors, including the adrenoceptors of the α and β group, the adenosine receptors, and the tachykinin receptors, are influenced by corticosteroids. Other studies reveal that the β_2-adrenoceptor polymorphism and codon 27 may play a role in asthma. Hall[112] demonstrated that the glutamate 27 homozygotes had a fourfold higher geometric mean methacholine provocative dose than individuals who were homozygous for the wild-type (glutamine 27) form of the receptor; heterozygotes had an intermediate value. A different study by Turki and co-workers[113] identified three polymorphic loci within the coding block of the β-adrenoceptor that alter amino acids at positions 16, 27, and 164, imparting specific biochemical and pharmacologic phenotypes to it. Glycine at position 16 imparts an accelerated agonist-promoted down-regulation of the receptor as compared with arginine and is significantly overrepresented in nocturnal asthmatics. Finally, Laing and associates[114] demonstrated a polymorphism in the gene for Clara cell secretory protein (*CC16*) that was linked to asthma. This was an A→G substitution at position 38 downstream from the transcription initiation site within the noncoding region of exon 1. Individuals who were homozygous wild type (AA) had a nearly 7-fold increased risk of developing asthma, compared with those who were homozygous for the polymorphism (GG). Heterozygous individuals had a 4.2-fold increased risk of developing asthma.

The Collaborative Study on the Genetics of Asthma[115] consisted of a genome-wide search in 140 families with two or more asthmatic siblings from three racial groups. Six significant genetic regions were identified from this study: 11p15 and 19q13 in whites, 5p15 and 17p11.1-q11.2 in blacks, and 2q33 and 21q21 in Hispanics. It, therefore, appears that race may be an important factor in the investigation of asthma genetics. Other studies isolated regions in chromosomes 5q23-31, 12q15-24.1, 19q13, and 21q21 as likely sites linked to asthma.[116] Given the overall findings, chromosomal loci (with their candidate genes) for asthma and atopy include 5q (IL-3, IL-4, IL-5, IL-9,

IL-13, GM-CSF, β_2-adrenoceptor), 6p (human leukocyte antigen [HLA] complex), 6p21.3 (TNF-α), 11q13 *MS4A2*, 12q (interferon gamma, nitric oxide synthase, mast cell growth factor), and 13q (esterase D, T-cell receptor / complex).[117]

Interestingly, individuals with heterozygote ΔF508 cystic fibrosis transmembrane conductance regulator (*CFTR*) mutation are less likely to have asthma in childhood and in early adult life.[118]

Emphysema and Chronic Fibrosing Lung Diseases

By standard light microscopic evaluation, emphysema and chronic fibrosing interstitial lung diseases are quite distinct from one another. Still, in terms of their molecular biology, both groups demonstrate imbalances of certain, and often complex, enzyme/substrate systems that lead to either production or destruction of the extracellular matrix. Given that this is the case, we discuss this group of diseases together but emphasize salient findings of each entity when appropriate.

The extracellular matrix, consisting of many separate components, governs the mechanics of the lungs. A short list of these components includes collagen, elastin, laminin, proteoglycan, fibronectin, thrombospondin, tenascin, osteonectin, integrin, matrix metalloproteinase, and fibrillin. Other extracellular matrix components may be found in excellent reviews.[119–121]

Several factors modulate the amount and type of extracellular matrix. Many of these modulators and substrates have been identified and are being investigated in clinicopathologic studies. For example, collagen, elastin, matrix metalloproteinases (MMPs), and their regulator tissue inhibitors of metalloproteinases (TIMPs) have been extensively investigated in lung disease. Likewise, signal pathways for appropriate matrix production/destruction are emerging.

Collagen is composed of three chains of similar or different amino acid composition. The chains have a high proportions of glycine, proline, and hydroxyproline triplet repeats, which is the predominant component[122]; other amino acids within a given chain form the subtype of the chain. The varying combination of α-chain subtypes produces the unique structure and properties of a given collagen. Collagen genes are located throughout the chromosomes, with most found on chromosomes 2, 6, 7, 17, and X. Only a few proteins contain collagen-like repeats,[123] namely, surfactant apolipoprotein-A[124] and surfactant apolipoprotein-D.[125]

There are at least 33 characterized collagens.[126–128] At least 11 of these are found in lung. The major subtypes in the interstitium of the lung are collagens I, III, V, and VI; collagens II, IX, and XI are present in cartilaginous structures of the airways. Collagen I and III are the most abundant and in the adult are present in a 2:1 ratio.[129] Collagen I gives a tissue tensile strength, and collagen III gives it compliance. Collagen IV is found in basement membranes, and collagen VI is a nonfibrillar collagen associated with microfibrils, where it forms filamentous structures.

Macrophages and neutrophils degrade collagens by releasing a host of proteinases, including MMPs, gelatinases (type IV collagenases), and stromeolysins (Tables 8–2 and 8–3).

The MMPs that are important in the pathogenesis of emphysema and fibrosing interstitial lung disease are MMP1 (interstitial collagenase), MMP2 (72-kDa gelatinase), MMP3 (stromeolysin-1), MMP8 (neutrophil collagenase), MMP9 (92-kDa gelatinase), and MMP10 (stromeolysin-2) (see Table 8–2). These enzymes are predominantly produced in fibroblasts, neutrophils, and macrophages, but normal mesenchymal cells can also synthesize MMPs constitutively or through stress-induced signals that include IL-1, PDGF, TNF-, TNF-, or TGF- (Fig. 8–1).[130] MMPs are secreted in inactive or precursor form. They are activated by plasmin, which itself is secreted as plasminogen, and by either tissue- or urokinase-type plasminogen activators (tPA and uPA, respectively), as well as MT1-MMP/MMP14 (membrane-type matrix metalloproteinase). Although it is difficult to see differences in tPA levels between normal and neoplastic lung cells, elevated expression of uPA and plasminogen activator inhibitor-1 (PAI-1) has been found in pulmonary neoplasia.[131–134]

TABLE 8–2

Pulmonary Metalloproteinases and Their Substrates

MMP Classification	Other Names	Substrates
MMP-1	Interstitial collagenase	Collagens I, II, III, VII, VIII, X
MMP-2	72-kd gelatinase, gelatinase A	Collagens IV, V, VII, X, XI
MMP-3	Stromeolysin-1	Collagens III, IV, V, IX, X, XI, procollagen
MMP-8	Neutrophil collagenase	Collagens I, II, III, VII, VIII, X
MMP-9	92-kDa gelatinase, gelatinase B	Collagens IV, V, VII, X, XI
MMP-10	Stromeolysin-2	Collagens III, IV, V, IX, X
MMP-11	Stromeolysin-3	Serpins
MT1-MMP		Progelatinase A, procollagenase 3

TABLE 8–3

Pulmonary Proteases and Antiproteases and Their Targets

Protease	Substrate
Neutrophil elastase	Elastin, collagens I, II, III, IV, fibronectin, laminin
Collagenase	Collagens I, II, III, VII, VIII, X, gelatin, fibronectin
Cathepsin G	Collagen IV, elastin, proteoglycans, fibronectin
Cathepsin B	Elastin
Plasminogen activator	Elastin Collagens
Gelatinase	Collagens IV, V, VII, X, XI
Antiprotease	**Target Enzyme**
TIMP	Collagenases, stromeolysins
α_1-Antitrypsin	Neutrophil elastase, cathepsin G
α_1-Antichymotrypsin	Cathepsin G
α_2-Macroglobulin	Most protease classes

TIMP, tissue inhibitor of metalloproteinases.

However, invasion may be more dependent on the balance of the proteases and their inhibitors rather than on their individual absolute levels.[134–136] This is evident because both the normal stroma, as well as tumor, produces a certain "level" of uPA; the balance of activator/inhibitor itself determines to what extent stroma is altered. Interestingly, both non–small cell and neuroendocrine carcinomas with high levels of uPA in their stroma rather than in their tumor cells have an increased frequency of lymph node metastases.[133, 134] Increased PAI-1 expression is likewise correlated with shorter survival in adenocarcinoma of lung,[134, 137] whereas elevated PAI-2 expression, which is expressed in stromal cells, is more likely to occur among node-negative lung cancer patients with elevated uPA expression. PAI may also be involved in bronchiectasis.[138] To complicate matters further, angiogenesis inducers, including TGF-β and basic fibroblast growth factor (bFGF), stimulate expression of both uPA and PAI-1. A second pathway of activation of MMP activation is through MT1-MMP, a transmembrane protein that enhances cellular invasion of reconstituted basement membrane that is expressed in invasive lung carcinoma cells.[139] In this light, a given cell may have the proteolytic activity localized to its cell membrane region and may be responsible for activation of extracellular proteases, thereby potentiating the invasive process.

Activated MMPs degrade substrates that are specific to each MMP (see Tables 8–2 and 8–3). Most non–small cell lung carcinomas reveal increased MMP expression.[140–144] Interestingly, MMP-3, MMP-9, MMP-11, and MT-MMP-1 are expressed in cells of squamous cell carcinoma and basaloid carcinoma, whereas matrilysin epithelial expression is predominantly found in adenocarcinomas.[140, 143] In neuroendocrine tumors of the lung, MMP-11 is frequently expressed in the stromal cells, whereas MMP-1 and MMP-3 are not expressed in the tumor cells.[131]

These degradative enzymes are held in check by either transcriptional control or inhibitors, including the broad-spectrum serum inhibitor α_2-macroglobulin and the zinc-binding endopeptidase tissue inhibitors of metalloproteinases (TIMPs) (see Fig. 8–1, Table 8–3). TIMP-1 and TIMP-2 are the major players in lung[130, 145] whereas TIMP-3 is found predominantly in placenta. In highly cross-linked collagen matrices, the neutrophil enzymes elastase and cathepsin G solubilize irreducible cross-links, enabling further proteolysis by collagenases.[146] Phagocytosis of collagen fragments, on the other hand, occurs after degradation by thiol proteases (cathepsins B and N) in the lysosomes. TIMPs inactivate MMPs through a 1:1 complex. TIMP-1 binds to the proenzyme form of MMP-9 (gelatinase B), whereas TIMP-2 binds to the proenzyme form of MMP-2 (gelatinase A). TIMP-3 binds to the extracellular matrix. The TIMPs are potent inhibitors found in the step to tumor invasion and metastasis in vivo.[147] However, several studies on human tissues have correlated high TIMP expression with poor prognosis, in particular with lymph node metastases and tumor recurrence among breast, colon, and bladder carcinoma cases.[148–150] TIMP-1 inhibits angiogenesis,[151] and TIMP-2 inhibits bFGF-stimulated proliferation of endothelial cells[152] but stimulates fibroblast proliferation through activation of cyclic AMP–dependent protein kinases.[153] The number of studies are, however, limited to draw useful conclusions about the relationship between TIMPs and outcome of lung carcinomas.

Collagen production is regulated at multiple levels, including mRNA transcription, splicing, translation, and degradation, post-translational modification, intracellular degradation of newly synthesized collagen, and extracellular degradation of collagen (both pre and post cross-linking).[154–157] Other factors regulating collagen synthesis and breakdown impact upstream of this process at the signal transduction level. Among these, protein kinase C may be an important factor in regulating the rate of procollagen transcription.[158] Cyclic AMP may also regulate collagen synthesis when activated by IL-1, TNF-α, and prostaglandin E_2.[159] Other factors affecting collagen levels include insulin, insulin-like growth factor-1, and tissue plasminogen activator, which increase collagen mRNA and procollagen synthesis.[160, 161] TGF-β increases mRNA and procollagen synthesis, decreases intracellular degradation and transcription of stromeolysin, and increases TIMP levels.[162–164] Endothelial cell growth factor, glucocorticoids, heparin, and interferon gamma decrease mRNA and procollagen synthesis.[165–167]

Elastin, which is only found in vertebrates,[168] gives tissues its compliance and extensibility. It is present in

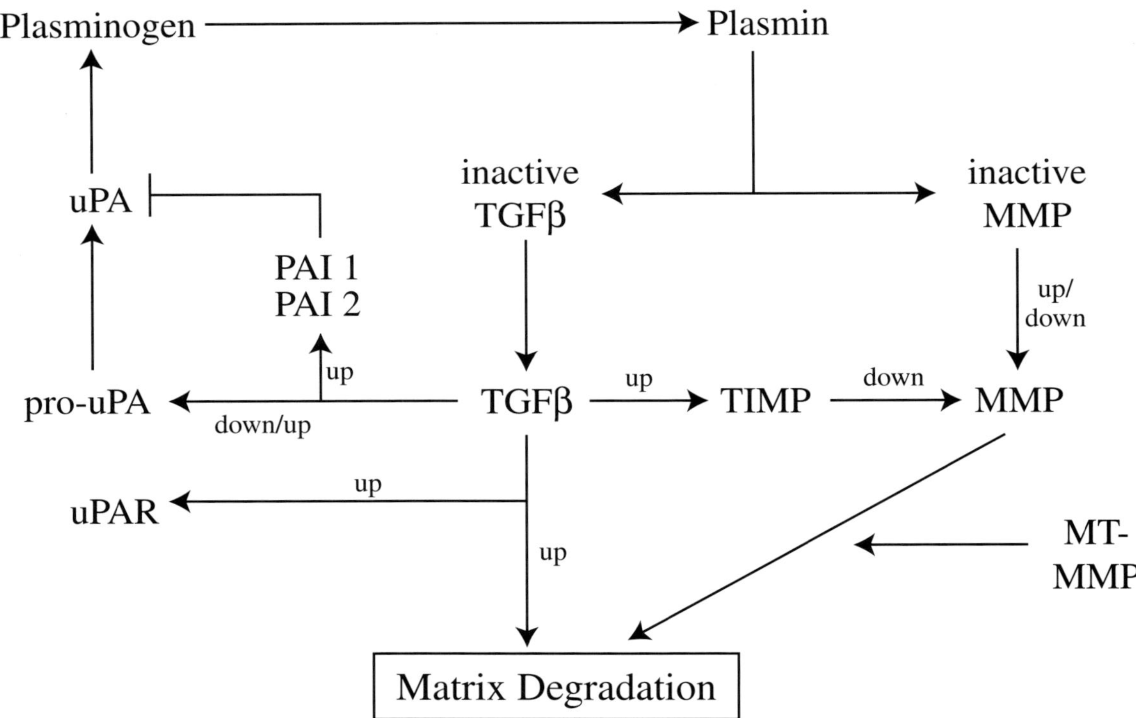

FIGURE 8–1
Matrix degradation and feedback regulation cascade. down, down-regulated; up, up-regulated.

lung tissue as a polymer lacking any ordered quaternary structure, but it is secreted as a monomer, tropoelastin, which, when deposited in the microfibrillar network, further undergoes cross-linking for stabilization through desmosin and isodesmosine. Unlike collagen, elastin is a single gene product. The coding gene for elastin is located on chromosome 7, and a pseudogene is present on chromosome 2. Through alternate splicing of RNA, at least five isoforms are produced.[169] When elastin is secreted as tropoelastin, it is thought to bind to a membrane glycoprotein called elastin receptor that helps to stabilize and promote the cross-linking between microfibrils. Lysine residues are converted to aldehydes by lysyl oxidase, generating the cross-links. In lung, three cells are apparently responsible for the formation of tropoelastase: arterial endothelial cells, smooth muscle cells, and the interstitial fibroblasts.[170–172]

Production and degradation of elastin is similar to that of collagen (see Table 8–3). Synthesis of tropoelastin is augmented by heparin and IGF-1[173, 174]; degradation is promoted through glucocorticoids, IL-1β, and TNF-α.[175–177] Soluble tropoelastin can be degraded by trypsin, chymotrypsin, thermolysin, cathepsin G, and stromeolysin, whereas cross-linked elastin is degraded by elastase.[178] Elastases are found in inflammatory cells, smooth muscle cells, and fibroblasts and are serine proteases.

Two other "classic" gene products that play a role in the breakdown of lung structure include $_1$-antitrypsin (A1AT) and α_1-antichymotrypsin (AACT). The liver is the site of most of the damage that occurs after loss of these gene products.

A1AT is a serine proteinase inhibitor, or "serpin," whose deficiency is associated with emphysema, possibly bronchiectasis, and liver disease. It is also the main inhibitor of elastase and cathepsin G. The gene encoding this protein is located on chromosome 14q31-32.3 and is inherited in an autosomal dominant fashion. Individuals who are either homozygotes or compound heterozygotes may have severe lung disease, whereas heterozygotes are predisposed to chronic obstructive lung disease. Evaluation of the gene is complicated by the fact that there are at least 75 "normal" variant alleles of the gene.[179–182]

Determination of the phenotype is obtained by performing thin-layer polyacrylamide gel electrophoresis at pH 4 to 5 and determining what type of inhibitor(s) is(are) present. By electrophoresis, the band slowest in migration is Z, the usual band is M, and the fastest migrating band is F. The second most common band is S, which falls between M and Z. Most individuals are homozygous for *M*, whereas the second most common is S. In persons who are homozygous *Z*, A1AT activity is reduced to 10% to 15% of the normal activity, whereas *MZ* phenotypes have approximately 60% of normal activity. Different mutations can affect the lung and other sites to differing extents. Phenotypic correlation falls into three categories: null mutation (no product), mutations causing an altered function of the gene, and mutations producing deficiency of the enzyme function. Thus, protease inhibitor (PI) Z and PI M(Malton) are deficiency mutations that are associated with both liver disease and emphysema. By contrast, PI S, M(Heerlen), M(Mineral Springs), M(Procida), M(Nichinan), I, null, and P(Lowell) are deficiency mutations that produce an increased risk for emphysema alone.[182]

Although electrophoresis remains the classic method of determining phenotype, other methods are now being employed to obtain genotype more directly. For example, a mutation in exon 5 of the α_1AT gene eliminates the *Bst*EII restriction endonuclease site, which allows quick determination of the mutation by PCR and restriction digestion.[183–185] If one needs to determine whether the Z band itself is present, an oligonucleotide probe has been used to determine the 342 GAG→AAG alteration.[186] Allele-specific PCR has also been found useful in determining five different mutation states in A1AT.[187] Finally, RFLP can also be used in evaluation of these genotypes. For example, Cox and co-workers,[188] studied RFLP in the A1AT gene and described PI and M subtypes using only this method.

Rodriguez-Cintron and associates[189] suggested that bronchiectasis should be considered part of the spectrum of pulmonary pathology encountered in patients with A1AT deficiency. They described a 21-year-old man with massive hemoptysis and homozygous *ZZ* A1AT deficiency; neither panlobular emphysema nor cirrhosis of the liver was present.

AACT, another serpin, is a plasma protease inhibitor synthesized in the liver. The gene has been localized to chromosome 14q32.1 by in situ hybridization.[190] It shares nucleic acid and protein sequence homology with A1AT.[191] AACT may constitute a gene cluster with A1AT because in situ hybridization shows that both map to the 14q31-q32.3 region.[190] Also, both genes are found in the same 360-kb *Mlu*I restriction fragment by pulsed-field gel electrophoresis.[192]

A study of AACT levels in 229 patients with liver disease showed 8 patients who had seronegative chronic active hepatitis and low AACT values.[193] Equally low AACT levels were among first-degree relatives of 1 of the 8 patients. Of this group, 3 had pulmonary disease and 6 had liver manifestations. The abnormal gene appeared to be inherited in an autosomal dominant manner with a frequency of 0.003.

Tsuda and associates[194] showed a variant AACT (Isehara-2) that had a 2-bp frameshift deletion from codon 391, resulting in elongation of the amino acid peptide chain by several amino acids. There are also two genetic variants associated with chronic obstructive pulmonary disease (COPD). The first of these, Bonn-1, was found in four related patients who shared a codon 229 CCT→GCT mutation, producing an alanine→proline amino acid substitution.[195, 196] The other variant, Bochum-1, has a codon CTG→CCG mutation. It was found in three generations of family members who had been afflicted with COPD.[196] Last, a polymorphism exists on the *AACC* gene, which when present along with *APOE*4*, significantly increases the risk for Alzheimer disease.[197]

The gene for α_2-macroglobulin *(A2M)* is located on 12p12.3-13.3. It consists of 32 exons with three transcription initiation sites and is a single copy gene in humans. It functions as a "universal" antiprotease, capable of inhibiting the majority of proteases.[198] Although the main source of A2M synthesis is the liver, adult and fetal fibroblasts and alveolar macrophages are also sources of synthesis.[199–201] Apart from rare case reports of A2M dysfunction in COPD, abnormalities of this protein have not been linked with any proteolytic lung disease.[202]

Emphysema is characterized by permanent enlargement of the air spaces distal to the bronchioles in the absence of obvious fibrosis.[203] Essentially, there is degradation of the matrix of the diseased lung, particularly the elastin of elastic fibers in the lung matrix.[204] Collagen degradation also occurs, although at a much lower rate. In this respect, the construction/destruction steady state continually ongoing in lung may be altered in favor of destruction. Two key factors may contribute to emphysema: A1AT deficiency[205] and cigarette smoke.[204] A1AT is one of the main inhibitors of elastase. Direct oxidation of lung tissues through cigarette smoke may damage elastin and collagen fibers directly and can recruit an acute inflammatory reaction.[206, 207] Neutrophils contain elastase, enabling the degradation of both elastin cross-links and collagen. Neutrophils can also inactivate A1AT and can generate hydrogen peroxide, leading to further degradation of the matrix.

Pulmonary interstitial fibrosis is the other extreme of the spectrum. It includes idiopathic pulmonary fibrosis, asbestosis, chemotherapeutic drug exposure, radiation-induced pulmonary fibrosis, pneumoconiosis, fibrosis resulting from diffuse alveolar damage (adult respiratory distress syndrome), and other fibrosing lung diseases. The commonly believed pathogenic sequence leading to fibrosis of the lung is pulmonary inflammation, subsequent fibroblast proliferation, and, ultimately, collagen deposition.[208, 209] As mentioned under collagen synthesis and degradation, TGF-β is a potent inducer of extracellular matrix[210] and it can raise the levels of TIMPs.[163] TGF-β localizes at sites of active matrix deposition.[211, 212] TGF-β's ability to induce cell proliferation depends on cellular ability to make and respond to PDGF.[213, 214] In addition, IGF-1, Epstein-Barr virus antibody titers,[215] and HLA type may play a role in lung fibrosis.[216–218] Myofibroblasts, which are mesenchymal cells that contain α-smooth muscle actin, desmin, and procollagen mRNA (as shown by IHC staining and in situ hybridization), may be responsible for the increased lung collagen gene expression in pulmonary fibrosis.[219–221] Some forms of pulmonary fibrosis also are considered to a heritable (so-called familial pulmonary fibrosis).[222, 223]

Although the histologic hallmark of interstitial fibrosis is fibrillar collagen deposition, proteoglycans (or acid mucopolysaccharides) appear to have a greater role in lung remodeling. Proteoglycans contain covalently attached glycosaminoglycan chains. They consist of four classes: chondroitin and dermatan sulfate, heparin and heparan sulfate, keratan sulfate, and hyaluronan. Increases in hyaluronan concentration have been found in patients with idiopathic pulmonary fibrosis, sarcoidosis, adult respiratory distress syndrome, and alveolar proteinosis.[224–226] Increased deposition of versican-like chondroitin sulfate proteoglycan has been found in hyaline membrane disease, and increased deposition of versican itself, which interacts with hyaluronan, has been found among idiopathic pulmonary fibrosis, organizing diffuse alveolar damage, and bronchiolitis obliterans with organizing pneumonia (BOOP).[227–229]

Goodpasture's syndrome (anti–glomerular basement membrane disease) is a type II cytotoxic antibody-mediated immune reaction characterized by crescentic glomerulonephritis and pulmonary alveolar hemorrhage. The autoantibody is directed against a major antigenic determinant (autoantigen) formed by the last 36 residues of the globular domain of the α5(IV) collagen, a component of basement membranes.[230–233] The HLA-B7 and HLA-DR2 haplotypes are expressed more commonly in these patients.[234] A rare familial group of patients with Goodpasture's disease also has been reported.[235, 236] Post-transplant autoantibodies to α5(IV) collagen are found in the X-linked form of Alport syndrome.[237] These patients probably develop autoantibodies to α5(IV) collagen because they lack this collagen chain in their own basement membrane, or show mutation in other collagen subtypes, and are exposed to it in the transplanted kidney. It is likely that there is heterogeneity in the pathogenesis of Goodpasture's syndrome and in the molecular aspects responsible for the binding of anti–basement membrane antibodies.[238]

Byssinosis is a form of reversible asthma-like lung disease caused by inhalation of cotton dust. The usual patients are cotton textile workers. In one study it was shown that A1AT, which neutralizes the enzymes released by neutrophils during the inflammatory response, can in fact be detrimental under certain circumstances. In particular, persons with the *MZ* phenotype of A1AT deficiency have an increased incidence of byssinosis, as compared with those with the *MM* phenotype (38% vs. 18%). *MZ* patients also have a slightly higher prevalence for familial allergy.

LYMPHOPROLIFERATIVE DISORDERS

Lymphoproliferative diseases of the lung span the gamut from reactive lymphoid processes, such as follicular bronchiolitis and lymphoid interstitial pneumonia, to malignant lymphomas, most frequently marginal zone B-cell lymphomas. These lymphoid processes are primarily B cell in type. There has been extensive molecular and IHC analysis of these diseases. Only two malignant lesions that are primarily found in lung are discussed here.

Angiocentric Immunoproliferative Lesion

Angiocentric immunoproliferative lesion, or lymphomatoid granulomatosis, was defined initially as an atypical lymphoproliferative process characterized by histologic features of angioinvasion and necrosis.[239] This disease, which is most common in older individuals, shows a nearly complete predilection for lung involvement in the form of nodules or masses, but it can affect the brain as well.

Histologically, the disease is characterized by a polymorphous lymphoid infiltrate composed of small lymphocytes, plasma cells, macrophages, and variable numbers of atypical mononuclear or multinuclear cells. This infiltrate is often necrotic and shows angioinvasion. Depending on the number of atypical cells, there is a histologic spectrum from low to high grade, with high-grade lesions showing clear-cut morphologic features of lymphoma, most commonly immunoblastic lymphoma. Most of the small lymphocytes in angiocentric immunoproliferative lesion are reactive with the T-cell CD4 and CD8 markers, initially suggesting that these lymphoid proliferations were of T-cell origin. However, a study by Guinee and associates[240] pointed to the contrary. Analysis by immunohistochemistry and in situ hybridization confirmed that the atypical cells are of B-cell (CD20+) phenotype and contain Epstein-Barr virus sequences, while the background small lymphocytes are T cells (CD45RO+) and lack this viral sequence. PCR analysis for immunoglobulin heavy-chain gene rearrangement also identified a monoclonal pattern in six of nine cases tested, whereas analysis for T-cell receptor γ-chain gene rearrangements was negative in three cases tested. Given these results, it appears that most cases of lymphomatoid granulomatosis involving the lung represent a proliferation of monoclonal Epstein-Barr virus–infected B cells with a prominent T-cell reaction. These tumors should therefore be reclassified as T cell–rich B-cell lymphomas.[240]

Marginal Zone B-Cell Lymphomas of Bronchus-associated Lymphoid Tissue (BALT)

Most lymphomas originating in lung are of low histologic grade. They are now recognized to be marginal zone B-cell lymphomas of BALT[241–243]; T-cell lymphomas are only rarely seen.[242] Marginal zone B-cell lymphomas present predominantly in elderly adults, with equal male and female distribution. Approximately 20% of marginal zone lymphomas with a lymphoplasmacytoid morphology have monoclonal protein in their serum; rare patients have cryoglobulinemia.[203, 243] The lymphoid infiltrate can be shown to be monoclonal by IHC staining in about 75% of cases.[242] Commonly expressed B-cell antigens include CD20, CD21, CD22, CD35, CD45RA, KB61, KB3, and Ki-B3. CD10 and CD5, present in follicular center cell lymphomas, are usually not expressed. Polyclonal plasma cells and reactive T cells usually are present surrounding the monoclonal B-cell foci.

GENE ALTERATIONS IN NEOPLASTIC DISEASES

Carcinogenesis is a multistep and multifactorial interchange of gene products. Some of these genes are relatively well understood, whereas others are only known to exist. Given that a certain gene may affect many of the lung tumors, and in different ways, the genes themselves are discussed first. The relevant alterations in a given tumor type are presented at the end of each gene discussion, highlighting how they affect the prognosis and differentiation, where needed. The major pathways governing molecular regulation of signal transduction, cell cycle genes, and so on, as well as an overall summary of tumor types and major gene functions, are listed at the end of the chapter.

DNA Damage, Susceptibility, and Repair

The initiating factor for most carcinogenesis is DNA damage by various mechanisms. Other factors that play a role are heritable gene alterations (e.g., Li-Fraumeni syndrome) and tumor susceptibility genes (discussed later). Both exogenous (environmental) and endogenous (e.g., genetic, hormonal) factors also appear to be involved in the ultimate progression to malignancy.

A large number of genes are responsible for the proper and correct maintenance of the genomic DNA and for its replication. Damage to the genomic DNA may be repaired, but failure of repair or cell death will further propagate this damage through cell division. The sensitized cell may or may not undergo additional insults or "hits," and it may finally become malignant. These changes may be rapid, or they may take many years for them to develop. The majority of theories of carcinogenesis favor the multi-hit hypothesis to explain the development of tumors.[244–247]

If this approach is correct, a single gene alteration does not usually cause a neoplasm to occur. Also, DNA damage should be defined as an occurrence wherein its outcome causes injury to the cell and, ultimately, the host if it goes unchecked. Therefore, polymorphisms are alterations in DNA that are not damaging yet are alterations in the base sequence deviating from the major "normal" population sequence. Similarly, such findings as di-, tri-, and tetranucleotide repeats and Alu segments, and so on, do not constitute DNA damage. Finally, a damaging event leading to neoplasia may depend on the time at which it occurs in the cell cycle. Depending on the period in which this damage happens, different outcomes may occur for a particular cell.[248]

MARKERS OF SUSCEPTIBILITY

An increased susceptibility to carcinogenesis can result from several factors. Some of these are metabolism of carcinogenic chemicals (uptake, activation, and detoxification), inherited or acquired alteration in oncogenes or tumor suppressor genes, and DNA repair mechanisms.

Metabolism of Carcinogenic Chemicals. A large number of compounds may affect the biologic properties of nucleic acids at the molecular level by interfering and binding to DNA bases, forming adducts. This property of chemicals may be useful in therapy for neoplasms, but when the propensity to modify and the inability to detoxify such adducts exists within an individual, the risk of mutagenesis and carcinogenesis is increased.

The gene status of certain cytochromes and detoxifiers conveys information regarding an individual's susceptibility to develop lung carcinoma. These include cytochrome P450 1A1 *(CYP1A1)*, P450 2E1 *(CYP2E1)*, P450 2D6 *(CYP2D6)*, glutathione-S-transferase M type *(GSTM1)* and P1 type *(GSTP1)*, and *N*-acetyltransferase *(NAT)*.

CYP1A1, primarily an inducible extrahepatic enzyme, is the gene product that produces aryl hydrocarbon hydroxylase, also known as benzo[a]pyrene hydroxylase. This protein initiates a multienzyme pathway that activates polycyclic aromatic hydrocarbons, including benzo[a]-pyrene. The benzo[a]pyrene metabolite epoxide is thought to bind to the N7 of guanine, causing alteration in base-pair reading and ultimately mutation. *CYP1A1* has an *Msp*I polymorphism,[249] located at the 264th base downstream from the poly A signal. Genotyping for the presence or absence of the *Msp*I site in the 3′ region reveals a predominant homozygous genotype, designated (A), a heterozygote (B), and a homozygous rare allele designated (C). Although the function of the *Msp*I polymorphism remains uncertain, a linked polymorphism in the heme-binding region in exon 7 at codon 462 (CYP1A1*2, m2) alters the protein structure by replacing an isoleucine with a valine,[250–252] evident on *Nco*I restriction digestion,[253] possibly producing an effect on the enzyme's catalytic activity.[252] In the Asian population, individuals with variant *CYP1A1* alleles are at increased risk of lung cancer. This risk is greater at lower smoking levels.[251, 254, 255] In Western countries, the "at risk" genotype is less frequent and no association with *CYP1A1* genotype has been observed to date.[253, 256, 257] The negative results may be caused by a lower frequency of the variant allele in Western countries.

The *CYP2E1* gene product metabolically activates several potential human carcinogens, including *N*-nitrosamines that are found in the environment and in cigarette smoke.[258] Some of the carcinogens can then be detoxified through the GSTM1 pathway.[259] Uematsu and colleagues[260] reported a positive association between a *Dra*I RFLP located in intron 6 of the *CYP2E1* gene and lung cancer in a Japanese population. This association has not been found in Western countries.[261–265] Still, because of the lower prevalence of variant allele in Western populations, these studies may lack sufficient statistical power to detect an effect.

GSTM1, a phase II enzyme, is one of a family of proteins that catalyze the conjugation of reduced glutathione to a variety of electrophilic compounds, including activated forms of many chemical carcinogens, and metabolites of benzo[a]pyrene.[266] GSTM1 detoxifies these metabolites, forming epoxides and hydroxylated forms. The null genotype has been associated with increased sister chromatid exchange,[267] mutations in a *Salmonella typhimurium* system,[268] and increase in polycyclic aromatic hydrocarbon–DNA adducts.[269] A deficient phenotype is caused by a homozygous null (deleted) *GSTM1* gene,[270] which is present in approximately 50% of the white population. The GSTM1 null phenotype may be increased among patients with lung cancer.[255, 270–273] Increased expression of GSTP1 in lung has been noted.[273a] Association of the codon 104 A > G polymorphism of *GSTP1* with null *GSTM1* was shown to increase DNA adduct formation and lung cancer risk among Norwegians.[273b]

CYP2D6 4-hydroxylates debrisoquine and sparteine in liver microsomes. CYP2D6 has a profound effect on the metabolic rate of many drugs.[274, 275] Metabolic rates vary among individuals, but the principal phenotypes that exist in the population are extensive metabolizers and poor metabolizers.[276,277] Several polymorphisms exist, the most common being CYP2D6*4, *5, *6, and *2.[278] Many studies find a correlation between higher CYP2D6 activity and an increased risk of bladder, stomach, and lung carcinoma.[279–283] People who are extensive metabolizers have a 4-fold increase in their risk of lung cancer, but the risk is probably dependent on race. Thus, blacks have a 4.5-fold risk, whereas whites have a 10.2-fold risk.[280] Poor metabolizers show little or no CYP2D6 proteins, owing to the aberrant splicing of the gene transcript.[284] These findings are however not as definitive as one would hope them to be. Additional studies in these directions need to be done. Analysis of the gene subtypes is performed by RFLP of PCR products.[282, 285]

NAT2 (acetyl-CoA:arylamine *N*-acetyltransferase, NAT2*4) is a cytosolic enzyme responsible for the bioactivation and deactivation of arylamine carcinogens.[286] RFLP fragments generated by *Msp*I, *Kpn*I, and *Bam*HI restriction enzymes define three different alleles of *NAT*, called M1, M2, and M3.[287] Subsequent studies have shown seven polymorphic sites; specific combinations determine the type of acetylation capacity.[288, 289] Individuals can be either slow acetylators or rapid acetylators. Slow acetylators are homozygous for the slow allele, whereas rapid acetylators are either heterozygotes or homozygous for the rapid allele. As with the other susceptibility genes, variations among races exist. The slow acetylator genotype is present with a frequency of 0.10 in the Japanese population, while its frequency is 0.72 in Americans and is as high as 0.90 in Mediterranean peoples.[290] Those who are slow acetylators are more prone to the deleterious effect of certain drugs, such as isoniazid, hydralazine, and procainamide. They are also more prone to bladder carcinoma.[291] By contrast, patients who have bronchogenic carcinoma are more likely to be fast acetylators.[279, 286, 288, 292] Still, extensive studies of lung carcinoma and NAT2 status remain to be performed. The analysis of NAT2 levels has been carried out by acetylation of certain caffeine metabolites,[293] as well as by RFLP.[288, 292]

Individuals with a high throughput from CYP1A1 and a low output from GSTM1 are subject to an accumulation of toxic phenols and epoxides from smoke. They also exhibit enhanced adduct formation with subsequent alteration of the coding TP53 strand (G:C→T:A). Ryberg and associates[294] and Kawajiri and co-workers[295] have reported associations between smoking, *CYP1A1* heterozygote/*GSTM1* null genotypes, and *TP53* transversion mutations. Both studies reveal a higher risk of developing lung cancer among those who have variant *CYP1A1* and *GSTM1* null genotypes. Przygodzki and colleagues[296] found that *TP53* mutation and positive p53 IHC staining are more likely to occur among those patients with non–small cell lung cancer who had a variant *CYP1A1*. These patients were more likely to have mutations in exon 8 and transition mutations at CpG sites in the *TP53* gene. Furthermore, younger, lighter smokers with lung cancer are more likely to be variant CYP1A1.[276, 296] It may be that CYP1A1 activation contributes to lung cancer through P53 inactivation.[296]

Inherited Alteration of Tumor Suppressor Genes and Oncogenes. The genetic predisposition to cancer can be influenced by the inheritance of mutated tumor suppressor genes. Two examples of this are the inheritance of a mutation of a single allele of the *TP53* gene in Li-Fraumeni syndrome and of the retinoblastoma *(RB1)* gene in hereditary retinoblastoma. Alteration of the single remaining wild-type gene produces complete inactivation of the gene and is the basis for the "two-hit" hypothesis of Knudsen.[297] These patients are therefore more susceptible to carcinomas because one mutation already exists and the second "hit" is all that is needed to complete inactivation of the gene. A study of 4101 relatives of patients with retinoblastoma found a 10-fold increase of nonocular cancers in carriers of the mutant gene and a 15-fold increase in lung cancers, in particular small cell lung cancer.[298] However, when one looks for evidence of a similar increased risk for lung cancer when there are mutations of another tumor suppressor gene, the *TP53* gene, one is disappointed. Although a large percentage of lung cancers show *TP53* mutations within the tumor, patients with the Li-Fraumeni syndrome do not have an increased rate of *TP53*-mutated lung carcinoma relative to control cases. Furthermore, most lung carcinomas that show *TP53* mutations do not have a somatic mutation for *TP53*.[299, 300] Finally, although inherited polymorphic alleles of the *RAS* oncogene[301] and of the *TP53* gene[302] have been associated with lung carcinoma, the association is not great.

DNA Repair Mechanisms. Mutations in DNA can be spontaneous or caused by exogenous or endogenous carcinogens. There are at least five different pathways for repair of mutated DNA: base excision, recombination repair, nucleotide excision repair, mismatch repair, and direct damage reversal. Mutations in some of these repair mechanisms (in particular *MLH1* and *MSH2*) can play a role in explaining failure to repair DNA alteration. Such cells are dubbed "mutator phenotypes," in that they acquire mutations at a much higher frequency than do normal cells.

Base excision repair involves the removal of altered DNA bases by glycosylases. Numerous proteins of the DNA repair machinery finally produce correction of the mutation. This mechanism is the usual one employed to repair DNA adduct formation.

Recombination repair involves strand exchange of homologous DNA duplexes. It usually occurs after ionizing radiation or chemotherapy (e.g., with cisplatin), which causes double-strand breaks. The initial steps required for repair in this situation are still unclear, but poly(ADP-ribose) produced by poly(ADP-ribose) transferase and by topoisomerase I[303–305] are likely candidates. Topoisomerase I is usually detected at elevated levels in transcriptionally active regions of DNA. Radiation-induced activation of poly(ADP-ribose) transferase inhibits topoisomerase I by adenosine diphosphate ribosylation and therefore interferes with DNA replication. Through this method, time is made for DNA repair.

Nucleotide excision repair involves formation of nicks in both DNA strands upstream and downstream of modified base(s). The DNA damage is usually caused by either ultraviolet photoproducts, cross-linking drugs, or bulky carcinogen adducts.[306–308] Helicases unwind the DNA strands to enable DNA machinery to complete its tasks.[309] This is usually performed by ERCC1, HSSB, XPA, ERCC4, TFIIH, ERCC2, XPC, and XPG.[310, 311] The resultant gap is patched by DNA polymerases δ and ε and by proliferating cell nuclear antigen. The broken strands are then sealed with DNA ligase.

Mismatch repair corrects the mistakes that happen during DNA synthesis and recombination. This type of repair usually occurs after spontaneous deamination of 5-methylcytosine. Spontaneous hydrolysis of the amino group of 5-methylcytosine yields thymine, or a C→T mutation, usually at CpG sites. Approximately 30% of all single nucleotide mutations are of this type. Alternately, mismatch repairs may be seen in stretches of DNA sequence where there are frequent sequence repeats (e.g., CACACACACA). Mismatch may arise from mutations of the *MSH2* (on 2p22) and *MLH1* (on 3p21.3-p23) genes, responsible for recognizing mismatched nucleotides and initialization of protein repair complex formation, respectively. Other genes within this group include *MSH3* (on 5q11-q13), *MSH6/GTBP* (on 2p16), *PMS1* (on 2q32), and *PMS2* (on 7p22). Benachenhou and co-workers[312] studied both tumor and non-tumor samples from 31 patient with non–small cell lung cancers, looking for loss of heterozygosity (LOH) and microsatellite instability at 34 markers linked to the listed genes. Chromosomal regions 3p21 and 5q11-q13 were found to be hemizygously deleted in 55% and 42% of the patients, respectively. Sixty-five percent of the patients who showed deletions at *MLH1* also had deletions at *MSH3*. The consequence of these allelic losses are still unknown, but the lack of inactivating mutation might explain that replication error, the hallmark of mismatch repair genes inactivation in cancer cells, was quasi-absent in tumors. Therefore, *MLH1* and *MSH3* genes could potentially be involved in lung tumorigenesis.

Direct damage reversal is a repair function wherein O^6-alkylguanine-DNA alkyltransferase can remove adducts from DNA in a single step. The adducts are removed from the O^6 position of guanine and the O^4 position of thymine, thereby restoring the original DNA base.[313, 314] If they are not repaired, O^6-alkylguanine causes G→A mutation, whereas O^4-alkylthymine causes T→C mutation. Alkylating carcinogens, such as alkylnitrosourea, methylating agents (e.g., procarbazine), and chloroethylating agents (e.g., carmustine or lomustine) are the responsible culprits.[313]

DOMINANT ONCOGENES

Dominant oncogenes are genes whose overexpression will ultimately contribute to the formation of malignancy (Fig. 8–2).

MYC

Background. Members of the MYC family of proteins share a number of protein motifs that are found in regulators of gene transcription. *L-MYC* (*MYCL1* on 1p32; *MYCLK1* on 7p15) was one of the first genes to be found in lung cancers,[315] where it was found to be expressed in both small cell and non–small cell lung carcinomas. During early development, its expression is restricted to the brain, lung, and kidney.[316] *MYCN* (on 2p24.1) and *MYCL1*, like *MYC* (on 8q24), contain adjacent basic region, helix-loop-helix, and leucine zipper

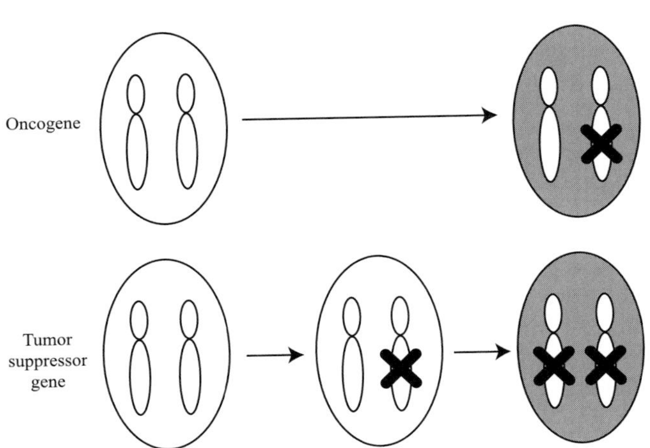

FIGURE 8–2
Oncogene and tumor suppressor mutations in tumorigenesis. Oncogenes require a single hit to be activated. Both alleles need to be lost for tumor suppressor genes to be activated.

TABLE 8–4
MYC and LMYC Overexpression and Gene Modulation

Activated by Overexpression	Repressed by Overexpression
CDC25	Cyclin D1
CDC2	Collagen genes
Dihydrofolate reductase	Neural cell adhesion molecules
Heat shock protein 70	Lymphocyte function–related antigen (LFA-1)
Plasminogen activator inhibitor-1	Major histocompatibility complex class I antigens
Adenovirus E4	

motifs, which characterize this family of DNA-binding proteins. Other genes of the family include *SMYC, RMYC, BMYC,* and the inactive *LMYCψ* pseudogene. MYC, MYCL1, and MYCN are proteins that form heterodimers with MAX and have a high affinity for the core binding sequence CACGTG motif (E box MYC sites)[317]; heterodimerization through the E box is responsible for transactivation.[318] MAX is homologous to the helix-loop-helix regions and leucine zipper regions of MYC, but it lacks the transactivation domain.[319, 320] The constitutively highly expressed MAD and MXI1 keep MAX in check by dimerization with it; neither can dimerize with MYC.[321, 322] The short-lived MYC protein responds to growth signals, whereas MAD and MXI1 are expressed with cell differentiation induction.[323, 324] Therefore, MYC-MAX dimers are present in proliferating cells, whereas MAD-MAX and MXI1-MAX are present in differentiated cells. MYC can also heterodimerize with the transcription initiation factor TFII-I and with the TATA-binding protein.[325] The association with TFII-I leads to inhibition of complex formation with TATA-binding protein and transcription initiation.[326, 327]

MYC has a role in cell cycle regulation and apoptosis (see Fig. 8–6, Table 8–4). In particular, high levels of MYC correlate with accelerated growth, whereas low levels correlate with differentiation. Transcription of CDC25, which is the phosphatase that mediates the activation of cyclin-dependent kinases, is directly activated by MYC-MAX.[328] The transactivating domain of MYC interacts with the retinoblastoma protein (RB1), and with the RB1-related protein P107,[329, 330] and is the same region that the TATA-binding protein binds to MYC.[331] Overall, MYC may have the ability to induce entry into the cell cycle. P107 and the D-cyclins act at the G_1/S transition, blocking progression; MYC can overcome the P107-mediated arrest, possibly by saturating the available P107.[332] MYC also represses expression of cyclin D1 at the transcription initiation phase.[333] Apoptosis is accelerated through sustained expression of MYC in hematopoietic cells.[334] MYC may accelerate cell death; however, it appears that this is mediated by functional p53.[335] MYC-induced apoptosis is associated with elevated expression of cyclin A and cyclin E and may be mediated by ornithine decarboxylase.[336, 337]

Activation of MYC in cancer appears to be accomplished through proviral insertion, chromosomal translocation, and gene amplification. Although point mutations occur in the *MYC* genes, they are rare; elevated expression of MYC appears to be the principal pathway.[338] In addition, *MYCL1* has two polymorphisms that produce three different genotypes (*LL, LS,* and *SS*).[339, 340] Altered MYC expression occurs in several tumor types, in particular small cell carcinoma of lung.[341] When *MYC* is amplified, as evidenced through in situ hybridization, 50% of cases show transcribed messenger RNA (mRNA), but 20% of cases show translation of the mRNA, as noted by IHC staining of frozen tissues.[342]

Clinicopathology. Ten percent to 44% of primary small cell lung carcinomas tumors contain amplified or overexpressed copies of one of the three *MYC* proto-oncogenes.[343–345] Specifically, *MYC, MYCL1,* and *MYCN* occur in 11% to 44%, 5% to 30%, and 6% to 25% of cases, respectively. Johnson and associates[346] compiled 15 different studies of *MYC* copy number data comprising 291 small cell lung cancer cases (183 tumors, 108 tumor cell lines). Thirty-five (32%) of 108 small cell lung cancer cell lines from patients had *MYC* gene family amplification (16 *MYC,* 7 *MYCN,* and 12 *MYCL1*); 20% of tumors from patients with small cell lung cancers had *MYC* family amplification (3 *MYC,* 13 *MYCN,* and 18 *MYCL1*). There were similar *MYC* copy numbers in the tumors themselves as in the cell lines established from them. However, Noguchi and colleagues[347] reported that 2 of 11 amplified cases had heterogenous expression of MYC. One primary tumor had areas with and without *MYCN* amplification in the primary tumor, and its metastases also showed variability of gene expression. The second case had no amplification of *MYCL1* in the primary tumor, but metastatic lesions showed amplification. Occasionally, DNA amplification of *MYC* genes is associated with DNA rearrangements with the *RLF* locus owing to intrachromosomal *MYCL1* rearrangements in small cell lung cancer.[343] The structurally similar rearrangements are probably caused by a highly repetitive region upstream of the *MYCL* gene and result in the formation of a chimeric RLF-MYCL1 fusion protein. The *RLF-MYCL1* fusion places the regulatory region and (at least) the first exon of RLF upstream of the *MYCL1* gene. In the characterized cases, the fusion gene has also been involved in DNA amplification.[348]

Gazzeri and associates[349] found *TP53* alterations in 66% of lung carcinomas (52% of neuroendocrine carcinomas and 75% of non–small cell lung carcinomas). MYC was found to be activated in 24% (10/42) of the neuroendocrine tumors and 48% (33/69) of the non–small cell lung carcinomas using Southern and Northern blot techniques. In addition, *MYCL1* and *MYCN* genes were also activated in 26% of neuroendocrine carcinomas. No correlation was found between *TP53* mutations and *MYC* activation in small cell or non–small cell lung cancers, but their association was significantly more frequent in the latter than in the former. The results indicate that the *TP53* and *MYC* gene alterations are important but represent independent occurrences in the development of lung tumors. Bia and associates[350] also found that *MYC* family genes may be used for prognostication purposes. In a series of 30 lung tumors with *TP53* alterations, *MYC* gene overexpression was found in 63% of stage III tumors and 76% of cases with stage III and relapse. Only 27% of patients without *MYC* gene overexpression had stage II tumors and only 22% without it relapsed.

Among small cell carcinoma cell lines, Plummer and colleagues[351] found that cell lines expressing the *KIT* gene also expressed either the *MYCL1* or *MYCN* gene product. In contrast, cell lines expressing *MYC* did not express *KIT*. They concluded that an autocrine growth loop might exist between *KIT* and *MYCL1* or *MYCN* in small cell lung cancers. Other investigators note, however, that usually a single *MYC* gene family member appears to be deregulated.[352, 353]

In contrast, non–small cell lung carcinomas show amplification or overexpression of the MYC family of genes in only 10% of cases[345, 354]; *MYC, MYCL1*, and *MYCN* are seen in approximately 10%, 2%, and 0% of cases, respectively. The highest level of expression is found among squamous cell carcinomas where MYC and MYCL1 overexpression is evident, whereas MYCN is typically not present.[355] Polly and associates,[356] using a type 2 pneumocyte–related cell culture model of mouse pulmonary adenocarcinoma that is known to contain an A→G transition in the second base position of codon 61 of the *KRAS* gene, examined molecular alteration in other oncogenes. The study found a twofold increase in *MYC* mRNA levels and transcription levels in the malignant cell lines (C4SE9 and NULB5) as compared with the nonmalignant cells (C4E10). More importantly, the *MYC* gene transcription levels in benign C4E10 cells were much higher in comparison to the other genes examined. Similar high levels of *MYC* gene expression levels were also seen in type 2 pneumocytes in normal mouse lung. The investigators did not find any major DNA rearrangements or amplifications between C4E10 cells and either C4SE9 or NULB5 cell lines. These findings suggest that high expression levels of MYC before *KRAS* alteration may predispose type 2 pneumocytes to transformation. This may be supported by the finding that all *MYC* family members can cooperate with an activated *RAS* gene to transform normal cells in culture and rat embryo fibroblasts.[357, 358]

In other studies, MYC gene family amplification was associated with shortened overall survival[346, 359] and was more likely to be found in cell lines established from patients who previously received chemotherapy.[359] The findings may be supported by a different study[355] involving examination of *MYC* gene family expression levels in normal and non–small cell carcinoma lung samples. In non-neoplastic lung, *MYC* expression was strongest in bronchial epithelium basal cells and hyperplastic alveolar type 2 pneumocytes, which are potential progenitor cells for bronchopulmonary epithelium and their tumors. Other investigations of tumor cell lines from chemotherapy-treated treated patients having small cell lung cancer with *MYC* amplification have been associated with shortened survival and more aggressive tumor morphology[359–361]; a 10-fold *MYC* amplification also correlated with shortened survival. Although p-glycoprotein may be associated with chemotherapy resistance in small cell lung cancers, it is not associated with *MYCN* expression.[362] Finally, in Japanese lung cancer patients, the presence of an *Eco*RI restriction site polymorphism between the second and third exons of the *MYCL1* gene appears to be associated with poor prognosis and lymph node metastasis. In a follow-up study of American patients, this restriction site was more frequent in African Americans (0.71) than in whites (0.49), thus making the allelic frequency in African Americans similar to that of the Japanese.[363]

RAS

Background. The *RAS* (rat sarcomas) family of oncogenes is made up of highly conserved *KRAS2* (on 12p12.1), *NRAS* (on 1p13), and *HRAS1* (on 11p15.5) genes, which code for 21-kDa membrane–associated proteins of the "small" guanosine triphosphatase (GTPase) family. *KRAS1* and *HRAS2* are inactive pseudogenes. The predominant form of *RAS* altered in lung cancers is *KRAS*, which will be the *RAS* type discussed in this section unless otherwise noted. The *RAS* family comprises about 50 currently known genes, including members of *NRASL1*, *NRASL2*, *NRASL3*, *RHOA*, *RHOB* and *RHOC*, *RAC1* and *RAC2*, *RRAS*, *RAL RAP1A*, *RAB2*, and *GEM*. The *RAS* family genes have homology to the α subunit of heterotrimeric G proteins. Sequence homology of these proteins separates them into three families: RAS, RHO/RAC, and RAB. The *RAS* genes normally bind guanosine triphosphate (GTP) and guanosine diphosphate (GDP), and they play an important role in signal transduction. They are membrane-bound GTPases that convert extracellular signals to intracellular effects by the way of pathway(s), thereby mediating control of cell growth and regulating cytoskeletal actin and membrane trafficking. The RHO/RAC proteins are involved in cytoskeletal organization, whereas RAB is involved in regulation of intracellular vesicular transport.[364]

The response signals that are transduced through RAS originate from different sources. One of them is dimerization and phosphorylation of receptor tyrosine kinase (PDGF or EGF), which in turn binds adapter molecules (SHC or GRB2) and a guanine nucleotide exchange factor (SOS) mediating the transfer of phosphate.[365] Another pathway for RAS is through the seven-helix transmembrane receptor inducing the tyrosine phosphorylation of Shc through G protein βγ subunits.[366] A third possible pathway is through a focal adhesion kinase–related tyrosine kinase called PTK2, which can also phosphorylate SHC and is activated by calcium ions and by protein kinase C.[367]

Once RAS is activated to the GTP-bound state, it recruits the cytoplasmically located 74-kDa serine threonine kinase called c-RAF1.[368, 369] RAF1 is stabilized by 14–3–3 protein,[370–373] which helps in binding of RAF1 with RAS, allowing further propagation of signal. The next kinase in this cascade is the mitogen-activated protein kinase-kinase (MAPKK or MEK), which after several other steps ultimately ends in "mitogen activation."[374–376] One other partially solved pathway for signaling from activated RAS is through phosphatidylinositol 3-kinase (PI 3-kinase) p110 subunit, a guanine nucleotide exchange factor for the Ral GTPase named RalGDS, a RalGDS-related protein, and Rin1.[377–382] These pathways are still under investigation, as are the more and ever complex pathways that the small GTPases have made for themselves. Ultimately, when the signal is passed down to either RAF1 or PI 3-kinase, the 120-kDa protein GTPase-activating protein (GAP) shuts down the activated RAS, returning it to the GDP state (Fig. 8–3).[383, 384] Essentially, two GAP proteins exist: P120GAP and NF1GAP. P120GAP possesses SRC homology domains SH2 and SH3 through which it can associate with tyrosine-phosphorylated proteins, whereas NF1GAP cannot; different activated RAS com-

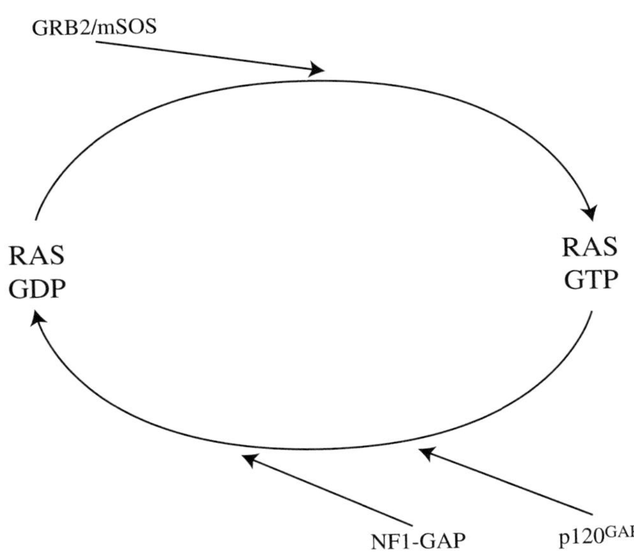

FIGURE 8–3
RAS–GDP/GTP cycle. RAS activation requires GRB2 and mSOS to be activated. RAS is cycled back to a GDP state through GAP and by NF1. GDP, guanosine diphosphate; GTP, guanosine triphosphate.

plexes can have distinct cellular targets.[385] Whereas GAP functions in response to signal activation, neurofibromatosis gene 1 *(NF1)* appears to control the basal RAS activity. Excellent overviews of the RAS systems may be gained from Macara and colleagues[365] and Marshall and co-workers.[386] A brief overview of the signaling pathway may be seen in Figure 8–4.

Oncogenic *RAS* stimulates activity of protein kinase C and activates transcription of cyclin D1, *FOS*, *JUN*, *JUNB*, *MDR1*, *MYC*, *TGFA*, *TGFB*, and ornithine decarboxylase-1.[387, 388] In addition, oncogenic *RAS* can markedly up-regulate vascular endothelial growth factor (VEGF); RAS may therefore contribute to tumor growth by indirectly promoting angiogenesis.[389] PDGF receptor, fibronectin genes, MYOD1, and myogenin are repressed by oncogenic RAS.[387] RAS can directly interact with RAF1, RalGDS, and phosphatidylinositol-2-OH kinase.[377, 390, 391] Continuous expression of RAS can also cause apoptosis when protein kinase C is down-regulated.[392] RAS-dependent apoptosis can, however, be prevented through BCL2, which is phosphorylated in a RAS-dependent manner and associates with it.[392]

Mutation of *KRAS*, the most commonly altered *RAS* in non–small cell lung tumors, produces a reduction in its GTPase activity. RAS is thereby constitutively activated. *HRAS* and *NRAS* mutations are not found in non–small cell carcinoma of lung.[393–397] It is therefore not surprising that histologic subtypes cannot be correlated with either *KRAS*, *HRAS*, or *NRAS* mutation status.[398] *KRAS* mutations predominantly occur in codons 12 and 13 of exon 1 and less frequently in codon 61 (and rarely 59) of exon 2.[397, 399–404] In smokers, most of the codon 12 mutations show a G→T transversion,

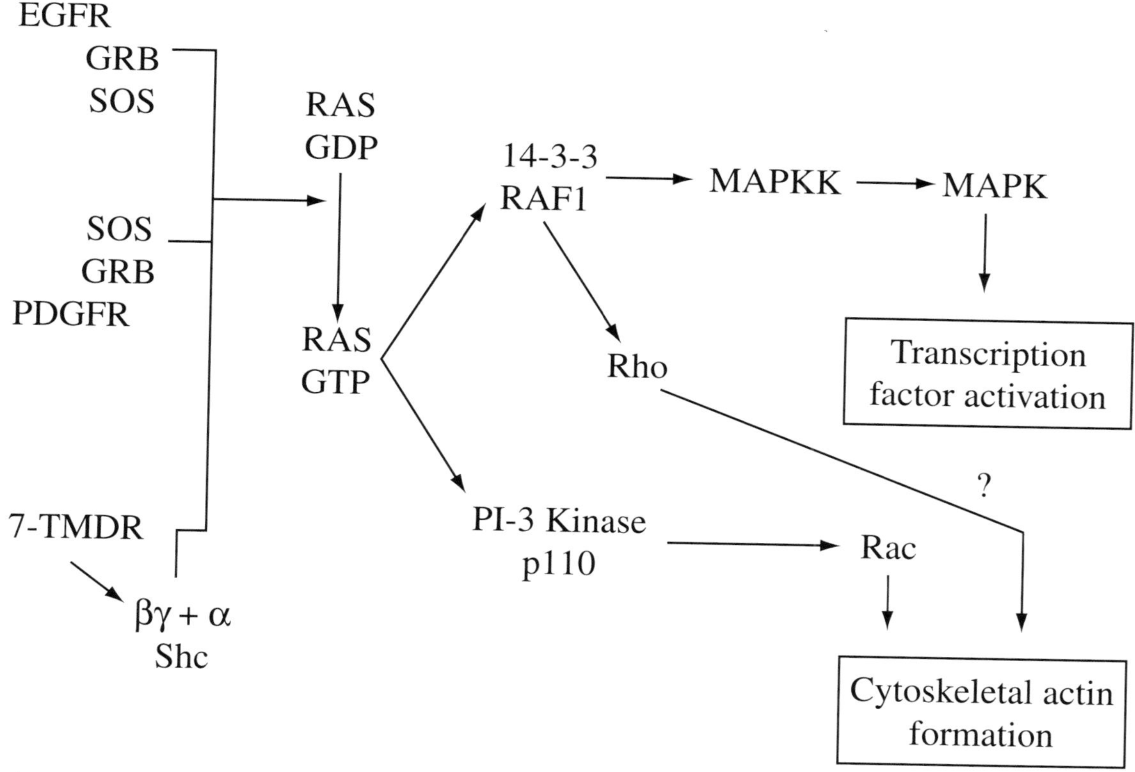

FIGURE 8–4
RAS signal transduction cascade. Among the several end points in this cascade are transcription factor activation and the promotion of actin formation.

whereas nonsmokers have G→A transition mutations in its first two bases.

Analysis of *RAS* mutation in persons exposed to radon do not demonstrate *KRAS*, *HRAS*, or *NRAS* mutations if they are nonsmokers.[405–407] Smoking appears to have a synergistic effect on the frequency of *RAS* mutations.[405]

Despite the absence of *HRAS* mutations among lung carcinomas, a large case-control study of whites and African Americans found the presence of a rare *Msp*I restriction endonuclease polymorphism in *HRAS* that conferred a relative risk for lung cancer of 2.0 for whites and 3.2 for African Americans.[408] Also, in non–small cell lung cancers, hypomethylation of CCGG sites in the 3′ region and allelic loss can occur, even though *HRAS* mutations are not evident.[409]

RAS mutation rates differ among smokers and nonsmokers. Smokers are more likely than nonsmokers to have *KRAS* mutations (30% vs. 10%).[398, 410–412] Also, smokers usually have G→T transversions (possibly through DNA-adduct formation), whereas nonsmokers most often have G→A transitions (spontaneous mutation). Interestingly, the *KRAS* mutation rate in lung cancers resected from patients who had stopped smoking for at least 10 years was similar to that in cancers of current smokers.[411] This further lends support to the use of sputum for *KRAS* analysis among smokers.[400]

RAS mutations have been analyzed by direct sequencing of PCR product, RFLP, single-stranded conformational polymorphism, denaturing gradient gel electrophoresis, allele-specific oligonucleotide hybridization, and enrichment-PCR. In the last of these, a *Bst*NI restriction enzyme site is introduced when the sequence is normal.[393, 395, 405, 413–416]

Clinicopathology. *KRAS* mutations occur in 25% to 50% of non–small cell carcinomas of lung.[397, 400–404] However, whereas 20% to 50% of adenocarcinomas have *KRAS* mutations,[400–402] only 1% to 10% of squamous cell carcinomas and large cell carcinomas[393, 417, 418] have them.[395, 397, 403] Pleomorphic (spindle and giant cell) carcinomas of lung have a 9% *KRAS* mutation rate.[413] Bronchioloalveolar carcinomas demonstrate a 30% to 40% mutation rate; of the subtypes, the mucinous variant is frequently mutated, whereas the nonmucinous type is mutated at a much lower rate.[419, 420] One additional feature that needs to be kept in mind is that epithelial proliferations away from lung carcinoma may demonstrate *KRAS* mutations.[412, 421] Thus, atypical adenomatous hyperplasia can show *KRAS* mutations and are currently deemed premalignant.[422] Small cell carcinomas of lung and other neuroendocrine tumors, including carcinoid tumors and atypical carcinoid tumors, usually lack *KRAS* mutations.[395, 396, 423]

Generally, for early stage cancers, *KRAS* mutations portend poor prognosis, with shorter survival and recurrence of tumor.[393, 398, 404, 417, 424, 425] Slebos and associates[425] found that these patients tend to have smaller and less well differentiated tumors and have overall worse survival (37% survival at 36 months in *RAS*-mutated patients versus 68% in patients with wild-type *RAS*). Likewise, *HRAS* alterations, if and when present, portend shorter overall survival.[344]

Epidermal Growth Factor Receptor Family

Background. The epidermal growth factor receptor family is one of tyrosine kinase receptors. The gene family includes *ERBB (EGFR), ERBB2 (HER2, neu), ERBB3 (HER3)*, and *ERBB4 (HER4)*. *EGFR*, located on 7p13-p12, is found widely expressed in body tissues, except in hematopoietic tissues. EGFR can heterodimerize with each of the other family members, producing different patterns of transphosphorylation.[426] Ligands capable of binding to EGFR include EGF, TGF-α, amphiregulin, and heregulin, to name a few.[427, 428] The activated EGFR phosphorylates the RAS-GTPase–activating protein (GAP)[429] and stimulates protein tyrosine phosphatase activity directed toward the EGFR itself and ERBB2.[430] Activated EGFR can also bind to phosphatidylinositol-3 kinase and phospholipase 3γ.[431, 432]

ERBB2, located on 17q21-q22, has approximately 80% homology to *EGFR*, and is likewise widely distributed on the plasma membranes of diverse cells of the body. ERBB2 is activated by differentially spliced neuregulins, also called heregulin and NEU differentiation factor (NDF).[433] ERBB2 can also form heterodimers with the other family members.[434–436] Ligand binding to ERBB2 can also activate the RAS-GTP pathway.[431] *ERBB3*, located on 12q13, is transcribed in lung and respiratory tract, kidney and urinary tract, brain, and stomach; it is not present in the lymphoid cells and muscle cells.[437] ERBB3 is 44% homologous to EGFR in the extracellular domain and 60% homologous in the tyrosine kinase domain. *ERBB4*, located on 2q33.3-34, is selectively expressed in brain, heart, and kidney, with low levels in other organs, including the lungs.

The methods used to identify *EGFR* and ERBB2 in lung cancers are immunohistochemistry, immunoprecipitation, and mRNA expression.

Clinicopathology. EGFR is commonly overexpressed, amplified, or mutated in several human tumors, including glioblastoma, breast carcinoma, and lung. In non–small cell carcinoma of lung, high levels of mRNA expression occur,[438] with similar findings seen both by immunoprecipitation and immunohistochemistry. Approximately 70% of squamous cell carcinomas, 40% of adenocarcinomas, and 0% of small cell carcinomas are positive for the receptor.[439–441] Among adenocarcinomas, overexpression of EGFR correlates with slightly worse survival.[442, 443] Amphiregulin, an EGFR ligand, when overexpressed, is also correlated with worse survival.[442] However, patients with large cell neuroendocrine carcinomas that overexpress EGFR do not appear to have shortened survival or poor response to chemotherapy.[444] Small cell lung carcinomas do not have alterations in EGFR, except, in vitro, where cell lines from invasive small cell carcinomas show elevated expression of EGFR.[445]

The expression of ERBB2 is present in both small and non–small cell carcinomas of lung. The difference of expression, though, is negligible versus abundant in small cell versus non–small cell lung carcinomas, respectively.[446, 447] Non–small cell lung carcinomas, and, in particular adenocarcinomas, show amplification/overexpression in 25% to 56% of cases.[439, 441, 448] Patients with stage I adenocarcinoma and *ERBB2* overexpression had a significantly higher incidence of early tumor recurrence.[449] It also appears that ERBB2 is elevated in the early stages of carcinogenesis, and where it can be identified by enzyme-linked immunosorbent assay techniques on serum.[450] Also, ERBB2 expression is more likely to be seen in lung cancers from women than men.[451] Non–small cell lung cancer cases, which express ERBB2, do so at levels higher than that found in normal bronchiolar epithelium; overexpression of ERBB2 in pulmonary adenocarcinomas usually predicts shorter overall survival.[439] This is particularly true when the receptor ligand is TGF-β, thereby completing the autocrine loop. Autocrine stimulation by NDF may likewise exist.[452]

Tateishi and co-workers[443] investigated the expression of both EGFR and the ERBB2 proteins in lung cancer. Expression of both EGFR and ERBB2 was significantly more frequent among patients with metastasis. The 5-year survival rates based on EGFR status alone were not significantly different; however, there was a significant difference in 5-year survival in patients whose tumors were ERBB2 positive versus those whose tumors were ERBB2 negative (0% and 52%, respectively). Of the EGFR-positive cases, the 5-year survival rates of patients with ERBB2 positivity and negativity were 33% and 59%, respectively. Furthermore, when ERBB2 was expressed in patients with tumors having mutated *KRAS*, survival was poor.[453]

ERBB3 appears to be overexpressed in non–small cell carcinomas,[442] in particular squamous cell carcinoma (28%), followed by adenocarcinoma (15%), and large cell carcinoma of lung (10%).[454] Patients with stage III and IV disease with high ERBB3 expression survived significantly shorter time periods than did patients with low ERBB3 expression.[454]

MDM2

Background. Murine double-minute 2 *(MDM2)* is a 90-kDa proto-oncogene located on 12q14.3-q15. It is oncogenic when amplified or overexpressed. It can bind to both wild-type and mutated p53 protein[455] through the amino terminus of p53.[299] Overexpression of MDM2 overcomes wild-type p53–mediated suppression and transcriptional transactivation in cells in an autoregulatory loop.[456, 457] MDM2 also appears to regulate the RB1 pathway; one way is through the binding of MDM2 to the DP1 protein of the DP1/E2F1 heterodimer,[458] thereby increasing the dimer's transcriptional activity (Fig. 8–5). A second way MDM2 functions is through a stable interaction between MDM2 and RB1 protein, whereby MDM2 overcomes the transcriptional inactivity brought by RB1 protein on the DP1/E2F heterodimer.[459] By inactivating p53 and promoting cell cycling through enhanced E2F activity, MDM2 is indeed oncogenic. IHC analysis of cells for MDM2 reveals predominantly nuclear localization, but Golgi and cytoplasmic staining may also be present.[455, 460]

Clinicopathology. Sarcomas are the tumors most likely to overexpress MDM2,[461] but lung carcinomas can do it as well. The MDM2 overexpression in lung carcinoma appears, at times, to be caused by increased transcription, rather than *MDM2* amplification.[462, 463] Fifty-four percent of non–small cell lung cancers show both p53 and MDM2 overexpression; only 7% had MDM2 overexpression alone. There may be a slight predilection for overexpression of MDM2 in adenocarcinoma of lung.[464, 465] In contrast, p53-immunopositive squamous cell carcinomas that were negative for *TP53* mutations did not overexpress MDM2.[463, 466] Also, CDKN2A was shown to bind MDM2 and prevent degradation of p53.[466a] Clearly, additional work needs to be done to better understand the MDM2/p53 phenomenon.

RAF1

Background. The gene for the cytoplasmic serine/threonine kinase RAF1 is located on 3p25. *RAF1* is expressed ubiquitously. Other members of the *RAF* family include RAFA1 (on Xp11.2), which is located primarily in the urogenital system, and RAFB1 (on 7q33–36), which is located in the brain, testes, and hematopoietic cell lines. RAF1 exists in a complex with heat shock protein HSP90, which is necessary for that protein's cellular localization.[369] Serine-phosphorylated RAF1 also associates with the SH2 domains of SRC, tubulin, and members of the 14–3–3 protein family (14–3–3β and 14–3–3ζ).[467] The dimeric form of 14–3–3 co-segregates with RAF to the plasma membrane and is able to promote RAF1 oligomerization, which promotes RAF1 activation through a RAS-dependent pathway (see Fig. 8–4).[370–372, 468] Activated RAS binds to RAF1, inducing conformational alteration and displacement of 14–3–3ζ from the amino terminus.[469] RAF1 also interacts with the Gβ2 subunit of the heterotrimeric G proteins[470] and can also bind to and phosphorylate

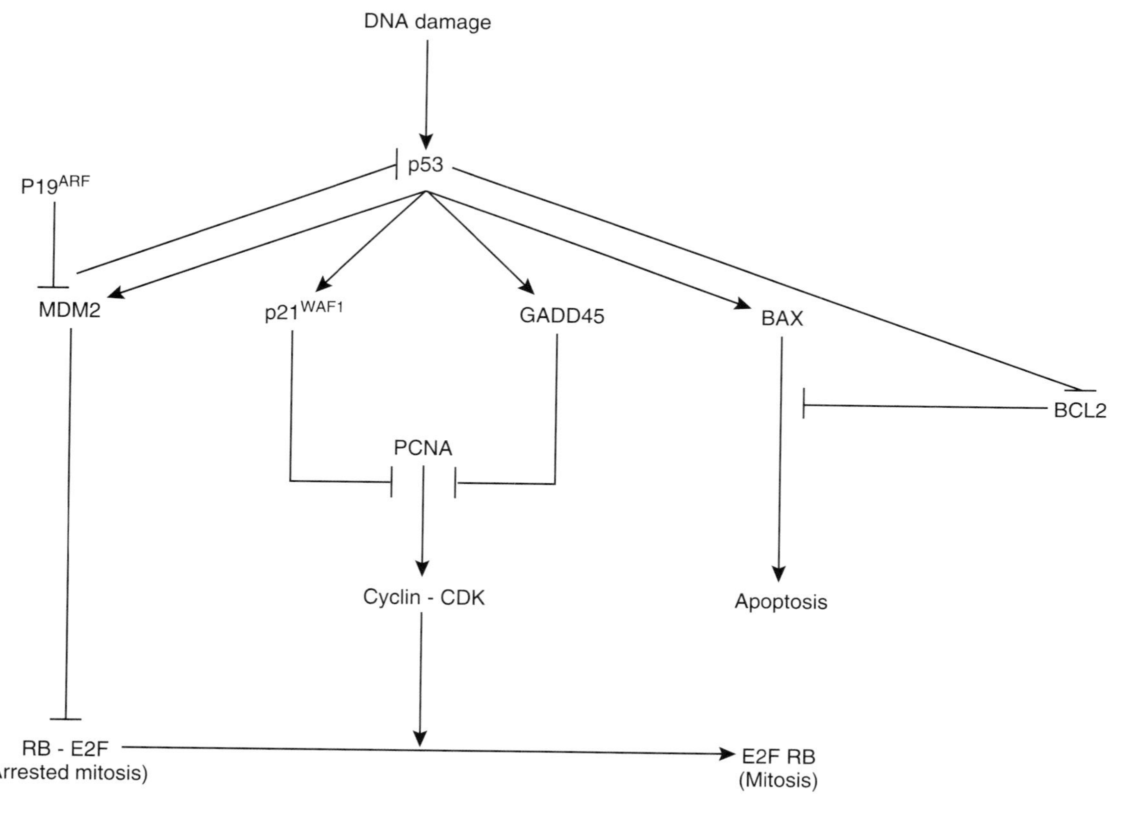

FIGURE 8–5
TP53 cascade of cell cycle arrest and apoptosis.

CDC25B.[471] RAF1 can, however, be activated in a RAS- and 14–3–3–independent manner.[472] RAF1 has a critical role in response to many growth factors, including EGF, PDGF, insulin, IL-1 and IL-2, granulocyte-macrophage colony-stimulating factor, tissue plasminogen activator, thrombin, FMS, SRC, SIS, HRAS, and polyoma middle T antigen.[473–477] Downstream activation through RAF1 includes MAP kinase kinase (MAPKK or MEK), MAPK (ERK1 and ERK2), FOS, and JUN.[368, 478–483]

Clinicopathology. High levels of *RAF1* expression occur in tumor cell lines or cell lines derived from human samples of small cell and non–small lung cancers.[344, 484, 485] Mutations of *RAF1* have also been found in murine neuroendocrine tumors,[486] but this result has not been confirmed by others.[487, 488] An analysis of human neuroendocrine tumors, including carcinoid, atypical carcinoid, large cell neuroendocrine carcinoma, and small cell lung carcinoma, was likewise unable to identify mutation alterations in *RAF1*.[423]

TUMOR SUPPRESSOR GENES

Tumor suppressor genes, or recessive oncogenes, are genes in which alterations of both alleles contribute to the formation of neoplasia. Rare inherited diseases, like the Li-Fraumeni syndrome or familial retinoblastoma, contain genetically inherited damage to one allele. Therefore, all cells in these cases will have germline alterations. Alteration of the second allele contributes to neoplasia. This may explain why the inherited diseases are usually multifocal. In the general population, however, both alleles would need to be altered for malignancy to ensue (see Fig. 8–2).

Retinoblastoma

Background. The retinoblastoma *(RB1)* gene, localized on chromosome 13q14.2, was the first tumor suppressor gene recognized.[489] It was the study of retinoblastoma that led to the "two-hit" hypothesis,[297, 490] which states that both the maternal and paternal copies of the gene must be inactivated for tumor to develop. The *RB1* gene consists of 26 exons in which exon 1 contains a 5′ untranslated region. The gene codes for a 105-kDa protein that functions as a nuclear phosphoprotein binding to double-stranded DNA in a non–sequence-specific manner. The protein also functions as a signal transducer, in that it is a major gateway that several proteins use to induce or arrest cell cycle. The carboxyl-terminal domain is required for the growth suppressive function of the RB1 protein. Lastly, RB1 protein plays a role in the apoptotic process.[491]

RB1 shows homology with P107 and the transcription factor TFIIB.[492, 493] RB2 encodes for P130, which is the E1A-associated protein that can bind to cyclins A and E.[494, 495] The P107 and P130 proteins are more similar to each other than to RB1. A distinguishing factor between them is the presence of a "spacer" region that is located between the binding pocket, the latter of which is present in all of the subtypes. This spacer region enables the proteins to associate with cyclin A/CDK2 or cyclin E/CDK2 kinase.[496, 497]

Cyclin-dependent kinases (CDKs), along with the appropriate cyclins, are the regulators of RB1 protein (Fig. 8–6). The D-cyclins (D1, D2 and D3), when induced by mitogens, complex with either CDK4 or CDK6.[498–500] Cyclin D1 has proto-oncogenic activity and, when expressed at high levels, will shorten the G_1 timeframe of a cell.[501, 502] Cyclin D/CDK4 and cyclin D/CDK6 preferentially phosphorylate RB1 protein.[503] Cyclin D has a protein motif on its amino terminus, enabling it to bind to the RB1 protein pocket region. Additional information may be found in the sections on CDKs and cyclins in this chapter. The E1A adenovirus protein, SV40 T antigen, and human papillomavirus (HPV) E7 proteins have remarkably conserved regions among themselves and the pocket region of RB1.[504–506] It is through this region that the RB1 protein is inactivated and the release of cell cycle is brought on. Cyclins E and A, with CDK2, also release the RB1 protein–dependent cell cycle arrest.[507, 508]

RB1 protein exerts its effect on proliferation by regulating the transcriptional activity of E2F; it also interacts with several other proteins (Table 8–5).[509, 510] The release of this ubiquitous transcription factor binds to DNA and up-regulates transcription. E2F (on 20q11) has a downstream effect on several genes, including dihydrofolate reductase, thymidylate synthase, and DNA polymerase α, *MYC*, *MYB*, *CDC2*, and cyclin A.[511, 512] E2F binds to the pocket region of RB1 protein, preferentially when RB1 protein is hypophosphorylated.[513] All RB1 family members bind with E2F. The E2F family consists of five homologous proteins, labeled E2F1 through E2F5[514]; E2F1 through E2F3 bind preferentially to RB1 protein, whereas E2F4 and E2F5 bind to either P107 or P130.[515–524]

Release of E2F is accomplished by phosphorylation of RB1 protein. RB1 protein phosphorylation occurs through cyclin/CDK complex in G_1 phase, through cyclin E/CDK2, which operates at the initiation of S phase, and through cyclin A/CDK2, which operates in S and G_2 phases.[525] Also, P107 and P130/E2F complexes occur during different times in the cell cycle. P107/E2F complex is found predominantly during the S phase, the P130/E2F complex is found late in G_1, whereas RB1 protein/E2F complex is found in G_1 and S phases.[497, 520] Lastly, E2F is a heterodimer consisting of E2F and DP family member 1 through 3.[514, 518, 519, 523] Phosphorylation of certain DP subtypes may be important in down-regulating transcription of specific genes during the later stages of the cell cycle.

The CDKN2A protein family can interact specifically with CDK4A and CDK6, thereby blocking D-type

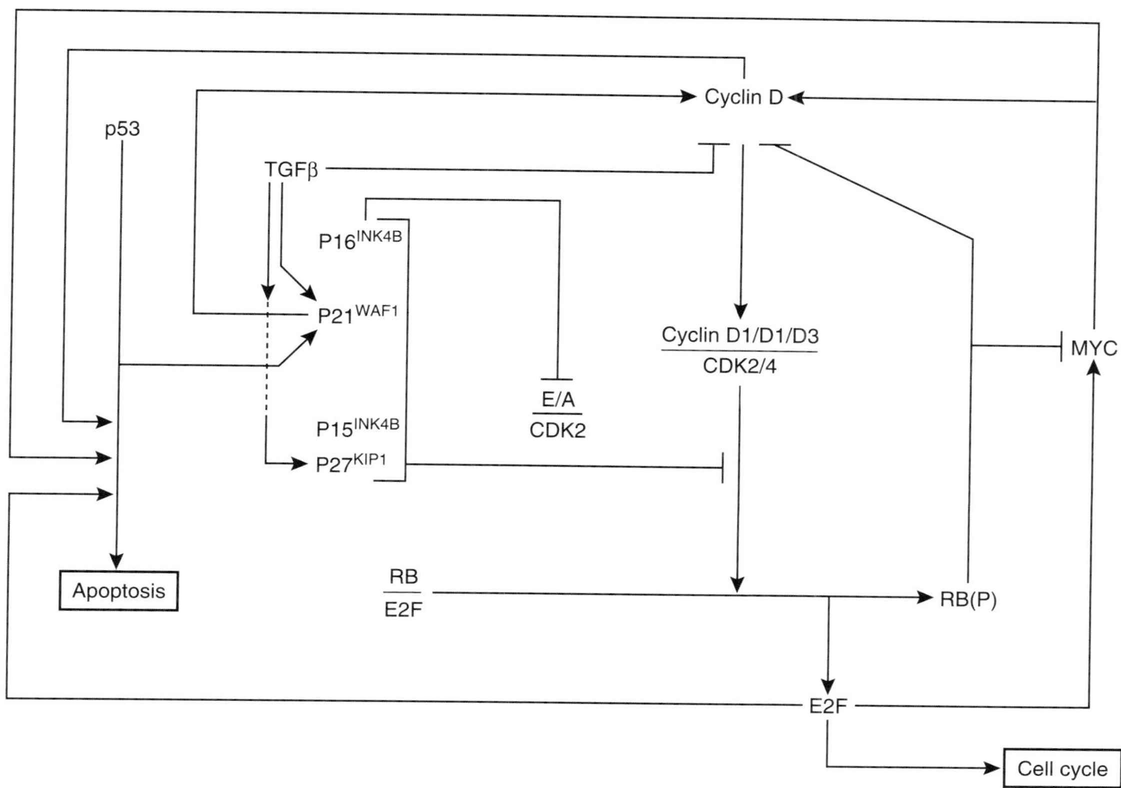

FIGURE 8–6
Cyclin/CDK feedback regulation cascade. End products in this cascade include promotion of cell cycle, or apoptosis.

cyclins only and causing G_1 arrest. The INK4A protein family relies on the presence of functional RB1 protein to function properly.[512] CDK activity may also be influenced by the level of cyclin D; overexpression may inappropriately phosphorylate RB1 protein and release the cell from G_1 arrest. More on the subject of INK4A is presented in the appropriate subsection.

As previously mentioned, MDM2 is associated with the RB1 pathway, as well as with p53 pathways (see Fig. 8–5). Binding of overamplified MDM2 can inactivate p53, and MDM2 can bind to the DP1 subcomponent of the E2F protein and increase transcriptional activity of E2F/DP1.[458] Furthermore, MDM2 may interact with RB1 protein and can overcome the RB1 protein/E2F binding.[459] Therefore, inactivation of p53 with release and stimulation of E2F will release the cell from G_1 arrest and possibly lead to carcinogenesis. A similar situation is used by oncogenic viruses, whereby inactivation of p53 and E2F release through competition with RB1 protein is the rule[526]; E1A, SV40 T antigen, or HPV E7 may disassociate the RB1 protein/E2F complex.[527–529] p53 inactivation is important in this scenario, because overexpression of E2F can in itself lead to p53-dependent apoptosis.[526] RB1 protein also protects the cell from apoptosis. Furthermore, RB1 protein may be essential for differentiation of cells, as is evident among RB −/− mouse embryos, which die before the 16th day of gestation, demonstrating prominent hematopoietic and neuronal terminal maturational defects as well as a high level of inappropriate apoptosis.[530]

The destination to carcinoma along the RB1 trail runs along many pathways (see Fig. 8–6). Overexpression of cyclin D, alterations in INK4A oncogenic viruses, *MDM2* overexpression, and simply mutation of *RB1* itself, either individually or in combination, can produce cancer. Although *E2F* and *DP1* are "oncogenic," no mutations or other alterations of these genes have been presented to date.

Mutations can affect any portion of the *RB1* gene. Blanquet and associates[531] sequenced all exons, introns,

TABLE 8–5

Proteins Associating with Retinoblastoma Protein

Cellular	Viral
E2F1, E2F2, E2F3	Human papillomavirus E7
DP1, DP2, DP3	Epstein-Barr virus nuclear antigens 2 and 5
D cyclins	Adenovirus E1A
MYC, NMYC	SV40 large T antigen
MDM2	
ABL	
CDC2	
ATF2 transcription factor	

and the promotor region in 232 cases of hereditary and nonhereditary retinoblastoma. They found mutations scattered throughout the *RB1* gene but preferentially within exons 3, 8, 18, and 19. Mutations in this region hinder E2F binding, thereby making E2F constitutively active. Other more rare alterations include hypermethylation of the 5′ region of the gene, which inhibits the binding of certain transcription factors,[532] and the C706 to F706 mutation in a small cell lung carcinoma cell line, which resulted in inability to bind SV40 T antigen or adenovirus E1A protein but retained the capacity to bind with MYC.[533, 534] Additional approaches to testing for presence or absence of the gene involve evaluation for LOH, Southern and Northern blots, and use of RFLP.[535, 536]

Clinicopathology. Among non–small cell lung carcinomas, LOH at the *RB1* locus is seen in approximately 30% of cases,[537–539] but only 15% to 35% of the cases showing a loss of RB1 protein expression.[537, 538, 540, 541] LOH does not consistently correlate with loss of RB1 protein.[537] Mutations among non–small cell lung carcinomas have been detected; however, too few cases have been analyzed to reliably support the findings.[539] Squamous cell carcinoma appears more likely to have LOH at the *RB1* locus than adenocarcinoma.[539] Among the squamous cell carcinomas that have LOH, one third of them had *RB1* gene alteration, as detected by single-stranded conformational polymorphism (SSCP). It also appears that squamous cell carcinomas lose their immunoreactivity to RB1 protein as they become more undifferentiated.[540] No mutations, to date, have been found among the *P107* and *P130* genes in non–small cell lung cancers.

In contrast, small cell carcinomas have frequent changes in the *RB1* locus; 90% of small cell carcinomas show LOH,[542, 543] and aberrant or absent RB1 protein expression is seen in approximately 90% of these cases.[542, 544–546] Homozygous deletions and rearrangements are detected in 13% to 18% of cases.[542, 544, 547] Point mutations, when present, usually occur in the pocket of the gene.[548] Both alleles of the gene are altered in small cell carcinomas, be it by point mutations, deletion, or chromosomal loss.[548] Still, in the majority of the cases studied, the inactivation of the remaining allele is rather unknown.[542, 544, 547, 549]

Among the other members of the neuroendocrine family, loss or altered expression of RB1 protein is more frequently observed in high-grade neuroendocrine lung carcinoma, including large cell neuroendocrine carcinoma as well as small cell carcinoma, than in typical and atypical carcinoids (82% vs. 11%, respectively).[550] All of the small cell carcinomas showed either rearrangement of the gene, point mutation, or low mRNA expression. In comparison, half of the large cell neuroendocrine carcinomas had these alterations.[550] Methylation of the 5′ CpG island was not evident in any of these cases. Among carcinoids in this study, only one case (11%) had low mRNA expression as the sole alteration. Others have found up to 20% of cases of atypical carcinoids to have RB1 protein expression alterations among typical and atypical carcinoids.[545, 551] It therefore appears that RB1 inactivation, although rare, can be seen among the lower-grade neuroendocrine carcinoma group.[550]

In terms of survival, patients with small cell carcinomas in which RB1 protein is not detectable have shorter survival that those who have detectable protein.[552] Interestingly, though, presence or absence of RB1 protein expression in non–small cell carcinoma has a questionable effect on survival.[538]

Finally, patients with familial *RB1* alteration are more prone to acquire small cell carcinoma at an earlier age.[553] Furthermore, relatives of patients with retinoblastoma have a 15-fold increase in acquiring small cell carcinoma of lung.[298]

TP53

Background. The tumor suppressor gene *TP53*, located on 17p13.1, is a 393 amino acid nuclear phosphoprotein that is ubiquitously expressed in cells. The gene was originally thought to be an oncogene[554] because of its ability to perform as a "dominant oncogene" when mutated. What led to its identification was an increased LOH of probes detecting an RFLP site on the short arm of chromosome 17.[543]

TP53 has numerous functions. In general, these include cell cycle arrest through the p21^{WAF1}-cyclin D1-CDK4-RB1 pathway or promotion of apoptosis through the CDKN1A-BAX/BCL2 pathway.[555–558] Therefore, *TP53* acts to suppress genetic instability (see Fig. 8–5).[559]

Delays in the cycle give the cell time to repair DNA damage before it undergoes DNA synthesis or mitosis. Failure in repairing this damage results in propagation of mutations and increased accumulation of genetic damage. The DNA binding transactivation that p53 possesses mediates downstream effector genes. For example, the *GADD45* (growth arrest on DNA damage) gene is induced in response to ionizing radiation but it is dependent on wild-type p53 for its effect.[560] GADD45 binds to PCNA, which is involved in both growth arrest and repair.[561] GADD45 stimulates DNA excision repair, and it inhibits entry in S phase. A second p53-induced gene is CDKN1A,[562] which inhibits CDKs that are required for the G_1/S transition.[563] Therefore, the p53-mediated G_1 checkpoint can be overcome several different ways, beginning with *TP53* mutation, as well as other upstream and downstream alterations. Epigenetic inactivation of p53 through stabilization of p53 protein by viral oncoprotein (SV40, adenovirus E1B), inactivation of p53 by HPV E6 protein leading to ubiquitin degradation, or inactivation by *MDM2* amplification are also seen in some lung cancers.[462, 463, 564]

If DNA damage is irreparable, apoptosis ensues (see Figs. 8–5 and 8–6). Increased levels of p53, as seen in growth arrest caused by DNA damage or cell stress, lead to apoptosis. p53 is also able to suppress transformation by many different oncogenes.[565] The apoptotic response requires the sequence-specific transactivating domain and carboxyl-terminal regulatory domains to be intact.[566] Two proapoptotic genes that p53 transcriptionally activates are *BAX* and *IGFBP3* (IGF-binding protein 3).[567] The homodimer BAX is the main effector of apoptosis, which is executed through the caspase (cysteine-aspartic acid–specific proteinase) pathway. This homodimer is opposed by heterodimerization with BCL2 or other family members of the BCL2 family, including $BclX_L$ and MCL1. BCL2 can block p53-mediated apoptosis, and BCL2 itself is negatively regulated by p53.[568] IGFBP3 blocks IGF1 mitotic signaling through interaction of its tyrosine kinase receptor. Other pathways for apoptosis include HPV E7 binding to RB1, allowing release of E2F1, which induce p53-dependent apoptosis. Cyclin D1 up-regulation and MYC activation likewise induces p53-mediated apoptosis.

Several proteins and sequences can bind with p53 (Tables 8–6 and 8–7). In normal cells, the concentration of p53 protein is kept low because of its short half-life of approximately 20 minutes,[569] maintained through rapid ubiquitin-mediated breakdown. In tumor cells, the level of p53 protein is raised severalfold, principally owing to the extended half-life of the mutant form, which approaches 4 hours.[570]

p53 functions by binding specifically to double-stranded DNA. The amino terminus is responsible for the transactivating function, directing it to promoter sequences located near p53-binding sites in the DNA.[571, 572] This transactivation function is ameliorated in mutated p53 protein, as well as by adenovirus E1B, HPV-16 E6 protein, and SV40 T antigen (see Table 8–6).[573, 574] Binding of MDM2 also inhibits p53 transactivation.[575] MDM2 expression is itself induced by p53, as seen following ultraviolet irradiation,[576] which may be an autoregulatory activity within normal cells.[577] *MDM2* amplification may override this p53 growth control. MDM2 also binds to E2F1 and stimulates E2F1/DP1 transcriptional activity. Therefore, MDM2 can block p53 and cause cell proliferation through stimulation of the S phase factor E2F1/DP1.[458] p53 also regulates gene expression encoding for products that regulate proteolytic degradation of the extracellular matrix. p53 represses transcription of the urokinase-type and tissue-type plasminogen activators through non-DNA binding mechanisms and activates transcription in the plasminogen activator inhibitor type 1 (PAI-1).[578] The p53 protein can also act to promote the reannealing of complementary DNA strands, thereby inhibiting helicase activity[579] and replication, and can suppress transcription from a wide variety of promoters in a non–sequence-specific manner.[580] Wild-type p53 has sequence-specific DNA binding activity that is strongly enhanced by factors on its carboxyl-terminal regulatory domain; oligomerization of p53 is necessary for this activity.[581, 582] However, monomeric wild-type p53 expresses transactivation activity, although it cannot increase expression of CDKN1A; it can, however, block transformation by HPV E7 and RAS.[583] Finally, wild-type p53 also possesses an Mg^{2+}-dependent 3′ to 5′ DNA exonuclease activity.[584]

Mutations within the *TP53* gene generally occur within the central DNA binding domain; approximately 85% of all mutations noted fall into the highly conserved domains of the gene, that is, exons 5 through 8.[299, 585] Hotspot codon mutations include 175, 248, 249, 273, and 282.[585] These hotspot residues lie in the region that either are directly in contact with the DNA (e.g., 248, 273) or stabilize the three-dimensional structure of the protein (e.g., 175, 249).[586] Variation in hotspot distribution occurs from organ to organ.[299] In lung, the hotspot sites include residues 157, 248, 249, and 273. Most of the mutations are of the missense type, but deletions and

TABLE 8–6

Proteins Associating with p53

Cellular	Viral
p53	Adenovirus type 5 E1B 55 kDa
MDM2	SV40 large T antigen
Heat shock protein 70	Epstein-Barr virus nuclear antigen 5
Protein kinase C	Hepatitis B virus X protein
Replication protein A	Cytomegalovirus IE48 protein
ERCC2, 3, and 6 transcription factors	Human papillomavirus E6
E2F1 and DP1	
TAT-binding protein	
TFIIB and TFIID	
Casein kinase C	
WT1	
ATM	

TABLE 8–7

Sequences to Which P53 Binds

TP53 consensus binding site (El-Deiry)
MDM2 intron 1
CDKN1A
GADD45 intron 3
EGFR
BAX
bFGF
TGF-α
Thrombospondin-1
SV40 origin region
FAS/APO-1
Plasminogen activator inhibitor-1
IGF-BP3
HIV type 1

insertions can occur, leading to loss of p53 protein.[587] Some of the mutations abolish the transactivating potential (e.g., residues 141 and 175), whereas other substantially enhance it (e.g., residues 248 and 273).[588]

Immunohistochemistry for p53 protein can be quickly performed with several antibodies targeted against different portions of the p53 protein and, in addition, to either wild-type p53, mutant, or both forms. In an excellent review, Tenaud and associates[589] discussed eight different p53 antibodies and conditions for antigen retrieval. This and other studies support the use of citrate buffer with microwave antigen retrieval for all p53 immunohistochemistry studies. Among the antibodies available, CM1, DO-7, DO-1, Pab1801, BP53.12, and PAb240 antibodies are mentioned most often. Antibodies CM1, DO-7, DO-1, Pab1801, and BP53.12 recognize both wild-type and mutant p53 expression, whereas PAb240 recognizes only mutant protein.

Clinicopathology. As mentioned, wild-type p53 protein is usually quickly degraded, whereas mutant forms have much longer half-lives. This leads to the interesting result that when a tumor stains with antibody to p53, a mutated form of p53 is generally present, in turn suggesting a mutated *TP53* gene. Because of this, and because of the availability of a stain against mutated p53 protein, one may be tempted to perform immunohistochemistry exclusively on a tumor to determine whether the *TP53* gene is mutated. In general, when more than 10% to 20% of tumor cells stain with antibody, the neoplasm will usually show a mutation by DNA analysis.[349, 590] Still, approximately 15% of *TP53* mutations are insertions or deletions, producing altered protein that may not stain, or the *TP53* mutations may yield no protein at all. These cases generate the false-negative results by immunohistochemistry.

Another question is what intensity and distribution of staining is needed for a case to be termed positive? It appears that cases with intense reactivity to p53 antibodies will likely be mutated by sequence analysis[413, 423, 591]; these cases also usually display diffuse immunoreactivity. In contrast, weakly diffuse or focally staining tissues may or may not have mutated *TP53*. Intense staining of scattered, single nuclei in a predominantly negative section usually predicts wild-type p53 by sequence analysis.[423] Another source for error is binding of p53 with MDM2, SV40, HPV E6 proteins, replicating protein A, and HSP 70, which can inactivate wild-type p53, leading to accumulation of p53 in the cell and a "false-positive" staining result (see Table 8–6). Lastly, we postulate that focal or patchy p53 staining can occur when there is overexpression of wild-type p53 to counter other noxious stimuli and to allow the cell time to repair damaged DNA.[423] This may explain why one can see strong and focal immunoreactivity of single cells with probable DNA damage amid abundant normal cells; presumably p53 simply is functioning as a "molecular policeman" in this situation.[592, 593]

Given these caveats to the use of p53 IHC stains, this method remains an excellent quick screen for p53 alterations. Among the many findings in lung cancers, IHC detection of p53 protein overexpression in non–small cell lung carcinomas correlates with the degree of histologic differentiation,[594] lymph node metastasis,[595–597] reduced prognosis in stage I or II tumors,[598] and positive smoking history.[594] Small cell carcinomas, in particular, are frequently immunoreactive.[423, 599, 600] Small cell carcinomas and large cell neuroendocrine carcinomas stain diffusely for p53, whereas atypical carcinoids stain either in a patchy, focal, or negative fashion and carcinoids are negative.[423] Furthermore, the pattern of immunostain in atypical carcinoids may predict recurrence of tumor or aggressive course.[423]

TP53 mutations appear relatively early in the course of lung carcinogenesis. Analysis of preneoplastic lesions of the bronchus reveals a stepwise increase in mutations beginning from mild dysplasia and markedly increasing through carcinoma and invasion.[601–604] An extensive database of *TP53* alterations in lung and other tumors is available through the International Agency for Research on Cancer and the European Bioinformatics Institute (ftp://ftp.ebi.ac.uk/pub/databases/p53/ and http://www.iarc.fr/p53/index.html).[605] In addition, Greenblatt and colleagues,[299] in their landmark study, referenced and correlated the *TP53* mutations found in every organ system, as cited in the literature. Fifty-six percent of 897 lung carcinomas had point mutations in *TP53* exons 5 through 8. Hotspot mutation sites in lung include codons 157, 248, 249, and 273. The lowest mutation rate was found in adenocarcinomas (33%), a higher rate of mutations was found in large cell carcinomas (60%) and squamous cell carcinomas (65%), whereas the highest rate was present in small cell lung carcinomas (70% to 100%). In contrast, the mutation rate for carcinoid and atypical carcinoid tumors is zero,[423, 606] whereas that for large cell neuroendocrine carcinoma is 27%.[423] Classification criteria for the neuroendocrine tumors (which vary from author to author) play a key role in such analyses. Pleomorphic (spindle and giant cell) carcinoma of lung shows a surprisingly low mutation rate of 14%,[413] given the marked pleomorphism and bizarre-appearing giant cells of these tumors.

The most common *TP53* mutation types in lung carcinomas are G→T transversion mutations, encompassing 40% of all lung carcinomas.[299] However, when analyzing lung tumors by tumor type, adenocarcinomas have G→A transition mutations at non-CpG sites in 24% of cases and G→T transversion mutations in 23% of cases. In squamous cell, small cell, and large cell carcinomas, the predominant base alteration type is G→T transversion mutations, representing 45%, 46%, and 54% of mutation types, respectively. In addition, in smokers, the leading mutation type is the G→T transversion (31%), whereas nonsmokers predominantly show G→A transitions at non-CpG sites (56%); smokers have G→A transversion mutations at CpG site in only 16% of cases, and nonsmokers have G→T transversions in 13% of cases. G→A transversion mutations usually result from spontaneous deamination of either cytosine or 5-methylcytosine.[607, 608] G→T transversion mutations usually are the result of DNA-adduct formation of *N*-nitrosamines, benzo[a]pyrene, or other polycyclic aromatic hydrocarbons found in smoke.[609] Additional information regarding base alterations secondary to mutagens can be found in the section on DNA repair mechanisms.

Generally, *TP53* mutation correlates with poor prognosis and usually is a very good indicator for recurrence of disease and survival.[610] However, it is interesting that most lung adenocarcinomas are *TP53* wild type/MDM2 overexpressed; MDM2 functions on both the p53 pathway and RB1 pathway[462, 463]; this is discussed further in the *MDM2* section of this chapter. Conversely, the *TP53* mutational status of small cell carcinomas does not appear to correlate with survival[423, 611]; however, one study found all stage III and IV cases to have mutated *TP53*, whereas stage I and II cases had a 50% mutation rate.[612] Finally, serum antibodies to p53 have been found in 13% to 17% of lung cancer patients.[598, 613] Lung carcinoma patients with antibodies to p53 appear to have a better survival and performance status.

Lung cancer patients in which both *TP53* and *KRAS* genes are wild type do better than those who have only *KRAS* mutation, who in turn do better than those who have *TP53* mutations alone. Those who have both genes mutated fare worst (R. Przygodzki, personal comment). This observation appears to be supported in other organ systems as well.[591]

HPV 6, 11, 16, 18, 31, and 33 are identified in 30% of lung adenocarcinomas.[564] There is an inverse relationship between the finding of HPV and p53 accumulation; however, this association is not clearly present in squamous cell carcinoma. The binding of the HPV E6 protein to p53 inactivates p53 and leads to its degradation. Neither SV40 nor adenovirus has been shown to have a role in lung carcinomas.

Gender and race have an important impact on the type of *TP53* mutations. Guinee and co-workers[451] found G→T transversion mutations were more frequent in women than men (40% vs. 25%). Furthermore, the *TP53* arginine/proline polymorphic allele found in exon 4, codon 72, is more common in whites (0.71) than African Americans (0.50).[363] The allelic frequency for the *TP53* polymorphisms in whites is similar to that found in the Japanese population.[408] However, RFLP studies of lung cancer cases and COPD cases have found no association between these RFLPs and disease status.

Analysis of TP53 alterations generally entails initial p53 IHC staining and screening with subsequent analysis by PCR methodologies. Given that one needs to usually analyze at least exons 4 through 8, or 9, many investigators turn to single-stranded conformational polymorphism (SSCP) as an additional screening tool for mutation analysis.[614] SSCP will also miss mutations; it, therefore, needs to be performed at two different temperatures to be reliable.[615] Ultimately, it seems that the "gold standard" for the time being is sequence analysis of PCR products.

P73, a protein with considerable homology to p53, was mapped to chromosome 1p36.[613] P73 is capable of activating transcription response genes and inducing apoptosis in a manner similar to p53. The possible role(s) of P73 in lung carcinomas still needs to be determined.

APC, *MCC*, and *DCC*

Background. Adenomatous polyposis coli (APC), mutated in colorectal cancer (MCC), and deleted in colorectal carcinoma (DCC) tumor suppressor genes play a major role in colorectal tumorigenesis.[616] The *APC* and *MCC* genes are both located on chromosome 5q21, are therefore closely linked, and are ubiquitously present in cells. APC forms dimers through the leucine zipper region and associates with the E-cadherin binding proteins α- and β-catenin.[617, 618] Catenin/cadherin complexes mediate cell adhesion, signaling, and cytoskeletal anchoring. APC/catenin complexes play a role in cell growth regulation. APC also interacts with DLG, a tumor suppressor and progenitor of the membrane-associated guanylate kinase (MAGUK) family.[619]

Little is known about *MCC*, aside from the fact that essentially no germline mutations exist within *MCC*.[620, 621] Analyses reveal that loss of either *APC* or *MCC* alone is rare.[622]

The *DCC* gene, found on chromosome 18q21, is a member of the immunoglobulin gene family; it codes for a type I transmembrane glycoprotein, displaying fibronectin-like domains. It has homology to neural cell adhesion molecules (NCAMs).[623] Mutations and deletions are generally the rule for this group of genes; investigation for LOH is the usual methodology of choice.[624]

Clinicopathology. Deletions in the *APC* and *MCC* genes (5q) range from 29% to 81% in non–small cell carcinomas.[624–626] These cases have significantly worse survival, as well as increased mediastinal or hilar lymph node involvement.[624] There is no difference in the frequency of deletions between small and non–small cell carcinomas of lung.[625] Of interest, LOH for 5q in small cell carcinoma is more likely to be found in metastasis to lymph node, rather than in the primary malignancy.[625]

In contrast, LOH in *DCC* occurs at a much lower rate (14% of non–small cell carcinomas of lung) and does not correlate with either advanced stage or prognosis.[624]

CDK INHIBITORS

Background. These genes code for CDK inhibitors (see Figs. 8–5 and 8–6).

The 21-kDa CDK inhibitor CDKN1A (*WAF1*, *CIP1*), located on chromosome 6p21, is an important regulator of normal proliferation. CDKN1A expression is induced by wild-type, not mutant, p53 acting through a p53 response element, as well as non-p53 pathways.[562, 563] CDKN1A binds to and inhibits cyclin D/CDK4, E/CDK2, A/CDK2, and CDC2. In normal cells, CDKN1A functions in a complex with a cyclin, a CDK, and proliferating cell nuclear antigen (PCNA, a DNA-polymerase δ subunit). Therefore, CDKN1A blocks cell progression, directly inhibits PCNA-dependent DNA cycle replication (through inhibition of cyclin/CDK), blocks DNA polymerase activation by PCNA, and prevents PCNA/GADD45 interaction (see Fig. 8–5).[563, 627–629] The inhibition of CDK activity by CDKN1A inhibits RB1 protein phosphorylation, and therefore it inhibits E2F activation in late G_1 cell cycle phase; CDKN1A can also suppress E2F transactivating capability in an RB1-independent fashion.[630] CDKN1A may also be induced through other p53-independent pathways, including fibroblast growth factor, PDGF, tPA, IL-6, interferon gamma, TGF-β, and granulocyte colony-stimulating factor.[631–633]

CDKN1B (*KIP1*, *P27*, *ICK*, *PIC2*) is located on chromosome 12p13. CDKN1B activity is up-regulated by TGF-β, and it binds to cyclin D/CDK5 complexes. Rare polymorphisms have been identified among CDKN1B; however, most solid tumors lack them as well as mutations.[634–636]

CDKN1C (*KIP2*, *P57*) is localized to 11p15.5, a site that frequently shows LOH in many sarcomas but is rarely mutated in lung cancers. Paternal imprinting of CDKN1C can, however, occur (see later).

Inhibitors of CDK4 consist of several family members. CDKN2A and CDKN2B are located on chromosome 9p21, CDKN2C is on 1p32, and CDKN2D is on 19p13, all of which are sites that potentially could play a role in development of lung carcinomas. CDKN2A binds to CDK4 and CDK6 in competition with cyclin D to block CDK activity.[637–639] In effect, INK4A may down-regulate CDK4/CDK6 through activation of E2F after inactivation of RB1 protein by phosphorylation.[332] CDKN2A protein thereby blocks the action of CDKs and produces cell cycle arrest.[556] In contrast, loss of CDKN2A and RB1 and overexpression of cyclin D1 will promote cell cycling and may lead to tumorigenesis. The CDKN2A gene has been shown to encode a second protein through alternate splicing of the first exon, thereby producing CDKN2A. CDKN2A is likewise a growth suppressor. Germline inactivation of this gene predisposes to development of cancer in mice. Cell cycle arrest mediated by CDKN2A is through interaction with MDM2, and requires functional p53.[466a, 639b] CDK4B is activated by TGF-β and binds to CDK4 and CDK6, blocking cyclins D1, D2, and D3.[640, 641] Several deletion and point mutations exist in CDKN2B in solid tumors, including lung cancer.[642] Methylation at the 5′ CpG island has also been identified as an alternate mechanism of inactivation.[643, 644]

Clinicopathology. CDKN1A overexpression is correlated with good prognosis in non–small cell carcinomas.[645–647] There usually is no correlation between p53 and CDKN1A IHC staining in these cases, nor is there a correlation with smoking status, *TP53* mutation status, or sex of patient.[645] Both adenocarcinomas and squamous cell carcinomas show IHC staining for CDKN1A in approximately the same percentages, which range from 30% to 57%.[645, 647] Also, the higher the grade of the malignancy, the lower the percentage of tumor cell immunostain for CDKN1A.[645, 646] Takeshima and associates[645] noted heterogeneous staining in adenocarcinomas, characterized by stronger staining of the peripheries of the tumors than in their centers. Intense CDKN1A immunostaining correlates with better survival.[647, 648] Komiya and colleagues[647] ascribes better survival to patients with squamous cell carcinomas that have intense CDKN1A immunostaining; however, this finding was not seen in adenocarcinomas. Small cell carcinoma evaluations for CDKN1A expression rarely show abnormalities. One report noted 19% of small cell lung cancers were positive by immunohistochemistry; 75% of these cases were immunostain negative for p53 and MDM2.

CDKN1B in high-grade non–small cell carcinomas appears to undergo increased degradation, in that the labeling index is much lower among tumor cells in comparison to normal tissues.[650–652] In comparison, small cell lung cancers show intense staining for CDKN1B.[651] Although the number of studies is limited, it appears that there may be a correlation between staining and poor survival.[650, 651] Lastly, Wang and co-workers[653] also concluded that there is a correlation of overexpression of CDKN1B with apoptosis.

As to the CDKN1C (KIP2) gene, because the paternal allele is methylated, maternal allele inactivation might lead to tumorigenesis through augmented cell cycle progression.[654] This is exactly the case found in lung cancers, because 85% of lung cancer cases have selective loss of the maternal allele.[655]

In lung cancers, CDKN2A alterations are mainly restricted to non–small cell lung carcinomas.[656–658] Loss of CDKN2A protein expression occurs in 37% to 67% of non–small cell carcinomas.[659–662] These cases must have intact RB1 expression. It appears that among non–small cell carcinomas, CDKN2A abnormalities are the most common mechanism for inactivation of the RB1/cyclin D1/CDK4/CDKN2A cell cycle control pathway; in small cell lung carcinomas, direct RB1 inactivation appears to be the more likely approach. A link between IHC staining for INK4A and prognosis is still questionable; currently, studies reveal no consistent relationship.[660, 661] Homozygous deletions appear to be the mechanism of alteration; yet the frequency of this finding varies among studies, ranging from 9% to 39%.[639, 642, 658, 663, 664] Methylation of the gene is found in 28% of CDKN2A-negative non–small cell cancers.[644] Mutations in CDKN2A are low in frequency, ranging from 0% to 8%; most are frameshift or nonsense mutations. However, rare missense mutation is also likely.[642, 657, 665–667] Interestingly, of non–small cell carcinomas that are negative by IHC staining for CDKN2A, 48% had deletion of the *INK4A* gene, 33% had methylation of the gene, and 14% had frameshift or missense mutations.[668] It appears, therefore, that many of the cases that are negative for CDKN2A by IHC methods indeed have genetic alterations. Furthermore, the use of HIFN-α and D9S171 microsatellite markers, which immediately flank the CDKN2A locus, have been found to be lost in 23% of informative non–small cell carcinomas.[669] By using the STS markers c5.1 and RN1.1 found in the genes coding for CDKN2A and CDKN2B, respectively, approximately 30% had either a homozygous or hemizygous deletion at c5.1 not at RN1.1.[669] Okamoto and associates[657] found a relatively low rate of mutations/deletions or insertions in the CDKN2A gene sequence; however, these mutations were seen only among the metastatic non–small cell carcinomas. None of the primary non–small cell carcinomas, as well as small cell carcinomas, were affected.

Epigenetic hypermethylation of the 5′ CpG islands is suggested to cause functional down-regulation of CDKN2A in lung cancers lacking mutation of this gene.[644] Finally, there is a C > A polymorphism in codon 31 of CDKN1A, which may be associated with development of lung cancer.[669a]

NF1/NF2

Background. Mutations in the neurofibromatosis-1 *(NF1)* gene are detected in neurofibromatosis type 1. This gene is one of the most common autosomal dominant genes leading to predisposition to cancer seen in humans: It affects about 1 in 2000 people.[670] *NF1* is localized to 17q11.2, and the alternately expressed gene product (type 2) is likewise widely expressed.[671] The protein shows homology to, and plays a role with, GAP protein in down-regulating activated RAS protein[672, 673] (see Fig. 8–3 and *RAS* for further explanation). It has a higher affinity for activated RAS than GAP itself does; however, NF1's specific activity is much lower than that of GAP. Furthermore, mutations, when identified, are usually outside of the GAP domain in *NF1* and they almost exclusively occur in neurofibromas. Loss of function mutation in *NF1* and activating mutations of *RAS* appear to be mutually exclusive.[674]

Neurofibromatosis type 2 *(NF2)* gene is characterized by the development of bilateral vestibular schwannomas. It affects the population at a lower rate than neurofibromatosis type 1, that is, approximately 1 in 30,000 individuals.[675] *NF2* is localized to chromosome 22q12, which is predominantly present in muscle and Schwann cells.[676] The gene product "merlin" (moesin-ezrin-radixin–like protein) shares a 45% amino acid identity with cytoskeleton-associated proteins and is a member of the erythrocyte band 4.1 protein.[677] It appears that merlin may be involved in signaling growth inhibitory pathways.[678]

Clinicopathology. Deletions and inactivating mutations occur in the germline and in neoplasms in NF1 familial-associated tumors.[679, 680] The *NF1* gene is always inherited as a mutant allele, unlike the *RB1* gene. Heterozygosity of *NF1* is found in benign neurofibromas and schwannomas, which suggests that different levels of the encoded protein may result in growth advantage, whereas complete loss of the gene may be involved in progression of the tumor. *NF1* mRNA and protein expression appear to be increased in all grades of astrocytomas through a positive feedback loop by RAS, which is constitutively activated in these tumors.[681] Several sites and types of mutations have been detected, including deletions and frameshift mutations, mainly causing premature termination.[682–686] In comparison, *NF2* functions as a recessive tumor suppressor gene, necessitating its loss for tumor occurrence. Most common mutations among *NF2* cause premature termination and occur at five CGA codons; inframe deletions as well as missense mutations likewise occur.[687, 688]

Koh and co-workers described two different *NF1* transcripts generated by alternate splicing in the region corresponding to the gene's GAP related domain, as evident in small cell lung carcinoma cell lines.[689] Examination of cell cultures for the ratios of the different mRNAs expressed revealed 66% type I mRNA expression, which correlated with a high DOPA-decarboxylase activity, whereas 33% expressed the type II mRNA, which showed lowered NCAM levels.

Tran and colleagues[690] using non–small cell lung tumors, reintroduced a gene named *DAL1* (differentially expressed in adenocarcinoma of the lung), a member of the *NF2* superfamily of genes, into nonexpressing cell lines. *DAL1* was shown to suppress tumor growth. More importantly, significantly reduced expression (> 50%) of *DAL1* was measured in 39 primary non–small cell lung carcinoma tumors as compared with patient-matched normal lung tissue. IHC staining with a polyclonal anti-DAL1 antibody localized the protein to the plasma membrane, particularly at cell-cell contact points, a pattern seen of other members of the protein 4.1 superfamily including ezrin and NF2. The data suggest DAL1 is a novel membrane-associated protein with a potential role in origin and progression of lung cancer. *NF2*, in another study, appears to be mutated in mesothelioma, rather than in lung cancer.[691]

WT1

Background. Deletions and point mutations of the *WT1* gene, located on chromosome 11p13, and of the *WT2* gene on 11p15, are found in patients with Wilms' tumor and in those with Denys-Drash syndrome, which predisposes to Wilms' tumor. The 10-exon gene containing two alternative splicing events can produce four alternative gene products.[692] The protein product is 46 to 49 kDa and is a zinc finger protein with 4 zinc finger motifs that also contains a proline-glutamine–rich region.[693] Given these structures, it has the ability to bind to a specific DNA sequence and is a potent repressor of EGR1-mediated transcription.[694] Usually, the mutation deletion is small, but large deletions of the short arm of chromosome 11 are possible. *WT1* has been associated with desmoplastic small round cell tumor, through the t(11;22)(p13;q12) fusion of *EWS* and *WT1* genes,[695] producing a strong activator of transcription from the IGF-1 receptor promoter.[696] In addition, a number of genes have been identified to contain potential WT1 binding sequences, including *BCL2, IGF2, MYC, TGFB, EGFR*, and ornithine decarboxylase. PDGFA and EGFR are strongly repressed by WT1. Various isoforms of WT1 can interact between each other; germline mutations that give rise to the Denys-Drash syndrome do so by antagonizing transcriptional repression by wild-type WT1. Therefore, like p53, WT1 can exhibit a dominant negative effect.

Clinicopathology. It is known that chromosome 11 is one of many site of deletion in lung carcinomas.[598, 697–703] The deletions in lung cancers are usually located to 11p13 and 11p15, with a bias toward 11p13 deletions.[702, 704] The site 11p13 contains a locus for the catalase gene, the *WT1* gene, and the chain of follicle-stimulating hormone. Seventy-six percent to 95% of non–small cell carcinomas of lung show deletion of the catalase gene,[704, 705] whereas 38% of non–small cell carcinomas have a deletion of the *WT1* gene. No additional alterations in the remaining *WT1* gene have been identified.[704] Furthermore, all non–small cell carcinomas studied noted lack mRNA for the catalase gene. From this, it is possible that the catalase gene may play a major role in progression of non–small cell carcinomas.[705] On the other hand, *HRAS* is also located at 11p15; however, the mutation rates of *HRAS* among non–small cell lung carcinoma are so infrequent as to raise questions about a major role for *HRAS* involvement.[697] Finally, a study involving non–small cell cancer cell lines treated with radon α particles revealed numerous chromosomal aberrations, including changes at 11p15.[698]

VHL

The von Hippel-Lindau gene, located on chromosome 3p25, is associated with hemangioblastomas of the brain, spinal cord, and retina; renal cell carcinoma; and small cell carcinoma.[706] *VHL* alteration in these tumors occurs through mutation (or methylation) of one allele and deletion of the other allele. *VHL* mutation is potentially a candidate in lung carcinogenesis because frequent chromosome 3p deletions are seen in lung cancers.[707–713] When the *VHL* gene was studied by SSCP in a series of cell lines of small cell carcinomas, non–small cell carcinomas of lung, carcinoid tumors, and mesotheliomas, Sekido and colleagues[714] found a point mutation in codon 177 (Gly→Asp). Still, another study found no mutations in 24 non–small cell and 7 small cell carcinomas.[706] Overall, it appears that *VHL* mutations may not play an important role in pulmonary carcinogenesis. Hypermethylation of the normally unmethylated CpG island in the 5′ region of VHL, as seen in renal carcinomas,[715] is not evident in lung carcinomas.

FRA3B/FHIT

Background. One of the most active of the inducible common fragile sites within the human genome is *FRA3B*, which is located within the short arm of chromosome 3.[716] Study of such fragile sites is important because they are induced by agents that alter DNA replication, are involved in sister chromatid exchanges and interchromosomal and intrachromosomal rearrangements, and, as expected, are highly conserved during evolution.[717, 718] Ohta and colleagues identified genomic sequences within the YAC clone 850A6 that overlap the chromosome 3 breakpoint and *FRA3B*, and they characterized the *FHIT* gene within a region that was partially deleted in tumors of the aerodigestive tract, as well as from other sites.[719] HPV 16 may also play a role in this region; an area of frequent breaks within *FRA3B* coincides with a spontaneous HPV 16 integration site.[720]

This fragile histidine triad, or *FHIT*, gene is a candidate tumor suppressor gene that shows deletion alterations in renal, gastrointestinal, and lung tumors.[719] The gene is located on chromosome 3p14.2, a frequent site of deletions of many tumors, including both small cell and non–small cell carcinomas of lung.[420, 536, 543, 721–723] The FHIT protein has a 69% homology to a *Saccharomyces pombe* enzyme, diadenosine 5′,5‴ P1,P4-tetraphosphate asymmetric hydrolase. The *FHIT* locus is composed of 10 exons, with three 5′ untranslated exons centromeric to the renal carcinoma-associated 3p14.2 breakpoint and the remaining exons telomeric to this translocation breakpoint. The open reading frame begins in exon 5 and ends in exon 9. Exon 5 falls with the region of homozygous deletion.

Clinicopathology. Studies show that 76% of lung carcinomas lack *FHIT* alleles when evaluated by sequencing and LOH analyses. Furthermore, 80% of small cell and 40% of non–small cell carcinomas of lung had abnormal mRNA in this study.[721] Deletions of alleles were also found in nontumorous bronchial epithelium, lung, and trachea of cancer patients, but these cells also displayed wild-type FHIT transcripts.[724] Gross deletions were evident in the *FHIT* gene; the most common ones spanned exons 3 to 7, 3 to 9, 4 to 8, and 4 to 9. Exon 8 deletions were suggested as being tumor specific[725]; however, this possibility seems unlikely because there is an absence of wild-type transcripts and mutation patterns of the type seen in "classic" tumor suppressor genes.[724] Insertions of various lengths of DNA, either between or replacing exons, are likewise observed in the altered *FHIT* allele.[719] LOH at three microsatellite markers internal to the *FHIT* gene are typically used; two are located at the fragile region (D3S1300, D3S4103), and one is at the telomeric 3′ region of the gene (D3S1234).

ADDITIONAL RELEVANT TOPICS

BCL2 Family

Background. The *BCL2* (B-cell leukemia/lymphoma-2) gene, located on chromosome 18q21, received its initial and well-deserved fame through analysis of B-cell leukemia and non-Hodgkin's follicular lymphomas.[726, 727]

BCL2 is one of the members of a family of cell death regulators; its expression inhibits apoptosis (see Fig. 8–5, Table 8–8). BCL2 has been localized to the mitochondrial membrane[728] and the nuclear membrane.[729] In B cells, it inhibits depletion of calcium stores in the endoplasmic reticulum, secondary to H_2O_2.[730] Much of this current work has been done on *Caenorhabditis elegans*, and homologues between *C. elegans* and human genes have been found; ced9 is homologous to *BCL2*, whereas ced3 is homologous to IL-1 – converting enzyme (ICE). ICE is a cysteine protease that processes IL-1 during inflammatory responses and is a critical upstream regulator of apoptosis.[731, 732]

BCL2 can be found as a homodimer, or it can heterodimerize with $BCLX_L$, $BCLX_S$, or BAX.[733, 734] BAX (on 14q22-q24) can also heterodimerize with $BCLX_L$, and overexpression of BAX can accelerate apoptosis.

TABLE 8–8

BCL Family Members

Protein	Apoptosis	Interacting Proteins
BCL2	Suppresses	BAX, BAK
$BCLX_L$	Suppresses	BAX, BAK
$BCLX_S$	Promotes	BAX, BAK
BAD	Promotes	BCL2, $BCLX_L$
BAX	Promotes	BCL2, $BCLX_L$, E1B 19 kDa
BAK	Promotes	BCL2, $BCLX_L$, E1B 19 kDa
EBV BHRF1	Suppresses	BCL2 homologue
E1B 19 kDa	Suppresses	BAX, BAK

The competitive dimerization of these gene products ultimately regulates whether promotion or suppression of apoptosis occurs. This hypothesis is supported by a study of p53-deficient mice, in which elevated bcl-2 expression was accompanied with a decreased Bax expression; however, when p53 was introduced ectopically, it down-regulated bcl-2 expression and up-regulated Bax expression.[568] This response may be due to a p53-negative response element present in the 5′ upstream promoter of BCL2.[568] $BCLX_L$ inhibits cell death after growth factor withdrawal.[735, 736] The truncated form of $BCLX_L$ is $BCLX_S$. $BCLX_S$ inhibits the ability of BCL2 or $BCLX_L$ to increase survivability after growth factor withdrawal. BCL2 and $BCLX_L$ prevent p53-induced apoptosis.[737, 738] Radiation can induce increased numbers of mutations among expressors of BCL2 and $BCLX_L$.[739]

Fibroblasts that overexpress both MYC and BCL2 have diminished apoptosis[740, 741]; cells overexpressing MYC alone would normally undergo apoptosis. The RAS pathway, through IL-3, can induce expression of BCL2 and $BCLX_L$, thereby preventing apoptosis[742]; RRAS can also bind with BCL2.[743] The p53-binding protein 53BP2 also interacts with BCL2 to halt G_2/M cell cycle progression.[744] TGF-β and p53 can suppress BCL2; p53 alone is capable of activating BAX.[555, 568, 745] Cells expressing high levels of wild-type p53 show increased levels of BAX and decreased levels of BCL2, which, as previously mentioned, would suggest that p53 may transcriptionally regulate these genes.[568, 745] Increased p53 levels also include activation of IGF-BP3, which is suggested as having a pro-apoptotic effect.

Clinicopathology. The finding of BCL2 protein in non–small cell lung carcinomas by IHC staining may be linked to increased survival.[746–751] Silvestrini and associates[746] investigated 128 adenocarcinoma and 101 squamous cell carcinomas in patients with stage I through stage IIIa disease. They noted that the probability of relapse-free survival at 6 years was greater for patients with BCL2-positive tumors (74%) than for those with BCL2-negative tumors (57%). This was mainly evident for the subgroups of patients with stage IIIa tumors, squamous cell carcinoma, or moderately/poorly differentiated carcinomas. When p53 immunopositivity was taken into account, worse outcome is found among those with BCL2-positive/p53-positive adenocarcinoma and squamous cell carcinoma.[747, 748, 752] This finding was likewise supported in a study of 99 lung carcinomas,[753] which found better survival among BCL2-positive stage I cancer patients than in BCL2-positive/p53-positive cases. Still, several investigations concluded that no correlation exists between BCL2 immunopositivity alone and survival.[754–756] Several of these studies have omitted investigation of BAX alongside BCL2, which may have better correlation to outcome, especially among neuroendocrine lung tumors,[757] as will be discussed later. It appears that either *TP53* mutation or up-regulation of BCL2 expression adequately modify the pro-apoptotic pathway in non–small cell lung carcinomas, and that BCL2-positive tumors are less aggressive.

Among non–small cell carcinomas, detection of BCL2 immunoreactivity is found in 12% to 44% of adenocarcinomas, in 25% to 58% of squamous cell carcinomas, and in 38% to 47% of large cell carcinomas of lung, depending on the IHC staining criteria used.[750, 751, 754] In several studies, squamous cell carcinomas were more likely than adenocarcinomas to be BCL2 positive.[747, 755] Squamous metaplasia and dysplasia appear to be nonreactive. Interestingly, Fontanini and associates noted development of, or death caused by, metastatic disease among patients in which BCL2 protein expression was low.[748]

Small cell carcinomas, on the other hand, have a high percentage of BCL2 immunopositivity, ranging from 69% up to 95% of cases.[756–761] Most reports, aside from rare studies, do find a survival difference between BCL2-positive and BCL2-negative cases.[750, 761] Among high-grade neuroendocrine tumors, including small cell carcinoma and large cell neuroendocrine carcinoma, p53 was immunopositive and mutated in 50% of the cases, whereas overexpression of BCL2 and low expression of BAX was present in 90% of the cases.[757] In contrast, low-grade neuroendocrine tumors, such as carcinoid tumors, were immunonegative and wild type for p53, had rare overexpression of BCL2, and had intense and diffuse overexpression of BAX in 15% of cases. BCL2:BAX ratios in favor of BAX in these tumors are correlated with longer survival.[757] These findings may again support the p53-mediated up-regulation of BCL2.[568]

There is a sparsity of direct gene analysis of the *BCL2* gene family in lung cancer. One notable study finds aberrant hypermethylation of a site within *BCL2* that has been found among non–small cell lung carcinomas, in particular adenocarcinomas, without any known association to *BCL2* expression.[762] Allelic loss at the *BCL2* locus was also seen in 40% of adenocarcinomas in this study. Further study is warranted, especially in light of recent findings suggesting that BCL2 may be converted to BAX-like death effectors by the caspase family of cysteine proteases.

Cyclin-Dependent Kinases and Cyclins

Background. The human cyclin family consists of eight major subtypes, labeled A through H. The cyclins regulating the G_1 phase of the cell cycle include cyclins D1 through D3, C, and E; cyclin A is present during the S and G_2 phase, whereas cyclin B is present during the G_2 phase.[525] Because most of the cancer studies deal with the G_1/S phases of the cell cycle, we limit this overview to the relevant cyclins, in particular the D1 through D3 cyclins.

The CDKs are a family of 12 proteins with extensive homology to CDC2; they are activated by specific association with cyclins, and in the G_1/S phase include CDK2, CDK4, CDK5, and CDK6. Most of the CDKs are present in excess amount within cells; the most abundantly present is CDK4 (on 12q13). The general cascade of activation starts with cyclin D/CDK4 and proceeds as follows: cyclin D/CDK4 → cyclin D/CKD6 → cyclin E/CDK2 → cyclin A/CDK2 → cyclin A/CDC2 → cyclin B → CDC2. Many of the CDKs are activated through binding of CDK-activating kinase (CAK, CDK7), which moves a segment of the CDK molecule outward, thereby exposing its catalytic cleft.[763, 764] Full activation of CDK is generated by phosphorylation of a specific threonine on CDK2 or CDK4 by CAK.[765, 766] Induction of CDK4 is blocked in dominant negative forms of CDK2, but not by CDK6.

The G_1 phase cell cyclins are rate-limiting controllers of G_1 phase progression. The D-cyclins (D1, PRAD1–11q13; D2–12p13; D3–6p21) are able to activate CDK2, CDK4, CDK5, and CDK6. The D-cyclins are important for RB1 protein regulation; cyclin D1/CDK4 in particular, as well as cyclin E/CDK2 and cyclin A/CDK2, phosphorylate RB1 protein and release the E2F/DP1 from RB1 protein.[503, 525] Increased cyclin D1 expression promotes earlier RB1 protein phosphorylation and an accelerated transition through G_1.[501, 502] One needs to stress that functional RB1 protein is required to arrest the cell cycle; therefore, cells whose RB1 protein is made nonfunctional through mutation or virus oncoprotein binding do not need cyclin D1 or CDK4.[767] Furthermore, cyclin D1 is down-regulated in cells with nonfunctional RB1 protein, whereas hypophosphorylated RB1 protein stimulates cyclin D1 expression (see Fig. 8–6).[768] Also, induction of $P21^{WAF1}$ through P53 forces hypophosphorylation of RB1 protein and induction of cyclin D1 synthesis.[769] Inhibition of the cyclin/CDK complexes is mediated through the CDK inhibitors that have already been mentioned, including CDKN1A, CDKN1B, CDKN1C, and CDKN2A. These inhibitors bind to cyclin/CDK complexes. Several molecules of the inhibitor are required to block the kinase activity.[770] Cyclin D1 activity can also be down-regulated by TGF-β (see Fig. 8–6). Furthermore, ubiquitin-mediated degradation of the short-lived cyclins D and E also limits their exposure in the cell cycle.[498, 771] In contrast, the stable cyclins A and B are specifically degraded in mitosis through ubiquitin ligase.[772, 773] Inactivation of the cyclin/CDK complexes also involves the CDC25 phosphatases. In contrast, CDC25, which is activated by the MYC: MAX heterodimer, activates CDKs.[328]

Understandably, there are several possible routes to release G_1 arrest in mutated cells (see Figs. 8–5 and 8–6). They include overexpression of cyclin D[502]; alterations in CDKN2A disabling its inhibitory action on cyclin D/CDK4; alterations in CDKN1A, CDKN1B, and CDKN1C enabling phosphorylation of RB1 protein by cyclin D/CDK4; repressed expression of cyclin D1 by MYC[333]; and mutations in *RB1* itself. Aside from cyclin

D and CDK4 alterations, the other variables are discussed in their appropriate subsections.

The cyclin D group is proto-oncogenic; in fact, cyclin D1 was originally identified as the *PRAD1* or *BCL1* oncogene found in the 11:14 translocation of lymphomas and leukemias.[774] Translocations within the cyclin D1 gene have not yet been found among lung tumors. CDKs have been found to contain point mutations in melanomas but not in gliomas, where overamplification is more likely.[775–777] Overexpression or amplification of cyclin D is likewise the more common pathway found among lung carcinomas. In the end, there are more mechanisms of altering the cyclins/CDK pathway itself then there are alterations among cyclin/CDK.

Clinicopathology. Rare studies investigating cyclin D1 expression in small cell lung carcinomas reveal overexpression in up to 20% of cases.[659, 778, 779] In contrast, non–small cell lung carcinomas show overexpression of cyclin D1 in most of the cases.[780–782] This not too surprising, because loss of RB1 protein function is frequently observed in small cell lung carcinomas; the lack of a negative feedback loop through functional RB1 will result in a decreased cyclin D1 expression.[768, 780] Interestingly though, concomitant overexpression of cyclin D1 and RB1 protein alteration can occur.[778] Overexpression of cyclin D1 is also associated with poorer histologic grade of the tumor and reduced incidence of local relapse. By contrast, cases lacking expression have a ninefold increase in tumor relapse.[783] The overexpression of cyclin D1 is seen regardless of non–small cell tumor subtype,[784] but one study found overexpression significantly to occur more often among adenocarcinomas.[779] Adenocarcinoma patients lacking cyclin D1 overexpression had a significantly shorter overall survival.[779] Also, patients who show overexpression of cyclin D and lack of RB1 protein expression have an increased incidence of local relapse and shorter event-free survival.[785]

Aberrant DNA Methylation

DNA methylation involves the modification of cytosine residues within CpG dinucleotides, which tend to cluster in "islands" at the 5′ end of many genes. These changes are epigenetic; methylation silences the gene expression, whereas unmethylated genes tend to be active. Through methylation, transcription factors are unable to bind to DNA, and the chromatin structure is altered into an inactive form. Methylation also plays an important role in mediating genomic imprinting, which is defined as gamete-specific modifications of DNA rendering different expression of the maternal or paternal alleles, depending on which is modified. Therefore, not only loss of a single allele, but which (imprinted or not) plays an important role in inappropriate gene expression. As an example of this, the loss of insulin-like growth factor 2 (*IGF2*) imprinting on chromosome 11p15 has been found in certain lung cancers.[785a] Furthermore, hypermethylation is a mechanism through which down-regulation of wild-type function of genes, i.e., tumor suppressor genes, may be silenced, effectively making them as "nonfunctional" as if they had undergone deletion or mutation. Hypermethylation appears to be an approach to CDKN2A inactivation,[644] in particular among non–small cell lung carcinomas. This is supported by the greater percentage for lack of CDKN2A protein expression as compared to CDKN2A mutations in non–small cell lung carcinomas. Among small cell lung carcinomas, there is evidence for regional hypermethylation in chromosome 3p, yet greater specific as to which gene(s) are likely candidates are still missing.[785b] Other genes that might also be affected by promotor methylation in both non–small cell and small cell lung carcinomas include *FHIT, RASSF1A, ECAD, HCAD, MGMT GSTP1, DPAK, AVC, CDKN2A,* and *RARB*, and possibly *TP53*.[785c–f]

Telomerase Activation

Vertebrates have specific structures at their chromosome ends named telomeres. They are composed of 5 to 15 kb pairs of hexomeric repeats (TTAGGG). In normal somatic cells, there is progressive loss of these telomeric repeats during normal cell division, which leads ultimately to senescence, thereby governing normal cellular aging and mortality. Germ cells and stem cells compensate for this telomere loss by expressing a telomerase activity that replaces these repeats at the chromosome ends. In this approach, these latter cells are "immortal," whereas the former cells are not.

Up to 80% of non–small cell lung carcinomas and all small cell lung carcinomas express high levels of telomerase activity as detected using the telomere-replication amplification protocol (TRAP).[785g, 785h] Further work is, however, required on the expression profiles of specific catalytic subunits in lung cancer.

Carbohydrate Antigens

The carbohydrate antigens predominantly investigated in lung carcinomas include the blood group antigens, neural cell adhesion molecule (NCAM), and fucosyl-G_{M1} ganglioside.

Loss of ABO blood group antigens, group A in particular, is associated with non–small cell carcinomas and with a poorer prognosis.[786–790] Strong expression of α1,3-fucosyltransferase gene type IV and VIII is correlated with significantly decreased survival among lung cancer patients.[791] Tanaka and colleagues[792] found that the expression of Lewis Y antigen is more likely among better differentiated non–small cell lung cancers and that 5-year survival is significantly better among patients with Le(y) expression, than among those without it (78.2% vs. 59.7%, respectively). Le(y) expression and survival is not significantly different between stage I and II non–small cell carcinomas.[793] On the other hand, expression of Le(x) is significantly correlated with metastatic potential,[794–797] and it can be used as a potential preoperative screening tool.[798] Likewise, pleural carcinomatosis secondary to pulmonary adenocarcinoma is associated with an increase in Le(x) levels when compared with pleural effusions secondary to benign conditions as well as metastatic adenocarcinoma other than from lung origin.[799]

NCAM and fucosyl-G_{M1} ganglioside are frequently expressed in small cell lung carcinomas, whereas α-fucosyl-, α-mannosyl-, and α-glucosyl-specific receptors are more frequently found in non–small cell carcinomas and are usually absent in small cell carcinomas.[800, 801] NCAM is detected in the serum of lung cancer patients; it is more likely to be found among patients with small cell lung cancer.[802–805]

DIAGNOSTIC IMMUNOPATHOLOGY

Immunohistochemistry is not routinely used in the classification of most lung tumors. Still, occasions arise in which antibody studies can be employed to support a diagnosis or aid in subclassification of a tumor. These occasions can be divided into five broad areas: differential diagnosis of anaplastic/pleomorphic carcinomas of lung; differential diagnosis of pulmonary adenocarcinoma metastatic to pleura versus mesothelioma; identification of neuroendocrine neoplasms; differential diagnosis of primary versus metastatic disease; and diagnosis of unusual primary lung tumors. In what follows, we first review IHC staining of the major subtypes of lung cancer so that the reader can become familiar with the surprisingly broad array of antibodies with which these tumors stain. Next, we summarize several uncommon tumors of lung in which IHC staining can play an important adjunctive role in diagnosis. We finish with an evaluation of the use of the antibody technique in the other diagnostically difficult areas just noted.

Immunohistochemical Staining of Major Histologic Subtypes of Lung Cancer

SQUAMOUS CELL CARCINOMA

Squamous cell carcinomas by definition show intercellular bridges and/or foci of keratinization.[806] They stain for both high- and low-molecular-weight keratins.[807–811] Staining for high-molecular-weight keratins (mol. wt. 63,000 daltons) occurs in areas of squamous differentiation; by contrast, it is usually not seen in adenocarcinomas.[812] Involucrin is found in 100% of squamous cell carcinomas but also can be found in up to 21% of other non–small cell carcinomas.[813] Other antigens that are often present in squamous cell carcinomas are epithelial membrane antigen (EMA), carcinoembryonic antigen (CEA), Leu-M1, and human milk fat globule (HMFG-2). Squamous cell carcinomas can also sometimes express S-100 protein, vimentin, neurofilament protein, synaptophysin, and even desmin.

ADENOCARCINOMA

These malignant tumors are characterized histologically by glandular differentiation evident by the presence of acini, tubules, papillae, bronchioloalveolar pattern, or lepidic growth or by a solid pattern of growth with mucin production. They usually express low-molecular-weight and sometimes high-molecular-weight keratins; when high-molecular-weight keratins are expressed, the tumor may have a mixed adenosquamous phenotype. EMA, CEA, HFMG-2, Leu-M1, and B72.3 are also often expressed. Of these, CEA is the most frequently encountered: it is positive in over 90% of cases (personal observations). Differentiation antigens, such as secretory component and surfactant apoprotein, have been reported in 65% and in 33% to 50% of adenocarcinomas, respectively.[814, 815] Linnoila and coworkers[816] reported the peripheral cell differentiation markers, Clara cell 10-kDa protein and surfactant-associated protein A, in approximately 40% of adenocarcinomas and in a smaller percentage of other non–small cell carcinomas; they are only rarely present in adenocarcinomas from extrapulmonary sites. Other antibodies useful to mark primary adenocarcinomas of lung are thyroid transcription factor-1 (TTF-1), cytokeratins 7 and 20, and villin. In particular, adenocarcinomas of lung are generally cytokeratin 7 positive but cytokeratin 20 negative. They are also villin positive. TTF-1 stains adenocarcinomas of lung and thyroid, but it does not generally stain adenocarcinomas from other sites.

BRONCHIOLOALVEOLAR CARCINOMA

These tumors are well-differentiated adenocarcinomas that grow along the walls of preexisting alveoli in the periphery of lung, without evidence of stromal, pleural, or lymphatic/lymph node spread.[806] IHC stains are not necessary for diagnosis, but they are useful for distinguishing these tumors from metastatic adenocarcinomas in lung (see later). Nonmucinous bronchioloalveolar carcinomas often stain for the peripheral cell differentiation markers Clara cell 10-kDa protein, surfactant-associated protein A, cytokeratin 7, and TTF-1.

LARGE CELL CARCINOMA

The World Health Organization defines this tumor as an undifferentiated malignant epithelial tumor that lacks the cytologic features of small cell carcinoma and that fails to show either squamous or glandular differentiation at the light microscopic level.[806] The tumor is therefore a diagnosis of exclusion. These neoplasms show a heterogeneous phenotype by electron microscopy, with areas of squamous (approximately 18%), glandular (34%), adenosquamous (19%), or neuroendocrine differentiation (14%); only 14% are truly undifferentiated.[203] A few mucin droplets can be seen in large cell carcinomas in mucicarmine stains.

Large cell carcinomas express keratin, as demonstrated by a cocktail of keratin monoclonal antibodies or by the broadly specific monoclonal antibody CAM 5.2 (directed against cytokeratins 8 and 18), in 50% to 75% of cases. They express EMA in over 50% of cases and CEA in 50% to 66% of cases. Other less frequently encountered antigens include vimentin, present in less than 50% of cases, and B72.3, present in less than 25% of cases.[203] Neuron-specific enolase (NSE) can be seen in up to two thirds of non–small cell carcinomas.[806] About 20% of the tumors stain with surfactant-associated apoprotein and Clara cell 10-kDa protein.

SMALL CELL CARCINOMA

Small cell carcinoma is a high-grade carcinoma composed of small cells with characteristic scant cytoplasm, finely granular nuclear chromatin, absent or scant nucleoli, ill-defined cell borders, and numerous mitoses. The cells are oval, round, or spindle shaped.[806] They are usually less than the diameter of three resting lymphocytes; still, occasionally, and particularly in open biopsy specimens from lung or metastatic sites, small cell carcinomas can have more ample cytoplasm. These tumors, formerly called intermediate cell type small cell carcinoma, are now termed small cell carcinomas, because they behave in a manner similar to standard small cell carcinomas.[806]

Keratin cocktails containing AE1/AE3 and CAM 5.2 stain a variable but generally high percentage of these tumors, depending on the size of the biopsy specimen. For example, in one study based on paraffin sections, 100% of small cell carcinomas in open lung biopsy specimens were positive for keratins AE1/AE3, whereas 95% of those in transbronchial lung biopsy specimens stained[817] (see Table 8–8). A granular or cytoplasmic dot pattern of immunoreactivity has been seen in some small cell carcinomas of lung (and is classically seen in Merkel cell carcinomas of skin). Two other carcinomatous epitopes, Ber-EP4 and CEA, can also be detected in a majority of the tumors (Table 8–9).

A long list of neuroendocrine antigens have been detected in small cell carcinomas (Table 8–10).[203] The most important general neuroendocrine markers in tissue sections are chromogranin (staining 23% to 78% of tumors),[818, 819] synaptophysin (staining 39% to 74% of tumors),[820, 821] and Leu-7 (staining 22% to 59% of tumors).[820, 821] The results from one study using these stains in paraffin sections of transbronchial and open lung biopsy specimens are shown in Table 8–9. From this, chromogranin appears to be the most sensitive marker, staining approximately 50% of small cell carcinomas in transbronchial biopsy specimens, followed by Leu-7 and synaptophysin.[817] Staining of tumor cells may be patchy, so that the stains have greater sensitivity in larger specimens (e.g., 60% staining for chromogranin in open lung biopsy specimens). NSE, although second in sensitivity to chromogranin, is both too focal and

TABLE 8–9

Results of Immunohistochemical Staining of Transbronchial and Open Lung Biopsies for Small Cell Carcinoma

Marker	Transbroncial Biopsy	Open-Lung Biopsy
Epithelial Markers		
AE1/AE3	100%	100%
Epithelial membrane antigen	100%	95%
Ber-EP4	100%	NA
Carcinoembryonic antigen	95%	55%
Neuroendocrine Markers		
Chromogranin	47%	60%
Leu-7	24%	40%
Synaptophysin	19%	5%
Neuron-specific enolase	33%	60%

Data from Guinee DG Jr, Fishback NF, Koss MN, et al: The spectrum of immunohistochemical staining of small-cell lung carcinoma in specimens from transbronchial and open-lung biopsies. Am J Clin Pathol 1994;102:406–412.

TABLE 8–10

Neuroendocrine Markers Detected in Small Cell Carcinomas of Lung

General
Neuron-specific enolase
Chromogranin
Leu-7
Synaptophysin
[met]enkephalin; leu-enkephalin
S-100 protein
Vimentin

Hormonal Markers
Corticotropin
Alpha–melanocyte-stimulating hormone
Bombesin
Calcitonin
Corticotropin-releasing hormone
Gastrin
Glucagon
Growth hormone–releasing factor
Human chorionic gonadotropin-alpha
Insulin
Pancreatic polypeptide
Serotonin
Somatostatin
Vasoactive intestinal peptide

Other
NCAM

Data from Colby, TV, Koss MN, Travis WD: Tumors of the lower respiratory tract. *In* Rosai J (ed): Atlas of Tumor Pathology, vol 13. Washington, DC, Armed Forces Institute of Pathology, 1995.

too unspecific (being seen in a substantial subset [60%] of non–small cell carcinomas) for use in a diagnostic setting.[822] Overall, staining of one or more markers in the panel was positive in 75% to 80% of biopsy specimens, a frequency similar to the frequency of finding neuroendocrine granules in small cell carcinomas by electron microscopy.[817] These results suggest the important point that the diagnosis of small cell carcinoma is a light microscopic one and that up to 20% of cases can be negative for IHC markers of neuroendocrine differentiation.

Specific hormonal markers may be positive in a small percentage of cases. In the study alluded to earlier, the most sensitive was bombesin, present in about 45% of cases; focal staining for adrenocorticotropic hormone was seen in about 15% of cases.[817]

Immunohistochemical Staining of Miscellaneous Lung Tumors

Certain less frequently encountered tumors show distinctive IHC staining patterns, which may serve as an adjunct to diagnosis.

SALIVARY GLAND TUMORS

Adenoid Cystic Carcinoma. This tumor shows the immunoprofile of myoepithelial tumors, with strong reactivity for CAM 5.2, vimentin, actin, and sometimes S-100 protein. Less certain in adenoid cystic carcinomas primary in the lung is staining for glial fibrillary acidic protein (GFAP), an antigen commonly found in the myoepithelial tumors of salivary glands. A similar pattern of staining is seen in the rare pleomorphic adenomas of the lung: CAM 5.2 stains tubules and glands, whereas the spindle and stellate cells of the myxoid matrix are decorated by antibodies to S-100 protein, actin, vimentin, and GFAP.

Myoepithelioma. This is a very rare pulmonary tumor, somewhat more common in the salivary glands and breast, consisting of islands of proliferated myoepithelial cells, without ductular elements.[823] The tumor cells react to S-100 protein and actin, but not to keratin, features that aid in separating the tumor from spindle cell carcinomas on the one hand and smooth muscle tumors on the other.

NEUROENDOCRINE TUMORS

Carcinoid Tumors. Carcinoid tumors in lung are neuroendocrine tumors of low malignancy that show organoid, trabecular, palisading ribbon, or rosette patterns of growth, and they are composed of cytologically uniform cells. Necrosis is absent, and mitoses are less than 2/10 high-powered fields of viable tumor (2/mm^2). Most, but not all, carcinoid tumors show reactivity to low-molecular-weight keratins. Chromogranin antibodies stain most tumors, followed in frequency by antibodies to synaptophysin and Leu-7. Markers for more specific hormones, such as adrenocorticotropic hormone and growth hormone–releasing hormone, can also be used in specific circumstances when ectopic hormone production is suspected. Atypical carcinoids can show more focal immunoreactivity for chromogranin than typical carcinoids.

Carcinoid tumors, such as paragangliomas, can show reactivity for S-100 protein in sustentacular cells. If the differential diagnosis in a given case is between carcinoid tumor and paraganglioma, then positive staining for keratin supports carcinoid tumor but negative staining does not completely exclude the diagnosis. *A note of caution:* paragangliomas of the lung, as opposed to the mediastinum, are extremely rare; most such neuroendocrine neoplasms in lung are carcinoid tumors.

Large Cell Neuroendocrine Carcinoma. This is a large cell carcinoma of high histologic grade characterized by neuroendocrine morphologic appearance, namely, organoid, trabecular, palisade, or rosette-like growth formation.[203, 806] As opposed to atypical carcinoids, which show mitotic counts of 2/10 high-powered fields of viable tumor (2/mm^2), large cell neuroendocrine carcinomas show mitotic rates greater than 10/10 high-powered fields, and often more than 40/10 high-powered fields.

By definition, these tumors stain for one or more neuroendocrine markers, as shown in Table 8–11.[203, 806] They also express the epithelial markers keratin and CEA. Carcinoid tumors, including atypical carcinoids, which are in the differential diagnosis of large cell neuroendocrine carcinoma, generally show more diffuse and more intense staining of neoplastic cells for chromogranin than do large cell neuroendocrine carcinomas.[806]

Well-Differentiated Fetal Adenocarcinoma. This tumor is one in which the glands composing the neoplasm are primitive or embryonal in appearance, hence the term *fetal adenocarcinoma.*[806, 824] Well-differentiated fetal adenocarcinomas have a distinctive epithelium. They show tubules or complex glands and are composed of glycogen-rich clear columnar cells that lack cilia and that resemble fetal lung tubules, which can be seen between 10 and 16 weeks' gestation. A distinctive feature is the presence of morules at the gland bases in 86% to 100% of cases. Morular cells in most cases show a striking abnormality in the form of optically clear nuclei.

The differential diagnosis is usually clear cell adenocarcinoma of adult type and carcinoid tumor. IHC stains can be helpful in the differential diagnosis, because these fetal-appearing glandular tumors express focal neuroendocrine differentiation. In particular, chromogranin and NSE are general neuroendocrine markers readily demonstrated in most of these tumors, but not in clear cell adenocarcinomas.[824, 825] At the same time, the extent of chromogranin staining is very focal, as opposed to the generally more extensive and intense staining of carcinoids. In particular, chromogranin A and NSE are present in a few glandular epithelial cells and, more abundantly, in morules in 64% to 72% of cases.[824, 826] A number of more specific amine and polypeptide hormones can also be identified in the cytoplasm of glandular epithelial cells and sometimes in the morules. These include calcitonin and gastrin-releasing peptide, bombesin, leucine enkephalin and methionine enkephalin, synaptophysin, somatostatin, and serotonin.[824, 826] Morules also stain with antibody to NCAM. The suggestion has been made that the morules resemble neuroepithelial bodies, based on their histologic appearance and staining for neuroendocrine markers. One other interesting finding is that biotin can be demonstrated in the optically clear nuclei of morules by immunohistochemistry.[826]

TABLE 8–11

Immunohistochemical Staining for Large Cell Neuroendocrine Carcinoma

Antigen	% Cases Staining
Neuron-specific enolase	100
Chromogranin	80
Leu-7	40
Synaptophysin	40
Bombesin	40
Keratin	100
Carcinoembryonic antigen	100

Data from Colby TV, Koss MN, Travis WD: Tumors of the lower respiratory tract. In Rosai J (ed): Atlas of Tumor Pathology, vol 13. Washington, DC, Armed Forces Institute of Pathology, 1995.

TUMORS OR LESIONS OF UNDETERMINED HISTOGENESIS

Sclerosing Hemangioma. This is an unusual benign tumor characterized by bland epithelioid cells that grow within the pulmonary interstitium.[806] The tumor is characterized to a varying extent by papillae, sclerotic areas, solid areas, and hemorrhagic patterns, in which red blood cells are present within alveolar spaces. Xanthoma cells, cholesterol clefts, and hemosiderin can be present. Cuboidal cells overlie the papillary structures, and they appear to be reactive type 2 cells. In most cases, the histologic appearance is distinctive enough to allow a ready diagnosis; in smaller biopsy specimens and when the histology is atypical, IHC stains can be used to support the diagnosis. In particular, the interstitial cells within the papillae and sometimes forming cellular sheets stain for EMA on a regular basis and for other epithelial markers, such as low-molecular-weight keratin, less frequently.[827, 828] A recent supportive finding is the presence of an IHC marker of peripheral epithelial cells of lung, TTF-1, in the nuclei of the proliferating cells.

Benign Clear Cell Tumor. These rare benign tumors, also called "sugar tumors," show cells with clear or eosinophilic cytoplasm containing abundant glycogen.[806] The cells surround thin-walled blood vessels without a muscle coat. The histogenesis of these cells is disputed.

By electron microscopy, the cells contain abundant cytoplasmic glycogen, including lysosomal glycogen.

The differential diagnosis is metastatic renal cell carcinoma. Recently, it has been shown that IHC staining can be of great aid in confirming the histologic impression. Benign clear cell tumors stain diffusely and intensely with antibodies to HMB-45, as well as HMB-50, cathepsin B, and CD34 but do not stain for keratin.[806, 829–831] The cells are also focally reactive to S-100 protein. This immunoprofile is distinctive enough to allow ready separation from renal cell carcinoma and clear cell carcinoma of the lung. Of interest, rare melanosomes can be found by electron microscopy.

Granular Cell Tumor. These rare, generally endobronchial tumors, are histologically similar to their counterparts in other parts of the body. Their IHC profile is supportive of the diagnosis. It includes, most strikingly, staining for S-100 protein, cathepsin B, myelin-associated protein, myelin-basic protein, and NSE.[832]

Pulmonary Langerhans Cell Histiocytosis. This lesion is characterized by a bilateral multinodular, generally peribronchial, and interstitial proliferation of Langerhans cells with ill-defined cell borders, a reniform vesicular nucleus, and a moderate amount of cytoplasm.[806] Generally, these Langerhans cells have numerous admixed eosinophils. In small biopsy specimens or largely sclerosed lesions, IHC studies can be of aid in diagnosis, in that Langerhans cells typically stain for S-100 protein[833] and often express O10 (CD1a) antigen in paraffin sections.[834] Furthermore, one study of bronchoalveolar lavage samples from children with multifocal Langerhans cell showed that CD1a-positive cells were greater than 5% (average, 30%) of the lavage cell population, a frequency significantly greater than in other lung diseases.[835]

Lymphangioleiomyomatosis (LAM). This widespread interstitial lesion in lung in women, generally of child-bearing age, is characterized by immature short spindle cells that resemble smooth muscle.[806] The disease can be a manifestation of tuberous sclerosis in women. The lesion is associated with cystic changes of varying degree in the lung, which can, in turn, cause spontaneous pneumothorax. The lesional cells can be found as small nodules in the walls of the cysts and adjacent to pulmonary venules, leading to postcapillary obstruction and hemorrhage/hemosiderosis.

The characteristic spindle cells are usually easy to diagnose, but, in some cases, distinction from smooth muscle in honeycombing fibrosis may produce difficulties; IHC studies can therefore be of aid in differential diagnosis. Although the spindle cells stain for smooth-muscle actin, the epithelioid cells seen in LAM react with monoclonal antibody to HMB-45, which recognizes a glycoprotein, gp100, and which is the differential diagnostic stain of choice.[836]

Intrapulmonary Fibrous Tumor. These tumors consist of spindle fibroblastic cells that fail to show a specific pattern of growth. Ropy hyalinization is a characteristic feature.[806] The tumor is the intrapulmonary counterpart of localized fibrous tumors of the pleura, and they tend to be subpleural or adjacent to a fissure in location. Malignant fibrous tumors (of pleura) are characterized by increased mitoses (>4 mitoses/10 high-powered fields), necrosis, cellular pleomorphism, and increased size (>10 cm diameter).[806]

These tumors are now known to stain with the antibody CD34, but not with antibody to keratin. By contrast, CD34 does not stain fibrosarcomas, synovial sarcomas, or diffuse malignant sarcomatoid or desmoplastic mesotheliomas. Still, about 60% of hemangiopericytomas stain with CD34.[837, 838]

Immunohistochemistry in Selected Problem Areas of Differential Diagnosis of Lung Tumors

ATYPICAL ADENOMATOUS HYPERPLASIA

Atypical adenomatous hyperplasia refers to a focal lesion that is often 5 mm or less in diameter, in which alveoli or respiratory bronchioles are lined by monotonous cuboidal to low columnar epithelial cells with scant cytoplasm. These cells generally have mild atypia but occasionally they can show more significant atypia.[806] The lesions resemble bronchioloalveolar carcinoma and they often occur in the setting of established bronchioloalveolar carcinoma; however, they are much smaller in size and typically occur as incidental findings. Ultrastructurally, the cells of atypical adenomatous hyperplasia resemble either Clara cells or type 2 pneumocytes.

Although the diagnosis of atypical adenomatous hyperplasia is usually readily made by light microscopy and by knowledge of the small or insignificant size of the lesion radiographically or grossly, IHC study can be of aid in some cases. CEA, p53, and B72.3 are expressed in bronchioloalveolar carcinomas, but their staining is either questionable or absent in atypical adenomatous hyperplasia.[839, 840]

DIFFERENTIAL DIAGNOSIS OF SPINDLE CELL CARCINOMAS OF LUNG

Some lung carcinomas consist purely of spindled neoplastic cells; they have been termed *spindle cell* in the new World Health Organization classification of lung tumors.[806] These neoplasms are rare and are liable to be confused with sarcomas and, in particular, malignant fibrous histiocytoma. For example, Wick and associates[841] have reported three cases of sarcomatoid carcinoma with "inflammatory" features, that is, a tumor with only modest nuclear pleomorphism, limited mitoses, and areas of keloidal type collagen, as well as an admixture of lymphocytes and plasma cells. These tumors invite comparison with inflammatory fibrosarcoma.

In these cases, IHC stains for keratin and other epithelial markers are the keys to the differential diagnosis. They are positive in 75% to 100% of spindle cell or pleomorphic carcinomas; stains for other markers, such as EMA, CEA, or Ber-EP4, are positive in a smaller percentage of these tumors.[842–844] One must be aware that spindle cell carcinomas frequently coexpress vimentin.

Thus, it would seem that a panel of antibodies, including combined high- and low-molecular-weight keratins, CEA, EMA, and Ber-EP4, is useful for demonstrating epithelial differentiation. Unfortunately, lack of immunogenicity, variability of fixation, and differences between IHC laboratories can yield inconclusive results in some cases. Also, although most sarcomas fail to show keratin, or show it weakly, certain spindle cell sarcomas do express it. These sarcomas include leiomyosarcomas (at times), malignant peripheral nerve sheath tumors, and monophasic synovial sarcomas. Also, sarcomas with epithelioid appearances, such as epithelioid sarcomas and epithelioid angiosarcomas, can express keratins. A careful review of the histology is always the first element toward making the correct diagnosis. It is also helpful to keep in mind that carcinomas account for 97.8% of all invasive lung malignancies, whereas sarcomas account for only 0.13%.[203]

DIFFERENTIAL DIAGNOSIS OF DIFFUSE MALIGNANT MESOTHELIOMA

IHC staining is now a key method for establishing the diagnosis of diffuse malignant mesothelioma. There are two facets to its use: in the diagnosis of diffuse malignant fibrous mesothelioma (so-called desmoplastic mesothelioma) and in the diagnosis of diffuse malignant epithelial mesothelioma.

Desmoplastic mesotheliomas can be mistaken for spindle cell sarcomas on the one hand and for reactive fibrosing pleuritis on the other. Desmosplastic mesotheliomas diffusely and reasonably strongly express low-molecular-weight keratin (CAM 5.2), whereas most spindle cell sarcomas either do not express keratin at all or express it only weakly or focally. The only exceptions to this are metastatic leiomyosarcomas and synovial sarcomas, which more diffusely express keratin. Still, the histologic appearance of these tumors is reasonably distinctive. Also, diffuse expression of smooth muscle-specific antibodies in leiomyosarcomas aids in differential diagnosis.

Keratin can also serve to highlight the pattern of the spindle cell proliferation in a mesothelial process, a feature that is important in distinguishing diffuse malignant fibrous mesothelioma from reactive fibrosing pleuritis.[845] In malignant tumors, the keratin stain decorates a disorganized, most often storiform, pattern of spindle cells, as well as cells that are invasive into the subjacent fat or lung. In reactive fibrosing pleuritis, by contrast, the keratin stain shows fascicles of mesothelial cells arranged parallel to the pleural surface. (One must be cautious not to interpret tangential cuts of the pleura, which can show an apparently disorganized pattern.)

A variety of antibodies have been used in distinguishing adenocarcinoma in pleura and diffuse epithelioid mesothelioma, but there is disagreement concerning the sensitivity and specificity of individual antibodies that stain. One issue is the percentage of a given tumor that should stain with an antibody before the result is called "positive." In our view, at least 5% of the relevant cells[846] should show reactivity. In addition, background staining of neutrophils may present a problem in interpretation of stains for polyclonal CEA when the antibody is not adsorbed.

Antibodies to CEA, Leu-M1 (CD15), B72.3, and Ber-EP4 stain 58% to 96%, 61% to 100%, 30% to 84%, and 87% of adenocarcinomas, respectively in a variety of studies[847–852] (Table 8–12). In our experience and in another recent study, polyclonal CEA was the single most sensitive antibody for diagnosing adenocarcinomas, staining from 92% to 97% of cases; this antibody is followed by B72.3 (44% to 90%), Ber-EP4 (56%), and Leu-M1 (50% to 77%).[852, 853] Monoclonal CEA (such as clone T84.66 developed in the Beckman Research Institute at the City of Hope National Medical Center) is more specific but less sensitive. Other monoclonal antibodies may have different results.

Wick and associates[851] have claimed that over 90% of pulmonary adenocarcinomas react with Leu-M1. We and others[852, 853] have found lower frequencies of reaction with antibody to Leu-M1, but it must be admitted that the stain, although less sensitive than CEA, is quite specific; however, rarely there can be false-positive staining of cells containing phagocytosed Leu-M1–positive leukocytes.[850] In addition, the pattern of stains is usually focal and this can be problematic in small biopsy specimens or cytologic preparations.[850]

Ber-EP4 is a sensitive marker for carcinomas from a variety of sites, with 87% of tumors showing diffuse membranous staining of tumor cells.[849, 850] Still, it has poor specificity, with up to 20% to 30% of mesotheliomas showing focal reactivity; therefore, with this antibody, diffuse staining is more meaningful in establishing a diagnosis of adenocarcinoma than focal staining.

TABLE 8–12

Immunohistochemical Stains for the Differential Diagnosis of Diffuse Malignant Epithelioid Mesothelioma and Adenocarcinoma

	Adenocarcinoma	Mesothelioma
Carcinomatous Epitopes		
Carcinoembryonic antigen	+	±
Leu-M1	+	−
B72.3	+	−
Ber-EP4+	±	+
Mesotheliomatous Epitopes		
Calretinin	−	+
CK 5/6	−	+

In general, the highest combined yield of sensitivity and specificity for adenocarcinomas (100% specificity and 88% sensitivity) is reached by having two positive immunostains, particularly those against CEA and B72.3, in a battery of stains including Leu-M1 and Ber-EP4.[852] If these two immunostains are negative, the specificity and sensitivity for mesothelioma is 99% and 91%, respectively.[852]

Two potentially very interesting antigens that may be of use in identifying adenocarcinomas of lung are surfactant protein B (pro-SP-B) precursor and TTF-1. The former is selectively expressed in respiratory epithelium, whereas the latter, a nuclear stain, is found in thyroid cells and in peripheral airway epithelium. In a study of 370 primary lung carcinomas, pro-SP-B stained 57% of adenocarcinomas and 20% of pulmonary large cell carcinomas whereas antibody to TTF-1 stained 76% of adenocarcinomas and 26% of large cell carcinomas. None of the 95 mesotheliomas stained with either of the antibodies, indicating that they may be of use to expand the battery of stains used against carcinomas.[854]

The antibody panels just described are used to identify carcinomatous epitopes. There have been attempts to use other antigens, such as keratins, EMA, vimentin, and actin as differential stains, but these have been generally of questionable effectiveness, at best. Keratin and EMA may produce overlapping patterns of staining between adenocarcinomas and mesotheliomas, making these stains less useful.[850, 855] High-molecular-weight keratins are present in a reasonably large proportion of malignant epithelial mesotheliomas, but adenocarcinomas can occasionally coexpress both high- and low-molecular-weight keratin.[848] EMA stains about 75% of mesotheliomas in a membranous (with or without cytoplasmic) pattern, whereas it stains adenocarcinomas principally in a cytoplasmic pattern, but there can be overlap in the patterns in paraffin-fixed tissues (21% of adenocarcinomas show both patterns). The most interesting keratin stain is cytokeratin 5/6, which is present in diffuse malignant epithelioid mesotheliomas but apparently not in adenocarcinomas[856]; still, it is also present in other types of carcinomas that can involve the pleura, such as squamous cell carcinomas.[855]

It is of interest that epithelioid mesotheliomas express muscle-specific actin, but not smooth muscle actin, whereas adenocarcinomas of lung are generally negative for these immunoreactants. However, these antibodies should not be viewed as differential stains. Malignant mesotheliomas also coexpress both keratin and vimentin in 50% of cases; adenocarcinomas coexpress vimentin in about 10% of cases.

Virtually all investigators agree that it would be of value to have a mesothelioma-directed antibody, and there have been a number of attempts to develop one. A recent candidate is HBME-1.[857, 858] This antibody stains most (85%) epithelioid mesotheliomas (although it does not stain sarcomatoid mesotheliomas), but the antibody also stains 14% to 70% of adenocarcinomas, albeit less conspicuously.[855, 857, 858]

Another candidate antibody is that directed against N-cadherin, which is a cell-to-cell adhesion molecule manifested by mesothelial cells, as opposed to E-cadherin, which is expressed by lung epithelial cells. All histologic subtypes of mesotheliomas express N-cadherin, whereas no adenocarcinomas do, but these IHC stains can only be done on frozen tissues, not formalin-fixed, paraffin-embedded material, nor are they currently available commercially.[859, 860]

Perhaps the antigen that shows the greatest promise as a mesothelioma marker in paraffin sections is calretinin (see Table 8–12). It has been suggested that the combination of calretinin and the carcinomatous marker E-cadherin gives high specificity (91% for mesothelioma; 100% for adenocarcinoma) and sensitivity (100% for mesothelioma; 91% for adenocarcinoma) in the differential diagnosis.[860]

In practice, at the Armed Forces Institute of Pathology, we use antibodies to a combination of carcinomatous epitopes—CEA, Leu-M1, Ber-EP4, and B72.3—and antibodies to the "mesotheliomatous" epitopes calretinin and CK5/6 to attempt to classify epithelioid or biphasic mesotheliomas correctly.

DIFFERENTIAL DIAGNOSIS OF DISTORTED NEUROENDOCRINE NEOPLASMS

IHC stains are of particular use in the differential diagnosis of crushed bronchial biopsy specimens in which distinction of small cell carcinoma or carcinoid tumor from either distorted lymphoid infiltrates or crushed non–small cell carcinoma is important. Antibodies to keratin and Ber-EP4 are most sensitive to establish an epithelial phenotype in the differential diagnosis of small cell carcinoma and lymphoma; EMA and CEA are less sensitive markers in this situation.[817] Rarely (less than 5% of cases), a small cell carcinoma is entirely negative for epithelial markers[817]; on occasion, carcinoids also fail to stain with antibodies to keratin. By contrast, staining for common leukocyte antigen supports crushed lymphocytes. The neuroendocrine battery, when positive, can be of aid in suggesting small cell, but its frequency of staining is at most 75% to 80% and in small biopsy specimens even less.[817]

Carcinoid tumors can be difficult to distinguish from small cell carcinomas in small or crushed tissue fragments. In this differential diagnosis, staining for p53 suggests small cell carcinomas whereas carcinoids lack staining for p53.[423]

DIFFERENTIAL DIAGNOSIS OF PRIMARY VERSUS METASTATIC ADENOCARCINOMA

IHC staining is being systematically explored as a means of distinguishing adenocarcinomas primary in lung from adenocarcinomas metastatic to lung. Antibodies to pulmonary surfactant apoprotein or protein A stain 33% to 65% of lung adenocarcinomas but generally do not stain metastatic tumors in lung.[814, 815] However, these antibodies are not yet commercially available.

An antibody of great interest is TTF-1, which has been mentioned briefly earlier in the setting of the problem of distinguishing adenocarcinoma from mesothelioma. This antibody stains thyroid carcinomas, but it also stains about 95% of pulmonary small cell carcinomas and approximately 75% of non–small cell lung carcinomas, including 75% to 100% of adenocarcinomas and 26% of large cell carcinomas.[854, 861] Because it is so frequently associated with peripheral airway cell neoplasms, TTF-1 has been used to distinguish adenocarcinomas of lung origin from adenocarcinomas from other sites. In one study, two thirds of adenocarcinomas from lung metastatic to brain showed TTF-1 nuclear staining, whereas primary tumors from breast and small numbers of tumors from colon, prostate, kidney, paranasal sinuses, and melanoma were negative.[862] Larger series of these studies are needed to evaluate the sensitivity and specificity of TTF-1 in this setting, but our preliminary experience with the antibody as a differential stain for determining whether adenocarcinomas present in lung are of pulmonary or extrapulmonary (e.g., breast or colon) origin seems hopeful.

Cytokeratin subsets have been advocated as a method of favoring adenocarcinoma or "non–small cell" carcinoma of lung over metastasis.[863] This is of particular importance in the differential diagnosis of primary lung adenocarcinoma and colonic adenocarcinoma. Adenocarcinomas of lung origin express cytokeratin 7 but are generally (but not always) negative for cytokeratin 20. By contrast, adenocarcinomas of colon are usually, although not always, cytokeratin 20 positive and cytokeratin 7 negative (Table 8–13).

TABLE 8–13

Cytokeratin Subsets in Adenocarcinomas of Different Primary Sites

Primary Site	CK7	CK20
Lung	+	−(+)
Colon	−(+)	+(−)
Breast	+	−
Pancreas	+	−/+
Renal cell, clear cell type	−	−
Endometrium	+	−
Ovary (serous)	+	−
Prostate	−	−

+, stain present; −, no staining present.
Unpublished data from E. Torlakovic.

Monoclonal anti-CEA helps identify pulmonary adenocarcinomas and enteric adenocarcinomas, if the pattern of reactivity is also taken into account.[864] Also, the presence of gross cystic disease fluid protein (GCDFP-15), estrogen receptor protein (ERP), or S-100 protein favors a breast primary lesion over a lung primary lesion.[864, 865]

CONCLUSION

Lung carcinomas appear to acquire a variety of mutations of oncogenes, tumor suppressor genes, and other stimulatory/loss of inhibition factors. In addition, tumor susceptibility genes arrange the setting in which all other factors can augment or reduce the likelihood of cancer. The knowledge of which genes can undergo alteration, and at what stage of carcinogenesis they are key, will enable us to better predict tumor aggressiveness, survival, and recurrence. Given the likelihood of gene therapy, we may yet see the day when a genetic profile obtained from frozen or paraffin-embedded tissue will dictate the viral/genetic therapy required for cure. For the time being, the laying down of a molecular pathology and IHC foundation for human ailments will certainly yield more rapid approaches to the diagnostics and prognostics of disease.

Acknowledgments

RMP would like to thank his wife Eva, children Isabela and Roman, parents Matthew and Irena, and dear friends Mike and Alina Orwicz for their never-ending support, love, and help through all times.

REFERENCES

1. Kwiatkowski DJ, Harpole DH Jr, Godleski J, et al: Molecular pathologic substaging in 244 stage I non–small-cell lung cancer patients: Clinical implications. J Clin Oncol 1998;16:2468–2477.
2. Komaki R, Milas L, Ro JY, et al: Prognostic biomarker study in pathologically staged N1 non–small cell lung cancer. Int J Radiat Oncol Biol Phys 1998;40:787–796.
3. Sekido Y, Fong KM, Minna JD: Progress in understanding the molecular pathogenesis of human lung cancer. Biochim Biophys Acta 1998;1378:F21–F59.
4. Graziano SL: Non–small cell lung cancer: Clinical value of new biological predictors. Lung Cancer 1997; 17(Suppl 1):S37–S58.
5. Leslie KO, Colby TV: Pathology of lung cancer. Curr Opin Pulm Med 1997;3:252–256.
6. Strauss GM: Prognostic markers in resectable non-small cell lung cancer. Hematol Oncol Clin North Am 1997;11:409–434.
7. Shackney SE, Shankey TV: Common patterns of genetic evolution in human solid tumors. Cytometry 1997; 29:1–27.

8. Greenblatt MS, Harris CC: Molecular genetics of lung cancer. Cancer Surv 1995;25:293–313.
9. Tsui LC: The cystic fibrosis transmembrane conductance regulator gene. Am J Respir Crit Care Med 1995;151(3 Pt 2):S47–S53.
10. Gazdar AF: Molecular markers for the diagnosis and prognosis of lung cancer. Cancer 1992;69(6 Suppl): 1592–1599.
11. Hasday JD, McCrea KA: Inherited predisposition to lung cancer. Occup Med 1992;7:227–240.
12. Iman DS, Harris CC: Oncogenes and tumor suppressor genes in human lung carcinogenesis. Crit Rev Oncog 1991;2:161–171.
13. Zhong S, Howie AF, Ketterer B, et al: Glutathione S-transferase mu locus: Use of genotyping and phenotyping assays to assess association with lung cancer susceptibility. Carcinogenesis 1991;12:1533–1537.
14. Van Zandwijk N, Van't Veer LJ: The role of prognostic factors and oncogenes in the detection and management of non-small-cell lung cancer. Oncology (Huntington) 1998;12(1 Suppl 2):55–59.
15. Birrer MJ: Translational research and epithelial carcinogenesis: Molecular diagnostic assays now—molecular screening assays soon? J Natl Cancer Inst 1995;87: 1041–1043.
16. Fokstuen S, Bottani A, Medeiros PFV, et al: Laryngeal atresia type III (glottic web) with 22q11.2 microdeletion: Report of three patients. Am J Med Genet 1997;70: 130–133.
17. Stoler JM, Ladoulis M, Holmes LB: Anterior laryngeal webs and 22q11 deletions. Am J Med Genet 1998; 79:152.
18. Strakowski SM, Butler MG, Cheek JW, et al: Familial laryngeal web in three generations with probable autosomal dominant transmission. Dysmorph Clin Genet 1988;2:9–12.
19. Schinzel A: The ulnar-mammary syndrome: An autosomal dominant pleiotropic gene. Clin Genet 1987;32: 160–168.
20. Hall JG, Pallister PD, Clarren SK, et al: Congenital hypothalamic hamartoblastoma, hypopituitarism, imperforate anus, and postaxial polydactyly—a new syndrome? I. Clinical, causal, and pathogenetic considerations. Am J Med Genet 1980;7:47–74.
21. Thomas HM, Todd PJ, Heaf D, Fryer AE: Recurrence of Pallister-Hall syndrome in two sibs. J Med Genet 1994;31:145–147.
22. Holder TM, Cloud DT, Lewis JE, Pilling GB: Esophageal atresia and tracheoesophageal fistula. Pediatrics 1964;35:542–549.
23. Quan L, Smith DW: Vertebral defects, anal atresia, T-E fistula with esophageal atresia, radial and renal dysplasia: A spectrum of associated defects. J Pediatr 1973;82: 104–107.
24. Khoury MJ, Cordero JF, Greenberg F, et al: A population study of the VACTERL association: Evidence for its etiologic heterogeneity. Pediatrics 1983;71: 815–820.
25. Porteous MEM, Cross I, Burn J: VACTERL with hydrocephalus: One end of the Fanconi anemia spectrum of anomalies? Am J Med Genet 1992;43:1032–1034.
26. Sommer A, Harmel R, Zwick D: Multiple congenital anomalies: Fanconi pancytopenia syndrome? Proc Greenwood Genet Center 1989;8:188–190.
27. Froster UG, Wallner SJ, Reusche E, et al: VACTERL with hydrocephalus and branchial arch defects: Prenatal, clinical, and autopsy findings in two brothers. Am J Med Genet 1996;62:169–172.
28. Hendren WH, McKee DM: Lobar emphysema of infancy. J Pediatr Surg 1966;1:24–39.
29. Sloan H: Lobar obstructive emphysema in infancy treated by lobectomy. J Thorac Cardiovasc Surg 1953;26:1–20.
30. Wall MA, Eisenberg JD, Campbell JR: Congenital emphysema in a mother and daughter. Pediatrics 1982; 70:131–133.
31. Rutledge J, Jensen P: Acinar dysplasia: A new form of pulmonary maldevelopment. Hum Pathol 1986;17: 1290–1293.
32. Stocker JT, Madewell JE, Drake RM: Congenital cystic malformation of the lung: Classification and morphologic spectrum. Hum Pathol 1977;8:155–177.
33. Stocker JT: Congenital and developmental diseases. *In* Dail DH, Hammar SP (eds): Pulmonary Pathology. New York, Springer, 1994, pp 174–180.
34. Ciancimino R, Monserrino P: Prenatal diagnosis of pulmonary cystic dysplasia associated with a polymorphic variant of chromosome 19: A clinical case. Minerva Ginecol 1995;47:455–459.
35. Collins FS, Drumm ML, Cole JL, et al: Construction of a general human chromosome jumping library, with application to cystic fibrosis. Science 1987;235: 1046–1049.
36. Rommens JM, Iannuzzi MC, Kerem B, et al: Identification of the cystic fibrosis gene: Chromosome walking and jumping. Science 1989;245:1059–1065.
37. Riordan JR, Rommens JM, Kerem B, et al: Identification of the cystic fibrosis gene: Cloning and characterization of complementary DNA. Science 1989;245: 1066–1073.
38. Kerem B, Rommens JM, Buchanan JA, et al: Identification of the cystic fibrosis gene: Genetic analysis. Science 1989;245:1073–1080.
39. Welsh MJ, Ramsey BW, Accurso, Cutting GR: Cystic fibrosis. *In* Scriver CR, Beaudet AL, Sly WS, Valle D (eds): The Metabolic and Molecular Basis of Inherited Diseases, edn. 8. New York, McGraw-Hill, pp 5121–5188.
40. Iannuzzi MC, Collins FS: Reverse genetics and cystic fibrosis. Am J Respir Cell Mol Biol 1990;2:309–316.
41. Quinton PM: Cystic fibrosis: A disease in electrolyte transport. FASEB J 1990;4:2709–2717.
42. Population variation of common cystic fibrosis mutations. The Cystic Fibrosis Genetic Analysis Consortium. Hum Mutat 1994;4:167–177.
43. Quinton PM: Chloride impermeability in cystic fibrosis. Nature 1983;301:421–422.
44. Knowles M, Gatzy J, Boucher R: Relative ion permeability of normal and cystic fibrosis nasal epithelium. J Clin Invest 1983;71:1410–1417.
45. Widdicombe JH, Welsh MJ, Finkbeiner WE: Cystic fibrosis decreases the apical membrane chloride permeability of monolayers cultured from cells of tracheal

epithelium. Proc Natl Acad Sci USA 1985;82: 6167–6171.
46. Eiberg H, Mohr J, Schmiegelow K, et al: Linkage relationships of paraoxanase (PON) with other markers: Indication of PON–cystic fibrosis synteny. Clin Genet 1985;28:265–271.
47. Tsui LC, Buchwald M, Barker D, et al: Cystic fibrosis locus defined by a genetic linked polymorphic DNA marker. Science 1985;230:1054–1957.
48. Wainwright BJ, Scambler PJ, Schmidtke J, et al: Localization of cystic fibrosis locus to human chromosome 7cen-q22. Nature 1985;318:384–385.
49. White R, Woodward S, Leppert M, et al: A closely linked genetic marker for cystic fibrosis. Nature 1985; 318:382–384.
50. Park M, Gonzatti-Haces M, Dean M, et al: The *met* oncogene: A new member of the tyrosine kinase family and a marker for cystic fibrosis. Cold Spring Harb Symp Quant Biol 1986;51(Pt 2):967–975.
51. Lemna WK, Feldman GL, Kerem B, et al: Mutation analysis for heterozygote detection and the prenatal diagnosis of cystic fibrosis. N Engl J Med 1990;322:291–296.
52. Smith AN, Barth ML, McDowell TL, et al: A regulatory element in intron 1 of the cystic fibrosis transmembrane conductance regulator gene. J Biol Chem 1996;271: 9947–9954.
53. Deuchars KL, Ling V: P-glycoprotein and multidrug resistance in cancer chemotherapy. Semin Oncol 1989; 16:156–165.
54. Anderson MP, Gregory RJ, Thompson S, et al: Demonstration that CFTR is a chloride channel by alteration of its anion selectivity. Science 1991;253:202–205.
55. Rich DP, Gregory RJ, Anderson MP, et al: Effect of deleting the R domain on CFTR-generated chloride channels. Science 1991;253:205–207.
56. Pier GB, Grout M, Zaidi TS, et al: Role of mutant CFTR in hypersusceptibility of cystic fibrosis patients to lung infection. Science 1996;271:64–67.
57. Pier GB, Grout M, Zaidi T, et al: *Salmonella typhi* uses CFTR to enter intestinal epithelial cells. Nature 1998; 393:79–82.
58. Rodman DM, Zamudio S: The cystic fibrosis heterozygote--advantage in surviving cholera? Med Hypotheses 1991;36:253–258.
59. Baxter PS, Goldhill J, Hardcastle J, et al: Accounting for cystic fibrosis. Nature 1988;335:211.
60. Romeo G, Devoto M, Galietta LJ: Why is the cystic fibrosis gene so frequent? Hum Genet 1989;84:1–5.
61. Serre JL, Simon-Bouy B, Mornet E, et al: Studies of RFLP closely linked to the cystic fibrosis locus throughout Europe lead to new considerations in populations genetics. Hum Genet 1990;84:449–454.
62. Dawson DB, Cummins LA, Schaid DJ, et al: Carrier identification of cystic fibrosis by recombinant DNA techniques. Mayo Clin Proc 1989;64:325–334.
63. Gradient of distribution in Europe of the major CF mutation and of its associated haplotype. European Working Group of CF Genetics. Hum Genet 1990;85: 436–445.
64. Cutting GR, Kasch LM, Rosensein BJ, et al: A cluster of cystic fibrosis mutations in the first nucleotide-binding fold of the cystic fibrosis conductance regulator protein. Nature 1990;346:366–369.
65. Estivill X, Chillon M, Casals T, et al: Delta F508 gene deletion in cystic fibrosis in southern Europe. Lancet 1989;2:1404.
66. Kerem B, Buchanan JA, Durie P, et al: DNA marker haplotype association with pancreatic sufficiency in cystic fibrosis. Am J Hum Genet 1989;44:827–834.
67. Kerem E, Corey M, Kerem B, et al: The relation between genotype and phenotype in cystic fibrosis-analysis of the most common mutation (delta-F508). N Engl J Med 1990;323:1517–1522.
68. Santis G, Osborne L, Knight RA, Hodson ME: Linked marker haplotypes and the delta F508 mutation in adults with mild pulmonary disease and cystic fibrosis. Lancet 1990;335:1426–1429.
69. Sheppard DN, Rich DP, Ostedgaard LS, et al: Mutations in *CFTR* associated with mild-disease-form Cl- channels with altered pore properties. Nature 1993; 362:160–164.
70. Fulmer SB, Schwiebert EM, Morales MM, et al: Two cystic fibrosis transmembrane conductance regulator mutations have different effects on both pulmonary phenotype and regulation of outwardly rectified chloride currents. Proc Natl Acad Sci USA 1995;92: 6832–6836.
71. Cutting GR, Kasch LM, Rosenstein BJ, et al: Two patients with cystic fibrosis, nonsense mutations in each cystic fibrosis gene, and mild pulmonary disease. N Engl J Med 1990;323:1685–1689.
72. Ivaschenko TE, White MB, Dean M, Baranov CS: A deletion of two nucleotides in exon 10 of the *CFTR* gene in a Soviet family with cystic fibrosis causing early infant death. Genomics 1991;10:298–299.
73. Gan KH, Veeze HJ, van den Ouweland AM, et al: A cystic fibrosis mutation associated with mild lung disease. N Engl J Med 1995;333:95–99.
74. Savov A, Angelicheva D, Balassopoulou A, et al: Double mutant alleles: Are they rare? Hum Mol Genet 1995;4: 1169–1171.
75. Highsmith WE Jr, Burch LH, Zhou Z, et al: A novel mutation in the cystic fibrosis gene in patients with pulmonary disease but normal sweat chloride concentrations. N Engl J Med 1994;331:974–980.
76. Macek M Jr, Mackova A, Hamosh A, et al: Identification of common cystic fibrosis mutations in African-Americans with cystic fibrosis increases the detection rate to 75%. Am J Hum Genet 1997;60:1122–1127.
77. Dork T, El-Harith EH, Stuhrmann M, et al: Evidence for a common ethnic origin of cystic fibrosis mutation 3120 + 1G→A in diverse populations [letter]. Am J Hum Genet 1998;63:656–662.
78. El-Harith E-HA, Stuhrmann M, Dork T, et al: PCR-based analysis of cystic fibrosis mutations specific for Saudi patients. Saudi Med J 1998;19:148–152.
79. Kerem E, Kalman YM, Yahav Y, et al: Highly variable incidence of cystic fibrosis and different mutation distribution among different Jewish ethnic groups in Israel. Hum Genet 1995;96:193–197.
80. Casals T, Ramos MD, Gimenez J, et al: High heterogeneity for cystic fibrosis in Spanish families: 75 mutations

account for 90% of chromosomes. Hum Genet 1997; 101:365–370.

81. Hammond KB, Abman SH, Sokol RJ, Accurso FJ: Efficacy of statewide neonatal screening for cystic fibrosis by assay of trypsinogen concentrations [see comments]. N Engl J Med 1991;325:769–774.
82. Ferec C, Verlingue C, Parent P, et al: Neonatal screening for cystic fibrosis: Result of a pilot study using both immunoreactive trypsinogen and cystic fibrosis gene mutation analyses. Hum Genet 1995;96:542–548.
83. Rommens J, Kerem BS, Greer W, et al: Rapid nonradioactive detection of the major cystic fibrosis mutation. Am J Hum Genet 1990;46:395–396.
84. Barany F: Genetic disease detection and DNA amplification using cloned thermostable ligase. Proc Natl Acad Sci USA 1991;88:189–193.
85. Martinelli RA, Arruda JC, Dwivedi P: Chemiluminescent hybridization-ligation assays for delta F508 and delta I507 cystic fibrosis mutations. Clin Chem 1996;42:14–18.
86. Cuppens H, Marynen P, De Boeck C, Cassiman JJ: Detection of 98.5% of the mutations in 200 Belgian cystic fibrosis alleles by reverse dot-blot and sequencing of the complete coding region and exon/intron junctions of the *CFTR* gene. Genomics 1993;18:693–697.
87. Hajra A, Sorenson RC, La Du BN: Detection of human DNA mutations with nonradioactive, allele-specific oligonucleotide probes. Pharmacogenetics 1992;2: 78–88.
88. Rady M, D'Alcamo E, Seia M, et al: Simultaneous detection of fourteen Italian cystic fibrosis mutations in seven exons by reverse dot-blot analysis. Mol Cell Probes 1995;9:357–360.
89. Kawasaki ES, Chehab FF: Analysis of gene sequences by hybridization of PCR-amplified DNA to covalently bound oligonucleotide probes: The reverse dot-blot method. Methods Mol Biol 1994;28:225–236.
90. Grody WW, Cutting GR, Klinger KW, et al: Laboratory Standards and guidelines for population-based cystic fibrosis carrier screening. Genet Med 2001; 3:149–154.
91. Highsmith WE Jr, Friedman KJ: The molecular pathology of cystic fibrosis: A clinical laboratory perspective. *In* Farkus D (ed): Molecular Biology and Pathology: A Guidebook for Quality Control. New York, Academic, 1993.
92. Highsmith WE Jr: The molecular pathology of cystic fibrosis. *In* Heim R, Silverman L (eds): Diagnosing Human Disease in the Clinical Laboratory. Durham, NC, Carolina Academic, 1994.
93. Wall J, Cai S, Chehab FF: A 31-mutation assay for cystic fibrosis testing in the clinical molecular diagnostics laboratory. Hum Mutat 1995;5:333–338.
94. Chehab FF, Wall J: Detection of multiple cystic fibrosis mutations by reverse dot blot hydridization: A technology for carrier screening. Hum Genet 1992;89:163–168.
95. Boushey HA, Nichols J: Asthma mortality. West J Med 1987;147:314–320.
96. Dolovich J, Hargreave F: The asthma syndrome: Inciters, inducers, and host characteristics. Thorax 1981;36: 641–643.
97. Vercelli D, Jabara HH, Arai K, Geha RS: Induction of human IgE synthesis requires interleukin 4 and T/B cell interactions involving the T cell receptor/CD3 complex and MHC class II antigens. J Exp Med 1989;169: 1295–1307.
98. Eiberg H, Lind P, Mohr J, Nielsen LS: Linkage relationship between the human immunoglobulin-E polymorphism and marker system [abstract]. Cytogenet Cell Genet 1985;40:622.
99. Cookson WOCM, Sharp PA, Faux JA, Hopkin JM: A gene for atopy (allergic asthma and rhinitis) located on 11q12–13 [abstract]. Cytogenet Cell Genet 1989;51: 979.
100. Cympany P, Welsh K, MacCochrane G, et al: Genetic analysis using DNA polymorphism of the linkage between chromosome 11q13 and atopy and bronchial hyperresponsiveness to methacholine. J Allergy Clin Immun 1992;89:619–628.
101. van Herwerden L, Harrap SB, Wong ZY, et al: Linkage of high-affinity IgE receptor gene with bronchial hyperreactivity, even in absence of atopy [see comments]. Lancet 1995;346:1262–1265.
102. De Sanctis GT, Merchant M, Beier DR, et al: Quantitative locus analysis of airway hyperresponsiveness in A/J and C57BL/6J mice. Nat Genet 1995;11: 150–154.
103. Postma DS, Bleeker ER, Amelung PJ, et al: Genetic susceptibilty to asthma: Bronchial hyperresponsiveness coinherited with a major gene for atopy. N Engl J Med 1995;333:894–900.
104. Hasday JD, McCrea KA, Meltzer SS, Bleeker ER: Dysregulation of airway cytokine expression in chronic obstructive pulmonary disease and asthma. Am J Respir Crit Care Med 1994;150(5 pt 2):S54–S58.
105. Gosset P, Tillie-Leblond I, Janin A, et al: Expression of E-selectin, ICAM-1 and VCAM-1 on bronchial biopsies from allergic and non-allergic asthmatic patients. Int Arch Allergy Immunol 1995;106:69–77.
106. Ohkawara Y, Yamauchi K, Maruyama N, et al: In situ expression of the cell adhesion molecules in bronchial tissues from asthmatics with air flow limitation: In vivo evidence of VCAM-1/VLA-4 interaction in selective eosinophil infiltration. Am J Respir Cell Mol Biol 1995;12:4–12.
107. Aubert JD, Dalal BI, Bai TR, et al: Transforming growth factor beta 1 gene expression in human airways. Thorax 1994;49:225–232.
108. Hamid Q, Springall DR, Riveros-Moreno V, et al: Induction of nitric oxide synthase in asthma. Lancet 1993;342:1510–1513.
109. Lilly CM, Bai TR, Shore SA, et al: Neuropeptide content of lungs from asthmatic and nonasthmatic patients. Am J Respir Crit Care Med 1995;151(2 pt 1): 548–553.
110. Bottazzo GF, Lendrum R: Separate autoantibodies to human pancreatic glucagon and somatostatin cells. Lancet 1976;11:873–876.
111. Liggett SB, Levi R, Metzger H: G-protein coupled receptors, nitric oxide, and the IgE receptor in asthma. Am J Respir Crit Care Med 1995;152:394–402.
112. Hall IP, Wheatley A, Wilding P, Liggett SB: Association of Glu 27 beta 2-adrenoceptor polymorphism with lower airway reactivity in asthmatic subjects. Lancet 1995;345: 1213–1214.

113. Turki J, Pak J, Green SA, et al: Genetic polymorphisms of the beta 2-adrenergic receptor in nocturnal and non-nocturnal asthma: Evidence that Gly16 correlates with the nocturnal phenotype. J Clin Invest 1995;95:1635–1641.
114. Laing IA, Goldblatt J, Eber E, et al: A polymorphism of the *CC16* gene is associated with an increased risk of asthma. J Med Genet 1998;35:463–467.
115. A genome-wide search for asthma susceptibility loci in ethnically diverse populations. The Collaborative Study on the Genetics of Asthma (CSGA). Nat Genet 1997; 15:389–392.
116. Ober C, Cox NJ, Abney M, et al: Genome-wide search for asthma susceptibility loci in a founder population. The Collaborative Study on the Genetics of Asthma. Hum Mol Genet 1998;7:1393–1398.
117. Holgate ST: Asthma genetics: Waiting to exhale. Nature Genet 1997;15:227–229.
118. Schroeder SA, Gaughan DM, Swift M: Protection against bronchial asthma by CFTR delta F508 mutation: A heterozygote advantage in cystic fibrosis. Nat Med 1995;1:703–705.
119. Lin CQ, Bissell MJ: Multi-faceted regulation of cell differentiation by extracellular matrix. FASEB J 1993;7:737–743.
120. Venstrom KA, Reichardt LF: Extracellular matrix 2: Role of extracellular matrix molecules and their receptors in the nervous system. FASEB J 1993;7: 996–1003.
121. Har-El R, Tanzer ML: Extracellular matrix 3: Evolution of the extracellular matrix in invertebrates. FASEB J 1993;7:1115–1123.
122. Gay S, Miller EJ: What is collagen, what is not? Ultrastruct Pathol 1983;4:365–377.
123. Rooney SA, Young SL, Mendelson CR: Molecular and cellular processing of lung surfactant. FASEB J 1994;8:957–967.
124. Hawgood S: Pulmonary surfactant apoproteins: A review of protein and genomic structure. Am J Physiol 1989;257:L13–L22.
125. Rust K, Grosso L, Zhang V, et al: Human surfactant protein D: SP-D contains a C-type lectin carbohydrate recognition domain. Arch Biochem Biophys 1991;290: 116–126.
126. van der Rest M, Garrone R: Collagen family of proteins. FASEB J 1991;5:2814–2823.
127. Kielty CM, Hopkinson I, Grant ME: The collagen family: Structure, assembly and organisation. *In* Royce PM, Steinman B (eds): Connective Tissue and Its Heritable Disorders. New York, Wiley-Liss, 1993, pp 103–147.
128. Miller EJ, Gay S: The collagens: An overview. *In* Cunningham LW, Frederiksen DW (eds): Methods in Enzymology. New York, Academic, 1987, pp 3–41.
129. Kirk JME, Heard BE, Kerr I, et al: Quantitation of types I and III collagen in biopsy lung samples from patients with cryptogenic fibrosing alveolitis. Collagen Relat Res 1984;4:169–182.
130. Matrisian LM: The matrix-degrading metalloproteinases. BioEssays 1992;14:455–463.
131. Bolon I, Gouyer V, Devouassoux M, et al: Expression of c-ets-1, collagenase 1, and urokinase-type plasminogen activator genes in lung carcinomas. Am J Pathol 1995;147:1298–1310.
132. Pappot H, Hoyer-Hansen G, Ronne E, et al: Elevated plasma levels of urokinase plasminogen activator receptor in non-small cell lung cancer patients. Eur J Cancer 1997;33:867–872.
133. Pedersen H, Brunner N, Francis D, et al: Prognostic impact of urokinase, urokinase receptor, and type 1 plasminogen activator inhibitor in squamous and large cell lung cancer tissue. Cancer Res 1994;54: 4671–4675.
134. Pedersen H, Grondahl-Hansen J, Francis D, et al: Urokinase and plasminogen activator inhibitor type 1 in pulmonary adenocarcinoma. Cancer Res 1994; 54:120–123.
135. Markus G, Takita H, Camiolo SM, et al: Content and characterization of plasminogen activators in human lung tumors and normal lung tissue. Cancer Res 1980; 40:841–848.
136. Nagayama M, Sato A, Hayakawa H, et al: Plasminogen activators and their inhibitors in non–small cell lung cancer: Low content of type 2 plasminogen activator inhibitor associated with tumor dissemination. Cancer 1994;73:1398–1405.
137. Pavey SJ, Marsh NA, Ray MJ, et al: Changes in plasminogen activator inhibitor-1 levels in non–small cell lung cancer. Boll Soc Ital Biol Sper 1996;72: 331–340.
138. Sepper R, Konttinen YT, Buo L, et al: Potentiative effects of neutral proteinases in an inflamed lung: Relationship of neutrophil procollagenase (proMMP-8) to plasmin, cathepsin G and tryptase in bronchiectasis in vivo. Eur Respir J 1997;10:2788–2793.
139. Sato H, Takino T, Okada Y, et al: A matrix metalloproteinase expressed on the surface of invasive tumour cells. Nature 1994;370:61–65.
140. Bolon I, Devouassoux M, Robert C, et al: Expression of urokinase-type plasminogen activator, stromelysin 1, stromelysin 3, and matrilysin genes in lung carcinomas. Am J Pathol 1997;150:1619–1629.
141. Urbanski SJ, Edwards DR, Maitland A, et al: Expression of metalloproteinases and their inhibitors in primary pulmonary carcinomas. Br J Cancer 1992;66: 1188–1194.
142. Muller D, Breathnach R, Engelmann A, et al: Expression of collagenase-related metalloproteinase genes in human lung or head and neck tumours. Int J Cancer 1991;48: 550–556.
143. Polette M, Nawrocki B, Gilles C, et al: MT-MMP expression and localisation in human lung and breast cancers. Virchows Arch 1996;428:29–35.
144. Anderson IC, Sugarbaker DJ, Ganju RK, et al: Stromelysin-3 is overexpressed by stromal elements in primary non–small cell lung cancers and regulated by retinoic acid in pulmonary fibroblasts. Cancer Res 1995;55: 4120–4126.
145. Stetler-Stevenson WG, Krutzsch HC, Liotta LA: Tissue inhibitor of metalloproteinase (TIMP-2): A new member of the metalloproteinase inhibitor family. J Biol Chem 1989;264:17374–17378.
146. Mays PK, McAnulty RJ, Laurent GJ: Age-related changes in lung collagen metabolism: A role for degra-

dation in regulating lung collagen production. Am Rev Respir Dis 1989;140:410–416.

147. Ogata Y, Itoh Y, Nagase H: Steps involved in activation of the pro-matrix metalloproteinase 9 (progelatinase B)-tissue inhibitor of metalloproteinases-1 complex by 4-aminophenylmercuric acetate and proteinases. J Biol Chem 1995;270:18506–18511.

148. Grignon DJ, Sakr W, Toth M, et al: High levels of tissue inhibitor of metalloproteinase-2 (TIMP-2) expression are associated with poor outcome in invasive bladder cancer. Cancer Res 1996;56:1654–1659.

149. Zeng ZS, Cohen AM, Zhang ZF, et al: Elevated tissue inhibitor of metalloproteinase 1 RNA in colorectal cancer stroma correlates with lymph node and distant metastases. Clin Cancer Res 1995;1:899–906.

150. Visscher DW, Hoyhtya M, Ottosen SK, et al: Enhanced expression of tissue inhibitor of metalloproteinase-2 (TIMP-2) in the stroma of breast carcinomas correlates with tumor recurrence. Int J Cancer 1994;59:339–344.

151. Moses MA, Langer R: A metalloproteinase inhibitor as an inhibitor of neovascularization. J Cell Biochem 1991;47:230–235.

152. Murphy AN, Unsworth EJ, Stetler-Stevenson WG: Tissue inhibitor of metalloproteinases-2 inhibits bFGF-induced human microvascular endothelial cell proliferation. J Cell Physiol 1993;157:351–358.

153. Corcoran ML, Stetler-Stevenson WG: Tissue inhibitor of metalloproteinase-2 stimulates fibroblast proliferation via a cAMP-dependent mechanism. J Biol Chem 1995;270:13453–13459.

154. Wu CH, Walton CM, Wu GY: Propeptide-mediated regulation of procollagen synthesis in IMR-90 human lung fibroblast cell cultures. J Biol Chem 1991; 266–267.

155. Katayama K, Seyer JM, Raghow R, Kang AH: Regulation of extracellular matrix production by chemically synthesized subfragments of type I collagen carboxy peptide. Biochemistry 1991;266:2983–2987.

156. Wu CH, Donovan CB, Wu GY: Evidence for pretranslational regulation of collagen synthesis by procollagen peptides. J Biol Chem 1986;261: 10482–10484.

157. Aycock RS, Raghow R, Stricklin GP, et al: Post-transcriptional inhibition of collagen and fibronectin synthesis by a synthetic homolog of a portion of the carboxyl-terminal propeptide of human type I collagen. J Biol Chem 1986;261:14355–14360.

158. Goldstein RH, Fine A, Farnsworth LJ, et al: Phorbol ester-induced inhibition of collagen accumulation by human lung fibroblasts. J Biol Chem 1990;265: 13623–13628.

159. Elias JA, Gustilo K, Baeder W, Freundlich B: Synergistic stimulation of fibroblast prostaglandin production by recombinant interleukin-1 and tumor necrosis factor. J Immunol 1987;138:3812–3816.

160. Golstein RH, Poliks CF, Pilch PF, et al: Stimulation of collagen formation by insulin and insulin-growth factor I in cultures of human lung fibroblasts. Endocrinology 1989;124:964–970.

161. Pardes JB, Takagi H, Martin TA, et al: Decreased levels of alpha 1(I) procollagen mRNA in dermal fibroblasts grown on fibrin gels and in response to fibrinopeptide B. J Cell Physiol 1995;162:9–14.

162. Matrisian LM, Hogan BLM: Growth factor–regulated proteases and extracellular matrix remodeling during mammalian development. Curr Top Dev Biol 1990; 24:219–259.

163. Edwards DR, Murphy G, Reynolds JJ, et al: Transforming growth factor beta modulates the expression of collagenase and metalloproteinase inhibitor. EMBO J 1987;6:1899–1904.

164. Raghow R, Postlethwaite AE, Keski-Oja J, et al: Transforming growth factor beta increases steady-state levels of type I procollagen and fibronectin messenger RNAs post-transcriptionally in cultured human dermal fibroblasts. J Clin Invest 1987;79:1285–1288.

165. Cockayne D, Sterling KM, Shull S, et al: Glucocorticoids decrease the synthesis of type I procollagen mRNAs: Biochemistry 1986;25:3202–3209.

166. Tan EM, Dodge GR, Sorger T, et al: Modulation of extracellular matrix gene expression by heparin and endothelial cell growth factor in human smooth muscle cells. Lab Invest 1991;64:474–482.

167. Clark JG, Dedon TF, Wayner EA, Carter WG: Effects of interferon-gamma on expression of cell surface receptors for collagen and deposition of newly synthesized collagen by cultured human lung fibroblasts. J Clin Invest 1989;83:1505–1511.

168. Sage H, Gray WR: Studies on the evolution of elastin: I. Phylogenetic distribution. Comp Biochem Physiol 1979;64B:313–327.

169. Fazio MJ, Olsen DR, Kauh EA, et al: Cloning of full-length elastin cDNAs from a human skin fibroblast recombinant cDNA library: Further elucidation of alternative splicing utilizing exon-specific oligonucleotides. J Invest Dermatol 1988;91:458–464.

170. Campagnone R, Regan J, Rich CB, et al: Pulmonary fibroblasts: A model system for studying elastin synthesis. Lab Invest 1987;56:224–230.

171. Noguchi A, Reddy R, Kursar JD, et al: Smooth muscle isoactin and elastin in fetal bovine lung. Exp Lung Res 1989;15:537–552.

172. Mecham RP, Madaras J, McDonald JA, Ryan U: Elastin production by cultured calf pulmonary artery endothelial cells. J Cell Physiol 1983;116:282–288.

173. Noguchi A, Nelson T: IGF-1 stimulates tropoelastin synthesis in neonatal rat pulmonary fibroblasts. Pediatr Res 1991;30:248–251.

174. McGowan SE, Liu R, Harvey CS: Effects of heparin and other glycosaminoglycans on elastin production by cultured neonatal rat lung fibroblasts. Arch Biochem Biophys 1993;302:322–331.

175. Kahari VM, Chen YQ, Bashir MM, et al: Tumor necrosis factor-alpha down-regulates human elastin gene expression: Evidence for the role of AP-1 in the suppression of promoter activity. J Biol Chem 1992;267: 26134–26141.

176. Burnett W, Finnigan-Bunick A, Yoon K, Rosenbloom J: Analysis of elastin gene expression in the developing chick aorta using cloned elastin cDNA. J Biol Chem 1982;257:1569–1572.

177. Berk JL, Franzblau C, Goldstein RH: Recombinant interleukin-1 beta inhibits elastin formation by a

neonatal rat lung fibroblast subtype. J Biol Chem 1991; 266:3192–3197.

178. Starcher BC: Elastin and the lung. Thorax 1986;412: 577–585.

179. Brantly M, Nukiwa T, Crystal RG: Molecular basis of alpha-1-antitrypsin deficiency. Am J Med 1988;84: 13–31.

180. Crystal RG, Brantly ML, Hubbard RC, et al: The alpha 1-antitrypsin gene and its mutations: Clinical consequences and strategies for therapy. Chest 1989; 95:196–208.

181. Crystal RG: The alpha 1-antitrypsin gene and its deficiency states. Trends Genet 1989;5:411–417.

182. Crystal RG: Alpha-1-antitrypsin deficiency, emphysema, and liver disease: Genetic basis and strategies for therapy. J Clin Invest 1990;85:1343–1352.

183. Nukiwa T, Brantly M, Garver R, et al: Evaluation of "at-risk" alpha-1-antitrypsin genotype SZ with synthetic oligonucleotide gene probes. J Clin Invest 1986;77:528–537.

184. Nukiwa T, Satoh K, Brantly ML, et al: Identification of a second mutation in the protein-coding sequence of the Z type alpha-1-antitrypsin gene. J Biol Chem 1986;261:15989–15994.

185. Nukiwa T, Brantly ML, Ogushi F, et al: Characterization of the gene and protein of the common alpha-1-antitrypsin normal M2 allele. Am J Hum Genet 1988; 43:322–330.

186. Kidd VJ, Wallace RB, Itakura K, Woo SL: Alpha 1-antitrypsin deficiency detection by direct analysis of the mutation in the gene. Nature 1983;304:230–234.

187. Okayama H, Curiel DT, Brantly ML, et al: Rapid, nonradioactive detection of mutations in the human genome by allele-specific amplification. J Lab Clin Med 1989;114:105–113.

188. Cox DW, Billingsley GD, Mansfield T: DNA restriction-site polymorphisms associated with the alpha-1-antitrypsin gene. Am J Hum Genet 1987;41:891–906.

189. Rodriguez-Cintron W, Guntupalli K, Fraire AE: Bronchiectasis and homozygous (P1ZZ) alpha 1-antitrypsin deficiency in a young man [see comments]. Thorax 1995;50: 424–425.

190. Rabin M, Watson M, Kidd V, et al: Regional location of alpha 1-antichymotrypsin and alpha 1-antitrypsin genes on human chromosome 14. Somat Cell Mol Genet 1986;12:209–214.

191. Chandra T, Stackhouse R, Kidd VJ, et al: Sequence homology between human alpha-1-antichymotrypsin, alpha-1-antitrypsin, and antithrombin III. Biochemistry 1983;22:5055–5061.

192. Sefton L, Kelsey G, Kearney P, et al: A physical map of the human *PI* and *AACT* genes. Genomics 1990;7: 382–388.

193. Eriksson S, Lindmark B, Lilia H: Familial alpha-1-antichymotrypsin deficiency. Acta Med Scand 1986; 220:447–453.

194. Tsuda M, Sei Y, Yamamura M, et al: Detection of a new mutant alpha-1-antichymotrypsin in patients with occlusive-cerebrovascular disease. FEBS Lett 1992; 304:66–68.

195. Poller W, Faber J-P, Scholz S, et al: Mis-sense mutation of alpha-1-antichymotrypsin gene associated with chronic lung disease [letter]. Lancet 1992;339:1538.

196. Poller W, Faber J-P, Weidinger S, et al: A leucine-to-proline substitution causes a defective alpha-1-antichymotrypsin allele associated with familial obstructive lung disease. Genomics 1993;17:740–743.

197. Kamboh MI, Sanghera DK, Ferrell RE, DeKosky ST: APOE*4-associated Alzheimer's disease risk is modified by alpha-1-antichymotrypsin polymorphism. Nat Genet 1995;10:286–288.

198. Travis J, Salvesen GS: Human plasma proteinase inhibitors. Annu Res Biochem 1983;52:655–709.

199. Brissenden JE, Cox DW: Alpha 2-macroglobulin production by cultured human fibroblasts. Somat Cell Genet 1982;8:289–305.

200. Munck Petersen C, Christiansen BS, Heickendorff L, Ingerslev J: Synthesis and secretion of alpha-2-macroglobulin by human hepatocytes in culture. Eur J Clin Invest 1988;18:543–548.

201. Mosher DF, Wing DA: Synthesis and secretion of alpha2-macroglobulin by cultured human fibroblasts. J Exp Med 1976;143:462–467.

202. Poller W, Barth J, Voss B: Detection of an alteration of the alpha 2-macroglobulin gene in a patient with chronic lung disease and serum alpha 2-macroglobulin deficiency. Hum Genet 1989;83:93–96.

203. Colby TV, Koss MN, Travis WD: Tumors of the lower respiratory tract. *In* Rosai J (ed): Atlas of Tumor Pathology, 3rd ed, vol 13. Washington, DC, Armed Forces Institute of Pathology, 1995.

204. Shock A, Laurent GJ: Leukocytes and pulmonary disorders: Mobilization, activation and role in pathology. Mol Aspects Med 1990;11:425–526.

205. Hutchison DCS: Natural history of alpha-1-antitrypsin deficiency. Am J Med 1988;84(Suppl. 6A):13–31.

206. Riley DJ, Kerr JS: Oxidant injury of the extracellular matrix: Potential role in the pathogenesis of pulmonary emphysema. Lung 1985;163:1–13.

207. Janoff A: Biochemical links between cigarette smoking and pulmonary emphysema. J Appl Physiol 1983;55: 285–293.

208. Thet LA, Parra SC, Shelbourne JD: Sequential changes in lung morphology during the repair of acute oxygen-induced lung injury in adult rats. Exp Lung Res 1986; 11:209–228.

209. Thrall RS, Barton RW, D'Amato DA, Sulavik SB: Differential cellular analysis of bronchioloalveolar lavage fluid obtained at various stages during the development of bleomycin-induced pulmonary fibrosis in the rat. Am Rev Respir Dis 1982;126:488–492.

210. Khalil N, O'Connor RN, Unruh HW, et al: Increased production and immunohistochemical localization of transforming growth factor-beta in idiopathic pulmonary fibrosis. Am J Respir Cell Mol Biol 1991;5:155–162.

211. Broekelmann TJ, Limper AH, Colby TV, McDonald JA: Transforming growth factor beta 1 is present at sites of extracellular matrix gene expression in human pulmonary fibrosis. Proc Natl Acad Sci USA 1991;88: 6642–6646.

212. Raghow R, Irish P, Kang AH: Coordinate regulation of transforming growth factor beta gene expression and cell proliferation in hamster lungs undergoing bleomycin-induced pulmonary fibrosis. J Clin Invest 1989;84: 1836–1842.

213. Martinet Y, Rom WN, Grotendorst GR, et al: Exaggerated spontaneous release of platelet-derived growth factor by alveolar macrophages from patients with idiopathic pulmonary fibrosis. N Engl J Med 1987;317: 202–209.
214. Kelley J: Cytokines of the lung. Am Rev Respir Dis 1990;141:765–788.
215. Wangoo A, Shaw RJ, Diss TC, et al: Cryptogenic fibrosing alveolitis: lack of association with Epstein-Barr virus infection. Thorax 1997;51:888–891.
216. Crystal RG, Fulmer JD, Roberts WC, et al: Idiopathic pulmonary fibrosis: Clinical, histologic, radiologic, physiologic scintigraphic, cytologic and biochemical aspects. Ann Intern Med 1976;85:769–788.
217. Briggs DC, Vaughan RW, Welsh KI, et al: Immunogenetic prediction of pulmonary fibrosis in systemic sclerosis. Lancet 1991;338:661–662.
218. Turton CWG, Morris LM, Lawler SD, Turner-Warwick M: HLA in cryptogenic fibrosing alveolitis. Lancet 1978;78:507–508.
219. Kuhn C, McDonald JA: The roles of the myofibroblast in idiopathic pulmonary fibrosis: Ultrastructural and immunohistochemical features of sites of active extracellular matrix synthesis. Am J Pathol 1991; 138:1257–1265.
220. Zhang K, Gharaee-Kermani M, McGarry B, Phan SH: In situ hybridization analysis of rat lung alpha 1(I) and alpha 2(I) collagen gene expression in pulmonary fibrosis induced by endotracheal bleomycin injection. Lab Invest 1994;70:192–202.
221. Zhang K, Rekhter MD, Gordon D, Phan SH: Myofibroblasts and their role in lung collagen gene expression during pulmonary fibrosis: A combined immunohistochemical and in situ hybridization study. Am J Pathol 1994;145:114–125.
222. Bitterman PB, Rennard SI, Keogh BA, et al: Familial idiopathic pulmonary fibrosis: Evidence of lung inflammation in unaffected family members. N Engl J Med 1986;314:1343–1347.
223. Musk AW, Zilko PJ, Manners P, et al: Genetic studies in familial fibrosing alveolitis: Possible linkage with immunoglobulin allotypes (Gm). Chest 1986;89: 206–210.
224. Hallgren R, Eklund A, Engstrom-Laurent A, Schmekel B: Hyaluronate in bronchoalveolar lavage fluid: A new marker in sarcoidosis reflecting pulmonary disease. BMJ 1985;290:1778–1781.
225. Hallgren R, Samuelsson T, Laurent TC, Modig J: Accumulation of hyaluronan in the lung in adult respiratory distress syndrome. Am Rev Respir Dis 1989;139:682–687.
226. Sahu S, Lynn WS: Hyaluronic acid in the pulmonary secretions of patients with alveolar proteinosis. Inflammation 1978;3:149–158.
227. Juul SE, Kinsella MG, Wight TN, Hodson WA: Alterations in nonhuman primate *(M. nemestrina)* lung proteoglycans during normal development and acute hyaline membrane disease. Am J Respir Cell Mol Biol 1993; 8:299–310.
228. Bensadoun ES, Burke AK, Hogg JC, Roberts CR: Proteoglycan deposition in pulmonary fibrosis. Am J Respir Crit Care Med 1996;154:1819–1828.
229. Bensadoun ES, Burke AK, Hogg JC, Roberts CR: Proteoglycans in granulomatous lung diseases. Eur Respir J 1997;10:2731–2737.
230. Turner N, Mason PJ, Brown R, et al: Molecular cloning of the human Goodpasture antigen demonstrates it to be the alpha-3 chain of type IV collagen. J Clin Invest 1992;89:592–601.
231. Kalluri R, Gunwar S, Reeders ST, et al: Goodpasture syndrome: Localization of the epitope for the autoantibodies to the carboxyl-terminal region of the alpha 3(IV) chain of basement membrane collagen. J Biol Chem 1991;266:24018–24024.
232. Gunwar S, Ballester F, Kalluri R, et al: Glomerular basement membrane: Identification of dimeric subunits of the noncollagenous domain (hexamer) of collagen IV and the Goodpasture antigen. J Biol Chem 1991;266: 15318–15324.
233. Gunwar S, Bejarano PA, Kalluri R, et al: Alveolar basement membrane: Molecular properties of the noncollagenous domain (hexamer) of collagen IV and its reactivity with Goodpasture autoantibodies [see comments]. Am J Respir Cell Mol Biol 1991;5:107–112.
234. Rees AJ, Peters DK, Amos N, et al: The influence of HLA-linked genes on the severity of anti-GBM antibody-mediated nephritis. Kidney Int 1984;26:1145.
235. Gossain VV, Gerstein AR, Jones AW: Goodpasture's syndrome: A familial occurrence. Am Rev Respir Dis 1972;105:621–624.
236. D'Apice AJF, Kincaid-Smith P, Becker GJ, et al: Goodpasture's syndrome in identical twins. Ann Intern Med 1978;88:61–62.
237. Kalluri R, van den Heuvel LP, Smeets HJM, et al: A *COL4A3* gene mutation and post-transplant anti-alpha-3(IV) collagen alloantibodies in Alport syndrome. Kidney Int 1995;47:1199–1204.
238. Yoshioka K, Iseki T, Okada M, et al: Identification of Goodpasture antigens in human alveolar basement membrane. Clin Exp Immunol 1988;74:419–424.
239. Liebow AA, Carrington CR, Friedman PJ: Lymphomatoid granulomatosis. Hum Pathol 1972;3:457–558.
240. Guinee D Jr, Jaffe E, Kingma D, et al: Pulmonary lymphomatoid granulomatosis: Evidence for a proliferation of Epstein-Barr virus–infected B lymphocytes with a prominent T-cell component and vasculitis. Am J Surg Pathol 1994;18:753–764.
241. Cordier JF, Chailleux E, Lauque D, et al: Primary pulmonary lymphomas: A clinical study of 70 cases in nonimmunocompromised patients. Chest 1993;103: 201–208.
242. Li G, Hansmann ML, Zwingers T, Lennert K: Primary lymphomas of the lung: Morphological, immunohistochemical and clinical features. Histopathology 1990;16: 519–531.
243. Koss MN: Pulmonary lymphoid disorders. Semin Diagn Pathol 1995;12:158–171.
244. Sugimura T: Multistep carcinogenesis: A 1990s perspective. Science 1992;258:603.
245. Harris CC: Chemical and physical carcinogenesis: Advances and perspectives for the 1990s. Cancer Res 1991;51(18 Suppl):5023s–5044s.
246. Kaye FJ: Lung cancer. In Cossman J (ed): Molecular Genetics in Cancer Diagnosis. New York, Elsevier, 1990.

247. Weinstein IB: The origins of human cancer: Molecular mechanisms of carcinogenesis and their implications for cancer prevention and treatment. Cancer Res 1988; 48:4135.

248. Kaufmann WK, Paules RS: DNA damage and cell cycle checkpoints. FASEB J 1996;10:238–247.

249. Kawajiri K, Nakchi K, Imai K, et al: Identification of genetically high risk individuals to lung cancer by DNA polymorphisms of the cytochrome *P450IA1* gene. FEBS Lett 1990;263:131–133.

250. Cascorbi I, Brockmoller J, Roots I: A *C4887A* polymorphism in exon 7 of human *CYP1A1:* Population frequency, mutation linkages, and impact on lung cancer susceptibility. Cancer Res 1996;56:4965–4969.

251. Kawajiri K, Fujii-Kuriyama Y: P450 and human cancer. Jpn J Cancer Res 1991;82:1325–1335.

252. Hayashi S, Watanabe J, Nakachi K, Kawajiri K: Genetic linkage of lung cancer-associated MspI polymorphisms with amino acid replacement in the heme binding region of the human cytochrome *p450Ia1* gene. J Biochem (Tokyo) 1991;110:407–411.

253. Shields PG, Bowman ED, Harrington AM, et al: Polycyclic aromatic hydrocarbon-DNA adducts in human lung and cancer susceptibility genes. Cancer Res 1993;53:3486–3492.

254. Nakachi K, Imai K, Hayashi S, et al: Genetic susceptibility to squamous cell carcinoma of the lung in relation to cigarette smoking dose. Cancer Res 1991;51: 5177–5180.

255. Nakachi K, Imai K, Hayashi S, Kawajiri K: Polymorphisms of the *CYP1A1* and glutathione S-transferase genes associated with susceptibility to lung cancer in relation to cigarette dose in a Japanese population. Cancer Res 1993;53:2994–2999.

256. Hirvonen A, Husgafvel PK, Karjalainen A, et al: Point-mutational MspI and Ile-Val polymorphisms closely linked in the *CYP1A1* gene: Lack of association with susceptibility to lung cancer in a Finnish study population. Cancer Epidemiol Biomarkers Prev 1992;1:485–489.

257. Tefre T, Ryberg D, Haugen A, et al: Human *CYP1A1* (cytochrome P(1)450) gene: Lack of association between the Msp I restriction fragment length polymorphism and incidence of lung cancer in a Norwegian population. Pharmacogenetics 1991;1:20–25.

258. Nebert DW: The Ah locus: Genetic differences in toxicity, cancer, mutation, and birth defects. Crit Rev Toxicol 1989;20:153–174.

259. Kato S, Bowman ED, Harrington AM, et al: Human lung carcinogen-DNA adduct levels mediated by genetic polymorphisms in vivo. J Natl Cancer Inst 1995;87: 902–907.

260. Uematsu F, Kikuchi H, Motomiya M, et al: Association between restriction fragment length polymorphism of the human cytochrome *P450IIE1* gene and susceptibility to lung cancer. Jpn J Cancer Res 1991;82:254–256.

261. Wu X, Shi H, Jiang H, et al: Associations between cytochrome *P4502E1* genotype, mutagen sensitivity, cigarette smoking and susceptibility to lung cancer. Carcinogenesis 1997;18:967–973.

262. Hirvonen A, Husgafvel-Pursiainen K, Anttila S, et al: The human *CYP2E1* gene and lung cancer: DraI and RsaI restriction fragment length polymorphisms in a Finnish study population. Carcinogenesis 1993;14: 85–88.

263. Kato S, Shields PG, Caporaso NE, et al: Analysis of cytochrome P450 2E1 genetic polymorphisms in relation to human lung cancer. Cancer Epidemiol Biomarkers Prev 1994;3:515–518.

264. Kato S, Shields PG, Caporaso NE, et al: Cytochrome *P450IIE1* genetic polymorphisms, racial variation, and lung cancer risk. Cancer Res 1992;52:6712–6715.

265. Persson I, Johansson I, Bergling H, et al: Genetic polymorphism of cytochrome *P4502E1* in a Swedish population: Relationship to incidence of lung cancer. FEBS Lett 1993;319:207–211.

266. Mannervik B, Danielson UH: Glutathione transferases—structure and catalytic activity. CRC Crit Rev Biochem 1988;23:283–337.

267. van Poppel G, de Vogel N, van Balderen PJ, Kok FJ: Increased cytogenetic damage in smokers deficient in glutathione S-transferase isozyme Mu. Carcinogenesis 1992;13:303–305.

268. Bartsch H, Petruzzelli S, De Flora S, et al: Carcinogen metabolism and DNA adducts in human lung tissues as affected by tobacco smoking or metabolic phenotype: A case-control study on lung cancer patients. Mutat Res 1991;250:103–114.

269. Shields PG, Caporaso NE, Falk RT, et al: Lung cancer, race, and a *CYP1A1* genetic polymorphism. Cancer Epidemiol Biomarkers Prev 1993;2:481–485.

270. Seidegard J, Pero RW, Miller DG, Beattie EJ: A glutathione transferase in human leukocytes as a marker for the susceptibility to lung cancer. Carcinogenesis 1986;7:751–753.

271. McWilliams JE, Sanderson BJ, Harris EL, et al: Glutathione S-transferase M1 (GSTM1) deficiency and lung cancer risk. Cancer Epidemiol Biomarkers Prev 1995;4:589–594.

272. Seidegard J, Pero RW, Markowitz MM, et al: Isoenzyme(s) of glutathione transferase (class Mu) as a marker for the susceptibility to lung cancer: A follow up study. Carcinogenesis 1990;11:33–36.

273. Hirvonen A, Husgafvel-Pursiainen K, Anttila S, Vainio H: The *GSTM1* null genotype as a potential risk modifier for squamous cell carcinoma of the lung. Carcinogenesis 1993;14:1479–1481.

273a. Hayes JD, Pulford DJ: The glutathione S-transferase supergene family: regulation of GST and the contribution of the isoenzymes to cancer chemoprevention and drug resistance. Crit Rev Biochem Mol Biol 1995;30: 445–600.

273b. Ryberg D, Skaug V, Hewer A, et al: Genotypes of the glutathione transferase M1 and P1 and their significance for lug DNA adduct levels and cancer risk. Carcinogenesis 1997;18:1285–1289.

274. Tucker GT: Clinical implications of genetic polymorphism in drug metabolism. J Pharm Pharmacol 1994; 46(Suppl 1):417–424.

275. Wolf CR, Smith CAD, Forman D: Metabolic polymorphisms in carcinogen metabolising enzymes and cancer susceptibility. Br Med Bull 1994;50:718–731.

276. Kawajiri K, Nakachi K, Imai K, et al: The *CYP1A1* gene and cancer susceptibility. Crit Rev Oncol Hematol 1993;14:77–87.

277. Nebert DW: The role of genetics and drug metabolism in human cancer risk. Mutat Res 1991;247:267–281.
278. Meyer UA, Zanger UM: Molecular mechanisms of genetic polymorphisms of drug metabolism. Annu Rev Pharmacol Toxicol 1997;37:269–296.
279. Roots I, Brockmoller J, Drakoulis N, Loddenkemper R: Mutant genes of cytochrome P-450IID6, glutathione S-transferase class Mu, and arylamine N-acetyltransferase in lung cancer patients. Clin Investig 1992;70: 307–319.
280. Caporaso NE, Tucker MA, Hoover RN, et al: Lung cancer and the debrisoquine metabolic phenotype. J Natl Cancer Inst 1990;82:1264–1272.
281. Caporaso N, Hayes RB, Dosemeci M, et al: Lung cancer risk, occupational exposure, and the debrisoquine metabolic phenotype. Cancer Res 1989;49: 3675–3679.
282. Hirvonen A, Husgafvel-Pursiainen K, Anttila S, et al: PCR-based *CYP2D6* genotyping for Finnish lung cancer patients. Pharmacogenetics 1993;3:19–27.
283. Ayesh R, Idle JR, Ritchie JC, et al: Metabolic oxidation phenotypes as markers for susceptibiltiy to lung cancer. Nature 1984;312:169–170.
284. Gonzalles FJ, Skoda RC, Kimura S, et al: Molecular characterization of the common human deficiency in metabolism of debrisoquine and other drugs. Nature 1988;331:442–446.
285. Heim M, Meyer UA: Genotyping of poor metabolisers of debrisoquine by allele-specific PCR amplification. Lancet 1990;336:529–532.
286. Lee EJD, Zhao B, Moochhala SM, Ngoi SS: Frequency of mutant *CYP1A1*, *NAT2* and *GSTM1* alleles in a normal Chinese population. Pharmacogenetics 1994;4: 355–358.
287. Blum M, Demierre A, Grant DM, et al: Molecular mechanism of slow acetylation of drugs and carcinogens in humans. Proc Natl Acad Sci USA 1991;88: 5237–5241.
288. Cascorbi I, Drakoulis N, Brockmoller J, et al: Arylamine N-acetyltransferase (NAT2) mutations and their allelic linkage in unrelated Caucasian individuals: Correlation with phenotypic activity. Am J Hum Genet 1995;57:581–592.
289. Cascorbi I, Brockmoller J, Bauer S, et al: NAT2*12A (803A→G) codes for rapid arylamine N-acetylation in humans. Pharmacogenetics 1996;6:257–259.
290. Nebert DW, Petersen DD, Fornace AJ Jr: Cellular responses to oxidative stress: The [Ah] battery as a paradigm. Health Perspect 1990;88:13–25.
291. Hanssen HP, Agarwal DP, Goedde HW, et al: Association of N-acetyltransferase polymorphism and environmental factors with bladder carcinogenesis. Eur Urol 1985;11:263–266.
292. Cascorbi I, Brockmoller J, Mrozikiewicz PM, et al: Homozygous rapid arylamine N-acetyltransferase (NAT2) genotype as a susceptibility factor for lung cancer. Cancer Res 1996;56:3961–3966.
293. Grant DM, Tang BK, Kalow W: Variability in caffeine metabolism. Clin Pharmacol Ther 1983;33: 591–602.
294. Ryberg D, Hewer A, Phillips DH, Haugen A: Different susceptibility to smoking-induced DNA damage among male and female lung cancer patients. Cancer Res 1994;54:5801–5803.
295. Kawajiri K, Hidetaka E, Nakachi K, et al: Association of *CYP1A1* germ line polymorphisms with mutations of the *p53* gene in lung cancer. Cancer Res 1996;56:72–76.
296. Przygodzki RM, Bennett WP, Guinee DG Jr, et al: *p53* mutation spectrum in relation to *GSTM1*, *CYP1A1* and *CYP2E1* in surgically treated patients with non–small cell lung cancer. Pharmacogenetics 1998;8:503–511.
297. Knudsen AG: Antioncogenes and human cancer. Proc Natl Acad Sci USA 1993;90:10914–10921.
298. Sanders BM, Jay M, Draper GJ, Roberts EM: Non-ocular cancer in relatives of retinoblastoma patients. Br J Cancer 1989;60:358–365.
299. Greenblatt MS, Bennett WP, Hollstein M, Harris CC: Mutations in the *p53* tumor suppressor gene: Clues to cancer etiology and molecular pathogenesis. Cancer Res 1994;54:4855–4878.
300. Chiba I, Takahashi T, Nau MM, et al: Mutations in the *p53* gene are frequent in primary, resected non-small cell lung cancer. Lung Cancer Study Group. Oncogene 1990;5:1603–1610.
301. Weston A, Vineis P, Caporaso NE, et al: Racial variation in the distribution of Ha-*ras*-1 alleles. Mol Carcinog 1991;4:265–268.
302. Weston A, Perrin LS, Forrester K, et al: Allelic frequency of a *p53* polymorphism in human lung cancer. Cancer Epidemiol Biomarkers Prev 1992;1:481–483.
303. Oshita F, Fujiwara Y, Saijo N: Radiation sensitivities in various anticancer-drug–resistant human lung cancer cell lines and mechanism of radiation cross-resistance in a cisplatin-resistant cell line. J Cancer Res Clin Oncol 1992;119:28–34.
304. Althaus FR, Richter C: ADP-ribosylation of proteins: Enzymology and biological significance. Mol Biol Biochem Biophys 1987;37:1.
305. Krupitza G, Crutti P: ADP-ribosylation of ADPR-transferase and topoisomerase I in intact mouse epidermal cell JB6. Biochemistry 1989;28:2034.
306. Roy R, Adamczewski JP, Seroz T, et al: The MO15 cell cycle kinase is associated with the TFIIH transcription-DNA repair factor. Cell 1994;79:1093–1101.
307. Feaver WJ, Svejstrup JQ, Henry NL, Kornberg RD: Relationship of CDK-activating kinase and RNA polymerase II CTD kinase TFIIH/TFIIK. Cell 1994;79: 1103–1109.
308. Huang J-C, Svoboda DL, Reardon JT, Sancar A: Human nucleotide excision nuclease removes thymine dimers from DNA by incising the 22nd phosphodiester bond 5′ and the 6th phosphodiester bond 3′ to the photodimer. Proc Natl Acad Sci USA 1992;89:3664.
309. Coverley D, Kenny MK, Munn M, et al: Requirement for the replication protein SSB in human DNA excision repair. Nature 1991;349:538–541.
310. Hanawalt PC: DNA repair comes of age. Mutat Res 1995;336:101–113.
311. Sancar A: Mechanisms of DNA excision repair. Science 1994;266:1954–1956.
312. Benachenhou N, Guiral S, Gorska-Flipot I, et al: High resolution deletion mapping reveals frequent allelic losses at the DNA mismatch repair loci hMLH1 and

hMSH3 in non–small cell lung cancer. Int J Cancer 1998; 77:173–180.
313. Pegg AE, Dolan ME, Moschel RC: Structure, function, and inhibition of O6-alkylguanine-DNA alkyltransferase. Prog Nucleic Acid Res Mol Biol 1995;51:167–223.
314. Saffhill R, Margison GP, O'Connor PJ: Mechanisms of carcinogenesis induced by alkylating agents. Biochim Biophys Acta 1985;823:111–145.
315. Nau MM, Carney DN, Battey J, et al: Amplification, expression and rearrangement of c-*myc* and n-*myc* oncogenes in human lung cancer. Curr Top Microbiol Immunol 1984;113:172–177.
316. Zimmerman K, Yancopoulos G, Collum R, et al: Differential expression of *myc* family genes during murine development. Nature 1986;319:780–783.
317. Ma A, Moroy T, Collum R, et al: DNA binding by N- and L-Myc proteins. Oncogene 1993;8:1093–1098.
318. Reddy CD, Dasgupta P, Saikumar P, et al: Mutational analysis of Max: Role of basic, helix-loop-helix/leucine zipper domains in DNA binding, dimerization and regulation of Myc-mediated transcriptional activation. Oncogene 1992;7:2085–2092.
319. Prendergast GC, Lawe D, Ziff EB: Association of Myn, the murine homolog of max, with c-Myc stimulates methylation-sensitive DNA binding and *ras* cotransformation. Cell 1991;65:395–407.
320. Blackwood EM, Eisenman RN: Max: a helix-loop-helix zipper protein that forms a sequence-specific DNA-binding complex with Myc. Science 1991;251: 1211–1217.
321. Zervos AS, Gyuris J, Brent R: Mxi1, a protein that specifically interacts with Max to bind Myc-Max recognition sites [published erratum appears in Cell 1994;79: following 388]. Cell 1993;72:223–232.
322. Ayer DE, Kretzner L, Eisenman RN: Mad: A heterodimeric partner for Max that antagonizes Myc transcriptional activity. Cell 1993;72:211–222.
323. Ayer DE, Eisenman RN: A switch from Myc:Max to Mad:Max heterocomplexes accompanies monocyte/ macrophage differentiation. Genes Dev 1993;7: 2110–2119.
324. Larsson LG, Pettersson M, Oberg F, et al: Expression of mad, mxi1, max, and c-myc during induced differentiation of hematopoietic cells: Opposite regulation of mad and c-myc. Oncogene 1994;9:1247–1252.
325. Maheswaran S, Lee H, Sonenshein GE: Intracellular association of the protein product of the c-*myc* oncogene with the TATA-binding protein. Mol Cell Biol 1994;14:1147–1152.
326. Roy AL, Malik S, Meisterernst M, Roeder RG: An alternative pathway for transcription initiation involving TFII–I. Nature 1993;365:355–359.
327. Roy AL, Carruthers C, Gutjahr T, Roeder RG: Direct role for Myc in transcription initiation mediated by interactions with TFII–I. Nature 1993;365:359–361.
328. Galaktionov K, Chen X, Beach D: CDC25 cell-cycle phosphatase as a target of c-myc. Nature 1996;382: 511–517.
329. Rustgi AK, Dyson N, Bernards R: Amino-terminal domains of c-myc and N-myc proteins mediate binding to the retinoblastoma gene product. Nature 1991;352: 541–544.
330. Beijersbergen RL, Hijmans EM, Zhu L, Bernards R: Interaction of c-Myc with the pRb-related protein p107 results in inhibition of c-Myc–mediated transactivation. EMBO J 1994;13:4080–4086.
331. Hateboer G, Timmers HT, Rustgi AK, et al: TATA-binding protein and the retinoblastoma gene product bind to overlapping epitopes on c-Myc and adenovirus E1A protein. Proc Natl Acad Sci USA 1993;90: 8489–8493.
332. Sherr CJ, Roberts JM: Inhibitors of mammalian G1 cyclin-dependent kinases. Genes Dev 1995;9: 1149–1163.
333. Philipp A, Schneider A, Vasrik I, et al: Repression of cyclin D1: A novel function of MYC. Mol Cell Biol 1994;14:4032–4043.
334. Williams GT: Programmed cell death: Apoptosis and oncogenesis. Cell 1991;65:1097–1098.
335. Hermeking H, Eick D: Mediation of c-Myc–induced apoptosis by p53. Science 1994;265:2091–2093.
336. Packham G, Cleveland JL: Ornithine decarboxylase is a mediator of c-Myc–induced apoptosis. Mol Cell Biol 1994;14:5741–5747.
337. Jansen-Durr P, Meichle A, Steiner P, et al: Differential modulation of cyclin gene expression by MYC. Proc Natl Acad Sci USA 1993;90:3685–3689.
338. Symonds G, Hartshorn A, Kennewell A, et al: Transformation of murine myelomonocytic cells by *myc:* Point mutations in v-*myc* contribute synergistically to transforming potential. Oncogene 1989;4:285–294.
339. Young J, Buttenshaw R, Butterworth L, et al: Association of the SS genotype of the L-*myc* gene and loss of 18q sequences with a worse clinical prognosis in colorectal cancers. Oncogene 1994;9:1053–1056.
340. Chernitsa OI, Togo AV, Shutkin VA, et al: S allele of the L-*myc* oncogene is associated with lung cancer metastases in patients from Moldova. Vopr Onkol 1998;44:33–36.
341. Gazdar AF, Carney DN, Nau MM, Minna JD: Characterization of variant subclasses of cell lines derived from small cell lung cancer having distinctive biochemical, morphological, and growth properties. Cancer Res 1985;45:2924–2930.
342. Tervahauta AI, Syrjanen SM, Kallio PJ, Syrjanen KJ: Immunohistochemistry, in situ hybridization and polymerase chain reaction (PCR) in detecting c-myc expression in human malignancies. Anticancer Res 1992;12: 1005–1011.
343. Makela TP, Saksela K, Alitalo K: Amplification and rearrangement of L-Myc in human small-cell lung cancer. Mutat Res 1992;276:307–315.
344. Hajj C, Akoum R, Bradley E, et al: DNA alterations at proto-oncogene loci and their clinical significance in operable non-small cell lung cancer. Cancer 1990;66: 733–739.
345. Shiraishi M, Noguchi M, Shimosato Y, Sekiya T: Amplification of protooncogenes in surgical specimens of human lung carcinomas. Cancer Res 1989;49: 6474–6479.
346. Johnson BE, Brennan JF, Ihde DC, Gazdar AF: myc family DNA amplification in tumors and tumor cell lines from patients with small-cell lung cancer. Monogr Natl Cancer Inst 1992;13:39–43.

347. Noguchi M, Hirohashi S, Hara F, et al: Heterogenous amplification of *myc* family oncogenes in small cell lung carcinoma. Cancer 1990;66:2053–2058.
348. Makela TP, Shiraishi M, Borrello MG, et al: Rearrangement and co-amplification of L-myc and rlf in primary lung cancer. Oncogene 1992;7(3):405–9.
349. Gazzeri S, Brambilla E, Caron de Fromentel C, et al: *p53* genetic abnormalities and *myc* activation in human lung carcinoma. Int J Cancer 1994;58:24–32.
350. Bai F, Matsui T, Ohtani-Fujita N, et al: Promoter activation and following induction of the *p21/WAF1* gene by flavone is involved in G1 phase arrest in A549 lung adenocarcinoma cells. FEBS Lett 1998;437:61–64.
351. Plummer H, Catlett J, Leftwich J, et al: c-*myc* expression correlates with suppression of c-*kit* protooncogene expression in small cell lung cancer cell lines. Cancer Res 1993;53:4337–4342.
352. Kiefer PE, Bepler G, Kubasch M, Havemann K: Amplification and expression of proto-oncogenes in human small cell lung cancer cell lines. Cancer Res 1987;47:6236–6242.
353. Nau MM, Brooks BJ Jr, Carney DN, et al: Human small-cell lung cancers show amplification and expression of the n-*myc* gene. Proc Natl Acad Sci USA 1986; 83:1092–1096.
354. Yokota J, Wada M, Yoshida T, et al: Heterogeneity of lung cancer cells with respect to the amplification and rearrangement of *myc* family oncogenes. Oncogene 1988;2:607–611.
355. Broers JL, Viallet J, Jensen SM, et al: Expression of c-*myc* in progenitor cells of the bronchopulmonary epithelium and in a large number of non-small cell lung cancers. Am J Respir Cell Mol Biol 1993;9:33–43.
356. Polly P, Nicholson RC: High levels of c-*myc* gene expression precede point mutational activation of Ki-*ras* in mouse lung cancer. Cancer Lett 1994;76: 87–92.
357. Birrer MJ, Segal S, DeGreve J, et al: L-*myc* cooperates with *ras* to transform primary rat embryo fibroblasts. Mol Cell Biol 1988;8:2573–2668.
358. Yancopoulos GP, Nisen PD, Tesfaye A, et al: N-*myc* can cooperate with *ras* to transform normal cells in culture. Proc Natl Acad Sci USA 1985;82:5455–5459.
359. Brennan J, O'Connor T, Makuch RW, et al: Myc family DNA amplification in 107 tumors and tumor cell lines from patients with small cell lung cancer treated with different combination chemotherapy regimens. Cancer Res 1991;51:1708–1712.
360. Johnson BE, Makuch RW, Simmons AD, et al: *myc* family DNA amplification in small cell lung cancer patients' tumors and corresponding cell lines. Cancer Res 1988;48:5163–5166.
361. Johnson BE, Battey J, Linnoila I, et al: Changes in the phenotype of human small cell lung cancer cell lines after transfection and expression of the c-*myc* proto-oncogene. J Clin Invest 1986;78:525–532.
362. Volm M: P-glycoprotein associated expression of c-fos and c-jun products in human lung carcinomas. Anticancer Res 1993;13:375–378.
363. Weston A, Ling-Cawley HM, Caporaso NE, et al: Determination of the allelic frequencies of an L-*myc* and a *p53* polymorphism in human lung cancer. Carcinogenesis 1994;15:583–587.
364. Boguski MS, McCormick F: Proteins regulating Ras and its relatives. Nature 1993;366:643–654.
365. Macara IC, Lounbury KM, Richards SA, et al: The Ras superfamily of GTPases. FASEB J 1996;10:625–630.
366. Van Blesen T, Hawes BE, Luttrell DK, et al: Receptor-tyrosine-kinase and G-beta-gamma-mediated MAP kinase activation by a common signaling pathway. Nature 1995;376:781–784.
367. Lev S, Moreno H, Martinez R, et al: Protein kinase PYK2 involved in Ca^{2+}-induced regulation of ion channel and MAP kinase functions. Nature 1995;376: 737–745.
368. Vojtek AB, Hollenberg SM, Cooper JK: Mammalian Ras interacts with the serine/threonine kinase Raf. Cell 1993;74:205–214.
369. Schulte TW, Blagosklonny MV, Ingui C, Neckers L: Disruption of the Raf-1-Hsp90 molecular complex results in destabilization of Raf-1 and loss of Raf-1-Ras association. J Biol Chem 1995;270:24585–24588.
370. Li S, Janosch P, Tanji M, et al: Regulation of Raf-1 kinase activity by the 14–3–3 family of proteins. EMBO J 1995;14:685–696.
371. Freed E, Symons M, Macdonald SG, et al: Binding of 14–3–3 proteins to the protein kinase Raf and effects on its activation. Science 1994;265:1713–1716.
372. Luo Z, Tzivion G, Belshaw PJ, et al: Oligomerization activates c-Raf-1 through a Ras-dependent mechanism. Nature 1996;383:181–185.
373. Morrison D: 14–3–3: Modulators of signaling proteins? Science 1994;266:56–57.
374. Kyriakis JM, App H, Zhang X-F, et al: Raf-1 activates MAP kinase-kinase. Nature 1992;358:417–421.
375. de Vries-Smits AM, Burgering BM, Leevers SJ, et al: Involvement of p21ras in activation of extracellular signal-regulated kinase 2. Nature 1992;357: 602–604.
376. Cook SJ, Rubinfeld B, Albert I, McCormick F: RapV12 antagonizes Ras-dependent activation of ERK1 and ERK2 by LPA and EGF in Rat-1 fibroblasts. EMBO J 1993;12:3475–3485.
377. Rodriguez-Viciana P, Warne PH, Dhand R, et al: Phosphatidylinositol-3-OH kinase as a direct target of Ras. Nature 1994;370:527–532.
378. Han L, Colicelli J: A human protein selected for interference with Ras function interacts directly with Ras and competes with Raf1. Mol Cell Biol 1995;15: 1318–1323.
379. Kikuchi A, Demo SD, Ye Z-H, et al: RalGDS family members interact with the effector loop of ras p21. Mol Cell Biol 1994;14:7483–7491.
380. Franke TF, Yang SI, Chan TO, et al: The protein kinase encoded by the Akt proto-oncogene is a target of the PDGF-activated phosphatidylinositol 3-kinase. Cell 1995;81:727–736.
381. Klinghoffer RA, Duckworth B, Valius M, et al: Platelet-derived growth factor–dependent activation of phosphatidylinositol 3-kinase is regulated by receptor binding of SH2-domain–containing proteins which influence Ras activity. Mol Cell Biol 1996;16: 5905–5914.

382. Satoh T, Fantl WJ, Escobedo JA, et al: Platelet-derived growth factor receptor mediates activation of ras through different signaling pathways in different cell types. Mol Cell Biol 1993;13:3706–3713.
383. Marshall MS: The effector interactions of p21ras. Trends Biochem Sci 1993;18:250–254.
384. Katz ME, McCormick F: Signal transduction from multiple Ras effectors. Curr Opin Genet Dev 1997;7: 75–79.
385. McCormick F: Coupling of ras p21 signaling and GTP hydrolysis by GTPase activating proteins. Philos Trans R Soc Lond B Biol Sci 1992;336:43–47; discussion 47–48.
386. Marshall MS: Ras target proteins in eukaryotic cells. FASEB J 1995;9:1311–1318.
387. Sistonen L, Holtta E, Makela TP, et al: The cellular response to induction of the p21 c-Ha-*ras* oncoprotein includes stimulation of *jun* gene expression. EMBO J 1989;8:815–822.
388. Winston JT, Coats SR, Wang YZ, Pledger WJ: Regulation of the cell cycle machinery by oncogenic ras. Oncogene 1996;12:127–134.
389. Rak J, Mitsuhashi Y, Bayko L, et al: Mutant *ras* oncogenes upregulate VEGF/VPF expression: Implications for induction and inhibition of tumor angiogenesis. Cancer Res 1995;55:4575–4580.
390. Wolthuis RM, Bauer B, van't Veer LJ, et al: RalGDS-like factor (Rlf) is a novel Ras and Rap 1A–associating protein. Oncogene 1996;13:353–362.
391. Russell M, Lange-Carter CA, Johnson GL: Direct interaction between Ras and the kinase domain of mitogen-activated protein kinase kinase kinase (MEKK1). J Biol Chem 1995;270:11757–11760.
392. Chen CY, Faller DV: Direction of p21ras-generated signals towards cell growth or apoptosis is determined by protein kinase C and Bcl-2. Oncogene 1995;11: 1487–1498.
393. Cho JY, Kim JH, Lee YH, et al: Correlation between K-*ras* gene mutation and prognosis of patients with non–small cell lung carcinoma. Cancer 1997;79:462–467.
394. Lung ML, Wong M, Lam WK, et al: Incidence of *ras* oncogene activation in lung carcinomas in Hong Kong. Cancer 1992;70:760–763.
395. Mitsudomi T, Viallet J, Mulshine JL, et al: Mutations of *ras* genes distinguish a subset of non–small cell lung cancer cell lines from small cell lung cancer cell lines. Oncogene 1991;6:1353–1362.
396. Kashii T, Mizushima Y, Monno S, et al: Gene analysis of K-, H-*ras*, *p53*, and retinoblastoma susceptibility genes in human lung cancer cell lines by the polymerase chain reaction/single-strand conformation polymorphism method. J Cancer Res Clin Oncol 1994; 120:143–148.
397. Carbone DP, Minna JD: The molecular genetics of lung cancer. Adv Intern Med 1992;37:153–171.
398. Rodenhuis S, Slebos RJ: Clinical significance of *ras* oncogene activation in human lung cancer. Cancer Res 1992;52(9 Suppl):2665s–2669s.
399. Barbacid M: *Ras* genes. Ann Rev Biochem 1987;67: 779–827.
400. Mao L, Hruban RH, Boyle JO, et al: Detection of oncogene mutations in sputum precedes diagnosis of lung cancer. Cancer Res 1994;54:1634–1637.
401. Mills NE, Fishman CL, Rom WN, et al: Increased prevalence of K-*ras* oncogene mutations in lung adenocarcinoma. Cancer Res 1995;55:1444–1447.
402. Reynolds SH, Anna CK, Brown KC, et al: Activated proto-oncogenes in human lung tumors from smokers. Proc Natl Acad Sci USA 1991;88:1085–1089.
403. Rodenhuis S, Slebos RJ, Boot AJ, et al: Incidence and possible clinical significance of K-*ras* oncogene activation in adenocarcinoma of the human lung. Cancer Res 1988;48:5738–5741.
404. Mitsudomi T, Steinberg SM, Oie HK, et al: *Ras* gene mutations in non–small cell lung cancers are associated with shortened survival irrespective of treatment intent. Cancer Res 1991;51:4999–5002.
405. Vahakangas KH, Samet JM, Metcalf RA, et al: Mutations of *p53* and *ras* genes in radon-associated lung cancer from uranium miners. Lancet 1992;339: 576–580.
406. McDonald JW, Taylor JA, Watson MA, et al: *p53* and K-*ras* in radon-associated lung adenocarcinoma. Cancer Epi Biomarkers Prev 1995;4:791–793.
407. Hei TK, Piao CQ, Willey JC, et al: Malignant transformation of human bronchial epithelial cells by radon-simulated alpha-particles. Carcinogenesis 1994; 15:431–437.
408. Weston A, Caporaso NE, Perrin LS, et al: Relationship of H-*ras*-1, L-*myc*, and *p53* polymorphisms with lung cancer risk and prognosis. Environ Health Perspect 1992;98:61–67.
409. Vachtenheim J, Horakova I, Novotna H: Hypomethylation of CCGG sites in the 3′ region of H-*ras* protooncogene is frequent and is associated with H-*ras* allele loss in non–small cell lung cancer. Cancer Res 1994;54: 1145–1148.
410. Husgafvel-Pursiainen K, Hackman P, Ridanpaa M, et al: K-*ras* mutations in human adenocarcinoma of the lung: Association with smoking and occupational exposure to asbestos. Int J Cancer 1993;53:250–256.
411. Westra WH, Slebos RJ, Offerhaus GJ, et al: K-*ras* oncogene activation in lung adenocarcinomas from former smokers: Evidence that K-*ras* mutations are an early and irreversible event in the development of adenocarcinoma of the lung. Cancer 1993;72: 432–438.
412. Clements NC Jr, Nelson MA, Wymer JA, et al: Analysis of K-*ras* gene mutations in malignant and nonmalignant endobronchial tissue obtained by fiberoptic bronchoscopy. Am J Respir Crit Care Med 1995;152: 1374–1378.
413. Przygodzki RM, Koss MN, Moran CA, et al: Pleomorphic (giant and spindle cell) carcinoma is genetically distinct from adenocarcinoma and squamous cell carcinoma by K-*ras*-2 and *p53* analysis. Am J Clin Pathol 1996;106:487–492.
414. Silini EM, Bosi F, Pellegata NS, et al: K-*ras* gene mutations: An unfavorable prognostic marker in stage I lung adenocarcinoma. Virchows Arch 1994;424*(4)*: 367–373.
415. Suzuki Y, Orita M, Shiraishi M, et al: Detection of *ras* gene mutations in human lung cancers by single-strand conformation polymorphism analysis of polymerase chain reaction products. Oncogene 1990;5:1037–1043.

416. Ohshima S, Shimizu Y, Takahama M: Detection of c-Ki-*ras* gene mutation in paraffin sections of adenocarcinoma and atypical bronchioloalveolar cell hyperplasia of human lung. Virchows Arch 1994;424:129–134.
417. Rosell R, Li S, Skacel Z, et al: Prognostic impact of mutated K-*ras* gene in surgically resected non–small cell lung cancer patients. Oncogene 1993;8:2407–2412.
418. Kitagawa Y, Wong F, Lo P, et al: Overexpression of Bcl-2 and mutations in *p53* and K-*ras* in resected human non–small cell lung cancers. Am J Respir Cell Mol Biol 1996;15:45–54.
419. Marchetti A, Buttitta F, Pellegrini S, et al: Bronchioloalveolar lung carcinomas: K-*ras* mutations are constant events in the mucinous subtype. J Pathol 1996; 179:254–259.
420. Marchetti A, Pellegrini S, Bertacca G, et al: *FHIT* and *p53* gene abnormalities in bronchioloalveolar carcinomas: Correlations with clinicopathological data and K-*ras* mutations. J Pathol 1998;184:240–246.
421. Nelson MA, Wymer J, Clements N Jr: Detection of K-*ras* gene mutations in non-neoplastic lung tissue and lung cancers. Cancer Lett 1996;103:115–121.
422. Westra WH, Baas IO, Hruban RH, et al: K-*ras* oncogene activation in atypical alveolar hyperplasias of the human lung. Cancer Res 1996;56:2224–2228.
423. Przygodzki RM, Finkelstein SD, Langer JC, et al: Analysis of *p53*, K-*ras*-2, and C-*raf*-1 in pulmonary neuroendocrine tumors: Correlation with histologic subtype and clinical outcome. Am J Pathol 1996;148:1531–1541.
424. Sugio K, Ishida T, Yokoyama H, et al: *Ras* gene mutations as a prognostic marker in adenocarcinoma of the human lung without lymph node metastasis. Cancer Res 1992;52:2903–2906.
425. Slebos RJ, Kibbelaar RE, Dalesio O, et al: K-*ras* oncogene activation as a prognostic marker in adenocarcinoma of the lung. N Engl J Med 1990;323:561–565.
426. Riese DJ II, van Raaij TM, Plowman GD, et al: The cellular response to neuregulins is governed by complex interactions of the erbB receptor family [published erratum appears in Mol Cell Biol 1996;16:735]. Mol Cell Biol 1995;15:5770–5776.
427. Laurence DJ, Gusterson BA: The epidermal growth factor: A review of structural and functional relationships in the normal organism and in cancer cells. Tumour Biol 1990;11:229–261.
428. Carpenter G: Receptors for epidermal growth factor and other polypeptide mitogens. Annu Rev Biochem 1987;56:881–914.
429. Filhol O, Chambaz EM, Gill GN, Cochet C: Epidermal growth factor stimulates a protein tyrosine kinase which is separable from the epidermal growth factor receptor. J Biol Chem 1993;268:26978–26982.
430. Hernandez-Sotomayor SM, Arteaga CL, Soler C, Carpenter G: Epidermal growth factor stimulates substrate-selective protein-tyrosine-phosphatase activity. Proc Natl Acad Sci USA 1993;90:7691–7695.
431. Segatto O, Pelicci G, Giuli S, et al: Shc products are substrates of erbB-2 kinase. Oncogene 1993;8:2105–2112.
432. Zhu G, Decker SJ, Saltiel AR: Direct analysis of the binding of Src-homology 2 domains of phospholipase C to the activated epidermal growth factor receptor. Proc Natl Acad Sci USA 1992;89:9559–9563.
433. Dobashi K, Davis JG, Mikami Y, et al: Characterization of a neu/c-erbB-2 protein–specific activating factor. Proc Natl Acad Sci USA 1991;88:8582–8586.
434. Carraway KL III, Cantley LC: A *neu* acquaintance for erbB3 and erbB4: A role for receptor heterodimerization in growth signaling. Cell 1994;78:5–8.
435. Dougall WC, Qian X, Peterson NC, et al: The *neu* oncogene: Signal transduction pathways, transformation mechanisms and evolving therapies. Oncogene 1994;9:2109–2123.
436. Karunagaran D, Tzahar E, Beerli RR, et al: ErbB-2 is a common auxiliary subunit of NDF and EGF receptors: Implications for breast cancer. EMBO J 1996;15: 254–2564.
437. Prigent SA, Lemoine NR, Hughes CM, et al: Expression of the c-erbB-3 protein in normal human adult and fetal tissues. Oncogene 1992;7:1273–1278.
438. Kaseda S, Ueda M, Ozawa S, et al: Expression of epidermal growth factor receptors in four histologic cell types of lung cancer. J Surg Oncol 1989;42:16–20.
439. Kern JA, Schwartz DA, Nordberg JE, et al: p185neu expression in human lung adenocarcinomas predicts shortened survival. Cancer Res 1990;50: 5184–5187.
440. Schneider PM, Hung MC, Chiocca SM, et al: Differential expression of the c-erbB-2 gene in human small cell and non-small cell lung cancer. Cancer Res 1989;49:4968–4971.
441. Weiner DB, Nordberg J, Robinson R, et al: Expression of the *neu* gene–encoded protein (P185neu) in human non–small cell carcinomas of the lung. Cancer Res 1990;50:421–425.
442. Fontanini G, De Laurentiis M, Vignati S, et al: Evaluation of epidermal growth factor–related growth factors and receptors and of neoangiogenesis in completely resected stage I–IIIA non–small-cell lung cancer: Amphiregulin and microvessel count are independent prognostic indicators of survival. Clin Cancer Res 1998;4:241–249.
443. Tateishi M, Ishida T, Kohdono S, et al: Prognostic influence of the co-expression of epidermal growth factor receptor and c-erbB-2 protein in human lung adenocarcinoma. Surg Oncol 1994;3:109–113.
444. Graziano SL, Kern JA, Herndon JE, et al: Analysis of neuroendocrine markers HER2 and CEA before and after chemotherapy in patients with stage IIIA non–small cell lung cancer: A Cancer and Leukemia Group B study. Lung Cancer 1998;21:203–211.
445. Damstrup L, Rude Voldborg B, Spang-Thomsen M, et al: In vitro invasion of small-cell lung cancer cell lines correlates with expression of epidermal growth factor receptor. Br J Cancer 1998;78:631–640.
446. Brandt-Rauf PW, Pincus MR, Carney WP: The c-erbB-2 protein in oncogenesis: Molecular structure to molecular epidemiology. Crit Rev Oncog 1994;5: 313–329.
447. Hynes NE, Stern DF: The biology of erbB-2/neu/HER-2 and its role in cancer. Biochim Biophys Acta 1994;1198: 165–184.
448. Shi D, He G, Cao S, et al: Overexpression of the c-ErbB-2/Neu-encoded p185 protein in primary lung cancer. Mol Carcinog 1992;5:213–218.

449. Hsieh CC, Chow KC, Fahn HJ, et al: Prognostic significance of HER-2/neu overexpression in stage I adenocarcinoma of lung. Ann Thorac Surg 1998;66: 1159–1163; discussion 1163–1164.
450. Brandt-Rauf PW, Luo JC, Carney WP, et al: Detection of increased amounts of the extracellular domain of the c-erbB-2 oncoprotein in serum during pulmonary carcinogenesis in humans. Int J Cancer 1994;56: 383–386.
451. Guinee DG Jr, Travis WD, Trivers GE, et al: Gender comparisons in human lung cancer: Analysis of *p53* mutations, anti-p53 serum antibodies and C-erbB-2 expression. Carcinogenesis 1995;16:993–1002.
452. Rachwal WJ, Bongiorno PF, Orringer MB, et al: Expression and activation of erbB-2 and epidermal growth factor receptor in lung adenocarcinomas. Br J Cancer 1995; 72:56–64.
453. Kern JA, Slebos RJ, Top B, et al: C-erbB-2 expression and codon 12 K-*ras* mutations both predict shortened survival for patients with pulmonary adenocarcinomas. J Clin Invest 1994;93:516–520.
454. Yi ES, Harclerode D, Gondo M, et al: High c-erbB-3 protein expression is associated with shorter survival in advanced non–small cell lung carcinomas. Mod Pathol 1997;10:142–148.
455. Wiethege T, Voss B, Muller KM: Detection of MDM2 proto-oncogene in paraffin embedded human bronchial epithelium. J Cancer Res Clin Oncol 1994;120: 252–255.
456. Wu X, Bayle JH, Olson D, Levine AJ: The p53-mdm-2 autoregulatory feedback loop. Genes Dev 1993;7: 1126–1132.
457. Barak Y, Juven T, Haffner R, Oren M: mdm2 expression is induced by wild type p53 activity. EMBO J 1993;12:461–468.
458. Martin K, Trouche D, Hagemeier C, et al: Stimulation of E2F1/DP1 transcriptional activity by MDM2 oncoprotein. Nature 1995;375:691–694.
459. Xiao ZX, Chen J, Levine AJ, et al: Interaction between the retinoblastoma protein and the oncoprotein MDM2. Nature 1995;375:694–698.
460. Maxwell SA: Selective compartmentalization of different mdm2 proteins within the nucleus. Anticancer Res 1994;14:2541–2547.
461. Ladanyi M, Cha C, Lewis R, et al: *MDM2* gene amplification in metastatic osteosarcoma. Cancer Res 1993;53: 16–18.
462. Pacinda SJ, Ledet SC, Gondo MM, et al: p53 and MDM2 immunostaining in pulmonary blastomas and bronchogenic carcinomas. Hum Pathol 1996;27:542–546.
463. Gorgoulis VG, Rassidakis GZ, Karameris AM, et al: Immunohistochemical and molecular evaluation of the *mdm-2* gene product in bronchogenic carcinoma. Mod Pathol 1996;9:544–554.
464. Marchetti A, Buttitta F, Pellegrini S, et al: *mdm2* gene amplification and overexpression in non–small cell lung carcinomas with accumulation of the p53 protein in the absence of *p53* gene mutations. Diagn Mol Pathol 1995;4:93–97.
465. Higashiyama M, Doi O, Kodama K, et al: *MDM2* gene amplification and expression in non–small-cell lung cancer: Immunohistochemical expression of its protein is a favourable prognostic marker in patients without p53 protein accumulation. Br J Cancer 1997;75: 1302–1308.
466. Swafford DS, Nikula KJ, Mitchell CE, Belinsky SA: Low frequency of alterations in *p53*, K-*ras*, and *mdm2* in rat lung neoplasms induced by diesel exhaust or carbon black. Carcinogenesis 1995;16:1215–1221.
466a. Zhang Y, Xiong Y, Yarbrough WG: ARF promotes MDM2 degradation and stabilizes p53: ARF-INK4a locus deletion impairs both the Rb and p53 tumor suppressor pathways. Cell 1998;92:725–734.
467. Cleghon V, Morrison DK: Raf-1 interacts with Fyn and Src in a non-phosphotyrosine-dependent manner. J Biol Chem 1994;269:17749–17755.
468. Farrar MA, Alberol I, Perlmutter RM: Activation of the Raf-1 kinase cascade by coumermycin-induced dimerization. Nature 1996;383:178–181.
469. Rommel C, Radziwill G, Lovric J, et al: Activated Ras displaces 14–3–3 protein from the amino terminus of c-Raf-1. Oncogene 1996;12:609–619.
470. Pumiglia KM, LeVine H, Haske T, et al: A direct interaction between G-protein beta gamma subunits and the Raf-1 protein kinase. J Biol Chem 1995;270: 14251–14254.
471. Galaktionov K, Lee AK, Eckstein J, et al: CDC25 phosphatases as potential human oncogenes. Science 1995;269:1575–1577.
472. Michaud NR, Fabian JR, Mathes KD, Morrison DK: 14–3–3 is not essential for Raf-1 function: Identification of Raf-1 proteins that are biologically activated in a 14–3–3- and Ras- independent manner. Mol Cell Biol 1995;15:3390–3397.
473. Kovacina KS, Yonezawa K, Brautigan DL, et al: Insulin activates the kinase activity of the Raf-1 proto-oncogene by increasing its serine phosphorylation. J Biol Chem 1990;265:12115–12118.
474. Morrison DK, Kaplan DR, Escobedo JA, et al: Direct activation of the serine/threonine kinase activity of Raf-1 through tyrosine phosphorylation by the PDGF beta-receptor. Cell 1989;58:649–657.
475. Blackshear PJ, Haupt DM, App H, Rapp UR: Insulin activates the Raf-1 protein kinase. J Biol Chem 1990; 265:12131–12134.
476. App H, Hazan R, Zilberstein A, et al: Epidermal growth factor (EGF) stimulates association and kinase activity of Raf-1 with the EGF receptor. Mol Cell Biol 1991;11:913–919.
477. Kolch W, Heidecker G, Kochs G, et al: Protein kinase C alpha activates RAF-1 by direct phosphorylation. Nature 1993;364:249–252.
478. Kyriakis JM, Force TL, Rapp UR, et al: Mitogen regulation of c-Raf-1 protein kinase activity toward mitogen-activated protein kinase-kinase. J Biol Chem 1993;268:16009–16019.
479. Howe LR, Leevers SJ, Gomez N, et al: Activation of the MAP kinase pathway by the protein kinase raf. Cell 1992;71:335–342.
480. Dent P, Haser W, Haystead TA, et al: Activation of mitogen-activated protein kinase kinase by v-Raf in NIH 3T3 cells and in vitro. Science 1992;257: 1404–1407.
481. Huang W, Alessandrini A, Crews CM, Erikson RL: Raf-1 forms a stable complex with Mek1 and activates

Mek1 by serine phosphorylation. Proc Natl Acad Sci USA 1993;90:10947–10951.

482. Muslin AJ, MacNicol AM, Williams LT: Raf-1 protein kinase is important for progesterone-induced *Xenopus* oocyte maturation and acts downstream of mos. Mol Cell Biol 1993;13:4197–4202.

483. Stokoe D, MacDonald SG, Cadwallader K, et al: Activation of Raf as a result of recruitment of the plasma membrane. Science 1994;264:1463–1467.

484. Graziano SL, Cowan BY, Carney DN, et al: Small cell lung cancer cell line derived from a primary tumor with a characteristic deletion of 3p. Cancer Res 1987;47: 2148–2145.

485. Stanton VP Jr, Cooper GM: Activation of human raf transforming genes by deletion of normal amino-terminal coding sequences. Mol Cell Biol 1987;7:1171–1179.

486. Storm SM, Rapp UR: Oncogene activation: c-*raf*-1 gene mutations in experimental and naturally occurring tumors. Toxicol Lett 1993;67:201–210.

487. Miwa W, Yasuda J, Yashimak K, et al: Absence of activating mutations of the RAF1 protooncogene in human lung cancer. Biol Chem Hoppe-Seyler 1994; 375:705–709.

488. Nickell-Brady C, Hahn FF, Finch GL, Belinsky SA: Analysis of K-*ras*, *p53* and c-*raf*-1 mutations in beryllium-induced rat lung tumors. Carcinogenesis 1994; 15:257–262.

489. Friend SH, Bernards R, Rogelj S, et al: A human DNA segment with properties of the gene that predisposes to retinoblastoma and osteosarcoma. Nature 1986;323: 643–646.

490. Knudson AG: Mutation and cancer: Statistical study of retinoblastoma. Proc Natl Acad Sci USA 1971;68: 820–823.

491. Chen WD, Otterson GA, Lipkowitz S, et al: Apoptosis is associated with cleavage of a 5 kDa fragment from RB which mimics dephosphorylation and modulates E2F binding. Oncogene 1997;14:1243–1248.

492. Zhu L, van den Heuvel S, Helin K, et al: Inhibition of cell proliferation by p107, a relative of the retinoblastoma protein. Genes Dev 1993;7:1111–1125.

493. Ewen ME, Xing YG, Lawrence JB, Livingston DM: Molecular cloning, chromosomal mapping, and expression of the cDNA for p107, a retinoblastoma gene product-related protein. Cell 1991;66:1155–1164.

494. Li Y, Graham C, Lacy S, et al: The adenovirus E1A-associated 130-kD protein is encoded by a member of the retinoblastoma gene family and physically interacts with cyclins A and E. Genes Dev 1993;7: 2366–2377.

495. Mayol X, Grana X, Baldi A, et al: Cloning of a new member of the retinoblastoma gene family *(pRb2)* which binds to the E1A transforming domain. Oncogene 1993;8:2561–2566.

496. Lees E, Faha B, Dulic V, et al: Cyclin E/cdk2 and cyclin A/cdk2 kinases associate with p107 and E2F in a temporally distinct manner. Genes Dev 1992;6: 1874–1885.

497. Cobrinik D, Whyte P, Peeper DS, et al: Cell cycle–specific association of E2F with the p130 E1A-binding protein. Genes Dev 1993;7:2392–2404.

498. Matsushime H, Roussel MF, Ashmun RA, Sherr CJ: Colony-stimulating factor 1 regulates novel cyclins during the G1 phase of the cell cycle. Cell 1991;65: 701–713.

499. Xiong Y, Zhang H, Beach D: D type cyclins associate with multiple protein kinases and the DNA replication and repair factor PCNA. Cell 1992;71:505–514.

500. Meyerson M, Harlow E: Identification of G1 kinase activity for cdk6, a novel cyclin D partner. Mol Cell Biol 1994;14:2077–2086.

501. Quelle DE, Ashmun RA, Shurtleff SA, et al: Overexpression of mouse D-type cyclins accelerates G1 phase in rodent fibroblasts. Genes Dev 1993;7: 1559–1571.

502. Hinds PW, Dowdy SF, Eaton EN, et al: Function of a human cyclin gene as an oncogene. Proc Natl Acad Sci USA 1994;91:709–713.

503. Kato J, Matsushime H, Hiebert SW, et al: Direct binding of cyclin D to the retinoblastoma gene product (pRb) and pRb phosphorylation by the cyclin D-dependent kinase CDK4. Genes Dev 1993;7:331–342.

504. Whyte P, Buchkovich KJ, Horowitz JM, et al: Association between an oncogene and an anti-oncogene: The adenovirus E1A proteins bind to the retinoblastoma gene product. Nature 1988;334:124–129.

505. Dyson N, Howley PM, Munger K, Harlow E: The human papillomavirus-16 E7 oncoprotein is able to bind to the retinoblastoma gene product. Science 1989;243:934–937.

506. DeCaprio JA, Ludlow JW, Figge J, et al: SV40 large tumor antigen forms a specific complex with the product of the retinoblastoma susceptibility gene. Cell 1988;54:275–283.

507. Sherr CJ: Mammalian G1 cyclins. Cell 1993;73: 1059–1065.

508. Hinds PW, Mittnacht S, Dulic V, et al: Regulation of retinoblastoma protein functions by ectopic expression of human cyclins. Cell 1992;70:993–1006.

509. Zamanian M, La Thangue NB: Adenovirus E1A prevents the retinoblastoma gene product from repressing the activity of a cellular transcription factor. EMBO J 1992;11:2603–2610.

510. Hiebert SW, Chellappan SP, Horowitz JM, Nevins JR: The interaction of RB with E2F coincides with an inhibition of the transcriptional activity of E2F. Genes Dev 1992;6:177–185.

511. Nevins JR: E2F: A link between the Rb tumor suppressor protein and viral oncoproteins. Science 1992;258: 424–429.

512. Weinberg RA: The retinoblastoma protein and cell cycle control. Cell 1995;81:323–330.

513. Chellappan SP, Hiebert S, Mudryj M, et al: The E2F transcription factor is a cellular target for the RB protein. Cell 1991;65:1053–1061.

514. Lam EW, La Thangue NB: DP and E2F proteins: Coordinating transcription with cell cycle progression. Curr Opin Cell Biol 1994;6:859–866.

515. Kaelin WG Jr, Krek W, Sellers WR, et al: Expression cloning of a cDNA encoding a retinoblastoma-binding protein with E2F-like properties. Cell 1992;70:351–364.

516. Helin K, Lees JA, Vidal M, et al: A cDNA encoding a pRB-binding protein with properties of the transcription factor E2F. Cell 1992;70:337–350.

517. Shan B, Zhu X, Chen PL, et al: Molecular cloning of cellular genes encoding retinoblastoma-associated pro-

teins: Identification of a gene with properties of the transcription factor E2F. Mol Cell Biol 1992;12: 5620–5631.

518. Hijmans EM, Voorhoeve PM, Beijersbergen RL, et al: E2F-5, a new E2F family member that interacts with p130 in vivo. Mol Cell Biol 1995;15:3082–3089.
519. Buck V, Allen KE, Sorensen T, et al: Molecular and functional characterisation of E2F-5, a new member of the E2F family. Oncogene 1995;11:31–38.
520. Lees JA, Saito M, Vidal M, et al: The retinoblastoma protein binds to a family of E2F transcription factors. Mol Cell Biol 1993;13:7813–7825.
521. Beijersbergen RL, Kerkhoven RM, Zhu L, et al: E2F-4, a new member of the E2F gene family, has oncogenic activity and associates with p107 in vivo. Genes Dev 1994;8:2680–2690.
522. Ginsberg D, Vairo G, Chittenden T, et al: E2F-4, a new member of the E2F transcription factor family, interacts with p107. Genes Dev 1994;8:2665–2679.
523. Vairo G, Livingston DM, Ginsberg D: Functional interaction between E2F-4 and p130: Evidence for distinct mechanisms underlying growth suppression by different retinoblastoma protein family members. Genes Dev 1995;9:869–881.
524. Sardet C, Vidal M, Cobrinik D, et al: E2F-4 and E2F-5, two members of the E2F family, are expressed in the early phases of the cell cycle. Proc Natl Acad Sci USA 1995;92:2403–2407.
525. Sherr CJ: Cancer cell cycles. Science 1996;274: 1672–1677.
526. Wu X, Levine AJ: p53 and E2F-1 cooperate to mediate apoptosis. Proc Natl Acad Sci USA 1994;91: 3602–3606.
527. Chellappan S, Kraus VB, Kroger B, et al: Adenovirus E1A, simian virus 40 tumor antigen, and human papillomavirus E7 protein share the capacity to disrupt the interaction between transcription factor E2F and the retinoblastoma gene product. Proc Natl Acad Sci USA 1992;89: 4549–4553.
528. Hamel PA, Gill RM, Phillips RA, Gallie BL: Transcriptional repression of the E2-containing promoters EIIaE, c-myc, and RB1 by the product of the *RB1* gene. Mol Cell Biol 1992;12:3431–3438.
529. Pagano M, Durst M, Joswig S, et al: Binding of the human E2F transcription factor to the retinoblastoma protein but not to cyclin A is abolished in HPV-16–immortalized cells. Oncogene 1992;7:1681–1686.
530. Wang JY, Knudsen ES, Welch PJ: The retinoblastoma tumor suppressor protein. Adv Cancer Res 1994;64: 25–85.
531. Blanquet V, Turleau C, Gross-Morand MS, et al: Spectrum of germline mutations in the *RB1* gene: A study of 232 patients with hereditary and non-hereditary retinoblastoma. Hum Molec Genet 1995;4:383–388.
532. Ohtani-Fujita N, Fujita T, Aoike A, et al: CpG methylation inactivates the promoter activity of the human retinoblastoma tumor-suppressor gene. Oncogene 1993;8:1063–1067.
533. Ray SK, Arroyo M, Bagchi S, Raychaudhuri P: Identification of a 60-kilodalton Rb-binding protein, RBP60, that allows the Rb-E2F complex to bind DNA. Mol Cell Biol 1992;12:4327–4333.
534. Kaye FJ, Kratzke RA, Gerster JL, Horowitz JM: A single amino acid substitution results in a retinoblastoma protein defective in phosphorylation and oncoprotein binding. Proc Natl Acad Sci USA 1990;87: 6922–6926.
535. Johnson BE, Sakaguchi AY, Gazdar AF, et al: Restriction fragment length polymorphism studies show consistent loss of chromosome 3p alleles in small cell lung cancer patients' tumors. J Clin Invest 1988;82: 502–507.
536. Naylor SL, Johnson BE, Minna JD, Sakaguchi AY: Loss of heterozygosity of chromosome 3p markers in small-cell lung cancer. Nature 1987;329:451–454.
537. Gouyer V, Gazzeri S, Brambilla E, et al: Loss of heterozygosity at the RB locus correlates with loss of RB protein in primary malignant neuro-endocrine lung carcinomas. Int J Cancer 1994;58:818–824.
538. Reissmann PT, Koga H, Takahashi R, et al: Inactivation of the retinoblastoma susceptibility gene in non–small-cell lung cancer. The Lung Cancer Study Group. Oncogene 1993;8:1913–1919.
539. Sachse R, Murakami Y, Shiraishi M, et al: DNA aberrations at the retinoblastoma gene locus in human squamous cell carcinomas of the lung. Oncogene 1994;9: 39–47.
540. Higashiyama M, Doi O, Kodama K, et al: Retinoblastoma protein expression in lung cancer: An immunohistochemical analysis. Oncology 1994;51:544–551.
541. Xu HJ, Hu SX, Cagle PT, et al: Absence of retinoblastoma protein expression in primary non–small cell lung carcinomas. Cancer Res 1991;51:2735–2739.
542. Hensel CH, Hsieh CL, Gazdar AF, et al: Altered structure and expression of the human retinoblastoma susceptibility gene in small cell lung cancer. Cancer Res 1990; 50:3067–3072.
543. Horowitz JM, Park SH, Bogenmann E, et al: Frequent inactivation of the retinoblastoma anti-oncogene is restricted to a subset of human tumor cells. Proc Natl Acad Sci USA 1990;87:2775–2779.
544. Yokota J, Akiyama T, Fung YK, et al: Altered expression of the retinoblastoma *(RB)* gene in small-cell carcinoma of the lung. Oncogene 1988;3:471–475.
545. Cagle PT, el-Naggar AK, Xu HJ, et al: Differential retinoblastoma protein expression in neuroendocrine tumors of the lung: Potential diagnostic implications. Am J Pathol 1997;150:393–400.
546. Shimizu E, Coxon A, Otterson GA, et al: RB protein status and clinical correlation from 171 cell lines representing lung cancer, extrapulmonary small cell carcinoma, and mesothelioma. Oncogene 1994;9:2441–2448.
547. Harbour JW, Lai SL, Whang-Peng J, et al: Abnormalities in structure and expression of the human retinoblastoma gene in SCLC. Science 1988;241:353–357.
548. Mori N, Yokota J, Akiyama T, et al: Variable mutations of the *RB* gene in small-cell lung carcinoma. Oncogene 1990;5:1713–1717.
549. Rygaard K, Sorenson GD, Pettengill OS, et al: Abnormalities in structure and expression of the retinoblastoma gene in small cell lung cancer cell lines and xenografts in nude mice. Cancer Res 1990;50:5312–5317.
550. Gouyer V, Gazzeri S, Bolon I, et al: Mechanism of retinoblastoma gene inactivation in the spectrum of

neuroendocrine lung tumors. Am J Respir Cell Mol Biol 1998;18:188–196.

551. Barbareschi M, Girlando S, Mauri FA, et al: Tumour suppressor gene products, proliferation, and differentiation markers in lung neuroendocrine neoplasms. J Pathol 1992;166:343–350.

552. Xu HJ, Quinlan DC, Davidson AG, et al: Altered retinoblastoma protein expression and prognosis in early-stage non–small-cell lung carcinoma. J Natl Cancer Inst 1994;86:695–699.

553. Leonard RCF, MacKay T, Brown A, et al: Small-cell lung cancer after retinoblastoma. Lancet 1988;2:1503.

554. Finlay C, Hinds P, Levine AJ: The *p53* protooncogene can act as a suppressor of transformation. Cell 1989;57: 1083–1093.

555. Haldar S, Negrini M, Monne M, et al: Down-regulation of bcl-2 by p53 in breast cancer cells. Cancer Res 1994;54:2095–2097.

556. Hunter T Pines J. Cyclins and cancer II: Cyclin D and cdk inhibitors come of age. Cell 1994;79:573–582.

557. Vogelstein B, Kinzler KW: p53 function and dysfunction. Cell 1992;70:523–526.

558. Yonish RE, Resnitzky D, Lotem J, et al: Wild-type p53 induces apoptosis of myeloid leukaemic cells that is inhibited by interleukin-6. Nature 1991;353:345–347.

559. Livingstone LR, White A, Sprouse J, et al: Altered cell cycle arrest and gene amplification potential accompany loss of wild type *p53* alleles. Cell 1992;70:923–935.

560. Kastan MB, Zhan Q, el-Deiry WS, et al: A mammalian cell cycle checkpoint pathway utilizing p53 and GADD45 is defective in ataxia-telangiectasia. Cell 1992;71:587–597.

561. Smith ML, Chen IT, Zhan Q, et al: Interaction of the p53-regulated protein GADD45 with proliferating cell nuclear antigen. Science 1994;266:1376–1380.

562. El-Deiry WS, Tokino T, Velculescu VE, et al: WAF1, a potential mediator of p53 tumor suppression. Cell 1993;75:817–825.

563. Harper JW, Adami GR, Wei N, et al: The p21 Cdk-interacting protein Cip1 is a potent inhibitor of G1 cyclin-dependent kinases. Cell 1993;75:805–816.

564. Soini Y, Nuorva K, Kamel D, et al: Presence of human papillomavirus DNA and abnormal p53 protein accumulation in lung carcinoma. Thorax 1996;51: 887–883.

565. Michalowitz D, Halvey O, Oren M: Conditional inhibition of transformation and of cell proliferation by a temperature-sensitive mutant of p53. Cell 1990;62: 671–680.

566. Chen X, Ko LJ, Jayaraman L, Prives C: p53 levels, functional domains, and DNA damage determine the extent of the apoptotic response of tumor cells. Genes Dev 1996;10:2438–2451.

567. Buckbinder L, Talbott R, Velasco-Miguel S, et al: Induction of the growth inhibitor IGF-binding protein 3 by p53. Nature 1995;377:646–649.

568. Miyashita T, Krajewski S, Krajewska M, et al: Tumor suppressor *p53* is a regulator of *bcl-2* and *bax* gene expression in vitro and in vivo. Oncogene 1994;9: 1799–1805.

569. Reich NC, Levine AJ: Growth regulation of a cellular tumor antigen, p53, in nontransformed cells. Nature 1984;308:199.

570. Finlay CA, Hinds PW, Tan TH, et al: Activating mutations for transformation by *p53* produce a gene product that forms an hsc70-p53 complex with an altered half-life. Mol Cell Biol 1988;8:531–539.

571. Fields S, Jang SJ: Presence of a potent transcription activating sequence in the p53 protein. Science 1990; 249:1046–1049.

572. Raycroft L, Wu HY, Lozano G: Transcriptional activation by wild type but not transforming mutants of the *p53* anti-oncogene. Science 1990;249:1049–1051.

573. Band V, Dalal S, Delmolino L, Androphy EJ: Enhanced degradation of p53 protein in HPV-6 and BPV-1 E6-immortalized human mammary epithelial cells. EMBO J 1993;12:1847–1852.

574. Mietz JA, Unger T, Huibregtse JM, Howley PM: The transcriptional transactivation function of wild-type p53 is inhibited by SV40 large T-antigen and by HPV-16 E6 oncoprotein. EMBO J 1992;11:5013–5020.

575. Haines DS, Landers JE, Engle LJ, George DL: Physical and functional interaction between wild-type p53 and mdm2 proteins. Mol Cell Biol 1994;14:1171–1178.

576. Perry ME, Piette J, Zawadzki JA, et al: The *mdm-2* gene is induced in response to UV light in a p53-dependent manner. Proc Natl Acad Sci USA 1993;90: 11623–11627.

577. Juven T, Barak Y, Zauberman A, et al: Wild type p53 can mediate sequence-specific transactivation of an internal promoter within the *mdm2* gene. Oncogene 1993;8: 3411–3416.

578. Kunz C, Pebler S, Otte J, von der Ahe D: Differential regulation of plasminogen activator and inhibitor gene transcription by the tumor suppressor *p53*. Nucleic Acids Res 1995;23:3710–3717.

579. Oberosler P, Hloch P, Ramsperger U, Stahl H: *p53*-catalyzed annealing of complementary single-stranded nucleic acids. EMBO J 1993;12:2389–2396.

580. Ragimov N, Krauskopf A, Navot N, et al: Wild-type but not mutant p53 can repress transcription initiation in vitro by interfering with the binding of basal transcription factors to the TATA motif. Oncogene 1993; 8:1183–1193.

581. Hainaut P, Hall A, Milner J: Analysis of p53 quaternary structure in relation to sequence-specific DNA binding. Oncogene 1994;9:299–303.

582. Stenger JE, Tegtmeyer P, Mayr GA, et al: p53 oligomerization and DNA looping are linked with transcriptional activation. EMBO J 1994;13:6011–6020.

583. Tarunina M, Grimaldi M, Ruaro E, et al: Selective loss of endogenous p21waf1/cip1 induction underlies the G1 checkpoint defect of monomeric p53 proteins. Oncogene 1996;13:589–598.

584. Mummenbrauer T, Janus F, Muller B, et al: p53 protein exhibits 3′-to-5′ exonuclease activity. Cell 1996; 85: 1089–1099.

585. Hollstein M, Sidransky D, Vogelstein B, Harris CC: *p53* mutations in human cancers. Science 1991;253:49–53.

586. Ludes-Meyers JH, Subler MA, Shivakumar CV, et al: Transcriptional activation of the human epidermal growth factor receptor promoter by human p53. Mol Cell Biol 1996;16:6009–6019.

587. Jego N, Thomas G, Hamelin R: Short direct repeats flanking deletions, and duplicating insertions in *p53* gene in human cancers. Oncogene 1993;8:209–213.

588. Miller CW, Chumakov A, Said J, et al: Mutant p53 proteins have diverse intracellular abilities to oligomerize and activate transcription. Oncogene 1993;8: 1815–1824.
589. Tenaud C, Negoescu A, Labat-Moleur F, et al: p53 immunolabeling in archival paraffin-embedded tissues: Optimal protocol based on microwave heating for eight antibodies on lung carcinomas. Mod Pathol 1994;7:853–859.
590. Nishio M, Koshikawa T, Kuroishi T, et al: Prognostic significance of abnormal p53 accumulation in primary, resected non–small-cell lung cancers. J Clin Oncol 1996;14:497–502.
591. Finkelstein SD, Przygodzki R, Pricolo VE, et al: Prediction of biologic aggressiveness in colorectal cancer by p53/K-ras-2 topographic genotyping. Molec Diag 1996;1:5–28.
592. Lane DP: p53, guardian of the genome. Nature 1992; 358:15–16.
593. Lane DP: p53 and human cancers. Br Med Bull 1994;50: 582–599.
594. Westra WH, Offerhaus GJ, Goodman SN, et al: Overexpression of the *p53* tumor suppressor gene product in primary lung adenocarcinomas is associated with cigarette smoking. Am J Surg Pathol 1993;17:213–220.
595. Dalquen P, Sauter G, Torhorst J, et al: Nuclear p53 overexpression is an independent prognostic parameter in node-negative non–small cell lung carcinoma. J Pathol 1996;178:53–58.
596. Brambilla E, Gazzeri S, Moro D, et al: Immunohistochemical study of p53 in human lung carcinomas. Am J Pathol 1993;143:199–210.
597. Fontanini G, Bigini D, Vignati S, et al: p53 expression in non–small cell lung cancer: Clinical and biological correlations. Anticancer Res 1993;13:737–742.
598. Minna JD: The molecular biology of lung cancer pathogenesis. Chest 1993;103(4 Suppl):449S–456S.
599. D'Amico D, Carbone D, Mitsudomi T, et al: High frequency of somatically acquired p53 mutations in small-cell lung cancer cell lines and tumors. Oncogene 1992; 7:339–346.
600. Takahashi T, Takahashi T, Suzuki H, et al: The *p53* gene is very frequently mutated in small-cell lung cancer with a distinct nucleotide substitution pattern. Oncogene 1991;6:1775–1778.
601. Bennett WP, Colby TV, Travis WD, et al: p53 protein accumulates frequently in early bronchial neoplasia. Cancer Res 1993;53:4817–4822.
602. Harris CC, Hollstein M: Clinical implications of the *p53* tumor suppressor gene. N Engl J Med 1993;329: 1318–1327.
603. Walker C, Robertson LJ, Myskow MW, et al: *p53* expression in normal and dysplastic bronchial epithelium and in lung carcinomas. Br J Cancer 1994;70: 297–303.
604. Fontanini G, Vignati S, Bigini D, et al: Human non–small cell lung cancer: p53 protein accumulation is an early event and persists during metastatic progression [see comments]. J Pathol 1994;174:23–31.
605. Hainaut P, Soussi T, Shomer B, et al: Database of *p53* gene somatic mutations in human tumors and cell lines: Updated compilation and future prospects. Nucleic Acids Res 1997;25:151–157.
606. Iggo R, Gatter K, Bartek J, et al: Increased expression of mutant forms of *p53* oncogene in primary lung cancer. Lancet 1990;335:675–679.
607. Holliday R, Grigg GW: DNA methylation and mutation. Mutat Res 1993;285:61–67.
608. Ehrlich M, Zhang XY, Inamdar NM: Spontaneous deamination of cytosine and 5-methylcytosine residues in DNA and replacement of 5-methylcytosine residues with cytosine residues. Mutat Res 1990;238:277–286.
609. Ronai ZA, Gradia S, Peterson LA, Hecht SS: G to A transitions and G to T transversions in codon 12 of the Ki-*ras* oncogene isolated from mouse lung tumors induced by 4-(methylnitrosamino)-1-(3-pyridyl)-1-butanone (NNK) and related DNA methylating and pyridyloxobutylating agents. Carcinogenesis 1993;14: 2419–2422.
610. Mitsudomi T, Oyama T, Kusano T, et al: Mutations of the *p53* gene as a predictor of poor prognosis in patients with non-small-cell lung cancer. J Natl Cancer Inst 1993;85:2018–2023.
611. Lohmann D, Putz B, Reich U, et al: Mutational spectrum of the *p53* gene in human small-cell lung cancer and relationship to clinicopathological data. Am J Pathol 1993;142:907–915.
612. Sameshima Y, Matsuno Y, Hirohashi S, et al: Alterations of the *p53* gene are common and critical events for the maintenance of malignant phenotypes in small-cell lung carcinoma. Oncogene 1992;7:451–457.
613. Mack U, Ukena D, Montenarh M, Sybrecht GW: Serum anti-p53 antibodies in patients with lung cancer. Oncol Rep 2000;7:669–674.
613a. Kaghad M, Bonnet H, Yang A, et al: Monoallelically expressed gene related to p53 at 1p36, a region frequently deleted in neuroblastoma and other human cancers. Cell 1997;90:809–819.
614. Hensel CH, Xiang RH, Sakaguchi AY, Naylor SL: Use of the single strand conformation polymorphism technique and PCR to detect *p53* gene mutations in small cell lung cancer. Oncogene 1991;6:1067–1071.
615. Welsh JA, Castren K, Vahakangas KH: Single-strand conformation polymorphism analysis to detect *p53* mutations: Characterization and development of controls. Clin Chem 1997;43:2251–2255.
616. Fearon ER, Jones PA: Progressing toward a molecular description of colorectal cancer development. FASEB J 1992;6:2783–2790.
617. Nagase H, Nakamura Y: Mutations of the APC (adenomatous polyposis coli) gene. Hum Mutat 1993; 2:425–434.
618. Su LK, Vogelstein B, Kinzler KW: Association of the APC tumor suppressor protein with catenins. Science 1993;262:1734–1737.
619. Matsumine A, Ogai A, Senda T, et al: Binding of APC to the human homolog of the *Drosophila* discs large tumor suppressor protein [see comments]. Science 1996;272:1020–1023.
620. Fearon ER: Genetic alterations underlying colorectal tumorigenesis. Cancer Surv 1992;12:119–136.
621. Bourne HR: Colon cancer: Suppression with a difference [news]. Nature 1991;353:696–697.
622. Cooper CA, Bubb VJ, Smithson N, et al: Loss of heterozygosity at 5q21 in non-small cell lung cancer: A

frequent event but without evidence of APC mutation. J Pathol 1996;180:33–37.
623. Edelman GM: Morphoregulatory molecules. Biochemistry 1988;27:3533.
624. Fong KM, Zimmerman PV, Smith PJ: Tumor progression and loss of heterozygosity at 5q and 18q in non-small cell lung cancer. Cancer Res 1995;55:220–223.
625. Hosoe S, Ueno K, Shigedo Y, et al: A frequent deletion of chromosome 5q21 in advanced small cell and non–small cell carcinoma of the lung. Cancer Res 1994;54: 1787–1790.
626. Ashton-Rickardt PG, Wyllie AH, Bird CC, et al: *MCC*, a candidate familial polyposis gene in 5q.21, shows frequent allele loss in colorectal and lung cancer. Oncogene 1991;6:1881–1886.
627. Chen IT, Smith ML, O'Connor PM, Fornace AJ Jr: Direct interaction of Gadd45 with PCNA and evidence for competitive interaction of Gadd45 and p21Waf1/Cip1 with PCNA. Oncogene 1995;11:1931–1937.
628. Waga S, Hannon GJ, Beach D, Stillman B: The p21 inhibitor of cyclin-dependent kinases controls DNA replication by interaction with PCNA. Nature 1994; 369:574–578.
629. Kearsey JM, Coates PJ, Prescott AR, et al: Gadd45 is a nuclear cell cycle regulated protein which interacts with p21Cip1. Oncogene 1995;11:1675–1683.
630. Dimri GP, Nakanishi M, Desprez PY, et al: Inhibition of E2F activity by the cyclin-dependent protein kinase inhibitor p21 in cells expressing or lacking a functional retinoblastoma protein. Mol Cell Biol 1996; 16:2987–2997.
631. Zeng YX, el-Deiry WS: Regulation of $p21^{WAF1/CIP1}$ expression by p53-independent pathways. Oncogene 1996;12:1557–1564.
632. Sheikh MS, Li XS, Chen JC, et al: Mechanisms of regulation of *WAF1/Cip1* gene expression in human breast carcinoma: Role of p53-dependent and independent signal transduction pathways. Oncogene 1994;9: 3407–3415.
633. Sheikh MS, Rochefort H, Garcia M: Overexpression of p21WAF1/CIP1 induces growth arrest, giant cell formation and apoptosis in human breast carcinoma cell lines. Oncogene 1995;11:1899–1905.
634. Stegmaier K, Takeuchi S, Golub TR, et al: Mutational analysis of the candidate tumor suppressor genes *TEL* and *KIP1* in childhood acute lymphoblastic leukemia. Cancer Res 1996;56:1413–1417.
635. Pietenpol JA, Bohlander SK, Sato Y, et al: Assignment of the human p27Kip1 gene to 12p13 and its analysis in leukemias. Cancer Res 1995;55:1206–1210.
636. Ponce-Castaneda MV, Lee MH, Latres E, et al: p27Kip1: Chromosomal mapping to 12p12-12p13.1 and absence of mutations in human tumors. Cancer Res 1995;55:1211–1214.
637. Larsen CJ: p16INK4a: A gene with a dual capacity to encode unrelated proteins that inhibit cell cycle progression. Oncogene 1996;12:2041–2044.
638. Kamb A, Gruis NA, Weaver-Feldhaus J, et al: A cell cycle regulator potentially involved in genesis of many tumor types. Science 1994;264:436–440.
639. Nobori T, Miura K, Wu DJ, et al: Deletions of the cyclin-dependent kinase-4 inhibitor gene in multiple human cancers. Nature 1994;368:753–756.
639a. Quelle DE, Zindy F, Ashmun RA, Sherr CJ: Alternative reading frames of the INK4a tumor-suppressor gene encoded two unrelated proteins capable of inducing cell cycle arrest. Cell 1995;83:993–1000.
639b. Pomerantz J, Schreiber-Agus N, Liegois NJ, et al: The Ink4a tumor-suppressor gene product p19Arf, interacts with MDM2 and neutralizes MDM2's inhibition of p53. Cell 1998;92:713–723.
640. Li JM, Nichols MA, Chandrasekharan S, et al: Transforming growth factor beta activates the promoter of cyclin-dependent kinase inhibitor p15INK4B through an Sp1 consensus site. J Biol Chem 1995;270: 26750–26753.
641. Hannon GJ Beach D: p15INK4B is a potential effector of TGF-beta-induced cell cycle arrest. Nature 1994; 371:257–261.
642. Nakagawa K, Conrad NK, Williams JP, et al: Mechanism of inactivation of CDKN2 and MTS2 in non-small cell lung cancer and association with advanced stage. Oncogene 1995;11:1843–1851.
643. Ookawa K, Shiseki M, Takahashi R, et al: Reconstitution of the *RB* gene suppresses the growth of small-cell lung carcinoma cells carrying multiple genetic alterations. Oncogene 1993;8:2175–2181.
644. Merlo A, Herman JG, Mao L, et al: 5′ CpG island methylation is associated with transcriptional silencing of the tumour suppressor *p16/CDKN2/MTS1* in human cancers. Nat Med 1995;1:686–692.
645. Takeshima Y, Yamasaki M, Nishisaka T, et al: *p21WAF1/CIP1* expression in primary lung adenocarcinomas: Heterogeneous expression in tumor tissues and correlation with p53 expression and proliferative activities. Carcinogenesis 1998;19:1755–1761.
646. Hayashi H, Miyamoto H, Ito T, et al: Analysis of p21Waf1/Cip1 expression in normal, premalignant, and malignant cells during the development of human lung adenocarcinoma. Am J Pathol 1997;151: 461–70.
647. Komiya T, Hosono Y, Hirashima T, et al: p21 expression as a predictor for favorable prognosis in squamous cell carcinoma of the lung [in process citation]. Clin Cancer Res 1997;3:1831–1835.
648. Caputi M, Esposito V, Baldi A, et al: p21waf1/cip1mda-6 expression in non–small-cell lung cancer: Relationship to survival. Am J Respir Cell Mol Biol 1998;18:213–217.
649. Stefanaki K, Rontogiannis D, Vamvouka C, et al: Immunohistochemical detection of bcl2, p53, mdm2 and p21/waf1 proteins in small-cell lung carcinomas. Anticancer Res 1998;18:1689–1695.
650. Esposito V, Baldi A, De Luca A, et al: Prognostic role of the cyclin-dependent kinase inhibitor p27 in non-small cell lung cancer. Cancer Res 1997;57: 3381–3385.
651. Yatabe Y, Masuda A, Koshikawa T, et al: p27KIP1 in human lung cancers: Differential changes in small cell and non-small cell carcinomas. Cancer Res 1998;58: 1042–1047.
652. Kawana H, Tamaru J, Tanaka T, et al: Role of p27Kip1 and cyclin-dependent kinase 2 in the proliferation of non–small cell lung cancer. Am J Pathol 1998;153: 505–513.

653. Wang X, Gorospe M, Huang Y, Holbrook NJ: p27Kip1 overexpression causes apoptotic death of mammalian cells. Oncogene 1997;15:2991–2997.
654. Hatada I, Mukai T: Genomic imprinting of p57KIP2, a cyclin-dependent kinase inhibitor, in mouse. Nat Genet 1995;11:204–206.
655. Kondo M, Matsuoka S, Uchida K, et al: Selective maternal-allele loss in human lung cancers of the maternally expressed *p57KIP2* gene at 11p15.5. Oncogene 1996; 12:1365–1368.
656. Washimi O, Nagatake M, Osada H, et al: In vivo occurrence of p16 (MTS1) and p15 (MTS2) alterations preferentially in non-small cell lung cancers. Cancer Res 1995;55:514–517.
657. Okamoto A, Hussain SP, Hagiwara K, et al: Mutations in the *p16INK4/MTS1/CDKN2*, *p15INK4B/MTS2*, and *p18* genes in primary and metastatic lung cancer. Cancer Res 1995;55:1448–1451.
658. Kelley MJ, Nakagawa K, Steinberg SM, et al: Differential inactivation of CDKN2 and Rb protein in non–small-cell and small-cell lung cancer cell lines. J Natl Cancer Inst 1995;87:756–761.
659. Shapiro GI, Edwards CD, Kobzik L, et al: Reciprocal Rb inactivation and p16INK4 expression in primary lung cancers and cell lines. Cancer Res 1995;55: 505–509.
660. Kratzke RA, Greatens TM, Rubins JB, et al: Rb and p16INK4a expression in resected non–small cell lung tumors. Cancer Res 1996;56:3415–3420.
661. Sakaguchi M, Fujii Y, Hirabayashi H, et al: Inversely correlated expression of p16 and Rb protein in non–small cell lung cancers: An immunohistochemical study. Int J Cancer 1996;65:442–445.
662. Geradts J, Kratzke RA, Niehans GA, Lincoln CE: Immunohistochemical detection of the cyclin-dependent kinase inhibitor 2/multiple tumor suppressor gene 1 (CDKN2/MTS1) product p16INK4A in archival human solid tumors: Correlation with retinoblastoma protein expression. Cancer Res 1995;55:6006–6011.
663. Okamoto A, Demetrick DJ, Spillare EA, et al: Mutations and altered expression of p16INK4 in human cancer. Proc Natl Acad Sci USA 1994;91: 11045–11049.
664. Cairns P, Polascik TJ, Eby Y, et al: Frequency of homozygous deletion at p16/CDKN2 in primary human tumours. Nat Genet 1995;11:210–212.
665. Marchetti A, Buttitta F, Pellegrini S, et al: Alterations of P16 (MTS1) in node-positive non–small cell lung carcinomas. J Pathol 1997;181:178–182.
666. de Vos S, Miller CW, Takeuchi S, et al: Alterations of CDKN2 (p16) in non–small cell lung cancer. Genes Chromosomes Cancer 1995;14:164–170.
667. Cairns P, Mao L, Merlo A, et al: Rates of *p16 (MTS1)* mutations in primary tumors with 9p loss [letter; comment]. Science 1994;265:415–417.
668. Gazzeri S, Gouyer V, Vour'ch C, et al: Mechanisms of p16INK4A inactivation in non–small cell lung cancers. Oncogene 1998;16:497–504.
669. Packenham JP, Taylor JA, White CM, et al: Homozygous deletions at chromosome 9p21 and mutation analysis of *p16* and *p15* in microdissected primary non-small cell lung cancers. Clin Cancer Res 1995;1:687–690.
669a. Sjalander A, Birgander R, Rannug A, et al: Association between the p21 codon 31 A1 (arg) allele and lung cancer. Human Heredity 1996;46:221–225.
670. Colman SD, Wallace MR: Neurofibromatosis type 1. Eur J Cancer 1994;13:1974–1981.
671. Andersen LB, Ballester R, Marchuk DA, et al: A conserved alternative splice in the von Recklinghausen neurofibromatosis *(NF1)* gene produces two neurofibromin isoforms, both of which have GTPase-activating protein activity. Mol Cell Biol 1993;13:487–495.
672. Xu GF, O'Connell P, Viskochil D, et al: The neurofibromatosis type 1 gene encodes a protein related to GAP. Cell 1990;62:599–608.
673. Xu GF, Lin B, Tanaka K, et al: The catalytic domain of the neurofibromatosis type 1 gene product stimulates *ras* GTPase and complements IRA mutants of *S. cerevisiae*. Cell 1990;63:835–841.
674. DeClue JE, Papageorge AG, Fletcher JA, et al: Abnormal regulation of mammalian p21ras contributes to malignant tumor growth in von Recklinghausen (type 1) neurofibromatosis. Cell 1992;69:265–273.
675. Thomas G, Merel P, Sanson M, et al: Neurofibromatosis type 2. Eur J Cancer 1994;13:1981–1987.
676. den Bakker MA, Riegman PH, Hekman RA, et al: The product of the *NF2* tumour suppressor gene localizes near the plasma membrane and is highly expressed in muscle cells. Oncogene 1995;10:757–763.
677. Trofatter JA, MacCollin MM, Rutter JL, et al: A novel moesin-, ezrin-, radixin-like gene is a candidate for the neurofibromatosis 2 tumor suppressor [published erratum appears in Cell 1993;75:826]. Cell 1993;72:791–800.
678. Takeshima H, Izawa I, Lee PS, et al: Detection of cellular proteins that interact with the *NF2* tumor suppressor gene product. Oncogene 1994;9:2135–2144.
679. Wallace MR, Marchuk DA, Andersen LB, et al: Type 1 neurofibromatosis gene: Identification of a large transcript disrupted in three NF1 patients [published erratum appears in Science 1990;250:1749]. Science 1990; 249:181–186.
680. Viskochil D, Buchberg AM, Xu G, et al: Deletions and a translocation interrupt a cloned gene at the neurofibromatosis type 1 locus. Cell 1990;62:187–192.
681. Gutmann DH, Giordano MJ, Mahadeo DK, et al: Increased neurofibromatosis 1 gene expression in astrocytic tumors: Positive regulation by p21-ras. Oncogene 1996;12:2121–2127.
682. Valero MC, Velasco E, Moreno F, Hernandez-Chico C: Characterization of four mutations in the neurofibromatosis type 1 gene by denaturing gradient gel electrophoresis (DGGE). Hum Mol Genet 1994;3: 639–641.
683. Hutter P, Antonarakis SE, Delozier-Blanchet CD, Morris MA: Exon skipping associated with A→G transition at +4 of the IVS33 splice donor site of the neurofibromatosis type 1 *(NF1)* gene. Hum Mol Genet 1994;3:663–665.
684. Purandare SM, Lanyon WG, Connor JM: Characterisation of inherited and sporadic mutations in neurofibromatosis type-1. Hum Mol Genet 1994;3:1109–1115.
685. Heim RA, Kam-Morgan LN, Binnie CG, et al: Distribution of 13 truncating mutations in the neurofibromatosis 1 gene. Hum Mol Genet 1995;4:975–981.

686. Ainsworth P, Rodenhiser D, Stuart A, Jung J: Characterization of an intron 31 splice junction mutation in the neurofibromatosis type 1 *(NF1)* gene. Hum Mol Genet 1994;3:1179–1181.

687. Bourn D, Carter SA, Mason S, et al: Germline mutations in the neurofibromatosis type 2 tumour suppressor gene. Hum Mol Genet 1994;3:813–816.

688. Sainz J, Figueroa K, Baser ME, et al: High frequency of nonsense mutations in the *NF2* gene caused by C to T transitions in five CGA codons. Hum Mol Genet 1995; 4:137–139.

689. Koh T, Yokota J, Ookawa K, et al: Alternative splicing of the neurofibromatosis 1 gene correlates with growth patterns and neuroendocrine properties of human small-cell lung-carcinoma cells. Int J Cancer 1995;60: 843–847.

690. Tran YK, Bogler O, Gorse KM, et al: A novel member of the NF2/ERM/4.1 superfamily with growth suppressing properties in lung cancer. Cancer Res 1999; 59:35–43.

691. Sekido Y, Pass HI, Bader S, et al: Neurofibromatosis type 2 (NF2) gene is somatically mutated in mesothelioma but not in lung cancer. Cancer Res 1995;55: 1227–1231.

692. Haber DA, Sohn RL, Buckler AJ, et al: Alternative splicing and genomic structure of the Wilms tumor gene *WT1*. Proc Natl Acad Sci USA 1991;88:9618–9622.

693. Rauscher FJd, Morris JF, Tournay OE, et al: Binding of the Wilms' tumor locus zinc finger protein to the EGR-1 consensus sequence. Science 1990;250:1259–1262.

694. Madden SL, Cook DM, Rauscher FJ III: A structure-function analysis of transcriptional repression mediated by the WT1, Wilms' tumor suppressor protein. Oncogene 1993;8:1713–1720.

695. Ladanyi M, Gerald W: Fusion of the *EWS* and *WT1* genes in the desmoplastic small round cell tumor. Cancer Res 1994;54:2837–2840.

696. Karnieli E, Werner H, Rauscher FJ III, et al: The IGF-I receptor gene promoter is a molecular target for the Ewing's sarcoma-Wilms' tumor 1 fusion protein. J Biol Chem 1996;271:19304–19309.

697. Pitterle DM, Jolicoeur EM, Bepler G: Hot spots for molecular genetic alterations in lung cancer. In Vivo 1998;12:643–658.

698. Weaver DA, Hei TK, Hukku B, et al: Cytogenetic and molecular genetic analysis of tumorigenic human bronchial epithelial cells induced by radon alpha particles. Carcinogenesis 1997;18:1251–1257.

699. Petersen I, Petersen S: Towards a genetic-based classification of lung cancer. Anal Cell Pathol 2001;22: 111–121.

700. Harris CC, Reddel R, Pfeifer A, et al: Role of oncogenes and tumour suppressor genes in human lung carcinogenesis. IARC Sci Publ 1991;105:294–304.

701. Gerhard DS, Lawrence E, Wu J, et al: Isolation of 1001 new markers from human chromosome 11, excluding the region of 11p13–p15.5, and their sublocalization by a new series of radiation-reduced somatic cell hybrids. Genomics 1992;13:1133–1142.

702. Ludwig CU, Raefle G, Dalquen P, et al: Allelic loss on the short arm of chromosome 11 in non–small-cell lung cancer. Int J Cancer 1991;49:661–665.

703. Skinner MA, Vollmer R, Huper G, et al: Loss of heterozygosity for genes on 11p and the clinical course of patients with lung carcinoma. Cancer Res 1990;50: 2303–2306.

704. Volm M, Rittgen W: Cellular predictive factors for the drug response of lung cancer. Anticancer Res 2000;20: 3449–3458.

705. Shipman R, Schraml P, Colombi M, Ludwig CU: Allelic deletion at chromosome 11p13 defines a tumor suppressor region between the catalase gene and D11S935 in human non–small cell lung carcinoma. Int J Oncol 1998;12:107–111.

706. Schmidt L, Tory K, Chen F, et al: Frequent and specific mutation of the von Hippel-Lindau tumor suppressor gene in sporadic renal cell carcinoma [meeting abstract]. In Proc Annu Meet Am Assoc Cancer Res 1994.

707. Beroud C, Joly D, Gallou C, et al: Software and database for the analysis of mutations in the *VHL* gene. Nucleic Acids Res 1998;26:256–258.

708. Hung J, Kishimoto Y, Sugio K, et al: Allele-specific chromosome 3p deletions occur at an early stage in the pathogenesis of lung carcinoma. JAMA 1995;273: 1908.

709. Todd S, Roche J, Hahner L, et al: YAC contigs covering an 8-megabase region of 3p deleted in the small-cell lung cancer cell line U2020. Genomics 1995;25: 19–28.

710. Carritt B, Kok K, van den Berg A, et al: A gene from human chromosome region 3p21 with reduced expression in small cell lung cancer. Cancer Res 1992;52: 1536–1541.

711. Murata Y, Tamari M, Takahashi T, et al: Characterization of an 800 kb region at 3p22-p21.3 that was homozygously deleted in a lung cancer cell line. Hum Mol Genet 1994;3:1341–1344.

712. Cheng JQ, Crepin M, Hamelin R: Loss of heterozygosity on chromosomes 1p, 3p, 11p, and 11q in human non-small cell lung cancer. Serono Symp Publ Raven 1990;78:357–364.

713. Thiberville L, Bourguignon J, Metayer J, et al: Frequency and prognostic evaluation of 3p21-22 allelic losses in non–small-cell lung cancer. Int J Cancer 1995;64:371–377.

714. Sekido Y, Bader S, Latif F, et al: Molecular analysis of the von Hippel-Lindau disease tumor suppressor gene in human lung cancer cell lines. Oncogene 1994;9: 1599–1604.

715. Herman JG, Latif F, Weng Y, et al: Silencing of the *VHL* tumor-suppressor gene by DNA methylation in renal carcinoma. Proc Natl Acad Sci USA 1994;91: 9700–9704.

716. Glover TW, Berger C, Coyle J, Echo B: DNA polymerase alpha inhibition by aphidicolin induces gaps and breaks at common fragile sites in human chromosomes. Hum Genet 1984;67:136–142.

717. Heubner K, Garrison PN, Barnes LD, Croce CM: The role of the *FHIT/FRA3B* locus in cancer. Annu Rev Genet 1998;32:7–31.

718. Schmid M, Ott G, Haaf T, Scheres JM: Evolutionary conservation of fragile sites induced by 5-azacytidine and 5-azadeoxycytidine in man, gorilla, and chimpanzee. Hum Genet 1985;71:342–350.

719. Ohta M, Inoue H, Cotticelli MG, et al: The *FHIT* gene, spanning the chromosome 3p14.2 fragile site and renal carcinoma-associated t(3;8) breakpoint, is abnormal in digestive tract cancers. Cell 1996;84: 587–597.
720. Wilke CM, Hall BK, Hoge A, et al: FRA3B extends over a broad region and contains a spontaneous HPV16 integration site: Direct evidence for the coincidence of viral integration sites and fragile sites. Hum Mol Genet 1996;5:187–195.
721. Sozzi G, Veronese ML, Negrini M, et al: The *FHIT* gene 3p14.2 is abnormal in lung cancer. Cell 1996;85:17–26.
722. Sozzi G, Pastorino U, Moiraghi L, et al: Loss of FHIT function in lung cancer and preinvasive bronchial lesions. Cancer Res 1998;58:5032–5037.
723. Yokoyama S, Yamakawa K, Tsuchiya E, et al: Deletion mapping on the short arm of chromosome 3 in squamous cell carcinoma and adenocarcinoma of the lung. Cancer Res 1992;52:873–877.
724. Fong KM, Biesterveld EJ, Virmani A, et al: FHIT and FRA3B 3p14.2 allele loss are common in lung cancer and preneoplastic bronchial lesions and are associated with cancer-related FHIT cDNA splicing aberrations. Cancer Res 1997;57:2256–2267.
725. Barnes LD, Garrison PN, Siprashvill Z, et al: Fhit, a putative tumor suppressor in humans, is a dinucleoside 5′,5‴-P1,P3-triphosphate hydrolase. Biochemistry 1996;35:11529–11535.
726. Yunis JJ, Oken MM, Kaplan ME, et al: Distinctive chromosomal abnormalities in histologic subtypes of non-Hodgkin's lymphoma. N Engl J Med 1982;307: 1231–1236.
727. Tsujimoto Y, Finger LR, Yunis J, et al: Cloning of the chromosome breakpoint of neoplastic B cells with the t(14;18) chromosome translocation. Science 1984;226: 1097–1099.
728. Hockenbery D, Nunez G, Milliman C, et al: Bcl-2 is an inner mitochondrial membrane protein that blocks programmed cell death. Nature 1990;348:334–336.
729. Lu QL, Hanby AM, Nasser Hajibagheri MA, et al: Bcl-2 protein localizes to the chromosomes of mitotic nuclei and is correlated with the cell cycle in cultured epithelial cell lines. J Cell Sci 1994;107:363–371.
730. Distelhorst CW, Lam M, McCormick TS: Bcl-2 inhibits hydrogen peroxide-induced ER Ca^{2+} pool depletion. Oncogene 1996;12:2051–2055.
731. Shimizu S, Eguchi Y, Kamiike W, et al: Bcl-2 expression prevents activation of the ICE protease cascade. Oncogene 1996;12:2251–2257.
732. Shimizu S, Eguchi Y, Kamiike W, et al: Bcl-2 blocks loss of mitochondrial membrane potential while ICE inhibitors act at a different step during inhibition of death induced by respiratory chain inhibitors. Oncogene 1996;13:21–29.
733. Farrow SN, Brown R: New members of the Bcl-2 family and their protein partners. Curr Opin Genet Dev 1996; 6:45–49.
734. Sato T, Hanada M, Bodrug S, et al: Interactions among members of the Bcl-2 protein family analyzed with a yeast two-hybrid system [published erratum appears in Proc Natl Acad Sci USA 1995;92:2016]. Proc Natl Acad Sci USA 1994;91:9238–9242.
735. Boise LH, Gonzalez-Garcia M, Postema CE, et al: bcl-x, a bcl-2-related gene that functions as a dominant regulator of apoptotic cell death. Cell 1993;74:597–608.
736. Fang W, Rivard JJ, Mueller DL, Behrens TW: Cloning and molecular characterization of mouse bcl-x in B and T lymphocytes. J Immunol 1994;153:4388–4398.
737. Chiou SK, Rao L, White E: Bcl-2 blocks p53-dependent apoptosis [published erratum appears in Mol Cell Biol 1994;14:4333]. Mol Cell Biol 1994;14: 2556–2563.
738. Wang Y, Szekely L, Okan I, et al: Wild-type p53-triggered apoptosis is inhibited by bcl-2 in a v-myc–induced T-cell lymphoma line. Oncogene 1993;8: 3427–3431.
739. Cherbonnel-Lasserre C, Gauny S, Kronenberg A: Suppression of apoptosis by Bcl-2 or Bcl-xL promotes susceptibility to mutagenesis. Oncogene 1996;13: 1489–1497.
740. Fanidi A, Harrington EA, Evan GI: Cooperative interaction between c-*myc* and *bcl-2* proto-oncogenes. Nature 1992;359:554–556.
741. Bissonnette RP, Echeverri F, Mahboubi A, Green DR: Apoptotic cell death induced by c-*myc* is inhibited by *bcl-2*. Nature 1992;359:552–4.
742. Chen CY, Faller DV: Phosphorylation of Bcl-2 protein and association with p21Ras in Ras-induced apoptosis. J Biol Chem 1996;271:2376–2379.
743. Fernandez-Sarabia MJ, Bischoff JR: Bcl-2 associates with the ras-related protein R-ras p23. Nature 1993; 366:274–275.
744. Naumovski L, Cleary ML: The p53-binding protein 53BP2 also interacts with Bc12 and impedes cell cycle progression at G2/M. Mol Cell Biol 1996;16: 3884–3892.
745. Selvakumaran M, Lin HK, Miyashita T, et al: Immediate early up-regulation of bax expression by p53 but not TGF beta 1: A paradigm for distinct apoptotic pathways. Oncogene 1994;9:1791–1798.
746. Silvestrini R, Costa A, Lequaglie C, et al: Bcl-2 protein and prognosis in patients with potentially curable non–small-cell lung cancer. Virchows Arch 1998;432: 441–444.
747. Athanassiadou P, Dosios T, Petrakakou E, et al: p53 and bcl-2 protein expression in non–small-cell lung carcinoma. Diagn Cytopathol 1998;19:255–259.
748. Fontanini G, Vignati S, Bigini D, et al: Bcl-2 protein: A prognostic factor inversely correlated to p53 in non–small-cell lung cancer. Br J Cancer 1995;71: 1003–1007.
749. Walker C, Robertson L, Myskow M, Dixon G: Expression of the BCL-2 protein in normal and dysplastic bronchial epithelium and in lung carcinomas. Br J Cancer 1995;72:164–169.
750. Ritter JH, Dresler CM, Wick MR: Expression of bcl-2 protein in stage T1N0M0 non–small cell lung carcinoma. Hum Pathol 1995;26:1227–1232.
751. Pezzella F, Turley H, Kuzu I, et al: bcl-2 protein in non–small-cell lung carcinoma [see comments]. N Engl J Med 1993;329:690–694.
752. Brambilla E, Gazzeri S, Lantuejoul S, et al: p53 mutant immunophenotype and deregulation of p53 transcription pathway (Bcl2, Bax, and Waf1) in precursor bron-

chial lesions of lung cancer. Clin Cancer Res 1998;4: 1609-1618.

753. Ohsaki Y, Toyoshima E, Fujiuchi S, et al: bcl-2 and p53 protein expression in non–small cell lung cancers: Correlation with survival time. Clin Cancer Res 1996; 2:915–920.

754. Anton RC, Brown RW, Younes M, et al: Absence of prognostic significance of bcl-2 immunopositivity in non–small cell lung cancer: Analysis of 427 cases. Hum Pathol 1997;28:1079–1082.

755. Fleming MV, Guinee DG Jr, Chu WS, et al: Bcl-2 immunohistochemistry in a surgical series of non–small cell lung cancer patients. Hum Pathol 1998;29: 60–64.

756. Sirzen F, Zhivotovsky B, Nilsson A, et al: Higher spontaneous apoptotic index in small cell compared with non-small cell lung carcinoma cell lines; lack of correlation with Bcl-2/Bax. Lung Cancer 1998;22:1–13.

757. Brambilla E, Negoescu A, Gazzeri S, et al: Apoptosis-related factors p53, Bcl2, and Bax in neuroendocrine lung tumors. Am J Pathol 1996;149:1941–1952.

758. Kaiser U, Schilli M, Haag U, et al: Expression of bcl-2 protein in small cell lung cancer. Lung Cancer 1996;15: 31–40.

759. Yan JJ, Chen FF, Tsai YC, Jin YT: Immunohistochemical detection of Bcl-2 protein in small cell carcinomas. Oncology 1996;53:6–11.

760. Jiang SX, Sato Y, Kuwao S, Kameya T: Expression of bcl-2 oncogene protein is prevalent in small cell lung carcinomas. J Pathol 1995;177:135–138.

761. Higashiyama M, Doi O, Kodama K, et al: High prevalence of bcl-2 oncoprotein expression in small cell lung cancer. Anticancer Res 1995;15:503–505.

762. Nagatake M, Osada H, Kondo M, et al: Aberrant hypermethylation at the bcl-2 locus at 18q21 in human lung cancers. Cancer Res 1996;56:1886–1891.

763. Jeffrey PD, Russo AA, Polyak K, et al: Mechanism of CDK activation revealed by the structure of a cyclin A-CDK2 complex. Nature 1995;376:313–320.

764. De Bondt HL, Rosenblatt J, Jancarik J, et al: Crystal structure of cyclin-dependent kinase 2. Nature 1993; 363:595–602.

765. Motokura T, Keyomarsi K, Kronenberg HM, Arnold A: Cloning and characterization of human cyclin D3, a cDNA closely related in sequence to the PRAD1/ cyclin D1 proto-oncogene. J Biol Chem 1992;267: 20412–20415.

766. Xiong Y, Menninger J, Beach D, Ward DC: Molecular cloning and chromosomal mapping of CCND genes encoding human D-type cyclins. Genomics 1992;13: 575–584.

767. Lukas J, Bartkova J, Rohde M, et al: Cyclin D1 is dispensable for G1 control in retinoblastoma gene–deficient cells independently of cdk4 activity. Mol Cell Biol 1995;15:2600–2611.

768. Spitkovsky D, Steiner P, Gopalkrishnan RV, et al: The role of p53 in coordinated regulation of cyclin D1 and p21 gene expression by the adenovirus E1A and E1B oncogenes. Oncogene 1995;10:2421–2425.

769. Chen X, Bargonetti J, Prives C: p53, through p21 (WAF1/CIP1), induces cyclin D1 synthesis. Cancer Res 1995;55:4257–4263.

770. Zhang H, Hannon GJ, Beach D: p21-containing cyclin kinases exist in both active and inactive states. Genes Dev 1994;8:1750–1758.

771. Deshaies RJ, Chau V, Kirschner M: Ubiquitination of the G1 cyclin Cln2p by a Cdc34p-dependent pathway. EMBO J 1995;14:303–312.

772. Hershko A, Ganoth D, Sudakin V, et al: Components of a system that ligates cyclin to ubiquitin and their regulation by the protein kinase cdc2. J Biol Chem 1994;269: 4940–4946.

773. King RW, Peters JM, Tugendreich S, et al: A 20S complex containing CDC27 and CDC16 catalyzes the mitosis-specific conjugation of ubiquitin to cyclin B. Cell 1995;81:279–288.

774. de Boer CJ, Loyson S, Kluin PM, et al: Multiple breakpoints within the BCL-1 locus in B-cell lymphoma: Rearrangements of the cyclin D1 gene. Cancer Res 1993;53:4148–4152.

775. Guldberg P, Kirkin AF, Gronbaek K, et al: Complete scanning of the CDK4 gene by denaturing gradient gel electrophoresis: A novel missense mutation but low overall frequency of mutations in sporadic metastatic malignant melanoma. Int J Cancer 1997; 72:780–783.

776. Gao L, Liu L, van Meyel D, et al: Lack of germ-line mutations of CDK4, p16(INK4A), and p15(INK4B) in families with glioma. Clin Cancer Res 1997;3: 977–981.

777. He J, Allen JR, Collins VP, et al: CDK4 amplification is an alternative mechanism to *p16* gene homozygous deletion in glioma cell lines. Cancer Res 1994;54: 5804–5807.

778. Schauer IE, Siriwardana S, Langan TA, Sclafani RA: Cyclin D1 overexpression vs. retinoblastoma inactivation: Implications for growth control evasion in non–small cell and small cell lung cancer. Proc Natl Acad Sci USA 1994;91:7827–7831.

779. Nishio M, Koshikawa T, Yatabe Y, et al: Prognostic significance of cyclin D1 and retinoblastoma expression in combination with p53 abnormalities in primary, resected non–small cell lung cancers. Clin Cancer Res 1997; 3:1051–1058.

780. Marchetti A, Doglioni C, Barbareschi M, et al: Cyclin D1 and retinoblastoma susceptibility gene alterations in non–small cell lung cancer. Int J Cancer 1998;75: 187–192.

781. Tanaka H, Fujii Y, Hirabayashi H, et al: Disruption of the RB pathway and cell-proliferative activity in non-small-cell lung cancers. Int J Cancer 1998;79:111–115.

782. Betticher DC, Heighway J, Thatcher N, Hasleton PS: Abnormal expression of CCND1 and RB1 in resection margin epithelia of lung cancer patients. Br J Cancer 1997;75:1761–1768.

783. Betticher DC, Heighway J, Hasleton PS, et al: Prognostic significance of CCND1 (cyclin D1) overexpression in primary resected non–small-cell lung cancer. Br J Cancer 1996;73:294–300.

784. Caputi M, De Luca L, Papaccio G, et al: Prognostic role of cyclin D1 in non–small cell lung cancer: An immunohistochemical analysis. Eur J Histochem 1997;41:133–138.

785. Betticher DC, White GR, Vonlanthen S, et al: G1 control gene status is frequently altered in resectable

non–small cell lung cancer. Int J Cancer 1997;74: 556–562.

785a. Suzuki H, Ueda R, Takahashi T: Altered imprinting in lung cancer. Nature 1994;6:332–333.

785b. Makos M, Nelkin BD, Lerman MI, et al: Distinct hypermethylation patterns occur at altered chromosome loci in human lung and colon cancer. Proc Natl Acad Sci USA 1992;89:1929–1933.

785c. Dammann R, Li C, Yoon JH, et al: Epigenetic inactivation of a RAS association domain family protein from the lung tumour suppressor locus 3p21.3. Nat Genet 2000;25:315–319.

785d. Zochbauer-Muller S, Fong KM, Maitra A, et al: 5′ CpG island methylation of the FHIT gene is correlated with loss of gene expression in lung and breast cancer. Cancer Res 2001;61:3581–3585.

785e. Zochbauer-Muller S, Fong KM, Virmani AK, et al: Aberrant promoter methylation of multiple genes in non–small cell lung cancers. Cancer Res 2001;61: 249–255.

785f. Burbee DG, Forgacs E, Zochbauer-Muller S, et al: Epigenetic inactivation of RASSF1A in lung and breast cancers and malignant phenotype supression. J Natl Cancer Inst 2001;93:691–699.

785g. Hiyama K, Hiyama E, Ishioka S, et al: Telomerase activity in small cell and non–small cell lung cancers. J Natl Cancer Inst 1995;87:895–902.

785h. Albanell J, Lonardo F, Rusch V, et al: High telomerase activity in primary lung cancers: association with increased cell proliferation rates and advanced pathologic stage. J Natl Cancer Inst 997;89:1609–1615.

786. Graziano SL, Tatum AH, Gonchoroff NJ, et al: Blood group antigen A and flow cytometric analysis in resected early-stage non–small cell lung cancer. Clin Cancer Res 1997;3:87–93.

787. Miyake M, Taki T, Hitomi S, Hakomori S: Correlation of expression of H/Le(y)/Le(b) antigens with survival in patients with carcinoma of the lung. N Engl J Med 1992;327:14–18.

788. Kawai T, Suzuki M, Kase K, Ozeki Y: Expression of carbohydrate antigens in human pulmonary adenocarcinoma. Cancer 1993;72:1581–1587.

789. Alvarez-Fernandez E, Carretero-Albinana L: Expression of blood group antigens by normal bronchopulmonary tissues and common norms of pulmonary carcinomas. Arch Pathol Lab Med 1991;115:42–49.

790. Lee JS, Ro JY, Sahin AA, et al: Expression of blood-group antigen A—a favorable prognostic factor in non-small-cell lung cancer. N Engl J Med 1991;324:1084–1090.

791. Ogawa J, Inoue H, Koide S: Expression of alpha-1,3-fucosyltransferase type IV and VII genes is related to poor prognosis in lung cancer. Cancer Res 1996;56: 325–329.

792. Tanaka F, Miyahara R, Ohtake Y, et al: Lewis Y antigen expression and postoperative survival in non–small cell lung cancer. Ann Thorac Surg 1998;66:1745–1750.

793. Mehdi SA, Tatum AH, Newman NB, et al: Prognostic significance of Lewis y antigen in resected stage I and II non–small cell lung cancer. Chest 1998;114: 1309–1315.

794. Satoh H, Ishikawa H, Kamma H, et al: Elevated serum sialyl Lewis X-i antigen levels in non–small cell lung cancer with lung metastasis. Respiration 1998;65: 295–298.

795. Fukuoka K, Narita N, Saijo N: Increased expression of sialyl Lewis(x) antigen is associated with distant metastasis in lung cancer patients: Immunohistochemical study on bronchofiberscopic biopsy specimens. Lung Cancer 1998;20:109–116.

796. Kim YJ, Borsig L, Varki NM, Varki A: P-selectin deficiency attenuates tumor growth and metastasis. Proc Natl Acad Sci USA 1998;95:9325–9330.

797. Ogawa J, Tsurumi T, Yamada S, et al: Blood vessel invasion and expression of sialyl Lewisx and proliferating cell nuclear antigen in stage I non–small cell lung cancer: Relation to postoperative recurrence. Cancer 1994;73: 1177–1183.

798. Satoh H, Ishikawa H, Yamashita YT, et al: Predictive value of preoperative serum sialyl Lewis X-i antigen levels in non–small cell lung cancer. Anticancer Res 1998;18:2865–2868.

799. Ishikawa H, Satoh H, Kamma H, et al: Elevated sialyl Lewis X-i antigen levels in pleural effusions in patients with carcinomatous pleuritis. Intern Med 1997;36: 685–689.

800. Nilsson O: Carbohydrate antigens in human lung carcinomas. APMIS Suppl 1992;27:149–161.

801. Kayser K, Gabius HJ, Ciesiolka T, et al: Histopathologic evaluation of application of labeled neoglycoproteins in primary bronchus carcinoma. Hum Pathol 1989;20: 352–360.

802. Lynch DF Jr, Hassen W, Clements MA, et al: Serum levels of endothelial and neural cell adhesion molecules in prostate cancer. Prostate 1997;32:214–220.

803. Niklinski J, Furman M: Clinical tumour markers in lung cancer. Eur J Cancer Prev 1995;4:129–138.

804. Ledermann JA, Pasini F, Olabiran Y, Pelosi G: Detection of the neural cell adhesion molecule (NCAM) in serum of patients with small-cell lung cancer (SCLC) with limited or extensive disease, and bone-marrow infiltration. Int J Cancer Suppl 1994;8:49–52.

805. Broers JL, Ramaekers FC: Differentiation markers for lung-cancer subtypes: A comparative study of their expression in vivo and in vitro. Int J Cancer Suppl 1994;8:134–137.

806. Travis WD, Colby TV, Corrin B, et al: Histologic Typing of Lung And Pleural Tumors, 3rd ed. World Health Organization International Histological Classification of Tumours. Berlin, Springer, 1999.

807. Gatter KC, Dunnill MS, Heryet A, Mason DY: Human lung tumours: Does intermediate filament co-expression correlate with other morphological or immunocytochemical features? Histopathology 1987;11: 705–714.

808. Gatter KC, Dunnill MS, Pulford KA, et al: Human lung tumours: A correlation of antigenic profile with histological type. Histopathology 1985;9:805–823.

809. Hammar S: The use of electron microscopy and immunohistochemistry in the diagnosis and understanding of lung neoplasms. Clin Lab Med 1987;7:1–30.

810. Hammar SP, Bolen JW, Bockus D, et al: Ultrastructural and immunohistochemical features of common lung tumors: An overview. Ultrastruct Pathol 1985;9: 283–318.

811. Said J: Immunohistochemistry of lung tumors. Lung Biol Health Dis 1990;44:635–651.
812. Linnoila RI, Aisner SC: Pathology of lung cancer: An exercise in classification. *In* Johnson BE, Johnson DH (eds): Lung Cancer. New York, Wiley-Liss, 1995, pp 73–95.
813. Said JW, Nash G, Sassoon AF, et al: Involucrin in lung tumors: A specific marker for squamous differentiation. Lab Invest 1983;49:563–568.
814. Dempo K, Satoh M, Tsuji S, et al: Immunohistochemical studies on the expression of pulmonary surfactant apoproteins in human lung carcinomas using monoclonal antibodies. Pathol Res Pract 1987;182:669–675.
815. Kawai T, Torikata C, Suzuki M: Immunohistochemical study of pulmonary adenocarcinoma. Am J Clin Pathol 1988;89:455–462.
816. Linnoila RI, Jensen SM, Steinberg SM, et al: Peripheral airway cell marker expression in non–small cell lung carcinoma: Association with distinct clinicopathologic features [see comments]. Am J Clin Pathol 1992; 97:233–243.
817. Guinee DG Jr, Fishback NF, Koss MN, et al: The spectrum of immunohistochemical staining of small-cell lung carcinoma in specimens from transbronchial and open-lung biopsies. Am J Clin Pathol 1994;102: 406–414.
818. Shy SW, Lee WH, Chou MC, et al: Small cell lung carcinoma: Clinicopathological, immunohistochemical, and ultrastructural study. J Surg Oncol 1990;45: 146–161.
819. Bonato M, Cerati M, Pagani A, et al: Differential diagnostic patterns of lung neuroendocrine tumours: A clinico-pathological and immunohistochemical study of 122 cases. Virchows Arch A Pathol Anat Histopathol 1992; 420:201–211.
820. Linnoila RI, Mulshine JL, Steinberg SM, et al: Neuroendocrine differentiation in endocrine and nonendocrine lung carcinomas. Am J Clin Pathol 1988;90: 641–652.
821. Travis WD, Linnoila RI, Tsokos MG, et al: Neuroendocrine tumors of the lung with proposed criteria for large-cell neuroendocrine carcinoma: An ultrastructural, immunohistochemical, and flow cytometric study of 35 cases. Am J Surg Pathol 1991;15:529–553.
822. Said JW, Vimadalal S, Nash G, et al: Immunoreactive neuron-specific enolase, bombesin, and chromogranin as markers for neuroendocrine lung tumors. Hum Pathol 1985;16:236–240.
823. Strickler JG, Hegstrom J, Thomas MJ, Yousem SA: Myoepithelioma of the lung. Arch Pathol Lab Med 1987;111:1082–1085.
824. Koss MN, Hochholzer L, O'Leary T: Pulmonary blastomas. Cancer 1991;67:2368–2381.
825. Nakatani Y, Dickersin GR, Mark EJ: Pulmonary endodermal tumor resembling fetal lung: A clinicopathologic study of five cases with immunohistochemical and ultrastructural characterization. Hum Pathol 1990;21: 1097–1107.
826. Nakatani Y, Kitamura H, Inayama Y, Ogawa N: Pulmonary endodermal tumor resembling fetal lung: The optically clear nucleus is rich in biotin. Am J Surg Pathol 1994; 18:637–642.
827. Satoh Y, Tsuchiya E, Weng SY, et al: Pulmonary sclerosing hemangioma of the lung: A type II pneumocytoma by immunohistochemical and immunoelectron microscopic studies. Cancer 1989;64:1310–1317.
828. Yousem SA, Wick MR, Singh G, et al: So-called sclerosing hemangiomas of lung: An immunohistochemical study supporting a respiratory epithelial origin [published erratum appears in Am J Surg Pathol 1989;13: 337]. Am J Surg Pathol 1988;12:582–590.
829. Gaffey MJ, Mills SE, Zarbo RJ, et al: Clear cell tumor of the lung: Immunohistochemical and ultrastructural evidence of melanogenesis [see comments]. Am J Surg Pathol 1991;15:644–653.
830. Gaffey MJ, Mills SE, Ritter JH: Clear cell tumors of the lower respiratory tract. Semin Diagn Pathol 1997;14: 222–232.
831. Lantuejoul S, Isaac S, Pinel N, et al: Clear cell tumor of the lung: An immunohistochemical and ultrastructural study supporting a pericytic differentiation. Mod Pathol 1997;10:1001–1008.
832. Deavers M, Guinee D, Koss MN, Travis WD: Granular cell tumors of the lung: Clinicopathologic study of 20 cases. Am J Surg Pathol 1995;19:627–635.
833. Travis WD, Borok Z, Roum JH, et al: Pulmonary Langerhans cell granulomatosis (histiocytosis X): A clinicopathologic study of 48 cases. Am J Surg Pathol 1993; 17:971–986.
834. Emile JF, Wechsler J, Brousse N, et al: Langerhans' cell histiocytosis: Definitive diagnosis with the use of monoclonal antibody O10 on routinely paraffin-embedded samples. Am J Surg Pathol 1995;19:636–641.
835. Refabert L, Rambaud C, Mamou-Mani T, et al: Cd1a-positive cells in bronchoalveolar lavage samples from children with Langerhans cell histiocytosis. J Pediatr 1996;129:913–915.
836. Matsumoto Y, Horiba K, Usuki J, et al: Markers of cell proliferation and expression of melanosomal antigen in lymphangioleiomyomatosis. Am J Respir Cell Mol Biol 1999;21:327–336.
837. van de Rijn M, Rouse RV: CD34: A review. Appl Immunohistochem 1994;2:71–80.
838. Chan JKC: Vascular tumors with a prominent spindle cell component. Curr Diagn Pathol 1997;4:76–90.
839. Barekman CL, Adair CF: Immunohistochemistry of pneumocytes in hyperplasia and neoplasia. Appl Immunohistochem 1996;4:61–65.
840. Kitamura H, Kameda Y, Nakamura N, et al: Atypical adenomatous hyperplasia and bronchoalveolar lung carcinoma: Analysis by morphometry and the expressions of p53 and carcinoembryonic antigen. Am J Surg Pathol 1996;20:553–562.
841. Wick MR, Ritter JH, Nappi O: Inflammatory sarcomatoid carcinoma of the lung: Report of three cases and clinicopathologic comparison with inflammatory pseudotumors in adult patients. Hum Pathol 1995;26: 1014–1021.
842. Ro JY, Chen JL, Lee JS, et al: Sarcomatoid carcinoma of the lung: Immunohistochemical and ultrastructural studies of 14 cases. Cancer 1992;69:376–386.
843. Matsui K, Kitagawa M, Miwa A: Lung carcinoma with spindle cell components: Sixteen cases examined by immunohistochemistry. Hum Pathol 1992;23:1289–1297.

844. Fishback NF, Travis WD, Moran CS, et al: Pleomorphic (spindle/giant cell) carcinoma of the lung: A clinicopathologic correlation of 78 cases. Cancer 1994;73:2936–2945.
845. Bolen JW, Hammar SP, McNutt MA: Reactive and neoplastic serosal tissue: A light-microscopic, ultrastructural, and immunocytochemical study. Am J Surg Pathol 1986; 10:34–47.
846. Warnock ML, Stoloff A, Thor A: Differentiation of adenocarcinoma of the lung from mesothelioma: Periodic acid-Schiff, monoclonal antibodies B72.3, and Leu M1. Am J Pathol 1988;133:30–38.
847. Ordonez NG: The immunohistochemical diagnosis of mesothelioma: Differentiation of mesothelioma and lung adenocarcinoma. Am J Surg Pathol 1989; 13:276–291.
848. Otis CN, Carter D, Cole S, Battifora H: Immunohistochemical evaluation of pleural mesothelioma and pulmonary adenocarcinoma: A bi-institutional study of 47 cases. Am J Surg Pathol 1987;11:445–456.
849. Sheibani K, Shin SS, Kezirian J, Weiss LM: Ber-EP4 antibody as a discriminant in the differential diagnosis of malignant mesothelioma versus adenocarcinoma. Am J Surg Pathol 1991;15:779–784.
850. Sheibani K: Immunopathology of malignant mesothelioma [editorial; comment]. Hum Pathol 1994;25: 219–220.
851. Wick MR, Loy T, Mills SE, et al: Malignant epithelioid pleural mesothelioma versus peripheral pulmonary adenocarcinoma: A histochemical, ultrastructural, and immunohistologic study of 103 cases. Hum Pathol 1990;21:759–766.
852. Brown RW, Clark GM, Tandon AK, Allred DC: Multiple-marker immunohistochemical phenotypes distinguishing malignant pleural mesothelioma from pulmonary adenocarcinoma [see comments]. Hum Pathol 1993;24:347–354.
853. Koss M, Travis W, Moran C, Hochholzer L: Pseudomesotheliomatous adenocarcinoma: A reappraisal. Semin Diagn Pathol 1992;9:117–123.
854. Khoor A, Whitsett JA, Stahlman MT, et al: Utility of surfactant protein B precursor and thyroid transcription factor 1 in differentiating adenocarcinoma of the lung from malignant mesothelioma. Hum Pathol 1999;30:695–700.
855. Miettinen M, Kovatich AJ: HBME-1: A monoclonal antibody useful in the differential diagnosis of mesothelioma, adenocarcinoma, and soft tissue and bone tumors. Appl Immunohistochem 1995;3:115–122.
856. Clover J, Oates J, Edwards C: Anti-cytokeratin 5/6: A positive marker for epithelioid mesothelioma. Histopathology 1997;31:140–143.
857. Bateman AC, al-Talib RK, Newman T, et al: Immunohistochemical phenotype of malignant mesothelioma: Predictive value of CA125 and HBME-1 expression. Histopathology 1997;30:49–56.
858. Attanoos RL, Goddard H, Gibbs AR: Mesothelioma-binding antibodies: Thrombomodulin, OV 632 and HBME-1 and their use in the diagnosis of malignant mesothelioma. Histopathology 1996;29:209–215.
859. Peralta Soler A, Knudsen KA, Jaurand MC, et al: The differential expression of N-cadherin and E-cadherin distinguishes pleural mesotheliomas from lung adenocarcinomas [see comments]. Hum Pathol 1995;26: 1363–1369.
860. Leers MP, Aarts MM, Theunissen PH: E-cadherin and calretinin: A useful combination of immunochemical markers for differentiation between mesothelioma and metastatic adenocarcinoma. Histopathology 1998;32: 209–216.
861. Folpe AL, Gown AM, Lamps LW, et al: Thyroid transcription factor-1: Immunohistochemical evaluation in pulmonary neuroendocrine tumors. Mod Pathol 1999; 12:5–8.
862. Bohinski RJ, Bejarano PA, Balko G, et al: Determination of lung as the primary site of cerebral metastatic adenocarcinomas using monoclonal antibody to thyroid transcription factor-1. J Neurooncol 1998;40:227–231.
863. Wang NP, Zee S, Zarbo RJ, et al: Coordinate expression of cytokeratins 7 and 20 defines unique subsets of carcinomas. Appl Immunohistochem 1995;3:99–107.
864. Raab SS, Berg LC, Swanson PE, Wick MR: Adenocarcinoma in the lung in patients with breast cancer: A prospective analysis of the discriminatory value of immuno-histology [see comments]. Am J Clin Pathol 1993; 100:27–35.
865. Askin FB: Something old? Something new? Second primary or pulmonary metastasis in the patient with known extrathoracic carcinoma [editorial; comment]. Am J Clin Pathol 1993;100:4–5.

AGNES FOGO
LILIANE STRIKER

9

Kidney

Renal biopsies are a relatively new technique for diagnosis of diseases affecting the kidney and have only been used in the past 30 years. Recognition of renal diseases has advanced from the medieval "pisse prophets" and their uroscopy divinations to the clinical insights by Bright and others regarding the nature of diseases leading to "dropsy." The advent of immunofluorescence and electron microscopic examination has aided in unraveling many aspects of renal lesions. However, many diseases may share a similar histologic lesion and the same disease may present as different morphologic manifestations. For example, the lesion of focal segmental glomerular sclerosis (FSGS) occurs as the major abnormality in a variety of diseases, including idiopathic nephrotic syndrome, human immunodeficiency virus (HIV) nephropathy, sickle cell–associated renal disease, obesity-associated glomerulopathy, and heroin-associated nephropathy. However, this lesion can also be superimposed in immune complex diseases such as membranous glomerulonephritis and IgA nephropathy.[1] Lupus nephritis, on the other hand, is not a single lesion but implies a complex set of underlying pathogenic events resulting in lesions as diverse as mild mesangial glomerulonephritis versus a necrotizing crescentic and proliferative process.

In this chapter we review recent advances in molecular, immunohistochemical, and quantitative methods for examination of the kidney. The focus is on new findings that shed light not only on recognition of lesions and have implications for diagnosis and pathogenesis of renal disease but also give information regarding prognosis and potential response to therapy.

TRANSPLANT PATHOLOGY

Rejection

Although light microscopic changes currently are the renal tissue parameter that correlates best with clinical outcomes, these studies may be inadequate to differentiate the specific cause of a lymphoplasmacytic infiltrate in the transplant. Studies of various cytokines have shed light on possible underlying mechanisms for the infiltrate that may aid in diagnosis, understanding pathogenesis, and/or providing additional targets for therapy.[2] The cytokine RANTES (*r*egulated upon *a*ctivation, *n*ormal *T* cell *e*xpressed and *s*ecreted) attracts memory T lymphocytes, monocytes, and eosinophils. RANTES was not expressed in immediate post-transplant biopsy specimens or in native kidneys of patients with cyclosporine nephrotoxicity. However, in renal transplants with mononuclear cell infiltrate, RANTES messenger RNA (mRNA) was found in infiltrating mononuclear cells and renal tubular epithelium. The RANTES protein localized to mononuclear cells, tubular epithelium, and vascular endothelium.[3] Expression of RANTES may therefore be useful in diagnosis.

Other cytokines that may play roles in pathologic processes in the transplant have also been investigated. In one study of 24 transplant patients, a sensitive in situ hybridization protocol was described that used riboprobes of very high specific radioactivity capable of detecting fewer than five copies of a specific mRNA per cell. These in situ hybridization results were achieved on 4-μm formaldehyde-fixed, paraffin-embedded renal biopsy material.[4] In patients with clinically defined acute rejection episodes, increased interleukin (IL)-2 and IL-6 mRNA expressions were detected by in situ hybridization. These results were verified by reverse transcriptase/polymerase chain reaction (RT-PCR) amplification on portions of the tissue.

Increased IL-6 has also been demonstrated on tubular cells, mesangial cells, and interstitial monocytes and macrophages in acute rejection. Serum levels of IL-6 showed high sensitivity (84%) and specificity (85%) for acute rejection when viral disease was not present. Confounding factors were found to be the presence of acute tubular necrosis and cytomegalovirus (CMV) disease, both common conditions affecting the allograft. However, in another study, analysis of cytokine expression by RT-PCR showed no differences for IL-1β, IL-6, tumor necrosis factor-α, IL-2, or IL-2 receptor in rejecting versus non-rejecting samples. Expression of cytotoxic T lymphocyte–specific serine protease was increased in rejecting samples, although one renal carcinoma control also had high transcript levels.[5] Thus, the use of IL-6 is limited by its lack of sensitivity and specificity in those situations.[6–8] Of note, the RT-PCR method used in some of these studies does not allow for rigorous *quantitation* of expression of each gene, and interpretation based on relative amounts of gene expressions must be made with caution.

An elegant study investigated presence or absence of interferon gamma (IFN-γ) expression by RT-PCR on renal allograft fine-needle aspirates. Patients with a clinical diagnosis of acute rejection showed presence of IFN-γ expression, whereas those with acute tubular necrosis or cyclosporine toxicity did not have detectable IFN-γ. Of note, two patients showed detectable IFN-γ preceding the clinically recognizable acute rejection, suggesting that IFN-γ expression could be predictive of rejection.[9]

The differentiation of origin of cells infiltrating the transplant has been studied by flow cytometric analysis. In a large series of 132 post-transplantation biopsies, numbers of HLA-DR-positive kidney tubular cells, total lymphocytes, T suppressor/cytotoxic cells, and natural killer cells increased during rejection. There were corresponding low numbers of suppressor/inducer and T suppressor cells during rejection, with reemergence of these latter cells with successful antirejection therapy.[10] Cells shed in the urine have been immunostained for CD25 to assess the immune responses in the graft.[11] Patterns of specific subsets of T cells appear to reflect the activity of the rejection process and may therefore be useful both in diagnosis of rejection and assessing response to therapy. Up-regulated macrophage migration inhibitory factor (MIF) was associated with macrophage and T-cell infiltration and correlated with severity of acute rejection.[12]

E-selectin and vascular cell adhesion molecule-1 (VCAM-1) were found on endothelial cells of renal allografts, as in the normal kidney, whereas tubular cells in the rejecting graft expressed markedly enhanced VCAM-1 and intercellular adhesion molecule-1 (ICAM-1).[13] Acute rejection was highly correlated with ICAM-1 and VCAM-1.[14] The potential importance of these up-regulated adhesion molecules in the rejection process is underscored by a recent phase 1 trial using antibodies to CD54 (ICAM-1). In patients achieving adequate monoclonal antibody levels, there was associated decrease in delayed graft function and rejection.[15] The expression of VCAM-1 in vessels correlated with arteritis changes in renal allografts.[16] However, therapy with antibodies directed only against adhesion molecules appears not sufficient to prevent acute rejection episodes, perhaps reflecting more severe rejection represented by vascular involvement. Current research indicates that combinations of anti-adhesion molecule antibodies and immunosuppression will be most effective.[17]

Specific differentiation of mechanism of injury may be possible based on new research studies on human biopsy tissues. C4D staining in peritubular capillaries has been shown to closely correlate with mechanisms of humoral rejection and may aid in making this diagnosis.[18] Specific up-regulation of endothelin-1, RANTES, and monocyte chemoattractant protein-1 (MCP-1) in tubular epithelial cells was associated with cyclosporine nephrotoxicity.[19] Differentiation of some causes of fibrosis may be possible based on preliminary studies suggesting increased interstitial collagen I and III in cyclosporine-induced fibrosis, contrasting to increased laminin-β2 and COL4A3 in proximal tubular basement membranes in chronic rejection.[20]

Localization of injury to specific tubular segments may provide new insights into pathogenesis. Although proximal tubules are known to be most susceptible to ischemic injury, and are thought to be the target for rejection responses, the most pronounced tubulitis in acute rejection was found in the distal convoluted tubule and cortical collecting system. Specific antibodies and lectins may aid in identifying tubule segments, especially in states of injury in which standard morphologic and anatomic criteria may not be adequate to differentiate specific nephron segments (see later). These new advances indicate that detection of cytokines, adhesion molecules, and other markers may aid in defining the etiology of inflammatory processes in the transplant and also provide markers of response to therapy.

Viral infection

Infectious agents in tissue may be identified by characteristic morphology of the organism, by typical tissue response, or by immunostaining and molecular methods. CMV infection in the transplant usually is diagnosed by culture and/or serology. However, these methods require longer time periods and may not be as sensitive or specific as direct detection of virus in the tissue by new methodologies. The use of a biotinylated, nonradioactive probe for in situ hybridization for detection of CMV was found to be a sensitive and rapid method for diagnosis. Positive results were confirmed by immunofluorescence and culture.[21] Detection of CMV in settings other than the transplant may also be important. Both immunocytochemistry and in situ hybridization have detected CMV in AIDS patients. Positivity was mostly within glomeruli. Of interest, most cells staining positively by either method did not show typical CMV inclusions, although 8 of the 10 cases studied in one series did contain typical Cowdry type A intranuclear CMV inclusions elsewhere in the specimen.[22] These findings indicate that these enhanced methods of CMV detection are more sensitive than light microscopy.

The feasibility of detecting very early-stage CMV infection, before cytopathic changes are detectable, has also been addressed by applying PCR techniques to renal allograft biopsies.[23] Primers from the late antigen region of CMV were used. Three of 21 nephrectomy samples showed CMV-specific amplified products by PCR. Only 1 of these samples showed CMV inclusion bodies. In a series of 16 renal biopsy specimens, three specimens showed positive CMV PCR products, with one showing viral inclusions. All patients with positive PCR cells showed positive CMV culture and/or serum conversions. None of the patients with negative samples showed clinical or serologic evidence of CMV infection. These studies would suggest that PCR in renal allografts is more sensitive then histologic examination and provides more rapid diagnosis than viral culture for CMV infection.

The diagnosis of Epstein-Barr virus (EBV) infection is increasingly being recognized as a cause of renal and systemic lymphoproliferative disorders in renal transplant recipients. Those patients who develop primary EBV infection and also receive potent antilymphocyte preparation are most at risk for post-transplant lymphoproliferative disorder. In the transplant, the suppression of cytotoxic T cells is thought to underlie EBV infection, which then is postulated to result in B-cell proliferation. These B-cell clones may then result in oligoclonal or monoclonal tumors, collectively called post-transplantation lymphoproliferative disorders. In addition to identification of EBV, studies of oligoclonality of lymphocytes may be useful in classifying these lesions.[24] Differentiation from rejection is crucial because effective treatment for these lymphoproliferative diseases includes decreased immunosuppression. In one study, direct immunofluorescence, immunoperoxidase, and in situ hybridization showed similar sensitivity in detection of EBV. Early detection of EBV infection may identify patients at high risk for lymphoproliferative disorders and may direct choice of immunosuppression.

Other renal lesions have also been reported with EBV infection. A renal transplant patient with negative EBV serology showed EBV infection of the graft by in situ hybridization and PCR. Severe widespread glomerular mesangiolysis was present.[25] Polyoma virus has now emerged as major infection in the transplant. Diagnosis is made by detection of viral cytopathic change, a pleomorphic infiltrate, and positive immunostaining.

In summary, these new molecular approaches offer the advantage of faster diagnosis than culture and greater sensitivity than routine histology for detection of viruses.

NATIVE KIDNEY DISEASE

Tests of Diagnostic Value

Diagnosis of both acute and chronic glomerular diseases relies on integrated interpretation of light microscopy, immunofluorescence, and electron microscopy, and correlation with the clinical setting. The vast majority of cases can be classified into described histologic categories using these techniques; however, a small percentage remain unclassified. Most of these cases are of chronic end-stage processes in which little insight into specific diagnosis has been gained by new techniques. New insights into pathogenesis have, however, emerged. In this section we review these diagnostic and prognostic implications.

Complement/Immune Diseases

Occasionally, inadequate tissue is preserved from frozen sections for standard immunofluorescence techniques, the cornerstone of the workup of the renal biopsy. Immunohistochemistry for detection of complement by the avidin-biotin-peroxidase method has shown results equivalent to indirect immunofluorescence and superior to direct immunofluorescence.[26] Examination of a component of immune injury, C3 mRNA, has also been examined by PCR on renal biopsy tissues. Expression of the C3 mRNA was increased in those patients with immune-complex glomerulonephritis and/or cell-mediated interstitial nephritis but not in patients with nonimmune glomerular injury.[27]

IgA staining may be seen both in mesangiopathic glomerulonephritis (Berger's disease) and lupus glomerulonephritis. C1q staining may provide useful information in differentiating these two processes. In one study, C1q was absent or scanty in IgA nephropathy, in contrast to the situation in lupus glomerulonephritis. Differentiation of these two diseases was highly accurate in a large series of patients based on the following diagnostic criteria for IgA nephropathy: greater than 2+ IgA staining, other immunoglobulins not present in greater intensity, and the presence of less than 2+ C1q staining.[28]

These studies indicate that more specific determination of complement activation will give added insights into mechanisms of disease. Molecular approaches can determine whether complement originates from renal cells and which specific molecules are present. This knowledge may offer new target sites for future therapies.

Thin Basement Membrane Lesion/Alport Syndrome

Diagnosis of thin basement membranes is based on morphometric measurements. Normal thickness in adults from one laboratory was 373 ± 42 nm in men versus 326 ± 45 nm in women.[29] It is imperative that each laboratory determines normal basement membrane thicknesses after their particular processing. In adults, several series showed high sensitivity and specificity for the diagnosis of thin basement membranes using glomerular basement membrane (GBM) thickness less than 250 nm as the cutoff.[30–33] In another laboratory with higher normal range, a cutoff of 330 nm was used.[34] In children, the diagnosis of thin basement membranes is more difficult than in adults, because GBM increases in thickness with normal maturation. Although it has been suggested that a cutoff of 250 nm be used, we and others have found that this range has a great overlap with normal.[35–38] More appropriate cutoffs for diagnosis of thin basement membranes in children are based on normal values for each age group. In our laboratory, we found a range of GBM thickness in normal children from about 110 nm at age 1 year to 222 ± 14 in 7-year olds. Gender also influenced GBM thickness in one study.[39] In yet another study, greater variability was found, with mean $\pm$ 2 SD ranges from 100 to 340 nm at 1 year of age to 190 to 440 nm at 9 years or older.[40] These findings underscore the need for carefully performed controls before morphometric data are analyzed and interpreted.

Of note, thin basement membranes are found in benign familial hematuria but may also be present in some kindreds with Alport syndrome even at advanced stages, in female carriers of classic, X-linked Alport syndrome, and at early stages of classic Alport or in autosomal forms of Alport syndrome, rather than the classic, lamellated, basketweaving appearance of the GBM by electron microscopy that is diagnostic of Alport syndrome.[41, 42] Thus, the presence of thin GBM cannot be taken as a specific indicator of benign familial hematuria.

The mutation in the classic form of Alport sundrome has been identified as the α5 (IV) collagen chain *(COL4A5)*. The rare autosomal recessive form of Alport syndrome was found to result from mutations of α3 or α4 type IV collagen genes *(COL4A3* or *COL4A4)* in several families. The organs involved reflect sites where these collagen chains are normally expressed. Thus α3, α4, and α5 type IV collagen chains are normally restricted to the kidney, eye, and ear. The abnormal α5 appears to prevent incorporation of α3 and α4 into the normal triple helical collagen monomers. These monomers normally form collagen dimers or tetramers, the building blocks of the basement membrane.

Skin or renal biopsy staining to demonstrate the absence of α5 type IV collagen has been suggested as a tool to distinguish patients with Alport syndrome from those with other causes of hematuria, who are expected to show normal α5 type IV collagen staining.[42, 43] Interestingly, staining of α3 and α4 type IV collagen was also abnormal in patients with severe classic Alport syndrome, supporting that the molecular defect in one of the type IV collagen chains results in defective incorporation of the other chains in the heterotrimer of the GBM. Thus, the co-absence of α3 and α5 is a major diagnostic clue to the diagnosis of Alport syndrome, because it has so far not been described in other glomerular diseases, including thin basement membrane nephropathy (thought to represent "benign familial hematuria"). However, the sensitivity and specificity of skin or renal biopsy immunofluorescence studies in the diagnosis of Alport syndrome has not been proven, and occasional cases with Alport syndrome clinically and by renal biopsy showed apparent normal α5 type IV pattern of skin immunofluorescence staining. About 20% of male classic Alport patients and affected homozygous autosomal recessive Alport patients show faint or even normal staining of the GBM for α3 and α5.[41] Thus, the absence of α5 type IV in the skin biopsy appears to be helpful in indicating a basement membrane abnormality, but an apparent normal staining pattern in either skin or kidney does not definitively rule out Alport syndrome.

The possible continuum of Alport syndrome with some cases of apparent benign familial hematuria with thin basement membranes further complicates interpretation of staining patterns. An α4 type IV collagen gene mutation segregated with hematuria in a kindred with apparent benign hematuria.[43] The index patient had electron microscopic changes typical of Alport syndrome by renal biopsy at age 5 years, that is, areas of lamellation alternating with areas of thinning. This boy's parents both had microscopic hematuria and family histories of benign hematuria without progression in any members. In contrast, the boy developed proteinuria at age 16 years. These findings suggest that this patient may have inherited a disorder manifest by hematuria from both parents, resulting in a more severe phenotype. Furthermore, the findings in this kindred suggest the possibility that autosomal recessive Alport disease and "benign familial hematuria/thin basement membrane disease" may be the severe and mild forms of different molecular defects in the same gene.

Abnormal GBM may coexist with other renal disorders. Of special interest is the occurrence of thin GBM in patients with diabetes mellitus with urinary abnormalities.[44] The diagnosis of thin GBM was made based on segmental (20% to 49% of loops involved) or diffuse (> 50% of loops involved) thinning of the GBM, using 200 nm as the cutoff. These patients also had areas of GBM thickening, proportional to mesangial matrix increase and duration of diabetes. Careful examination and measurement of GBM in multiple loops is necessary to detect the coexistence of thin GBM lesion and diabetic changes.

Collagen Type III Glomerulopathy

Immunohistochemistry for interstitial type III and type IV collagen associated with sclerosing processes may be particularly useful to ascertain the stage of disease (see later). Such assessment may also be useful in diagnosis. A recently described hereditary nephropathy is characterized by increased collagen type III in glomeruli of children with progressive glomerular disease, hypertension, and the nephrotic syndrome. Histologically, the glomeruli showed diffuse increase in mesangial matrix and widened capillary walls. There was fibrillar collagen within the matrix, identified as collagen type III by immunohistochemistry. An association of this collagen abnormality with hemolytic-uremic syndrome in some patients or their siblings suggests a link to some familial cases of hemolytic-uremic syndrome. Transmission in these kindreds appeared to be autosomal recessive.[45]

Fibronectin Glomerulopathy

This rare, familial disease manifests as a membranoproliferative type pattern by light microscopy, with variable immunoglobulin staining by immunofluorescence. The mesangial/subendothelial deposits have vague or fibrillary substructure and stain intensely for fibronectin.[46]

Renal Disease in Dysproteinemias

AMYLOID AND FIBRILLARY GLOMERULONEPHRITIS

Morphometric evaluation of fibrils has been suggested to differentiate between amyloid (10–12 nm diameter) and nonamyloid fibrillary glomerulopathy (range, 14–20 nm diameter).[47] However, we have found significant overlap and suggest that Congo red staining remains the gold standard for diagnosis of the β-pleated sheet arrangement that defines amyloid. In cases of amyloidosis, the underlying biochemical abnormality leading to deposition of fibrillary material may be obvious in some patients and may require additional investigation in others. Even in patients with typical Congo red–positive amyloid fibrils, differentiation of AA versus AL amyloid may be of diagnostic and prognostic significance in searching for associated potentially treatable disease. Such differentiation may be done on cases with substantial amyloid deposition by performing Congo red staining on 7-μm thick sections followed by permanganate treatment. Sections treated in this way will maintain amyloid staining characteristics by Congo red for AA but not for AL.[48] Immunofluorescence with specific antibodies against AA amyloid and light-chain components may also be used. Both frozen-section and formalin-fixed paraffin methods have been studied. Concordance of identification of amyloid subtype with clinical and laboratory data was 88% in one series of 50 cases using the frozen-section technique.[49] When formalin-fixed tissue was used in a smaller series, all 11 cases of secondary amyloidosis but only 5 of 8 cases of primary amyloidosis were identified by antibody staining.[50] Immunoelectron microscopy has successfully identified amyloid A fibrils in five patients with known AA amyloid.[51] Of interest, the λ_{VI} class appears to be particularly amyloidogenic and amyloid P glycoprotein must also be present for amyloid protein to deposit in the glomeruli.[52]

Recent studies have more fully characterized lesions in patients with Congo red–negative amyloid-like deposits, so-called fibrillary glomerulonephritis. The fibrillary deposits in this disorder stain predominantly for the IgG4 subclass, not typical of other immune complex diseases.[53] However, the immunoglobulin deposits are not monoclonal, and these patients typically do not have dysproteinemias. Although the etiology and pathogenesis remain obscure, elegant studies by Yang and coworkers identified amyloid P component in fibrils of patients with fibrillary glomerulonephritis.[52] Further studies of the involved protein-forming fibrils may elucidate pathogenesis and direct therapies.

LIGHT CHAIN NODULAR GLOMERULOSCLEROSIS

Immunostaining for κ and λ light chains is helpful in understanding pathogenesis and classification of dysproteinemia-related diseases. The fibrillary β-pleated sheets of amyloid related to dysproteinemias are more commonly composed of λ light chain (see earlier). In contrast, monoclonal κ light chains in particular can form granular, that is, nonfibrillar, deposits. These deposits may result in a nodular glomerulosclerosis with a strong resemblance to diabetic nephropathy by light microscopy. Careful electron microscopic examination, in combination with immunofluorescent staining, is necessary for diagnosis of light-chain nodular glomerulosclerosis. Immunoelectron microscopy has confirmed the κ component of the granular deposits within tubular basement membranes as well as in glomeruli in most cases.[54] Amyloid P component is absent in the granular light-chain deposits in light-chain nodular glomerulosclerosis.[55] Although exceedingly rare, lambda light-chain deposits can cause similar lesions. Although these studies show progress in our understanding of factors leading to deposition of fibrils in the kidney, clearly further detailed characterization is necessary. Advances in immunoelectron microscopy are promising and may allow more precise diagnoses and classification.

HEAVY-CHAIN DEPOSITION DISEASE

Monoclonal immunoglobulin deposition disease (MIDD) has been proposed to include light-chain deposition disease and those deposition diseases with the same pathologic appearance, including heavy-chain deposition disease (HCDD).[56] Thus, amyloid, although it may be composed of light chains, is classified separately based on the differing mechanisms likely underlying fibrillar deposits in amyloid versus the amorphous precipitates common to MIDD. Heavy-chain deposits may coexist with light-chain deposits or be the sole component in HCDD. Tubular deposits are prominent, predominantly around distal tubules and Henle's loop, and can be visualized by periodic acid–Schiff stain as refractile ribbon-like material along the outer tubular basement membrane. Glomeruli are more variably involved but typically show nodular glomerulosclerosis with little cellularity within the nodules. Immunofluorescence stains in a smooth pattern for monotypic immunoglobulin. The deposits are finely or coarsely granular by electron microscopy. Multiple myeloma is the most common underlying disorder, but it may appear to be nonsecretory in up to 30% of patients. Studies have revealed abnormalities in light- and heavy-chain variable regions in MIDD and HCDD. Immunofluorescence with specific monoclonal antibodies for heavy- and light-chain components can aid in diagnosis and understanding of pathogenesis.[56]

Hepatitis B and C Virus

Membranous glomerulonephritis is associated with hepatitis B infection. Immunoelectron microscopy has identified Hb_e antigen as the main hepatitis B virus antigen involved in renal deposits in these cases. Viral transcripts for hepatitis B have been detected in glomerular cells and renal tubular cells by in situ hybridization.[57] Rheumatoid factors that are commonly present in these patients make it technically difficult to establish the role of hepatotropic viruses in these immune-complex diseases. The rheumatoid factors may be present in deposited immune complexes and nonspecifically bind immunoreagents directed against the viral antigens. Therefore, $F(ab')_2$ preparations of immunoreagents must be used for both the immunofluorescence and immunoelectron microscopy localization studies.[58]

Membranous glomerulonephritis has also been reported, albeit rarely, in association with hepatitis C infection. Hepatitis C virus has been detected in tissue (i.e., liver) by in situ hybridization and PCR.[59, 60] In two patients with known hepatitis C infection after bone marrow transplant, renal biopsy was done for nephrotic syndrome. Hepatitis C virus genome was detected by PCR performed on the RNA extracted from the paraffin-embedded biopsy specimen, requiring fifteen 5-μm sections. In situ hybridization studies of these biopsy specimens did not detect hepatitis C virus. Morphologic examination showed stage I membranous glomerulonephritis. It is possible that the virus was present in too low amount to be detected by in situ hybridization whereas PCR appears to be a sensitive method of detecting the virus. Whether hepatitis C is causal in this form of renal disease has not been established.[61] Direct demonstration of hepatitis C virus antigens in the immune deposits has not yet been accomplished.[62]

A high percentage of patients with membranoproliferative glomerulonephritis (MPGN) are infected with hepatitis C, demonstrated by PCR and/or serologic tests. Conversely, patients with hepatitis C not infrequently have renal disease.[63, 64] Cryoglobulins may form in response to hepatitis C infection and thus cause renal disease. Hepatitis C virus, when it affects the kidney, typically is associated with increased mesangial cellularity with positive immunofluorescence for IgG, IgM, and C_3 in an MPGN-like pattern. In the United States, it is estimated that 10% to 20% of cases of previously "idiopathic" MPGN may be related to hepatitis C virus. In Japan, over half of MPGN cases may be related to hepatitis C.[65]

The underlying cause of MPGN has important implications both for treatment and long-term prognosis. If hepatitis C is shown to be the underlying cause of MPGN, clinically significant hepatic disease may develop. Even transplantation must be evaluated in light of possible infection of the graft with the virus. Currently, no cure or long-term effective treatment is available. Although interferon therapy has reduced manifestations of disease, relapses were frequent once interferon therapy was stopped.[64]

HIV Virus

HIV nephropathy is manifest by FSGS with marked tubular dilatation and numerous reticular aggregates by electron microscopy. However, one must note that detection of the HIV genome in renal tissue does not per se allow diagnosis of HIV nephropathy. Thus, HIV genome was found in the kidney tissue of both HIV-infected patients with nephrotic-range proteinuria and in HIV-infected patients with no evidence of nephropathy.[66, 67] Whether HIV is present in only inflammatory cells or also infects resident glomerular cells is controversial, with carefully performed in situ hybridization and immunohistochemical studies failing to demonstrate viral signal within renal parenchymal cells.[68]

IgA nephropathy has also been reported in patients with HIV infection.[67] Of note, a positive HIV serum test in a patient with IgA nephropathy does not establish a causal relationship. However, the use of molecular biology techniques has established with high probability that IgA directed against HIV antigens is causally implicated in IgA nephropathy in a small group of patients. In these patients with HIV infection and apparent immune-mediated IgA glomerulonephritis, antibodies eluted from renal biopsies were found to react with HIV antigens from circulating immune complexes. Such approaches may become useful in defining an etiologic agent in immune-mediated diseases in this group of patients. The presence of reticular aggregates, a feature of HIV-associated FSGS, in apparent IgA nephropathy would suggest that HIV infection be included in the differential. Of note, lupus nephritis also shows numerous reticular aggregates by electron microscopy; this finding is by no means specific for HIV infection. The prognosis of HIV-associated IgA nephropathy has not been shown to be different from "idiopathic" IgA nephropathy as yet. If evidence emerges that there indeed is a difference in prognosis, more specific molecular analysis of tissue might be indicated for precise diagnosis and potential treatment. In this regard, special caution in interpreting molecular data from tissue homogenates is appropriate, because positivity with this method does not differentiate between parenchymal versus circulating cell infection.

Cytomegalovirus

A recent report has linked CMV to restenosing lesions after coronary angioplasty. CMV was detected by in situ hybridization and immunostaining of smooth muscle cells cultured from atherectomy specimens and correlated highly with increased p53 expression in these lesions. A CMV product was also found to inhibit normal p53 function, which may impact on cell turnover and thus contribute to the development of vascular lesions. These studies suggest that CMV, in addition to its direct impact on the immunocompromised host, may have important impact on scarring processes.[69] These mechanisms may be present not only in atherosclerosis but also in vascular scarring in kidneys and in other organs. If such a link is established by further studies, early detection of CMV, or other potential fibrogenic viruses, may direct specific therapies against ongoing proliferation of these viruses to impact on chronic scarring processes.

Tubulointerstitial Disease

Tubulointerstitial lesions may appear similar after exposure to various heavy metals. Specific histologic features include lead inclusions, visualized as particles by periodic acid–Schiff stain, or copper inclusions stained by rubeanic acid. Microprobe spectrum analysis is a more direct method of assessing tissue levels.[70] This technique allows identification of most atomic elements by specific emission and can be focused on the specific inclusion particle in question. However, care must be taken to avoid confusion with elements of processing metals or grid metals used for electron microscopy. Specific characterization and identification of heavy metals may lead to new understanding of etiology of many cases of "chronic renal failure" and have important consequences, not only for diagnosis, but also for public health and environmental safety policies.

Chronic interstitial nephritis is a nonspecific lesion that may be associated with exposure to nonsteroidal anti-inflammatory drugs. Studies have suggested that interstitial mucin, detected by Alcian blue/periodic acid–Schiff stain is an indicator of toxicity to these drugs.[71] This stain may allow more specific determination of underlying etiology of chronic interstitial nephritis lesions.

Differentiation of etiology of casts present in tubulointerstitial disease may occasionally be accomplished by light microscopic examination. Bilirubin casts seen with severe liver failure have typical greenish gold casts. Myoglobin casts are often reddish brown, whereas hemoglobin casts are more red. However, sometimes distinct pigmentation is not present. Immunostaining may then be helpful, using specific antibodies directed against myoglobin or hemoglobin. Likewise, immunohistochemistry may define the specific nature of casts with surrounding syncytial reaction in myeloma kidney.

In a study of acute tubular necrosis (ATN), most tubules with regenerating morphologic features in native kidneys showed distal phenotype marking. In transplants with ATN, particularly after treatment with cyclosporine, there was an equal distribution of distal and proximal tubules with apparent regenerating change.[72] These findings suggest that different mechanisms of injury affect ATN in different clinical settings. *Tetragonolobus purpureas* and *Phaseolus vulgaris* erythroagglutinin lectins are specific proximal tubule markers, whereas the distal nephron can be identified with antibody to epithelial membrane antigen, low-molecular-weight cytokeratin (AE1/AE3), or the lectin *Arachnis hypogaea*. The thick ascending limb of Henle can be specifically identified by its staining with antibody to Tamm-Horsfall protein.[73] Using these techniques, Nadasdy and colleagues have shown that typical atrophic tubule segments in the end-stage kidney originate largely from proximal tubules, whereas those tubules appearing thyroidized were of distal origin.[73] These authors have found most consistent results using the *T. purpureas* lectin and antibody to epithelial membrane antigen as proximal and distal markers, respectively. Specific distribution of nephron injury may then ultimately be used as an indicator of pathogenesis and for diagnosis of specific causes.

Tests of Prognostic Significance

The pisse prophets examined urine with the aid of uroscopy charts, smelling, and even tasting, to divine patients' prognosis. In modern times, nephrologists also utilized serum and urine findings to assess prognosis and evaluate response to treatment in patients with renal diseases.[74] The advent of percutaneous renal biopsies resulted in a new classification of renal diseases, based on histologic criteria.[75, 76] Expectations were that renal biopsy histologic analysis would give not only a diagnosis but also a stage of renal disease and prognostic and therapeutic response information.[77] However, recognition and classification based on the limited number of histologic lesions within the kidney's repertoire in response to injury may represent no more than different stages of these relatively limited glomerular responses caught at various stages of their evolution. In this section we review recent developments aimed at defining stages of injury by new approaches to the renal biopsy.

Interstitial Fibrosis

Many studies have attempted to define morphologic changes that correlate with renal function at time of biopsy or, of greater importance clinically, could predict functional outcome. However, even efforts to define structural injury of glomeruli that mirrors the patient's glomerular filtration rate have been fraught with difficulty. This should not be surprising, because both hemodynamic adaptation and glomerular growth may allow increased filtration and thus serve to normalize glomerular filtration rate, even with advanced glomerulosclerosis. Therefore, in studies with varied renal diseases, glomerular sclerosis was a less sensitive indicator of renal function than tubulointerstitial fibrosis.[78–80] Furthermore, the extent of tubulointerstitial damage was a predictor of subsequent renal failure in one study of children with FSGS.[81]

These findings may relate to the imprecise determination of areas of sclerosis affecting the glomerulus. The focal segmental pattern of sclerosis typical of many progressive glomerular diseases cannot be accurately assessed on a single section. In one retrospective serial section study, small peripheral lesions in patients with idiopathic FSGS were associated with a tendency to better clinical outcome than lesions also involving central areas of the glomerulus.[82] Whether these patterns have predictive value remains to be tested prospectively. This serial section analysis also importantly showed that intact glomeruli remain even in moderately advanced disease. Of note, more glomeruli were free of sclerosis in children at the time of diagnostic biopsy than in adults. This has important implications for intervention and potential response to therapy.

Laborious and time-consuming serial section analysis has been necessary to accurately assess total glomerular scarring. Scoring interstitial lesions on a single section may be a more sensitive indicator than assessing single section glomerular lesions, because the affected interstitial parenchyma is a sample representing a larger number and larger proportion of nephrons. It is possible that confocal microscopy, allowing optical serial sectioning of glomeruli, may in the future provide a more sensitive method of assessment and detection of focal segmental lesions.

Increased transforming growth factor-β (TGF-β) has been proposed as a marker and mediator of fibrosis, and its expression correlates with extent of fibrosis.[83] Chronic tubulointerstitial damage also correlated with expression of connective growth tissue factor (CTGF), which mediates TGF-β effects.[84] TGF-β receptor up-regulation was increased in areas of adhesions and sclerosis.[85]

Crescentic Glomerulonephritis

In crescentic glomerulonephritis, responsiveness to therapy may be determined by severity of crescentic lesions. Rupture was associated with fibrous crescent formation and sclerosis.[86, 87] This rupture may be seen with silver stain or can be detected by antibodies to basement membrane collagens. Studies have further identified up-regulated ICAM-1 in glomerular endothelial cells corresponding to early infiltration by polymorphonuclear leukocytes and associated with crescentic lesions.[88] Experimental evidence suggests that capsular rupture triggers periglomerular leukocytic infiltration, composed of T cells and IL-2 receptor–positive cells and surrounding macrophages. Insights into specific stage of crescents may thus be useful in establishing possible responsiveness of lesions, especially if the site of Bowman's space rupture cannot be determined by serial section analysis of histologic material.

Studies of human crescentic glomerulonephritis demonstrated increased expression of macrophage inflammatory protein (MIP)-1α and monocyte chemoattractant protein (MCP)-1 via the chemokine receptor CCR5. Locally produced MIP-1α appeared to be involved in the development of cellular crescents via CCR5, whereas MCP-1 was increased in the phase of fibrocellular or fibrous crescents.[89] Additional immunohistochemical and in situ hybridization studies indicated that resident renal cells as well as infiltrating cells produce CC chemokines and may thus regulate macrophage and T-cell recruitment.[90] Crescents also showed evidence of local activation of the coagulation system, with increased tissue factor and plasminogen activator inhibitor-1 (PAI-1) mainly expressed by resident cells.[91]

Lupus Nephritis

Early efforts focused on more precise quantification of severity and extent of injury to assess evolution of lesions and response to therapy. Such classifications were used for lupus nephritis. We developed a chronicity index[92] to semiquantitatively estimate the amount of chronic damage in patients with lupus nephritis, complementing the activity index initially developed by Pirani.[93] Histologic features of sclerosis and interstitial fibrosis were major indicators of chronicity, whereas cellular crescents, necrosis, and proliferation were markers of activity. The semiquantitative findings of chronicity and activity were useful in examining large groups of patients and defining groups with worse prognosis. A study reported by Schwartz and associates found little value for individual patients, however, by using this scoring system.[94] Furthermore, in the nonacademic setting, reproducibility was only moderate for chronicity and activity indices.[95] However, other studies found that cellular crescents and interstitial fibrosis were signs of poor prognosis, providing additional outcome prediction over clinical data alone.[96] The presence of one or more chronicity markers in a given renal biopsy specimen was also associated with a poor prognosis. These variable results using semiquantitative or subjective scoring systems have led to efforts to use quantitative morphometric assessments of severity of lesions.[95]

Diabetic Nephropathy

The use of morphometric quantitative methods to define glomerular diseases was initially introduced to study diabetic nephropathy. The Minnesota group established correlations between the severity of renal disease, assessed by the amount of urinary albumin and the proportion of the glomerular tufts occupied by the mesangium (the so-called index of mesangial expansion).[97] For any morphometric evaluation, nonbiased sampling methods must be used. Using such techniques, Østerby and colleagues found more variable structural abnormalities in diabetic patients with normal albumin excretion rate than those with elevated albumin excretion rate, who had thicker glomerular basement membranes and increased mesangial matrix and cell volume.[98] The higher variability in the group with normal albumin excretion rate may, in part, reflect preclinical glomerulopathy, although identification of specific morphologic indicators for development of overt nephropathy have not yet been identified.

Although diagnosis of diabetic nephropathy is accomplished by standard renal biopsy techniques, the very early changes that might correlate with subsequent progression to diabetic nephropathy in the subset of diabetic patients who develop this complication are not clearly defined. A series of 17 patients with diabetes and persistent microalbuminuria were found to show thickened basement membranes compared with controls (595 vs. 305 nm), mild mesangial volume fraction expansion (0.22 vs. 0.19) and also increased mesangial matrix volume fraction (0.13 vs. 0.09).[98] Another series involving a smaller number of older patients showed variable lesions with microalbuminuria at the time of biopsy.[99, 100] It is not yet established whether mesangial expansion or other morphologic changes are reliable markers of long-term progression. In addition, although the lesions in type I and type II diabetes may be caused by a similar pathogenetic mechanism, they exhibit significant morphologic differences. For instance, whereas glomerular hypertrophy is present in type I diabetes mellitus, the glomerular volume remains normal in type II diabetics. There are no long-term studies establishing whether the degree and/or presence of glomerular hypertrophy has a predictive value, per se, in type I diabetes.[101] Careful quantitation of abnormalities, coupled with molecular techniques, may allow better understanding of the stage of the disease at time of biopsy. The effect of therapy on the components of abnormalities may also be more carefully assessed by molecular analysis of biopsy specimens.

Elevated expression of TGF-β has been found in numerous animal models associated with renal scarring.[102] Glomerular TGF-β expression was increased in patients with overt diabetic nephropathy compared with biopsy specimens in patients with nonprogressive renal disease (minimal change disease and thin basement membrane disease).[103] Quantity of staining correlated with the severity of glomerular sclerosis. A note of caution is in order, however, in extrapolating directly from animal models to human disease. The predictive value of enhanced growth factor expression has not been determined in any human disease, although many animal studies have shown an association of up-regulation of various growth factors, including TGF-β, basic fibroblast growth factor (bFGF), and platelet-derived growth factor (PDGF) at various stages with injury.[1, 103, 104] In diabetes, there was also increased matrix metalloprotease-3, tissue inhibitor of metalloproteinase-1 (TIMP-1), and PAI-1 associated with sclerosis, suggesting an imbalance of matrix degradation and synthesis.[105, 106] PAI-1 is increased in human thrombotic and vascular sclerotic disease and promotes both thrombosis and fibrosis by inhibiting fibrinolysis and proteolysis.[107]

"Minimal Change Disease"—Focal Segmental Glomerulosclerosis

Our early studies of factors involved with progression of glomerular diseases led to the hypothesis that glomerular enlargement could be a marker for aberrant growth factor expression, ultimately leading to scarring of the kidney. In our study of pediatric patients with apparent minimal change disease, we found that those patients who subsequently developed overt FSGS indeed had larger glomeruli than either normal age-matched controls or patients with typical minimal change disease who had benign clinical courses and, on resampling, also had minimal change disease (Fig. 9–1). These findings were confirmed in a study by the Minnesota group.[108] A sensitive cutoff index was found for glomerular area greater than 150% of age-matched control. In our laboratory, this corresponded to glomerular diameters of more than 118 μm as a cutoff in the pediatric age group younger than 5 years

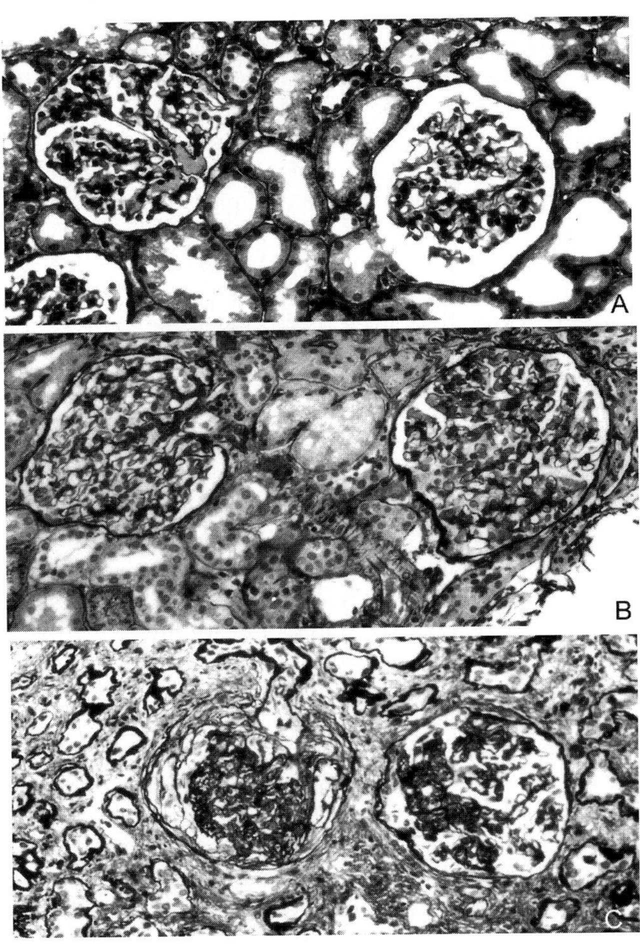

FIGURE 9–1
Glomerular size in focal segmental glomerular sclerosis (FSGS) versus minimal change disease (MCD). *A* and *B*, Initial biopsy specimens from patients with apparent MCD. The 5-year-old girl's initial biopsy specimen in *B* was indistinguishable from the age-matched typical MCD in *A*, except for marked glomerular enlargement. *C*, The girl's subsequent biopsy specimen, 50 months later, showed FSGS (Jones' silver stain, ×160). (From Fogo A, Hawkins EP, Berry PL, et al: Glomerular hypertrophy in minimal change disease predicts subsequent progression to focal glomerular sclerosis. Kidney Int 1990;38:115–123.)

of age, compared with normal diameter of 95 μm in this age group.[109] Of note, other conditions that could predispose to glomerular enlargement must be excluded, because it is our view that it is not glomerular enlargement per se that causes glomerulosclerosis. Rather, glomerular enlargement is taken as a sign of aberrant growth factors that are pathogenic.[1] Conditions associated with enlarged glomeruli include solitary kidney, congenital cyanotic heart disease, and marked obesity (all of which may, interestingly, be associated with FSGS).

Analysis of individual glomeruli in patients with FSGS and in animal models showed a biphasic relationship between glomerular size and scarring. Thus, early sclerosis was characterized by increasing glomerular size whereas the final end-stage hyalinized glomerulus was smaller.[1] Of interest, this association of increased glomerular size and early pathogenetic events of glomerular sclerosis was also seen in the setting of recurrent FSGS in the transplant. Therefore, children who received an adult transplant who did not develop FSGS in their transplants did not show increased glomerular size over the initial months after transplantation. In contrast, those children who developed recurrent FSGS had marked, abnormal glomerular growth, preceding overt manifestation of FSGS.[110] These findings may be useful in earlier recognition of recurrent FSGS and also in understanding underlying mechanisms.

Similarly, adult patients with existing FSGS had significantly larger glomerular size than adult patients with minimal change disease. In patients with glomerular tip lesions in which prognosis is thought to be similar to that of minimal change disease, glomerular enlargement was not found.[111] Thus, in cases of nephrotic syndrome without evident segmental glomerular sclerosis, patients with normal glomerular size appear to have a good prognosis. In contrast, those patients with markedly enlarged glomerular size have a high risk of subsequent progression to overt FSGS.

Extensive foot process effacement is a shared characteristic of minimal change disease and FSGS. Decreased expression of the adhesion protein dystroglycan, a major binding protein for laminin, agrin, and perlecan, was present in minimal change disease but not in FSGS. This test might thus be useful in differentiating between minimal change disease and FSGS in cases in which the segmental sclerotic lesion is not sampled. These findings also suggest different pathogenic mechanisms in foot process injury in minimal change disease and FSGS.[112]

Chronic Renal Disease

Different population groups also show varying risks for progression. We have explored the participation of growth factors in development of the glomerular sclerotic lesions. We also examined whether abnormal glomerular size distribution could account for population differences in severity and incidence of progressive renal disease. Kidneys from African American and white normal adults who died suddenly were assessed morphometrically. Subjects were matched for body mass index, age, and gender. Average glomerular size in African Americans was significantly greater than in whites. Of note, the distribution, while Gaussian in African Americans, showed a biphasic distribution in whites (Fig. 9–2). We speculate that the subpopulation of whites with larger glomeruli may have increased risk for progressive renal disease, comparable to the African American population.[113] Currently, studies are underway to investigate whether differences in genotype

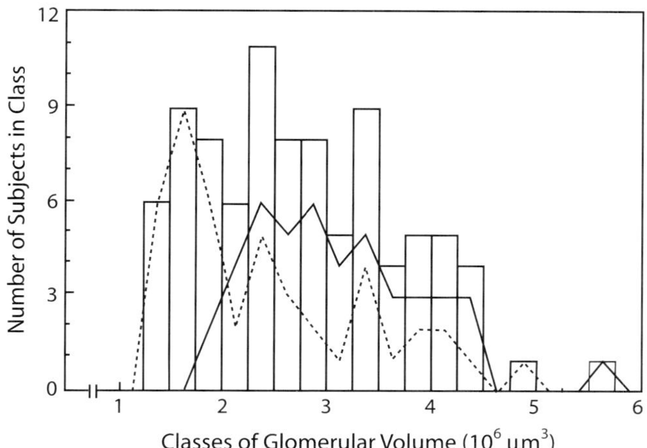

FIGURE 9–2
Distribution of mean glomerular volume values in African Americans (n = 45, solid line) and whites (n = 45, *dotted line*). Values from the total population are shown by the open bars. Each size class is identified by the lowest glomerular volume value. (From Pesce C, Schmidt K, Fogo A: Glomerular size and the incidence of renal disease in African Americans and Caucasians. J Nephrol 1994;7:355–358.)

Competitive PCR on 1/10 Normal Glomerulus for mα$_1$IV Collagen

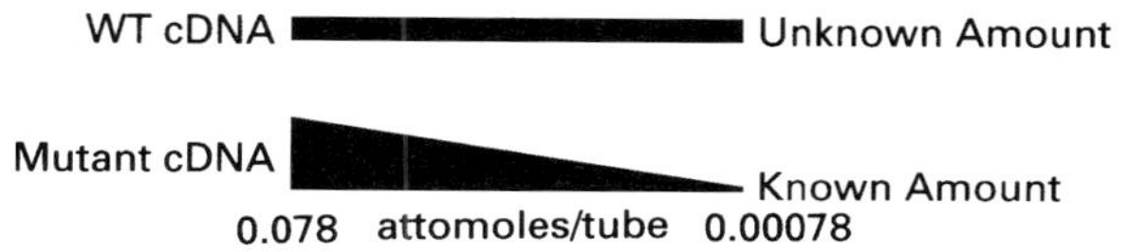

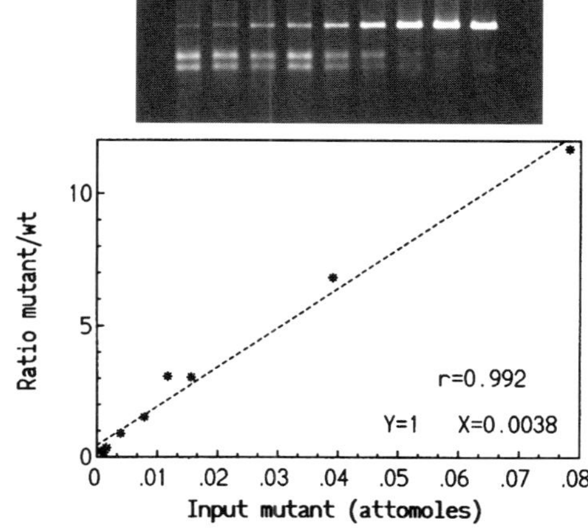

FIGURE 9–3
Competitive PCR for 1 type IV collagen in one tenth of a normal mouse glomerulus. Each tube has added unknown amount of wild-type (WT) complementary DNA (cDNA) and known amounts of mutant cDNA (*top*). Mutants were constructed to differ from WT by adding a *BclI* restriction enzyme site. The *middle panel* shows the resulting ethidium bromide–stained gel after PCR amplification. After PCR, the PCR products were exposed to *BclI*, and WT and mutant bands were analyzed by densitometry. The graph shows the ratio of mutant to WT density, versus the amount of mutant cDNA per tube. Amount of cDNA in the unknown sample is then calculated from the equivalence point (y = 1).

and/or glomerular number may underlie this difference in size.

STAGE OF INJURY

Cells and Cytokines

Specific investigation of phenotype of renal cells may define more precisely the stage of injury. Thus, the presence of α-actin in mesangial cells is an indicator of a myofibroblast phenotype. This cell type is associated with wound healing and repair and has increased matrix-producing capability.[114]

Studies have started mapping human renal biopsy specimens for expression of various cytokines that have been implicated in progressive renal disease. These observations include increased PDGF in proliferative glomerulonephritides but not in those processes that do not show proliferation such as minimal change disease.[115] Numerous studies in IgA nephropathy have applied immunohistochemical and in situ hybridization methodologies, implicating fibrinogen, VCAM-1, and monocytes in segmental necrotizing lesions.[116] Expression of PDGF-AB/BB paralleled the severity of proliferative changes in IgA nephropathy,[117] and proliferative lesions in IgA nephropathy and vasculitic lesions were associated with up-regulation with IL-10.[118] As of yet, the delineation of these cytokines has not yielded diagnostic information. Advances in this area may, however, lead to new predictors of course of disease. The development of in situ RT-PCR to quantitate mRNA from small numbers of microdissected glomeruli has provided a basis for assessing aberrant cytokine and collagen production in human biopsy specimens (Fig. 9–3). This technique offers the advantage that a small portion of a diagnostic biopsy specimen be used without sacrificing standard information for diagnosis. The tissue can then yield important information regarding markers of injury or progression. Indeed, clinical observations have shown that not only are different diseases variable in their rates of progression, but also individual patients show marked heterogeneity in disease progression. Thus, only a portion of patients with, for example, diabetes mellitus or IgA nephropathy develop progressive glomerulosclerosis. Recent efforts have been directed at identifying those at risk for progression both by analysis of genetic susceptibilities and by molecular analysis of kidney tissue. Patients with IgA nephropathy with aspecific deletion polymorphism (D/D) of the angiotensin-converting enzyme were more likely to show progression than those with the insertion (I/I) genotype.[119] Investigation of genotypes of candidate genes from archival renal biopsy material will yield much information in this rapidly developing area. Future advances may map not only risk for progression (from DNA analyses) but ultimately rate of progression and the current molecular stage of disease in individual patients from mRNA profiles of key mediators of progression.

Matrix Accumulation

The ultimate anatomic feature of glomerulosclerosis is the accumulation of connective tissue in the glomerulus.[87] Possible mechanisms could relate to increased matrix production or decreased matrix degradation.[120, 121] Although in vivo evidence is yet lacking, in vitro evidence supports that mRNA levels indeed parallel protein levels for one key extracellular matrix component, namely, α1 type IV collagen.[122] Type IV collagen mRNA is a major component of the normal glomerulus that accumulates in most instances of progressive human and experimental glomerulosclerosis. Type IV collagen mRNA is not detectable in kidneys of normal adults by in situ hybridization, although it is normally expressed during development.[123] Thus, the detection of glomerular mRNA could serve as a prognostic indicator of glomerulosclerosis. To be able to quantitate such expression, we developed a technique of in situ reverse transcription, PCR analysis (RT-PCR)[124] with a competitive assay,[125] applied to individual microdissected glomeruli. We were able to reproducibly measure mRNA levels in the attomolar range (10^{18}),[126] allowing detection of mRNA from one tenth of a glomerulus (see Fig. 9–3). The quantitative method that we chose is based on the introduction in each PCR reaction tube of a defined amount of a mutated complementary DNA (cDNA) that competes with the primers on an equimolar basis.[125] The amount of cDNA in a sample can be calculated as the amount at which there is an equal ratio between the test cDNA and the amount of mutant template. Studies in mice showed close correspondence between the occurrence of sclerosis and the mRNA and immunofluorescence levels for α1 and α2 type IV collagens.

In another mouse strain transgenic for bovine growth hormone (bGH), sclerosis is prominent, with increased type IV collagen, laminin, and heparan sulfate proteoglycan by immunofluorescence microscopy.[122] Type IV collagen mRNA was increased most in glomeruli[127] and less in cortex.[128] Type I collagen, an interstitial collagen not expressed in normal conditions, was also increased, similar to human diabetic nephropathy. Of note, this marked increase in collagen mRNA was already evident early when sclerosis was minimal. These findings suggest that this increase in collagen mRNA may not merely mirror existing sclerosis but may also have a predictive value early in the disease. There was also a marked increase in glomerular cell turnover (fourfold) by ^{3}H-thymidine labeling index, predominantly caused by cells in the mesangial regions.[129] Markers for cell proliferation, such as Ki-67, PCNA, and bromodeoxyuridine, can be detected by immunocytochemistry.[130] Apoptosis may de detected not only by classic apoptotic bodies but also by in situ end-labeling techniques that detect the characteristic fragmented DNA. Alterations in apoptosis have been reported in human glomerular diseases.[131] Interestingly, this increased turnover and increased extracellular matrix mRNA persisted at the same high levels even in terminal lesions, suggesting that remodeling, with both cell proliferation and cell death or apoptosis, persists at late stages of glomerular scarring, a finding that may have important therapeutic implications in humans.

These findings have been further examined in a nonprogressive transgenic model, in which bGH also carries a mutation in the third α helix (M11). Levels of α1 type IV collagen are 2.6 times higher than those in normal mice,[132] but they never reach the elevation (8- to 10-fold) observed in the bGH mice.[127] These observations suggest that the slope of progression of a given type of glomerulosclerosis is parallel to that of extracellular matrix mRNA. Thus, it should be possible to define genes of predictive value for progression (see Fig. 9–1). The postulate that gene activation reaches a maximum elevation early in the course of a disease will have to be further examined. Studies of other models and, mostly, of multiple human diseases will establish whether this concept can be extended to many forms of glomerular disease.

Studies of Human Glomeruli

Nephrectomy specimens in adult patients undergoing surgery for cancer were assessed. Approximately half the patients with renal cancer show glomeruli with increased mesangial matrix.[126] Patients with glomerulosclerosis showed a significant elevation (mean, 3.8-fold) of collagen type IV mRNA compared with patients without glomerulosclerosis. The two patients with most severe sclerosis also had the highest levels of collagen type IV gene expression, an observation consistent with our experimental data suggesting that late sclerosis is still an active process and thus could potentially be manipulated.

Matrix accumulation is also affected by rate of degradation. The metalloproteinase PUMP-1, which can degrade collagen, has been found to be expressed in human proliferative glomerulonephritis but not in normal glomeruli.[133] Genes that are implicated in basement membrane degradation, *TIMP1* and *TIMP2* and *PAI1*, have also been assessed in human tissue.[106,107,134] *TIMP1* and *TIMP2* genes were expressed in normal human glomeruli and were up-regulated in tissue from patients with glomerulosclerosis. PA1-1 also correlates tightly with sclerosis in experimental models of sclerosis and in human diseases and is implicated in inhibition of fibrinolysis and proteolysis.[107] Thus, degradation of collagen may be impaired in concert with up-regulation of matrix-producing genes, both promoting sclerosis. Possible therapies in the future could be targeted at either of these mechanisms. The balance of these processes might provide an index of possible therapeutic efficacy long before changes would be manifest by light microscopy or by functional assessment.

RENAL TUMORS

Diagnosis

RENAL CELL CARCINOMA

Immunohistologic studies have revealed that renal cell carcinomas can be derived from proximal or distal convoluted tubules or collecting ducts. The majority of clear cell carcinomas originate from proximal convoluted tubules, whereas most tumors in the classic "granular" category react with distal convoluted tubular or collecting duct markers. Thus, immunostaining to identify nephron segment antigenic markers may be a useful adjunct to classification by histologic means. Whether this also has prognostic implication has not been defined.

A monoclonal antibody, ERY-1, which reacts with erythrocytes, erythroid precursor cells, and embryonal yolk sac in normal liver and kidney has been reported to stain neoplastic cells of the clear cell renal and yolk sac carcinoma. Reactivity has not been reported in other epithelial or mesenchymal neoplasms by the authors of the study. For undifferentiated neoplasms, this might prove to be a useful marker of possible renal cell origin.[135]

Immunocytochemical studies of renal cell carcinomas showed positive staining for IL-4 receptor in one small series. Positivity was also seen in primary cultures of renal cell carcinoma tumor cells. The positivity of IL-4 expression was confirmed by flow cytometric analysis.[136] This marker may serve as a diagnostic marker, as well as a target to specifically direct therapeutic agents to tumor cells by use of chemotherapeutic agents linked to antibody to IL-4.

Differentiation of benign renal cortical adenomas from renal cell carcinomas, while classically based on size less than 3 cm, is not accurate. Thus, even Bell's original paper showed a tumor smaller than this size that had metastasized.[137] A newer classification based on cytoplasmic appearance differentiates clear cell, chromophobe, chromophilic, and spindle-shaped forms. The clear cell type is typified by abundant lipid and glycogen. The chromophobe type has abundant pale cytoplasm with a fine reticular appearance and strong positivity with Hale's colloidal iron. Chromophilic tumors contain abundant mitochondria and have densely granular cytoplasm. Whether each of these subtypes has distinct clinical implication has not yet been determined.[138] Of note, oncocytomas, characterized by a benign prognosis, are distinct from the chromophobe tumors by their lack of staining with Hale's colloidal iron. In addition, oncocytomas frequently demonstrate loss of chromosomes 1 and Y; these cytogenetic changes may be useful in the differential diagnosis.[139]

Subtypes of renal cell carcinoma are associated with abnormalities of different chromosomes. Most nonpapillary clear cell renal carcinomas are associated with loss of tumor suppressor genes on the short arm of chromosome 3. Different suppressor genes are affected in various forms of renal cell carcinoma. The 3p13-p14 locus appears affected in familial renal cell carcinomas, whereas sporadic renal cell carcinomas show an abnormality in the suppressor gene at 3p21-p24. Yet another site, 3p25-p26, is altered in von Hippel-Lindau syndrome. The VHL tumor suppressor gene has recently been identified as causal in this disease. Papillary renal cell carcinoma, corresponding most often to a chromophil cell type, is associated with abnormalities of chromosome 7, 16, 17, or Y.[140] Trisomy for chromosomes 7 and 17 is common in this tumor. Increased number of chromosomal abnormalities may herald a more aggressive course. Thus, small tubulopapillary lesions with a morphologic appearance of "adenoma" may manifest only trisomy for chromosomes 7 and 17, in contrast to the multiple additional chromosomal aberrations in typical papillary carcinomas. Chromophobe carcinomas have unusual and multiple chromosomal abnormalities, most often involving loss of seven chromosomes (1, 2, 6, 10, 13, 17, 21).[141, 142] Flow cytometric studies evaluating DNA ploidy have shown a correlation of grade of tumor with ploidy. However, even diploid tumors may show progression.

WILMS' TUMOR

Wilms' tumor is frequently associated with nephrogenic rest, a precursor tissue that can remain dormant, regress, or lead to the development of tumor. Polysialic acid represents an oncodevelopmental antigen detected in both embryonic human kidney and Wilms' tumor. In a comparative immunohistochemical study, no staining for polysialic acid was found in a variety of other tumors, including clear cell sarcomas of kidney, renal cell carcinomas, Ewing's sarcomas, hepatoblastomas, rhabdomyosarcomas, and various carcinomas. Within Wilms' tumor, the blastemal cells and epithelial components were positive whereas the stroma did not stain.[143]

Two suppressor genes are thought to be involved in genesis of Wilms' tumor. The *WT1* and *WT2* genes are both located on the short arm of chromosome 11. Mutations of *WT1* have been identified in patients with Wilms' tumor in association with other syndromal abnormalities. The *WT1* gene codes for a protein with characteristics typical of DNA binding transcription factors with four zinc finger domains at the carboxyl terminus mediating DNA binding. The *WT1* transcript has two alternative splice sites resulting in four distinct mRNA species.[144] Although homology with the early growth response gene family exists, the predominant form of *WT1* mRNA does not bind to the EGR-1 site.[145] Because WT1 is normally expressed in the developing kidney in condensed blastema renal vesicle and early glomerulus, especially in the podocyte, detection of WT1 cannot per se invoke a diagnosis of Wilms' tumor.[146] However, a correlation between the relative abundance of WT1 messenger RNA and histologic type of Wilms' tumor has been found, with predominantly blastemal types expressing higher levels of WT1 versus predominantly stromal or heterologous differentiated Wilms' tumors.[144]

Many different point mutations in Wilms' tumor have been found to involve the zinc finger domains, particularly in exon 9. Evidence indicates that mutations in *WT1* are not sufficient per se to cause tumor genesis. A second somatic mutation at the same disease locus is thought to be necessary. Imprinting is also thought to be involved in tumor genesis, in that the maternal allele is nearly always preferentially lost when heterozygosity at 11p is lost in Wilms' tumor. This imprinting does not, however, involve the *WT1* locus.[147, 148] The *WT2* locus is a candidate for a second mutation and may be involved in imprinting. Duplication of the 11p15 *WT2* locus with inheritance of two copies of the paternal gene has been linked to Beckwith-Wiedemann syndrome. In contrast, *WT2* loss has been described in Wilms' tumor.[149]

The insulin-like growth factor-2 (IGF-2) embryonal growth inducing gene *(IGF2)* resides at the *WT2* 11p15 site and has been intensively studied. The *IGF2* gene remains a candidate as a tumor promoter, in addition to the possibility of an as yet unidentified tumor suppressor.[150] In some Wilms' tumors, both maternal and paternal alleles of *IGF2* are expressed, whereas normally only the paternal allele is constitutively expressed. Further advances in PCR-amplified in situ hybridization may allow detection of these specific mutations.

Prognosis

RENAL CELL CARCINOMA

The immunohistochemistry score for the proliferation marker Ki-67 correlated well with histologic grading in a series of 93 patients with renal cell carcinoma.[151] Nuclear morphometry and cellular DNA content may both be useful tools to identify populations with high risk for micrometastases where adjuvant therapy may be useful.[152] In one series, patients with tumor nuclear area of less then 35 μm^2 have a good prognosis, contrasting to patients with larger nuclear areas who had a poor prognosis (17.2% 5-year survival in the latter versus 96.7% 5-year survival in the former).[153] Other factors including nuclear perimeter, major diameter, nucleolar area, nuclear shape factor, and nuclear size showed lesser degrees of prognostic value.

Two molecular biologic features have shown some evidence of prognostic significance. Patients whose tumors demonstrate *KRAS* amplification appear to have a poorer prognosis than those without.[154] In addition, immunohistochemical staining for p53 is associated with poor survival in patients with early-stage renal cell carcinoma.[155]

Microchip gene array analysis has been applied to renal cell carcinoma analysis, showing frequent vimentin gene expression in clear cell carcinoma (51%) and papillary renal cell carcinoma (61%) but rare expression in chromophobe RCC (4%) and oncocytomas (12%). Furthermore, vimentin expression was significantly associated with poor patient prognosis, independent of grade and stage.[156]

WILMS' TUMOR

In addition to molecular markers, recent evaluation of Wilms' tumor by morphometric techniques has been used to assess prognosis in these patients. Nuclear morphometry, evaluating nuclear roundness, ellipticity, convexity, and bending energy, accurately separated the groups, predicting children who would respond to therapy. However, all nine patients in this small study had favorable histologic disease and the validity of these parameters for other histologic appearances of Wilms' tumor has not been tested.[157]

In an analysis of a larger series of Wilms' tumors (175 cases), DNA characteristics were investigated by flow cytometry from paraffin-embedded material. The technique was successful in 73 of the cases. Aneuploidy was only seen in seven tumors. Ploidy analyses have indicated that diploid and aneuploid tumors have better response to therapy than tetraploid tumors. In addition, advanced stage, female gender, a lower number of cells in the synthetic phase, and lower proliferative index predicted worse prognosis.[158] The results may reflect greater chemotherapy sensitivity in tumors with high cell turnover.

In addition, possible interactions of *TP53* mutations with *WT1* and *IGF2* genes have been proposed. However, so far *TP53* mutations have not clearly distinguished cases of Wilms' tumors with favorable versus anaplastic features.[159] Identification of other specific gene markers may elucidate mechanisms of abnormal growth in these neoplasms. As gene therapy evolves, manipulations of specific genes may even be used to effect regression of these tumors.

PERSPECTIVES

The presence or magnitude of expression of certain proteins can be diagnostic and/or prognostic. Assessment of protein expression can be done by immunohistochemistry or molecular studies. In situ hybridization is difficult to quantify and may be insufficiently sensitive to detect small amounts of mRNA. The advantages of this technique are that specific cell types involved in mRNA expression may be identified, especially with novel double-staining techniques. Increased sensitivity of riboprobes may also produce more sensitive detection. Renal biopsy tissue is insufficient to allow mRNA analysis by Northern blotting. PCR can be difficult to interpret quantitatively, owing to the potential for errors that reflects the high degree of sensitivity to small variations in the sample and protocol. Recent advances with competitive PCR, using the elegant approach of constructing mutant cDNA templates as controls, have partly overcome these difficulties. Advances with implications for prognosis have also been made in morphometric studies both of progressive renal diseases and neoplasms. New insights into genetic abnormalities underlying development of renal tumors allows for more precise classification, and perhaps more effectively targeted therapies. New approaches may also provide insights into the pathogenesis of end-stage glomerular disease. For instance, although many data suggest a role of growth factors, such as TGF-β and PDGF in glomerular disease, their exact role in humans has not been elucidated.[1, 103, 104, 160] New quantitative methods of assessing such potential markers of stages of disease on small amounts of tissue will allow more readily the direct transfer of knowledge obtained from animal experimentation to human disease. Laser capture microdissection allows specific isolation of portions of tissue that may then be analyzed for DNA and/or RNA content. This technique has been successful in analyzing gene expression from even fragments of a single glomerulus.[161] Microdissection techniques have been applied to fresh kidney biopsy specimens, yielding adequate RNA using silica gel–based membrane spin technology for competitive RT-PCR. The method was also used successfully in biopsy specimens frozen for more then 10 years at 70°C.[162] Most recently, novel techniques have been used to detect expression of transcription factors with Southwestern histochemistry, allowing cell type specific localization of such nuclear factors.[163]

The next stage of insights in diagnosis of diseases affecting the kidney will lie in application of these advances made in the areas of immunohistochemistry and with the explosion of molecular and quantitative techniques. The goals of these techniques will be to not merely define a lesion but also to gain insights into specific pathogenesis, provide prognostic information at early stages of disease, and predict the response to, and direct, therapy in a more precise manner.

Acknowledgments

Dr. Agnes Fogo is a recipient of an Established Investigator Award from the American Heart Association.

REFERENCES

1. Fogo A, Ichikawa I; Glomerular Growth Promoter; the Common Channel to Glomerulosclerosis. In Mitch WE (ed): The Progressive Nature of Renal Disease. New York, Churchill Livingstone, 1992, pp 23–54.
2. Gray DW, Richardson A, Hughes D, et al: A prospective, randomized, blind comparison of three biopsy techniques in the management of patients after renal transplantation. Transplantation 1992;53:1226–1232.
3. Pattison J, Nelson PJ, Huie P, et al: RANTES chemokine expression in cell-mediated transplant rejection of the kidney. Lancet 1994;343:209–211.
4. Tovey MG, Deglise-Favre A, Schoevaert D: Differential in situ expression of cytokine genes in human renal transplantation. Kidney Int Suppl 1993;39:S129–S132.
5. Lipman ML, Stevens AC, Bleackley RC, et al: The strong correlation of cytotoxic T lymphocyte–specific serine protease gene transcripts with renal allograft rejection. Transplantation 1992;53:73–79.
6. Raasveld MH, Bloemena E, Wilmink JM, et al: Interleukin-6 and neopterin in renal transplant recipients: A longitudinal study. Transpl Int 1993;6:89–94.
7. Raasveld MH, Weening JJ, Kerst JM, et al: Local production of interleukin-6 during acute rejection in human renal allografts. Nephrol Dial Transplant 1993; 8:75–78.
8. Yoshimura N, Oka T, Kahan BD: Sequential determinations of serum interleukin 6 levels as an immunodiagnostic tool to differentiate rejection from nephrotoxicity in renal allograft recipients. Transplantation 1991;51: 172–176.
9. Nast CC, Zuo XJ, Prehn J, et al: Gamma-interferon gene expression in human renal allograft fine-needle aspirates. Transplantation 1994;57:498–502.
10. Totterman TH, Hanas E, Bergstrom R, et al: Immunologic diagnosis of kidney rejection using FACS analysis of graft-infiltrating functional and activated T and NK cell subsets. Transplantation 1989;47:817–823.
11. Kyo M, Mihatsch MJ, Gudat F, et al: Renal graft rejection or cyclosporin toxicity? Early diagnosis by a combination of Papanicolaou and immunocytochemical staining of urinary cytology specimens. Transpl Int 1992;5:71–76.
12. Lan HY, Yang N, Brown FG, et al: Macrophage migration inhibitory factor expression in human renal allograft rejection. Transplantation 1998;66:1465–1471.
13. Brockmeyer C, Ulbrecht M, Schendel DJ, et al: Distribution of cell adhesion molecules (ICAM-1, VCAM-1, ELAM-1) in renal tissue during allograft rejection. Transplantation 1993;55:610–615.
14. Andersen CB: Acute kidney graft rejection morphology and immunology. APMIS Suppl 1997;67:1–35.
15. Haug CE, Colvin RB, Delmonico FL, et al: A phase I trial of immunosuppression with anti-ICAM-1 (CD54) mAb in renal allograft recipients. Transplantation 1993;55:766–772.
16. Briscoe DM, Pober JS, Harmon WE, Cotran RS: Expression of vascular cell adhesion molecule-1 in human renal allografts. J Am Soc Nephrol 1992;3: 1180–1185.

17. Heemann UW, Tullius SG, Schumann V, Tilney NL: Neutrophils and macrophages are prominent in the pathophysiology of chronic rejection of rat kidney allografts. Transplant Proc 1993;25:937–938.
18. Collins AB, Schneeberger EE, Pascual MA, et al: Complement activation in acute humoral renal allograft rejection: Diagnostic significance of C4d deposits in peritubular capillaries. J Am Soc Nephrol 1999;10: 2208–2214.
19. Benigni A, Bruzzi I, Mister M, et al: Nature and mediators of renal lesions in kidney transplant patients given cyclosporine for more than one year. Kidney Int 1999; 55:674–685.
20. Abrass CK, Berfield AK, Stehman-Breen C, et al: Unique changes in interstitial extracellular matrix composition are associated with rejection and cyclosporine toxicity in human renal allograft biopsies. Am J Kidney Dis 1999;33:11–20.
21. Murer L, Zacchello G, Basso G, et al: Early and rapid diagnosis of CMV infection by nonradioactive in situ hybridization in pediatric kidney transplant recipients. Nephron 1992;60:25–29.
22. Nadasdy T, Miller KW, Johnson LD, et al: Is cytomegalovirus associated with renal disease in AIDS patients? Mod Pathol 1992;5:277–282.
23. Chen YT, Mercer GO, Cheigh JS, Mouradian JA: Cytomegalovirus infection of renal allografts: Detection by polymerase chain reaction. Transplantation 1992;53: 99–102.
24. Cockfield SM, Preiksaitis JK, Jewell LD, Parfrey NA: Post-transplant lymphoproliferative disorder in renal allograft recipients: Clinical experience and risk factor analysis in a single center. Transplantation 1993;56: 88–96.
25. Nadasdy T, Park CS, Peiper SC, et al: Epstein-Barr virus infection–associated renal disease: Diagnostic use of molecular hybridization technology in patients with negative serology. J Am Soc Nephrol 1992;2:1734–1742.
26. Yamashina M, Takami T, Kanemura T, et al: Immunohistochemical demonstration of complement components in formalin-fixed and paraffin-embedded renal tissues. Lab Invest 1989;60:311–316.
27. Sacks SH, Zhou W, Andrews PA, Hartley B: Endogenous complement C3 synthesis in immune complex nephritis. Lancet 1993;342:1273–1274.
28. Jennette JC: The immunohistology of IgA nephropathy. Am J Kidney Dis 1988;12:348–352.
29. Steffes MW, Barbosa J, Basgen JM, et al: Quantitative glomerular morphology of the normal human kidney. Lab Invest 1983;49:82–86.
30. Abe S, Amagasaki Y, Iyori S, et al: Thin basement membrane syndrome in adults. J Clin Pathol 1987;40:318–322.
31. Basta-Jovanovic G, Venkataseshan VS, Gil J, et al: Morphometric analysis of glomerular basement membranes (GBM) in thin basement membrane disease (TBMD). Clin Nephrol 1990;33:110–114.
32. Pettersson E, Tornroth T, Wieslander J: Abnormally thin glomerular basement membrane and the Goodpasture epitope. Clin Nephrol 1990;33:105–109.
33. Tiebosch AT, Frederik PM, van Breda V, et al: Thin-basement-membrane nephropathy in adults with persistent hematuria. N Engl J Med 1989;320:14–18.
34. Dische FE, Anderson VE, Keane SJ, et al: Incidence of thin membrane nephropathy: Morphometric investigation of a population sample. J Clin Pathol 1990;43: 457–460.
35. Gauthier B, Trachtman H, Frank R, Valderrama E: Familial thin basement membrane nephropathy in children with asymptomatic microhematuria. Nephron 1989;51:502–508.
36. Lang S, Stevenson B, Risdon RA: Thin basement membrane nephropathy as a cause of recurrent haematuria in childhood. Histopathology 1990;16:331–337.
37. Tina L, Jenis E, Jose P, et al: The glomerular basement membrane in benign familial hematuria. Clin Nephrol 1982;17:1–4.
38. Vogler C, McAdams AJ, Homan SM: Glomerular basement membrane and lamina densa in infants and children: An ultrastructural evaluation. Pediatr Pathol 1987;7:527–534.
39. Shindo S, Yoshimoto M, Kuriya N, Bernstein J: Glomerular basement membrane thickness in recurrent and persistent hematuria and nephrotic syndrome: Correlation with sex and age. Pediatr Nephrol 1988;2:196–199.
40. Morita M, White RH, Raafat F, et al: Glomerular basement membrane thickness in children: A morphometric study. Pediatr Nephrol 1988;2:190–195.
41. Pirson Y: Making the diagnosis of Alport's syndrome. Kidney Int 1999;56:760–775.
42. Kashtan CE: Alport syndrome: Is diagnosis only skin-deep? [editorial]. Kidney Int 1999;55:1575–1576.
43. Lemmink HH, Nillesen WN, Mochizuki T, et al: Benign familial hematuria due to mutation of the type IV collagen alpha4 gene. J Clin Invest 1996;98: 1114–1118.
44. Matsumae T, Fukusaki M, Sakata N, et al: Thin glomerular basement membrane in diabetic patients with urinary abnormalities. Clin Nephrol 1994;42:221–226.
45. Gubler MC, Dommergues JP, Foulard M, et al: Collagen type III glomerulopathy: A new type of hereditary nephropathy. Pediatr Nephrol 1993;7:354–360.
46. Strom EH, Banfi G, Krapf R, et al: Glomerulopathy associated with predominant fibronectin deposits: A newly recognized hereditary disease. Kidney Int 1995;48:163–170.
47. Fogo A, Qureshi N, Horn RG: Morphologic and clinical features of fibrillary glomerulonephritis versus immunotactoid glomerulopathy. Am J Kidney Dis 1993;22: 367–377.
48. Striker LJ, Olson JL, Striker GE: The Renal Biopsy, ed 2. Philadelphia, WB Saunders, 1990.
49. Gallo GR, Feiner HD, Chuba JV, et al: Characterization of tissue amyloid by immunofluorescence microscopy. Clin Immunol Immunopathol 1986;39:479–490.
50. Van de Kaa CA, Hol PR, et al: Diagnosis of the type of amyloid in paraffin wax embedded tissue sections using antisera against human and animal amyloid proteins. Virchows Arch A Pathol Anat Histopathol 1986;408: 649–664.
51. Linke RP, Huhn D, Casanova S, Donini U: Immunoelectron microscopic identification of human AA-type amyloid: Exploration of various monoclonal AA-antibodies, methods of fixation, embedding and of other parameters for the protein–A gold method. Lab Invest 1989;61: 691–697.

52. Yang GC, Nieto R, Stachura I, Gallo GR: Ultrastructural immunohistochemical localization of polyclonal IgG, C3, and amyloid P component on the Congo red–negative amyloid-like fibrils of fibrillary glomerulopathy. Am J Pathol 1992;141:409–419.
53. Iskandar SS, Falk RJ, Jennette JC: Clinical and pathologic features of fibrillary glomerulonephritis. Kidney Int 1992;42:1401–1407.
54. Herrera GA: Ultrastructural immunolabeling: A general overview of techniques and applications. Ultrastruct Pathol 1992;16:37–45.
55. Gallo G, Picken M, Frangione B, Buxbaum J: Nonamyloidotic monoclonal immunoglobulin deposits lack amyloid P component. Mod Pathol 1988;1:453–456.
56. Preud'homme JL, Aucouturier P, Touchard G, et al: Monoclonal immunoglobulin deposition disease (Randall type): Relationship with structural abnormalities of immunoglobulin chains [editorial]. Kidney Int 1994;46: 965–972.
57. Lai KN, Ho RT, Tam JS, Lai FM: Detection of hepatitis B virus DNA and RNA in kidneys of HBV related glomerulonephritis. Kidney Int 1996;50:1965–1977.
58. Johnson RJ, Couser WG: Hepatitis B infection and renal disease: Clinical, immunopathogenetic and therapeutic considerations. Kidney Int 1990;37:663–676.
59. Nouri AK, Sallie R, Sangar D, et al: Detection of genomic and intermediate replicative strands of hepatitis C virus in liver tissue by in situ hybridization. J Clin Invest 1993;91:2226–2234.
60. Nuovo GJ, Lidonnici K, MacConnell P, Lane B: Intracellular localization of polymerase chain reaction (PCR)-amplified hepatitis C cDNA. Am J Surg Pathol 1993;17:683–690.
61. Davda R, Peterson J, Weiner R, et al: Membranous glomerulonephritis in association with hepatitis C virus infection. Am J Kidney Dis 1993;22:452–455.
62. Davis CL, Gretch DR, Carithers RL: Hepatitis C virus in renal disease. Curr Opin Nephrol Hypertens 1994;3: 164–173.
63. Johnson RJ, Gretch DR, Yamabe H, et al: Membranoproliferative glomerulonephritis associated with hepatitis C virus infection. N Engl J Med 1993;328: 465–470.
64. Johnson RJ, Willson R, Yamabe H, et al: Renal manifestations of hepatitis C virus infection. Kidney Int 1994;46:1255–1263.
65. Yamabe H, Johnson RJ, Gretch DR, et al: Hepatitis C virus infection and membranoproliferative glomerulonephritis in Japan. J Am Soc Nephrol 1995;6:220–223.
66. Kimmel PL, Phillips TM, Ferreira-Centeno A, et al: HIV-associated immune-mediated renal disease. Kidney Int 1993;44:1327–1340.
67. Kimmel PL, Ferreira-Centeno A, Farkas-Szallasi T, et al: Viral DNA in microdissected renal biopsy tissue from HIV infected patients with nephrotic syndrome. Kidney Int 1993;43:1347–1352.
68. Eitner F, Cui Y, Hudkins KL, et al: Chemokine receptor CCR5 and CXCR4 expression in HIV-associated kidney disease. J Am Soc Nephrol 2000;11:856–867.
69. Speir E, Modali R, Huang ES, et al: Potential role of human cytomegalovirus and p53 interaction in coronary restenosis. Science 1994;265:391–394.
70. Hutchinson TE, Somlyo AP: Microprobe Analysis of Biological Systems. New York, Academic Press, 1981.
71. Dowling JP, Agar JW: Diclofenac-associated interstitial mucinosis. Nephrol Dial Transplant 1991;6:595–598.
72. Nadasdy T, Laszik Z, Blick KE, et al: Human acute tubular necrosis: A lectin and immunohistochemical study. Hum Pathol 1995;26:230–239.
73. Nadasdy T, Laszik Z, Blick KE, et al: Tubular atrophy in the end-stage kidney: A lectin and immunohistochemical study. Hum Pathol 1994;25:22–28.
74. Addis T: Glomerular Nephritis: Diagnosis and Treatment. New York, Macmillan, 1948.
75. Brun C, Raaschou F: The results of 500 percutaneous renal biopsies. Arch Intern Med 1958;102:716–721.
76. Habib R, Kleinknecht C: The primary nephrotic syndrome of childhood: Classification and clinicopathologic study of 406 cases. *In* Sommers SC (ed): Kidney Pathology Decennial. New York, Appleton-Century-Crofts, 1975.
77. Morel-Maroger L: The value of renal biopsy. Am J Kidney Dis 1982;1:244–248.
78. Schainuck LI, Striker GE, Cutler RE, Benditt EP: Structural-functional correlations in renal disease: II. The correlations. Hum Pathol 1970;1:631–641.
79. Striker GE, Schainuck LI, Cutler RE, Benditt EP: Structural-functional correlations in renal disease: I. A method for assaying and classifying histopathologic changes in renal disease. Hum Pathol 1970;1:615–630.
80. Risdon RA, Sloper JC, De Wardener HE: Relationship between renal function and histological changes found in renal-biopsy specimens from patients with persistent glomerular nephritis. Lancet 1968;2:363–366.
81. Mongeau JG, Robitaille PO, Clermont MJ, et al: Focal segmental glomerulosclerosis (FSG) 20 years later: From toddler to grown up. Clin Nephrol 1993;40:1–6.
82. Fogo A, Glick AD, Horn SL, Horn RG: Is focal segmental glomerulosclerosis really focal? Distribution of lesions in adults and children. Kidney Int 1995;47: 1690–1696.
83. Peters H, Noble NA, Border WA: Transforming growth factor-beta in human glomerular injury. Curr Opin Nephrol Hypertens 1997;6:389–393.
84. Horiuchi S, Endo T, Shimoji H, et al: Goblet cell carcinoid of the appendix endoscopically diagnosed and examined with p53 immunostaining. J Gastroenterol 1998;33:582–587.
85. Yamamoto T, Watanabe T, Ikegaya N, et al: Expression of types I, II, and III TGF-beta receptors in human glomerulonephritis. J Am Soc Nephrol 1998;9:2253–2261.
86. Boucher A, Droz D, Adafer E, Noel LH: Relationship between the integrity of Bowman's capsule and the composition of cellular crescents in human crescentic glomerulonephritis. Lab Invest 1987;56:526–533.
87. Morel-Maroger SL, Killen PD, Chi E, Striker GE: The composition of glomerulosclerosis: I. Studies in focal sclerosis, crescentic glomerulonephritis, and membranoproliferative glomerulonephritis. Lab Invest 1984;51: 181–192.
88. Hill PA, Lan HY, Nikolic-Paterson DJ, Atkins RC: The ICAM-1/LFA-1 interaction in glomerular leukocytic accumulation in anti-GBM glomerulonephritis. Kidney Int 1994;45:700–708.

89. Wada T, Furuichi K, Segawa-Takaeda C, et al: MIP-1alpha and MCP-1 contribute to crescents and interstitial lesions in human crescentic glomerulonephritis. Kidney Int 1999;56:995–1003.
90. Cockwell P, Howie AJ, Adu D, Savage CO: In situ analysis of C-C chemokine mRNA in human glomerulonephritis. Kidney Int 1998;54:827–836.
91. Grandaliano G, Gesualdo L, Ranieri E, et al: Tissue factor, plasminogen activator inhibitor-1, and thrombin receptor expression in human crescentic glomerulonephritis. Am J Kidney Dis 2000;35:726–738.
92. Morel-Maroger L, Mery JP, Droz D, et al: The course of lupus nephritis: Contribution of serial renal biopsies. Adv Nephrol Necker Hosp 1976;6:79–118.
93. Pirani CL: The reproducibility of semiquantitative analyses of renal histology. Nephron 1964;1:230–237.
94. Schwartz MM, Lan SP, Bernstein J, et al: Role of pathology indices in the management of severe lupus glomerulonephritis. Lupus Nephritis Collaborative Study Group. Kidney Int 1992;42:743–748.
95. Wernick RM, Smith DL, Houghton DC, et al: Reliability of histologic scoring for lupus nephritis: A community-based evaluation. Ann Intern Med 1993;119: 805–811.
96. Austin HA, Boumpas DT, Vaughan EM, Balow JE: Predicting renal outcomes in severe lupus nephritis: Contributions of clinical and histologic data. Kidney Int 1994;45:544–550.
97. Mauer SM, Steffes MW, Ellis EN, et al: Structural-functional relationships in diabetic nephropathy. J Clin Invest 1984;74:1143–1155.
98. Østerby R: Renal pathology in diabetes mellitus. Curr Opin Nephrol Hypertens 1993;2:475–483.
99. Bangstad HJ, Osterby R, Dahl-Jorgensen K, et al: Early glomerulopathy is present in young, type 1 (insulin-dependent) diabetic patients with microalbuminuria. Diabetologia 1993;36:523–529.
100. Chavers BM, Bilous RW, Ellis EN, et al: Glomerular lesions and urinary albumin excretion in type I diabetes without overt proteinuria. N Engl J Med 1989;320: 966–970.
101. Breyer JA: Diabetic nephropathy in insulin-dependent patients. Am J Kidney Dis 1992;20:533–547.
102. Ketteler M, Noble NA, Border WA: Increased expression of transforming growth factor-beta in renal disease. Curr Opin Nephrol Hypertens 1994;3:446–452.
103. Border WA, Ruoslahti E: Transforming growth factor-beta in disease: The dark side of tissue repair. J Clin Invest 1992;90:1–7.
104. Floege J, Burns MW, Alpers CE, et al: Glomerular cell proliferation and PDGF expression precede glomerulosclerosis in the remnant kidney model. Kidney Int 1992;41:297–309.
105. Suzuki D, Miyazaki M, Jinde K, et al: In situ hybridization studies of matrix metalloproteinase-3, tissue inhibitor of metalloproteinase-1 and type IV collagen in diabetic nephropathy. Kidney Int 1997;52:111–119.
106. Paueksakon P, Revelo MP, MaL-J, et al: Microangiopathic injury and augmented PA1-1 in human diabetic nephropathy. Kidney Int (in press).
107. Fogo AB: The role of angiotensin II and plasminogen activator inhibitor-1 in progressive glomerulosclerosis. Am J Kidney Dis 2000;35:179–188.
108. Vats AN, Basgen JM, Steffes MW, et al: Mean glomerular volume (GV) in minimal change nephrotic syndrome (MCNS), focal segmental glomerulosclerosis (FSGS), normal children and adults [abstract]. J Am Soc Nephrol 1994;5:797.
109. Fogo A, Hawkins EP, Berry PL, et al: Glomerular hypertrophy in minimal change disease predicts subsequent progression to focal glomerular sclerosis. Kidney Int 1990;38:115–123.
110. Fogo A, Hawkins EP, Verani R, et al: Focal segmental glomerulosclerosis (FSGS) in renal transplantation is associated with marked glomerular hypertrophy [abstract]. J Am Soc Nephrol 1991;2:797.
111. Jennette JC, Marquis A, Falk RJ, et al: Glomerulomegaly in focal segmental glomerulosclerosis (FSGS) but not minimal change glomerulopathy (MCG) [abstract]. Lab Invest 1990;62:48A.
112. Regele HM, Fillipovic E, Langer B, et al: Glomerular expression of dystroglycans is reduced in minimal change nephrosis but not in focal segmental glomerulosclerosis. J Am Soc Nephrol 2000;11:403–412.
113. Pesce C, Schmidt K, Fogo A: Glomerular size and the incidence of renal disease in African Americans and Caucasians. J Nephrol 1994;7:355–358.
114. Johnson RJ, Floege J, Yoshimura A, et al: The activated mesangial cell: A glomerular "myofibroblast"? J Am Soc Nephrol 1992;2(10 Suppl):S190–S197.
115. Nabeshima K, Yohimura A, Inui K, et al: Relationship of PDGF B-chain mRNA expression identified by in situ hybridization (ISH) and disease severity in various human glomerular diseases [abstract]. J Am Soc Nephrol 1993;4:777.
116. Ferrario F, Rastaldi MP, Napodano P: Morphological features in IgA nephropathy. Ann Med Interne (Paris) 1999;150:108–116.
117. Niemir ZI, Stein H, Noronha IL, et al: PDGF and TGF-beta contribute to the natural course of human IgA glomerulonephritis. Kidney Int 1995;48: 1530–1541.
118. Niemir ZI, Ondracek M, Dworacki G, et al: In situ up-regulation of IL-10 reflects the activity of human glomerulonephritides. Am J Kidney Dis 1998;32:80–92.
119. Yoshida H, Mitarai T, Kawamura T, et al: Role of the deletion of polymorphism of the angiotensin converting enzyme gene in the progression and therapeutic responsiveness of IgA nephropathy. J Clin Invest 1995;96: 2162–2169.
120. Nakamura T, Ebihara I, Shirato I, et al: Modulation of basement membrane component gene expression in glomeruli of aminonucleoside nephrosis. Lab Invest 1991; 64:640–647.
121. Ledbetter S, Copeland EJ, Noonan D, et al: Altered steady-state mRNA levels of basement membrane proteins in diabetic mouse kidneys and thromboxane synthase inhibition. Diabetes 1990;39:196–203.
122. Doi T, Striker LJ, Kimata K, et al: Glomerulosclerosis in mice transgenic for growth hormone: Increased mesangial extracellular matrix is correlated with kidney mRNA levels. J Exp Med 1991;173:1287–1290.
123. Laurie GW, Horikoshi S, Killen PD, et al: In situ hybridization reveals temporal and spatial changes in cellular expression of mRNA for a laminin receptor, laminin,

and basement membrane (type IV) collagen in the developing kidney. J Cell Biol 1989;109:1351–1362.

124. Moriyama T, Murphy HR, Martin BM, Garcia-Perez A: Detection of specific mRNAs in single nephron segments by use of the polymerase chain reaction. Am J Physiol 1990;258(5 Pt 2):F1470–F1474.

125. Gilliland G, Perrin S, Blanchard K, Bunn HF: Analysis of cytokine mRNA and DNA: Detection and quantitation by competitive polymerase chain reaction. Proc Natl Acad Sci U S A 1990;87:2725–2729.

126. Peten EP, Striker LJ, Carome MA, et al: The contribution of increased collagen synthesis to human glomerulosclerosis: A quantitative analysis of alpha 2IV collagen mRNA expression by competitive polymerase chain reaction. J Exp Med 1992;176:1571–1576.

127. Peten EP, Striker LJ, Garcia-Perez A, Striker GE: Studies by competitive PCR of glomerulosclerosis in growth hormone transgenic mice. Kidney Int Suppl 1993;39:S55–S58.

128. Ihm CG, Lee GS, Nast CC, et al: Early increased renal procollagen alpha 1(IV) mRNA levels in streptozotocin induced diabetes. Kidney Int 1992;41:768–777.

129. Pesce CM, Striker LJ, Peten E, et al: Glomerulosclerosis at both early and late stages is associated with increased cell turnover in mice transgenic for growth hormone. Lab Invest 1991;65:601–605.

130. Nadasdy T, Laszik Z, Blick KE, et al: Proliferative activity of intrinsic cell populations in the normal human kidney. J Am Soc Nephrol 1994;4:2032–2039.

131. Szabolcs MJ, Ward L, Buttyan R, et al: Apoptosis elucidated by labeling for DNA fragmentation in human renal biopsies [abstract]. Lab Invest 1994;70:160A.

132. Yang CW, Striker LJ, Kopchick JJ, et al: Glomerulosclerosis in mice transgenic for native or mutated bovine growth hormone gene. Kidney Int Suppl 1993; 39:S90–S94.

133. Marti HP, McNeil L, Thomas G, et al: Molecular characterization of a low-molecular-mass matrix metalloproteinase secreted by glomerular mesangial cells as PUMP-1. Biochem J 1992;285:899–905.

134. Carome MA, Striker LJ, Peten EP, et al: Human glomeruli express TIMP-1 mRNA and TIMP-2 protein and mRNA. Am J Physiol 1993;264:F923–F929.

135. Nadji M, Matsuo S, Ganjei P, et al: Monoclonal antibody ERY-1 identifies an antigen in erythroid cells, hepatocellular and renal cell carcinomas. Acta Haematol 1988;79:68–71.

136. Varricchio F, Obiri NI, Haas GP, Puri RK: Immunostaining of interleukin-4 receptor on human renal cell carcinoma. Lymphokine Cytokine Res 1993;12: 465–469.

137. Bell ET: A classification of renal tumors with observations on the frequencies of various types. J Urol 1938; 39:238–243.

138. Thoenes W, Storkel S, Rumpelt HJ: Histopathology and classification of renal cell tumors (adenomas, oncocytomas, and carcinomas): The basic cytological and histopathological elements and their use for diagnostics. Pathol Res Pract 1986;181:125–143.

139. Heim S, Mitelman F, Helm S, Mitelman F (eds): Cancer Cytogenetics. New York, Wiley-Liss, 1995; pp 350–368.

140. Ruckle HC, Torres VE, Richardson RL, Zincke H: Renal tumors. Curr Opin Nephrol Hypertens 1993;2: 201–210.

141. Kovacs G: Molecular differential pathology of renal cell tumours. Histopathology 1993;22:1–8.

142. Kovacs G: The value of molecular genetic analysis in the diagnosis and prognosis of renal cell tumours. World J Urol 1994;12:64–68.

143. Roth J, Brada D, Blaha I, et al: Evaluation of polysialic acid in the diagnosis of Wilms' tumor: A comparative study on urinary tract tumors and non-neuroendocrine tumors. Virchows Arch B Cell Pathol Incl Mol Pathol 1988;56:95–102.

144. Clapp WL, Abrahamson DR: Regulation of kidney organogenesis: Homeobox genes, growth factors, and Wilms tumor. Curr Opin Nephrol Hypertens 1993;2: 419–429.

145. Bickmore WA, Oghene K, Little MH, et al: Modulation of DNA binding specificity by alternative splicing of the Wilms tumor *wt1* gene transcript. Science 1992;257: 235–237.

146. Pritchard-Jones K, Fleming S, Davidson D, et al: The candidate Wilms' tumour gene is involved in genitourinary development. Nature 1990;346:194–197.

147. Little MH, Dunn R, Byrne JA, et al: Equivalent expression of paternally and maternally inherited *WT1* alleles in normal fetal tissue and Wilms' tumours. Oncogene 1992;7:635–641.

148. Zhang Y, Tycko B: Monoallelic expression of the human H19 gene. Nat Genet 1992;1:40–44.

149. Junien C, Henry I: Genetics of Wilms' tumor: A blend of aberrant development and genomic imprinting [editorial]. Kidney Int 1994;46:1264–1279.

150. DeChiara TM, Robertson EJ, Efstratiadis A: Parental imprinting of the mouse insulin-like growth factor II gene. Cell 1991;64:849–859.

151. Kaiser U, Hansmann ML, Papadopoulos I: Does the immunophenotype of renal cell carcinoma correlate with its clinical stage? Urol Int 1991;47:194–198.

152. Thrasher JB, Paulson DF: Prognostic factors in renal cancer. Urol Clin North Am 1993;20:247–262.

153. Gutierrez JL, Val-Bernal JF, Garijo MF, et al: Nuclear morphometry in prognosis of renal adenocarcinoma. Urology 1992;39:130–134.

154. Kozma L, Kiss I, Nagy A, et al: Investigation of c-*myc* and k-*ras* amplification in renal clear cell adenocarcinoma. Cancer Lett 1997;111:127–131.

155. Uhlman DL, Nguyen PL, Manivel JC, et al: Association of immunohistochemical staining for p53 with metastatic progression and poor survival in patients with renal cell carcinoma. J Natl Cancer Inst 1994;86:1470–1475.

156. Moch H, Schraml P, Bubendorf L, et al: High-throughput tissue microarray analysis to evaluate genes uncovered by cDNA microarray screening in renal cell carcinoma. Am J Pathol 1999;154:981–986.

157. Partin AW, Walsh AC, Epstein JI, et al: Nuclear morphometry as a predictor of response to therapy in Wilms tumor: A preliminary report. J Urol 1990;144: 952–954.

158. Barrantes JC, Muir KR, Toyn CE, et al: Thirty-year population-based review of childhood renal tumours with an assessment of prognostic features including tumour DNA characteristics. Med Pediatr Oncol 1993; 21:24–30.

159. Coppes MJ, Haber DA, Grundy PE: Genetic events in the development of Wilms' tumor. N Engl J Med 1994; 331:586–590.

160. Striker LJ, Peten EP, Elliot SJ, et al: Mesangial cell turnover: Effect of heparin and peptide growth factors. Lab Invest 1991;64:446–456.

161. Kohda Y, Murakami H, Moe OW, Star RA: Analysis of segmental renal gene expression by laser capture microdissection. Kidney Int 2000;57:321–331.

162. Eikmans M, Baelde HJ, De Heer E, Bruijn JA: Processing renal biopsies for diagnostic mRNA quantification: Improvement of RNA extraction and storage conditions. J Am Soc Nephrol 2000;11:868–873.

163. Hernandez-Presa MA, Gomez-Guerrero C, Egido J: In situ non-radioactive detection of nuclear factors in paraffin sections by Southwestern histochemistry. Kidney Int 1999;55:209–214.

TIMOTHY J. O'LEARY
DENNIS M. FRISMAN

10

Testes, Bladder, and Prostate

TRANSITIONAL CELL TUMORS OF THE URINARY BLADDER

Transitional cell carcinoma of the urinary bladder is frequently multifocal and has an incidence of approximately 50,000 cases per year in the United States.[1] Most tumors are papillary lesions with a high likelihood of recurrence after treatment but only about a 20% likelihood of becoming invasive. A smaller group of high-grade in situ carcinomas are much more likely to invade and metastasize.

Cytogenetics and Molecular Genetics

Most cytogenetic studies have focused on papillary tumors. Although abnormalities of chromosome 1 are found in nearly half of cases of transitional cell tumors of the bladder, the changes are variable and found throughout both the p and q arms. Trisomy 7 and monosomy 9 are also common and are frequently noted as the sole cytogenetic change,[2] but it is not certain that either abnormality contributes to the neoplastic process. Chromosomes 3, 5, and 10 are also frequently abnormal; chromosomes 6, 8, 11, 13, 17, 18, X, and Y less frequently demonstrate abnormalities.[2] Comparative genomic hybridization (CGH) studies suggest that the earliest cytogenetic abnormality is deletion of 9q.[3] Deletions of 9p and 11p and gains of 1q and 8q frequently follow as the cancer progresses, with gains of 5p and 20q occurring frequently in tumors that are at stage pT2–4.[3–7] No specific genetic changes are seen in metastases that are not found in primary tumors.[8]

Loss of heterozygosity (LOH) studies confirm the importance of chromosome 9 deletions; at least 95% of all bladder tumors demonstrate LOH at some place on this chromosome.[9, 10] Chromosomal losses on chromosome 9p21 are also seen in normal bladder mucosa, however, demonstrating the need for caution in interpreting allelic deletion studies from this site.[11] Other regions of frequent loss include 1p, 3p, 4q, 11p, 13q, and 17p.[1, 12] The strongest evidence that any of these regions contains a tumor suppressor gene important in the pathogenesis of bladder carcinoma is that the tumorigenic phenotype of immortalized human urothelial cells is suppressed by the introduction of chromosome region 3p13-21.2.[13] Allelic deletion at 13q also appears likely to be of pathogenetic significance, because these deletions typically involve the retinoblastoma gene (*RB1*), which is frequently altered in high-grade/stage tumors,[14, 15] and are frequently associated with loss of the *RB1* gene product.[16]

High-level gene amplifications are typically found in advanced disease and have been reported for cyclin D1,[17] *EMS1*,[17] *MYC*,[18] *ERBB2* (*HER2/neu*),[19] *BCL1*,[20] *INT2*,[20] and *HST*.[20] In addition, CGH studies have reported uncharacterized high-level amplifications at 1p32, 3p21-24, 3q24, 4q26, 8q21-qter, 10p13-14, 11q13-22, 12q13-24, 13q21-31, 17q22, 17q22-23, 18p11, 18q22, and 22q11-13.[20–23] Whether these amplifications are important in the pathogenesis of these tumors or are rather a reflection of genetic instability in advanced cancers remains to be determined.

Mutations of the *TP53* gene occur in 20% to 40% of bladder cancers.[24–26] Although mutations are found more frequently in aggressive tumors, *TP53* gene sequence analysis does not appear to be prognostic information beyond that provided by tumor stage alone.[27] Both point mutations and deletions have also been observed in the *CDKN2* gene; these genetic alterations appear to be an early event in bladder carcinogenesis.[28–30] Similarly, mutations of the *RB1* gene are found with similar frequency (approximately 30% of cases) in early and late bladder carcinomas, suggesting that *RB1* gene alteration is also an early event.

Cytometry

Cytometric studies confirm the presence of aneuploid DNA populations in over half of papillary bladder carcinomas[31]; cytometric techniques contribute little prognostic information beyond that afforded by tumor stage, however.[31, 32] Limited interinstitutional reproducibility of flow cytometric methods further limits the clinical use of these techniques.[33]

Immunohistochemical Methods

Immunohistochemical assessments of the tumor suppressor gene products RB1 and p53 have shown prognostic value in univariate analysis but have not contributed significant information beyond that provided by histologic and clinical parameters.[24, 34–36] Conflicting results have been reported regarding the use of immunohistochemical staining for BCL2, PCNA, Ki-67 (MIB1), NME1 (nm23), and ERBB2.[37–46] Taken together, the results of these studies do not provide a basis for routine use of any of these immunohistochemical assays for routine assessment of bladder carcinomas.

Immunohistochemistry is seldom required for diagnosis of transitional cell tumors but may occasionally be helpful in the characterization of metastatic disease. The immunohistochemical characteristics of transitional cell carcinoma are briefly summarized in Table 10–1.

ADENOCARCINOMA OF THE PROSTATE

Adenocarcinoma of the prostate is the leading cancer of males in developed countries, but it remains poorly understood. Histologic grading, tumor size, capsular invasion, and patient race and age are all somewhat useful in predicting which tumors will remain indolent and which are likely to metastasize; yet there is no combination of variables that reliably predicts outcome for most prostate cancers. For this reason there has been a substantial effort to discern cytogenetic and molecular genetic mechanisms involved in disease progression and to use this information to develop new laboratory tests.

TABLE 10–1

Immunohistochemical Staining Characteristics of Transitional Cell Carcinoma

Antigen	Percentage of Cases Demonstrating Immunoreactivity
Cytokeratin 7	100
CA 15-3	87–100
Epithelial membrane antigen	87–100
Cytokeratin 20	68–90
CA 19-9	58–83
CD 117	43–82
Carcinoembryonic antigen (polyclonal)	24–39

Cytogenetics and Molecular Genetics

Cytogenetic studies have been hampered by the fact that stromal cells, frequently admixed with malignant cells, may grow preferentially in cell culture systems, which actually seem to select against cytogenetically abnormal clones.[47–49] Only about one third of cases demonstrate structural abnormalities—most commonly involving chromosomal regions on 1p, 1q, 2p, 2q, 7q, and 10q.[47] Numerical abnormalities, including duplication of chromosome 7 and deletion of the Y chromosome, have also been reported.[47] Fluorescence in situ hybridization studies suggest that tumors with chromosome 7 anomalies tend to behave more aggressively than do other prostate tumors.[50] This may reflect a propensity to chromosome 7 aneuploidy in proliferative prostatic lesions in general, because trisomy 7 is a frequent finding in benign prostatic hypertrophy.[51] The chromosome 10q changes may be more significant, because deletion of 10q24 has been reported as the sole cytogenetic anomaly in several cases.[52]

CGH reveals many cytogenetic abnormalities not appreciated in conventional karyotypes.[53] Losses of chromosome 8p are observed in almost 80% of cases, often in association with gains of 8q and losses of 13q, 16p, 16q, 17p, 17q, 20q, and Y.[54, 55] Tumors from African-American patients, which on average behave more aggressively than do those from white Americans, showed significantly more frequent gains of 4q25-28.[55] Other regions of the genome show no differences.[56] Gains in 13q12-13 have been seen with increased frequency in androgen-independent tumors,[57] but the relationship of these changes to alterations of the Xq androgen receptor is unclear.

CGH has also demonstrated a novel mechanism for the development of androgen independence in prostate cancer. Although tumors seldom demonstrate abnormalities in Xq11-13—the region in which the androgen receptor gene is found—amplifications in this region develop frequently in recurrences that occur during androgen deprivation therapy.[58] This suggests that therapy selects for clones in which amplification of the androgen receptor gene has occurred. This result has been confirmed by fluorescence in situ hybridization experiments.[59]

LOH studies confirm the importance of 8p deletion in prostate cancer[60–62]; tumors having deletions in this region appear to have higher metastatic potential than those without.[63] Deletions of 8p12-21 are also frequently noted in prostatic intraepithelial neoplasia,[64] as are deletions on chromosomes 5 and 16.[65] A wide variety of other sites of allelic loss have been reported, including 3p24-26 and 3p22-12,[66] 6q14-21,[67, 68] 9p21 (the region of the *CDKN2A* tumor suppressor gene),[69] both 10p loci and 10q22-24 (the site of the *PTEN* gene),[70, 71] 11p15, p11-12 (a region that contains the putative metastasis suppressor gene *KAI1*), q22, q23-24,[72, 73] 12p12-13 (site of the *CDKN1B* and *ETV6* genes),[74] 13q14.3,[75–78] 16q22-24,[79–81] 17q21-23 (a region that includes the *BRCA1* and *NME1* genes),[82–84] and 21q.[65] Many of these chromosomal alterations are more frequently observed in advanced cancers, but it is unclear whether any particular deletion promotes cancer aggressiveness or whether some of the deletions instead reflect a propensity to genetic instability in aggressive cancers. Genetic instability, in the form of *microsatellite instability,* has been frequently observed in prostate cancers.[85–88] Microsatellite alterations are significantly more common in advanced cancers than in early tumors. Whether this represents de novo development of microsatellite instability during tumor progression or clonal expansion of genetically unstable cells that were present but undetectable at early stages is uncertain.

Amplifications of *MYC,*[89] *ERBB2,*[89] *INT2,*[89] and AR (androgen receptor)[59, 90, 91] genes are frequently reported in late-stage tumors but less frequently in early-stage tumors.[92] Although amplification of the androgen receptor gene may contribute to loss of hormonal responsiveness in prostate cancer, the clinical significance of this and other gene amplifications remains uncertain.

Somatic mutations occur in a large number of genes, including *HRAS,*[93] *NRAS,*[93] *KRAS,*[93, 94] *AR,*[95, 96] *RB1,*[97, 98] *TP53,*[99, 100] *PTEN,*[101, 102] *MXI1,*[103] and *BRCA1.*[104] For the most part, these mutations are infrequent in early cancers and more common in more advanced cancers. The clinical use of these observations remains uncertain, although it is clear that mutations in the androgen receptor gene, together with amplifications of this gene (see earlier), contribute to the development of androgen independence in prostate cancers.

Many cancers demonstrate activity of the enzyme telomerase, which is normally not present in quiescent epithelial cells. Eighty percent to 90% of prostatic adenocarcinomas demonstrate telomerase activity,[105–107] as do about 15% of high-grade prostatic intraepithelial neoplasia.[108] Studies on benign prostate have yielded conflicting results. Most studies show telomerase activity in less than 10% to 15% of benign hypertrophic prostates[105–107, 109]; others have seen telomerase activity in over one third of benign cases.[110] Although it seems likely that telomerase activity provides a sensitive indicator of malignant potential, there is no evidence that suggests that it provides clinically relevant data beyond that which is available by morphologic examination.

Serial analysis of gene expression[110a, 110b] and complementary DNA microarray[110c–110f] techniques have identified a number of genes that are differentially expressed in normal prostate and prostatic carcinoma. Although it seems likely that these large-scale gene expression analysis techniques will provide better understanding of the pathogenesis and treatment of prostate cancer, practical application of these techniques in the practice of pathology remains in the future.

About 10% of patients with prostate cancer appear to have a genetic predisposition.[111] Linkage analysis has suggested a variety of potential sites for tumor susceptibility genes on chromosome 1, including 1q42-43,[111] 1q24-25,[112–115] 1p36[116] and Xq27-28.[117, 118]

Early Diagnosis and Molecular Staging

When prostate cancer is diagnosed as a result of an abnormal digital rectal examination or elevated serum prostate-specific antigen (PSA), it may already be quite advanced. In addition, prediction of likely outcome (and hence appropriate treatment) is often difficult when based only on clinical information and gross and microscopic morphology. Molecular diagnosis and staging of prostate cancer, using cancer cell–specific reverse transcriptase/polymerase chain reaction (RT-PCR) assays, provide promising approaches by which to diagnose more patients whose disease is early in development, as well as to identify those whose disease is metastatic at the time of initial diagnosis or surgery.[119] RT-PCR assays for PSA messenger RNA (mRNA) may be used to identify prostate cells in ejaculate and urethral washings but do not discriminate between normal and cancerous cells.[120] Long-term follow-up studies suggest that identification of PSA mRNA in blood, pelvic lymph nodes, or bone marrow identifies a population that is at risk of biochemical recurrence,[121–126] but the results of these investigations are not uniform.[127, 128] Prostate biopsy itself increases the likelihood of a positive RT-PCR result[129, 130]; the RT-PCR test demonstrates significant spillage of prostate cells during the process of radical prostatectomy.[131, 132] The finding of PSA mRNA in bone marrow seems to have the most consistently adverse effect on prognosis, but even this approach should be considered investigational.

Flow and Image Cytometry

A large number of investigators have studied the clinical use of flow and image cytometry in the assessment of prostatic carcinoma. Aneuploid tumors have generally been associated with shorter survival.[133–138] In some studies this survival difference has been independent of either tumor stage or histologic grade, but in others it has been found to provide information only for low-grade tumors[139] or for tumors presenting at an advanced stage.[140] Studies comparing the utility of S-phase fraction with that of ploidy have found the former to be superior.[141] Nevertheless, it remains uncertain whether either ploidy or S-phase fraction provides sufficient prognostic information beyond that afforded by grade and stage to warrant its routine use.[141]

Immunohistochemical Methods

Immunohistochemical assessment of proliferation markers has been proposed as an alternative to flow and image cytometry for predicting outcome in prostate and other cancers. Immunohistochemical assessments of MIB1 (Ki-67) and PCNA have both been employed, although MIB1 staining appears to be more easily interpreted in routine use.[142] There is some evidence that PCNA staining provides independent prognostic information in T1–2 M0 stage tumors[143]; similarly, there is evidence suggesting that the Ki-67 labeling index (as determined by MIB1 staining) carries prognostic information beyond that associated with stage and grade.[144–148] Convincing tests of the relative clinical use of cytometric and immunohistochemical methods for assessing cellular proliferation are not available.

Immunohistochemical assessment of p53 accumulation has also been investigated as a predictor of outcome. Several studies have demonstrated that p53 staining is associated with shorter survival of patients with prostatic carcinoma and that it is independent of age, race, stage, and grade,[149–153] but other studies have failed to demonstrate prognostic significance for p53.[154, 155] This may reflect the considerable heterogeneity in the technical methods by which immunohistochemical stains for p53 are performed and assessed and emphasizes the need for independent validation of prognostic utility when importing "home brew" assays for immunohistochemical prognostic markers into a new laboratory setting.

Because the diagnosis of prostatic adenocarcinoma is usually straightforward on morphologic grounds alone, immunohistochemical assessment is most commonly used to identify the site of origin of metastatic disease. Typical staining patterns of prostatic adenocarcinoma may be found in Table 10–2.

TABLE 10–2

Immunohistochemical Staining Characteristics of Prostatic Adenocarcinoma

Antigen	Percentage of Cases Demonstrating Immunoreactivity
AE1/AE3	100
Androgen receptor	100
CD57	100
Prostatic acid phosphatase	91–100
Prostate-specific antigen	91–99
CAM 5.2	84–100
AE1	74–100
CA 15-3	64–92
E-cadherin	60–85
B72.3	53–71
Chromogranin B	34–69
Carcinoembryonic antigen (polyclonal)	20–49
Chromogranin A	21–37
Epithelial membrane antigen	8–44
Cytokeratin type 20	14–36
Cytokeratin type 7	6–42
CD117	6–35
Cytokeratin—high molecular weight (polyclonal)	4–11
CA 19-9	1–11
CA 125	0–5
CD31	0
S-100	0

TESTICULAR GERM CELL TUMORS

The most common cytogenetic aberration in testicular germ cell tumors (including both seminomas and nonseminomatous germ cell tumors) is isochromosome 12p, found in 70% to 80% of cases[52, 156–158]; other recurrent structural abnormalities are uncommon.[157, 159] Even in the absence of i(12p), an increase in the number of 12p sequences is found.[160] Thus, it is not surprising that the finding of i(12p) does not convey information regarding any distinctive tumor behavior patterns.[156] Rather, an increase in 12p copy number is seen once in situ malignant transformation is observed in testicular germ cells[161]; amplification of chromosome 12p sequences apparently leads to deregulated overexpression of cyclin D2, a cell cycle G_1/S checkpoint regulator.[162, 163] When found in other tumors, one must keep in mind the possibility that the tumor ultimately arose from a malignant germ cell clone.[164–166]

CGH studies demonstrate a variety of losses (predominantly on chromosomes 4, 5, 11, 13q, and 18q) and gains (1q, 7, 8, 12, 14q, 15q, 21q, and 22q).[167, 168] Amplification of chromosome 12p11.1-12p12.1 is the most common finding and can be used to help establish a germ cell origin for a tumor of unknown primary site.[168, 169] LOH studies have identified two regions of frequent allelic deletion on chromosome 12—12q13 and 12q22[170, 171]; these studies have yet to identify specific tumor suppressor genes associated with the development of testicular germ cell tumors. LOH studies have also identified frequent allelic deletion in the regions of 1p13, 1p22, 1p31.3-32.2,[172] 18q21 (the site of the *DCC* gene),[173] 5p15.1-5p15.2, 5q11, and 5q34-35.[174] These sites (particularly those on chromosomes 1 and 18) have frequently been implicated as sites of potential tumor suppressor genes in other tumors.

NRAS mutations in codons 12 and 61 are found in about one third of germ cell tumors[175]; mutations of *KRAS* and *HRAS* are less common. Mutations of *TP53* have not been seen by most investigators,[176] although some authors have found mutations in as many as two thirds of cases in which microdissection was performed to isolate cells representing carcinoma in situ.[177]

TABLE 10–3
Immunohistochemical Staining Characteristics of Testicular Tumors

Antigen	Percentage of Cases Demonstrating Immunoreactivity			
	Seminoma	*Embryonal Carcinoma*	*Choriocarcinoma*	*Yolk Sac Tumor*
α_1-Antitrypsin	0–10	3–18	14–52	20–64
α-Fetoprotein	0	21–42	0	66–87
AE1/AE3	15–40	100	?	?
CAM 5.2	2–10	100	?	100
CD30	3–16	79–92	?	5–32
CD57	7–26	0–11	0	?
CD74	0	0	0	0
Carcinoembryonic antigen (polyclonal)	0	0–8	?	10–39
Chromogranin A	0	0	0	0
Cytokeratin (pan)	6–19	61–81	100	34–62
Epithelial membrane antigen	0–3	0–8	38–71	0–11
Human chorionic gonadotropin-β	2–13	14–32	100	0
M2A	100	?	?	?
Neuron-specific enolase	74–93	70–91	26–66	44–86
Placental alkaline phosphatase	85–93	74–86	35–61	34–56
S-100	0	0	0	0–11
Vimentin	21–39	9–25	?	14–38

Mutations of *KIT*, a gene that codes for a tyrosine kinase receptor that binds stem cell factor, have also been identified in seminoma[178]; expression of KIT is also seen immunohistochemically in most seminomas,[179] as well as in most testicular germ cells.[180]

Approximately 40% of testicular germ cell tumors are classified as seminomas. Since the advent of multidrug chemotherapy, an overall cure rate of over 90% is achieved for all stages of presentation. Studies of prognostic factors are, not surprisingly, uncommon. Although similarly high survival rates are seen for stage I nonseminomatous germ cell tumors (embryonal carcinoma, choriocarcinoma), high-stage disease is more typically associated with 5-year survival rates of around 50% for these histologic types. In these patients, it appears that high levels of proliferative activity (as assessed by S-phase fraction) may be associated with reduced survival.[181]

Histologic diagnosis of primary germ cell tumors is generally straightforward, but proper diagnosis of metastatic disease is frequently aided by immunohistochemical characterization. Some immunohistochemical staining characteristics of testicular cancers are shown in Table 10–3.

REFERENCES

1. Cairns P, Sidransky D, Vogelstein B, Kinzler KW (eds): The Genetic Basis of Human Cancer. New York, McGraw-Hill, 1998, pp 639–645.
2. Heim S, Mitelman F: Tumors of the urinary tract. In Heim S, Mitelman F (eds): Cancer Cytogenetics. New York, Wiley-Liss, 1995, pp 350–368.
3. Bruch J, Wohr G, Hautmann R, et al: Chromosomal changes during progression of transitional cell carcinoma of the bladder and delineation of the amplified interval on chromosome arm 8q. Genes Chromosomes Cancer 1998;23:167–174.
4. Richter J, Jiang F, Gorog JP, et al: Marked genetic differences between stage pTa and stage pT1 papillary bladder cancer detected by comparative genomic hybridization. Cancer Res 1997;57:2860–2864.
5. Richter J, Beffa L, Wagner U, et al: Patterns of chromosomal imbalances in advanced urinary bladder cancer detected by comparative genomic hybridization. Am J Pathol 1998;153:1615–1621.
6. Simon R, Burger H, Brinkschmidt C, et al: Chromosomal aberrations associated with invasion in papillary superficial bladder cancer. J Pathol 1998;185:345–351.
7. Zhao J, Richter J, Wagner U, et al: Chromosomal imbalances in noninvasive papillary bladder neoplasms (pTa). Cancer Res 1999;59:4658–4661.
8. Hovey RM, Chu L, Balazs M, et al: Genetic alterations in primary bladder cancers and their metastases. Cancer Res 1998;58:3555–3560.
9. Aveyard JS, Skilleter A, Habuchi T, Knowles MA: Somatic mutation of PTEN in bladder carcinoma. Br J Cancer 1999;80:904–908.
10. Stadler WM, Olopade OI: The 9p21 region in bladder cancer cell lines: Large homozygous deletion inactivate the *CDKN2, CDKN2B* and *MTAP* genes. Urol Res 1996;24:239–244.
11. Baud E, Catilina P, Boiteux JP, Bignon YJ: Human bladder cancers and normal bladder mucosa present the same

hot spot of heterozygous chromosome-9 deletion. Int J Cancer 1998;77:821–824.

12. Fletcher JA: Renal and Bladder Cancers. *In* Wolman SR, Sell S (eds): Human Cancer Cytogenetic Markers. Totawa, NJ, Humana, 1997, pp 169–202.
13. Klingelhutz AJ, Wu SQ, Huang J, Reznikoff CA: Loss of 3p13-p21.2 in tumorigenic reversion of a hybrid between isogeneic nontumorigenic and tumorigenic human uroepithelial cells. Cancer Res 1992;52: 1631–1634.
14. Miyamoto H, Shuin T, Torigoe S, et al: Retinoblastoma gene mutations in primary human bladder cancer. Br J Cancer 1995;71:831–835.
15. Cairns P, Proctor AJ, Knowles MA: Loss of heterozygosity at the RB locus is frequent and correlates with muscle invasion in bladder carcinoma. Oncogene 1991; 6:2305–2309.
16. Xu HJ, Cairns P, Hu SX, et al: Loss of RB protein expression in primary bladder cancer correlates with loss of heterozygosity at the RB locus and tumor progression. Int J Cancer 1993;53:781–784.
17. Bringuier PP, Tamimi Y, Schuuring E, Schalken J: Expression of cyclin D1 and EMS1 in bladder tumours; relationship with chromosome 11q13 amplification. Oncogene 1996;12:1747–1753.
18. Christoph F, Schmidt B, Schmitz-Drager BJ, Schulz WA: Over-expression and amplification of the c-*myc* gene in human urothelial carcinoma. Int J Cancer 1999;84: 169–173.
19. Coombs LM, Pigott DA, Sweeney E, et al: Amplification and over-expression of c-erbB-2 in transitional cell carcinoma of the urinary bladder. Br J Cancer 1991;63: 601–608.
20. Proctor AJ, Coombs LM, Cairns JP, Knowles MA: Amplification at chromosome 11q13 in transitional cell tumours of the bladder. Oncogene 1991;6:789–795.
21. Voorter C, Joos S, Bringuier PP, et al: Detection of chromosomal imbalances in transitional cell carcinoma of the bladder by comparative genomic hybridization. Am J Pathol 1995;146:1341–1354.
22. Savelieva E, Belair CD, Newton MA, et al: 20q gain associates with immortalization: 20q13.2 amplification correlates with genome instability in human papillomavirus 16 E7 transformed human uroepithelial cells. Oncogene 1997;14:551–560.
23. Koo SH, Kwon KC, Ihm CH, et al: Detection of genetic alterations in bladder tumors by comparative genomic hybridization and cytogenetic analysis. Cancer Genet Cytogenet 1999;110:87–93.
24. Bernardini S, Adessi GL, Billerey C, et al: Immunohistochemical detection of p53 protein overexpression versus gene sequencing in urinary bladder carcinomas. J Urol 1999;162:1496–1501.
25. Esrig D, Spruck CH, Nichols PW, et al: p53 nuclear protein accumulation correlates with mutations in the *p53* gene, tumor grade, and stage in bladder cancer. Am J Pathol 1993;143:1389–1397.
26. Vet JA, Bringuier PP, Poddighe PJ, et al: *p53* mutations have no additional prognostic value over stage in bladder cancer. Br J Cancer 1994;70:496–500.
27. Vet JA, Bringuier PP, Schaafsma HE, et al: Comparison of p53 protein overexpression with *P53* mutation in bladder cancer: Clinical and biologic aspects. Lab Invest 1995;73:837–843.
28. Balazs M, Carroll P, Kerschmann R, et al: Frequent homozygous deletion of cyclin-dependent kinase inhibitor 2 (MTS1, p16) in superficial bladder cancer detected by fluorescence in situ hybridization. Genes Chromosomes Cancer 1997;19:84–89.
29. Orlow I, LaRue H, Osman I, et al: Deletions of the INK4A gene in superficial bladder tumors: Association with recurrence. Am J Pathol 1999;155:105–113.
30. Wu WJ, Kakehi Y, Chang SF, et al: Genetic alterations of the p16 gene in urothelial carcinoma in Taiwanese patients. BJU Int 2000;85:143–149.
31. Blomjous CE, Schipper NW, Vos W, et al: Comparison of quantitative and classic prognosticators in urinary bladder carcinoma: A multivariate analysis of DNA flow cytometric, nuclear morphometric and clinicopathological features. Virchows Arch A Pathol Anat Histopathol 1989;415:421–428.
32. Fossa SD, Berner AA, Jacobsen AB, et al: Clinical significance of DNA ploidy and S-phase fraction and their relation to p53 protein, c-erbB-2 protein and HCG in operable muscle-invasive bladder cancer. Br J Cancer 1993;68:572–578.
33. Coon JS, Deitch AD, de Vere W, et al: Interinstitutional variability in DNA flow cytometric analysis of tumors. The National Cancer Institute's Flow Cytometry Network experience. Cancer 1988;61:126–130.
34. Lipponen PK, Liukkonen TJ: Reduced expression of retinoblastoma (Rb) gene protein is related to cell proliferation and prognosis in transitional-cell bladder cancer. J Cancer Res Clin Oncol 1995;121:44–50.
35. al-Abadi H, Nagel R, Neuhaus P: Immunohistochemical detection of p53 protein in transitional cell carcinoma of the bladder in correlation to DNA ploidy and pathohistological stage and grade. Cancer Detect Prev 1998;22:43–50.
36. Gao JP, Uchida T, Wang C, et al: Relationship between *p53* gene mutation and protein expression: Clinical significance in transitional cell carcinoma of the bladder. Int J Oncol 2000;16:469–475.
37. Vollmer RT, Humphrey PA, Swanson PE, et al: Invasion of the bladder by transitional cell carcinoma: Its relation to histologic grade and expression of p53, MIB-1, c-erb B-2, epidermal growth factor receptor, and bcl-2. Cancer 1998;82:715–723.
38. Wu TT, Chen JH, Lee YH, Huang JK: The role of bcl-2, p53, and ki-67 index in predicting tumor recurrence for low grade superficial transitional cell bladder carcinoma. J Urol 2000;163:758–760.
39. Shiina H, Igawa M, Nagami H, et al: Immunohistochemical analysis of proliferating cell nuclear antigen, p53 protein and nm23 protein, and nuclear DNA content in transitional cell carcinoma of the bladder. Cancer 1996;78:1762–1774.
40. Glick SH, Howell LP, White RW: Relationship of p53 and bcl-2 to prognosis in muscle-invasive transitional cell carcinoma of the bladder. J Urol 1996;155:1754–1757.
41. Inagaki T, Ebisuno S, Uekado Y, et al: PCNA and p53 in urinary bladder cancer: Correlation with histological findings and prognosis. Int J Urol 1997;4:172–177.
42. Li B, Kanamaru H, Noriki S, et al: Reciprocal expression of bcl-2 and p53 oncoproteins in urothelial dysplasia

and carcinoma of the urinary bladder. Urol Res 1998;26: 235–241.
43. Nakopoulou L, Vourlakou C, Zervas A, et al: The prevalence of bcl-2, p53, and Ki-67 immunoreactivity in transitional cell bladder carcinomas and their clinicopathologic correlates. Hum Pathol 1998;29:146–154.
44. Lee SE, Chow NH, Chi YC, et al: Expression of c-erbB-2 protein in normal and neoplastic urothelium: Lack of adverse prognostic effect in human urinary bladder cancer. Anticancer Res 1994;14:1317–1324.
45. Nakanishi K, Kawai T, Suzuki M, Torikata C: Growth factors and oncogene products in transitional cell carcinoma. Mod Pathol 1996;9:292–297.
46. Sato K, Moriyama M, Mori S, et al: An immunohistologic evaluation of C-erbB-2 gene product in patients with urinary bladder carcinoma. Cancer 1992;70:2493–2498.
47. Brothman AR, Williams BJ: Prostate cancer. *In* Wolman SR, Sell S (eds): Human Cytogenetic Cancer Markers. Totawa, NJ, Humana, 1997, pp 223–246.
48. Jones E, Zhu XL, Rohr LR, et al: Aneusomy of chromosomes 7 and 17 detected by FISH in prostate cancer and the effects of selection in vitro. Genes Chromosomes Cancer 1994;11:163–170.
49. Konig JJ, Teubel W, van Dongen JW, et al: Tissue culture loss of aneuploid cells from carcinomas of the prostate. Genes Chromosomes Cancer 1993;8:22–27.
50. Alcaraz A, Takahashi S, Brown JA, et al: Aneuploidy and aneusomy of chromosome 7 detected by fluorescence in situ hybridization are markers of poor prognosis in prostate cancer. Cancer Res 1994;54:3998–4002.
51. Aly MS, Cin PD, Van de Voorde W, Van Poppel H, et al: Chromosome abnormalities in benign prostatic hyperplasia. Genes Chromosomes Cancer 1994;9:227–233.
52. Heim S, Mitelman F: Tumors of the Male Genital Organs. *In* Heim S, Mitelman F (eds): Cancer Cytogenetics, 2nd ed. New York, Wiley-Liss, 1995, pp 408–421.
53. Verma RS, Manikal M, Conte RA, Godec CJ: Chromosomal basis of adenocarcinoma of the prostate. Cancer Invest 1999;17:441–447.
54. Cher ML, MacGrogan D, Bookstein R, et al: Comparative genomic hybridization, allelic imbalance, and fluorescence in situ hybridization on chromosome 8 in prostate cancer. Genes Chromosomes Cancer 1994;11: 153–162.
55. Cher ML, Bova GS, Moore DH, et al: Genetic alterations in untreated metastases and androgen-independent prostate cancer detected by comparative genomic hybridization and allelotyping. Cancer Res 1996;56: 3091–3102.
56. Cher ML, Lewis PE, Banerjee M, et al: A similar pattern of chromosomal alterations in prostate cancers from African-Americans and Caucasian Americans. Clin Cancer Res 1998;4:1273–1278.
57. Hyytinen ER, Thalmann GN, Zhau HE, et al: Genetic changes associated with the acquisition of androgen-independent growth, tumorigenicity and metastatic potential in a prostate cancer model. Br J Cancer 1997; 75:190–195.
58. Visakorpi T, Hyytinen E, Koivisto P, et al: In vivo amplification of the androgen receptor gene and progression of human prostate cancer. Nat Genet 1995;9: 401–406.
59. Koivisto P, Kononen J, Palmberg C, et al: Androgen receptor gene amplification: A possible molecular mechanism for androgen deprivation therapy failure in prostate cancer. Cancer Res 1997;57:314–319.
60. Bova GS, Carter BS, Bussemakers MJ, et al: Homozygous deletion and frequent allelic loss of chromosome 8p22 loci in human prostate cancer. Cancer Res 1993; 53:3869–3873.
61. Cheng L, Bostwick DG, Li G, et al: Allelic imbalance in the clonal evolution of prostate carcinoma. Cancer 1999; 85:2017–2022.
62. Vocke CD, Pozzatti RO, Bostwick DG, et al: Analysis of 99 microdissected prostate carcinomas reveals a high frequency of allelic loss on chromosome 8p12-21. Cancer Res 1996;56:2411–2416.
63. Liu QY, Wang LF, Miao SY, Catterall JF: Expression and characterization of a novel human sperm membrane protein. Biol Reprod 1996;54:323–330.
64. Emmert-Buck MR, Vocke CD, Pozzatti RO, et al: Allelic loss on chromosome 8p12-21 in microdissected prostatic intraepithelial neoplasia. Cancer Res 1995;55: 2959–2962.
65. Saric T, Brkanac Z, Troyer DA, et al: Genetic pattern of prostate cancer progression. Int J Cancer 1999;81: 219–224.
66. Dahiya R, McCarville J, Hu W, et al: Chromosome 3p24-26 and 3p22-12 loss in human prostatic adenocarcinoma. Int J Cancer 1997;71:20–25.
67. Cooney KA, Wetzel JC, Consolino CM, Wojno KJ: Identification and characterization of proximal 6q deletions in prostate cancer. Cancer Res 1996;56:4150–4153.
68. Srikantan V, Sesterhenn IA, Davis L, et al: Allelic loss on chromosome 6q in primary prostate cancer. Int J Cancer 1999;84:331–335.
69. Perinchery G, Bukurov N, Nakajima K, et al: High frequency of deletion on chromosome 9p21 may harbor several tumor-suppressor genes in human prostate cancer. Int J Cancer 1999;83:610–614.
70. Ittmann M: Allelic loss on chromosome 10 in prostate adenocarcinoma. Cancer Res 1996;56:2143–2147.
71. Trybus TM, Burgess AC, Wojno KJ, et al: Distinct areas of allelic loss on chromosomal regions 10p and 10q in human prostate cancer. Cancer Res 1996;56:2263–2267.
72. Dahiya R, McCarville J, Lee C, et al: Deletion of chromosome 11p15, p12, q22, q23-24 loci in human prostate cancer. Int J Cancer 1997;72:283–288.
73. Maraj BH, Leek JP, Carr IM, Markham AF: Identification of a novel microsatellite marker tightly linked to the *KAI-1* gene for predicting prostate cancer progression. Eur Urol 2000;37:228–233.
74. Kibel AS, Freije D, Isaacs WB, Bova GS: Deletion mapping at 12p12-13 in metastatic prostate cancer. Genes Chromosomes Cancer 1999;25:270–276.
75. Afonso A, Emmert-Buck MR, Duray PH, et al: Loss of heterozygosity on chromosome 13 is associated with advanced stage prostate cancer. J Urol 1999;162:922–926.
76. Hyytinen ER, Frierson HFJ, Boyd JC, et al: Three distinct regions of allelic loss at 13q14, 13q21-22, and 13q33 in prostate cancer. Genes Chromosomes Cancer 1999;25:108–114.
77. Ueda T, Emi M, Suzuki H, et al: Identification of a I-cM region of common deletion on 13q14 associated with

human prostate cancer. Genes Chromosomes Cancer 1999;24:183–190.

78. Yin Z, Spitz MR, Babaian RJ, et al: Limiting the location of a putative human prostate cancer tumor suppressor gene at chromosome 13q14.3. Oncogene 1999;18: 7576–7583.
79. Elo JP, Harkonen P, Kyllonen AP, et al: Loss of heterozygosity at 16q24.1-q24.2 is significantly associated with metastatic and aggressive behavior of prostate cancer. Cancer Res 1997;57:3356–3359.
80. Latil A, Cussenot O, Fournier G, et al: Loss of heterozygosity at chromosome 16q in prostate adenocarcinoma: Identification of three independent regions. Cancer Res 1997;57:1058–1062.
81. Li C, Berx G, Larsson C, et al: Distinct deleted regions on chromosome segment 16q23-24 associated with metastases in prostate cancer. Genes Chromosomes Cancer 1999;24:175–182.
82. Chekmareva MA, Hollowell CM, Smith RC, et al: Localization of prostate cancer metastasis-suppressor activity on human chromosome 17. Prostate 1997;33:271–280.
83. Gao X, Zacharek A, Grignon DJ, et al: Localization of potential tumor suppressor loci to a 2 Mb region on chromosome 17q in human prostate cancer. Oncogene 1995; 11:1241–1247.
84. Gao X, Zacharek A, Salkowski A, et al: Loss of heterozygosity of the *BRCA1* and other loci on chromosome 17q in human prostate cancer. Cancer Res 1995;55: 1002–1005.
85. Egawa S, Uchida T, Suyama K, et al: Genomic instability of microsatellite repeats in prostate cancer: Relationship to clinicopathological variables. Cancer Res 1995; 55:2418–2421.
86. Rohrbach H, Haas CJ, Baretton GB, et al: Microsatellite instability and loss of heterozygosity in prostatic carcinomas: Comparison of primary tumors, and of corresponding recurrences after androgen-deprivation therapy and lymph-node metastases. Prostate 1999;40: 20–27.
87. Suzuki H, Komiya A, Aida S, et al: Microsatellite instability and other molecular abnormalities in human prostate cancer. Jpn J Cancer Res 1995;86:956–961.
88. Uchida T, Wada C, Wang C, et al: Microsatellite instability in prostate cancer. Oncogene 1995;10: 1019–1022.
89. Fournier G, Latil A, Amet Y, et al: Gene amplifications in advanced-stage human prostate cancer. Urol Res 1995;22:343–347.
90. Koivisto P, Visakorpi T, Kallioniemi OP: Androgen receptor gene amplification: A novel molecular mechanism for endocrine therapy resistance in human prostate cancer. Scand J Clin Lab Invest Suppl 1996;226:57–63.
91. Koivisto P, Kolmer M, Visakorpi T, Kallioniemi OP: Androgen receptor gene and hormonal therapy failure of prostate cancer. Am J Pathol 1998;152:1–9.
92. Latil A, Baron JC, Cussenot O, et al: Oncogene amplifications in early-stage human prostate carcinomas. Int J Cancer 1994;59:637–638.
93. Anwar K, Nakakuki K, Shiraishi T, et al: Presence of *ras* oncogene mutations and human papillomavirus DNA in human prostate carcinomas. Cancer Res 1992; 52:5991–5996.
94. Capella G, Cronauer-Mitra S, Pienado MA, Perucho M: Frequency and spectrum of mutations at codons 12 and 13 of the c-K-*ras* gene in human tumors. Environ Health Perspect 1991;93:125–131.
95. Barrack ER: Androgen receptor mutations in prostate cancer. Mt Sinai J Med 1996;63:403–412.
96. Culig Z, Hobisch A, Hittmair A, et al: Androgen receptor gene mutations in prostate cancer: Implications for disease progression and therapy. Drugs Aging 1997;10: 50–58.
97. Bookstein R, Rio P, Madreperla SA, et al: Promoter deletion and loss of retinoblastoma gene expression in human prostate carcinoma. Proc Natl Acad Sci USA 1990;87:7762–7766.
98. Kubota Y, Fujinami K, Uemura H, et al: Retinoblastoma gene mutations in primary human prostate cancer. Prostate 1995;27:314–320.
99. Meyers FJ, Gumerlock PH, Chi SG, et al: Very frequent *p53* mutations in metastatic prostate carcinoma and in matched primary tumors. Cancer 1998;83:2534–2539.
100. Bookstein R, MacGrogan D, Hilsenbeck SG, et al: *p53* is mutated in a subset of advanced-stage prostate cancers. Cancer Res 1993;53:3369–3373.
101. Cairns P, Okami K, Halachmi S, et al: Frequent inactivation of *PTEN/MMAC1* in primary prostate cancer. Cancer Res 1997;57:4997–5000.
102. Dong JT, Sipe TW, Hyytinen ER, et al: *PTEN/MMAC1* is infrequently mutated in pT2 and pT3 carcinomas of the prostate. Oncogene 1998;17:1979–1982.
103. Eagle LR, Yin X, Brothman AR, et al: Mutation of the *MXI1* gene in prostate cancer. Nat Genet 1995;9: 249–255.
104. Uchida T, Wang C, Sato T, et al: *BRCA1* gene mutation and loss of heterozygosity on chromosome 17q21 in primary prostate cancer. Int J Cancer 1999;84:19–23.
105. Kallakury BV, Brien TP, Lowry CV, et al: Telomerase activity in human benign prostate tissue and prostatic adenocarcinomas. Diagn Mol Pathol 1997;6:192–198.
106. Lin Y, Uemura H, Fujinami K, et al: Telomerase activity in primary prostate cancer. J Urol 1997;157:1161–1165.
107. Lin Y, Uemura H, Fujinami K, et al: Detection of telomerase activity in prostate needle-biopsy samples. Prostate 1998;36:121–128.
108. Koeneman KS, Pan CX, Jin JK, et al: Telomerase activity, telomere length, and DNA ploidy in prostatic intraepithelial neoplasia (PIN). J Urol 1998;160:1533–1539.
109. Takahashi C, Miyagawa I, Kumano S, Oshimura M: Detection of telomerase activity in prostate cancer by needle biopsy. Eur Urol 1997;32:494–498.
110. Scates DK, Muir GH, Venitt S, Carmichael PL: Detection of telomerase activity in human prostate: A diagnostic marker for prostatic cancer? Br J Urol 1997;80: 263–268.
110a. Argani P, Iacobuzio-Donahue C, Ryu B, et al: Mesothelin is overexpressed in the vast majority of ductal adenocarcinomas of the pancreas: Identification of a new pancreatic cancer marker by serial analysis of gene expression (SAGE). Clin Cancer Res 2001;7:3862–3868.
110b. Waghray A, Schober M, Feroze F, et al: Identification of differentially expressed genes by serial analysis of gene expression in human prostate cancer. Cancer Res 2001;61:4283–4286.

110c. Chaib H, Cockrell EK, Rubin MA, Macoska JA: Profiling and verification of gene expression patterns in normal and malignant human prostate tissues by cDNA microarray analysis. Neoplasia 2001;3:43–52.
110d. Svaren J, Ehrig T, Abdulkadir SA et al: EGR1 target genes in prostate carcinoma cells identified by microarray analysis. Biol Chem 2000;275:38524–38531.
110e. Xu J, Stolk JA, Zhang X, et al: Identification of differentially expressed genes in human prostate cancer using subtraction and microarray. Cancer Res 2000; 60:1677–1682.
110f. Bubendorf L, Kolmer M, Kononen J, et al: Hormone therapy failure in human prostate cancer: Analysis by complementary DNA and tissue microarrays. J Natl Cancer Inst 1999;91:1758–1764.
111. Berthon P, Valeri A, Cohen-Akenine A, et al: Predisposing gene for early-onset prostate cancer, localized on chromosome 1q42.2-43. Am J Hum Genet 1998;62: 1416–1424.
112. Cooney KA, McCarthy JD, Lange E, et al: Prostate cancer susceptibility locus on chromosome 1q: A confirmatory study. J Natl Cancer Inst 1997;89:955–959.
113. Gronberg H, Xu J, Smith JR, et al: Early age at diagnosis in families providing evidence of linkage to the hereditary prostate cancer locus *(HPC1)* on chromosome 1. Cancer Res 1997;57:4707–4709.
114. Gronberg H, Smith J, Emanuelsson M, et al: In Swedish families with hereditary prostate cancer, linkage to the *HPC1* locus on chromosome 1q24-25 is restricted to families with early-onset prostate cancer. Am J Hum Genet 1999;65:134–140.
115. Neuhausen SL, Farnham JM, Kort E, et al: Prostate cancer susceptibility locus *HPC1* in Utah high-risk pedigrees. Hum Mol Genet 1999;8:2437–2442.
116. Gibbs M, Stanford JL, McIndoe RA, et al: Evidence for a rare prostate cancer-susceptibility locus at chromosome 1p36. Am J Hum Genet 1999;64:776–787.
117. Xu J, Meyers D, Freije D, et al: Evidence for a prostate cancer susceptibility locus on the X chromosome. Nat Genet 1998;20:175–179.
118. Lange EM, Chen H, Brierley K, et al: Linkage analysis of 153 prostate cancer families over a 30-cM region containing the putative susceptibility locus HPCX. Clin Cancer Res 1999;5:4013–4020.
119. de la Taille A, Olsson CA, Katz AE: Molecular staging of prostate cancer: Dream or reality? Oncology 1999; 13:187–194.
120. Clements JA, Rohde P, Allen V, et al: Molecular detection of prostate cells in ejaculate and urethral washings in men with suspected prostate cancer. J Urol 1999; 161:1337–1343.
121. de la Taille A, Olsson CA, Buttyan R, et al: Blood-based reverse transcriptase polymerase chain reaction assays for prostatic specific antigen: Long-term follow-up confirms the potential utility of this assay in identifying patients more likely to have biochemical recurrence (rising PSA) following radical prostatectomy. Int J Cancer 1999;84:360–364.
122. Edelstein RA, Zietman AL, de las M, et al: Implications of prostate micrometastases in pelvic lymph nodes: An archival tissue study. Urology 1996;47:370–375.
123. Gao CL, Dean RC, Pinto A, et al: Detection of circulating prostate specific antigen expressing prostatic cells in the bone marrow of radical prostatectomy patients by sensitive reverse transcriptase polymerase chain reaction. J Urol 1999;161:1070–1076.
124. Ghossein RA, Rosai J, Scher HI, et al: Prognostic significance of detection of prostate-specific antigen transcripts in the peripheral blood of patients with metastatic androgen-independent prostatic carcinoma. Urology 1997;50:100–105.
125. Olsson CA, De Vries GM, Benson MC, et al: The use of RT-PCR for prostate-specific antigen assay to predict potential surgical failures before radical prostatectomy: Molecular staging of prostate cancer. Br J Urol 1996; 77:411–417.
126. Wood DPJ, Banerjee M: Presence of circulating prostate cells in the bone marrow of patients undergoing radical prostatectomy is predictive of disease-free survival. J Clin Oncol 1997;15:3451–3457.
127. Ellis WJ, Vessella RL, Corey E, et al: The value of a reverse transcriptase polymerase chain reaction assay in preoperative staging and followup of patients with prostate cancer. J Urol 1998;159:1134–1138.
128. Gao CL, Maheshwari S, Dean RC, et al: Blinded evaluation of reverse transcriptase-polymerase chain reaction prostate-specific antigen peripheral blood assay for molecular staging of prostate cancer. Urology 1999;53: 714–721.
129. Goldman HB, Israeli RS, Lerner JL, et al: Effect of prostate biopsy on the results of the PSA RT-PCR test. Urology 1998;52:1073–1078.
130. Moreno JG, O'Hara SM, Long JP, et al: Transrectal ultrasound-guided biopsy causes hematogenous dissemination of prostate cells as determined by RT-PCR. Urology 1997;49:515–520.
131. Moreno JG, Shenot PJ, Shupp-Byrne D, Gomella LG: Analysis of tumor spillage during radical prostatectomy using RT-PCR of prostate specific antigen. Tech Urol 1996;2:54–57.
132. Oefelein MG, Ignatoff JM, Clemens JQ, et al: Clinical and molecular followup after radical retropubic prostatectomy. J Urol 1999;162:307–310.
133. Adolfsson J, Ronstrom L, Hedlund PO, et al: The prognostic value of modal deoxyribonucleic acid in low grade, low stage untreated prostate cancer. J Urol 1990;144: 1404–1406.
134. Hittmair A, Rogatsch H, Mikuz G, Feichtinger H: Quantification of spermatogenesis by dual-parameter flow cytometry. Fertil Steril 1994;61:746–750.
135. Azua J, Romeo P, Valle J, Azua JJ: DNA quantification as a prognostic factor in prostatic adenocarcinoma. Anal Quant Cytol Histol 1996;18:330–336.
136. Azua J, Romeo P, Valle J, Azua JJ: Cytologic differentiation grade and malignancy DNA index in prostatic adenocarcinoma. Anal Quant Cytol Histol 1997;19:102–106.
137. Badalament RA, O'Toole RV, Young DC, Drago JR: DNA ploidy and prostate-specific antigen as prognostic factors in clinically resectable prostate cancer. Cancer 1991;67:3014–3023.
138. Blatstein LM, Ginsberg PC, Daskal I, Finkelstein LH: Flow cytometric determination of ploidy in prostatic

adenocarcinoma and its relation to clinical outcome. J Am Osteopath Assoc 1993;93:463–472.
139. Borre M, Hoyer M, Nerstrom B, Overgaard J: DNA ploidy and survival of patients with clinically localized prostate cancer treated without intent to cure. Prostate 1998;36:244–249.
140. Tinari N, Natoli C, Angelucci D, et al: DNA and S-phase fraction analysis by flow cytometry in prostate cancer: Clinicopathologic implications. Cancer 1993; 71:1289–1296.
141. Bratt O, Anderson H, Bak-Jensen E, et al: Metaphase cytogenetics and DNA flow cytometry with analysis of S-phase fraction in prostate cancer: Influence on prognosis. Urology 1996;47:218–224.
142. Hepburn PJ, Glynne-Jones E, Goddard L, et al: Cell proliferation in prostatic carcinoma: Comparative analysis of Ki-67, MIB-1 and PCNA. Histochem J 1995; 27:196–203.
143. Vesalainen SL, Lipponen PK, Talja MT, et al: Proliferating cell nuclear antigen and p53 expression as prognostic factors in T1-2M0 prostatic adenocarcinoma. Int J Cancer 1994;58:303–308.
144. Bubendorf L, Sauter G, Moch H, et al: Ki-67 labelling index: An independent predictor of progression in prostate cancer treated by radical prostatectomy. J Pathol 1996;178:437–441.
145. Feneley MR, Young MP, Chinyama C, et al: Ki-67 expression in early prostate cancer and associated pathological lesions. J Clin Pathol 1996;49:741–748.
146. Keshgegian AA, Johnston E, Cnaan A: Bcl-2 oncoprotein positivity and high MIB-1 (Ki-67) proliferative rate are independent predictive markers for recurrence in prostate carcinoma. Am J Clin Pathol 1998;110: 443–449.
147. Stattin P: Prognostic factors in prostate cancer. Scand J Urol Nephrol Suppl 1997;185:1–46.
148. Stattin P, Damber JE, Karlberg L, Bergh A: Cell proliferation assessed by Ki-67 immunoreactivity on formalin fixed tissues is a predictive factor for survival in prostate cancer. J Urol 1997;157:219–222.
149. Bauer JJ, Sesterhenn IA, Mostofi KF, et al: p53 nuclear protein expression is an independent prognostic marker in clinically localized prostate cancer patients undergoing radical prostatectomy. Clin Cancer Res 1995;1: 1295–1300.
150. Grignon DJ, Caplan R, Sarkar FH, et al: p53 status and prognosis of locally advanced prostatic adenocarcinoma: A study based on RTOG 8610. J Natl Cancer Inst 1997; 89:158–165.
151. Kuczyk MA, Serth J, Bokemeyer C, et al: The prognostic value of p53 for long-term and recurrence-free survival following radical prostatectomy. Eur J Cancer 1998; 34:679–686.
152. Stapleton AM, Zbell P, Kattan MW, et al: Assessment of the biologic markers p53, Ki-67, and apoptotic index as predictive indicators of prostate carcinoma recurrence after surgery. Cancer 1998;82:168–175.
153. Theodorescu D, Broder SR, Boyd JC, et al: p53, bcl-2 and retinoblastoma proteins as long-term prognostic markers in localized carcinoma of the prostate. J Urol 1997;158:131–137.
154. Berner A, Harvei S, Tretli S, et al: Prostatic carcinoma: A multivariate analysis of prognostic factors. Br J Cancer 1994;69:924–930.
155. Brooks JD, Bova GS, Ewing CM, et al: An uncertain role for *p53* gene alterations in human prostate cancers. Cancer Res 1996;56:3814–3822.
156. Bosl GJ, Ilson DH, Rodriguez E, et al: Clinical relevance of the i (12p) marker chromosome in germ cell tumors. J Natl Cancer Inst 1994;86:349–355.
157. van Echten J, Oosterhuis JW, Looijenga LH, et al: No recurrent structural abnormalities apart from i (12p) in primary germ cell tumors of the adult testis. Genes Chromosomes Cancer 1995;14:133–144.
158. Gibas Z, Prout GR, Pontes JE, Sandberg AA: Chromosome changes in germ cell tumors of the testis. Cancer Genet Cytogenet 1986;19:245–252.
159. Rodriguez E, Mathew S, Reuter V, et al: Cytogenetic analysis of 124 prospectively ascertained male germ cell tumors. Cancer Res 1992;52:2285–2291.
160. Meng FJ, Zhou Y, Giwercman A, et al: Fluorescence in situ hybridization analysis of chromosome 12 anomalies in semen cells from patients with carcinoma in situ of the testis. J Pathol 1998;186:235–239.
161. Murty VV, Chaganti RS: A genetic perspective of male germ cell tumors. Semin Oncol 1998;25:133–144.
162. Houldsworth J, Reuter V, Bosl GJ, Chaganti RS: Aberrant expression of cyclin D2 is an early event in human male germ cell tumorigenesis. Cell Growth Differ 1997; 8:293–299.
163. Chaganti RS, Houldsworth J: The cytogenetic theory of the pathogenesis of human adult male germ cell tumors. APMIS 1998;106:80–83.
164. Chaganti RS, Ladanyi M, Samaniego F, et al: Leukemic differentiation of a mediastinal germ cell tumor. Genes Chromosomes Cancer 1989;1:83–87.
165. Ilson DH, Motzer RJ, Rodriguez E, et al: Genetic analysis in the diagnosis of neoplasms of unknown primary tumor site. Semin Oncol 1993;20:229–237.
166. Motzer RJ, Rodriguez E, Reuter VE, et al: Molecular and cytogenetic studies in the diagnosis of patients with poorly differentiated carcinomas of unknown primary site. J Clin Oncol 1995;13:274–282.
167. Ottesen AM, Kirchhoff M, De-Meyts ER, et al: Detection of chromosomal aberrations in seminomatous germ cell tumours using comparative genomic hybridization. Genes Chromosomes Cancer 1997;20:412–418.
168. Mostert MM, van de Pol M, Olde WD, et al: Comparative genomic hybridization of germ cell tumors of the adult testis: Confirmation of karyotypic findings and identification of a 12p- amplicon. Cancer Genet Cytogenet 1996;89:146–152.
169. Summersgill B, Goker H, Osin P, et al: Establishing germ cell origin of undifferentiated tumors by identifying gain of 12p material using comparative genomic hybridization analysis of paraffin-embedded samples. Diagn Mol Pathol 1998;7:260–266.
170. Murty VV, Renault B, Falk CT, et al: Physical mapping of a commonly deleted region, the site of a candidate tumor suppressor gene, at 12q22 in human male germ cell tumors. Genomics 1996;35:562–570.
171. Murty VV, Houldsworth J, Baldwin S, et al: Allelic deletions in the long arm of chromosome 12 identify

sites of candidate tumor suppressor genes in male germ cell tumors. Proc Natl Acad Sci USA 1992;89: 11006–11010.

172. Mathew S, Murty VV, Bosl GJ, Chaganti RS: Loss of heterozygosity identifies multiple sites of allelic deletions on chromosome 1 in human male germ cell tumors. Cancer Res 1994;54:6265–6269.
173. Murty VV, Li RG, Houldsworth J, et al: Frequent allelic deletions and loss of expression characterize the DCC gene in male germ cell tumors. Oncogene 1994;9: 3227–3231.
174. Murty VV, Reuter VE, Bosl GJ, Chaganti RS: Deletion mapping identifies loss of heterozygosity at 5p15.1-15.2, 5q11 and 5q34-35 in human male germ cell tumors. Oncogene 1996;12:2719–2723.
175. Ganguly S, Murty VV, Samaniego F, et al: Detection of preferential NRAS mutations in human male germ cell tumors by the polymerase chain reaction. Genes Chromosomes Cancer 1990;1:228–232.
176. Guillou L, Estreicher A, Chaubert P, et al: Germ cell tumors of the testis overexpress wild-type p53. Am J Pathol 1996;149:1221–1228.
177. Kuczyk MA, Serth J, Bokemeyer C, et al: Alterations of the *p53* tumor suppressor gene in carcinoma in situ of the testis. Cancer 1996;78:1958–1966.
178. Tian Q, Frierson HFJ, Krystal GW, Moskaluk CA: Activating c-*kit* gene mutations in human germ cell tumors. Am J Pathol 1999;154:1643–1647.
179. Izquierdo MA, Van der Valk P, van Ark-Otte J, et al: Differential expression of the c-*kit* proto-oncogene in germ cell tumours. J Pathol 1995;177:253–258.
180. Strohmeyer T, Reese D, Press M, et al: Expression of the c-*kit* proto-oncogene and its ligand stem cell factor (SCF) in normal and malignant human testicular tissue. J Urol 1995;153:511–515.
181. Sledge GWJ, Eble JN, Roth BJ, et al: Relation of proliferative activity to survival in patients with advanced germ cell cancer. Cancer Res 1988;48:3864–3868.

DEBORAH DILLON
JOSÉ COSTA

11

Gastrointestinal System

During the past 15 years, our understanding of the pathogenesis of disease has rapidly expanded because of breakthroughs in molecular biology and biotechnology. Application of molecular genetics and advanced cell biology techniques to the study of human tumors and, especially, correlative studies of genetic changes with histopathology and the natural history of tumors have yielded important evidence supporting the central role that genetic alterations play in the pathogenesis of cancer. Much of the newly acquired knowledge has been applied to the diagnosis and prognosis of tumors and to assessment of the inherited and acquired risk of developing neoplasms.

Studies of gastrointestinal tumors suggest that both adenomas and carcinomas arise after mutational events occurring in somatic cells.[1] Because we know that the smallest observable lesions are clonal,[2] mutations (base substitutions, deletions, repeat length variations, amplifications, and translocations) become, in fact, markers of clonal cell populations and can be used to reconstruct clonal evolution. Mutations that promote clonal outgrowth are more likely to be significant for early diagnosis and for assessing prognosis than alterations that confer only a small growth advantage. Although the latter are likely to introduce relatively small modifications of the biologic properties of a clone, they can be used to define tumor progression more precisely or to compare and distinguish different subclones derived from the same tumor stem cell.

For the pathologist concerned with tumors, mutations can be exploited in the following settings: (1) to establish that a lesion is clonal (tumor vs. reactive pseudotumor); (2) to distinguish two synchronous tumors of the same histologic pattern; (3) to distinguish a metastasis from a second metachronous primary tumor; (4) to distinguish the origin of a metastasis when two similar primary tumors have been known to exist in the patient. Because DNA recombinant assays and polymerase chain reaction (PCR)-based techniques have revolutionized detection of mutations in tissues and cytologic samples, it is also possible (5) to detect early, very small, primary tumors; (6) to evaluate minimal residual disease; (7) to implement early detection of recurrence or second primary lesions in the same organ or site; and (8) to improve staging of tumors by assessing involvement of anatomic sites with enhanced sensitivity and accuracy.

For each histologic type of tumor known to harbor one or several genetic alterations, it is possible to imagine a number of different clinical scenarios in which the just-presented applications might be useful. In the gastrointestinal tract, we encounter tumors of the epithelium, the neuroendocrine system, the stroma, and the lymphoid tissue. Because several genetic alterations have been uncovered in these tumors, the quantity of new information of potential interest for patient management is considerable. In some instances, because of differences in methodology or in patient populations studied, results have been contradictory. It is, thus, necessary to assess the clinical use and cost efficiency of the new diagnostic and prognostic tests in a critical fashion. At the same time, it is important to standardize reagents and procedures and to provide practical guidelines for the conduct and interpretation of tests.

Recent studies of some of the common tumor types of the digestive system that are of potential practical interest to the pathologist are presented next.

ESOPHAGUS

Despite progress in therapy, carcinoma of the esophagus remains a tumor with somber prognosis. In the United States, cancer of the esophagus is responsible for approximately 8000 deaths per year. The natural history of esophageal squamous cell carcinoma (SCC) is one of extensive local growth with regional lymph node involvement and eventual widespread hematogenous dissemination. Because the tumor remains asymptomatic for a long interval, patients often present with relatively advanced tumors. Progression of SCC of the esophagus from the in situ to the invasive stage has been recorded to take 3 to 4 years.[3]

Only a small number of karyotypes have been obtained on carcinomas of the esophagus, and most of these have been incomplete. Cytogenetic abnormalities reported to occur in esophageal squamous cell carcinoma include loss of the Y chromosome and deletions of 2p, 4p, 7q, and 12p.[4] A newly established esophageal SCC cell line, HKESC-1, shows many structural chromosomal abnormalities, with breakpoints at 1p32, 7p22, 7q34, and 20q13.[5] Comparative genomic hybridization (CGH) studies have shown high-level amplifications in the regions of 8p23 (possibly involving *MYC*), 17q21 (possibly involving *ERBB2*), and 18p11.[6] Deletions have frequently been observed on 2q, 3p, 4q, 4p, 5q, 13q, and 18q.[6]

Of the genes known to be altered in SCC of the esophagus, *TP53* is most often found to be abnormal.[7] *TP53* mutations and/or p53 protein overexpression are reported to be present in up to 70% of esophageal SCCs.[8–12] It appears that *TP53* mutation is a relatively early event in esophageal carcinogenesis and that different *TP53* mutations may be present in multifocal preneoplastic lesions.[13] *TP53* mutations have even been detected in esophagitis adjacent to squamous cell carcinoma.[14] An unusual pattern of mutations in *TP53* has been noted, suggesting that the etiologic contribution of genotoxic factors might be complex and might associate a variety of endogenous and exogenous mutagenic exposures.[15] A high frequency of biallelic *TP53* mutations in esophageal squamous cell carcinomas with associated alterations in the transactivation of a number of cell cycle and apoptosis genes[16] supports the idea that *TP53* plays a central role in esophageal carcinogenesis.

Other genes that appear to be involved in the pathogenesis of esophageal squamous cell carcinoma are cell cycle regulators *RB1*, *CDKN1B*, *CDKN2A*, and *CCND1* (cyclin D1), the cell-cell adhesion molecule β-catenin, and heat shock protein HSP70.[17] In addition, loss of heterozygosity (LOH) can be detected in 43% of cases for *TP53*, 55% for the *APC* gene, 48% for the *MCC* gene, and 52% for the *RB1* gene.[18] LOH is even more frequent (69%) at the chromosome 17q tylosis-associated cancer susceptibility gene locus[19] and on 18q.[20] LOH at or around the *FHIT* gene has been described in 70% to 80% of primary esophageal tumors and appears to occur in association with heavy carcinogen exposure.[21, 22]

The contribution of molecular studies to the prognosis of SCC of the esophagus is not yet firmly established. Studies on the prognostic significance of *TP53* mutations in esophageal SCC have yielded conflicting results.[8, 10, 23, 24] Strong expression of the proliferation-regulating molecule p21WAF1 and weak expression of the apoptosis-regulating molecule BCLXL have been shown to be predictors of poor survival in both univariate and multivariate analyses.[25] Accumulation of cyclin D1, which is associated with accumulation of the retinoblastoma protein, also appears to be associated with adverse prognosis.[26]

Although the prognostic significance of each of these markers remains to be determined,[27] there is great promise for these markers in early detection strategies.[28] Preliminary data suggest that it might be useful to assess the *TP53* status in biopsy specimens obtained while screening populations known to be at increased risk for the development of esophageal cancer.[14] In addition, the fact that esophageal tumor metastases have been found to retain the identical *TP53* mutation present in the original tumor[29] allows mutations to serve as markers for clinical monitoring of patients whose primary tumors have been resected. Molecular profiles may also provide other clinically relevant information. Recent data comparing typical SCC of the esophagus with the aggressive basaloid variant have shown that this subtype bears a distinctive molecular signature, involving coactivation of MYC and BCL2, not seen in typical SCC.[30] This finding is consistent with the growing body of evidence in other tumor types that different molecular pathways may define subtypes of disease with different anticipated clinical behaviors.

Adenocarcinoma of the esophagus represents about 10% of the tumors of the esophagus, but its relative frequency appears to be increasing. Most esophageal adenocarcinomas arise in the context of chronic gastroesophageal reflux disease and the consequent development of columnar metaplasia (Barrett's esophagus). The fact that patients with Barrett's esophagus undergo routine surveillance endoscopy and biopsy has made this an excellent model system for the study of early events in neoplastic progression.

A common genetic event seen in both squamous cell carcinoma and adenocarcinoma of the esophagus is loss of the Y chromosome. The very high frequency of chromosome Y loss in adenocarcinoma, shown by interphase cytogenetics and in situ hybridization, suggests that this event is of pathogenetic significance.[31, 32] In one study of 30 esophageal adenocarcinomas using laser microdissection and CGH, gains on 8q (80%), 20q (60%), 2p, 7p, and 10q (47% each) were identified, with losses on the Y chromosome (76%), 4q (50%), 5q and 9p (43% each), 18q (40%), 7q (33%), and 14q (30%). High-level amplifications were seen on 8q23-qter, 8p12-pter, 7p11-14, 7q21-31, and 17q11-23. Many of these alterations were also identified in the associated metaplastic and dysplastic epithelium.[33]

Mutations in *TP53* and 17p allelic loss have been studied in adenocarcinomas and associated dysplastic lesions. *TP53* mutations have been detected in 70%, and 17p allelic loss has been detected in 80%, of esophageal adenocarcinomas.[34, 35] Most *TP53* mutations in esophageal adenocarcinomas are G→C to A→T base transitions at CpG dinucleotides, with the identical mutation detected both in tumor and in adjacent dysplastic Barrett's epithelium in a significant subset of cases.[34] In a study of 58 patients who had high-grade dysplasia without cancer, half had *TP53* mutations in their Barrett's segments.[36] Thus, *TP53* mutation is likely to be an early event in neoplastic progression of the metaplastic Barrett's epithelium. Successful long-term cultures established from Barrett's epithelium have shown *TP53* mutations and 17p LOH (three of four cases) in addition to abnormalities in *P16* (four of four cases) and 5q LOH (one of four cases).[37]

TP53 mutation and allelic loss appear also to be correlated with the development of aneuploidy in Barrett's esophagus.[38] In a prospective study of 62 patients, the presence of aneuploidy or increased 4N cell fractions on flow cytometry of premalignant Barrett's epithelium was predictive of subsequent progression to high-grade dysplasia or carcinoma.[39] The incorporation of molecular markers in prospective surveillance studies will be of great interest and will shed light on the value of *TP53* mutation and allelic loss as predictors of risk for developing malignancy.

Although *TP53* mutations are clearly an important event in the molecular pathogenesis of both squamous cell carcinomas and adenocarcinomas of the esophagus, it is interesting that the spectrum of *TP53* mutations found in the two cancers is quite different. Esophageal adenocarcinomas are characterized by a high frequency of G→A transitions at CpG dinucleotides, whereas mutations at A:T base pairs are considerably more frequent in esophageal squamous cell carcinomas.[34] These different mutational spectra may reflect different causes and, along with abnormalities in other genes, are likely part of distinct molecular pathways.[40]

One study of chromosome 17 LOH in 12 Barrett's adenocarcinomas has implicated LOH in multiple regions of chromosome 17 in the pathogenesis of this cancer. Using 41 microsatellite loci, six minimal regions on 17p and seven minimal regions on 17q have been determined.[41] Although these regions encompass known tumor suppressor genes *TP53* (17p13.1), *NFI* (17q11.2), and *BRCA1* (17q21.1), and a putative tumor suppressor gene at 17p13.3, it appears likely that other important tumor suppressor genes on chromosome 17 are also involved in the pathogenesis of esophageal adenocarcinoma.

Other genes known to be altered frequently in esophageal adenocarcinoma include *CDKN2A* and *FHIT*.[21, 22] LOH at the *CDKN2A* (*P16*) locus was noted in 89% of Barrett's adenocarcinomas but not in associated dysplasias; *CDKN2A* (*P16*) showed homozygous deletion in 3 of 12 cases in the same study and no evidence of mutation.[42] LOH at or around the *FHIT* locus appears to occur much more frequently in squamous cell carcinoma (80%) than in adenocarcinoma (44%), perhaps a reflection of the greater association of esophageal squamous cell carcinomas with exposure to environmental carcinogens.[22] The detection of these and other genes and gene products in biopsy specimens or in esophageal cell brushings could constitute valuable markers for cell populations at risk in early detection screening programs.

STOMACH

The incidence of gastric cancer is decreasing in the United States, but the stage of disease at diagnosis and survival after surgical resection have remained essentially unchanged.[43] An increase in the incidence of adenocarcinoma of the cardia is responsible for a leveling off of this generally downward trend during the past 2 decades.[44, 45] In about 10% of cases, the so-called lymphoepithelioma-like carcinomas, a link to Epstein-Barr virus infection can be identified,[46, 47] possibly involving expression of the transforming gene *BARF1*.[48] *Helicobacter pylori* infection has also been linked to the development of gastric adenocarcinoma[49, 50, 51, 52] and may be involved early in the neoplastic process.[53]

More than half of the cases of gastric adenocarcinoma with cytogenetic abnormalities show involvement of the region of 8q12; this often occurs as the reciprocal translocation t(3;8) (p21;q12).[4] Alterations of 3p that do not involve chromosome 8 are also common, and alterations of chromosome 12q13-15 are also known to occur. CGH demonstrates frequent losses on 3p21-23 (approximately 20% of cases) but does not demonstrate changes in the region of 8q12. Losses are also frequently seen at 5q14-22 (approximately 33%), 17p13 (approximately 50%), and 18q11-21 (33%) and on chromosome 19 (approximately 40%).[54] High-level amplifications are most commonly observed in the regions of *MYCN*, *MET*, *WNT2*, and *ERBB2* oncogenes.[55] LOH studies largely confirm the cytogenetic findings, demonstrating frequent deletions on chromosomes 1q, 5q, 13q, and 17p.[4, 56] LOH is also common at 11p15.5, a site that is often deleted in other tumors.[57] It appears that LOH at 17p is an early event in gastric carcinogenesis, whereas allelic loss at 5q typically occurs later in the course of the disease.[58] At least two different tumor suppressor genes (one of which is *APC*) appear to be involved in the 5q deletions.[59]

Research on DNA alterations and the molecular genetics of gastric tumors suggests that intestinal and diffuse types of gastric cancer are distinct entities at the molecular level. Whereas the diffuse type tends to appear de novo, the intestinal variety, arising from metaplastic epithelium, is more likely to show discrete genetic events correlating with progression. Conventional cytogenetic studies support the idea that there are fundamental differences between the two histologic types. Whereas only chromosome Y is lost in diffuse tumors, changes in chromosomes 20 and 13, as well as aneuploidy, are common in intestinal type tumors.[60] Examination of biopsy or resection specimens with interphase cytogenetics[31] promises to elucidate the question of separate genetic pathways for the main histologic types of gastric cancer. In restriction fragment length polymorphism analysis of 48 human gastric carcinomas, allelic loss on chromosome 17p appeared to be a common event in both histologic types. However, significant differences in allelic loss at other loci were found, with losses on chromosomes 1q, 5q, and 7p not detected in diffuse-type tumors.[56] Amplification and/or overexpression of *ERBB2* occurs in a subset of intestinal-type gastric cancers and is rare in tumors of the diffuse type.[61, 62] Mutations in β-catenin have been detected only in the well-differentiated intestinal-type gastric cancers (7 of 26) and not in tumors of the diffuse type (0 of 17).[63] Mutations in *TP53* are also more common in intestinal-type carcinomas than in cancers of the diffuse type.[64]

Molecular studies of cancer genes in gastric tumors and derivative cell lines have shown frequent alterations in both oncogenes and tumor suppressor genes, and potential clinical applications are beginning to emerge. Immunohistochemical membrane staining for the product of the oncogene *ERBB2* correlates with high-level gene amplifications in fluorescent in situ hybridization studies.[65] *ERBB2* is amplified and/or overexpressed in 10% to 20% of well-differentiated gastric carcinomas, correlating with poor survival[61, 62] and possibly related to invasion and nodal involvement.[66]

A number of abnormalities in the hepatocyte growth factor receptor MET have been described in gastric carcinomas. Gene amplification and/or overexpression occur in 10% and 46%, respectively, and correlate with depth of invasion and lymph node metastasis.[62] Furthermore, in multivariate analysis, overexpression of MET has proved to be an independent prognostic factor.[62] Activation of *MET* by rearrangement of *TPR-MET* is present in roughly half of gastric carcinomas. The presence of rearranged TPR-MET messenger RNA (mRNA) in tumor-free gastric tissues in patients with gastric cancer suggests that this is an early event in gastric carcinogenesis.[67] Thus, screening for *MET* abnormalities might be useful in the identification of individuals at risk for the development of gastric carcinoma.

The Kirsten-*ras (KRAS)* oncogene, often mutated in colorectal carcinoma, is seldom found to harbor mutations in gastric cancer.[68] Results showing overexpression of RAS p21 by immunohistochemistry are likely to reflect increased cell proliferation or to be due to metaplasia, because it is known that RAS p21 is strongly expressed in gastric intestinal metaplasia. Expression of MYC has also been studied in conjunction with other molecular alterations. Again, it is difficult to distinguish whether changes in *MYC* expression are secondary to increased cell proliferation or if they correspond to a fundamental lesion implicated in the causation of the tumors studied. Fluorescent in situ hybridization studies have demonstrated amplification of *MYC* in 15% of gastric cancers.[69] Gene amplifications have been shown to represent a relatively late event in gastric carcinogenesis,[70] and analysis for gene amplifications such as *MYC* may have a role in the pretreatment evaluation of small biopsy specimens. It has been suggested that in situ hybridization for *MYC* mRNA in biopsy tissue obtained from elevated gastric lesions could be a reliable aid in distinguishing between adenomas and well-differentiated carcinomas of the stomach of the elevated type.[71]

Alterations in tumor suppressor genes in gastric tumors and related lesions have been studied by several laboratories. *TP53* mutations have been demonstrated in up to two thirds of well-differentiated gastric carcinomas,[24, 35, 64, 72] occurring particularly in association with aneuploidy.[73] The spectrum of *TP53* mutations in gastric cancer is similar to that found in colorectal and esophageal carcinomas. Mutations, predominantly base transitions, are found both in early cancers and in advanced disease, but LOH at the 17p13 chromosomal region shows an increased incidence with advanced disease. These data suggest that mutated alleles acting in a dominant negative fashion contribute to the early stages of tumor development in the gastric mucosa.[74] There is a lack of agreement regarding the timing of *TP53* mutations, with some authors reporting *TP53* mutations at the adenoma stage.[75, 76] The incidence and spectrum of *TP53* mutations is similar in adenocarcinomas of the esophagus and the gastric cardia, suggesting a common pathogenesis,[24] and studies that have separated gastric carcinomas according to site have shown a significantly lower incidence of *TP53* mutations in subcardiac regions.[24, 64] *TP53* mutation is associated with poor prognosis.[24]

The recently described apoptosis inhibitor survivin is overexpressed in one third of cases of gastric carcinoma (60 of 174).[77] Expression of survivin is significantly higher in cases showing positive staining for p53 and BCL2 and in cases with a decreased apoptotic index. Thus, it appears likely that survivin plays a role in promoting cell survival in gastric cancer.

The candidate tumor suppressor gene *FHIT* (fragile histidine triad) has been mapped to the chromosomal region 3p14.2, a region showing frequent LOH in a number of human tumors, including gastric carcinomas.[78] The presence of *FHIT* alterations in the majority of gastric cancers suggests that alteration of a carcinogen-susceptible fragile region within the *FHIT* gene might be an early event in gastric carcinogenesis, as it is in lung cancer. Rearrangement of the *FHIT* gene and aberrant reverse transcriptase (RT)-PCR products has been detected in over 50% of gastric carcinomas, with almost 70% showing absent FHIT protein expression.[79] A study of 55 gastric cancers showed absence of FHIT protein to correlate with high tumor stage and grade and shortened survival[80]; thus, there may be a role for FHIT analysis in small biopsy specimens and surgical resection material.

Disruption of the APC–β-catenin–T-cell factor (Tcf)/lymphoid enhancer–binding factor pathway appears to play a role in gastric cancer, as well as in colorectal cancer. Mutations in the *APC* gene have been detected in a small number of gastric cancers[81] and in a larger number

(20%) of gastric adenomas.[82] Allelic loss at the *APC* locus is detected in a significant percentage of both intestinal and diffuse types of gastric cancer.[83] Somatic mutations in a portion of exon 3 coding for the glycogen synthase kinase 3β phosphorylation consensus region of the β-catenin gene have been detected in 7 of 43 gastric cancers, all of the intestinal type.[63] Both β-catenin and γ-catenin mutations are associated with constitutive Tcf transcriptional activation in gastric and pancreatic cancers.[84]

Microsatellite instability (MSI) is characteristic of tumors associated with the hereditary nonpolyposis colorectal carcinoma syndrome and is caused by multiple replication errors occurring during cell proliferation. Gastric carcinoma shows a high prevalence of MSI (30% to 40%),[85, 86, 87] yet mutations in DNA mismatch repair genes *MLH1* and *MSH2* have not been described. Methylation of the *MLH1* promoter was recently studied in a group of 65 gastric cancers. Hypermethylation of the *MLH1* promoter was strongly associated with MSI, supporting an epigenetic mechanism for defective mismatch repair in gastric carcinoma.[88]

Genes typically mutated in the microsatellite mutator phenotype gastrointestinal cancers include transforming growth factor- type II receptor *(TGFBR2)*, insulin-like growth factor 2 receptor *(IGF2R)*, and *BAX*.[86, 89] Caspase-5 has also been suggested as another target gene in the microsatellite mutator pathway, with mutations in an (A)10 repeat within its coding region present in 44% of gastric carcinomas.[90] Alterations in *BAX* and in *BAT26* have been associated particularly with tumors showing widespread MSI.[91]

Gastric cancers with a high degree of MSI have been associated with antral location, intestinal subtype, previous *Helicobacter pylori* infection, advanced stage, and lower incidence of lymph node metastasis.[86] However, the prognostic significance of MSI in gastric cancers is not entirely clear at this time, with many authors reporting a better prognosis[85, 92, 93] and others reporting no significant differences in survival.[87]

In addition to hypermethylation of the *MLH1* promoter in a subset of gastric carcinomas, methylation of *CDKN2A* also appears to play a role in the pathogenesis of some gastric carcinomas.[94] Deletions and mutations of *CDKN2A* and *CDKN2B* are not seen in gastric carcinomas.[95]

Genes that play a role in tumor invasion and metastasis are of interest because knowledge of their status in tumors may be of prognostic value. E-cadherin alleles are mutated and deleted in both cell lines[96] and tissue[96, 97, 98] derived from gastric carcinoma; mutation appears to be restricted to diffuse gastric carcinomas. The E-cadherin promoter has also been shown to undergo frequent hypermethylation, particularly in gastric tumors of the diffuse type, correlating with reduced tissue expression of E-cadherin.[99]

Certain characteristics of gastric adenocarcinoma are of interest because they can be exploited as specific markers of tumor cells. The first is an approximately 1.75-kb mRNA that encodes the CK20 form of cytokeratin.[100] This intermediate filament protein is a major constituent of enterocytes and goblet cells and is a marker for the epithelium of the gastric and intestinal mucosa. RT-PCR can enhance detection of this relatively specific message and allow identification of cells in abnormal anatomic locations and in the circulation.[101] Tissue inhibitor of matrix metalloproteinase-1 (TIMP-1) has also been used as a plasma marker in patients with gastric carcinoma and appears to correlate with serosal invasion and metastasis.[102] An additional marker that can distinguish distant tumor cells (when it is known to be present in the primary tumor) is the Epstein-Barr virus. EBV RNA can be detected with great sensitivity and specificity and has been shown to reside in the carcinoma cells and not in the noncancerous epithelium or in infiltrating lymphocytes.[103]

Molecular markers are also of interest in the diagnosis of lymphomas involving the gastric mucosa. The demonstration of clonality in a lymphoid cell population is helpful in establishing the diagnosis of lymphoma in cases with difficult morphologic features. With PCR-based protocols, endoscopic biopsy specimens can be assessed for clonality of B-cell receptors.[104, 105] Immunoglobulin gene rearrangement studies are also an excellent tool for the preoperative establishment of the extent of involvement of the gastric mucosa and for the early diagnosis of recurrence.[106]

Gastrointestinal stromal tumors (GIST) are characterized immunohistochemically by expression of the CD117 (KIT) and CD34 antigens; immunohistochemical expression of these antigens does not relate predictably to clinical behavior. Mutation of exon 11 of the *KIT* gene, a membrane-bound tyrosine kinase receptor, is associated with malignant behavior and reduced survival,[107, 108, 109] as is LOH in the region of chromosome 1p36.[110] Patients with aneuploid tumors by flow-cytometry have shorter survival than those with diploid tumors.[111]

COLON

Colorectal carcinoma provides a good example of how understanding the molecular pathogenesis of tumors improves our ability to provide better care to families and patients affected by this disease. In less than a decade, genes responsible for two major forms of inherited predisposition to colon cancer, as well as a cohort of genes involved in the causation of sporadic tumors, have been identified. In recent years, many of these genetic alterations have found practical applications along the lines described in the introductory paragraphs. Translation of progress in understanding into advances at the bedside has been facilitated by the fact that a good correlation exists between the natural history of colorectal carcinoma and the cumulative genetic alterations found in these neoplasms. As soon as a model of the sequential events became available, and especially when the model was refined, potential clinical applications could be intuitively derived (Fig. 11–1).

Karyotypic analysis of colorectal adenomas typically demonstrates only numerical aberrations—particularly gains of chromosomes 7, 8, 13, and 14; deletions of 1p36 are also frequent findings.[4] Carcinomas, in contrast, most frequently demonstrate deletions or rearrangements involving chromosome 17p (site of the *TP53* gene) and loss of chromosome 18.[4] A variety of other structural rearrangements are also commonly observed, and every chromosome except Y has been involved in recurrent structural rearrangements. Colon carcinomas that demonstrate structural chromosomal rearrangements are most frequently poorly differentiated, whereas well- and moderately well-differentiated tumors most frequently demonstrate either normal karyotypes or simple numerical aberrations.[112] CGH studies confirm this tendency to increased cytogenetic abnormality as neoplasia progresses,[113] with numerical aberration progressing to structural abnormality as tumors become more undifferentiated.

About 20% of all colorectal carcinomas are considered to be familial and likely the result of interactions of multiple genes and environmental factors. In a smaller proportion of cases, inherited mutations in single cancer susceptibility genes can be identified. Hereditary nonpolyposis colorectal cancer (HNPCC) is responsible for about 5% of all cases of colorectal cancer and involves inherited mutations in the DNA mismatch repair genes. Inherited mutations in the adenomatous polyposis coli (APC) gene are responsible for familial adenomatous polyposis (FAP), which accounts for less than 1% of all cases of colorectal cancer. An even smaller fraction of inherited cases are caused by Peutz-Jeghers syndrome and juvenile polyposis. Study of the genes involved in these inherited colorectal cancer syndromes has been important in elucidating the mechanisms and pathways of both inherited and sporadic colorectal cancer.

The gene for familial polyposis was identified in 1991.[114, 115, 116, 117] It is composed of 15 exons encoding a cytoplasmic protein of 2843 amino acids that interacts with β-catenin.[118] Inherited mutations of the gene result in loss of function of the gene product, and identical mutations can underlie various extracolonic phenotypes.[119] Formation of polyps requires inactivation of both alleles,[120] although it has been shown that truncated proteins, the product of mutations commonly encountered in FAP families, can interact with the wild-type protein. This finding suggests that the mutated gene may also act in a dominant negative fashion.[121] Mutations in defined regions of the gene can be correlated with specific phenotypes.[122, 123] At the same time, it is important to realize that studies in a murine model of FAP suggest the existence of modifier genes.[124] True nonallelic heterogeneity exists for syndromes close to FAP, and even for families with manifestations indistinguishable from FAP.[125] Sporadic mutations in the gene can be identified in extracolonic lesions seen either in FAP or Gardner's syndrome, such as desmoid tumors and adenomas of the ampulla of Vater.[126, 127]

Identification of the *APC* gene has made it possible to determine which individuals belonging to an afflicted kindred carry mutant alleles. This can be accomplished by a variety of strategies relying either on the identification of the precise mutation or using linkage analysis to establish whether a particular member of the kindred carries the mutated allele. It is of interest that such analyses can make use of paraffin-embedded archival tissues.[128]

Cells from some colon cancers with the clinicopathologic features of HNPCC[129] display numerous mutations throughout the genome (mutator phenotype).[130–133] When a new strand of DNA is synthesized during replication, errors that are not immediately corrected by the 3′ to 5′ exonuclease activity of DNA polymerase are corrected by a DNA mismatch repair system. Mutations in genes coding for proteins that participate in the mismatch repair system allow persistence of replication errors (mutations)

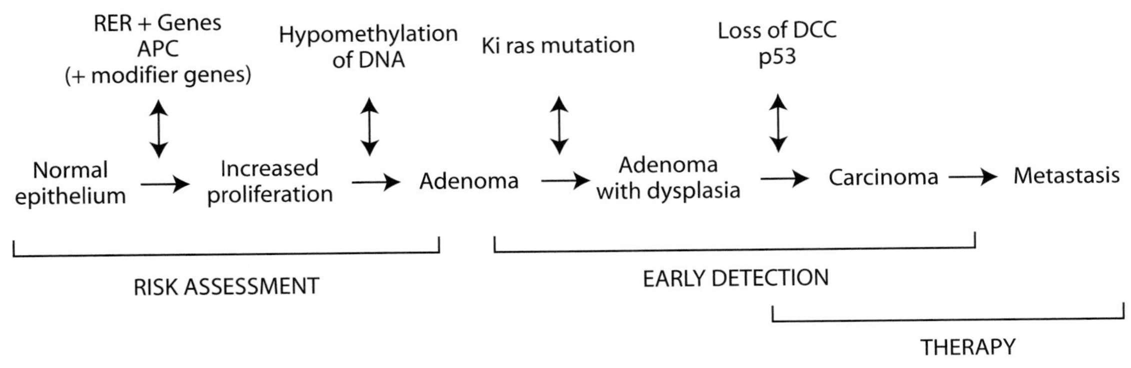

FIGURE 11–1
Model depicting cumulative genetic alterations found in colorectal carcinoma and their relationship to the natural history of these neoplasms.

that would otherwise be repaired. This results in MSI. Approximately 0.1% to 0.5% of the population carries a germline mutation in one of six mismatch repair genes (*MSH2*, *MSH6*, *MSH3*, *MLH1*, *PMS1*, or *PMS2*) that results in a substantial increase in the probability of developing cancer of the colon and rectum, endometrium, kidney, and other sites.[134] Up to 80% of people who harbor a mutation in one of the mismatch repair genes will develop colorectal cancer, accounting for approximately 5000 new colorectal cancer cases in the United States yearly[135]; up to 60% of women with inherited mutations in mismatch repair genes will develop endometrial cancer.[136]

Individuals who are members of HNPCC families may benefit from colonoscopic surveillance carried out as often as every 1 to 3 years. Such intensive surveillance is of proven value in reducing morbidity and mortality in HNPCC family members.[137, 138] Unfortunately, mismatch repair gene mutations cannot be identified in all families meeting even the strictest criteria for HNPCC.[135] Thus, mismatch repair gene sequencing is of limited use in selecting individual family members for intensive surveillance.[139]

Approximately 90% of colorectal cancers arising in individuals with HNPCC demonstrate MSI. If colorectal tumors from a family suspected of harboring HNPCC do not show MSI, it is unlikely that known repair gene defects are involved. Therefore, one may use the absence of MSI as a criterion to argue against, but not completely exclude, a diagnosis of HNPCC. Identification of MSI does little to support a diagnosis of HNPCC, however, because about 85% of colorectal cancers demonstrating MSI arise in patients who do not show mismatch repair gene defects.[140]

One of the windfalls of identifying genes responsible for hereditary forms of tumors is that often some of the same genes are found to be of pathogenetic significance in sporadic forms of the same tumor. The development of sporadic colorectal cancers appears to proceed along one of two molecular pathways,[141] one involving chromosomal instability and mutations in *APC*, *KRAS*, and/or *TP53* and the other characterized by MSI and mutations in genes such as *TGFBR2* and *BAX*.

The majority of sporadic colorectal carcinomas develop in association with widespread chromosomal instability, with multiple gains and losses and frequent aneuploidy. Mutations and/or allelic loss of one or more genes, including *APC*, *KRAS*, and *TP53*, are characteristic.[1] The *APC* gene appears to be an important gatekeeper in the development of sporadic colorectal cancers, with mutation occurring early in the process of carcinogenesis in over 75% of all colorectal tumors. It is clear that alteration of *APC* is rate limiting for adenoma formation.[142] *APC* codes for a cytoplasmic protein that can bind to and target β-catenin for degradation.[143] Mutant APC is defective in down-regulating transcriptional activation mediated by β-catenin and T-cell transcription factor 4 (Tcf-4).[144] The downstream targets of this pathway are not well described; however, *MYC* may be one of the genes activated by *APC* mutation.[145] *MYC* is overexpressed at both the RNA and protein levels during the development of colorectal tumors, yet gene amplifications or rearrangements have not been described.[146]

There are three human *RAS* genes, *HRAS*, *KRAS*, and *NRAS*, all of which code for 21-kd guanine nucleotide binding proteins involved in growth factor signaling via the MAP kinase pathway.[147] *RAS* genes are commonly mutated in many different tumor types, and *RAS* mutations are found in 40% to 50% of colorectal carcinomas, likely occurring at a relatively early stage of carcinogenesis.[148, 149, 150] Mutations in *RAS* interfere with the protein's ability to hydrolyze guanosine triphosphate and result in constitutive activation of the MAP-kinase signaling pathway. Most mutations are in *KRAS*, with about 80% being in codon 12 and the remainder in codons 13 or 61. Mutations in *NRAS*, codons 12, 13, and 61, have also been described to occur in colorectal carcinomas, but at a much lower frequency than *KRAS* mutations.[151] Mutations in *HRAS* have not been described.

Detailed studies using selective ultraviolet irradiation fractionation and PCR analysis show that adenoma growth and progression may include a stage in which multiple genetically distinct subclones for *KRAS* may be detected.[152] Because carcinomas are clonal for *RAS*, these data imply that the adenoma subclones harboring *KRAS* mutations are at selective advantage with respect to clones containing wild-type *KRAS* sequences. Of interest in this respect are data suggesting that *KRAS* mutations can be detected in 73% of aberrant crypt foci in colectomy specimens.[153] Given that slightly less than half of adenomas contain mutations of *KRAS*, it is likely that some of the aberrant crypt foci never progress to adenoma. The pathogenetic significance of aberrant crypt foci in the human is underscored by experiments in the rat that show that such foci can be induced with carcinogens causing colon carcinomas and that they harbor mutations in the *RAS* gene.[154]

Studies integrating histopathology and genotyping of colorectal tumors are likely to be of use in clinical decision making regarding therapy and prognosis.[155, 156] Specific mutations may, in addition, have specific prognostic significance. Colorectal tumors harboring mutations in *KRAS* other than GAT in codon 12 have been shown to be more likely to recur, either locally or as distant disease, than tumors with a *KRAS* wild-type sequence in codon 12 or those showing a GAT mutation.[157] A large international collaborative group (RASCAL) is studying the prognostic significance of specific *KRAS* mutations in colorectal cancer. In analysis of the first 2500 cases, mutation of *KRAS*, particularly codon 12 GTT, has been associated with an increased risk of tumor relapse and increased risk of death.[158] Data such as these support a role for routine genotyping of colorectal tumors; such information, for instance, might help identify the subgroup of Dukes' B patients at higher risk for recurrence.

The *TP53* gene, located on chromosome 17p, encodes a protein involved in cell cycle regulation and apoptosis. Point mutations in *TP53* are found in association with loss of the remaining wild-type allele in about half of all colorectal tumors but are infrequent in adenomas.[159] Most mutations occur within exons 5 to 8, with "hot spots" in exons 5, 7, and 8.[160] Alterations of the *TP53* gene have been found in preinvasive lesions.[161, 162] However, stabilization of the P53 protein is thought to play a crucial role in the aneuploid clonal divergence during the adenoma to carcinoma sequence[163] and perhaps to be causal in the transition from in situ to invasive carcinoma. In advanced carcinomas, the presence of *TP53* mutations appears to be related to the aggressiveness of the tumor and correlated with shortened survival.[156, 164, 165] p53 immunoreactivity in tumor cells has also been associated with poor prognosis; it has been suggested that cytoplasmic reactivity is of particular prognostic relevance,[166] a somewhat unexpected finding given the fact that p53 is a nuclear protein.

The remaining 15% of sporadic colorectal carcinomas progress along a pathway characterized by MSI and the acquisition of sporadic mutations in genes such as *TGFBR2*, *BAX*, *IGF2R*, *MSH3*, and *MSH6*. The main cause of MSI in sporadic colorectal cancer cases appears not to be mutations in the mismatch repair genes, as in HNPCC, but rather somatic *MLH1* promoter methylation,[167] Genes harboring simple repeat sequences in their coding regions are often inactivated by somatic frameshift mutations in microsatellite mutator phenotype colorectal cancers. *TGFBR2* is mutated within a polyadenine tract in a large percentage of colorectal cancers with MSI.[168, 169] About half of microsatellite mutator phenotype colorectal carcinomas have frameshift mutations in a tract of eight deoxyguanosines within the apoptosis promoting gene *BAX*.[170] The insulin-like growth factor 2 receptor gene *(IGF2R)* also contains several repetitive sequences within its coding region. Frameshift mutations in the poly(G)8 tract of *IGF2R* have also been described in colorectal cancers showing MSI.[89] Colorectal carcinomas showing MSI are generally diploid.

The different genetic alterations known to play a role in the progression of colorectal tumors will likely be used to assess the acquired risk of carcinoma. Both the total accumulation of genetic alterations as well as the order of their acquisition appear to be important in the development of colorectal carcinoma. Certain genetic alterations, in particular, mutations in *APC* and *KRAS*, are more often associated with early stages of the disease (adenoma, hyperplastic patch, dysplasia).[142, 171] The restricted range of possible mutation sites has greatly facilitated the development of efficient *RAS* mutation screening assays and early clinical applications. A growing number of studies indicate that it will be possible to exploit mutations in the *KRAS* gene to assess acquired risk. The ability to detect mutated *RAS* alleles in the stools of patients bearing adenomas and carcinomas[172–175] indicates that it might be possible to screen asymptomatic populations using this approach. Technical advances for detection of mutated alleles will make screening feasible, although the long-term efficacy and benefit remain to be demonstrated. It appears more realistic to think that assessment of acquired risk will be of interest in populations known to be at higher risk because of pre-existing conditions or lesions. Recent studies confirm earlier observations indicating that dysplastic lesions in ulcerative colitis harbor some of the genetic alterations found in colorectal cancer. LOH on chromosome 8p and mutations in *KRAS* and *TP53* have been reported in dysplastic lesions associated with carcinomas in ulcerative colitis.[162, 176] The dysplasia is not always of the same genotype as the carcinoma, and diverse genotypes can coexist in the same patient. It is likely that assessment of mutations or deletions in somatic cells from tissue or fluid specimens will become a powerful adjunct to conventional morphology. Screening of colonic lavage fluids has demonstrated a higher incidence of detectable mutations in *KRAS* and *TP53* in patients with long-standing ulcerative colitis than in control patients.[177] We also anticipate that the ability to quantitate the percentage of cells harboring mutations or deletions by fluorescent in situ hybridization, or to determine the percentage of mutated alleles present in a population of molecules cloned by PCR, will greatly enhance the assessment of acquired risk. Data are now beginning to emerge that support measurement of the frequency of mutated alleles in non-neoplastic ulcerative colitis tissues as an indicator of acquired cancer risk.[178]

Mutations in both *KRAS* and *TP53* genes can serve as specific tumor markers. Once the genotype of the primary tumor is known, micrometastases can be identified by detecting the mutation using protocols based on PCR, which can effectively detect tumor at the level of one tumor cell in a million. This approach has allowed detection of colon carcinoma cells in lymph nodes considered to be uninvolved and of tumor-associated genetic alterations in the circulation. A recent study of stage II colorectal carcinoma patients has found significantly decreased survival in patients with RT-PCR–detected lymph node micrometastases.[179] Similar approaches also allow detection of circulating tumor cells or non–cell-associated DNA in the peripheral blood.[180–183] There is a need for careful longitudinal studies to establish the significance and prognostic value of molecularly positive histologically negative lymph nodes and to determine the significance of circulating cells bearing the genotypic characteristics of a known primary tumor. Both *TP53* and *KRAS* mutations also serve well to establish synchronous tumors as originating from different clones and thus as independent lesions.[184, 185]

A number of other sporadic genetic alterations have been described in colorectal carcinoma, including alterations in cyclins, cyclin-dependent kinases and their inhibitors,[186, 187] growth factors and growth factor receptors,[188, 189] cell adhesion molecules,[190, 191] and extracellular matrix enzymes.[192, 193] Careful prospective trials are required to validate those markers and assays with the greatest promise for early successful clinical application.

PANCREAS

A great deal of progress has been made in identifying the molecular events important in the pathogenesis of pancreatobiliary neoplasms. Still, pancreatic carcinoma remains an aggressive disease with an extremely poor prognosis. Clinical applications that make use of new molecular targets to achieve earlier diagnosis hold hope for improved survival in this devastating disease.

Cytogenetic studies of pancreatic adenocarcinoma reveal frequent structural abnormalities of chromosome 1 (including both deletions of 1p and gains of 1q), chromosome 8 (8p losses and 8q gains), and 17 (mostly 17q gains).[4, 194] Gains of whole chromosome 20 and whole chromosome 7 are relatively common, as are losses of chromosomes 18, 13, 12, 17, and 6.[194] Abnormal karyotypes are found most frequently in poorly differentiated carcinomas. These findings differ somewhat from those of CGH studies, which most frequently show gains of 20q[195, 196] and losses of 8q, 9p, 15q, and 21q.[196] It seems likely that these differences are related to biases introduced in standard karyotype analysis by the requirement that tumor cells be successfully cultured. LOH studies most frequently demonstrate deletion of genetic information on 1p, 5q, 11q, 17p, and 18q.[4, 156, 197]

Point mutations in the *KRAS* gene are present in 80% to 90% of pancreatic adenocarcinomas.[198, 199, 200, 201] The majority of mutations are located in codon 12, with the remainder in codons 13 or 61. Mutations in *RAS* interfere with guanosine triphosphate hydrolysis and result in constitutive growth factor signaling via the MAP/kinase pathway. There is considerable evidence to support the idea that *KRAS* mutation is an early event in the pathogenesis of pancreatic carcinoma,[197, 202] occurring, at least in some cases, before evidence of morphologic atypicality.[203, 204] Although this fact calls for caution in the interpretation of diagnostic assays based on the presence of mutations in *KRAS*, it also makes *KRAS* an ideal molecular target for the earlier diagnosis of pancreatic carcinoma.

Almost all pancreatic carcinomas show inactivation of the cell cycle inhibitor CDKN2A. *CDKN2A* codes for a cyclin/cyclin dependent kinase inhibitor important in the control of cell cycle progression; inactivation results in loss of an important cell cycle checkpoint.[205] Three different mechanisms of inactivation of *CDKN2A* are seen in pancreatic carcinomas: homozygous deletion in about 40%, mutation of one allele and loss of the remaining wild-type allele in another 40%, and hypermethylation of the promoter in about 15%.[206, 207, 208] Microdissection studies of noninvasive pancreatic intraductal precursor lesions show that alterations of *CDKN2A* appear to affect a subset of intraductal lesions that have already sustained mutation in the *KRAS* gene.[204] Thus, perhaps alterations in *CDKN2A* may identify a group of lesions at even higher risk for the development of invasive malignancy. An immunohistochemical study of CDKN2A protein expression in pancreatic carcinoma has demonstrated shorter survival and a higher rate of metastasis associated with loss of CDKN2A expression.[209]

TP53 is inactivated in 50% to 70% of pancreatic carcinomas, primarily by point mutation of one allele coupled with loss of the remaining wild-type allele.[210–212] The p53 protein binds to DNA in a sequence-specific manner.[213] Tumor-associated mutations in *TP53* are found predominantly in this evolutionarily conserved DNA-binding domain.[210, 212, 214, 215] Most are missense mutations, with transitions predominating over transversions; almost one third affect the hot-spot codons 248, 273, and 282.[210, 212] Whereas *KRAS* mutations can be found in the early stages of formation of ductal carcinomas, mutations of the *TP53* gene are generally found in more advanced lesions.[211]

The *MADH4* has been described to be altered in about half of pancreatic carcinomas by homozygous deletion or by mutation of one allele and deletion of the other.[216–218] *MADH4* is located on chromosome 18q in the region of *DCC*, and appears to play a role in TGF-β signaling.[219]

There is growing evidence for alternate molecular pathways functioning in the pathogenesis of pancreatic carcinoma. Differences in *MADH4* expression between the intraductal papillary mucinous neoplasm (IPMN) variant of pancreatic carcinoma and typical ductal adenocarcinomas support the notion that IPMNs are fundamentally different tumors.[220] MSI has been described to occur in a small number of pancreatic carcinomas, in association with wild-type *KRAS* gene status and a medullary phenotype.[221] If these patients demonstrate better long-term survival than typical glandular pancreatic adenocarcinomas, preoperative molecular evaluation of biopsy or fine-needle aspiration samples might influence choice of therapy.

The development of refined imaging and sampling techniques has greatly improved access to this diagnostically difficult region and facilitated the acquisition of small tissue samples amenable to molecular analysis. The high incidence of *KRAS* mutation in pancreatic carcinomas, coupled with the relative ease of molecular analysis of this gene, has fostered the clinical use of mutations as markers for the presence of small numbers of tumor cells in diagnostic assays. Studies of pancreatic fine-needle aspirates,[222, 223, 224] pancreatic juice,[225, 226] duodenal fluid,[227] and stool[228] have demonstrated the potential use of molecular markers such as *KRAS* mutations in the diagnosis of pancreatobiliary cancers. In general, these studies show that genotyping is specific and suggest that it is a good adjunct to cytologic examination, especially when the morphology is equivocal.[229, 230] Circulating cells and soluble mutated *KRAS* alleles can also be detected in patients with pancreatic carcinoma.[225, 231, 232] Although the significance of this finding remains to be determined, preliminary results suggest that serial examination may prove useful in clinical monitoring for disease recurrence and progression.[233]

LIVER

Ninety-five percent of malignant tumors of the liver are epithelial, and the vast majority of these are hepatocellular carcinomas (HCCs). Relatively uncommon in the United States and western Europe, HCC is one of the most common malignant tumors worldwide, with an estimated 500,000 to 1 million new cases annually. Conditions associated with chronic hepatic injury predispose to the development of HCC. Iterative hepatocellular injury leads to sustained hyperplasia, which is thought to increase the susceptibility of hepatocytes to genetic damage.

Classic cytogenetic investigations suggest that loss of chromosomes 16, 1p, and 6q may be frequent events in the pathogenesis of hepatocellular carcinoma.[4] CGH studies have demonstrated frequent gains of 1q and 8q and losses of 4q and 13q.[234–237] Amplification of 11q12-13 is also common.[234, 236, 237] These findings are paralleled by those derived from LOH studies. LOH at a variety of loci is encountered frequently and correlates with the degree of histologic differentiation. In patients exposed to hepatitis B virus or hepatitis C virus, accumulation of genetic alterations in multiple tumor suppressor gene loci, especially 17p, 4q, and 8p, is involved in the progression of liver cancer. It also appears that LOH on 17p and 4q precede the other genetic alterations, suggesting a preferred order of accumulation of lesions.[238] Allelic loss at 8p is seen in no T1 stage tumors, 45% of stage T2 tumors, and 65% of stage T3/4 carcinomas. In addition, LOH on 8p also correlates with the degree of tumor differentiation.[239] A deletion on chromosome 5q35-qter has been found in patients with HCC not linked to cirrhosis. Because *APC* and *MCC*, two known tumor suppressor genes involved in the pathogenesis of colorectal carcinoma, reside in the same region, their status has been investigated and found to be unaltered.[240] Studies in cell lines derived from HCC suggest that abnormalities of the *RB1* gene are very rare in HCC.[241]

Mutations of the *TP53* gene in HCC were first described in tumors occurring in patients from high-risk areas such as China and South Africa. One piece of evidence indicating that carcinogens leave "footprints" was the consistent association of a G→T transversion at the third base in codon 249 of the gene with exposure to aflatoxins, whereas cases associated with hepatitis B virus infection exhibited a wider spectrum of mutations.[242] Interestingly, studies of site-specific adduct formation show that codon 249 is not the major site involved and suggest that aflatoxin may require additional mechanisms such as infection with hepatitis B for selection of the codon 249 mutants.[243] Detection of the *TP53* codon 249 serine mutation in plasma DNA has been strongly associated with hepatocellular carcinoma in patients in Gambia and shows promise for development as an early detection strategy in endemic regions.[244]

The precise role of hepatitis B virus in hepatic carcinogenesis is not yet completely elucidated. It can certainly be the cause of chronic hepatocyte injury, but it has also been suggested that the product of the hepatitis B virus X gene is important in the pathogenesis of hepatocellular carcinoma. The protein product encoded by the X open reading frame is a transcriptional activator that inhibits p53 function as an early event in carcinogenesis. The hepatitis B virus X protein exerts a variety of other effects on the cell, including the inhibition of repair of damaged hepatocyte DNA.[245]

TP53 mutations are seen in 30% to 50% of non–aflatoxin-associated hepatocellular carcinomas. *TP53* mutations appear to occur as a later event in the pathogenesis of hepatitis B and C virus–associated hepatocellular carcinomas and demonstrate a different spectrum of mutation sites from those seen in other tumors.[246, 247] Mutations in *TP53* have also been detected in angiosarcoma of the liver occurring in patients with occupational exposure to vinyl chloride.[248] A study of 184 hepatocellular carcinoma cases suggests that p53 protein and mRNA expression patterns correlate well with tumor size and behavior of the tumor,[249] indicating a possible prognostic role for p53 status in patients with HCC.

Another tumor suppressor gene with potential prognostic significance is E-cadherin, also commonly altered in hepatocellular carcinomas.[250, 251] Inactivation of the cell cycle inhibitor CDKN2A by homozygous deletion or promoter hypermethylation has been described in a substantial number (12 of 20 cases) of human hepatocellular carcinomas.[252] Somatic point mutations or deletions in the β-catenin gene have been found in eight of 31 (26%) human liver tumors and two hepatocellular carcinoma cell lines,[253] implicating disregulation of Wnt-wingless signaling in the pathogenesis of at least a subset of hepatocellular carcinomas.

CONCLUSION

Advances in cell biology and molecular genetics promise not only a much deeper understanding of the pathogenesis of tumors but also major advances in our capabilities to diagnose, predict the course of, and discover novel treatments for tumors. As discoveries are made and applications to the clinic are attempted, there is bound to be excitement, sometimes followed by disappointment. At the time of this writing, most of the laboratory procedures and tests described are not yet sufficiently well validated for routine clinical use. In addition, the laboratory assays are, in many instances, labor intensive and not yet automated. However, the clarity of results and precision of the techniques already available promise to answer, in an unequivocal fashion, many of the questions that today are intractable or resolved in a nonprecise and somewhat arbitrary way. Because many of these questions are raised by the pathologist, it behooves us to find the appropriate answers by applying sophisticated techniques to the analysis of tissues in a critical and cost-effective manner.

Acknowledgment

We are indebted to Rebekah Sue Harris for her help in the preparation of this manuscript.

REFERENCES

1. Fearon ER, Vogelstein B: A genetic model for colorectal tumorigenesis. Cell 1990;61:759–767.
2. Fearon ER, Hamilton SR, Vogelstein B: Clonal analysis of human colorectal tumors. Science 1987;238:193–197.
3. Guanrei Y, He H, Sungliang Q, Yuming C: Endoscopic diagnosis of 115 cases of early esophageal carcinoma. Endoscopy 1982;14:157–161.
4. Heim S, Mitelman F: Tumors of the Digestive Tract. *In* Cancer Cytogenetics. New York, Wiley-Liss, 1995, pp 325–349.
5. Hu Y, Lam KY, Wan TS, et al: Establishment and characterization of HKESC-1, a new cancer cell line from human esophageal squamous cell carcinoma. Cancer Genet Cytogenet 2000;118:112–120.
6. Moskaluk CA, Hu J, Perlman EJ: Comparative genomic hybridization of esophageal and gastroesophageal adenocarcinomas shows consensus areas of DNA gain and loss. Genes Chromosomes Cancer 1998;22:305–311.
7. Hollstein MC, Metcalf RA, Welsh JA, et al: Frequent mutation of the *p53* gene in human esophageal cancer. Proc Natl Acad Sci U S A 1990;87:9958–9961.
8. Flejou JF, Muzeau F, Potet F, et al: Overexpression of the *p53* tumor suppressor gene product in esophageal and gastric carcinomas. Pathol Res Pract 1994;190:1141–1148.
9. Liang YY, Esteve A, Martel-Planche G, et al: *p53* mutations in esophageal tumors from high-incidence areas of China. Int J Cancer 1995;61:611–614.
10. Coggi G, Bosari S, Roncalli M, et al: p53 protein accumulation and *p53* gene mutation in esophageal carcinoma: A molecular and immunohistochemical study with clinicopathologic correlations. Cancer 1997;79:425–432.
11. Olshan AF, Weissler MC, Pei H, Conway K: *p53* mutations in head and neck cancer: New data and evaluation of mutational spectra. Cancer Epidemiol Biomarkers Prev 1997;6:499–504.
12. Shi ST, Yang GY, Wang LD, et al: Role of *p53* gene mutations in human esophageal carcinogenesis: Results from immunohistochemical and mutation analyses of carcinomas and nearby non-cancerous lesions. Carcinogenesis 1999;20:591–597.
13. Wang LD, Zhou Q, Hong JY, et al: p53 protein accumulation and gene mutations in multifocal esophageal precancerous lesions from symptom free subjects in a high incidence area for esophageal carcinoma in Henan, China. Cancer 1996;77:1244–1249.
14. Mandard AM, Hainaut P, Hollstein M: Genetic steps in the development of squamous cell carcinoma of the esophagus. Mutat Res 2000;462:335–342.
15. Audrezet M, Robaszkiewicz M, Mercier B, et al: *TP53* gene mutation profile in esophageal squamous cell carcinomas. Cancer Res 1993;53:5745–5749.
16. Robert V, Michel P, Flaman JM, et al: High frequency in esophageal cancers of p53 alterations inactivating the regulation of genes involved in cell cycle and apoptosis. Carcinogenesis 2000;21:563–565.
17. Shiozaki H, Doki Y, Kawanishi K, et al: Clinical application of malignancy potential grading as a prognostic factor of human esophageal cancers. Surgery 2000;127:552–561.
18. Maesawa C, Tamura G, Suzuki Y, et al: Aberrations of tumor-suppressor genes (*p53*, *apc*, *mcc* and *Rb*) in esophageal squamous-cell carcinoma. Int J Cancer 1994;57:21–25.
19. von Brevern M, Hollstein MC, Risk JM, et al: Loss of heterozygosity in sporadic oesophageal tumors in the tylosis oesophageal cancer (TOC) gene region of chromosome 17q. Oncogene 1998;17:2101–2105.
20. Dolan K, Garde J, Gosney J, et al: Allelotype analysis of oesophageal adenocarcinoma: Loss of heterozygosity occurs at multiple sites. Br J Cancer 1998;78:950–957.
21. Mori M, Mimori K, Shiraishi T, et al: Altered expression of Fhit in carcinoma and precarcinomatous lesions of the esophagus. Cancer Res 2000;60:1177–1182.
22. Menin C, Santacatterina M, Zambon A, et al: Anomalous transcripts and allelic deletions of the *FHIT* gene in human esophageal cancer. Cancer Genet Cytogenet 2000;119:56–61.
23. Uchino S, Saito T, Inomata M, et al: Prognostic significance of the *p53* mutation in esophageal cancer. Jpn J Clin Oncol 1996;26:287–292.
24. Ireland AP, Shibata DK, Chandrasoma P, et al: Clinical significance of *p53* mutations in adenocarcinoma of the esophagus and cardia. Ann Surg 2000;231:179–187.
25. Sarbia M, Gabbert HE: Modern pathology: Prognostic parameters in squamous cell carcinoma of the esophagus. Recent Results Cancer Res 2000;155:15–27.
26. Roncalli M, Bosari S, Marchetti A, et al: Cell cycle–related gene abnormalities and product expression in esophageal carcinoma. Lab Invest 1998;78:1049–1057.
27. zur Hausen A, Sarbia M, Heep H, et al: Retinoblastoma-protein (pRb) expression and prognosis in squamous-cell carcinomas of the esophagus. Int J Cancer 1999;84:618–622.

28. Shamma A, Doki Y, Shiozaki H, et al: Cyclin D1 overexpression in esophageal dysplasia: A possible biomarker for carcinogenesis of esophageal squamous cell carcinoma. Int J Oncol 2000;16:261–266.
29. Ribeiro U, Safatle-Ribeiro AV, Posner MC, et al: Comparative *p53* mutational analysis of multiple primary cancers of the upper aerodigestive tract. Surgery 1996; 120:45–53.
30. Sarbia M, Loberg C, Wolter M, et al: Expression of Bcl-2 and amplification of c-*myc* are frequent in basaloid squamous cell carcinomas of the esophagus. Am J Pathol 1999;155:1027–1032.
31. Rao P, Mathew S, Lauwers G, et al: Interphase cytogenetics of gastric and esophageal adenocarcinomas. Diagn Mol Pathol 1993;2:264–268.
32. Hunter S, Gramlich T, Abbott K, Varma V: Y chromosome loss in esophageal carcinoma: An in situ hybridization study. Genes Chromosomes Cancer 1993;8:172–177.
33. Walch AK, Zitzelsberger HF, Bruch J, et al: Chromosomal imbalances in Barrett's adenocarcinoma and the metaplasia-dysplasia-carcinoma sequence. Am J Pathol 2000;156:555–566.
34. Gleeson CM, Sloan JM, McGuigan JA, et al: Base transitions at CpG dinucleotides in the *p53* gene are common in esophageal adenocarcinoma. Cancer Res 1995; 55:3406–3411.
35. Gleeson CM, Sloan JM, McManus DT, et al: Comparison of p53 and DNA content abnormalities in adenocarcinoma of the oesophagus and gastric cardia. Br J Cancer 1998;77:277–286.
36. Prevo LJ, Sanchez CA, Galipeau PC, Reid BJ: *p53*-mutant clones and field effects in Barrett's esophagus. Cancer Res 1999;59:4784–4787.
37. Palanca-Wessels MC, Barrett MT, Galipeau PC, et al: Genetic analysis of long-term Barrett's esophagus epithelial cultures exhibiting cytogenetic and ploidy abnormalities. Gastroenterology 1998;114:295–304.
38. Galipeau PC, Cowan DS, Sanchez CA, et al: 17p (*p53*) allelic losses, 4N (G2/tetraploid) populations, and progression to aneuploidy in Barrett's esophagus. Proc Natl Acad Sci U S A 1996;93:7081–7084.
39. Reid BJ, Blount PL, Rubin CE, et al: Flow-cytometric and histological progression to malignancy in Barrett's esophagus: Prospective endoscopic surveillance of a cohort [see comments]. Gastroenterology 1992;102: 1212–1219.
40. Montesano R, Hollstein M, Hainaut P: Molecular etiopathogenesis of esophageal cancers. Ann Ist Super Sanita 1996;32:73–84.
41. Dunn J, Garde J, Dolan K, et al: Multiple target sites of allelic imbalance on chromosome 17 in Barrett's oesophageal cancer. Oncogene 1999;18:987–993.
42. Gonzalez MV, Artimez ML, Rodrigo L, et al: Mutation analysis of the *p53*, *APC*, and *p16* genes in the Barrett's oesophagus, dysplasia, and adenocarcinoma. J Clin Pathol 1997;50:212–217.
43. Wanebo HJ, Kennedy BJ, Chmiel J, et al: Cancer of the stomach: A patient care study by the American College of Surgeons. Ann Surg 1993;218:583–592.
44. Longmire W. A current view of gastric cancer in the US. Ann Surg 1993;218:579–582.
45. Zheng T, Mayne S, Holford T, et al: The time trend and age-period-cohort effects on incidence of adenocarcinoma of the stomach in Connecticut from 1955–1989. J Cancer 1993;72:330–340.
46. Min KW, Holmquist S, Peiper SC, O'Leary TJ: Poorly differentiated adenocarcinoma with lymphoid stroma (lymphoepithelioma-like carcinomas) of the stomach: Report of three cases with Epstein-Barr virus genome demonstrated by the polymerase chain reaction. Am J Clin Pathol 1991;96:219–227.
47. Gulley ML, Pulitzer DR, Eagan PA, Schneider BG: Epstein-Barr virus infection is an early event in gastric carcinogenesis and is independent of bcl-2 expression and p53 accumulation. Hum Pathol 1996;27:20–27.
48. zur Hausen A, Brink AA, Craanen ME, et al: Unique transcription pattern of Epstein-Barr virus (EBV) in EBV-carrying gastric adenocarcinomas: Expression of the transforming *BARF1* gene. Cancer Res 2000;60: 2745–2748.
49. Hahm KB, Lee KJ, Kim JH, et al: *Helicobacter pylori* infection, oxidative DNA damage, gastric carcinogenesis, and reversibility by rebamipide. Dig Dis Sci 1998; 43:72S–77S.
50. Karttunen TJ, Genta RM, Yoffe B, et al: Detection of *Helicobacter pylori* in paraffin-embedded gastric biopsy specimens by in situ hybridization. Am J Clin Pathol 1996;106:305–311.
51. Palli D, Caporaso NE, Shiao YH, et al: Diet, *Helicobacter pylori*, and *p53* mutations in gastric cancer: A molecular epidemiology study in Italy. Cancer Epidemiol Biomarkers Prev 1997;6:1065–1069.
52. Wu MS, Shun CT, Wang HP, et al: Genetic alterations in gastric cancer: Relation to histological subtypes, tumor stage, and *Helicobacter pylori* infection. Gastroenterology 1997;112:1457–1465.
53. Correa P: *Helicobacter pylori* and gastric carcinogenesis. Am J Surg Pathol 1995;19:S37–S43.
54. Sakakura C, Mori T, Sakabe T, et al: Gains, losses, and amplifications of genomic materials in primary gastric cancers analyzed by comparative genomic hybridization. Genes Chromosomes Cancer 1999;24:299–305.
55. Nessling M, Solinas-Toldo S, Wilgenbus KK, et al: Mapping of chromosomal imbalances in gastric adenocarcinoma revealed amplified proto-oncogenes MYCN, MET, WNT2, and ERBB2. Genes Chromosomes Cancer 1998;23:307–316.
56. Sano T, Tsujino T, Yoshida K, et al: Frequent loss of heterozygosity on chromosomes 1q, 5q, and 17p in human gastric carcinomas. Cancer Res 1991;51: 2926–2931.
57. Baffa R, Negrini M, Mandes B, et al: Loss of heterozygosity for chromosome 11 in adenocarcinoma of the stomach. Cancer Res 1996;56:268–272.
58. Nishizuka S, Tamura G, Terashima M, Satodate R: Loss of heterozygosity during the development and progression of differentiated adenocarcinoma of the stomach. J Pathol 1998;185:38–43.
59. Tamura G, Ogasawara S, Nishizuka S, et al: Two distinct regions of deletion on the long arm of chromosome 5 in differentiated adenocarcinomas of the stomach. Cancer Res 1996;56:612–615.
60. Vollmers H, Stulle K, Dammrich J, et al: Characterization of four new gastric cancer cell lines. Virchows Arch B Cell Pathol Incl Mol Pathol 1993;63:335–343.

61. Uchino S, Tsuda H, Maruyama K, et al: Overexpression of c-*erbB-2* protein in gastric cancer: Its correlation with long-term survival of patients. Cancer 1993;72: 3179–3184.
62. Nakajima M, Sawada H, Yamada Y, et al: The prognostic significance of amplification and overexpression of c-*met* and c-*erb* B-2 in human gastric carcinomas [see comments]. Cancer 1999;85:1894–1902.
63. Park WS, Oh RR, Park JY, et al: Frequent somatic mutations of the beta-catenin gene in intestinal-type gastric cancer. Cancer Res 1999;59:4257–4260.
64. Tolbert D, Fenoglio-Preiser C, Noffsinger A, et al: The relation of *p53* gene mutations to gastric cancer subsite and phenotype. Cancer Causes Control 1999;10: 227–231.
65. Ishikawa T, Kobayashi M, Mai M, et al: Amplification of the c-*erbB-2* (HER-*2/neu*) gene in gastric cancer cells: Detection by fluorescence in situ hybridization. Am J Pathol 1997;151:761–768.
66. Mizutani T, Onda M, Tokunaga A, et al: Relationship of C-*erbB-2* protein expression and gene amplification to invasion and metastasis in human gastric cancer. Cancer 1993;72:2083–2088.
67. Yu J, Miehlke S, Ebert MP, et al: Frequency of *TPR-MET* rearrangement in patients with gastric carcinoma and in first-degree relatives. Cancer 2000;88:1801–1806.
68. Koshiba M, Ogawa O, Habuchi T, et al: Infrequent *ras* mutation in human stomach cancers. Jpn J Cancer Res 1993;84:163–167.
69. Hara T, Ooi A, Kobayashi M, et al: Amplification of c-*myc*, K-*sam*, and c-*met* in gastric cancers: Detection by fluorescence in situ hybridization. Lab Invest 1998;78: 1143–1153.
70. Amadori D, Maltoni M, Volpi A, et al: Gene amplification and proliferative kinetics in relation to prognosis of patients with gastric carcinoma. Cancer 1997;79: 226–232.
71. Tatsuta M, Iishi H, Baba M, et al: Expression of c-*myc* mRNA as an aid in histologic differentiation of adenoma from well differentiated adenocarcinoma in the stomach. Cancer 1994;73:1795–1799.
72. Hongyo T, Buzard GS, Palli D, et al: Mutations of the K-*ras* and *p53* genes in gastric adenocarcinomas from a high-incidence region around Florence, Italy. Cancer Res 1995;55:2665–2672.
73. Tamura G, Kihana T, Nomura K, et al: Detection of frequent *p53* gene mutations in primary gastric cancer by cell sorting and polymerase chain reaction single-strand conformation polymorphism analysis. Cancer Res 1991;51:3056–3058.
74. Renault B, van den Broek M, Fodde R, et al: Base transitions are the most frequent genetic changes at *P53* in gastric cancer. Cancer Res 1993;53:2614–2617.
75. Tohdo H, Yokozaki H, Haruma K, et al: *p53* gene mutations in gastric adenomas. Virchows Arch B Cell Pathol Incl Mol Pathol 1993;63:191–195.
76. Sakurai S, Sano T, Nakajima T: Clinicopathological and molecular biological studies of gastric adenomas with special reference to p53 abnormality. Pathol Int 1995; 45:51–57.
77. Lu CD, Altieri DC, Tanigawa N: Expression of a novel antiapoptosis gene, survivin, correlated with tumor cell apoptosis and p53 accumulation in gastric carcinomas. Cancer Res 1998;58:1808–1812.
78. Gemma A, Hagiwara K, Ke Y, et al: *FHIT* mutations in human primary gastric cancer. Cancer Res 1997;57: 1435–1437.
79. Baffa R, Veronese ML, Santoro R, et al: Loss of FHIT expression in gastric carcinoma. Cancer Res 1998;58: 4708–4714.
80. Capuzzi D, Santoro E, Hauck WW, et al: Fhit expression in gastric adenocarcinoma: Correlation with disease stage and survival. Cancer 2000;88:24–34.
81. Horii A, Nakatsuru S, Miyoshi Y, et al: The APC gene, responsible for familial adenomatous polyposis, is mutated in human gastric cancer. Cancer Res 1992;52: 3231–3233.
82. Tamura G, Maesawa C, Suzuki Y, et al: Mutations of the *APC* gene occur during early stages of gastric adenoma development. Cancer Res 1994;54:1149–1151.
83. Sugai T, Habano W, Nakamura S, et al: Correlation of histologic morphology and tumor stage with molecular genetic analysis using microdissection in gastric carcinomas. Diagn Mol Pathol 1998;7:235–240.
84. Caca K, Kolligs FT, Ji X, et al: Beta- and gamma-catenin mutations, but not E-cadherin inactivation, underlie T-cell factor/lymphoid enhancer factor transcriptional deregulation in gastric and pancreatic cancer. Cell Growth Differ 1999;10:369–376.
85. dos Santos NR, Seruca R, Constancia M, et al: Microsatellite instability at multiple loci in gastric carcinoma: Clinicopathologic implications and prognosis. Gastroenterology 1996;110:38–44.
86. Wu MS, Lee CW, Shun CT, et al: Clinicopathological significance of altered loci of replication error and microsatellite instability–associated mutations in gastric cancer. Cancer Res 1998;58:1494–1497.
87. Wirtz HC, Muller W, Noguchi T, et al: Prognostic value and clinicopathological profile of microsatellite instability in gastric cancer. Clin Cancer Res 1998;4: 1749–1754.
88. Fleisher AS, Esteller M, Wang S, et al: Hypermethylation of the *hMLH1* gene promoter in human gastric cancers with microsatellite instability. Cancer Res 1999;59: 1090–1095.
89. Ouyang H, Shiwaku HO, Hagiwara H, et al: The insulin-like growth factor II receptor gene is mutated in genetically unstable cancers of the endometrium, stomach, and colorectum. Cancer Res 1997;57:1851–1854.
90. Schwartz S Jr, Yamamoto H, Navarro M, et al: Frameshift mutations at mononucleotide repeats in caspase-5 and other target genes in endometrial and gastrointestinal cancer of the microsatellite mutator phenotype. Cancer Res 1999;59:2995–3002.
91. Yamamoto H, Itoh F, Fukushima H, et al: Frequent *Bax* frameshift mutations in gastric cancer with high but not low microsatellite instability. J Exp Clin Cancer Res 1999;18:103–106.
92. Oliveira C, Seruca R, Seixas M, Sobrinho-Simoes M: The clinicopathological features of gastric carcinomas with microsatellite instability may be mediated by mutations of different "target genes": a study of the *TGFbeta RII*, *IGFII R*, and *BAX* genes. Am J Pathol 1998;153: 1211–1219.

93. Iacopetta BJ, Soong R, House AK, Hamelin R: Gastric carcinomas with microsatellite instability: Clinical features and mutations to the TGF-beta type II receptor, IGFII receptor, and *BAX* genes. J Pathol 1999; 187:428–432.
94. Toyota M, Ahuja N, Suzuki H, et al: Aberrant methylation in gastric cancer associated with the CpG island methylator phenotype. Cancer Res 1999;59:5438–5442.
95. Lee YY, Kang SH, Seo JY, et al: Alterations of *p16INK4A* and *p15INK4B* genes in gastric carcinomas. Cancer 1997;80:1889–1896.
96. Tamura G, Sakata K, Nishizuka S, et al: Inactivation of the E-cadherin gene in primary gastric carcinomas and gastric carcinoma cell lines. Jpn J Cancer Res 1996;87: 1153–1159.
97. Berx G, Becker KF, Hofler H, van Roy F: Mutations of the human E-cadherin (*CDH1*) gene. Hum Mutat 1998;12:226–237.
98. Berx G, Nollet F, van Roy F: Dysregulation of the E-cadherin/catenin complex by irreversible mutations in human carcinomas. Cell Adhes Commun 1998;6: 171–184.
99. Tamura G, Yin J, Wang S, et al: E-Cadherin gene promoter hypermethylation in primary human gastric carcinomas. J Natl Cancer Inst 2000;92:569–573.
100. Moll R, Zimbelmann R, Goldschmidt M, et al: The human gene encoding cytokeratin 20 and its expression during fetal development and in gastrointestinal carcinomas. Differentiation 1993;53:75–93.
101. Chausovsky G, Luchansky M, Figer A, et al: Expression of cytokeratin 20 in the blood of patients with disseminated carcinoma of the pancreas, colon, stomach, and lung. Cancer 1999;86:2398–2405.
102. Yoshikawa T, Saitoh M, Tsuburaya A, et al: Tissue inhibitor of matrix metalloproteinase-1 in the plasma of patients with gastric carcinoma: A possible marker for serosal invasion and metastasis. Cancer 1999;86:1929–1935.
103. Oda K, Tamaru J, Takenouchi T, et al: Association of Epstein-Barr virus with gastric carcinoma with lymphoid stroma. Am J Pathol 1993;143:1063–1071.
104. Ono H, Kondo H, Saito D, et al: Rapid diagnosis of gastric malignant lymphoma from biopsy specimens: Detection of immunoglobulin heavy chain rearrangement by polymerase chain reaction. Jpn J Cancer Res 1993;84:813–817.
105. Sanchez L, Algara P, Villuendas R, et al: B-cell clonal detection in gastric low-grade lymphomas and regional lymph nodes: An immunohistologic and molecular study. Am J Gastroenterol 1993;88:413–419.
106. Fend F, Weyrer K, Drach J, et al: Immunoglobulin gene rearrangement in plasma cell dyscrasias: Detection of small clonal cell populations in peripheral blood and bone marrow. Leuk Lymphoma 1993;10:223–229.
107. Hirota S, Isozaki K, Moriyama Y, et al: Gain-of-function mutations of c-*kit* in human gastrointestinal stromal tumors. Science 1998;279:577–580.
108. Ernst SI, Hubbs AE, Przygodzki RM, et al: *KIT* mutation portends poor prognosis in gastrointestinal stromal/smooth muscle tumors. Lab Invest 1998;78:1633–1636.
109. Lasota J, Jasinski M, Sarlomo-Rikala M, Miettinen M: Mutations in exon 11 of c-*Kit* occur preferentially in malignant versus benign gastrointestinal stromal tumors and do not occur in leiomyomas or leiomyosarcomas. Am J Pathol 1999;154:53–60.
110. O'Leary T, Ernst S, Przygodzki R, et al: Loss of heterozygosity at 1p36 predicts poor prognosis in gastrointestinal stromal/smooth muscle tumors. Lab Invest 1999; 79:1461–1467.
111. Cunningham RE, Federspiel BH, McCarthy WF, et al: Predicting prognosis of gastrointestinal smooth muscle tumors: Role of clinical and histologic evaluation, flow cytometry, and image cytometry. Am J Surg Pathol 1993;17:588–594.
112. Bardi G, Pandis N, Mitelman F, et al: Karyotypic characteristics of colorectal tumors. *In* Wolman SR, Sell S (eds): Human Cytogenetic Cancer Markers. Totawa, NJ, Humana, 1997, pp 151–168.
113. Ried T, Knutzen R, Steinbeck R, et al: Comparative genomic hybridization reveals a specific pattern of chromosomal gains and losses during the genesis of colorectal tumors. Genes Chromosomes Cancer 1996;15:234–245.
114. Groden J, Thliveris A, Samowitz W, et al: Identification and characterization of the familial adenomatous polyposis coli gene. Cell 1991;66:589–600.
115. Joslyn G, Carlson M, Thliveris A, et al: Identification of deletion mutations and three new genes at the familial polyposis locus. Cell 1991;66:601–613.
116. Kinzler KW, Nilbert MC, Su LK, et al: Identification of FAP locus genes from chromosome 5q21. Science 1991;253:661–665.
117. Nishisho I, Nakamura Y, Miyoshi Y, et al: Mutations of chromosome 5q21 genes in FAP and colorectal cancer patients. Science 1991;253:665–669.
118. Peifer M: Cancer, catenins and cuticle pattern: A complex connection. Science 1993;262:1667–1668.
119. Paul P, Letteboer T, Gelbert L, et al: Identical *APC* exon 15 mutations result in a variable phenotype in familial adenomatous polyposis. Hum Mol Genet 1993;2:925–931.
120. Ichii S, Takeda S, Horii A, et al: Detailed analysis of genetic alterations in colorectal tumors from patients with and without familial adenomatous polyposis (FAP). Oncogene 1993;8:2399–2405.
121. Su LK, Johnson KA, Smith KJ, et al: Association between wild type and mutant *APC* gene products. Cancer Res 1993;53:2728–2731.
122. Olschwang S, Tiret A, Laurent-Puig P, et al: Restriction of ocular fundus lesions to a specific subgroup of *APC* mutations in adenomatous polyposis coli patients. Cell 1993;75:959–968.
123. Spirio L, Olschwang S, Groden J, et al: Alleles of the *APC* gene: An attenuated form of familial polyposis. Cell 1993;75:951–957.
124. Dietrich WF, Lander ES, Smith JS, et al: Genetic identification of Mom-1, a major modifier locus affecting Min-induced intestinal neoplasia in the mouse. Cell 1993;75:631–639.
125. Tops CM, van der Klift HM, van der Luijt RB, et al: Non-allelic heterogeneity of familial adenomatous polyposis. Am J Med Genet 1993;47:563–567.
126. Bapat B, Odze R, Mitri A, et al: Identification of somatic *APC* gene mutations in periampullary adenomas in a patient with familial adenomatous polyposis (FAP). Hum Mol Genet 1993;2:1957–1959.

127. Miyaki M, Konishi M, Kikuchi-Yanoshita R, et al: Coexistence of somatic and germ-line mutations of *APC* gene in desmoid tumors from patients with familial adenomatous polyposis. Cancer Res 1993;53:5079–5082.
128. Bapat B, Mitri A, Greenberg CR: Improved predictive carrier testing for familial adenomatous polyposis using DNA from a single archival specimen and polymorphic markers with multiple alleles. Hum Pathol 1993;24:1376–1379.
129. Vasen HF, Mecklin JP, Khan PM, Lynch HT: The International Collaborative Group on Hereditary Non-Polyposis Colorectal Cancer (ICG-HNPCC). Dis Colon Rectum 1991;34:424–425.
130. Ionov Y, Peinado MA, Malkhosyan S, et al: Ubiquitous somatic mutations in simple repeated sequences reveal a new mechanism for colonic carcinogenesis. Nature 1993;363:558–561.
131. Thibodeau SN, Bren G, Schaid D: Microsatellite instability in cancer of the proximal colon. Science 1993;260:816–819.
132. Aaltonen LA, Peltomaki P, Leach FS, et al: Clues to the pathogenesis of familial colorectal cancer. Science 1993;260:812–816.
133. Peltomaki P, Aaltonen LA, Sistonen P, et al: Genetic mapping of a locus predisposing to human colorectal cancer. Science 1993;260:810–812.
134. Lynch HT, Watson P, Shaw TG, et al: Clinical impact of molecular genetic diagnosis, genetic counseling, and management of hereditary cancer: II. Hereditary nonpolyposis colorectal carcinoma as a model. Cancer 1999;86:2457–2463.
135. Boland CR: Hereditary nonpolyposis colorectal cancer. *In* Vogelstein B, Kinzler KW (eds): The Genetic Basis of Human Cancer. New York, McGraw-Hill, 1998, pp 333–346.
136. Aarnio M, Sankila R, Pukkala E, et al: Cancer risk in mutation carriers of DNA-mismatch-repair genes. Int J Cancer 1999;81:214–218.
137. Jarvinen HJ, Mecklin JP, Sistonen P: Screening reduces colorectal cancer rate in families with hereditary nonpolyposis colorectal cancer. Gastroenterology 1995;108:1405–1411.
138. Syngal S, Weeks JC, Schrag D, et al: Benefits of colonoscopic surveillance and prophylactic colectomy in patients with hereditary nonpolyposis colorectal cancer mutations. Ann Intern Med 1998;129:787–796.
139. O'Leary TJ: Molecular diagnosis of hereditary nonpolyposis colorectal cancer. JAMA 1999;282:281–282.
140. Aaltonen LA: Molecular epidemiology of hereditary nonpolyposis colorectal cancer in Finland. Recent Results Cancer Res 1998;154:306–311.
141. Lengauer C, Kinzler KW, Vogelstein B: Genetic instability in colorectal cancers. Nature 1997;386:623–627.
142. Powell SM, Zilz N, Beazer-Barclay Y, et al: *APC* mutations occur early during colorectal tumorigenesis. Nature 1992;359:235–237.
143. Rubinfeld B, Souza B, Albert I, et al: Association of the *APC* gene product with beta-catenin. Science 1993;262:1731–1734.
144. Morin PJ, Sparks AB, Korinek V, et al: Activation of beta-catenin-Tcf signaling in colon cancer by mutations in beta-catenin or *APC* [see comments]. Science 1997;275:1787–1790.
145. He TC, Sparks AB, Rago C, et al: Identification of c-*MYC* as a target of the APC pathway [see comments]. Science 1998;281:1509–1512.
146. Sikora K, Chan S, Evan G, et al: c-*myc* oncogene expression in colorectal cancer. Cancer 1987;59:1289–1295.
147. Barbacid M: *ras* genes. Annu Rev Biochem 1987;56:779–827.
148. Bos JL, Fearon ER, Hamilton SR, et al: Prevalence of *ras* gene mutations in human colorectal cancers. Nature 1987;327:293–297.
149. Forrester K, Almoguera C, Han K, et al: Detection of high incidence of K-*ras* oncogenes during human colon tumorigenesis. Nature 1987;327:298–303.
150. Shaw P, Tardy S, Benito E, et al: Occurrence of Ki-*ras* and *p53* mutations in primary colorectal tumors. Oncogene 1991;6:2121–2128.
151. Spandidos DA, Glarakis IS, Kotsinas A, et al: *Ras* oncogene activation in benign and malignant colorectal tumours. Tumori 1995;81:7–11.
152. Shibata D, Schaeffer J, Li ZH, et al: Genetic heterogeneity of the c-K-*ras* locus in colorectal adenomas but not in adenocarcinomas. J Natl Cancer Inst 1993;85:1058–1063.
153. Pretlow TP, Brasitus TA, Fulton NC, et al: K-*ras* mutations in putative preneoplastic lesions in human colon. J Natl Cancer Inst 1993;85:2004–2007.
154. Vivona AA, Shpitz B, Medline A, et al: K-*ras* mutations in aberrant crypt foci, adenomas and adenocarcinomas during azoxymethane-induced colon carcinogenesis. Carcinogenesis 1993;14:1777–1781.
155. Finkelstein SD, Sayegh R, Christensen S, Swalsky PA: Genotypic classification of colorectal adenocarcinoma: Biologic behavior correlates with K-*ras*-2 mutation type. Cancer 1993;71:3827–3838.
156. Finkelstein SD, Przygodzki R, Pricolo VE, et al: Prediction of biologic aggressiveness in colorectal cancer by *p53*/K-*ras*-2 topographic genotyping. Mol Diagn 1996;1:5–28.
157. Benhattar J, Losi L, Chaubert P, et al: Prognostic significance of K-*ras* mutations in colorectal carcinoma. Gastroenterology 1993;104:1044–1048.
158. Andreyev HJ, Norman AR, Cunningham D, et al: Kirsten ras mutations in patients with colorectal cancer: The multicenter "RASCAL" study. J Natl Cancer Inst 1998;90:675–684.
159. Baker SJ, Preisinger AC, Jessup JM, et al: *p53* gene mutations occur in combination with 17p allelic deletions as late events in colorectal tumorigenesis. Cancer Res 1990;50:7717–7722.
160. Hainaut P, Hernandez T, Robinson A, et al: IARC Database of *p53* gene mutations in human tumors and cell lines: Updated compilation, revised formats and new visualisation tools. Nucleic Acids Res 1998;26:205–213.
161. Yin J, Harpaz N, Tong Y, et al: *p53* point mutations in dysplastic and cancerous ulcerative colitis lesions. Gastroenterology 1993;104:1633–1639.
162. Chaubert P, Benhattar J, Saraga E, Costa J: K-*ras* mutations and *p53* alterations in neoplastic and nonneoplastic lesions associated with long-standing ulcerative colitis. Am J Pathol 1994;144:767–775.

163. Carder P, Wyllie AH, Purdie CA, et al: Stabilised p53 facilitates aneuploid clonal divergence in colorectal cancer. Oncogene 1993; 8:1397–1401.
164. Hamelin R, Laurent-Puig P, Olschwang S, et al: Association of *p53* mutations with short survival in colorectal cancer. Gastroenterology 1994;106:42–48.
165. Kahlenberg MS, Stoler DL, Rodriguez-Bigas MA, et al: *p53* tumor suppressor gene mutations predict decreased survival of patients with sporadic colorectal carcinoma. Cancer 2000;88:1814–1819.
166. Bosari S, Viale G, Bossi P, et al: Cytoplasmic accumulation of p53 protein: An independent prognostic indicator in colorectal adenocarcinomas. J Natl Cancer Inst 1994;86:681–687.
167. Kuismanen SA, Holmberg MT, Salovaara R, et al: Genetic and epigenetic modification of *MLH1* accounts for a major share of microsatellite-unstable colorectal cancers. Am J Pathol 2000; 156:1773–1779.
168. Parsons R, Myeroff LL, Liu B, et al: Microsatellite instability and mutations of the transforming growth factor beta type II receptor gene in colorectal cancer. Cancer Res 1995;55:5548–5550.
169. Samowitz WS, Slattery ML: Transforming growth factor-beta receptor type 2 mutations and microsatellite instability in sporadic colorectal adenomas and carcinomas. Am J Pathol 1997;151:33–35.
170. Rampino N, Yamamoto H, Ionov Y, et al: Somatic frameshift mutations in the *BAX* gene in colon cancers of the microsatellite mutator phenotype. Science 1997; 275:967–969.
171. Jen J, Powell SM, Papadopoulos N, et al: Molecular determinants of dysplasia in colorectal lesions. Cancer Res 1994;54:5523–5526.
172. Sidransky D, Tokino T, Hamilton SR, et al: Identification of *ras* oncogene mutations in the stool of patients with curable colorectal tumors. Science 1992;256:102–105.
173. Ratto C, Flamini G, Sofo L, et al: Detection of oncogene mutation from neoplastic colonic cells exfoliated in feces. Dis Colon Rectum 1996;39:1238–1244.
174. Villa E, Dugani A, Rebecchi AM, et al: Identification of subjects at risk for colorectal carcinoma through a test based on K-*ras* determination in the stool [see comments]. Gastroenterology 1996;110:1346–1353.
175. Machiels BM, Ruers T, Lindhout M, et al: New protocol for DNA extraction of stool. Biotechniques 2000;28: 286–290.
176. Greenwald BD, Harpaz N, Yin J, et al: Loss of heterozygosity affecting the *p53*, *Rb*, and *MCC/APC* tumor suppressor gene loci in dysplastic and cancerous ulcerative colitis. Cancer Res 1992;52:741–745.
177. Lang SM, Stratakis DF, Heinzlmann M, et al: Molecular screening of patients with long standing extensive ulcerative colitis: Detection of *p53* and Ki-*ras* mutations by single strand conformation polymorphism analysis and differential hybridisation in colonic lavage fluid. Gut 1999;44:822–825.
178. Hussain SP, Amstad P, Raja K, et al: Increased *p53* mutation load in noncancerous colon tissue from ulcerative colitis: A cancer-prone chronic inflammatory disease. Cancer Res 2000;60:3333–3337.
179. Liefers GJ, Cleton-Jansen AM, van de Velde CJ, et al: Micrometastases and survival in stage II colorectal cancer [see comments]. N Engl J Med 1998;339: 223–228.
180. Kopreski MS, Benko FA, Kwee C, et al: Detection of mutant K-*ras* DNA in plasma or serum of patients with colorectal cancer. Br J Cancer 1997;76:1293–1299.
181. Anker P, Lefort F, Vasioukhin V, et al: K-*ras* mutations are found in DNA extracted from the plasma of patients with colorectal cancer. Gastroenterology 1997; 112:1114–1120.
182. Mayall F, Jacobson G, Wilkins R, Chang B: Mutations of *p53* gene can be detected in the plasma of patients with large bowel carcinoma. J Clin Pathol 1998;51:611–613.
183. Kopreski MS, Benko FA, Borys DJ, et al: Somatic mutation screening: Identification of individuals harboring K-*ras* mutations with the use of plasma DNA. J Natl Cancer Inst 2000;92:918–923.
184. Terunuma H, Hayakashi T, Tsuneyoshi T, et al: Mutational heterogeneity among individual tumors in a case of multiple primary malignancy of the colon. Jpn J Clin Oncol 1993;23:350–355.
185. Koness RJ, King TC, Schechter S, et al: Synchronous colon carcinomas: Molecular-genetic evidence for multicentricity. Ann Surg Oncol 1996;3:136–143.
186. Arber N, Hibshoosh H, Moss SF, et al: Increased expression of cyclin D1 is an early event in multistage colorectal carcinogenesis. Gastroenterology 1996;110:669–674.
187. Loda M, Cukor B, Tam SW, et al: Increased proteasome-dependent degradation of the cyclin-dependent kinase inhibitor p27 in aggressive colorectal carcinomas [see comments]. Nat Med 1997;3:231–234.
188. Kapitanovic S, Radosevic S, Kapitanovic M, et al: The expression of p185(HER-2/neu) correlates with the stage of disease and survival in colorectal cancer. Gastroenterology 1997;112:1103–1113.
189. Tsushima H, Kawata S, Tamura S, et al: High levels of transforming growth factor beta 1 in patients with colorectal cancer: Association with disease progression. Gastroenterology 1996;110:375–382.
190. Hiscox S, Jiang WG: Expression of E-cadherin, alpha, beta and gamma-catenin in human colorectal cancer. Anticancer Res 1997;17:1349–1354.
191. Gold JS, Reynolds AB, Rimm DL: Loss of p120ctn in human colorectal cancer predicts metastasis and poor survival. Cancer Lett 1998;132:193–201.
192. Murray GI, Duncan ME, O'Neil P, et al: Matrix metalloproteinase-1 is associated with poor prognosis in colorectal cancer. Nat Med 1996;2:461–462.
193. Itoh F, Yamamoto H, Hinoda Y, Imai K: Enhanced secretion and activation of matrilysin during malignant conversion of human colorectal epithelium and its relationship with invasive potential of colon cancer cells. Cancer 1996;77:1717–1721.
194. Griffin CA: Pancreatic exocrine tumors. *In* Wolman SR, Sell S (eds): Human Cytogenetic Cancer Markers. Totawa, NJ, Humana, 1997, pp 403–423.
195. Fukushige S, Waldman FM, Kimura M, et al: Frequent gain of copy number on the long arm of chromosome 20 in human pancreatic adenocarcinoma. Genes Chromosomes Cancer 1997;19:161–169.
196. Mahlamaki EH, Hoglund M, Gorunova L, et al: Comparative genomic hybridization reveals frequent gains of 20q, 8q, 11q, 12p, and 17q, and losses of 18q, 9p,

and 15q in pancreatic cancer. Genes Chromosomes Cancer 1997;20:383–391.
197. Sugio K, Molberg K, Albores-Saavedra J, et al: K-*ras* mutations and allelic loss at 5q and 18q in the development of human pancreatic cancers. Int J Pancreatol 1997;21:205–217.
198. Almoguera C, Shibata D, Forrester K, et al: Most human carcinomas of the exocrine pancreas contain mutant c-K-*ras* genes. Cell 1988;53:549–554.
199. Smit VT, Boot AJ, Smits AM, et al: *KRAS* codon 12 mutations occur very frequently in pancreatic adenocarcinomas. Nucleic Acids Res 1988;16:7773–7782.
200. Grunewald K, Lyons J, Frohlich A, et al: High frequency of Ki-*ras* codon 12 mutations in pancreatic adenocarcinomas. Int J Cancer 1989;43:1037–1041.
201. Hruban RH, van Mansfeld AD, Offerhaus GJ, et al: K-*ras* oncogene activation in adenocarcinoma of the human pancreas: A study of 82 carcinomas using a combination of mutant-enriched polymerase chain reaction analysis and allele-specific oligonucleotide hybridization. Am J Pathol 1993;143:545–554.
202. Yanagisawa A, Ohtake K, Ohashi K, et al: Frequent c-Ki-*ras* oncogene activation in mucous cell hyperplasias of pancreas suffering from chronic inflammation. Cancer Res 1993;53:953–956.
203. Tada M, Ohashi M, Shiratori Y, et al: Analysis of K-*ras* gene mutation in hyperplastic duct cells of the pancreas without pancreatic disease [see comments]. Gastroenterology 1996;110:227–231.
204. Moskaluk CA, Hruban RH, Kern SE: *p16* and K-*ras* gene mutations in the intraductal precursors of human pancreatic adenocarcinoma. Cancer Res 1997;57: 2140–2143.
205. Hara E, Smith R, Parry D, et al: Regulation of p16CDKN2 expression and its implications for cell immortalization and senescence. Mol Cell Biol 1996; 16:859–867.
206. Caldas C, Hahn SA, da Costa LT, et al: Frequent somatic mutations and homozygous deletions of the *p16 (MTS1)* gene in pancreatic adenocarcinoma [published erratum appears in Nat Genet 1994;8:410]. Nat Genet 1994;8:27–32.
207. Bartsch D, Shevlin DW, Tung WS, et al: Frequent mutations of *CDKN2* in primary pancreatic adenocarcinomas. Genes Chromosomes Cancer 1995;14:189–195.
208. Schutte M, Hruban RH, Geradts J, et al: Abrogation of the Rb/p16 tumor-suppressive pathway in virtually all pancreatic carcinomas. Cancer Res 1997;57:3126–3130.
209. Hu YX, Watanabe H, Ohtsubo K, et al: Frequent loss of p16 expression and its correlation with clinicopathological parameters in pancreatic carcinoma. Clin Cancer Res 1997;3:1473–1477.
210. Redston MS, Caldas C, Seymour AB, et al: *p53* mutations in pancreatic carcinoma and evidence of common involvement of homocopolymer tracts in DNA microdeletions. Cancer Res 1994;54:3025–3033.
211. Scarpa A, Capelli P, Mukai K, et al: Pancreatic adenocarcinomas frequently show *p53* gene mutations. Am J Pathol 1993;142:1534–1543.
212. Weyrer K, Feichtinger H, Haun M, et al: *p53*, Ki-*ras*, and DNA ploidy in human pancreatic ductal adenocarcinomas. Lab Invest 1996;74:279–289.
213. Kern SE, Kinzler KW, Bruskin A, et al: Identification of *p53* as a sequence-specific DNA-binding protein. Science 1991;252:1708–1711.
214. Rall CJ, Yan YX, Graeme-Cook F, et al: Ki-*ras* and *p53* mutations in pancreatic ductal adenocarcinoma. Pancreas 1996;12:10–17.
215. Ruggeri BA, Huang L, Berger D, et al: Molecular pathology of primary and metastatic ductal pancreatic lesions: Analyses of mutations and expression of the *p53*, *mdm-2*, and *p21/WAF-1* genes in sporadic and familial lesions. Cancer 1997;79:700–716.
216. Hahn SA, Schutte M, Hoque AT, et al: *DPC4*, a candidate tumor suppressor gene at human chromosome 18q21.1 [see comments]. Science 1996;271:350–353.
217. Hahn SA, Hoque AT, Moskaluk CA, et al: Homozygous deletion map at 18q21.1 in pancreatic cancer. Cancer Res 1996;56:490–494.
218. Schutte M, Hruban RH, Hedrick L, et al: *DPC4* gene in various tumor types. Cancer Res 1996;56: 2527–2530.
219. Grau AM, Zhang L, Wang W, et al: Induction of p21waf1 expression and growth inhibition by transforming growth factor beta involve the tumor suppressor gene *DPC4* in human pancreatic adenocarcinoma cells. Cancer Res 1997;57:3929–3934.
220. Iacobuzio-Donahue CA, Klimstra DS, Adsay NV, et al: Dpc-4 protein is expressed in virtually all human intraductal papillary mucinous neoplasms of the pancreas: Comparison with conventional ductal adenocarcinomas. Am J Pathol 2000;157:755–761.
221. Goggins M, Offerhaus GJ, Hilgers W, et al: Pancreatic adenocarcinomas with DNA replication errors (RER+) are associated with wild-type K-*ras* and characteristic histopathology: Poor differentiation, a syncytial growth pattern, and pushing borders suggest RER+. Am J Pathol 1998;152:1501–1507.
222. Shibata D, Almoguera C, Forrester K, et al: Detection of c-K-*ras* mutations in fine needle aspirates from human pancreatic adenocarcinomas. Cancer Res 1990; 50:1279–1283.
223. Tada M, Omata M, Ohto M: Clinical application of *ras* gene mutation for diagnosis of pancreatic adenocarcinoma. Gastroenterology 1991;100:233–238.
224. Urban T, Ricci S, Grange JD, et al: Detection of c-Ki-*ras* mutation by PCR/RFLP analysis and diagnosis of pancreatic adenocarcinomas [see comments]. J Natl Cancer Inst 1993;85:2008–2012.
225. Tada M, Omata M, Kawai S, et al: Detection of *ras* gene mutations in pancreatic juice and peripheral blood of patients with pancreatic adenocarcinoma. Cancer Res 1993;53:2472–2474.
226. Watanabe H, Sawabu N, Songur Y, et al: Detection of K-*ras* point mutations at codon 12 in pure pancreatic juice for the diagnosis of pancreatic cancer by PCR-RFLP analysis. Pancreas 1996;12:18–24.
227. Wilentz RE, Chung CH, Sturm PD, et al: K-*ras* mutations in the duodenal fluid of patients with pancreatic carcinoma. Cancer 1998;82:96–103.
228. Caldas C, Hahn SA, Hruban RH, et al: Detection of K-*ras* mutations in the stool of patients with pancreatic adenocarcinoma and pancreatic ductal hyperplasia. Cancer Res 1994;54:3568–3573.

229. Sturm PD, Rauws EA, Hruban RH, et al: Clinical value of K-*ras* codon 12 analysis and endobiliary brush cytology for the diagnosis of malignant extrahepatic bile duct stenosis. Clin Cancer Res 1999;5:629–635.
230. Dillon DA, Johnson CC, Topazian MD, et al: The utility of Ki-*ras* mutation analysis in the cytologic diagnosis of pancreatobiliary neoplasms [in process citation]. Cancer J 2000;6:294–301.
231. Sorenson GD, Pribish DM, Valone FH, et al: Soluble normal and mutated DNA sequences from single-copy genes in human blood. Cancer Epidemiol Biomarkers Prev 1994;3:67–71.
232. Mulcahy HE, Lyautey J, Lederrey C, et al: A prospective study of K-*ras* mutations in the plasma of pancreatic cancer patients. Clin Cancer Res 1998;4:271–275.
233. Yamada T, Nakamori S, Ohzato H, et al: Detection of K-*ras* gene mutations in plasma DNA of patients with pancreatic adenocarcinoma: Correlation with clinicopathological features. Clin Cancer Res 1998;4:1527–1532.
234. Kusano N, Shiraishi K, Kubo K, et al: Genetic aberrations detected by comparative genomic hybridization in hepatocellular carcinomas: Their relationship to clinicopathological features. Hepatology 1999;29:1858–1862.
235. Marchio A, Meddeb M, Pineau P, et al: Recurrent chromosomal abnormalities in hepatocellular carcinoma detected by comparative genomic hybridization. Genes Chromosomes Cancer 1997;18:59–65.
236. Sakakura C, Hagiwara A, Taniguchi H, et al: Chromosomal aberrations in human hepatocellular carcinomas associated with hepatitis C virus infection detected by comparative genomic hybridization. Br J Cancer 1999;80:2034–2039.
237. Wong N, Lai P, Lee SW, et al: Assessment of genetic changes in hepatocellular carcinoma by comparative genomic hybridization analysis: Relationship to disease stage, tumor size, and cirrhosis. Am J Pathol 1999;154:37–43.
238. Konishi M, Kikuchi-Yanoshita R, Tanaka K, et al: Genetic changes and histopathological grades in human hepatocellular carcinomas. Jpn J Cancer Res 1993;84:893–899.
239. Emi M, Fujiwara Y, Ohata H, et al: Allelic loss at chromosome band 8p21.3-p22 is associated with progression of hepatocellular carcinoma. Genes Chromosomes Cancer 1993;7:152–157.
240. Ding SF, Delhanty JD, Dooley JS, et al: The putative tumor suppressor gene on chromosome 5q for hepatocellular carcinoma is distinct from the *MCC* and *APC* genes. Cancer Detect Prev 1993;17:405–409.
241. Puisieux A, Galvin K, Troalen F, et al: Retinoblastoma and *p53* tumor suppressor genes in human hepatoma cell lines. FASEB J 1993;7:1407–1413.
242. Harris CC: *p53:* At the crossroads of molecular carcinogenesis and risk assessment. Science 1993;262:1980–1981.
243. Denissenko MF, Koudriakova TB, Smith L, et al: The p53 codon 249 mutational hotspot in hepatocellular carcinoma is not related to selective formation or persistence of aflatoxin B1 adducts. Oncogene 1998;17:3007–3014.
244. Kirk GD, Camus-Randon AM, Mendy M, et al: Ser-249 *p53* mutations in plasma DNA of patients with hepatocellular carcinoma from The Gambia. J Natl Cancer Inst 2000;92:148–153.
245. Arbuthnot P, Capovilla A, Kew M: Putative role of hepatitis B virus X protein in hepatocarcinogenesis: Effects on apoptosis, DNA repair, mitogen-activated protein kinase and JAK/STAT pathways [see comments]. J Gastroenterol Hepatol 2000;15:357–368.
246. Konishi M, Kikuchi-Yanoshita R, Tanaka K, et al: Genetic changes and histopathological grades in human hepatocellular carcinomas. Jpn J Cancer Res 1993;84:893–899.
247. Teramoto T, Satonaka K, Kitazawa S, et al: *p53* gene abnormalities are closely related to hepatoviral infections and occur at a late stage of hepatocarcinogenesis. Cancer Res 1994;54:231–235.
248. Hollstein M, Marion MJ, Lehman T, et al: *p53* mutations at A:T base pairs in angiosarcomas of vinyl chloride–exposed factory workers. Carcinogenesis 1994;15:1–3.
249. Hsu HC, Tseng HJ, Lai PL, et al: Expression of *p53* gene in 184 unifocal hepatocellular carcinomas: Association with tumor growth and invasiveness. Cancer Res 1993;53:4691–4694.
250. Slagle BL, Zhou YZ, Birchmeier W, Scorsone KA: Deletion of the E-cadherin gene in hepatitis B virus–positive Chinese hepatocellular carcinomas. Hepatology 1993;18:757–762.
251. Endo K, Ueda T, Ueyama J, et al: Immunoreactive E-cadherin, alpha-catenin, beta-catenin, and gamma-catenin proteins in hepatocellular carcinoma: Relationships with tumor grade, clinicopathologic parameters, and patients' survival. Hum Pathol 2000;31:558–565.
252. Jin M, Piao Z, Kim NG, et al: p16 is a major inactivation target in hepatocellular carcinoma. Cancer 2000;89:60–68.
253. de La Coste A, Romagnolo B, Billuart P, et al: Somatic mutations of the beta-catenin gene are frequent in mouse and human hepatocellular carcinomas. Proc Natl Acad Sci U S A 1998;95:8847–8851.

JACK H. LICHY
TIMOTHY J. O'LEARY

12

Breast and Female Reproductive Tract

BREAST CARCINOMA

Breast cancer is both the most common malignancy in women and the most extensively studied. A variety of cytogenetic abnormalities can be identified in breast cancers grown for short periods of time in culture. Breast cancers commonly demonstrate very complex karyotypes, including multiple monosomies, trisomies, and translocations.[1] However, cytogenetic analysis of breast cancers has not revealed any consistent, characteristic genetic alteration. Perhaps the most important finding from cytogenetic studies of breast cancer has been the frequent identification of multiple clones, sometimes bearing no discernible similarities.[2, 3]

Studies of sporadic breast cancer by comparative genomic hybridization (CGH) have identified several areas of recurrent gain or loss of chromosomal copy number. The most frequent alterations revealed by CGH of sporadic breast tumors were gains of 1q (67%) and 8q (49%).[4, 5] Recurrent gains were reported at 33 other chromosomal regions, with the most frequent being 5p12-14, 19q, 11q13-14, 16p, 17q12, 17q22-24, 19p, and 20q13. Interestingly, three of these loci contain genes known from earlier studies to be commonly amplified in breast cancer: cyclin D1 (*CCND1*) at 11q13, *HER2* at 17q12, and *MYC* at 8q. Recurrent losses were seen at 6q, 8p, 9p, 11p, 11q, 13q, 16q, 17p, 18q, and Xq. As is evident by comparison with Table 12–1, five of these loci correspond to sites of high-frequency loss of heterozygosity (LOH) detected by short tandem repeat analysis. Therefore, although the story is complex, there is reasonable concordance between regions identified as amplified or deleted by CGH and those identified by Southern blot or polymerase chain reaction (PCR)–based methods.

Clonal Heterogeneity in Breast Cancer

Several studies, based on cytogenetic methods, CGH, and LOH analysis, have reported observations of genetically divergent clones in breast cancer specimens. Cytogenetic analysis of tumor specimens grown for short periods of time in culture has provided evidence for the presence of apparently unrelated clones in half of the tumors analyzed.[2, 3, 6–9] Because no common genetic alteration among these distinct clones could be identified, these authors interpret their findings as evidence for a polyclonal origin of breast cancer.

In a study employing LOH analysis, genetically divergent clones were demonstrated in different foci of intraductal carcinoma microdissected from the same specimen.[10] Heterogeneity among invasive or metastatic components appeared to be rare, and all clones from any given tumor sample could be linked to a common precursor by loss of similar genetic markers, consistent with a monoclonal origin of the tumor (Fig. 12–1).

Further evidence for the existence and importance of genetic divergence in breast cancer came from a study based on CGH. In this study, asynchronous breast cancer metastases frequently were found to have little evidence of clonal relatedness to the primary tumor.[11] This group has also reported that CGH can sometimes reveal marked clonal divergence between intraductal and in situ foci.[12]

Loss of Heterozygosity in Morphologically Normal Breast Tissue

Although LOH is usually considered one of the many kinds of genetic abnormalities that occur during malignant transformation, several studies have identified LOH in morphologically normal breast epithelium. In one study, LOH was identified in normal terminal duct lobular units (TDLUs) adjacent to tumor.[13] LOH patterns in these TDLUs suggested that they are clonal precursors of the tumor. In another study using LOH analysis, Larson and associates demonstrated clonal genetic abnormalities in microdissected TDLUs from reduction mammoplasty specimens lacking histologic abnormalities.[14] Clonal chromosome aberrations have also been reported in benign lesions, including fibroadenoma, atypical hyperplasia, and intraductal papilloma,[15–19] as well as in benign

TABLE 12–1

Loci Showing High-Frequency Loss of Heterozygosity (LOH) with Candidate Tumor Suppressor Genes

Gene	Locus	LOH Frequency (%)
FHIT	3p	30–40
CDKN2A	9p21–22	50–60
CDKN1B	11p15	30–40
ATM	11p24	40–50
RB1, BRCA2	13q	30–40
E-Cadherin	16q	>50
TP53, other?	17p13	50–60
BRCA1, NME1	17q	30–40

Data from references 300–302.

epithelium in patients from breast cancer families[20] or at no increased risk of breast cancer.[14]

The significance of LOH in normal breast epithelium is unknown. It is possible that LOH may occur normally during the development of the breast, but additional studies using carefully microdissected foci of normal tissue will be needed to gain further insight into this issue.

Telomerase

Telomerase is an enzyme required for the maintenance of telomere length during DNA replication. Most benign cells do not express telomerase. Activation of telomerase expression may be a critical event in cellular immortalization. Whereas benign breast epithelium lacks expression of this enzyme, most carcinomas express telomerase. The level of expression in breast cancer varies over a wide range. High-level expression of telomerase has been associated with p53 protein accumulation, but not with *TP53* mutations, and with poor prognosis in node-negative breast cancers.[21]

Growth-Regulatory Signaling Pathways in Breast Cancer

Among the regulators of cell growth are extracellular stimuli, including hormones, growth factors, and cell

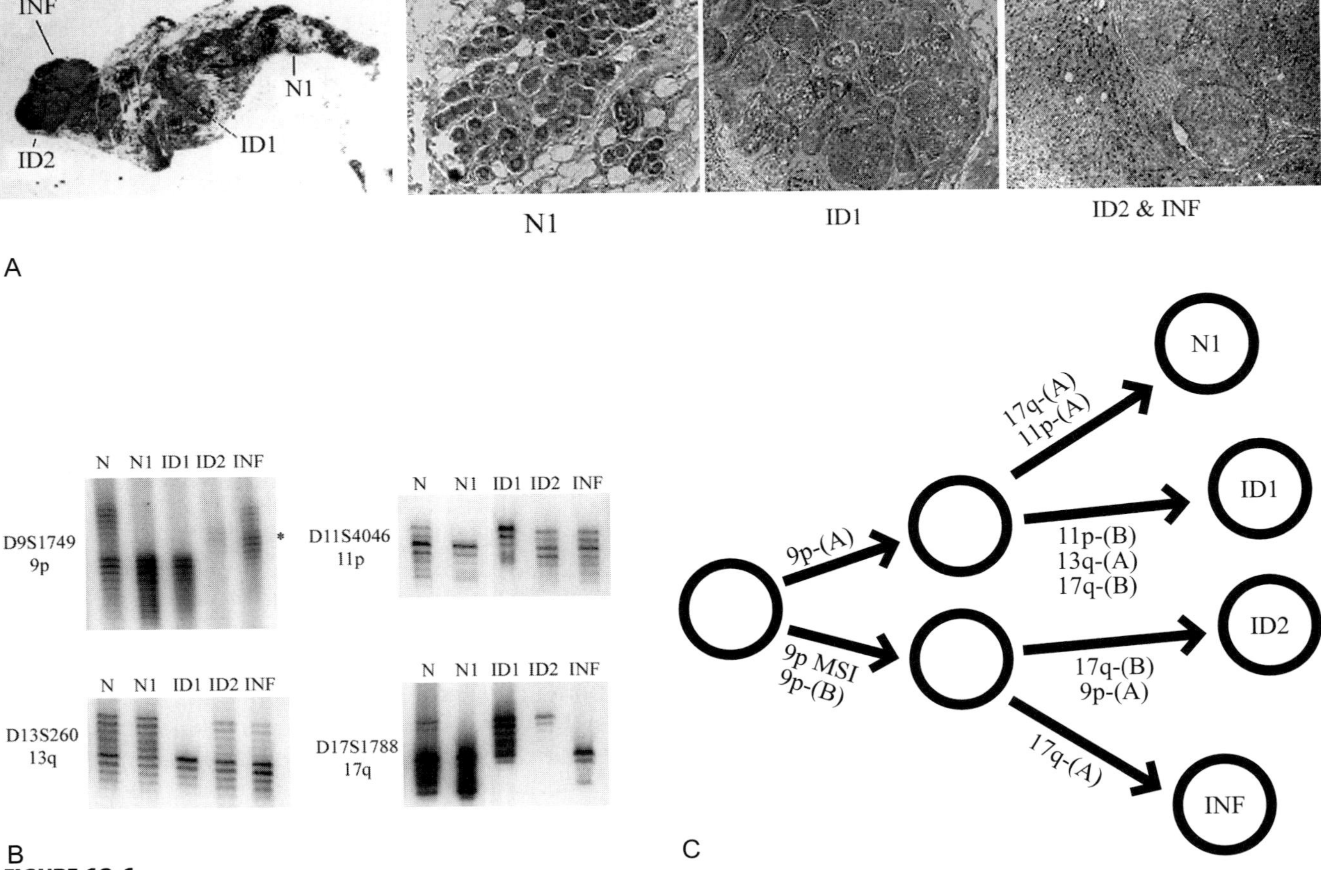

FIGURE 12–1
A, Histology. *B,* Loss of heterozygosity data obtained at the indicated loci. *C,* Clonal relationship between microdissected tumor components suggested by loss of heterozygosity data. ID1, locular carcinoma in situ; ID2, distinct focus of lobular carcinoma in situ; INF, infiltrating lobular carcinoma adjacent to ID2; N, benign axillary lymph node; N1, benign terminal duct-lobular unit.

surface molecules that mediate contact inhibition of cell growth. Such stimuli activate growth-regulatory signal transduction pathways. These pathways transmit the growth-regulatory signal by means of a series of proteins and small molecules (e.g., inositol triphosphate), often terminating in a kinase cascade that leads to the activation of downstream target molecules by phosphorylation. Among the targets of signaling pathways are transcription factors, which can alter the expression of large numbers of genes, and cytoskeletal components, which can alter cell morphology.

One class of mutations important in the pathogenesis of breast cancer results in the constitutive activation of a growth-regulatory signaling pathway. If the mutation results in activation of one of the proteins in the pathway, the gene encoding that protein is a *proto-oncogene* and the mutated form is an *oncogene*. If the mutation results in inactivation of an inhibitor of the pathway, then the coding gene is a *tumor suppressor gene*.

Many signaling pathways have been characterized. Although the overall workings of the signaling pathways are extremely complex, different pathways share common features. The best studied pathway, initiated by the binding of epidermal growth factor (EGF) to its receptor, is described here to help clarify the relationships between the types of proteins involved (Fig. 12–2). Interaction of EGF with its receptor at the cell membrane leads to receptor dimerization and autophosphorylation on a specific tyrosine residue. This phosphotyrosine, together with several adjacent amino acids, binds to an adapter molecule, GRB2. The GRB2 molecule consists almost entirely of domains involved in protein-protein interactions. The interaction of GRB2 with the EGF receptor brings another GRB2-bound protein, SOS, to the cell membrane. The SOS protein functions as an activator of RAS. Activated RAS in turn initiates a protein kinase cascade, activating sequentially protein kinases named MEK kinase (MEKK), MEK, and MAP kinase (or ERK for "extracellular signal–regulated kinase"). The targets of MAP kinase include the transcription factors and cytoskeletal components just mentioned.

This model provides a basis for understanding the complex network of interacting signaling pathways, involving multiple MEKKs, MEKs, and ERKs, many parallel pathways, and many variations on the scheme shown in the figure. Alterations of a growth-regulatory signal transduction pathway at any point could theoretically result in constitutive activation. Alterations of several components have been identified in breast cancer, as described in the following paragraphs.

ERBB2 AMPLIFICATION

The product of the *ERBB2* gene (also known as *HER2* and *neu*) is a 185-kd receptor localized to the cell membrane. The receptor is structurally related to the EGF receptor, and its ligand, heregulin, is an EGF-like molecule. The gene product is overexpressed in 25% to 30% of sporadic breast cancers, usually owing to gene amplification. Although results of studies have conflicted over the years, most studies find a correlation between overexpression of *ERBB2* and poor prognosis.[22] Furthermore, there is evidence that women whose breast cancers demonstrate *ERBB2* overexpression may benefit from more aggressive adjuvant chemotherapy.[23, 24] The importance of this gene in breast cancer diagnosis and treatment has continued to increase since the introduction of Herceptin, a monoclonal antibody directed against the *ERBB2* gene product, as a therapeutic agent. Whenever therapy with Herceptin is a consideration, a test for *ERBB2* overexpression is required. Although most laboratories use an immunohistochemical kit approved by the U.S. Food and Drug Administration for this test, considerable controversy has arisen as to whether a fluorescent in situ hybridization (FISH) assay for increased gene copy number might not be more appropriate[25]; such assays have been developed and appear to yield highly reproducible results.[26, 27] The best approach may be to use the immunohistochemical assay to "triage out" cases that are unlikely to demonstrate gene amplification, then to definitively identify amplification with FISH.[27]

RAS MUTATIONS

Mutation of the *HRAS*, *NRAS*, or *KRAS* genes occurs frequently in many types of tumors. In sporadic breast cancers, overexpression of RAS proteins has been observed in 67% of specimens.[28] In the same study, *KRAS* mutations were identified in 4 of 61 cases (6.5%).

PTEN MUTATIONS

The *PTEN* gene is mutated in Cowden's syndrome, a familial cancer syndrome associated with increased risk for breast cancer. The protein appears to function as an antagonist of signal transduction pathways involving inositol triphosphate. The gene is occasionally (2 of 54 cases analyzed) mutated in sporadic breast cancers.[29]

MKK4 MUTATIONS

In studies of sporadic breast cancer cases, most of the activating mutations identified affect either a receptor or one of the *RAS* genes. However, the kinase MKK4, functionally analogous to MEK, has been found to be homozygously deleted or mutated in 14% of cases (3 of 22). Interestingly, this particular MEK kinase appears to function in a signaling pathway structurally similar to the EGF-RAS-MAP kinase pathway, but with the opposite downstream effect, that is, growth inhibition rather than stimulation. Consequently, the growth stimulatory alteration of *MKK4* would be inactivation of both alleles, and therefore *MKK4* would be classified as a tumor suppressor gene.

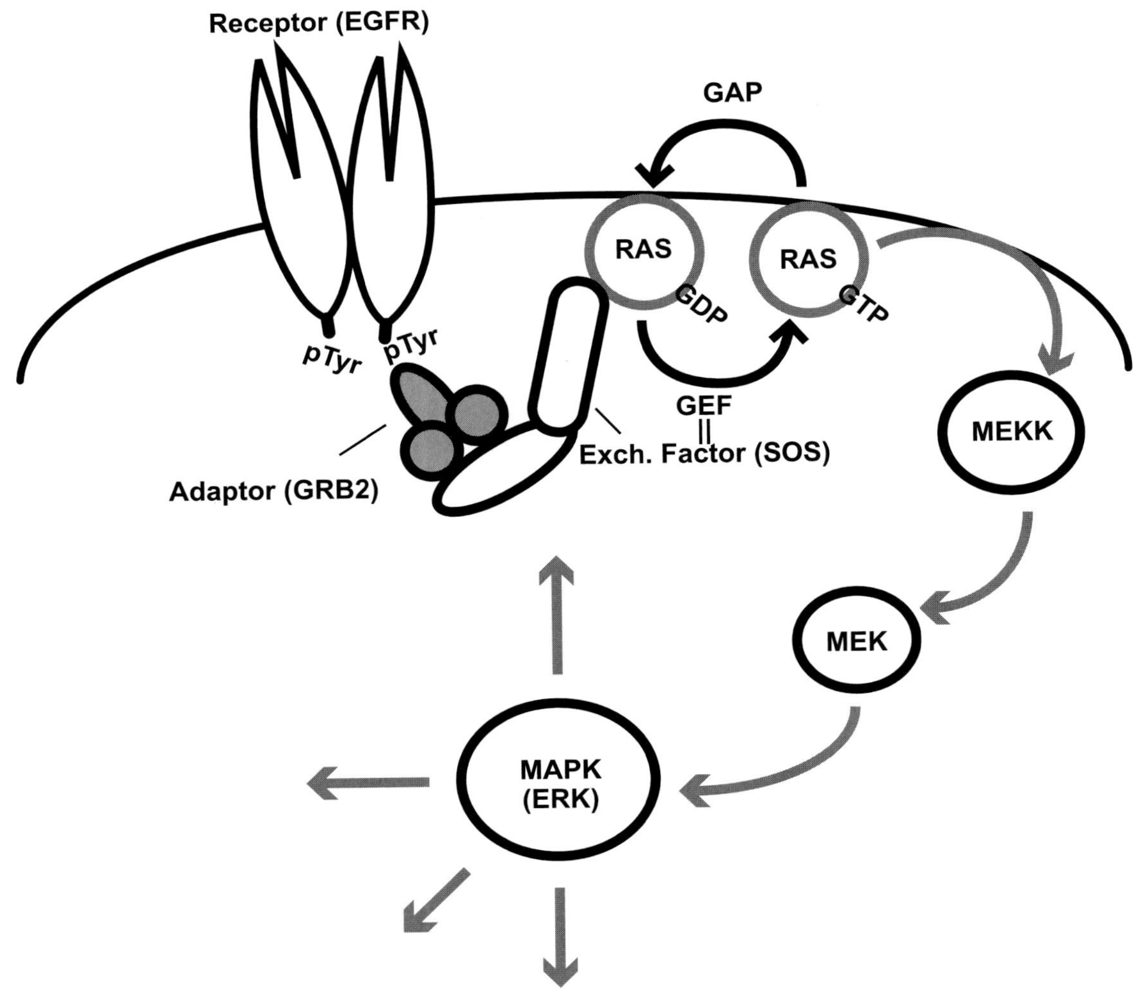

FIGURE 12–2
Schematic of components of EGF-Ras-MAPK signal transduction pathway. A transmembrane receptor protein (EGFR) interacts with an extracellular growth factor, leading to dimerization of the receptor and activation of its intracellular tyrosine kinase activity. The receptor autophosphorylates, creating a binding site for an SH2 domain of an adaptor protein. The SH3 domains of the adaptor interact with a GEF protein, recruiting it to the membrane, thereby allowing it to activate RAS by exchanging guanosine triphosphate (GTP) for guanosine diphosphate (GDP). RAS-GTP then activates the kinase MEKK, initiating a kinase cascade, leading to the sequential activation of the kinases MEK and MAPK by phosphorylation. MAPK, the final kinase in the pathway, phosphorylates multiple intracellular protein targets, as indicated by the *arrows,* some of which are the upstream components of the pathway, such as SOS. EGFR, epidermal growth factor receptor; pTyr, phosphotyrosine; GAP, GTPase activator protein; GEF, GTP exchange factor; MEKK, MEK kinase; MEK, MAP or ERK kinase; MAPK, MAP kinase; ERK, extracellular signal–regulated kinase.

Disorders of Cell Cycle Regulation in Breast Cancer

Another class of proteins that plays a role in breast cancer pathogenesis is the cell cycle regulators. Advancement from one stage of the cell cycle to the next requires specific events to occur. For example, progression from G_1 to S phase, a particularly important point of regulation in the cell cycle, requires synthesis of the proteins required for DNA replication. For this to happen, the transcription factors regulating these genes must be activated. But in G_1 phase, these are bound in an inactive form to other proteins. One of these is RB1, the 105-kd product of the tumor suppressor gene responsible for familial retinoblastoma. Activation of the RB1-associated transcription factors requires phosphorylation of the RB1 protein. One of the kinases that carries out this phosphorylation is cyclin-dependent kinase 4 (CDK4). If CDK4 is active, then RB1 can be phosphorylated, transcription factors activated, and the cell cycle can progress to S phase.

Disruption of the mechanisms that regulate CDK4 activity, the cyclins and CDK inhibitors, leads to abnormalities in cell cycle regulation in cancer. Cyclin D1 is necessary for CDK4 activity. Normally, cyclin D1 expression occurs only in late G_1, when CDK4 activity is needed. The kinase CDK4 is also subject to negative regulators. Activation of these negative regulators, which occurs in response to DNA damage, provides a "checkpoint" in the cell cycle.

Participants in the G1→S cell cycle checkpoint include several inhibitors of the CDKs, including the ATM protein (product of the gene responsible for ataxia-telangiectasia) and the tumor suppressor gene product p53. The p53 protein blocks entry into S phase in the presence of genomic damage. This allows time for DNA repair to occur before replication initiates. One mechanism of p53 action is through its activity as a transcription factor. Among the genes regulated by p53 is *CDKN1A*. Another gene, *CDKN2* (also named *P16INK4* for the 16-kd inhibitor of kinase 4), which also encodes a CDK inhibitor, plays a role in a wide variety of tumors, including breast cancer.

The use of flow cytometry in assessing breast cancer prognosis follows directly from the relationship between disruption of these regulatory pathways and clinical outcome in breast cancer patients. Numerous studies have demonstrated that patients with highly proliferative tumors (as demonstrated by high S-phase fractions) have a substantially poorer prognosis than those without[30, 31]; immunohistochemical assessment of cellular proliferation using MIB-1 staining appears to offer much of the same prognostic information at lower cost.[32–34]

RETINOBLASTOMA GENE

The frequency of retinoblastoma gene *(RB1)* mutations in breast cancer is not known. LOH at the *RB1* locus occurs in approximately 25% of cases, and reduced expression of the RB1 protein has been reported in 10% to 45% of breast tumors.[35]

CYCLIN D1 *(CCND1)*

Cyclin D1 gene amplification has been reported in 15% to 20% of sporadic breast cancers. Overexpression of the protein occurs in more than 40% of cases. Expression of the gene is regulated in part by hormones; consistent with this regulatory control, negativity for estrogen receptor correlates with reduced cyclin D1 expression.[35] Studies that relate cyclin D1 expression to prognosis have suggested that decreased expression may be associated with adverse outcome.[36, 37]

CDK INHIBITORS

In sporadic breast cancer, LOH at the *CDKN2A* gene locus occurs in more than 50% of cases.[38] Expression of the protein is often low or absent, but mutations in the structural gene are rare. Alteration in gene expression is thought to be related to the methylation status of the gene.

Overexpression of the CDK inhibitor *CDKN1A* is common. Conflicting reports in the literature have associated high tumor grade with either low- or high-level expression of this gene.

The CDK inhibitor *CDKN1B* (p27 Kip1) is frequently underexpressed in breast cancer. Low levels of this protein correlate with poor prognosis and an aggressive phenotype.

TP53 MUTATIONS

TP53 is mutated in approximately 40% of cases of sporadic breast cancer.[39–45] The nature of the mutations has been studied as a possible reflection of the etiology of the tumor.[46] The identification of excess G→T transversions over what would be expected by chance has led to the suggestion that environmental carcinogens might be involved in breast cancer. Some investigators have found an association between *TP53* mutation and high-frequency LOH in breast cancer,[47, 48] but others have not observed this.[49]

Mutations of *TP53* are associated with the presence of lymph node metastasis, *ERBB2* amplification, and lack of estrogen receptor expression.[50] Furthermore, *TP53* mutation seems to confer resistance to doxorubicin, one of the first-line chemotherapeutic drugs for breast cancer.[51] It is thus perhaps not surprising that women whose tumors demonstrate *TP53* mutation have a shorter time to disease recurrence, and shorter survival, than those whose tumors harbor wild-type *TP53*.[44] Mutation is frequently associated with immunohistochemically detectable accumulation of p53 protein. As a result, p53 overexpression, as assessed immunohistochemically, is also associated with decreased survival[50, 52–57]; some studies have suggested that it is second in importance only to axillary node status as a predictor of outcome.[58]

Cell Adhesion Defects in Breast Cancer

One of the important pathways of growth regulation regulates cell growth in response to cell-cell adhesion. Important components of this particular signaling pathway are the proteins E-cadherin and members of the catenin family. Mutations of the E-cadherin gene occur with high frequency in infiltrating lobular carcinoma of the breast and are usually associated with LOH of the other allele.[59–62] The gene is virtually never mutated in ductal carcinoma. Inactivation of E-cadherin results from truncation of the protein caused by mutation. The E-cadherin mutation may account for the discohesiveness of the cells of lobular carcinoma and the characteristic histologic pattern of infiltrating lobular carcinoma. Decreased expression of E-cadherin protein, as detected either immunohistochemically or by message quantitation, has been associated with adverse outcome.[63–65] These findings are primarily of academic interest, because the assays are technically difficult and not particularly suitable for routine use.

Angiogenesis

Thrombospondins 1 and 2 are extracellular matrix glycoproteins that modulate the growth of new blood vessels. They are secreted in larger amounts by breast cancer cells than by benign tissues, and thrombospondin secretion appears to correlate strongly with the amount of tumor vascularization.[66] In turn, there appears to be a striking correlation between the proliferation of intratumor blood vessels and metastasis in patients with breast cancer.[57, 67–72] These findings strongly suggest that angiogenesis inhibitors may prove useful in the management of patients with breast cancer.

Although microvessel density counts are in theory straightforward, requiring only identification of vessel walls by a suitable immunohistochemical marker (such as CD34) and stereologic computations, not all investigators have been able to confirm the prognostic utility of this technique.[73] This may reflect a lack of standardization in both immunohistochemical staining[74] and stereologic counting methods.[75]

Marker Genes of Potential Relevance to Breast Cancer Management

Because one of the goals of molecular pathology is to provide tests with high sensitivity for detecting small populations of malignant cells in a benign background, reverse transcriptase (RT–PCR) assays to detect the transcripts of several candidate genes have been designed and studied for the sensitivity and specificity of detecting small populations of malignant cells in a benign background. There has been considerable interest in developing such an assay as a means to detect breast cancer cells in biopsy specimens of sentinel lymph nodes. The ideal gene for such an assay would be one expressed only in breast cancer cells. At the least, the target gene should not be expressed in benign lymph nodes.

A promising candidate gene that has been described only recently encodes a 10-kd protein named mammaglobin.[76] The potential value of this gene as a tumor marker was supported by the results of a study that compared the sensitivity and specificity of seven different genes: cytokeratin 19, MUC1, maspin, vascular endothelial growth factor (VEGF), transforming growth factor-β, carcinoembryonic antigen (CEA), and mammaglobin.[77] The first five of these markers lacked the desired specificity; 30% to 100% of normal lymph nodes yielded positive results. However, CEA and mammaglobin were not detected in these benign specimens. In a panel of seven breast cancer cell lines, CEA and mammaglobin were detected in 71% and 100% of cases. In dilution experiments, the RT-PCR assay gave a positive result with as little as one tumor cell per 10^6 normal cells. The RT-PCR assay appears to be more sensitive than morphology in detecting micrometastases in lymph nodes. However, the clinical utility of detecting micrometastases remains to be proved.

Immunohistochemical Characteristics of Breast Carcinoma

Immunocytochemical analysis is not generally useful in the diagnosis of primary breast tumors (except for spindle cell neoplasms and mesenchymal tumors), but it may prove useful in the identification of a primary site for metastatic disease. Perhaps most common among these is differentiation of metastatic lung cancer from metastatic breast cancer. The antibodies directed against thyroid transcription factor 1 (TTF1) do not react with breast cancers but do react with approximately 70% of lung adenocarcinomas.[78] In contrast, antibodies to gross cystic disease fluid protein (GCDFP-15) react with fewer than 1% of lung adenocarcinomas but with 60% of breast cancers.[79] Finally, polyclonal antibodies directed against CEA react with nearly 90% of lung adenocarcinomas but only about 20% of breast cancers.[80] A brief summary of selected immunohistochemical characteristics of breast carcinoma is given in Table 12–2.

FIBROADENOMA

Karyotypes are available on only a few fibroadenomas.[15, 81–83] Although rearrangements of 1p, 12p, and trisomies 11 and 20 have been seen in more than one case, there is no evidence for consistent nonrandom change in either classic karyotypic studies[81] or by CGH.[84] Gross aneuploidy has not been observed in fibroadenomas, either by conventional cytogenetic methods or by flow and image cytometry.[85]

A variety of molecular alterations have been observed in fibroadenomas, including LOH on chromosome 3p,[86] microsatellite instability,[87] *TP53* mutation and overexpression,[88] and low-level expression of telomerase.[89–91] As yet, however, none of the findings point toward a molecular pathway for the pathogenesis of these benign lesions.

Although fibroadenomas are clinically benign, there is a histologically similar counterpart—*cystosarcoma phylloides* or *phylloides tumor*—that may on occasion behave aggressively. Even less is known about the pathogenesis of this lesion than about fibroadenoma. Diploid phylloides tumors appear to behave indolently, however, whereas those with an aneuploid cell population are likely to develop metastases.[85]

TABLE 12–2
Selected Immunohistochemical Staining Characteristics of Breast Carcinoma

Antigen	Percentage of Cases Demonstrating Immunoreactivity
Epithelial membrane antigen	98–100
CAM 5.2	95–100
Cytokeratin 7	94–100
AE1/AE3	92–100
BER-EP4	63–83
Cytokeratin 19	43–82
GCDFP-15	54–67
Carcinoembryonic antigen	51–63
S-100	28–52
Neuron-specific enolase	12–23
Cytokeratin 20	2–8

EPITHELIAL TUMORS OF THE UTERUS

Endometrial Carcinoma

Endometrial adenocarcinoma is a common tumor of older women. The most common cytogenetic abnormalities, found in 75% of cases, are gains of chromosome 1q by means of isochromosome formation or unbalanced translocation.[92] Rearrangement of 11q21-25 has been found in almost 20% of karyotypes demonstrating clonal abnormalities.[93] Gains of a complete copy of chromosomes 2, 7, 10, and 12 are also commonly reported, as is deletion of one copy of chromosome 22.[92, 93] CGH studies reveal cytogenetic abnormalities in about three fourths of specimens, including gains at 3q, 8q, 5p, 6p, and 1q.[94, 95] Losses at 4q, 15q, and 18q are found in less than 20% of cases. Endometrioid carcinomas show less extensive changes, and these are present in only about half of cases. Gains at 1q, 2q, and 8q predominate.[94] The substantial differences in cytogenetic findings suggest a different pathogenesis for these histologic types of tumor.

LOH studies demonstrate allelic deletion on 16q in approximately 40% of patients with endometrial carcinoma; allelic deletion is not seen in patients with endometrial hyperplasia.[96] LOH of chromosomes 2, 13, and 17 may also be detected in about 20% of cases.[97] Approximately 30% of endometrial carcinomas demonstrate LOH on chromosome 18q—the site of the *DCC* (deleted in colon carcinoma) gene,[98] and *DCC* gene alterations are found in about one fourth of cases.

Amplification and overexpression of the *ERBB2* (*HER2/neu*) oncogene is found in approximately 20% of endometrial carcinomas and is typically associated with high-grade tumors[99, 100]; amplification is associated with decreased survival, and is independent of stage, grade, and histologic type.[100] Amplification of *MYC* is found in about one third of endometrial carcinomas and also seems to be associated with higher tumor grade.[99] Not surprisingly, immunohistochemical evidence of ERBB2 overexpression is also associated with advanced disease,[101] but evidence for independent prognostic value is currently lacking. Immunohistochemical demonstration of a related tyrosine kinase receptor, EGFR (epidermal growth factor receptor) has, however, been shown to correlate with both metastasis and shortened survival in patients with endometrial carcinoma.[102]

Sequence analysis has demonstrated frequent *HRAS* gene alteration in endometrial carcinoma, with *KRAS* mutations of in about fifteen percent of specimens.[103–105] There does not appear to be a relationship between *RAS* mutation and survival, however.[105] Mutations of *TP53* are also common, being found in about 15% of early cancers and half of advanced cancers.[106] Immunohistochemical identification of *p53* overexpression is associated with a worse prognosis,[107, 108] at least in the case of papillary serous carcinoma.

Women in families demonstrating hereditary nonpolyposis colon cancer (HNPCC, Lynch syndrome) have a lifetime risk of endometrial cancer that is over 40%.[109] Endometrial carcinoma associated with HNPCC typically demonstrates microsatellite instability and is associated with mutations in the mismatch repair system.[110] Unfortunately, clearly pathogenic mutations can be identified in only about half of families with HNPCC, so molecular analysis is of limited use in detecting family members at increased risk of disease. Hence, careful surveillance for endometrial carcinoma should accompany colon cancer surveillance in women from HNPCC families.

The proliferation rate of endometrial carcinoma is an important factor in determining patient outcome. High expression of the Ki-67 proliferation antigen is associated with adverse outcome and appears to be more useful in predicting prognosis than does the S-phase fraction determined by flow cytometry.[111] Tumor cell aneuploidy is also a powerful prognostic factor that displaces tumor grade in multivariate survival analyses.[112, 113]

Although diagnosis of endometrial adenocarcinoma does not generally require the use of special techniques, immunohistochemical stains may occasionally prove helpful in determining the histogenesis of metastatic disease. The immunohistochemical staining of endometrial carcinoma is summarized in Table 12–3, although different histologic subtypes demonstrate somewhat distinctive immunohistochemical staining patterns.

Carcinoma of the Uterine Cervix

Cervical carcinoma typically develops only after a long period during which cytologic changes are present in the "transformation zone"—a region of the cervix in which columnar epithelium is replaced by metaplastic squamous epithelium. These cytologic changes, including such effects as an increased nucleus/cytoplasm ratio and condensation of nuclear chromatin, are referred to as "squamous intraepithelial neoplasia" or, in earlier literature, "dysplasia." The milder changes that are observed are called "low-grade squamous intraepithelial (LSIL) lesion," whereas the more dramatic changes that may develop are referred to as "high-grade squamous intraepithelial (HSIL) lesion." Recognition of these changes in exfoliated cervical cells, followed by effective treatment, is the basis for the success of the Papanicolaou smear in reducing cervical cancer mortality in developed countries. Most LSIL lesion regress spontaneously, however, and only about 1 case in 100 will progress to invasive cervical carcinoma. Regression of HSIL lesion is far less common, and many cases will progress to invasive carcinoma.

Karyotypic studies of cervical carcinoma have demonstrated common rearrangements of chromosome 1—either I(1q) or deletion of 1p; translocations of 1q to chromosome 17 are also frequent.[92] Chromosomes 2, 3, 4, 5, 6, 9, and 11 also demonstrate frequent karyotypic abnormalities,[92, 93] but no "characteristic" findings have been described. CGH studies suggest that gains of 3q are found in 35% of HSIL lesion and in 70% to 90% of invasive cervical carcinomas.[114, 115] Chromosome 3p, on the other hand, is lost in half the cases of invasive cervical carcinoma.[114] These cytogenetic findings have been amply confirmed by studies using microsatellite markers. Allelic deletion at 3p14 is found in 30% of LSIL, 50% of HSIL, and 75% of invasive cervical cancers.[116, 117] LOH is also frequently observed at 11q22-23 and 17p13.3.[118] LOH on 18q appears to be associated with decreased survival[119]; no specific gene has been associated with this loss.

TABLE 12–3

Selected Immunohistochemical Staining Characteristics of Endometrial Carcinoma

Antigen	Percentage of Cases Demonstrating Immunoreactivity
CA 15-3	100
CAM 5.2	100
Epithelial membrane antigen	91–100
CA 125	87–100
CK 7	86–100
Colon-specific antigen	83–100
Colon/ovary tumor antigen	76–97
CD44S	71–100
S-100	62–86
PRP	64–78
ERP	63–75
BCA-225	54–83
CA 19-9	52–73
Vimentin	36–61
CD44V6	23–67
Carcinoembryonic antigen (p)	5–16
CK20	0–10

Although *TP53* mutation may be associated with the evolution of a few cervical carcinomas,[120] the vast majority (about 90%) of these tumors result from the consequences of infection with human papillomaviruses (HPVs). A detailed discussion of the mechanisms by which HPVs cause cervical cancer is beyond the scope of this chapter. Nevertheless, it appears that proteins coded by the *E6* and *E7* genes of "high-risk" HPVs (types 16 and 18) can cause cellular transformation, apparently by binding to the p53 protein (E6) or the retinoblastoma protein (E7), thus disrupting DNA repair and cell cycle control pathways.[121–123] Survival appears to be shorter in patients with invasive cervical carcinomas who harbor HPV 18 rather than HPV 16[124,125]; survival is also shorter for patients who demonstrate integration of HPV into the carcinoma cell genome,[125–127] an event that appears to be particularly common in HPV 18 infections. Several HPVs that are commonly found in the genital tract (types 31, 33, 35, 45, 51, 52, and 56) have been associated with an intermediate risk of cervical cancer, whereas others (types 6, 11, 42, 43, and 44) are associated with a low cervical cancer risk. The various methods by which HPV infections can be diagnosed and typed are discussed in Chapter 17.

Mutations of *TP53* are uncommon in cervical cancer, but mutations of *HRAS*, *NRAS*, and *KRAS* have been frequently reported.[128–132] The significance of these findings to tumor pathogenesis is unknown, and there is no evidence that identification of *RAS* gene sequences carries prognostic information for patients with cervical cancer.

Large studies intended to demonstrate the clinical use of cytometric assessment of tumor aneuploidy or S-phase fraction have given conflicting results,[133–136] perhaps reflecting the highly variable experimental methods and approaches to interpretation. Studies of immunohistochemical proliferation markers, such as Ki-67 (MIB1) have not demonstrated use in predicting outcome.[137] For the most part, studies have also failed to find clinical use for p53 immunohistochemistry.[138–142] Although some studies have suggested that BCL2 positivity is associated with favorable prognosis,[143–145] other large studies have failed to confirm clinical use for BCL2 staining of cervical carcinoma.[146] Estrogen and progesterone receptors are expressed in 20% to 30% of cervical adenocarcinomas; expression is not associated with survival.[147] Immunohistochemical demonstration of *ERBB2* overexpression in cervical carcinoma has been associated with poor prognosis,[148–152] as has overexpression of the closely related tyrosine kinase receptor EGFR.[153] Other studies provide conflicting results, however, suggesting that differences in the way the assay is performed and interpreted may have a significant effect on the clinical use of this immunohistochemical test.[154] Demonstration of *ERBB2* amplification, while frequent in cervical cancer,[155, 156] has yet to be associated with clinical outcome.

Current theories of metastatic spread suggest that at least two elements—tumor-induced angiogenesis and tissue invasion—are required for tumors to metastasize. High levels of tumor-induced angiogenesis, as assessed by microvessel density, have been associated with poor survival in patients with adenocarcinoma of the cervix.[157] Its significance in squamous cell carcinoma is uncertain, because some studies have suggested prognostic importance[158] whereas others have not.[159] Failure to express *NME1 (NM23)* a putative "metastasis-suppressor" gene, has also been associated with metastasis and decreased survival,[148, 160] but *NME1* has not been proven to have independent prognostic value when information on tumor size, vessel invasion, and lymph node metastasis is available.[161] Finally, expression of matrix metalloproteinases (MMPs), such as MMP-9, although theoretically important in the process of metastasis, has not proven to be clinically useful as a prognostic marker.[162]

SMOOTH MUSCLE TUMORS OF THE UTERUS

Leiomyoma

Leiomyomas are frequently occurring, benign, monoclonal neoplasms that, nevertheless, result in considerable morbidity in the older female population.[163] Over 300 karyotypes from uterine leiomyomas have been reported,[92, 164–168] and clonal cytogenetic changes are observed in approximately one third of uterine leiomyomas that are cultured.[93] The most characteristic rearrangement is t(12;14)(q14–15;q23–24), which represents approximately 15% of all abnormalities. Deletion of the long arm of chromosome 7 is also frequently reported, as is trisomy 12.[169] A variety of less common abnormalities, including rearrangements of 1p and 6p, have been observed. Complex karyotypes are more frequently observed in hypercellular tumors and in those exhibiting mitotic figures. CGH studies have revealed genetic alterations in only a minority of cases—typically gains on chromosomes 14 and 19 and losses on chromosomes 1 and 4.[170] These studies provide no evidence for progression from leiomyoma to leiomyosarcoma.[170] This is somewhat surprising in view of the fact that classic karyotyping often reveals cytogenetic changes in leiomyosarcoma that are similar to those seen in leiomyoma.[93]

LOH studies have yet to demonstrate frequent allelic deletion in any region of the genome, save perhaps chromosome 7q, which demonstrates loss in from 9% to 34% of cases.[171–174] As yet, no specific gene in this region has been definitively linked to the development of leiomyoma, however.

Diagnosis of leiomyoma is straightforward, and immunohistochemical stains are almost never warranted in their evaluation. Table 12–4 delineates the immunohistochemical profile associated with these tumors and others originating from smooth muscle.

Leiomyosarcoma

In contrast to leiomyoma, leiomyosarcoma is an uncommon, but highly aggressive, malignancy. Few karyotypes are available for analysis, but clonal karyotypic abnormalities have been reported in half of these.[93] Chromosomes 1, 7, 10, and 17 are most frequently abnormal, but no single anomaly is commonly described.[92] CGH studies show both gains and losses, with the most common aberrations being gains on both arms of chromosome 1.[170] The significance of this finding is unknown. LOH studies demonstrate frequent allelic loss on both arms of chromosome 10, which is not seen in leiomyomas[175]; there does not appear to be any relationship between LOH and either outcome or morphologic features of malignancy. The hypothesis that cytogenetic alterations may have a relationship with outcome in patients with uterine smooth muscle tumors is bolstered, however, by the observation that patients whose leiomyosarcomas demonstrate aneuploidy or elevated S-phase fraction have a worse prognosis than those whose tumors do not demonstrate these findings.[176–179]

Gene sequence analysis has demonstrated *TP53* mutationsin about one third of uterine leiomyosarcomas,[180–183] but there is little evidence that these changes are etiologic. *HRAS* mutations have not been reported.[181]

TABLE 12–4

Selected Immunohistochemical Staining Characteristics of Uterine Smooth Muscle Tumors

Antigen	Percentage of Cases Demonstrating Immunoreactivity
Actin-HHF35	90–95
Actin-SM	88–94
Vimentin	83–90
Desmin	71–78
Estrogen receptor protein	41–83
CD68	30–47
AE1	13–32
α_1-Antichymotrypsin	10–28
CD99	9–28
CD34	11–21
CAM5.2	6–21
Keratin (pan)	6–15
HMB-45	2–14
S-100	3–9
CD5	0–12
CD31	0–4
CD57	0
Epithelial membrane antigen	0
Myoglobin	0
Factor VIII–related antigen	0

Leiomyosarcoma is usually easily distinguished from leiomyoma by a relative abundance of mitotic figures. Leiomyosarcoma generally demonstrates higher immunoreactivity for MIB1 (Ki-67) than does leiomyoma.[184] Patients whose tumors are diploid by flow cytometry have a better overall survival than do those whose tumors are aneuploid,[179] but neither ploidy nor proliferation rate is absolutely predictive of outcome in an individual patient.[185]

Gestational Trophoblastic Disease

Hydatidiform moles, their invasive counterparts, and choriocarcinoma represent a spectrum of neoplastic diseases that arise from products of conception "gone awry." The "complete mole" is characterized histologically by the absence of an embryo or fetus, conspicuous trophoblastic hyperplasia, and the formation of numerous large cisternae. The complete mole has a diploid chromosome complement that is entirely paternal in origin.[93, 186–188] In contrast, the "partial mole" is often associated with an embryo or fetus and a partially molar placenta; the partial mole typically has a triploid chromosome complement.[93,189] Because complete moles are much more likely to evolve into gestational choriocarcinoma than are partial moles, it is important to distinguish between the two, a process that can sometimes be aided considerably by flow or image cytometric determination of ploidy.[190–194] Interphase cytogenetic methods, such as FISH, provide an alternative approach for determining whether an abnormal chromosome number is present.[192, 195]

Gestational choriocarcinoma is a highly aggressive tumor that, fortunately, is usually responsive to chemotherapy.[196] Very few karyotypic results have been reported,[93, 197] and no general conclusions can be drawn. Neither CGH nor LOH studies have been reported.

Although *TP53* mutations have been reported in a hydatidiform mole,[198] there is no evidence for any specific genetic event in the evolution of gestational choriocarcinoma from complete moles. Complete moles and gestational choriocarcinomas both show stronger immunohistochemical staining for both the p53 protein and the *RB1* gene product than do partial moles,[199] suggesting the possibility of defects in cell cycle regulation or DNA repair. Similarly, complete moles and choriocarcinomas frequently overexpress MYC, ERBB2, and BCL2 when compared with partial moles.[200] Nevertheless, neither oncoprotein nor tumor suppressor gene expression appears to be useful in predicting which molar pregnancies will develop into persistent gestational trophoblastic disease (invasive mole or choriocarcinoma). Outcome of patients with choriocarcinoma is best predicted on the basis of clinical considerations alone.[201] Immunohistochemistry may occasionally prove useful in the characterization of metastatic diseases, however. The immunohistochemical profile of choriocarcinoma is thus shown in Table 12–5.

TUMORS OF THE OVARY

Sex Cord Stromal Tumors

A variety of neoplasms may develop from ovarian stroma, including tumors that secrete estrogens (granulosa-theca cell tumors) or androgens (Sertoli-Leydig cell tumors) or that demonstrate fibroblastic differentiation (fibroma-thecomas). These tumors are cytogenetically similar. The karyotypes are simple, typically exhibiting only numerical abnormalities. Of these, trisomy 12 is most frequent,[92, 202–204] although trisomy 14[205] and monosomy 22[206] have both been reported, as has a translocation, t(6;16).[207]

Although neither karyotypic analysis nor FISH studies have shown evidence of gross cytogenetic abnormalities, flow cytometry has demonstrated the presence of an aneuploid cell population in about one third of granulosa cell tumors.[208–212] The relationship between tumor aneuploidy and outcome is uncertain; patients with high S-phase fractions are at a significantly higher risk of recurrence, metastases, and death.[208, 209] The relationship between high S-phase fraction and reduced survival is buttressed by the finding that high mitotic index and high levels of Ki-67 expression are both associated with poor outcome.[213] In contrast, immunohistochemical staining for p53, MYC, HRAS, and ERBB2 provides no useful prognostic information.[213, 214]

Given the nonspecific cytogenetic findings, it is not surprising that virtually nothing is known regarding the molecular alterations underlying these tumors.[215, 216]

TABLE 12–5

Selected Immunohistochemical Staining Characteristics of Choriocarcinoma

Antigen	Percentage of Cases Demonstrating Immunoreactivity
β-Human chorionic gonadotropin (β-HCG)	100
Cytokeratin (pan)	100
Epithelial membrane antigen	38–71
Placental alkaline phosphatase	35–61
Neuron-specific enolase	26–66
α_1-Antitrypsin	14–52
Carcinoembryonic antigen (polyclonal)	5-33
Vimentin	0-9
α-Fetoprotein	0
S-100	0

Cystadenoma

Cytogenetic and molecular analysis of benign ovarian surface epithelial tumors has yielded limited insight into these tumors. Trisomy 12 has been found in four cystadenomas characterized by classic karyotyping[217]; a FISH study failed to confirm these findings in 20 tumors.[203] These results contrast to studies of mucinous cystadenomas that demonstrated chromosomal aberrations in nearly two thirds of cases by interphase cytogenetic methods.[218] CGH studies are not available. LOH has not been reported in studies of chromosomes 6q, 13p, 13q, 17p, nor 17q, although these regions are the frequent sites of alteration in ovarian carcinomas.[219, 220]

KRAS mutations have been reported in over half of both benign and malignant mucinous ovarian tumors[221]; in contrast, *KRAS* mutation is found only in about 20% of serous cystadenomas.[222] Microdissection of mucinous cystadenomas, followed by analysis of *KRAS* mutation patterns, demonstrates a heterogeneous distribution of cells demonstrating this mutation throughout the tumors.[223] These results suggest that although *KRAS* mutation is not the initial step in the pathogenesis of mucinous cystadenoma, it may be important in the development of the mucinous phenotype. *TP53* mutations have not been observed in ovarian cystadenomas,[224] nor is accumulation of p53 protein observed immunohistochemically.[225]

Serous Borderline Tumor

Borderline tumors of the ovary demonstrate cellular atypia and proliferation but, because they are not invasive, carry a much more favorable prognosis than other neoplasms of the ovarian surface epithelium. Only a few karyotypes have been reported[226, 227]; in several of the karyotypes, nonrandom cytogenetic abnormalities (trisomy 2, 7, and 12) have been observed; structural chromosomal changes were not reported. FISH studies confirm the frequent presence of trisomy 12 in these tumors[228, 229] and the occasional presence of trisomy 7.[203, 229] Trisomy 12 is uncommon in overtly malignant ovarian epithelial tumors and thus appears to be a relatively specific marker for tumors of low malignant potential. FISH studies of borderline tumors also suggest frequent loss of the telomeric region of chromosome 6, but this finding is also common in more aggressive ovarian malignancies.[230] Cytometric studies have shown that both euploid and grossly aneuploid borderline tumors occur and that ploidy is not predictive of clinical outcome.[231–234]

Only about 10% of borderline tumors demonstrate LOH at any site by microsatellite analysis.[220, 235–238] These studies do not suggest any specific locus as a site for a tumor-associated suppressor gene. X-inactivation studies suggest that these tumors are polyclonal in origin, in contrast to invasive serous tumors, which are monoclonal.[239] There is also evidence that many borderline tumors demonstrate inactivation (primarily by interstitial deletion) of one or more loci in the inactive copy of Xq.[219] This change is apparently not seen in invasive carcinomas, although deletions of Xq12 in the region of the androgen receptor are found in both borderline and invasive tumors. Mutations of *TP53* appear to be very uncommon,[240–243] but mutation of *KRAS* is reported in almost half of borderline tumors.[244] Methylation of the *CDKN2A* and *MYOD1* loci have, however, been observed in about half of the borderline tumors tested, suggesting that suppression of gene activity by this mechanism plays a role in the pathogenesis of these tumors.[241, 245, 246] Telomerase activity has also been observed in almost all borderline tumors,[247–249] although at lower levels than typically seen in invasive serous carcinomas.

Immunohistochemical studies suggest overexpression of p53 in fewer than 10% of cases.[250–252] In contrast, immunoreactivity for EGFR is common.[253] Nevertheless, the role of EGFR in the pathogenesis of borderline tumors remains obscure.

Cystadenocarcinoma

Although a large number of ovarian adenocarcinoma karyotypes have been analyzed and reported, most reported karyotypes are not accompanied by histologic classification. Furthermore, these karyotypes have, for the most part, been derived from abdominal effusions and thus represent a very late stage of ovarian neoplasia.[92] Most tumors have complex karyotypes; the most common numerical changes were losses of chromosome X, 22, 18, 14, 13, and 8; gains are far less common.[92, 254, 254–258] Rearrangements most commonly involve 19p13, 19q13, and 6q21. There is clearly no specific chromosomal rearrangement found in a significant percentage of cases, although the presence of a 19p+ marker chromosome is found in nearly half of all cases.[259] The aneuploidy observed in karyograms is also observed in two thirds of ovarian tumors by flow cytometry; there is some evidence that patients with euploid tumors have a somewhat better prognosis than those whose tumors are aneuploid.[260, 261]

CGH studies confirm the presence of frequent chromosomal gains of 1q, 2p, 7q, 8q, and 17q, with losses of 8p, 9p, and 13q most frequently reported.[262] There is some suggestion of karyotypic-cytogenetic correlation, but the number of specimens examined has been too small to draw definitive conclusions.

Immortalization occurs in some tumor systems by means of increased telomerase activity. Telomerase activity is found in virtually all ovarian carcinomas and borderline tumors but is not found in cystadenomas.[263]

Among the oncogenes for which amplification in ovarian carcinoma has been reported are *ERBB2*,[264] cyclin D1,[265] cyclin A,[265] and *MDM2*.[266] In contrast to breast carcinoma, there is no evidence that *ERBB2* amplification or overexpression influences survival in ovarian carcinoma[267]; it seems likely that useful prognostic information will come from determining amplification of other genes, because overall survival is so poor in ovarian cancers.

LOH studies have detected allelic deletions from chromosomes 3p, 4p, 6q, 8q, 11p, 12, 16, 17, and 19p.[92] Allelic deletion in the region of 11p15.4-11p15.5 has been associated with a poor prognosis[268]; this is a region in which allelic deletion is commonly found in a large variety of cancers. A variety of genes, including *DCC*, *KRAS2*, *TP53*, *BRCA1*, *BRCA2*, *CDKN2A*, and *LKB1* are found in the regions of reported deletions. Mutations of *TP53* are particularly frequent, occurring in approximately 30% of carcinomas.[269] The frequency of mutations increases with increasing tumor grade and stage; neither mutation nor p53 protein accumulation provides useful prognostic information.[269–271]

Mutations of *KRAS2* are particularly common in ovarian cystadenocarcinoma but are also frequently identified in cystadenomas and borderline tumors; they are significantly more common in mucinous tumors (75% of cases) than in other histologic subtypes (15% of cases).[272] *KRAS2* mutations are more common in mucinous tumors of low malignant potential than in mucinous cystadenocarcinomas, suggesting a different molecular pathogenesis.[273] The presence of *KRAS2* point mutations does not correlate with survival in serous tumors.[222]

Mutations of *DCC*, *LKB1*, *BRCA1*, *BRCA2*, and *CDKN2A* are rare in sporadic ovarian carcinoma.[274–277] Immunocytochemical investigations suggest that loss of DCC protein expression,[278] loss of E-cadherin protein expression,[279] and increased expression of vascular endothelial growth factor[280] may all be associated with decreased survival in patients with ovarian cancer, but these data must be considered preliminary. Interestingly, elevated expression of the metastasis suppressor protein NME1 has also been associated with decreased survival.[281] This is perplexing because NME1 is believed to inhibit metastasis in other tumor systems. Studies relating outcome to expression of proliferation markers, such as Ki-67 (MIB1), have provided inconclusive results.[282–284]

Immunocytochemical characterization of ovarian carcinoma is most useful when it proves necessary to distinguish tumors arising in the colon from those arising in the ovary. Immunocytochemical staining for CK7 and CEA is sufficient to correctly classify most cases.[285] Over 90% of all mucinous cystadenocarcinomas demonstrate CK7, compared with less than 20% of colon adenocarcinomas; CEA is expressed in twice as many colon cancers as mucinous ovarian cancers.[286]

CARCINOMA OF THE VULVA

Cytogenetic analysis of vulvar squamous cell carcinoma demonstrates complex karyotypic changes, including losses of 3cen-p14, 8q, 10q23-25, 18q22-23, 22q13, and Xp.[92, 287, 288] Tumors demonstrating complex karyotypes are more likely to be biologically aggressive than those demonstrating simpler cytogenetic findings. This finding is corroborated by flow-cytometric measurements, which show increased biologic aggressiveness in Paget's disease of the vulva that demonstrates aneuploidy.[289, 290] Cytometric evaluation of tumor DNA does not appear to provide independently useful prognostic information, however.[291]

Sequence analysis of the *TP53* tumor suppressor gene has given conflicting results, with some authors reporting frequent mutation and overexpression[106, 292, 293] and others reporting *TP53* alterations in a minority of tumors.[294, 295] Vulvar carcinomas are frequently associated with infection by "high-risk" HPV genotypes; binding of HPV proteins can lead to p53 inactivation in these tumors.[294, 295] It appears that *TP53* mutation confers a more aggressive phenotype on these tumors; *TP53* mutations are observed more frequently in tumors that have metastasized to regional lymph nodes than those that have not.[296]

CARCINOMA OF THE VAGINA

Tumors of the vagina are quite rare, but carcinoma (particularly clear cell carcinoma), sarcoma, and malignant melanoma may all occur in this site. Although cytogenetic analyses of some of these tumors has been performed, too few karyotypes are available to draw any general conclusions.[92, 287] Microsatellite instability is apparently common in clear cell carcinoma of the vagina, with virtually all diethylstilbestrol (DES)—associated tumors, and half of non–DES-associated tumors demonstrating microsatellite alterations.[297] Mutations of *KRAS*, *HRAS*, *WT1*, the estrogen receptor gene, and *TP53* have not been observed,[297, 298] although immunohistochemical staining for p53 protein may be found in most cases.[298, 299] The prognostic significance of this finding is unknown.

REFERENCES

1. Devilee P, Cornelisse CJ: Somatic genetic changes in human breast cancer. Biochim Biophys Acta 1994;1198: 113–130.
2. Teixeira MR, Pandis N, Bardi G, et al: Clonal heterogeneity in breast cancer: Karyotypic comparisons of multiple intra- and extra-tumorous samples from 3 patients. Int J Cancer 1995;63:63–68.
3. Teixeira MR, Pandis N, Bardi G, et al: Karyotypic comparisons of multiple tumorous and macroscopically normal surrounding tissue samples from patients with breast cancer. Cancer Res 1996;56:855–859.
4. Tirkkonen M, Tanner M, Karhu R, et al: Molecular cytogenetics of primary breast cancer by CGH. Genes Chromosomes Cancer 1998;21:177–184.

5. Nishizaki T, DeVries S, Chew K, et al: Genetic alterations in primary breast cancers and their metastases: Direct comparison using modified comparative genomic hybridization. Genes Chromosomes Cancer 1997; 19:267–272.
6. Heim S, Teixeira MR, Dietrich CU, Pandis N: Cytogenetic polyclonality in tumors of the breast. Cancer Genet Cytogenet 1997;95:16–19.
7. Teixeira MR, Pandis N, Bardi G, et al: Cytogenetic analysis of multifocal breast carcinomas: Detection of karyotypically unrelated clones as well as clonal similarities between tumour foci. Br J Cancer 1994;70: 922–927.
8. Pandis N, Heim S, Bardi G, et al: Chromosome analysis of 20 breast carcinomas: Cytogenetic multiclonality and karyotypic-pathologic correlations. Genes Chromosomes Cancer 1993;6:51–57.
9. Teixeira MR, Pandis N, Bardi G, et al: Discrimination between multicentric and multifocal breast carcinoma by cytogenetic investigation of macroscopically distinct ipsilateral lesions. Genes Chromosomes Cancer 1997; 18:170–174.
10. Fujii H, Marsh C, Cairns P, et al: Genetic divergence in the clonal evolution of breast cancer. Cancer Res 1996;56:1493–1497.
11. Kuukasjarvi T, Karhu R, Tanner M, et al: Genetic heterogeneity and clonal evolution underlying development of asynchronous metastasis in human breast cancer. Cancer Res 1997;57:1597–1604.
12. Kuukasjarvi T, Tanner M, Pennanen S, et al: Genetic changes in intraductal breast cancer detected by comparative genomic hybridization. Am J Pathol 1997;150: 1465–1471.
13. Deng G, Lu Y, Zlotnikov G, et al: Loss of heterozygosity in normal tissue adjacent to breast carcinomas. Science 1996;274:2057–2059.
14. Larson PS, De Las M, Cupples LA, et al: Genetically abnormal clones in histologically normal breast tissue. Am J Pathol 1998;152:1591–1598.
15. Petersson C, Pandis N, Rizou H, et al: Karyotypic abnormalities in fibroadenomas of the breast. Int J Cancer 1997;70:282–286.
16. Dietrich CU, Pandis N, Teixeira MR, et al: Chromosome abnormalities in benign hyperproliferative disorders of epithelial and stromal breast tissue. Int J Cancer 1995;60:49–53.
17. Kasami M, Vnencak-Jones CL, Manning S, et al: Loss of heterozygosity and microsatellite instability in breast hyperplasia: No obligate correlation of these genetic alterations with subsequent malignancy. Am J Pathol 1997;150:1925–1932.
18. Rosenberg CL, Larson PS, Romo JD, et al: Microsatellite alterations indicating monoclonality in atypical hyperplasias associated with breast cancer. Hum Pathol 1997;28: 214–219.
19. Rosenberg CL, De Las M, Huang K, et al: Detection of monoclonal microsatellite alterations in atypical breast hyperplasia. J Clin Invest 1996;98:1095–1100.
20. Petersson C, Pandis N, Mertens F, et al: Chromosome aberrations in prophylactic mastectomies from women belonging to breast cancer families. Genes Chromosomes Cancer 1996;16:185–188.
21. Roos G, Nilsson P, Cajander S, et al: Telomerase activity in relation to p53 status and clinico-pathological parameters in breast cancer. Int J Cancer 1998;79:343–348.
22. Reese DM, Slamon DJ: HER-2/neu signal transduction in human breast and ovarian cancer. Stem Cells 1997;15:1–8.
23. Thor AD, Berry DA, Budman DR, et al: erbB-2, p53, and efficacy of adjuvant therapy in lymph node-positive breast cancer. J Natl Cancer Inst 1998;90:1346–1360.
24. Muss HB, Thor AD, Berry DA, et al: c-erbB-2 expression and response to adjuvant therapy in women with node-positive early breast cancer [published erratum appears in N Engl J Med 1994 Jul 21;331(3): 211]. N Engl J Med 1994;330:1260–1266.
25. Nelson NJ: Experts debate value of HER2 testing methods [news]. J Natl Cancer Inst 2000;92:292–294.
26. Persons DL, Bui MM, Lowery MC, et al: Fluorescence in situ hybridization (FISH) for detection of *HER-2/neu* amplification in breast cancer: A multicenter portability study. Ann Clin Lab Sci 2000;30:41–48.
27. Wang S, Saboorian MH, Frenkel E, et al: Laboratory assessment of the status of Her-2/neu protein and oncogene in breast cancer specimens: Comparison of immunohistochemistry assay with fluorescence in situ hybridisation assays. J Clin Pathol 2000;53:374–381.
28. Miyakis S, Sourvinos G, Spandidos DA: Differential expression and mutation of the *ras* family genes in human breast cancer. Biochem Biophys Res Commun 1998;251:609–612.
29. Rhei E, Kang L, Bogomolniy F, et al: Mutation analysis of the putative tumor suppressor gene *PTEN/MMAC1* in primary breast carcinomas. Cancer Res 1997;57:3657–3659.
30. Bergers E, Baak JP, van Diest PJ, et al: Prognostic implications of different cell cycle analysis models of flow cytometric DNA histograms of 1,301 breast cancer patients: Results from the Multicenter Morphometric Mammary Carcinoma Project (MMMCP). Int J Cancer 1997;74:260–269.
31. Romero H, Schneider J, Burgos J, et al: S-phase fraction identifies high-risk subgroups among DNA-diploid breast cancers. Breast Cancer Res Treat 1996;38:265–275.
32. Bozzetti C, Nizzoli R, Camisa R, et al: Comparison between Ki-67 index and S-phase fraction on fine-needle aspiration samples from breast carcinoma. Cancer 1997;81:287–292.
33. Keshgegian AA, Cnaan A: Proliferation markers in breast carcinoma: Mitotic figure count, S-phase fraction, proliferating cell nuclear antigen, Ki-67 and MIB-1. Am J Clin Pathol 1995;104:42–49.
34. Ostrowski ML, Chakraborty S, Laucirica R, et al: Quantitative image analysis of MIB-1 immunoreactivity: A comparison with flow cytometric assessment of proliferative activity in invasive carcinoma of the breast. Anal Quant Cytol Histol 1995;17:15–24.
35. Jares P, Rey MJ, Fernandez PL, et al: Cyclin D1 and retinoblastoma gene expression in human breast carcinoma: Correlation with tumour proliferation and oestrogen receptor status. J Pathol 1997;182:160–166.
36. Gillett C, Smith P, Gregory W, et al: Cyclin D1 and prognosis in human breast cancer. Int J Cancer 1996; 69:92–99.
37. Pelosio P, Barbareschi M, Bonoldi E, et al: Clinical significance of cyclin D1 expression in patients with node-

positive breast carcinoma treated with adjuvant therapy. Ann Oncol 1996;7:695–703.

38. Brenner AJ, Aldaz CM: Chromosome 9p allelic loss and p16/CDKN2 in breast cancer and evidence of p16 inactivation in immortal breast epithelial cells. Cancer Res 1995;55:2892–2895.
39. Davidoff AM, Kerns BJ, Iglehart JD, Marks JR: Maintenance of p53 alterations throughout breast cancer progression. Cancer Res 1991;51:2605–2610.
40. Varley JM, Brammar WJ, Lane DP, et al: Loss of chromosome 17p13 sequences and mutation of *p53* in human breast carcinomas. Oncogene 1991;6:413–421.
41. Thompson AM, Anderson TJ, Condie A, et al: *p53* allele losses, mutations and expression in breast cancer and their relationship to clinicopathological parameters. Int J Cancer 1992;50:528–532.
42. Osborne RJ, Merlo GR, Mitsudomi T, et al: Mutations in the *p53* gene in primary human breast cancers. Cancer Res 1991;51:6194–6198.
43. Coles C, Condie A, Chetty U, et al: *p53* mutations in breast cancer. Cancer Res 1992;52:5291–5298.
44. Saitoh S, Cunningham J, De Vries EM, et al: *p53* gene mutations in breast cancers in midwestern US women: Null as well as missense-type mutations are associated with poor prognosis. Oncogene 1994;9:2869–2875.
45. Hartmann A, Blaszyk H, McGovern RM, et al: *p53* gene mutations inside and outside of exons 5–8: The patterns differ in breast and other cancers. Oncogene 1995;10:681–688.
46. Biggs PJ, Warren W, Venitt S, Stratton MR: Does a genotoxic carcinogen contribute to human breast cancer? The value of mutational spectra in unravelling the aetiology of cancer. Mutagenesis 1993;8:275–283.
47. Eyfjord JE, Thorlacius S, Steinarsdottir M, et al: *p53* abnormalities and genomic instability in primary human breast carcinomas. Cancer Res 1995;55:646–651.
48. Eyfjord JE, Thorlacius S, Valgardsdottir R, et al: *TP53* abnormalities and genetic instability in breast cancer. Acta Oncol 1995;34:663–667.
49. Deng G, Chen LC, Schott DR, et al: Loss of heterozygosity and *p53* gene mutations in breast cancer. Cancer Res 1994;54:499–505.
50. Andersen TI, Holm R, Nesland JM, et al: Prognostic significance of *TP53* alterations in breast carcinoma. Br J Cancer 1993;68:540–548.
51. Aas T, Borresen AL, Geisler S, et al: Specific *P53* mutations are associated with de novo resistance to doxorubicin in breast cancer patients. Nat Med 1996;2:811–814.
52. O'Malley FP, Saad Z, Kerkvliet N, et al: The predictive power of semiquantitative immunohistochemical assessment of *p53* and c-*erb* B-2 in lymph node-negative breast cancer. Hum Pathol 1996;27:955–963.
53. Visscher DW, Castellani R, Wykes SM, et al: Concurrent abnormal expression of *ERBB-2*, *EGFR*, and *p53* genes and clinical disease progression of breast carcinoma. Breast Cancer Res Treat 1993;28:261–266.
54. Thor AD, Moore DH II, Edgerton SM, et al: Accumulation of *p53* tumor suppressor gene protein: An independent marker of prognosis in breast cancers. J Natl Cancer Inst 1992;84:845–855.
55. Beck T, Weller EE, Weikel W, et al: Usefulness of immunohistochemical staining for p53 in the prognosis of breast carcinomas: Correlations with established prognosis parameters and with the proliferation marker, MIB-1. Gynecol Oncol 1995;57:96–104.
56. Eissa S, Khalifa A, el-Gharib A, et al: Multivariate analysis of DNA ploidy, p53, c-erbB-2 proteins, EGFR, and steroid hormone receptors for prediction of poor short term prognosis in breast cancer. Anticancer Res 1997;17:1417–1423.
57. Gasparini G, Weidner N, Bevilacqua P, et al: Tumor microvessel density, p53 expression, tumor size, and peritumoral lymphatic vessel invasion are relevant prognostic markers in node-negative breast carcinoma. J Clin Oncol 1994;12:454–466.
58. Barnes DM, Dublin EA, Fisher CJ, et al: Immunohistochemical detection of p53 protein in mammary carcinoma: An important new independent indicator of prognosis? Hum Pathol 1993;24:469–476.
59. Berx G, Cleton-Jansen AM, Nollet F, et al: E-cadherin is a tumour/invasion suppressor gene mutated in human lobular breast cancers. EMBO J 1995;14:6107–6115.
60. Berx G, Cleton-Jansen AM, Strumane K, et al: E-cadherin is inactivated in a majority of invasive human lobular breast cancers by truncation mutations throughout its extracellular domain. Oncogene 1996;13:1919–1925.
61. Berx G, Nollet F, van Roy F: Dysregulation of the E-cadherin/catenin complex by irreversible mutations in human carcinomas. Cell Adhes Commun 1998;6:171–184.
62. Vos CB, Cleton-Jansen AM, Berx G, et al: E-cadherin inactivation in lobular carcinoma in situ of the breast: An early event in tumorigenesis. Br J Cancer 1997;76:1131–1133.
63. Charpin C, Garcia S, Bonnier P, et al: Reduced E-cadherin immunohistochemical expression in node-negative breast carcinomas correlates with 10-year survival. Am J Clin Pathol 1998;109:431–438.
64. Guriec N, Marcellin L, Gairard B, et al: E-cadherin mRNA expression in breast carcinomas correlates with overall and disease-free survival. Invasion Metastasis 1996;16:19–26.
65. Siitonen SM, Kononen JT, Helin HJ, et al: Reduced E-cadherin expression is associated with invasiveness and unfavorable prognosis in breast cancer. Am J Clin Pathol 1996;105:394–402.
66. Bertin N, Clezardin P, Kubiak R, Frappart L: Thrombospondin-1 and -2 messenger RNA expression in normal, benign, and neoplastic human breast tissues: Correlation with prognostic factors, tumor angiogenesis, and fibroblastic desmoplasia. Cancer Res 1997;57:396–399.
67. Weidner N: Current pathologic methods for measuring intratumoral microvessel density within breast carcinoma and other solid tumors. Breast Cancer Res Treat 1995;36:169–180.
68. Weidner N, Gasparini G: Determination of epidermal growth factor receptor provides additional prognostic information to measuring tumor angiogenesis in breast carcinoma patients. Breast Cancer Res Treat 1994;29:97–107.
69. Weidner N: Tumor angiogenesis: Review of current applications in tumor prognostication. Semin Diagn Pathol 1993;10:302–313.
70. Weidner N, Folkman J, Pozza F, et al: Tumor angiogenesis: A new significant and independent prognostic indicator in early-stage breast carcinoma. J Natl Cancer Inst 1992;84:1875–1887.

71. Weidner N, Semple JP, Welch WR, Folkman J: Tumor angiogenesis and metastasis—correlation in invasive breast carcinoma. N Engl J Med 1991;324:1–8.
72. Bosari S, Lee AK, DeLellis RA, et al: Microvessel quantitation and prognosis in invasive breast carcinoma. Hum Pathol 1992;23:755–761.
73. Costello P, McCann A, Carney DN, Dervan PA: Prognostic significance of microvessel density in lymph node negative breast carcinoma. Hum Pathol 1995;26: 1181–1184.
74. Siitonen SM, Haapasalo HK, Rantala IS, et al: Comparison of different immunohistochemical methods in the assessment of angiogenesis: Lack of prognostic value in a group of 77 selected node-negative breast carcinomas. Mod Pathol 1995;8:745–752.
75. Hansen S, Grabau DA, Rose C, et al: Angiogenesis in breast cancer: A comparative study of the observer variability of methods for determining microvessel density. Lab Invest 1998;78:1563–1573.
76. Watson MA, Darrow C, Zimonjic DB, et al:. Structure and transcriptional regulation of the human mammaglobin gene, a breast cancer–associated member of the uteroglobin gene family localized to chromosome 11q13. Oncogene 1998;16:817–824.
77. Min CJ, Tafra L, Verbanac KM: Identification of superior markers for polymerase chain reaction detection of breast cancer metastases in sentinel lymph nodes. Cancer Res 1998;58:4581–4584.
78. Bejarano PA, Baughman RP, Biddinger PW, et al: Surfactant proteins and thyroid transcription factor-1 in pulmonary and breast carcinomas. Mod Pathol 1996;9: 445–452.
79. Perry A, Parisi JE, Kurtin PJ: Metastatic adenocarcinoma to the brain: An immunohistochemical approach. Hum Pathol 1997;28:938–943.
80. Brown RW, Campagna LB, Dunn JK, Cagle PT: Immunohistochemical identification of tumor markers in metastatic adenocarcinoma: A diagnostic adjunct in the determination of primary site. Am J Clin Pathol 1997;107:12–19.
81. Heim S, Mitelman F: Tumors of the breast. *In* Heim S, Mitelman F (eds): Cancer Cytogenetics. New York, Wiley-Liss, 1995, pp 369–388.
82. Ozisik YY, Meloni AM, Stephenson CF, et al: Chromosome abnormalities in breast fibroadenomas. Cancer Genet Cytogenet 1994;77:125–128.
83. Rohen C, Staats B, Bonk U, et al: Significance of clonal chromosome aberrations in breast fibroadenomas. Cancer Genet Cytogenet 1996;87:152–155.
84. Ried T, Just KE, Holtgreve-Grez H, et al: Comparative genomic hybridization of formalin-fixed, paraffin-embedded breast tumors reveals different patterns of chromosomal gains and losses in fibroadenomas and diploid and aneuploid carcinomas. Cancer Res 1995;55:5415–5423.
85. el-Naggar AK, Mackay B, Sneige N, Batsakis JG: Stromal neoplasms of the breast: A comparative flow cytometric study. J Surg Oncol 1990;44:151–156.
86. Euhus DM, Maitra A, Wistuba II, et al: Loss of heterozygosity at 3p in benign lesions preceding invasive breast cancer. J Surg Res 1999;83:13–18.
87. McCulloch RK, Sellner LN, Papadimitrou JM, Turbett GR: The incidence of microsatellite instability and loss of heterozygosity in fibroadenoma of the breast. Breast Cancer Res Treat 1998;49:165–169.
88. Millikan R, Hulka B, Thor A, et al: *p53* mutations in benign breast tissue. J Clin Oncol 1995;13:2293–2300.
89. Hiyama E, Gollahon L, Kataoka T, et al: Telomerase activity in human breast tumors. J Natl Cancer Inst 1996;88:116–122.
90. Poremba C, Bocker W, Willenbring H, et al: Telomerase activity in human proliferative breast lesions. Int J Oncol 1998;12:641–648.
91. Yashima K, Milchgrub S, Gollahon LS, et al: Telomerase enzyme activity and RNA expression during the multistage pathogenesis of breast carcinoma. Clin Cancer Res 1998;4:229–234.
92. Heim S, Mitelman F: Tumors of the female genital organs. *In* Heim S, Mitelman F (eds): Cancer Cytogenetics. New York, Wiley-Liss, 1995, pp 389–407.
93. Surti U, Hoffner L: Cytogenetic markers in selected gynecologic malignancies. *In* Wolman SR, Sell S (eds): Human Cytogenetic Cancer Markers. Totawa, NJ, Humana, 1997, pp 203–221.
94. Pere H, Tapper J, Wahlstrom T, et al: Distinct chromosomal imbalances in uterine serous and endometrioid carcinomas. Cancer Res 1998;58:892–895.
95. Sonoda G, du MS, Godwin AK, et al: Detection of DNA gains and losses in primary endometrial carcinomas by comparative genomic hybridization. Genes Chromosomes Cancer 1997;18:115–125.
96. Kihana T, Yano N, Murao S, et al: Allelic loss of chromosome 16q in endometrial cancer: Correlation with poor prognosis of patients and less differentiated histology. Jpn J Cancer Res 1996;87:1184–1190.
97. Tritz D, Pieretti M, Turner S, Powell D: Loss of heterozygosity in usual and special variant carcinomas of the endometrium. Hum Pathol 1997;28:607–612.
98. Ronnett BM, Burks RT, Cho KR, Hedrick L: *DCC* genetic alterations and expression in endometrial carcinoma. Mod Pathol 1997;10:38–46.
99. Monk BJ, Chapman JA, Johnson GA, et al: Correlation of C-*myc* and *HER-2/neu* amplification and expression with histopathologic variables in uterine corpus cancer. Am J Obstet Gynecol 1994;171:1193–1198.
100. Rolitsky CD, Theil KS, McGaughy VR, et al: *HER-2/neu* amplification and overexpression in endometrial carcinoma. Int J Gynecol Pathol 1999;18:138–143.
101. Berchuck A, Rodriguez G, Kinney RB, et al: Overexpression of *HER-2/neu* in endometrial cancer is associated with advanced stage disease. Am J Obstet Gynecol 1991;164(1 pt 1):15–21.
102. Khalifa MA, Mannel RS, Haraway SD, et al: Expression of *EGFR*, *HER-2/neu*, *P53*, and *PCNA* in endometrioid, serous papillary, and clear cell endometrial adenocarcinomas. Gynecol Oncol 1994;53:84–92.
103. Duggan BD, Felix JC, Muderspach LI, et al: Early mutational activation of the c-Ki-*ras* oncogene in endometrial carcinoma. Cancer Res 1994;54:1604–1607.
104. Mizuuchi H, Nasim S, Kudo R, et al: Clinical implications of K-*ras* mutations in malignant epithelial tumors of the endometrium. Cancer Res 1992;52:2777–2781.
105. Varras MN, Koffa M, Koumantakis E, et al: *Ras* gene mutations in human endometrial carcinoma. Oncology 1996;53:505–510.

106. Berchuck A, Kohler MF, Marks JR, et al: The *p53* tumor suppressor gene frequently is altered in gynecologic cancers. Am J Obstet Gynecol 1994;170(1 pt 1):246–252.
107. Bancher-Todesca D, Gitsch G, Williams KE, et al: p53 protein overexpression: A strong prognostic factor in uterine papillary serous carcinoma. Gynecol Oncol 1998;71:59–63.
108. King SA, Adas AA, LiVolsi VA, et al: Expression and mutation analysis of the *p53* gene in uterine papillary serous carcinoma. Cancer 1995;75:2700–2705.
109. Aarnio M, Sankila R, Pukkala E, et al: Cancer risk in mutation carriers of DNA-mismatch-repair genes. Int J Cancer 1999;81:214–218.
110. Weber TK, Conlon W, Petrelli NJ, et al: Genomic DNA-based *hMSH2* and *hMLH1* mutation screening in 32 Eastern United States hereditary nonpolyposis colorectal cancer pedigrees. Cancer Res 1997;57: 3798–3803.
111. Salvesen HB, Iversen OE, Akslen LA: Identification of high-risk patients by assessment of nuclear Ki-67 expression in a prospective study of endometrial carcinomas. Clin Cancer Res 1998;4:2779–2785.
112. Nordstrom B, Strang P, Lindgren A, et al: Carcinoma of the endometrium: Do the nuclear grade and DNA ploidy provide more prognostic information than do the FIGO and WHO classifications? Int J Gynecol Pathol 1996;15:191–201.
113. Dyas CH, Simmons TK, Ellis CN, et al: Effect of deoxyribonucleic acid ploidy status on survival of patients with carcinoma of the endometrium. Surg Gynecol Obstet 1992;174:133–136.
114. Kirchhoff M, Rose H, Petersen BL, et al: Comparative genomic hybridization reveals a recurrent pattern of chromosomal aberrations in severe dysplasia/carcinoma in situ of the cervix and in advanced-stage cervical carcinoma. Genes Chromosomes Cancer 1999;24:144–150.
115. Heselmeyer K, Schrock E, du MS, et al: Gain of chromosome 3q defines the transition from severe dysplasia to invasive carcinoma of the uterine cervix. Proc Natl Acad Sci USA 1996;93:479–484.
116. Chu TY, Shen CY, Lee HS, Liu HS: Monoclonality and surface lesion-specific microsatellite alterations in premalignant and malignant neoplasia of uterine cervix: A local field effect of genomic instability and clonal evolution. Genes Chromosomes Cancer 1999;24:127–134.
117. Jones MH, Nakamura Y: Deletion mapping of chromosome 3p in female genital tract malignancies using microsatellite polymorphisms. Oncogene 1992;7:1631–1634.
118. Kersemaekers AM, Hermans J, Fleuren GJ, van de Vijver MJ: Loss of heterozygosity for defined regions on chromosomes 3, 11 and 17 in carcinomas of the uterine cervix. Br J Cancer 1998;77:192–200.
119. Kersemaekers AM, Kenter GG, Hermans J, et al: Allelic loss and prognosis in carcinoma of the uterine cervix. Int J Cancer 1998;79:411–417.
120. Busby-Earle RM, Steel CM, Williams AR, et al: *p53* mutations in cervical carcinogenesis—low frequency and lack of correlation with human papillomavirus status. Br J Cancer 1994;69:732–737.
121. Chellappan S, Kraus VB, Kroger B, et al: Adenovirus E1A, simian virus 40 tumor antigen, and human papillomavirus E7 protein share the capacity to disrupt the interaction between transcription factor E2F and the retinoblastoma gene product. Proc Natl Acad Sci USA 1992;89:4549–4553.
122. Howley PM, Munger K, Werness BA, et al: Molecular mechanisms of transformation by the human papillomaviruses. Princess Takamatsu Symp 1989;20:199–206.
123. Howley PM, Scheffner M, Huibregtse J, Munger K: Oncoproteins encoded by the cancer-associated human papillomaviruses target the products of the retinoblastoma and *p53* tumor suppressor genes. Cold Spring Harb Symp Quant Biol 1991;56:149–155.
124. Burger RA, Monk BJ, Kurosaki T, et al: Human papillomavirus type 18: Association with poor prognosis in early stage cervical cancer. J Natl Cancer Inst 1996;88: 1361–1368.
125. Konya J, Veress G, Hernadi Z, et al: Correlation of human papillomavirus 16 and 18 with prognostic factors in invasive cervical neoplasias. J Med Virol 1995;46:1–6.
126. Kalantari M, Karlsen F, Kristensen G, et al: Disruption of the E1 and E2 reading frames of HPV 16 in cervical carcinoma is associated with poor prognosis. Int J Gynecol Pathol 1998;17:146–153.
127. Vernon SD, Unger ER, Miller DL, et al: Association of human papillomavirus type 16 integration in the E2 gene with poor disease-free survival from cervical cancer. Int J Cancer 1997;74:50–56.
128. Dokianakis DN, Sourvinos G, Sakkas S, et al: Detection of HPV and ras gene mutations in cervical smears from female genital lesions. Oncol Rep 1998;5:1195–1198.
129. Enomoto T, Inoue M, Perantoni AO, et al: K-*ras* activation in neoplasms of the human female reproductive tract. Cancer Res 1990;50:6139–6145.
130. Enomoto T, Inoue M, Perantoni AO, et al: K-*ras* activation in premalignant and malignant epithelial lesions of the human uterus. Cancer Res. 1991;51:5308–5314.
131. Grendys ECJ, Barnes WA, Weitzel J, et al: Identification of H, K, and N-*ras* point mutations in stage IB cervical carcinoma. Gynecol Oncol 1997;65:343–347.
132. Wong YF, Chung TK, Cheung TH, et al: Frequent ras gene mutations in squamous cell cervical cancer. Cancer Lett 1995;95:29–32.
133. Kristensen GB, Kaern J, Abeler VM, et al: No prognostic impact of flow-cytometric measured DNA ploidy and S-phase fraction in cancer of the uterine cervix: A prospective study of 465 patients. Gynecol Oncol 1995;57:79–85.
134. Lutgens LC, Schutte B, de Jong JM, Thunnissen FB: DNA content as prognostic factor in cervix carcinoma stage IB-III treated with radiotherapy. Gynecol Oncol 1994;54:275–281.
135. Strang P, Stendahl U, Bergstrom R, et al: Prognostic flow cytometric information in cervical squamous cell carcinoma: A multivariate analysis of 307 patients. Gynecol Oncol 1991;43:3–8.
136. Willen R, Himmelmann A, Langstrom-Einarsson E, et al: Prospective malignancy grading, flow cytometry DNA measurements and adjuvant chemotherapy for invasive squamous cell carcinoma of the uterine cervix. Anticancer Res 1993;13:1187–1196.
137. Avall-Lundqvist EH, Silfversward C, Aspenblad U, et al: The impact of tumour angiogenesis, p53 overexpression and proliferative activity (MIB-1) on survival in squamous cervical carcinoma. Eur J Cancer 1997;33:1799–1804.

138. Dellas A, Schultheiss E, Almendral AC, et al: Altered expression of mdm-2 and its association with p53 protein status, tumor-cell proliferation rate and prognosis in cervical neoplasia. Int J Cancer 1997;74:421–425.
139. Ebara T, Mitsuhashi N, Saito Y, et al: Prognostic significance of immunohistochemically detected p53 protein expression in stage IIIB squamous cell carcinoma of the uterine cervix treated with radiation therapy alone. Gynecol Oncol 1996;63:216–218.
140. Gitsch G, Kainz C, Joura E, Breitenecker G: Mutant p53 product in patients with stage III cervical cancer. Anticancer Res 1992;12:2241–2242.
141. Hunt CR, Hale RJ, Buckley CH, Hunt J: p53 expression in carcinoma of the cervix. J Clin Pathol 1996;49: 971–974.
142. Kainz C, Kohlberger P, Gitsch G, et al: Mutant *p53* in patients with invasive cervical cancer stages IB to IIB. Gynecol Oncol 1995;57:212–214.
143. Crawford RA, Caldwell C, Iles RK, et al: Prognostic significance of the bcl-2 apoptotic family of proteins in primary and recurrent cervical cancer. Br J Cancer 1998;78: 210–214.
144. Tjalma W, Weyler J, Goovaerts G, et al: Prognostic value of bcl-2 expression in patients with operable carcinoma of the uterine cervix. J Clin Pathol 1997;50:33–36.
145. Tjalma W, De Cuyper E, Weyler J, et al: Expression of bcl-2 in invasive and in situ carcinoma of the uterine cervix. Am J Obstet Gynecol 1998;178:113–117.
146. Uehara T, Kuwashima Y, Izumo T, et al: Expression of the proto-oncogene bcl-2 in uterine cervical squamous cell carcinoma: Its relationship to clinical outcome. Eur J Gynaecol Oncol 1995;16:453–460.
147. Fujiwara H, Tortolero-Luna G, Mitchell MF, et al: Adenocarcinoma of the cervix: Expression and clinical significance of estrogen and progesterone receptors. Cancer 1997;79:505–512.
148. Mandai M, Konishi I, Koshiyama M, et al: Altered expression of nm23-H1 and c-erbB-2 proteins have prognostic significance in adenocarcinoma but not in squamous cell carcinoma of the uterine cervix. Cancer 1995;75:2523–2529.
149. Nakano T, Oka K, Ishikawa A, Morita S: Correlation of cervical carcinoma c-erb B-2 oncogene with cell proliferation parameters in patients treated with radiation therapy for cervical carcinoma. Cancer 1997;79: 513–520.
150. Nishioka T, West CM, Gupta N, et al: Prognostic significance of c-erbB-2 protein expression in carcinoma of the cervix treated with radiotherapy. J Cancer Res Clin Oncol 1999;125:96–100.
151. Oka K, Nakano T, Arai T: c-erbB-2 oncoprotein expression is associated with poor prognosis in squamous cell carcinoma of the cervix. Cancer 1994;73:664–671.
152. Kihana T, Tsuda H, Teshima S, et al: Prognostic significance of the overexpression of c-erbB-2 protein in adenocarcinoma of the uterine cervix. Cancer 1994;73: 148–153.
153. Hale RJ, Buckley CH, Gullick WJ, et al: Prognostic value of epidermal growth factor receptor expression in cervical carcinoma. J Clin Pathol 1993;46:149–153.
154. Ndubisi B, Sanz S, Lu L, et al: The prognostic value of *HER-2/neu* oncogene in cervical cancer. Ann Clin Lab Sci 1997;27:396–401.
155. Mitra AB, Murty VV, Pratap M, et al: *ERBB2 (HER2/neu)* oncogene is frequently amplified in squamous cell carcinoma of the uterine cervix. Cancer Res 1994;54: 637–639.
156. Sharma A, Pratap M, Sawhney VM, et al: Frequent amplification of C-*erbB2 (HER-2/Neu)* oncogene in cervical carcinoma as detected by non-fluorescence in situ hybridization technique on paraffin sections. Oncology 1999;56:83–87.
157. Kaku T, Hirakawa T, Kamura T, et al: Angiogenesis in adenocarcinoma of the uterine cervix. Cancer 1998;83: 1384–1390.
158. Schlenger K, Hockel M, Mitze M, et al: Tumor vascularity—a novel prognostic factor in advanced cervical carcinoma. Gynecol Oncol 1995;59:57–66.
159. Rutgers JL, Mattox TF, Vargas MP: Angiogenesis in uterine cervical squamous cell carcinoma. Int J Gynecol Pathol 1995;14:114–118.
160. Sarac E, Ayhan A, Ertoy D, et al: *nm23* expression in carcinoma of the uterine cervix. Eur J Gynaecol Oncol 1998;19:312–315.
161. Kristensen GB, Holm R, Abeler VM, Trope CG: Evaluation of the prognostic significance of nm23/NDP kinase protein expression in cervical carcinoma: An immunohistochemical study. Gynecol Oncol 1996;61: 378–383.
162. Davidson B, Goldberg I, Kopolovic J, et al: Expression of matrix metalloproteinase-9 in squamous cell carcinoma of the uterine cervix-clinicopathologic study using immunohistochemistry and mRNA in situ hybridization. Gynecol Oncol 1999;72:380–386.
163. Hashimoto K, Azuma C, Kamiura S, et al: Clonal determination of uterine leiomyomas by analyzing differential inactivation of the X-chromosome–linked phosphoglycerokinase gene. Gynecol Obstet Invest 1995;40: 204–208.
164. Nibert M, Heim S: Uterine leiomyoma cytogenetics. Genes Chromosomes Cancer 1990;2:3–13.
165. Nilbert M, Heim S, Mandahl N, et al: Ring formation and structural rearrangements of chromosome 1 as secondary changes in uterine leiomyomas with t(12;14)(q14–15; q23–24). Cancer Genet Cytogenet 1988;36:183–90.
166. Nilbert M, Heim S, Mandahl N, et al: Complex karyotypic anomalies in a bizarre leiomyoma of the uterus. Genes Chromosomes Cancer 1989;1:131–134.
167. Rein MS, Friedman AJ, Barbieri RL, et al: Cytogenetic abnormalities in uterine leiomyomata. Obstet Gynecol 1991;77:923–926.
168. Sargent MS, Weremowicz S, Rein MS, Morton CC: Translocations in 7q22 define a critical region in uterine leiomyomata. Cancer Genet Cytogenet 1994;77:65–68.
169. Nilbert M, Heim S, Mandahl N, et al: Trisomy 12 in uterine leiomyomas: A new cytogenetic subgroup. Cancer Genet Cytogenet 1990;45:63–66.
170. Packenham JP, du MS, Schrock E, et al: Analysis of genetic alterations in uterine leiomyomas and leiomyosarcomas by comparative genomic hybridization. Mol Carcinog 1997;19:273–279.
171. Ishwad CS, Ferrell RE, Hanley K, et al: Two discrete regions of deletion at 7q in uterine leiomyomas. Genes Chromosomes Cancer 1997;19:156–160.
172. Mao X, Barfoot R, Hamoudi RA, et al: Allelotype of uterine leiomyomas. Cancer Genet Cytogenet 1999;114: 89–95.

173. Quade BJ, Pinto AP, Howard DR, et al: Frequent loss of heterozygosity for chromosome 10 in uterine leiomyosarcoma in contrast to leiomyoma. Am J Pathol 1999;154:945–950.
174. van der Heijden O, Chiu HC, Park TC, et al: Allelotype analysis of uterine leiomyoma: Localization of a potential tumor suppressor gene to a 4-cM region of chromosome 7q. Mol Carcinog 1998;23:243–247.
175. Quade BJ, Pinto AP, Howard DR, et al: Frequent loss of heterozygosity for chromosome 10 in uterine leiomyosarcoma in contrast to leiomyoma. Am J Pathol 1999;154:945–950.
176. Blom R, Guerrieri C, Stal O, et al: Leiomyosarcoma of the uterus: A clinicopathologic, DNA flow cytometric, p53, and mdm-2 analysis of 49 cases. Gynecol Oncol 1998;68:54–61.
177. Nordal RR, Kristensen GB, Kaern J, et al: The prognostic significance of stage, tumor size, cellular atypia and DNA ploidy in uterine leiomyosarcoma. Acta Oncol 1995;34:797–802.
178. Wolfson AH, Wolfson DJ, Sittler SY, et al: A multivariate analysis of clinicopathologic factors for predicting outcome in uterine sarcomas. Gynecol Oncol 1994;52:56–62.
179. Peters WA, Howard DR, Andersen WA, Figge DC: Deoxyribonucleic acid analysis by flow cytometry of uterine leiomyosarcomas and smooth muscle tumors of uncertain malignant potential. Am J Obstet Gynecol 1992;166:1646–1653.
180. de Vos S, Wilczynski SP, Fleischhacker M, Koeffler P: *p53* alterations in uterine leiomyosarcomas versus leiomyomas. Gynecol Oncol 1994;54(2):205–8.
181. Hall KL, Teneriello MG, Taylor RR, et al: Analysis of *Ki-ras*, *p53*, and *MDM2* genes in uterine leiomyomas and leiomyosarcomas. Gynecol Oncol 1997;65:330–335.
182. Jeffers MD, Farquharson MA, Richmond JA, McNicol AM: p53 immunoreactivity and mutation of the *p53* gene in smooth muscle tumours of the uterine corpus. J Pathol 1995;177:65–70.
183. Zhai YL, Kobayashi Y, Mori A, et al: Expression of steroid receptors, Ki-67, and p53 in uterine leiomyosarcomas. Int J Gynecol Pathol 1999;18:20–28.
184. Amada S, Nakano H, Tsuneyoshi M: Leiomyosarcoma versus bizarre and cellular leiomyomas of the uterus: A comparative study based on the MIB-1 and proliferating cell nuclear antigen indices, p53 expression, DNA flow cytometry, and muscle specific actins. Int J Gynecol Pathol 1995;14:134–142.
185. Tsushima K, Stanhope CR, Gaffey TA, Lieber MM: Uterine leiomyosarcomas and benign smooth muscle tumors: Usefulness of nuclear DNA patterns studied by flow cytometry. Mayo Clin Proc 1988;63:248–255.
186. Kajii T, Ohama K: Androgenetic origin of hydatidiform mole. Nature 1977;268:633–634.
187. Ohama K, Kajii T, Okamoto E, et al: Dispermic origin of XY hydatidiform moles. Nature 1981;292:551–552.
188. Kajii T, Kurashige H, Ohama K, Uchino F: XY and XX complete moles: Clinical and morphologic correlations. Am J Obstet Gynecol 1984;150:57–64.
189. Szulman AE, Surti U: The syndromes of partial and complete molar gestation. Clin Obstet Gynecol 1984;27:172–180.
190. Barclay ID, Dabbagh L, Babiak J, Poppema S: DNA analysis (ploidy) of molar pregnancies with image analysis on paraffin tissue sections. Am J Clin Pathol 1993;100:451–455.
191. Berezowsky J, Zbieranowski I, Demers J, Murray D: DNA ploidy of hydatidiform moles and nonmolar conceptuses: A study using flow and tissue section image cytometry. Mod Pathol 1995;8:775–781.
192. Cheville JC, Greiner T, Robinson RA, Benda JA: Ploidy analysis by flow cytometry and fluorescence in situ hybridization in hydropic placentas and gestational trophoblastic disease. Hum Pathol 1995;26: 753–757.
193. Fisher RA, Lawler SD, Ormerod MG, et al: Flow cytometry used to distinguish between complete and partial hydatidiform moles. Placenta 1987;8:249–256.
194. Fukunaga M, Endo Y, Ushigome S: Flow cytometric and clinicopathologic study of 197 hydatidiform moles with special reference to the significance of cytometric aneuploidy and literature review. Cytometry 1995;22:135–138.
195. van de Kaa CA, Nelson KA, Ramaekers FC, et al: Interphase cytogenetics in paraffin sections of routinely processed hydatidiform moles and hydropic abortions. J Pathol 1991;165:281–287.
196. Berkowitz RS, Goldstein DP: Gestational trophoblastic disease. Cancer 1995;76(Suppl 10):2079–2085.
197. Sasaki S, Katayama PK, Roesler M, et al: Cytogenetic analysis of choriocarcinoma cell lines. Nippon Sanka Fujinka Gakkai Zasshi 1982;34:2253–2256.
198. Chen CA, Chen YH, Chen TM, et al: Infrequent mutation in tumor suppressor gene *p53* in gestational trophoblastic neoplasia. Carcinogenesis 1994;15:2221–2223.
199. Fulop V, Mok SC, Genest DR, et al: p53, p21, Rb and mdm2 oncoproteins: Expression in normal placenta, partial and complete mole, and choriocarcinoma. J Reprod Med 1998;43:119–127.
200. Fulop V, Mok SC, Genest DR, et al: c-myc, c-erbB-2, c-fms and bcl-2 oncoproteins: Expression in normal placenta, partial and complete mole, and choriocarcinoma. J Reprod Med 1998;43:101–110.
201. Lurain JR, Casanova LA, Miller DS, Rademaker AW: Prognostic factors in gestational trophoblastic tumors: A proposed new scoring system based on multivariate analysis. Am J Obstet Gynecol 1991;164:611–616.
202. Leung WY, Schwartz PE, Ng HT, Yang-Feng TL: Trisomy 12 in benign fibroma and granulosa cell tumor of the ovary. Gynecol Oncol 1990;38:28–31.
203. Persons DL, Hartmann LC, Herath JF, et al: Fluorescence in situ hybridization analysis of trisomy 12 in ovarian tumors. Am J Clin Pathol 1994;102:775–779.
204. Shashi V, Golden WL, von Kap-Herr C, et al: Interphase fluorescence in situ hybridization for trisomy 12 on archival ovarian sex cord-stromal tumors. Gynecol Oncol 1994;55:349–354.
205. Gorski GK, McMorrow LE, Blumstein L, et al: Trisomy 14 in two cases of granulosa cell tumor of the ovary. Cancer Genet Cytogenet 1992;60:202–205.
206. Speleman, Dermaut B, De Potter CR, et al: Monosomy 22 in a mixed germ cell-sex cord-stromal tumor of the ovary. Genes Chromosomes Cancer 1997;19:192–194.
207. Verhest A, Nedoszytko B, Noel JC, et al: Translocation (6;16) in a case of granulosa cell tumor of the ovary. Cancer Genet Cytogenet 1992;60:41–44.

208. Jacoby AF, Young RH, Colvin RB, et al: DNA content in juvenile granulosa cell tumors of the ovary: A study of early- and advanced-stage disease. Gynecol Oncol 1992;46:97–103.
209. Klemi PJ, Joensuu H, Salmi T: Prognostic value of flow cytometric DNA content analysis in granulosa cell tumor of the ovary. Cancer 1990;65:1189–1193.
210. Roush GR, el-Naggar AK, Abdul-Karim FW: Granulosa cell tumor of ovary: A clinicopathologic and flow cytometric DNA analysis. Gynecol Oncol 1995;56: 430–434.
211. Suh KS, Silverberg SG, Rhame JG, Wilkinson DS: Granulosa cell tumor of the ovary: Histopathologic and flow cytometric analysis with clinical correlation. Arch Pathol Lab Med 1990;114:496–501.
212. Wabersich J, Fracas M, Mazzer S, et al: The value of the prognostic factors in ovarian granulosa cell tumors. Eur J Gynaecol Oncol 1998;19:69–72.
213. King LA, Okagaki T, Gallup DG, et al: Mitotic count, nuclear atypia, and immunohistochemical determination of Ki-67, c-myc, p21-ras, c-erbB2, and p53 expression in granulosa cell tumors of the ovary: Mitotic count and Ki-67 are indicators of poor prognosis. Gynecol Oncol 1996;61:227–232.
214. Horny HP, Marx L, Krober S, et al: Granulosa cell tumor of the ovary: Immunohistochemical evidence of low proliferative activity and virtual absence of mutation of the *p53* tumor-suppressor gene. Gynecol Obstet Invest 1999;47:133–138.
215. Fuller PJ, Verity K, Shen Y, et al: No evidence of a role for mutations or polymorphisms of the follicle-stimulating hormone receptor in ovarian granulosa cell tumors. J Clin Endocrinol Metab 1998;83: 274–279.
216. Shen Y, Mamers P, Jobling T, et al: Absence of the previously reported G protein oncogene (gip2) in ovarian granulosa cell tumors. J Clin Endocrinol Metab 1996; 81:4159–4161.
217. Pejovic T, Heim S, Mandahl N, et al: Trisomy 12 is a consistent chromosomal aberration in benign ovarian tumors. Genes Chromosomes Cancer 1990;2:48–52.
218. Diebold J, Siegert S, Baretton GB, et al: Interphase cytogenetic analysis of mucinous ovarian neoplasms. Lab Invest 1997;76:661–670.
219. Cheng PC, Gosewehr JA, Kim TM, et al: Potential role of the inactivated X chromosome in ovarian epithelial tumor development. J Natl Cancer Inst 1996;88: 510–518.
220. Kim TM, Benedict WF, Xu HJ, et al: Loss of heterozygosity on chromosome 13 is common only in the biologically more aggressive subtypes of ovarian epithelial tumors and is associated with normal retinoblastoma gene expression. Cancer Res 1994;54:605–609.
221. Cuatrecasas M, Villanueva A, Matias-Guiu X, Prat J: K-*ras* mutations in mucinous ovarian tumors: A clinicopathologic and molecular study of 95 cases. Cancer 1997;79:1581–1586.
222. Cuatrecasas M, Erill N, Musulen E, et al: K-*ras* mutations in nonmucinous ovarian epithelial tumors: A molecular analysis and clinicopathologic study of 144 patients. Cancer 1998;82:1088–1095.
223. Mandai M, Konishi I, Kuroda H, et al: Heterogeneous distribution of K-*ras*–mutated epithelia in mucinous ovarian tumors with special reference to histopathology. Hum Pathol 1998;29:34–40.
224. Teneriello MG, Ebina M, Linnoila RI, et al: *p53* and Ki-*ras* gene mutations in epithelial ovarian neoplasms. Cancer Res 1993;53:3103–3108.
225. Ioakim-Liossi A, Karakitsos P, Aroni K, et al: p53 protein expression and DNA ploidy in common epithelial tumors of the ovary. Acta Cytol 1997;41:1714–1718.
226. Crickard K, Marinello MJ, Crickard U, et al: Borderline malignant serous tumors of the ovary maintained on extracellular matrix: Evidence for clonal evolution and invasive potential. Cancer Genet Cytogenet 1986;23: 135–143.
227. Yang-Feng TL, Li SB, Leung WY, et al: Trisomy 12 and K-*ras*-2 amplification in human ovarian tumors. Int J Cancer 1991;48:678–681.
228. Lounis H, Mes-Masson AM, Dion F, et al: Mapping of chromosome 3p deletions in human epithelial ovarian tumors. Oncogene 1998;17:2359–2365.
229. Pejovic T, Iosif CS, Mitelman F, Heim S: Karyotypic characteristics of borderline malignant tumors of the ovary: Trisomy 12, trisomy 7, and r(1) as nonrandom features. Cancer Genet Cytogenet 1996;92:95–98.
230. Tibiletti MG, Bernasconi B, Furlan D, et al: Early involvement of 6q in surface epithelial ovarian tumors. Cancer Res 1996;56:4493–4498.
231. De Nictolis M, Montironi R, Tommasoni S, et al: Serous borderline tumors of the ovary: A clinicopathologic, immunohistochemical, and quantitative study of 44 cases. Cancer 1992;70:152–160.
232. De Nictolis M, Montironi R, Tommasoni S, et al: Benign, borderline, and well-differentiated malignant intestinal mucinous tumors of the ovary: A clinicopathologic, histochemical, immunohistochemical, and nuclear quantitative study of 57 cases. Int J Gynecol Pathol 1994;13:10–21.
233. Demirel D, Laucirica R, Fishman A, et al: Ovarian tumors of low malignant potential: Correlation of DNA index and S-phase fraction with histopathologic grade and clinical outcome. Cancer 1996;77:1494–1500.
234. Harlow BL, Fuhr JE, McDonald TW, et al: Flow cytometry as a prognostic indicator in women with borderline epithelial ovarian tumors. Gynecol Oncol 1993;50: 305–309.
235. Dodson MK, Hartmann LC, Cliby WA, et al: Comparison of loss of heterozygosity patterns in invasive low-grade and high-grade epithelial ovarian carcinomas. Cancer Res 1993;53:4456–4460.
236. Eccles DM, Russell SE, Haites NE, et al: Early loss of heterozygosity on 17q in ovarian cancer: The Abe Ovarian Cancer Genetics Group. Oncogene 1992;7:2069–2072.
237. Gallion HH, Powell DE, Morrow JK, et al: Molecular genetic changes in human epithelial ovarian malignancies. Gynecol Oncol 1992;47:137–142.
238. Saretzki G, Hoffmann U, Rohlke P, et al: Identification of allelic losses in benign, borderline, and invasive epithelial ovarian tumors and correlation with clinical outcome. Cancer 1997;80:1241–1249.
239. Lu KH, Bell DA, Welch WR, et al: Evidence for the multifocal origin of bilateral and advanced human serous borderline ovarian tumors. Cancer Res 1998;58:2328–2330.

240. Bellacosa A, de Feo D, Godwin AK, et al: Molecular alterations of the *AKT2* oncogene in ovarian and breast carcinomas. Int J Cancer 1995;64:280–285.
241. Fujita M, Enomoto T, Haba T, et al: Alteration of *p16* and *p15* genes in common epithelial ovarian tumors. Int J Cancer 1997;74:148–155.
242. Shigemasa K, Hu C, West CM, et al: p16 overexpression: A potential early indicator of transformation in ovarian carcinoma. J Soc Gynecol Investig 1997;4: 95–102.
243. Zheng J, Benedict WF, Xu HJ, et al: Genetic disparity between morphologically benign cysts contiguous to ovarian carcinomas and solitary cystadenomas. J Natl Cancer Inst 1995;87:1146–1153.
244. Mok SC, Bell DA, Knapp RC, et al: Mutation of K-*ras* protooncogene in human ovarian epithelial tumors of borderline malignancy. Cancer Res 1993;53: 1489–1492.
245. Cheng P, Schmutte C, Cofer KF, et al: Alterations in DNA methylation are early, but not initial, events in ovarian tumorigenesis. Br J Cancer 1997;75:396–402.
246. McCluskey LL, Chen C, Delgadillo E, et al: Differences in *p16* gene methylation and expression in benign and malignant ovarian tumors. Gynecol Oncol 1999;72: 87–92.
247. Oishi T, Kigawa J, Minagawa Y, et al: Alteration of telomerase activity associated with development and extension of epithelial ovarian cancer. Obstet Gynecol 1998;91:568–571.
248. Park TW, Riethdorf S, Riethdorf L, et al: Differential telomerase activity, expression of the telomerase catalytic sub-unit and telomerase-RNA in ovarian tumors. Int J Cancer 1999;84:426–431.
249. Wan M, Li WZ, Duggan BD, et al: Telomerase activity in benign and malignant epithelial ovarian tumors. J Natl Cancer Inst 1997;89:437–441.
250. Berchuck A, Kohle MF, Hopkins MP, et al: Overexpression of *p53* is not a feature of benign and early-stage borderline epithelial ovarian tumors. Gynecol Oncol 1994;52:232–236.
251. Klemi PJ, Takahashi S, Joensuu H, et al: Immunohistochemical detection of p53 protein in borderline and malignant serous ovarian tumors. Int J Gynecol Pathol 1994;13:228–233.
252. Koshiyama M, Konishi I, Mandai M, et al: Immunohistochemical analysis of p53 protein and 72-kDa heat shock protein (HSP72) expression in ovarian carcinomas: Correlation with clinicopathology and sex steroid receptor status. Virchows Arch 1995;425:603–609.
253. Ito K, Sasano H, Ozawa N, et al: Immunolocalization of epidermal growth factor receptor and c-erbB-2 oncogene product in human ovarian carcinoma. Int J Gynecol Pathol 1992;11:253–257.
254. Thompson FH, Emerson J, Alberts D, et al: Clonal chromosome abnormalities in 54 cases of ovarian carcinoma. Cancer Genet Cytogenet 1994;73:33–45.
255. Whang-Peng J, Knutsen T, Douglass EC, et al: Cytogenetic studies in ovarian cancer. Cancer Genet Cytogenet 1984;11:91–106.
256. Jenkins RB, Bartelt DJ, Stalboerger P, et al: Cytogenetic studies of epithelial ovarian carcinoma. Cancer Genet Cytogenet 1993;71:76–86.
257. Pejovic T, Heim S, Mandahl N, et al: Complex karyotypic anomalies, including an i(5p) marker chromosome, in malignant mixed mesodermal tumor of the ovary. Cancer Genet Cytogenet 1990;46:65–69.
258. Pejovic T, Heim S, Mandahl N, et al: Bilateral ovarian carcinoma: Cytogenetic evidence of unicentric origin. Int J Cancer 1991;47:358–361.
259. Pejovic T, Heim S, Mandahl N, et al: Consistent occurrence of a 19p+ marker chromosome and loss of 11p material in ovarian seropapillary cystadenocarcinomas. Genes Chromosomes Cancer 1989;1:167–171.
260. Kuhn W, Kaufmann M, Feichter GE, et al: DNA flow cytometry, clinical and morphological parameters as prognostic factors for advanced malignant and borderline ovarian tumors. Gynecol Oncol 1989;33:360–367.
261. Klemi PJ, Joensuu H, Kiilholma P, Maenpaa J: Clinical significance of abnormal nuclear DNA content in serous ovarian tumors. Cancer 1988;62:2005–2010.
262. Tapper J, Butzow R, Wahlstrom T, et al: Evidence for divergence of DNA copy number changes in serous, mucinous and endometrioid ovarian carcinomas. Br J Cancer 1997;75:1782–1787.
263. Wan M, Li WZ, Duggan BD, et al: Telomerase activity in benign and malignant epithelial ovarian tumors. J Natl Cancer Inst 1997;89:437–441.
264. Slamon DJ, Godolphin W, Jones LA, et al: Studies of the *HER-2/neu* proto-oncogene in human breast and ovarian cancer. Science 1989;244:707–712.
265. Courjal F, Louason G, Speiser P, et al: Cyclin gene amplification and overexpression in breast and ovarian cancers: Evidence for the selection of cyclin D1 in breast and cyclin E in ovarian tumors. Int J Cancer 1996;69: 247–253.
266. Courjal F, Cuny M, Rodriguez C, et al: DNA amplifications at 20q13 and MDM2 define distinct subsets of evolved breast and ovarian tumours. Br J Cancer 1996;74:1984–1989.
267. Fajac A, Benard J, Lhomme C, et al: c-*erbB2* gene amplification and protein expression in ovarian epithelial tumors: Evaluation of their respective prognostic significance by multivariate analysis. Int J Cancer 1995;64:146–151.
268. Eccles DM, Gruber L, Stewart M, et al: Allele loss on chromosome 11p is associated with poor survival in ovarian cancer. Dis Markers 1992;10:95–99.
269. Niwa K, Itoh M, Murase T, et al: Alteration of *p53* gene in ovarian carcinoma: Clinicopathological correlation and prognostic significance. Br J Cancer 1994;70:1191–1197.
270. Skomedal H, Kristensen GB, Abeler VM, et al: TP53 protein accumulation and gene mutation in relation to overexpression of MDM2 protein in ovarian borderline tumours and stage I carcinomas. J Pathol 1997;181: 58–165.
271. Eltabbakh GH, Belinson JL, Kennedy AW, et al: *p53* overexpression is not an independent prognostic factor for patients with primary ovarian epithelial cancer. Cancer 1997;80:892–898.
272. Enomoto T, Weghorst CM, Inoue M, et al: K-*ras* activation occurs frequently in mucinous adenocarcinomas and rarely in other common epithelial tumors of the human ovary. Am J Pathol 1991;139:777–785.
273. Chenevix-Trench G, Kerr J, Hurst T, et al: Analysis of loss of heterozygosity and *KRAS2* mutations in ovarian

neoplasms: Clinicopathological correlations. Genes Chromosomes Cancer 1997;18:75–83.

274. Wang ZJ, Churchman M, Campbell IG, et al: Allele loss and mutation screen at the Peutz-Jeghers *(LKB1)* locus (19p13.3) in sporadic ovarian tumours. Br J Cancer 1999;80:70–72.

275. Takahashi H, Behbakht K, McGovern PE, et al: Mutation analysis of the *BRCA1* gene in ovarian cancers. Cancer Res 1995;55:2998–3002.

276. Takahashi H, Chiu HC, Bandera CA, et al: Mutations of the *BRCA2* gene in ovarian carcinomas. Cancer Res 1996;56:2738–2741.

277. Shih YC, Kerr J, Liu J, et al: Rare mutations and no hypermethylation at the *CDKN2A* locus in epithelial ovarian tumours. Int J Cancer 1997;70:508–511.

278. Saegusa M, Machida D, Okayasu I: Loss of *DCC* gene expression during ovarian tumorigenesis: Relation to tumour differentiation and progression. Br J Cancer 2000;82:571–578.

279. Darai E, Scoazec JY, Walker-Combrouze F, et al: Expression of cadherins in benign, borderline, and malignant ovarian epithelial tumors: A clinicopathologic study of 60 cases. Hum Pathol 1997;28:922–928.

280. Hartenbach EM, Olson TA, Goswitz JJ, et al: Vascular endothelial growth factor (VEGF) expression and survival in human epithelial ovarian carcinomas. Cancer Lett 1997;121:169–175.

281. Srivatsa PJ, Cliby WA, Keeney GL, et al: Elevated nm23 protein expression is correlated with diminished progression-free survival in patients with epithelial ovarian carcinoma. Gynecol Oncol 1996;60:363–372.

282. Garzetti GG, Ciavattini A, Goteri G, et al: Ki67 antigen immunostaining (MIB 1 monoclonal antibody) in serous ovarian tumors: Index of proliferative activity with prognostic significance. Gynecol Oncol 1995;56:169–174.

283. McMenamin ME, O'Neill AJ, Gaffney EF: Extent of apoptosis in ovarian serous carcinoma: Relation to mitotic and proliferative indices, p53 expression, and survival. Mol Pathol 1997;50:242–246.

284. Viale G, Maisonneuve P, Bonoldi E, et al: The combined evaluation of p53 accumulation and of Ki-67 (MIB1) labelling index provides independent information on overall survival of ovarian carcinoma patients. Ann Oncol 1997;8:469–476.

285. Martinez-Zaguilan R, Martinez GM, Lattanzio F, Gillies RJ: Simultaneous measurement of intracellular pH and Ca^{2+} using the fluorescence of SNARF-1 and fura-2. Am J Physiol 1991;260:C297–C307.

286. Lagendijk JH, Mullink H, van Diest PJ, et al: Tracing the origin of adenocarcinomas with unknown primary using immunohistochemistry: Differential diagnosis between colonic and ovarian carcinomas as primary sites. Hum Pathol 1998;29:491–497.

287. Teixeira MR, Kristensen GB, Abeler VM, Heim S: Karyotypic findings in tumors of the vulva and vagina. Cancer Genet Cytogenet 1999;111:87–91.

288. Worsham MJ, Van Dyke DL, Grenman SE, et al: Consistent chromosome abnormalities in squamous cell carcinoma of the vulva. Genes Chromosomes Cancer 1991;3: 420–432.

289. Scheistroen M, Trope C, Kaern J, et al: DNA ploidy and expression of *p53* and C-*erbB-2* in extramammary Paget's disease of the vulva. Gynecol Oncol 1997;64: 88–92.

290. Cotton J, Kotylo PK, Michael H, et al: Flow cytometric DNA analysis of extramammary Paget's disease of the vulva. Int J Gynecol Pathol 1995;14:324–330.

291. Drew PA, al-Abbadi MA, Orlando CA, et al: Prognostic factors in carcinoma of the vulva: A clinicopathologic and DNA flow cytometric study. Int J Gynecol Pathol 1996;15:235–241.

292. Hietanen SH, Kurvinen K, Syrjanen K, et al: Mutation of tumor suppressor gene *p53* is frequently found in vulvar carcinoma cells. Am J Obstet Gynecol 1995;173: 1477–1482.

293. Milde-Langosch K, Albrecht K, Joram S, et al: Presence and persistence of HPV infection and *p53* mutation in cancer of the cervix uteri and the vulva. Int J Cancer 1995;63:639–645.

294. Kim YT, Thomas NF, Kessis TD, et al: *p53* mutations and clonality in vulvar carcinomas and squamous hyperplasias: Evidence suggesting that squamous hyperplasias do not serve as direct precursors of human papillomavirus–negative vulvar carcinomas. Hum Pathol 1996; 27:389–395.

295. Lee YY, Wilczynski SP, Chumakov A, et al: Carcinoma of the vulva: HPV and *p53* mutations. Oncogene 1994;9: 1655–1659.

296. Pilotti S, D'Amato L, Della TG, et al: Papillomavirus, *p53* alteration, and primary carcinoma of the vulva. Diagn Mol Pathol 1995;4:239–248.

297. Boyd J, Takahashi H, Waggoner SE, et al: Molecular genetic analysis of clear cell adenocarcinomas of the vagina and cervix associated and unassociated with diethylstilbestrol exposure in utero. Cancer 1996;77: 507–513.

298. Waggoner SE, Anderson SM, Luce MC, et al: p53 protein expression and gene analysis in clear cell adenocarcinoma of the vagina and cervix. Gynecol Oncol 1996; 60:339–344.

299. Waggoner SE, Anderson SM, Van Eyck S, et al: Human papillomavirus detection and p53 expression in clear-cell adenocarcinoma of the vagina and cervix. Obstet Gynecol 1994;84:404–408.

300. Ruppert JM, Wright M, Rosenfeld M, et al: Gene therapy strategies for carcinoma of the breast. Breast Cancer Res Treat 1997;44:93–114.

301. Brenner AJ, Aldaz CM: The genetics of sporadic breast cancer. Prog Clin Biol Res 1997;396:63–82.

302. Kerangueven F, Noguchi T, Coulier F, et al: Genome-wide search for loss of heterozygosity shows extensive genetic diversity of human breast carcinomas. Cancer Res 1997;57:5469–5474.

IRINA A. LUBENSKY
TIMOTHY J. O'LEARY

13

Endocrine System

The pathology of the endocrine/neuroendocrine system is complex. Many of the important endocrine diseases demonstrate biochemical defects without a direct morphologic correlate in the affected organ. In some cases, our knowledge of one endocrine organ predicts the presence of diseases in others, yet the predicted diseases are rarely diagnosed. For example, hyperplastic lesions are routinely diagnosed in all neuroendocrine organs, however, pituitary "hyperplasia," which is well recognized in animals[1] and for which there is evidence that it exists in humans,[2–4] is only rarely diagnosed in the pathology laboratory. Other well-recognized endocrine lesions, such as Reidel's struma of the thyroid, are poorly understood and may reflect a single morphologic manifestation of several different disease processes. To complicate the issue further, there is a lack of reliable working histopathologic classification of neuroendocrine tumors that would be applicable to the neuroendocrine tumors in all organs. In some organ systems, such as the gastrointestinal tract, the existing histopathologic classification of such tumors has been based on the function of the released hormone and is of limited usefulness. Furthermore, the morphologic criteria used in classification of the epithelial, nonendocrine neoplasms are not applicable to classification of the neuroendocrine tumors and do not predict the biologic behavior of these tumors. Thus, nuclear atypia and mitoses are common features of many benign endocrine tumors. In contrast, in the most frequent malignant tumor of the thyroid gland, papillary carcinoma, the diagnosis of malignancy is made based strictly on nuclear features (i.e., presence of nuclear overlap, clearing, and grooves), whereas nuclear atypia, mitoses, and necrosis are not usually seen in these tumors. The only definitive criteria for malignancy in most endocrine tumors remain local lymph node and distant metastases (pancreatic and gastrointestinal neuroendocrine tumors, lung carcinoid and adrenal pheochromocytoma) or vascular and/or capsular invasion (follicular thyroid carcinoma).

Recent discoveries of the genes for multiple endocrine neoplasia, type 1, in 1997, multiple endocrine neoplasia type 2, in 1993, and von Hippel-Lindau disease, in 1993, as well as molecular genetic studies of the neuroendocrine tumors in multiple endocrine syndromes and of sporadic counterpart tumors helped to shed light on the pathogenesis of parathyroid, pancreatic, gastrointestinal, pulmonary, adrenal, and thyroid endocrine neoplasms. In contrast, molecular pathogenesis of anterior pituitary tumors remains largely unknown.

In this chapter we focus attention on the diagnosis and molecular aspects of neuroendocrine and endocrine neoplasms and non-neoplastic disorders with which they may be confused. In addition, other diseases that give rise to pathologic specimens from endocrine organs are discussed. An excellent review that gives greater attention to non-neoplastic endocrine disorders has been written by Bower and Malchoff.[5]

HEREDITARY ENDOCRINE NEOPLASIA

Multiple Endocrine Neoplasia Type 1 (MEN 1)

MEN 1 is an autosomal dominant disorder characterized by the tumors of multiple parathyroid glands and anterior pituitary, duodenal gastrinomas, pancreatic neuroendocrine tumors (nonfunctioning, gastrinomas and insulinomas), and foregut carcinoids (thymic, lung, and gastric) (Table 13–1). Most of the endocrine tumors in MEN 1 are benign, except for gastrinoma and thymic carcinoid, which have a high malignant potential, and atypical lung carcinoid (low-grade neuroendocrine carcinoma). Mesenchymal tumors of MEN 1 include lipomas, facial angiofibromas, and smooth muscle tumors.[6–8] Follicular adenoma and papillary carcinoma of the thyroid and adrenal cortical hyperplasia/adenoma are seen with increased frequency in MEN 1 patients

TABLE 13–1

Major Patterns of Tissue Involvement in Multiple Endocrine Neoplasia (MEN) syndromes

Tissue	MEN 1	MEN 2A	MEN 2B
Parathyroid	Hyperplasia/adenoma—all four glands (99%)	Hyperplasia/adenoma (10%)	Normal
Thyroid	Adenoma/papillary/carcinoma (8%)	C-cell hyperplasia/medullary carcinoma (100%)	C-cell hyperplasia/medullary carcinoma (100%)
Adrenal	Adenoma/hyperplasia (16%)	Pheochromocytoma/medullary hyperplasia (50%)	Pheochromocytoma/medullary hyperplasia (50%)
Enteric ganglia	Normal	Normal	Hyperplasia (100%)
Pancreas/duodenum	Neuroendocrine tumor (80%)	Normal	Normal
Pituitary	Adenoma (47%)	Normal	Normal
Other features	Angiofibroma (88%) Collagenoma (72%) Lipoma (34%) Leiomyoma (2%) Carcinoid (16%)	Normal	Hypotonia, thick lips, other facial abnormalities

but are not part of the syndrome.[6] MEN 1 tumors are caused by a germline mutation of the *MEN1* tumor suppressor gene (chromosome 11q13) followed by a deletion of the wild-type allele.[9, 10] *MEN1* gene sequence predicted a novel protein, menin, which is localized predominantly in the nucleus.[11, 12] Its function is unknown, and it shows no protein homologies. *MEN1* mutations predict truncation of menin protein, causing functional inactivation. Inactivation-type mutations further support menin's predicted role as a tumor suppressor. *MEN1* germline mutations have been detected in over 90% of MEN 1 families and are found in 9 coding exons of the *MEN1* gene (Fig. 13–1).[13, 14] Germline mutation testing can give valuable information for MEN 1 family members and clinicians but does not need to be performed until age 18.[14] Parathyroid neoplasms that affect all four glands, and multiple duodenal and pancreatic gastrinomas that follow indolent but malignant course and metastasize to lymph nodes and liver, cannot be prevented. Sporadic counterpart tumors, gastrinoma (33%), insulinoma (17%), parathyroid adenoma (21%), lung carcinoid (36%), foregut carcinoids (15%), lipoma, and

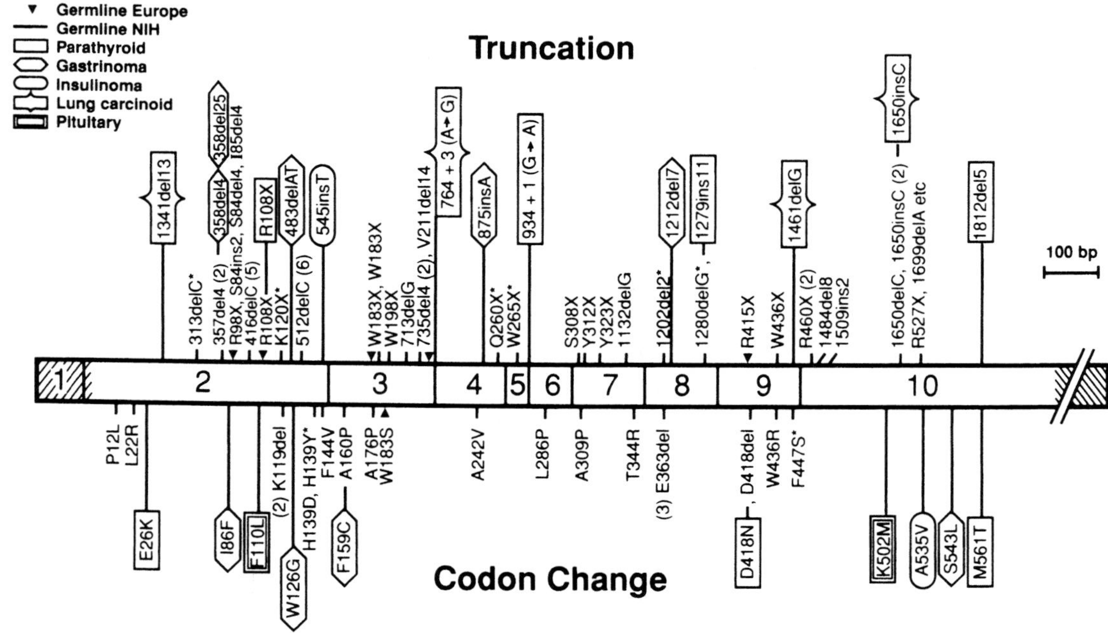

FIGURE 13–1

Germline and somatic mutations in the *MEN1* gene. (From Marx S, Spiegel AM, Skarulis MC, et al: Multiple endocrine neoplasia type 1: Clinical and genetic topics. Ann Intern Med 1998;129:484–494.)

angiofibroma often show somatic *MEN1* mutations.[14–17] Somatic *MEN1* mutation is the most common and/or only described gene mutation in sporadic gastrinoma, insulinoma, parathyroid adenoma, and lung carcinoid.[14] Somatic *MEN1* mutation is rare in sporadic pituitary adenoma (0% to 5%).[18]

Multiple Endocrine Neoplasia Type 2 (MEN 2)

The tumors of MEN 2 include medullary thyroid carcinoma (MTC)/C-cell hyperplasia, adrenal pheochromocytoma/medullary hyperplasia, and parathyroid adenoma/hyperplasia. Most MEN 2 cases result from a mutation in the *RET* proto-oncogene on chromosome 10q11.2.[19, 20] *RET* binds to a tyrosine kinase receptor and is thought to be involved not only in the pathogenesis of MEN 2 tumors but also in the tumorigenesis of sporadic papillary thyroid carcinoma. As a result of alternative splicing, *RET* codes for three slightly different polypeptides ranging from 1072 to 1114 amino acids; the protein product binds to glial-derived neurotropic factor (GDNF). Mutations apparently result in constitutional activation, but the precise cellular pathways affected by this activation have yet to be defined. There is a strong genotype/phenotype correlation in MEN 2 (see Table 13–1). For example, MEN 2B (developmental abnormalities followed by MTC and pheochromocytoma in the second and third decades) is associated with a Met918Thr mutation in over 90% of cases.[21] The mutational associations between various clinical patterns and *RET* mutational loci (hot spots) are included in Table 13–2. The strong association of specific mutational patterns with particular *RET* mutations suggests that the nature or extent of gene activation differs with the domain affected. Mutations in the cysteine-rich domain are believed to affect dimerization,[21] whereas the Met918Thr mutation is thought to affect the specificity of substrate binding to that of a cytoplasmic tyrosine kinase (Fig. 13–2). Interestingly, new mutations associated with MEN 2 invariably occur in the paternal allele.[22] Sequencing analysis is a reasonable approach to identification of a heritable trait on presentation of an apparently sporadic medullary carcinoma or pheochromocytoma, because sporadic *RET* mutations seldom affect the "hereditary hot spots" associated with MEN 2. Screening for germline *RET* mutations in MEN 2 family members is recommended at early age (5 years for MEN 2A; 1 year for MEN 2B; and 5 to 18 years for familial MTC).[14] Early surgical removal of the thyroid gland for malignant medullary tumor may prevent metastases and increase survival of MEN 2 patients. The absence of *RET* mutation in a patient with multiple pheochromocytomas should suggest the possibility of von Hippel-Lindau disease and be followed with *VHL* mutation analysis.[23] Although pheochromocytoma may occur as a part of von Recklinghausen's disease, it is rare and is seen in only 0.1% to 5.7% of such patients.[24] Sequencing analysis for the *NF1* gene in patients with pheochromocytoma is not usually recommended unless the suspicion for neurofibromatosis is high.

Hyperthyroidism/Jaw Tumor Syndrome (HPT/JT)

Hyperthyroidism/jaw tumor syndrome (HPT/JT) is a distinct autosomal dominant disorder in which multiple parathyroid adenomas or parathyroid carcinoma cause primary hyperthyroidism. Associated ossifying fibroma of the jaw is common. In addition, renal lesions, including renal hamartomas, Wilms' tumor, polycystic kidney disease, and degenerative cysts have been associated with the syndrome. The HPT/JT gene *(HRPT2)* has been mapped to chromosome 1q25-q31 but has not yet been identified.[25]

TABLE 13–2

Patterns of Gene Invovement in Hereditary Endocrine Syndromes

Syndrome	Locus	Gene/Codon	Gene/Domain Function
MEN 1	11q13	*MEN* 1	Unknown
MEN 2A	10q11.2	*RET* codons 609 611 618 620 634	Cysteine-rich
MEN 2B	10q11.2	*RET* Met918thr	Tyrosine kinase
Familial medullary carcinoma of thyroid	10q11.2	*RET* codons 768 804 634	Tyrosine kinase Cysteine-rich
Carney's syndrome	2p,17q	*PRKAR1A*	Protein kinase A RIα
Von Hippel-Lindau syndrome	3p	*VHL*	Elongin-binding
Hyperthyroidism–jaw tumor syndrome	1q21-32	?	?
Neurofibromatosis	17q	*NF1*	Down-regulator of oncogenic *RAS*

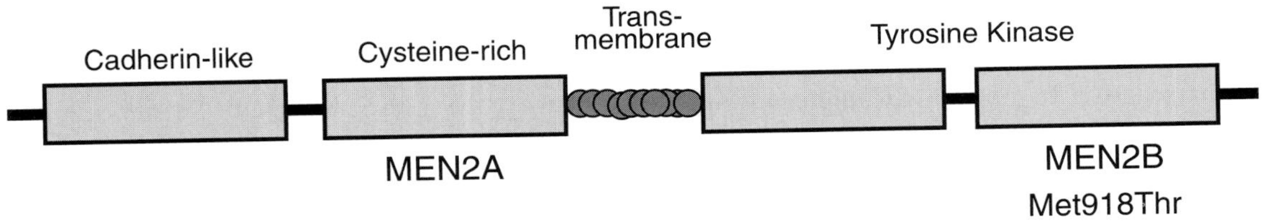

FIGURE 13–2
Structural features of the RET protein.

Carney's Complex (Carney's Syndrome)

Carney's complex is an autosomal dominant familial syndrome characterized by lentigenes (particularly on the vermilion border of the lips), atrial and dermal myxomas, acromegaly (growth hormone–producing pituitary adenoma), and Cushing's syndrome caused by pigmented nodular adrenal cortical disease.[26] Thyroid gland abnormalities, ranging from follicular hyperplasia to carcinoma, are also common.[27] Karyotype analysis has demonstrated multiple telomeric associations (tas) in myxomas and micronodular adrenals from several patients.[28] Linkage analysis has suggested a defect on chromosome 2p16 in some families.[29, 30] This region of chromosome 2p16 harbors the *MSH2* and *MSH6* genes.[29] Microsatellite analysis has demonstrated substantial pangenomic instability in Carney's syndrome patients; however, no increase in microsatellite length instability has been observed[28] and neither of the just-mentioned mismatch repair genes appear to be involved. The gene for Carney's complex on 2p16 has not yet been identified. Recently, a subset of Carney's complex families was found to have germline mutations in *PRKAR1A* tumor suppresson gene at 17 of 22–24.[30]

Von Hippel-Lindau Disease

Von Hippel-Lindau disease (VHL) is an autosomal dominant inherited disorder characterized by central nervous system hemangioblastomas (60%); retinal angiomas (40%); renal cysts and renal cell carcinomas (40%); cystic disease of the pancreas (35%), epididymis, broad ligament, and endolymphatic sac tumor of middle ear.[31] Pancreatic neuroendocrine tumors are nonfunctioning and occur in 12% to 17% of VHL patients. Functioning and nonfunctioning adrenal pheochromocytomas and extra-adrenal paragangliomas are seen in 12% of VHL patients.[32] The *VHL* gene on chromosome 3p25.5 functions as a tumor suppressor[33] and competes with the elongin A molecule to bind to elongins B and C, thus inhibiting RNA polymerase and transcription.[34, 35] There is a strong relationship between the type of mutation and the clinical phenotype. For example, T → C transitions at codon 505 result in VHL type 2 with familial predisposition to pheochromocytoma without renal cell carcinoma.[36]

ANTERIOR PITUITARY GLAND

Pituitary Adenoma

Pituitary adenomas are common neoplasms, constituting approximately 10% of intracranial tumors. They have been reported in up to 27% of patients in autopsy series.[37] Pituitary adenomas most commonly secrete prolactin (30% to 40% of cases), but nonfunctioning tumors (25% to 35%), somatotropinomas (10% to 15%), and adrenocorticotropic hormone [ACTH]-producing tumors (5% to 10%) are also relatively common.[38] Although most patients initially present with endocrine symptoms, a substantial number of them are diagnosed as a result of neurologic deficits caused by tumor expansion and local invasion.

For many years there has been an ongoing debate regarding the possible causes of pituitary tumorigenesis. Two main theories have prevailed: a hypothalamic hormone influence versus an intrinsic pituitary defect. In favor of the hypothalamic theory is the paradoxical pituitary hormone response to exogenous stimuli, the retention of a normal response to hypothalamic hormone stimulation, the presence of hypothalamic hormone transcripts in the pituitary, the development of adenomas in humans with growth hormone–releasing hormone (GHRH)-producing hypothalamic gangliocytomas and in mice transgenic for GHRH, and the rare cases of prolonged hypothyroidism or hypogonadism resulting in the development of a thyrotroph or gonadotroph adenoma.[39, 40] In favor of the intrinsic pituitary defect model is the documentation of monoclonal composition of pituitary adenomas using the X-chromosome inactivation technique.[41, 42] Nevertheless, few somatic defects in genes governing cell proliferation or hormone production have so far been identified in pituitary adenomas. Single base substitutions in the G_s protein have been implicated in the pathogenesis of a minority of growth hormone (GH)–producing adenomas.[43] Mutations in *RAS*[44–46] or *PKC*[47] genes have been identified in extremely rare cases. Mutations and overexpression of *ERBB2* are not found in these tumors.[48] Similarly, loss of tumor suppressor gene function as evidenced by mutations or deletions of the retinoblastoma *(RB1)* [49, 50] or *TP53* [51] genes are rarely present in pituitary neoplasms. The events leading to pituitary tumorigenesis remain to be elucidated and are likely to be distinct from those identified in other forms of neoplasia.

Pituitary adenomas occur sporadically and as a part of an inherited syndrome, MEN 1. The potential role of the *MEN1* gene in pituitary tumorigenesis was suggested by studies on 11q13 LOH in MEN 1–associated pituitary disease.[52, 53] Several such studies investigated the association of putative *MEN1* chromosomal locus deletions with sporadic pituitary adenomas and showed an overall 11q13 loss of heterozygosity (LOH) rate of 10% to 18%.[52] However, somatic mutations in the *MEN1* gene are exceedingly rare in sporadic pituitary adenomas and the *MEN1* gene inactivation does not represent a likely pathogenic mechanism in sporadic pituitary tumor development.[18]

Cytogenetic studies have demonstrated normal karyotypes in about half of tumors; numerical aberrations constitute most of the abnormalities.[54–58] Telomeric associations[54] and an inconsistent variety of other abnormalities have been observed in the remaining cases. Comparative genomic hybridization (CGH) studies demonstrate abnormalities in about three fourths of tumors. For the most part, these are copy number aberrations, but inconsistent deletions and amplifications have been observed on every chromosome.[59, 60] Allelic deletions have been observed at a variety of loci, including 11q13, 13q12–14, 10q, 9p, and 1p. Some authors showed that tumors demonstrating allelic deletion are more likely to be locally invasive than those that do not.[61, 62] Expression of the *CDKN2A* gene is dramatically reduced in most pituitary adenomas as a result of extensive methylation.[63]

Approximately 40% of growth-hormone producing pituitary adenomas (somatotropinomas) harbor an activated oncogene *(GSP)* due to mutation of the chromosome 20q13.2-13.3 guanine nucleotide binding protein GS *(GNAS1)*—a guanosine triphosphatase that couples adenylate cyclase to cell membrane hormone receptors.[52, 64–66] A number of mutations have been reported (most frequently, Arg201Cys, Arg201His, Gln227Leu, and Gln227Arg). Mutation causes constitutive activation of adenylate cyclase, apparently stimulating cell division[65] and increasing expression of prolactin and growth hormone.[67] Patients with adenomas expressing GSP are more likely to be successfully managed with a combination of surgery and octreotide than are those patients whose tumors do not demonstrate this defect.[68] Rare *GSP* mutations have also been seen in nonfunctioning pituitary tumors and corticotroph adenomas[69, 70]; their clinical significance in these tumors is unknown.

In addition to LOH at one or more genetic loci,[61, 71] a number of other molecular alterations have been reported to be associated with locally aggressive behavior in pituitary adenoma. Collagenase activity[72] and MYC protein expression[73] appear to be higher in locally invasive tumors than in more indolent varieties. Although the aggressive adenomas appear to demonstrate increased proliferation as reflected in immunohistochemical assays for Ki-67 (MIB1) and proliferating cell nuclear antigen (PCNA),[74–80] this finding is not confirmed using cytometric analysis.[81, 82] Because cytologic appearance of pituitary adenomas is not useful in predicting behavior,[83] use of these methods may be somewhat helpful in the clinical management of patients with pituitary adenomas, although they are limited by significant overlap between invasive and noninvasive groups of tumors.

Although immunohistochemical staining of the pituitary is used most commonly to verify the secretory product of a putative microadenoma, it may occasionally be necessary to differentiate pituitary adenoma from other tumors (e.g., craniopharyngioma, astrocytoma, metastatic carcinoma, and esthesioneuroblastoma) that may be found in the sellar region. When interpreting the results of hormone stains, one must remember that the presence of hormonal (particularly gonadotropin) immunoreactivity in the tumor does not necessarily imply a clinically functional adenoma.[84]

Pituitary Carcinoma

Although local invasion is common in recurrent pituitary adenomas,[74] frank pituitary carcinomas are quite rare. There are no published cytogenetic studies and a very limited number of molecular biologic investigations. Mutations of *RAS* and *TP53* have not been identified in primary pituitary carcinomas,[45, 46] although *RAS* mutations have been found in distant metastases,[45] and immunohistochemical staining for p53 protein is seen in 60% to 100% of primary pituitary carcinomas.[85, 86] Loss of the *RB1* gene locus and *RB1* gene expression have each been reported in single pituitary carcinomas,[87] whereas LOH at the *RB1* locus is uncommon in pituitary adenoma.[88] Very low levels of BCL2, BAX, and BCLX have been reported in pituitary carcinoma, suggesting a higher rate of apoptosis in carcinoma than in adenoma.[89] There is also evidence that a transcription factor, BRN3A, may be highly overexpressed in some of these tumors.[90] Most, but not all, pituitary carcinomas appear to be aneuploid.[86, 91] Most pituitary carcinomas demonstrate significant numbers of mitotic figures (mean, 2 mitoses per high-power field) and high MIB1 and PCNA indices.[86] Whether assessment of molecular biologic, immunohistochemical, or cytometric markers provides more diagnostically useful information in addition to mitotic index in predicting malignancy in the pituitary gland will require significantly larger studies than those that have been published to date.

Pituitary Hyperplasia

Pituitary hyperplasia, defined as a cell proliferation in response to a stimulus in contrast to the dysregulated cell proliferation of neoplasia, has been described. Hyperplasia of adenohypophysial cells in humans gives rise to clinical symptoms indistinguishable from manifestations of pituitary adenomas, and it is rarely diagnosed by a pathologist. Physiologic lactotroph hyperplasia during pregnancy is an example of a normal response to the hormonal environment.[92] Pathologic response to an abnormal excessive stimulus may cause pituitary hyperplasia in humans. Somatotroph or mammosomatotroph hyperplasia has been reported in patients with ectopic secretion of GHRH, in whom chronic stimulation results in proliferation of these subtypes of adenohypophysial cells but adenoma rarely develops.[93]

Corticotroph hyperplasia is associated with some cases of Cushing's disease[94, 95] and occurs in patients with untreated or inadequately treated Addison's disease.[96] The occurrence and pathogenesis of pituitary hyperplasia in hereditary syndrome settings has not been investigated.

PARATHYROID GLAND

Parathyroid disease usually comes to attention as a result of parathyroid hyperfunction and may be associated with bone loss. Hyperparathyroidism can be caused by a solitary adenoma or carcinoma, multiglandular hyperplastic or neoplastic parathyroid disease, or occur as a complication of chronic renal failure. Clinicopathologic correlation is crucial in the diagnosis and treatment of patients with hyperparathyroidism. Many cases of primary hyperparathyroidism are associated with the multiple endocrine neoplasia syndromes such as MEN 1, MEN 2, and HPT/JT. Once it has been determined that primary hyperparathyroidism is hereditary and perhaps associated with one of the multiple endocrine neoplasia syndromes, it is very important to determine if resection of a single gland will result in adequate treatment or whether multiple gland resection is required. When a single large gland is identified, it must be further established whether it represents an adenoma or carcinoma. Neither of these questions has an easy answer.

Parathyroid Hyperplasia

Parathyroid hyperplasia (diffuse and nodular) is defined as an absolute increase in parathyroid parenchymal cell mass resulting from proliferation of chief cells, oncocytic cells, and transitional oncocytic cells in *multiple* parathyroid glands. Hyperplastic parathyroid disease may arise spontaneously, in association with one of the hereditary endocrinopathies or in association with chronic renal failure. In spite of diverse causes, however, it has several common features. Interestingly, many "hyperplastic" proliferations that arise spontaneously[97–99] or in association with chronic renal failure[98, 100] were shown to be monoclonal. Nevertheless, polyclonal proliferations may also be observed in each of these settings. These results suggest that in many cases a polyclonal hyperplastic proliferation gives rise to a single dominant clone. Although initially thought to be a monoclonal process on the basis of 11q13 LOH analysis,[101] multiglandular parathyroid disease in the setting of MEN 1 has been shown to be polyclonal by X-chromosome inactivation analysis.[9] Based on combined 11q13 LOH and X-chromosome inactivation data, MEN 1–associated multiglandular parathyroid disease has been shown to arise from multiple independent neoplastic clones[9] and, therefore, should not be called "hyperplasia." In view of this fact, a current arbitrary clinicopathologic definition of "parathyroid hyperplasia" based on the number of glands (more than one) involved should be re-evaluated.

There are no reliable histologic or clinical criteria for proliferations in which clinical cure will be achieved by single gland resection from those for which multiple gland resection will be required.[102] The assessment of tumors for presence of a monoclonal versus polyclonal cell population, at least in the setting of MEN 1, does not appear to be useful.[9] Morphometric analysis fails to demonstrate differences between "hyperplasia" and "adenoma."[103] Furthermore, there is no immunohistochemical evidence (based on Ki-67/MIB1 staining) that cell proliferation rates differ between "hyperplasia" and adenoma.[104]

Parathyroid Adenoma

Adenomas are the cause of primary hyperparathyroidism about 85% of the time. Although one widely cited study suggested the possibility that many parathyroid adenomas are polyclonal hyperplastic proliferations,[97] most studies have both confirmed the monoclonal nature of parathyroid adenoma and even suggested the possibility that some lesions diagnosed as hyperplasias are, in fact, neoplastic.[97, 105]

A single karyotype has been reported, with a t(1;5)(p22;q32) as the sole clonal abnormality. CGH studies have demonstrated frequent deletions on chromosomes 1p, 1q, 6q, 9p, 9q, 11p, 11q, 13q, 15q, 17, and 22[106, 107] and gains on 16p and 19p.[108] In contrast, parathyroid carcinoma demonstrated deletions on chromosome 1p and chromosome 17 and gains on chromosome 5.[109] These findings do not resolve the question of whether a parathyroid carcinoma may evolve from an adenomatous proliferation.

Less than 10% of parathyroid adenomas involve a clonal rearrangement that combines the *PTH* gene on 11q15 with the *cyclin D1 (CCND1)* gene on 11q13.[110] The tumorigenic effect appears to result from unregulated transcription leading to overexpression of an otherwise normal transcript; there is no evidence for oncogenic mutation.[111]

Approximately 20% of sporadic adenoma cases demonstrate a somatic mutation of the *MEN1* gene accompanied by LOH on 11q13.[16] Such mutations represent the most common genetic abnormality described in parathyroid adenomas to date. LOH at 11q13, which is common in sporadic parathyroid adenomas,[112] does not appear to be related to *CCND1* function. A variety of other cell-cycle control genes have been investigated as a potential cause for parathyroid adenoma tumorigenesis, but no such genes have been demonstrated. Potential involvement of the putative *HRPT2* gene (1q25–31), which is thought to be associated with the autosomal dominant HPT/JT syndrome, needs to be investigated in sporadic adenomas.[25, 108, 113] Alternatively, one or more yet unidentified tumor suppressor genes that localize to distal 1p may be involved. LOH near the *BRCA2* locus has been observed in about 15% of cases.[88] Although the *RET* protein product was shown to be expressed in both MEN 2A parathyroid tumors and sporadic adenomas, *RET* mutations were not observed.[114–116]

Demonstration of parathyroid differentiation can be accomplished by immunohistochemical staining for parathyroid hormone (PTH). This may be particularly useful when the parathyroid is located in the thymus or thyroid gland; however, one must remember that ectopic PTH production by nonparathyroid tumors demonstrating neuroendocrine differentiation may occasionally complicate interpretation.[117]

Parathyroid Carcinoma

Although most cases of parathyroid carcinoma are sporadic, families with parathyroid carcinoma causing primary hyperthyroidism have been reported.[118] Cytogenetic studies of a parathyroid carcinoma from one such patient demonstrated reciprocal translocation between chromosomes 3 and 4, trisomy 7, and a pericentric inversion in chromosome 9 and no evidence of *RAS* mutation, *PTH* gene rearrangement, or allelic loss from chromosome 11q13.[118] LOH studies in tumors from another such family showed LOH on chromosomes 13q12.3-q32 in one adenoma and 9p21-p22 and 13q12.3-q32 in a second, but no changes in the carcinoma.[119] These localizations suggest possible involvement of the retinoblastoma and *BRCA2* genes. Parathyroid carcinoma is common in patients with familial HPT/JT syndrome. The putative HPT/JT gene *(HRPT2)* has been mapped to chromosome 1q25-q31 but has not been identified.[25]

PCR amplification and sequencing of the *RET* oncogene in a parathyroid gland from one patient with MTC and metastatic parathyroid carcinoma revealed a monoallelic germline Cys634Tyr mutation confirming the presence of MEN 2A. In addition, loss of tumor heterozygosity was seen on chromosomes 1, 2, 3p, 13q, and 16p.[120]

Immunohistochemical studies of the *RB1* gene product have demonstrated evidence of *RB1* gene inactivation in most parathyroid carcinomas, and only rarely in parathyroid adenomas; interpretation of the data is limited by very small numbers of patients.[121, 122] Similarly, the studies suggesting evidence that *TP53* mutation may be involved in the pathogenesis of some parathyroid carcinomas suffer from the same limitation.[123] CGH studies demonstrate frequent chromosomal deletions on chromosome 17 (site of the *TP53* gene) and chromosome 1p (site of the putative neuroblastoma suppressor gene), together with gains on chromosome 5.[106]

It is sometimes difficult to histologically differentiate between parathyroid adenoma and parathyroid carcinoma. Studies of the diagnostic and prognostic utility of flow and image cytometric DNA histogram analysis have yielded conflicting results. Although some studies suggest that parathyroid carcinomas are more likely to be aneuploid and demonstrate higher S-phase fractions than adenomas or hyperplasias,[124–126] other investigations suggest no use for cytometric analysis of parathyroid lesions.[127, 128] Larger studies are required to obtain definitive results. There are reports that suggest using immunohistochemical staining for Ki-67 (MIB1) to assess cell proliferation and correlate with benign versus malignant behavior of parathyroid tumors.[104, 129, 130] One report showed that carcinomas are more likely to demonstrate epidermal growth factor receptor (EGFR) messenger RNA (mRNA) than are adenomas.[131] Whether any ancillary method is more useful than a careful search for mitotic figures, necrosis, hyaline bands, and capsular and vascular invasion will require more extensive studies.

Although parathyroid carcinomas generally demonstrate PTH by immunocytochemical methods, the use of PTH antibodies as a diagnostic adjunct may be limited by the fact that ectopic PTH is commonly produced by lung carcinomas.[117]

THYROID GLAND

Autoimmune Thyroid Disease

Lymphocytic (Hashimoto's) thyroiditis and most cases of Graves' disease are autoimmune disorders with a striking predisposition toward females,[132, 133] particularly those with Turner's syndrome.[134–137] Linkage analyses have demonstrated an association between Graves' disease and loci on chromosomes Xq21.33-22 and 20q11.2[133, 138]; however, no specific genetic abnormalities have been identified. There appears to be a familial predisposition to these diseases[139]; autosomal dominant inheritance of antibodies to thyroid peroxidase, with reduced penetrance in males, has been suggested.[140]

Although Hashimoto's thyroiditis is associated with the development of MALT lymphomas, most gene rearrangement studies demonstrate that the infiltrating lymphocyte population is polyclonal.[141–144]

Hyperplastic (Adenomatoid) Nodules (Nodular Goiter)

The diagnosis of "adenomatoid nodule" is made more frequently than any other diagnosis on thyroid aspirates.[145] Cytogenetic studies have demonstrated a variety of abnormalities, including translocations involving chromosomes 1, 5, 19, and 22[146–149] as well as numerical abnormalities.[148, 149] Numerical chromosomal aberrations have also been observed by fluorescent in situ hybridization.[148] Approximately 10% of goiters exhibit abnormal numbers of chromosomes 7 and 12,[150] which roughly corresponds to the percentage demonstrating aneuploidy on DNA histograms obtained using flow or image cytometry.[151–153] One to two thirds of unencapsulated thyroid nodules appear to be monoclonal, thus blurring the traditional distinction between hyperplastic and neoplastic processes.[154–158] Whether karyotypic abnormality arises only from within monoclonal nodules has not been determined.

Although goiter is most often associated with iodine deficiency, hereditary forms have been described.[159–161] In at least one pedigree, inheritance has been linked to a putative gene on 14q.[160] However, it is a thyroglobulin defect (chromosome 8)[162–164] that is thought most likely to account for goiter development in most cases.

Mutation of the *RAS* oncogene[165, 166] and high levels of RAS protein expression have been reported in several nodular goiters.[167] Nevertheless, *RAS* mutations appear to be unusual events, and their relationship to the disease is uncertain.[168] Expression of *retTPC/PTC* , an activated form of the *RET* oncogene,[169] the *ETS1*-1 proto-oncogene,[170] and the *MET* oncogene[171] have all been reported.

Hyperplastic nodules invariably express thyroglobulin,[172] as well as cytokeratins 7, 8, 18, and 19.[173] The Leu-7 antigen is generally not detected in hyperplastic nodules, although it is found in about half of all papillary carcinomas, follicular carcinomas, and follicular adenomas.[174] About one third of nodular goiters express estrogen receptor protein,[175] and about one fourth express HMBE-1.[176] Staining for CD15 and CA19-9 is seen uncommonly.[176]

Follicular Adenoma

The distinction between follicular hyperplasia and follicular adenoma is obscured by the fact that hyperplastic nodules are frequently monoclonal, leading to the suggestion that follicular adenomas arise from a hyperplastic process. Solitary and encapsulated nodules are invariably monoclonal[154–156] and may harbor a variety of cytogenetic abnormalities. The abnormalities range from numerical changes[150, 177–185] to apparently nonrandom structural rearrangements, including t(2;3) (q12;p24),[160, 163, 168] t(5;19) (q13;q13),[160, 169] t(6;19) (q12;q13), t(10;19) (q22;p13 or q13), and t(8;14) (q13;q24.1) translocations.[186–188] The frequent rearrangement of chromosome 19q13 would seem to make this a particularly worthwhile target of molecular investigation,[183] because it is also observed in a follicular adenoma cell line.[189] As might be expected in a tumor frequently demonstrating numerical chromosomal aberrations, DNA aneuploidy is reproducibly detected by flow or image cytometry in 25% to 50% of follicular adenomas.[151, 153, 190–192] Thus, aneuploidy is more common than in hyperplastic nodules but less common than in follicular carcinomas.[193]

CGH studies demonstrate frequent gains of chromosomes 5, 7, 9, 12, 14, 17, 18, and 8; however, losses are occasionally seen on chromosome 22.[194] By using microsatellite markers, allelic loss in the Cowden locus (10q22-23) has been observed in about 25% of follicular adenomas.[195] Functional loss of the *PTEN/MMACI* gene, which codes for a dual specificity phosphatase, has been suggested.[196] LOH of 11q13, at the *MEN1* gene locus, is seen in about 20% of follicular adenomas[197]; however, the *MEN1* gene does not show somatic mutations in thyroid tumors. LOH at 7q31, which is common in follicular carcinoma, is relatively uncommon in follicular adenoma.[198] Microsatellite instability at several other loci has also been reported,[199] although no direct evidence for a mismatch repair enzyme defect exists.

The most common molecular abnormalities observed in thyroid adenomas are mutations of the thyroid-stimulating hormone receptor *(TSHR)* and *GSP*, each occurring in 5% to 10% of adenomas, or one third of functioning adenomas.[200–208] The prevalence of these mutations and the precise mechanisms by which these mutations contribute to the formation of adenomas are debated.[209–213] Such mutations are not observed in nonfunctioning adenomas and are thought not to be relevant to malignant transformation.[214]

Mutations of *KRAS* and *NRAS* oncogenes are uncommon in follicular adenomas,[215, 216] but mutations of *HRAS* may be observed in approximately 20% to 30% of cases.[217, 218] The relationship to tumor progression, if any, is uncertain. Mutations of *TP53* have not been observed,[219, 220] and inactivation of the *RB1* gene has not been implicated. Telomerase activity is reported to be present in the minority of follicular adenomas and is seen in the majority of follicular carcinomas[221]; however, there has been a significant interlaboratory variation in these findings.[222] Oncogene amplification has not been reported in follicular adenoma.

Some studies on morphometric assessment of thyroid nodules have demonstrated a progression of average nuclear size as one goes from hyperplastic nodule to follicular adenoma to follicular carcinoma.[223, 224] Thus, nuclear size, in combination with nuclear roundness, the identification of cellular aggregates, and observation of nuclear overlap has been proposed by some authors as useful criteria in discriminating adenomas from hyperplasias and carcinomas in fine-needle aspirates.[225, 226] The chromatin pattern of follicular adenomas, although similar to that of carcinomas, differs significantly from that of goiter.[227] The most important diagnostic criteria for differentiating follicular adenoma from follicular carcinoma of the thyroid (i.e., vascular and capsular invasion) cannot be assessed on fine-needle aspiration. Therefore, fine-needle aspiration diagnosis of follicular thyroid lesions can only be confirmed in an accurately evaluated surgical pathology specimen.

Thyroglobulin staining is virtually always observed in follicular adenomas; staining for milk fat globulin is seen in about half of cases.[228] The Leu-7 antigen may sometimes be useful in helping to differentiate between follicular carcinoma, in which staining is typically diffuse and strong, and follicular adenoma, in which staining, when present, is diffuse and weak.[229] Immunohistochemical staining for p53 is occasionally observed, despite the lack of evidence for involvement of *TP53* in the pathogenesis of these tumors.[230] Staining for BCL2 is frequent.[231]

Follicular Carcinoma

Karyotypic analysis of follicular carcinoma of the thyroid (FCT) has demonstrated considerable variation from case to case.[177, 178, 232–235] The karyotypic picture is not particularly useful at predicting clinical outcome, because many metastatic thyroid carcinomas demonstrate normal stem lines.[177] Both karyotypic abnormalities[233–235] and LOH[236] on chromosome 3p are common in FCT, suggesting the presence of a yet unknown gene at this locus that may be important in tumor progression. In addition, t(7;8) (p15;q24) and der(8)t(7;8) (p15;q24) have been observed in highly aggressive follicular carcinomas, suggesting that one or both of these chromosome breakpoints, or the translocation itself, may be involved in the unusually aggressive tumor behavior.[234] CGH studies frequently reveal gains of chromosomes 9, 17, and 18.[194] Loss of chromosome 22q is observed in approximately one half of cases, and loss of 1p occurs in about one third.[194] It seems surprising that deletions frequently observed using classic cytogenetic techniques have not been seen with CGH.

In addition to 3p,[236] allelic deletion has been observed occasionally on 10q22-23,[237] 11p,[197] 2p, and 2q.[238] Fifty percent of FCT demonstrate deletions on two or more chromosomal arms[239]; LOH studies have not demonstrated deletions at a rate higher than 33% at any chromosomal location.[239]

There is no evidence of *RB1* gene inactivation in FCT[240] despite the fact that deletions of *CDKN2A* and *CDKN2B*, both components of the retinoblastoma/cyclin-dependent kinase pathway, have been observed.[240] Activating point mutations in *HRAS*, *KRAS1*, and *NRAS* have also been demonstrated.[165, 216–218, 241, 242] The relationship of *RAS* mutation to tumor progression is debatable. Although *TP53* abnormalities are not seen in well-differentiated FCT, 40% of poorly differentiated FCTs show immunohistochemical evidence of overexpression,[243] and up to one third of poorly differentiated FTCs have *TP53* point mutations.[243–245] These findings suggest that *TP53* mutation results in dedifferentiation of previously established FCT and that assessment of *TP53* status could have prognostic use in these patients.[246] Unfortunately, studies that have directly compared the outcomes of patients whose tumors demonstrated immunohistochemical reactivity for *TP53* with those that did not have failed to demonstrate significant differences.[247] Similarly, whereas several studies have described the results of immunohistochemical analyses for PCNA[174, 230] and Ki-67,[248–250] none has demonstrated a role for these analyses in routine clinical diagnosis. Studies on various cell adhesion molecules have failed to demonstrate abnormalities in FCT.[251–254]

Tumor aneuploidy is frequently detected in FCT by image and flow cytometry[151, 193, 255, 256]; aneuploid cell populations demonstrate significantly higher S-phase fractions than do their diploid counterparts.[255] Nevertheless, neither DNA ploidy nor S-phase fraction provides prognostically useful information beyond that which has been available from histologic examination.[190, 193, 256] Although the diagnosis of FCT can generally be made on the basis of histology, immunohistochemical assessment is occasionally helpful in differential diagnosis with medullary carcinoma and in the examination of metastases. Thyroglobulin immunoreactivity is almost invariably present (Table 13–3), together with immunoreactivity for thyroid peroxidase, neuron-specific enolase, milk fat globulin HMFG2, and S-100.[228, 257–259] Vimentin, lactoferrin, and cytokeratin-19 immunoreactivity are each observed in about half of FCT,[172, 260, 261] but significant interlaboratory variation exists.[262] Leu-7 generally demonstrates a diffusely strong staining pattern, which may be useful in distinguishing FCT from follicular adenoma[263]; caution is advised, however, because interlaboratory differences in immunohistochemical techniques may result in significant differences in staining utility. Apparent differences in patterns of immunoreactivity are at best a weak adjunct in differentiating among thyroid neoplasms.

HÜRTHLE CELL TUMORS

Hürthle cell tumors are histologically, and to a degree clinically, unique follicular thyroid neoplasms. Although

TABLE 13–3

Thyroglobulin Immunoreactivity as a Function of Histologic Classification of Thyroid Tumors*

Diagnosis	Percentage of Cases Demonstrating Immunoreactivity
Anaplastic carcinoma	4–16
Follicular carcinoma	82–98
Medullary carcinoma	1–10
Papillary carcinoma	89–100

* There is generally a reciprocal relationship between staining for calcitonin and staining for thyroglobulin.

few cases have been studied, classic cytogenetic investigations of Hürthle cell tumors have demonstrated frequent numerical chromosomal abnormalities in the absence of other clonal changes.[177, 264] Three of five cases examined demonstrated a hemizygous deletion of the *PTEN* gene, a phosphatase gene localized to 10q22-23 that appears to have tumor-suppressor properties.[237] Hürthle cell tumors also demonstrate allelic deletions on chromosomes 1q, 2p, 3q, and 18q.[265, 266] When present, changes on 1q and 2p have been associated with malignant behavior,[265] a fact that has been exploited to assist in cytodiagnosis.[267] These changes are all similar to those that have been described in follicular neoplasms.

Hürthle cell tumors demonstrate a variety of changes at the molecular level, the significance of which is not understood. Immunohistochemical accumulation of p53 is seen in about half of Hürthle cell tumors[268, 269] but is not generally accompanied by *TP53* mutation.[269] Nevertheless, it has been suggested that tumors that are p53 protein positive and BCL2 negative are more likely to be clinically aggressive.[270] Mutations of *NRAS* and *HRAS* have both been reported, with an increased frequency of *NRAS* mutations in clinically aggressive tumors.[217, 271] Accumulation of mutated *RAS* can often be demonstrated immunohistochemically.[167, 272] A single *GSP* mutation (Arg201Cys) has been reported,[210] as has been a thyrotropin receptor gene mutation that constitutively activated cyclic adenosine monophosphate production, leading to thyrotoxicosis in a patient with Hürthle cell carcinoma.[273] Hürthle cell tumors frequently show immunohistochemical reactivity for TGFA (63%), TGFB (88%), IGF1 (88%), and MYCN (100%).[272]

E-cadherin is a calcium-dependent adhesion molecule necessary for normal epithelial function. In Hürthle cell tumors, E-cadherin immunoreactivity is reduced and distributed intracellularly rather than at the cell surface.[251] Loss of expression seems to result from hypermethylation of the E-cadherin 5′ CpG island.[274] The *MET* oncogene protein, a cell surface tyrosine kinase that serves as a receptor for hepatocyte growth factor, is observed immunohistochemically in 70% of these tumors (as well as in a large percentage of papillary carcinomas), but not in other thyroid neoplasms. Finally, Hürthle cell neoplasms demonstrate an unusual pattern of basement membrane laminin deposition, suggesting uncontrolled synthesis.[275] Taken together, these findings suggest that the clinical behavior of these neoplasms may be determined, at least in part, by alteration of intercellular interactions.

DNA histograms of Hürthle cell tumors frequently demonstrate aneuploidy, whether the tumors are benign or malignant.[276] There is no evidence that tumor cell aneuploidy is a useful prognostic factor.[276, 277]

Although the diagnosis of Hürthle cell tumors can generally be made on routinely stained sections, the immunohistochemical characteristics have, nevertheless, been described. Almost all cases express thyroglobulin[268]; approximately 30% of cases demonstrate progesterone receptor.[278] The expression of epithelial membrane antigen (EMA) and carcinoembryonic antigen (CEA) is variable.[268, 279]

Papillary Carcinoma

Papillary carcinoma of the thyroid (PCT) is the most common thyroid malignancy. Cytogenetic studies generally demonstrate simple karyotypes,[280] but inv(10) (q11;q21) has been described in a number of tumors.[179, 233, 264, 281, 282] Translocations involving this region of chromosome 10, t(5;10)(p15;q11))[233] and t(7,10) (q35;q21)[283] have also been reported. Inv(10) (q11;q21) fuses the tyrosine kinase domain of the *RET* proto-oncogene with a gene called *H4* to form a fusion oncogene called *PTC1*.[284] This fusion gene can be detected in about one fourth of papillary carcinomas.[285, 286] The hybrid gene product oligomerizes readily; this is a critical step for tyrosine kinase activation.[287] In addition, because expression of the fusion protein is driven by the *H4* gene promoter, and *H4* is normally expressed in thyroid, one might expect substantially increased levels of tyrosine kinase activity.[287] The t(10;17) translocation results in a fusion of *RET* with a regulatory subunit of cyclic adenosine phosphate–dependent protein kinase C (PKA) to form the *PTC2* chimera.[288] Cytogenetically undetectable paracentric inversion within 10q11.2 results in fusion of *RET* with *ELE1* to form the *PTC3* [289–291] and *PTC4* [292] chimeras. A *PTC5* chimera has also been detected but not described in detail.[293] The *PTC2-PTC55* chimeras together are found in about 5% of papillary carcinomas. Several other less common fusion products have also been described. *RET* rearrangements are particularly frequent in radiation-associated PTC.[294–296]

Oncogenic fusion of the *NTRK1* proto-oncogene (1q21-22) to the tropomyosin gene by intrachromosomal rearrangement has also been reported in PCT.[285,297] *NTRK1* rearrangement appears to be about half as frequent as *RET* rearrangement in the few published studies.[285,297]

It has been suggested that *RET* and *NTRK1* rearrangements are associated with an increased likelihood of lymph node metastasis in papillary carcinoma.[298, 299] If the data are confirmed, a role might exist for molecular diagnosis in a subgroup of PCT, which are otherwise easily identified on morphologic grounds.

A single CGH/spectral karyotyping study of radiation-associated PCT has shown structural alterations affecting identical chromosomes 1q, 2, 4q, 5q, 6p, 9, 10q, 12q, 13q, and 14q.[300] LOH has been demonstrated on chromosome 4q, 5p, 7p, and 11p by microsatellite methods[301] in some, but not all,[239] studies. Numerous studies on the role of *TP53* and *RAS* have failed to demonstrate a role for these genes in the pathogenesis of papillary carcinoma. Telomerase activity is observed in about half of cases.[302–304]

Akslen and Varhaug have presented results of a study that showed ERBB2 protein, estrogen receptor-related protein, S-phase, G_2M-phase, sex, age, histologic grade, and primary tumor extent are all of prognostic importance in univariate analysis of patient survival, but only male sex ($P = .017$), older age ($P = .00005$), and high-grade histologic features ($P = .006$) were associated independently with decreased survival.[305] A suggestion that loss of RB1 protein expression is associated with the development of distant metastases or recurrent disease[306] has not been confirmed. Similarly, diagnostic use for immunohistochemical assessment of PCNA or Ki-67 (MIB1) has yet to be established.

More than 90% of papillary carcinomas demonstrate thyroglobulin (see Table 13–3), at least focally, by immunohistochemical methods.[117, 257] Most cases also demonstrate CD117 (KIT),[307] CD44,[308, 309] CD57 (Leu7)[174, 310] cytokeratin,[311] HBME-1,[312] CD15,[312] and S-100.[313] CD57 staining may be particularly useful in differentiating the follicular variant of papillary carcinoma, which typically exhibits relatively strong staining, from follicular carcinoma, which is less frequently positive.[310]

Medullary Carcinoma

Medullary carcinoma (MTC), which is the only true neuroendocrine tumor of the thyroid gland, arises from thyroid C cells. Approximately 75% of cases appear to be sporadic, with most of the remaining cases being a manifestation of two multiple endocrine neoplasia syndromes (MEN 2A and 2B) and a few representing a familial MTC syndrome. Sporadic cases are generally unilateral, whereas hereditary medullary carcinomas are frequently bilateral and occur in a thyroid gland demonstrating significant C-cell hyperplasia. Only a few karyotypes from medullary carcinomas have been reported.[177, 178, 264, 314, 315] No characteristic cytogenetic pattern has been found. Cytogenetic characterization of long-established medullary carcinoma cell lines has demonstrated abnormalities at 9q and 3p,[316] but the relevance of this findings to in vivo tumors is uncertain. Tumor cell aneuploidy is detected by flow cytometry in approximately 40% of cases[256]; the clinical use of DNA cytometry is disputed in the literature.[256, 317]

Linkage studies have demonstrated that MEN 2 is caused by mutations in the *RET* oncogene; these mutations predispose to the various MEN 2–associated neoplasms, including MTC.[21] Similarly, linkage studies of familial medullary carcinoma syndrome demonstrate conclusively that this disease is caused by mutation at the site of the *RET (MEN2)* gene.[20, 318, 319] The location and nature of these mutations is important. Those associated with familial medullary carcinoma are *RET* Cys634Arg, Glu768Asp, or Leu804Val, whereas MEN 2A and 2B show a variety of other mutations (see Table 13–2).[21] The *RET* gene is a membrane-associated tyrosine kinase; MEN 2– and MTC–associated mutations result in constitutional activation of *RET*, but no clear picture of subsequent events has emerged.[21]

Approximately half of sporadic medullary carcinomas demonstrate somatic *RET* mutations.[320] For the most part, the locations more closely resemble those involved in MEN 2B (particularly Met918Thr),[321] although mutations at several MEN 2A loci are also found.[322] Deletions[322, 323] appear to predominate in the MEN 2A region. A minority of apparently sporadic medullary cancer cases are associated with germline *RET* mutations; estimates range from 1.5%[324] to nearly 30%.[325]

There has been limited investigation of other possible genetic alterations in MTC. LOH on chromosomes 1p and 22q has been reported.[326] Mutations of *TP53* are not seen in this tumor,[327] *RAS* mutations are rare,[328] and there is no evidence for loss of *RB1* gene activity.[329]

Patients with sporadic medullary carcinoma whose tumors have the Met918Thr mutation in the MEN 2B region appear to have a significantly worse prognosis than those whose tumors do not demonstrate this mutation.[330, 331] Although *MYCN* amplification is not seen in MTC, it has been reported that tumors that demonstrate *MYCN* protein in more than 10% of the cells appear to be significantly more aggressive than those that do not.[332] Medullary carcinomas demonstrating Leu-M1–positive cells are reported to have a significantly worse prognosis than those that are Leu-M1 negative.[333] PCNA staining does not appear to have prognostic use.[332] There has been no independent verification of the clinical use of any of these potential prognostic markers.

Immunohistochemical staining for thyrocalcitonin is the most valuable immunohistochemical adjunct for the diagnosis of MTC; almost 100% of cases demonstrate at least some staining.[117, 258] Ectopic production of thyrocalcitonin by neuroendocrine tumors of lung, pancreas, and colon is also common, however. Many MTCs also react with other neuroendocrine markers, including vasoactive intestinal peptide, ACTH,[334] neuron-specific enolase,[258, 335] and chromogranin.[336–338] They are positive for cytokeratins.[311, 339] Fewer than 20% of cases demonstrate epithelial membrane antigen and S-100.[258] The percentage of cases reacting with carcinoembryonic antigen depends on the precise antibody formulation employed,[340] but it may be up to 100%.[258] Rare cases may demonstrate thyroglobulin immunoreactivity.[341]

Anaplastic Carcinoma

Anaplastic carcinoma of the thyroid is an aggressive tumor that is characterized by a 1-year survival rate of approximately 10%.[342] The histologically aggressive features are associated with abundant karyotypic abnormality, but the few reported karyotypes have failed to reveal consistent cytogenetic anomalies.[233, 343, 344] The presence of double minutes in some tumors[343] suggests the possibility of oncogene amplification, but no specific examples have been reported. The karyotypic abnormality is mirrored by the observation of significant aneuploidy in a majority of DNA histograms obtained by either image[345] or flow cytometry.[346]

Activating mutations of *RAS* genes are uncommon in papillary carcinoma of the thyroid, common in follicular carcinoma, and found in 60% to 75% of anaplastic thyroid carcinomas.[218, 347] In addition to *RAS* activation, the most prominent molecular alteration in undifferentiated carcinoma of the thyroid is *TP53* mutation, which is found in a large majority of cases and sometimes in association with increased *MDM2* expression.[348] Although *TP53* mutation in itself is probably incapable of producing a malignant phenotype,[349] there is strong evidence of its association with tumor progression. Mutations of *TP53* are rare in well-differentiated papillary and follicular carcinomas[220, 350] but are increasingly common as tumors become progressively less differentiated.[243, 350, 351] Mutation of *TP53* is correlated with increased *BCL2* expression.[352] The importance of *TP53* mutation in progression is highlighted by the fact that introduction of wild-type p53 into thyroid carcinoma cell lines inhibits tumorigenic potential.[353] Activation of the *RET* oncogene, which is seen in papillary and medullary carcinomas of the thyroid, is rare or absent in anaplastic carcinoma.[286, 354] Loss of RB1 protein expression is also not seen in this tumor.[329]

The *NME1 (NM23)* gene product is thought to serve as a metastasis suppressor protein, and reduced expression is associated with metastatic behavior in some forms of cancer. Most workers have found decreased *NME1* expression in anaplastic carcinomas of the thyroid,[355, 356] although one paper reports a twofold increase.[357] It is possible that these apparently conflicting findings reflect differences in expression of different proteins, NME1 and NME2, arising from alternative splicing.

A number of other genetic abnormalities have been observed in small studies. Expression of E-cadherin, β-catenin, and γ-catenin has been nearly undetectable in virtually all anaplastic carcinomas of the thyroid.[358] Integrin-2 has been expressed in anaplastic carcinomas but not other thyroid tumors.[252] Telomerase activity has not been seen in anaplastic carcinoma.[222] All of the following have been reported: overexpression of *MYCN*, *PDGFA*, and *PDGFBB*[359]; mutation of the *APC* gene[360]; deletion of *PTEN*[237]; LOH in the region of the *CDKN2* gene[361]; production of oncofetal fibronectin[362]; production of the *ETS1* transcription factor[170]; and increased expression of *MYC*.[363]

Although both immunohistochemical and cytometry methods demonstrate high levels of proliferative activity in anaplastic carcinoma,[249, 256, 364] there is no evidence that routine assessment of proliferative activity provides useful prognostic information.[256]

The differentiation of anaplastic carcinoma of the thyroid from other undifferentiated neoplasms can be problematic. Most cases demonstrate vimentin, epithelial markers, and lactoferrin,[365–367] and thyroglobulin staining is rare (see Table 13–3).[368, 369] Some anaplastic carcinomas of the thyroid lack immunoreactivity for any of the differentiation antigens. This must be distinguished from global loss of immunoreactivity caused by overfixation or other factors by immunohistochemically staining for one of the proliferation markers, such as MIB1.

The thyroid frequently exhibits cytoplasmic biotin-like activity that may confuse the immunohistochemical analysis of thyroid lesions, particularly after "antigen-retrieval" procedures.[370]

ADRENAL GLAND

Hyperplastic Processes

Although most cases of adrenal hyperplasia probably represent a physiologic response to pituitary stimulation, as in the case of Cushing's disease, diffuse adrenal hyperplasia may occur as a process that is primary within the adrenal gland. Three of the most common causes of "intrinsic" adrenal hyperplasia are discussed here.

CONGENITAL ADRENAL HYPERPLASIA

Congenital adrenal hyperplasia is the morphologic outcome of a deficiency in one of the adrenal steroid biosynthetic pathways. In most cases it results from a 21-hydroxylase *(CYP21B)* deficiency that blocks conversion of 1-hydroxyprogesterone to 11-deoxycortisol. One of the most common consequences is excessive androgen production, resulting in inappropriate or premature virilization. The gene codes for a 494 amino acid cytochrome P450 protein; inactivation may result from point mutation, complete deletion, or recombination events (gene conversion) involving a nearby 21-hydroxylase pseudogene; gene conversion is by far the most common cause. Although the diagnosis may be made by linkage analysis, using the nearby human leukocyte antigen loci, direct mutation detection is straightforward and widely used.[371–374]

Less common causes of congenital adrenal hyperplasia are 3-hydroxysteroid dehydrogenase deficiency,[375] 17-hydroxyase deficiency,[376] 11-hydroxylase deficiency,[377] and mutation of the steroidogenic acute regulatory protein gene *(STAR)*. [378]

NODULAR HYPERPLASIA

ACTH-independent macronodular adrenal hyperplasia is a poorly understood cause of Cushing's syndrome. The lesions associated with this disease are usually bilateral and may be shown to have a polyclonal origin by X-inactivation analysis.[379] An Arg201Cys mutation in the guanine nucleotide binding protein GS *(GNAS1)* has been described in several patients[380, 381]; whether this is a rare or common finding has not been investigated. The occurrence of macronodular hyperplasia in association with multiple colon adenomas/carcinomas and *APC* mutation has also been reported.[382]

MICRONODULAR HYPERPLASIA

Most cases of micronodular adrenal cortical hyperplasia probably accompany Carney's complex, but both hereditary Cushing's syndrome–associated and hyperaldosteronism-associated adrenal micronodules have been reported in families that do not demonstrate any other elements of this syndrome.[383, 384]

Cortical Adenoma

Although most benign adrenal cortical tumors that are classified as adenomas are monoclonal, the demonstration of polyclonality in some of these tumors[379] suggests the possibility that some nodular hyperplastic lesions are being misdiagnosed as neoplasms. Cytogenetic abnormalities have been found in almost half the adrenal cortical adenomas that have been karyotyped, but no consistent changes have been noted.[385, 386] CGH studies have demonstrated no changes in small adenomas (<5 cm) but have shown inconsistent abnormalities in two larger tumors.[387] Studies using LOH methods have demonstrated that both 11q13 and 11p15 deletions, which are common in carcinomas, are much rarer in adrenal adenoma.[388, 389] The little sequence analysis data that are available suggest a relatively low frequency of *RAS* and *TP53* gene mutations,[390, 391] although there appears to be a subset of Taiwanese patients whose adenomas frequently show *TP53* abnormalities.[392]

In general, the distinction between benign and malignant adrenal cortical lesions is best made on clinical and histologic grounds.[393] There is some evidence that immunohistochemical assessment of cell proliferation, and DNA histogram analysis, may assist in identifying a subset of patients whose tumors are more likely to behave aggressively.[394–401]

Adrenal Cortical Carcinoma

Only a small number of karyotypic analyses have been performed in adrenal cortical carcinomas (ACC).[402–405] The cytogenetic picture is complex, and no consistent chromosomal abnormalities have been identified.

Not surprisingly, given the appearance of ACC among the constellation of tumors associated with Li-Fraumeni syndrome,[406] *TP53* gene mutations are relatively common, occurring in 20% to 30% of sporadic cases.[391, 407] Mutation is generally accompanied by immunohistochemical evidence of p53 accumulation.[391] Although LOH near the *MEN1* locus at 11q13 is frequent, occurring in about 60% of ACCs, somatic *MEN1* gene mutations are not detected in these tumors.[389, 408] LOH at the *RB1* gene locus is also frequent, occurring in up to 80% of cases, but it is not known whether *RB1* mutation occurs in this tumor.[409] Structural abnormalities of 11p15 (as assessed by LOH analysis) are also present in most of these tumors.[388] Mutations of *RAS* are observed in about 10% of adrenal carcinomas.[410] Analysis of LOH patterns may be useful in helping to distinguish between benign and malignant lesions, but this procedure is sufficiently laborious as to be impractical in the routine diagnostic laboratory. Assessment of telomerase activity would be more readily accomplished, but the study performed to date does not establish clinical utility in this neoplasm.[411]

The differentiation of benign adrenal cortical tumors from their malignant counterparts is sometimes difficult and can be only reliably based on the presence or development of distant metastases. Although immunohistochemical assessment of *RB1* does not assist in this discrimination, studies based on small numbers of patients suggest that immunohistochemical assessment of proliferation fraction (using MIB1) and immunohistochemical assessment of p53 accumulation may assist in the diagnosis of malignancy.[130, 395, 396] Patients whose tumors demonstrate D11 immunoreactivity have a higher survival rate and a lower likelihood of metastatic disease than those with tumors that have lost D11 immunoreactivity.[412] Nuclear DNA histogram analysis by flow or image cytometry is also somewhat helpful, because aneuploid tumors are typically more aggressive than those with "normal" histograms.[397–401]

Nevertheless, euploid tumors may behave aggressively and aneuploid tumors may remain indolent. It is uncertain whether any of these adjunct methods improve on the outcome prediction using a model incorporating clinical and histologic criteria (weight loss, broad fibrous bands, diffuse growth pattern, vascular invasion, tumor cell necrosis, and tumor mass).[393]

Although immunohistochemical assessment is seldom required to make a diagnosis, it may sometimes be necessary to distinguish this tumor from pheochromocytoma, renal cell carcinoma, or hepatocellular carcinoma. A typical profile of staining is shown in Table 13–4; a panel that may be helpful in distinguishing these four tumors is shown in Table 13–5. Differences in immunohistochemical procedures among laboratories may result in substantial interlaboratory variation, however.

Neuroblastoma

Neuroblastoma is the most common solid tumor of childhood. It has proven to be a sentinel for the kinds of contributions that molecular biology can make to the understanding, diagnosis, and treatment of malignant disease. For many years it has been known that neuroblastoma frequently demonstrates karyotypic abnormalities, particularly involving chromosome 1 or chromosome 2. Among the most frequent of these are "double minutes" (small fragments of DNA that segregate independently of the chromosomes during mitosis) and "homogeneously staining regions."[413] Analysis of neuroblastoma cell lines containing these karyotypic abnormalities indicated that a gene, *MYCN*, that codes for a nuclear transcription factor, was amplified (present in more than a normal number of copies) in virtually every line tested.[414] A nearby gene, *DDX*, is frequently coamplified.[415] This DNA amplification gave rise to both the double minutes and the homogeneously staining regions in the chromosome spreads. Further work demonstrated that *MYCN* amplification occurred in about one third of neuroblastomas removed surgically, and almost always in patients who had advanced disease.[416] Stage for stage, patients exhibiting *MYCN* amplification were shown to have a poorer prognosis than patients without *MYCN* amplification.[417, 418] In particular, patients who had stage II or stage III disease, but had more than 10 copies of the *MYCN* gene, had a much poorer prognosis than those with only a single copy or from 3 to 10 copies of the gene.[419] Patients with stage IV disease had a grim prognosis regardless of the degree of *MYCN* amplification, although those with a single copy of *MYCN* did somewhat better than those with many copies. The *MYCN* copy number appears to be stable throughout the course of disease and at different sites of tumor spread within a given patient.[417] Apparently, in situ hybridization can be used to estimate amplification of this oncogene. Several groups have demonstrated that the number of cells that demonstrate *MYCN* DNA and/or RNA by in situ hybridization correlates well with the average DNA copy number determined by filter hybridization methods.[420–422] This suggests that a relatively small percentage of tumor cells may contain a very high degree of *MYCN* amplification and that it is these cells that contribute somehow to the overall aggressiveness of the tumor. The mechanism by which gene amplification contributes to a poor prognosis is unclear, both because the function of the *MYCN* gene product is unknown and because the degree of *MYCN* amplification apparently does not correlate with *MYCN* mRNA expression.[423] It is possible that *MYCN* amplification is simply a reflection of abnormalities in a gene localizing to 1p36.

In addition to *MYCN* amplification, LOH in the region of 1p36 is frequent in neuroblastoma[424] and correlates with the presence of *MYCN* amplification; cytogenetic changes in 1p36 are found in approximately two thirds of neuroblastomas.[425] Considerable effort has gone into characterizing cytogenetic and molecular changes in this region of chromosome 1, but the "neuroblastoma suppressor gene" in this region has to date remained elusive.[426] It appears that in tumors with single copies of *MYCN*, maternal 1p36 alleles are preferentially lost, whereas in tumors with *MYCN* amplification, the paternal alleles are lost.[427] This suggests the possibility of more than one tumor suppressor gene near this locus. The paternal *MYCN* allele is preferentially amplified.[428] There is some evidence that karyotypic abnormalities involving the structure of the short arm of chromosome 1 are more important prognostic indicators than age, stage, or *MYCN* amplification.[429, 430] LOH at 1p36 is also, together with LOH at 7q, a very strong indicator of poor prognosis.[431]

TABLE 13–4

Immunoreactivity of Adrenal Cortical Carcinoma for Selected Antigens

Antigen	Percentage of Cases with Positive Reaction
Synaptophysin	72–97
D11	67–96
Vimentin	48–78
Keratin (pan)	5–22
AE 1	0–9
CAM 5.2	0–9
CK 19	0–9
Epithelial membrane antigen	0–6
Calcitonin	0
Chromogranin A	0
HMB-45	0
S-100	0
Somatostatin	0

TABLE 13–5

Immunohistochemical Panel for Distinguishing Adrenal Cortical Carcinoma, Hepatocelluar Carcinoma, Pheochromocytoma, and Renal Cell Carcinoma

	Percentage of Tumors Demonstrating Immunoreactivity			
Antigen	Adrenal Cortical Carcinoma	Hepatocellular Carcinoma	Pheochromocytoma	Renal Cell Carcinoma
AE1/AE3	0	10–29	Low	82–93
CAM 5.2	0–9	79–90	Low	59–75
Chromogranin A	0	Low	90–100	0
D11	67–96	Unknown	0	Unknown
Epithelial membrane antigen	0–6	24–43	0	88–97
Vimentin	48–78	3–10	28–52	50–68

* Results may demonstrate significant interlaboratory variation, depending on details of the immunohistochemical technique employed.

CGH studies have demonstrated that, in addition to *MYCN* amplification and chromosome 1p36 deletion, over half of neuroblastomas demonstrate chromosome 17 aberrations, as well as regional aberrations on 3q24-26, 11q, 12q, 13q, 14q, and 15q.[432–436] Mutations of *TP53* are rare, however, and the p53 regulatory pathway appears to be intact in neuroblastoma.[437–440] Microsatellite instability is also uncommon in neuroblastoma.[441]

Other methods have also proven somewhat useful in predicting the prognosis of patients with neuroblastoma. DNA aneuploidy, as determined by flow cytometry, appears to be a favorable prognostic factor, as does a low fraction of cells in the S + G_2M fractions of the cell cycle.[442–444] However, assessments of DNA ploidy convey no prognostic information beyond that provided by cytogenetic analysis of chromosome 1p or *MYCN* amplification.[445] Telomerase activity is seen in progressing tumors and is absent in nonprogressing tumors.[446] Nevertheless, it appears that telomerase activity is so strongly correlated with *MYCN* amplification and 1p deletion that it is unlikely to have independent prognostic value.[447] Expression of BCL2 protein in neuroblastoma also correlates with both *MYCN* amplification and unfavorable histology[448, 449] and is unlikely to have independent prognostic significance. Overexpression of *ERBB2* has been associated with an unfavorable outcome, as has immunohistochemical accumulation of p53 protein.[450] The latter finding is particularly surprising, in light of studies demonstrating that *TP53* mutation is rare and the p53 regulatory pathway intact. Assessment of proliferation marker Ki-S5 has also proven useful in a single small study.[451] Multivariate studies in which immunohistochemical assessments are analyzed together with cytogenetic and gene amplification data are required to determine if these immunocytochemical methods have any real value.

In the meantime, it is clear that cytogenetic assessment of the tumor and determination of *MYCN* amplification are powerful methods for both confirming the histologic diagnosis of difficult cases and for predicting the ultimate outcome for patients with neuroblastoma.

Although assessment of *MYCN* amplification and 1p36 chromosome abnormalities may assist in the diagnosis of neuroblastoma, they are sufficiently time consuming that one cannot practically wait for these results before rendering a diagnosis. The differential diagnosis of neuroblastoma includes the full spectrum of "small round blue cell tumors," including Ewing's sarcoma/peripheral neuroectodermal tumor (PNET), leukemia/lymphoma, and alveolar rhabdomyosarcoma. Immunohistochemical assessment is a valuable diagnostic adjunct; typical patterns of immunoreactivity are shown in Table 13–6. The NB 84 antibody,[452] though useful as part of this panel, also reacts with Ewing's sarcoma/PNET and does not assist much in distinguishing this group of tumors from neuroblastoma (Table 13–7).[452, 453]

Pheochromocytoma

Pheochromocytoma is a clinically and histologically distinctive tumor of the adrenal medulla. Most cases come to medical attention as a result of either hypertension or a family history of multiple endocrine neoplasia. The histologic diagnosis of pheochromocytoma is, in most cases, straightforward. Nevertheless, conventional morphologic criteria are insufficient to allow determination of malignant potential in pheochromocytoma.

There have been few classic cytogenetic investigations of pheochromocytoma. Three cases associated with von Hippel-Lindau disease demonstrated chromosome 3 rearrangements resulting in partial or total trisomy.[454] Chromosome 20 deletions have been reported in MEN 2 families. There is a seldom, if ever, observable change in 10q11, the site of the *RET* proto-oncogene.[455]

TABLE 13–6

Immunoreactivity of Neuroblastoma for Selected Antigens

Antigen	Percentage of Cases Demonstrating Immunoreactivity
NB-84	98–100
Neuron-specific enolase	79–94
Neurofilament protein	63–86
Chromogranin A	60–82
Synaptophysin	46–75
Vimentin	37–75
S-100	23–51
CD 57	0–20
Glial fibrillary acidic protein	0–12
Desmin	0–10
β_2-Microglobulin	0
CD 99	0

TABLE 13–8

Immunoreactivity of Pheochromocytoma for Selected Antigens

Antigen	Percentage of Cases Demonstrating Immunoreactivity
Synaptophysin	100
Chromogranin A	90–100
Neurofilament protein	85–98
BCL2	73–97
Glial fibrillary acidic protein	34–74
S-100*	33–61
Vimentin	28–52
Calcitonin	6–37
Keratin (pan)	9–27
Somatostatin	0–17
D11	0

* S-100 stains scattered sustentacular cells only.

Pheochromocytomas associated with MEN 2 invariably demonstrate the germline *RET* mutations on chromosome 10q11.2. The *RET* proto-oncogene is generally overexpressed in both familial and sporadic forms,[456, 457] and *RET* mutation is observed in about 20% of sporadic pheochromocytomas.[115, 458, 459] Mutations of the von Hippel-Lindau gene *(VHL)* appear to occur in fewer than 5% of cases.[460] *NF1* mutation is seen in 1% of neurofibromatosis type 1 pheochromocytomas. LOH studies suggest the possible participation of genes on chromosomes 1p, 3p, 11q, 17p, and 22q in the progression of both sporadic and hereditary pheochromocytomas.[326, 461–464] Neither *RAS* nor *TP53* gene mutations are common.[327, 328, 390] Both *MYC* and *FOS* genes may be constitutively overexpressed,[465] at least in some malignant pheochromocytomas,[466] but only a limited number of tumors have been investigated; oncogene amplification has not been reported.

Histologic criteria alone are insufficient to distinguish benign from malignant pheochromocytomas. Telomerase activity, as assessed by the telomerase repeat (TRAP) assay, appears to be elevated in the small number of malignant tumors investigated.[467] Flow cytometric investigations demonstrate aneuploid DNA histograms are rare even in benign pheochromocytomas,[468] although there is some evidence that tumors demonstrating an aneuploid DNA histogram are more likely to behave malignantly than those with a euploid histogram.[401, 469–472] Assessment of MIB1 immunoreactivity was proposed to help in predicting outcome[473]; S-100 immunoreactivity tends to be lost in malignancy.[473, 474]

Immunohistochemical assessment is seldom necessary in making a diagnosis of pheochromocytoma. Typical immunohistochemical results are summarized in Table 13–8. The spectrum of immunoreactivity differs little from that of extra-adrenal paragangliomas, with the exception of neurofilament protein (NFP), which is generally present in adrenal tumors is lacking in extra-adrenal ones. In addition to the expected constellation of neuroendocrine markers, ACTH, melanocyte-stimulating hormone, and β-endorphin are all frequently demonstrated in pheochromocytomas.[475]

TABLE 13–7

Reactivity of Monoclonal Antibody NB 84 for Various Tissues

Tissue	Percentage of Cases Demonstrating Immunoreactivity
Neuroblastoma	98–100
Medulloblastoma	27–63
Ewing's sarcoma/primitive neuroectodermal tumor	12–33
Intra-abdominal desmoplastic small cell tumor	14–70
Wilms' tumor	0–20
Lymphoblastic lymphoma	0
Alveolar rhabdomyosarcoma	0
Sarcoma botryoides	0

EXTRA-ADRENAL PARAGANGLIOMA

Paragangliomas arise from paraganglia in the sympathetic chain; 90% behave benignly. Carotid body tumors and glomus jugulare tumors are often considered as part of the disease spectrum. Although sporadic occurrence is not uncommon, many paragangliomas accompany either of two familial nonchromaffin paraganglioma syndromes mapping to two distinct imprinted genes in the region of 11q22.[476–479] Paragangliomas are also seen as part of Carney's triad[480] (gastric leiomyosarcoma/stromal tumor, pulmonary chondroma and extra-adrenal paraganglioma)[481] and occasionally in association with the von Hippel-Lindau syndrome.[482] In patients with Carney's triad, functioning extra-adrenal paragangliomas present at a young age—usually younger than 35 years. There does not appear to be a genetic predisposition, and no specific molecular abnormalities have been reported.

Relatively little cytogenetic information is available on sporadic paraganglioma. CGH of a sporadic paraganglioma demonstrated evidence of isochromosome 1q and low level gains in 4, 5, 6q, and 13q, with LOH on 1p.[483] A conflicting study suggested that LOH is restricted to 11q in patients with head and neck paragangliomas.[476]

Typical immunohistochemical findings for extra-adrenal paragangliomas are shown in Table 13–9. The reactivity profile is generally similar to that of pheochromocytoma, with the exception that NFP staining is significantly less frequent in extra-adrenal paragangliomas. S-100 and glial fibrillary acidic protein immunoreactivity appears to be lost in malignant tumors and may be a tool for assisting in the determination of malignant potential.[484, 485] Paragangliomas may stain for leu-enkephalin.[486]

On average, an increase in AgNOR (Silver-Stained Nucleolar Organizer Region) counts is associated with worse prognosis in paraganglioma, but a large overlap between benign and malignant cases limits the predictive value for an individual patient.[487] Flow cytometric determination of DNA aneuploidy is not predictive of outcome[488]; the role of S-phase fraction has not been determined. The value of immunohistochemical assessment of proliferation markers is also unknown.

TABLE 13–9

Immunoreactivity of Extra-adrenal Paragangliomas for Selected Antigens

Antigen	Percentage of Cases with Positive Reaction
Synaptophysin	91–100
S-100*	87–100
Neuron-specific enolase	85–100
Chromogranin A	74–95
Serotonin	68–95
Keratin (pan)	0–21
Neurofilament protein	0–21
Desmin	0
Glial fibrillary acidic protein	0

* S-100 stains scattered sustentacular cells only.

NEUROENDOCRINE TUMORS OF THE PANCREAS AND DUODENUM

Pancreatic neuroendocrine tumors (NET) may occur sporadically, or in association with MEN 1 (nonfunctioning/functioning) and VHL (nonfunctioning) syndromes. Sporadic duodenal and pancreatic NET are usually solitary, whereas MEN 1–associated neoplasms are characteristically multiple in the pancreas and duodenum. VHL-associated nonfunctioning NET are multiple and occur in the pancreas. Insulinomas and nonfunctioning NET are found exclusively in the pancreas, whereas the most common site for both sporadic and familial gastrinomas is the duodenum. Insulinomas usually follow a benign clinical course, whereas gastrinomas have high malignant potential, with regional lymph node or liver metastases developing in up to 90% of the cases. Sporadic NET may secrete any of a wide variety of gastrointestinal hormones, including insulin, gastrin, glucagon, somatostatin, vasoactive intestinal polypeptide, and pancreatic polypeptide. Insulinomas and gastrinomas constitute the vast majority of all NET.

In general, NET in MEN patients are discovered at a younger age than are sporadic tumors. Pancreatic NET and duodenal gastrinomas occur with frequency of 82% and 60%, respectively, in patients with familial MEN 1. The *MEN1* tumor suppressor gene on chromosome 11q13 is involved in the development of MEN 1–associated enteropancreatic NET. *VHL* gene alterations are responsible for the development of VHL-associated nonfunctioning pancreatic NET.[32]

Sporadic gastrinoma (33%) and insulinoma (17%) often show somatic *MEN1* mutations,[15] whereas somatic *VHL* gene mutations have not been documented in sporadic pancreatic NET.[489] Somatic *MEN1* mutation is the only described gene mutation in sporadic gastrinoma and insulinoma.

Insulinoma

Relatively few cytogenetic studies have been performed in insulinomas. Numerical chromosomal abnormalities are frequent.[490] A t(7;11) translocation has been identified in a single case; double minutes and marker chromosomes have also been observed.[491] Most insulinomas associated with MEN 1 demonstrate LOH of the wild-type allele at the *MEN1* gene locus on 11q13,[492, 493] whereas sporadic insulinomas demonstrate LOH at this site in approximately 50%.[15] Different deletion patterns may be observed in different enteropancreatic tumors in MEN 1 patients harboring more than a single insulinoma.[9] Somatic *MEN1* gene mutations are found in approximately 17% of sporadic insulinomas.[15]

Oncogene amplification has not been observed in insulinoma, and immunoreactivity for *MYC*, *MYCL1*, and *MYCN* are not observed in benign tumors.[494, 495]

Metastatic insulinomas demonstrate codon 12 *KRAS* point mutations in about two thirds of cases and may overexpress both MYC and p53 protein.[495, 496] Although *RB1* gene alterations have been observed in several cases,[497, 498] they do not appear to be common.[499]

In addition to demonstrating immunoreactivity for insulin, insulinomas may also demonstrate immunoreactivity for other pancreatic hormones. Immunohistochemical demonstration of synaptophysin and neuron-specific enolase, but not necessarily chromogranin, is also observed.[500] It has been reported that the α subunit of human chorionic gonadotropin (HCG) is expressed in one half to two thirds of malignant insulinomas but only in about 10% of benign tumors.[501] Other authors have failed to demonstrate increased frequency of α-HCG immunoreactivity in malignant cases.[502] Assessment of DNA ploidy by image cytometry is similarly unhelpful in establishing malignancy, although it has been reported that multiploid malignant tumors have a significantly worse prognosis than other pancreatic neuroendocrine tumors.[503–505]

Gastrinoma

Gastrinomas are the most common functioning NET associated with MEN 1, occurring in 60% of the patients. Both sporadic and MEN 1–associated gastrinomas are characterized by malignant but indolent clinical course; lymph node and/or liver metastases occur in 60% to 90% of patients at the time of presentation. Cytogenetic information is sparse, and no consistent karyotypic abnormalities have been identified.[506] Before the discovery of the *MEN1* gene, allelic deletions at 11q13 were detected by microsatellite analysis in approximately 40% of gastrinomas, whether MEN-associated or sporadic.[493, 507] After the identification of the *MEN1* gene, allelic deletions at the gene locus in sporadic gastrinomas have been detected at a rate of 93%.[15] Association with somatic *MEN1* gene mutation is found in 33% of sporadic gastrinomas.[15, 508, 509] The *MEN1* gene remains to be the only known gene to be linked to the development of the primary and metastatic gastrinoma.[510]

The *CDKN2A (p16* or *MTS1)* gene has been shown to be homozygously deleted in approximately 40% of gastrinomas and methylated in 60%, but small deletions and/or point mutations have not been identified. The relationship between *CDKN2A* alteration and *MEN1* alteration has yet to be explored. Neither *TP53* nor *RAS* alterations have been identified, but amplification of *ERBB2* appears to be virtually universal.[511]

Gastrinomas may demonstrate strong immunoreactivity for CD44; interestingly, there is a relative overproduction of alternatively spliced larger variants in comparison with other types of endocrine pancreatic tumors.[512] In addition, gastrinomas may demonstrate immunohistochemical reactivity for other pancreatic hormones, although usually only in a small minority of tumor cells.[513] Both benign and malignant gastrinomas express α-HCG; approximately 30% of malignant gastrinomas (and no benign gastrinomas) demonstrate ACTH protein or pro-opiomelanocortin (POMC) mRNA by in situ hybridization.[514]

Although experience is quite limited, there is some evidence that DNA flow cytometry is useful in predicting outcome of patients with sporadic gastrinomas; the presence of multiple stem line aneuploid tumors is associated with metastatic disease.[515]

Nesidioblastosis

Nesidioblastosis is a putative pancreatic islet cell abnormality characterized by an increase in the number of islets with irregular contours (particularly in close apposition with pancreatic ducts) and the presence of endocrine cells scattered in the acinar tissue. Image analytic studies cast doubt about the existence of morphologic abnormalities in pancreas of patients who have been given this diagnosis.[516] Careful reexamination of the pancreas of some patients given this diagnosis has revealed small discrete islet cell tumors; morphologic distinctions have also been made between focal islet cell hyperplasia and diffuse islet cell hyperplasia. Image analytic studies demonstrate the cells of nesidioblastosis to have a euploid DNA profile[517]; it has also been suggested that islet cell tumors simply represent the end of a spectrum of hyperplastic pancreatic endocrine disorders.[518]

Although nesidioblastosis is most frequently associated with hypoglycemia of infancy and childhood,[519] these anatomic findings are also frequently identified in the pancreas of adults with fully developed islet cell tumors.[520] Family studies demonstrate a linkage between 11p15 alleles and inheritance of familial hypoglycemia of infancy and childhood[521–524]; both autosomal dominant[525] and autosomal recessive[526] forms of this disorder occur. Patients with sporadic focal, but not diffuse, pancreatic islet cell hyperplasia demonstrate specific loss of maternal 11p15 alleles in the area of hyperplasia.[527] Mutations in the pancreatic cell sulfonylurea receptor gene *SUR* have been found in patients with hyperinsulinemia and hypoglycemia of infancy and childhood,[528–530] as have mutations in a potassium channel gene, *KCNJ11*.[531] Although these findings do not yet have routine diagnostic utility, they establish unequivocally that one or more forms of pancreatic nesidioblastosis exist as a distinct pathologic entity.

REFERENCES

1. Borrelli E, Sawchenko PE, Evans RM: Pituitary hyperplasia induced by ectopic expression of nerve growth factor. Proc Natl Acad Sci U S A 1992;89:2764–2768.
2. Gurnell M, Rajanayagam O, Barbar I, et al: Reversible pituitary enlargement in the syndrome of resistance to thyroid hormone. Thyroid 1998;8:679–682.

3. Horvath E, Kovacs K: Pituitary gland. Pathol Res Pract 1988;183:129–142.
4. McNicol AM: Current topics in neuropathology: Cushing's disease. Neuropathol Appl Neurobiol 1985;11: 485–494.
5. Bower BF, Malchoff CD: Molecular mechanisms of endocrine disorders. *In* Coleman WB, Tsongalis GJ (eds): Molecular Diagnostics for the Clinical Laboratorian. Totowa, NJ, Humana, 1997, pp 249–69.
6. Vortmeyer AO, Lubensky IA, Skarulis M, et al: Multiple endocrine neoplasia type 1: Atypical presentation, clinical course, and genetic analysis of multiple tumors. Mod-Pathol 1999;12:919–924.
7. Pack S, Turner ML, Zhuang Z, et al: Cutaneous tumors in patients with multiple endocrine neoplasia type 1 show allelic deletion of the *MEN1* gene. J Invest Dermatol 1998;110:438–440.
8. McKeeby JL, Li X, Zhuang Z, et al: Multiple biomyomas of the esophagus, lung and uterus in MEN1. Am J Pathol 2001;159:1121–1127.
9. Lubensky IA, Debelenko LV, Zhuang Z, et al: Allelic deletions on chromosome 11q13 in multiple tumors from individual MEN1 patients. Cancer Res 1996;56: 5272–5278.
10. Chandrasekharappa SC, Guru SC, Manickam P, et al: Positional cloning of the gene for multiple endocrine neoplasia type 1. Science 1997;276:404–407.
11. Guru SC, Goldsmith PK, Burns AL, et al: Menin, the product of the *MEN1* gene, is a nuclear protein. Proc Natl Acad Sci U S A 1998;95:1630–1634.
12. Huang SC, Zhuang Z, Weil RJ, et al: Nuclear/cytoplasmic localization of the multiple endocrine neoplasia type 1 gene product, menin. Lab Invest 1999;79: 301–310.
13. Agarwal SK, Kester MB, Debelenko LV, et al: Germline mutations of the *MEN1* gene in familial multiple endocrine neoplasia type 1 and related states. Hum Mol Genet 1997;6:1169–1175.
14. Marx SJ, Agarwal SK, Kester MB, et al: Multiple endocrine neoplasia type 1: Clinical and genetic features of the hereditary endocrine neoplasias. Recent Prog Horm Res 1999;54:397–438; discussion 438–439.
15. Zhuang Z, Vortmeyer AO, Pack S, et al: Somatic mutations of the *MEN1* tumor suppressor gene in sporadic gastrinomas and insulinomas. Cancer Res 1997;57: 4682–4686.
16. Heppner C, Kester MB, Agarwal SK, et al: Somatic mutation of the *MEN1* gene in parathyroid tumours. Nat Genet 1997;16:375–378.
17. Debelenko LV, Brambilla E, Agarwal SK, et al: Identification of *MEN1* gene mutations in sporadic carcinoid tumors of the lung. Hum Mol Genet 1997;6:2285–2290.
18. Zhuang Z, Ezzat SZ, Vortmeyer AO, et al: Mutations of the *MEN1* tumor suppressor gene in pituitary tumors. Cancer Res 1997;57:5446–5451.
19. Mulligan LM, Kwok JB, Healey CS, et al: Germ-line mutations of the *RET* proto-oncogene in multiple endocrine neoplasia type 2A. Nature 1993;363:458–460.
20. Donis-Keller H, Dou S, Chi D, et al: Mutations in the *RET* proto-oncogene are associated with MEN 2A and FMTC. Hum Mol Genet 1993;2:851–856.
21. Ponder BAJ: Multiple endocrine neoplasia type 2. *In* Vogelstein B, Kinzler KW (eds): The Genetic Basis of Human Cancer. New York, McGraw-Hill, 1998, pp 475–487.
22. Carlson KM, Bracamontes J, Jackson CE, et al: Parent-of-origin effects in multiple endocrine neoplasia type 2B. Am J Hum Genet 1994;55:1076–1082.
23. Neumann HP, Eng C, Mulligan LM, et al: Consequences of direct genetic testing for germline mutations in the clinical management of families with multiple endocrine neoplasia, type II. JAMA 1995;274:1149–1151.
24. Walther MM, Herring J, Enquist E, et al: von Recklinghausen's disease and pheochromocytomas. J Urol 1999; 162:1582–1586.
25. Szabo J, Heath B, Hill VM, et al: Hereditary hyperparathyroidism-jaw tumor syndrome: The endocrine tumor gene *HRPT2* maps to chromosome 1q21–q31. Am J Hum Genet 1995;56:944–950.
26. Carney JA, Gordon H, Carpenter PC, et al: The complex of myxomas, spotty pigmentation, and endocrine overactivity. Medicine (Baltimore) 1985;64:270–283.
27. Stratakis CA, Courcoutsakis NA, Abati A, et al: Thyroid gland abnormalities in patients with the syndrome of spotty skin pigmentation, myxomas, endocrine overactivity, and schwannomas (Carney complex). J Clin Endocrinol Metab 1997;82:2037–2043.
28. Stratakis CA, Jenkins RB, Pras E, et al: Cytogenetic and microsatellite alterations in tumors from patients with the syndrome of myxomas, spotty skin pigmentation, and endocrine overactivity (Carney complex). J Clin Endocrinol Metab 1996;81:3607–3614.
29. Stratakis CA, Carney JA, Lin JP, et al: Carney complex, a familial multiple neoplasia and lentiginosis syndrome: Analysis of 11 kindreds and linkage to the short arm of chromosome 2. J Clin Invest 1996;97:699–705.
30. Kirschner LS, Carney JA, Pack SD, et al: Mutations of the gene encoding the protein kinase A type 1-α regulatory subunit in patients with the Carney complex. Nature Genetics 2000;26:89–92.
31. Maddock IR, Moran A, Maher ER, et al: A genetic register for von Hippel-Lindau disease. J Med Genet 1996; 33:120–127.
32. Lubensky IA, Pack S, Ault D, et al: Multiple neuroendocrine tumors of the pancreas in von Hippel-Lindau disease patients: Histopathological and molecular genetic analysis. Am J Pathol 1998;153:223–231.
33. Latif F, Tory K, Gnarra J, et al: Identification of the von Hippel-Lindau disease tumor suppressor gene. Science 1993;260:1317–1320.
34. Duan DR, Pause A, Burgess WH, et al: Inhibition of transcription elongation by the VHL tumor suppressor protein. Science 1995;269:1402–1406.
35. Kibel A, Iliopoulos O, DeCaprio JA, Kaelin WGJ: Binding of the von Hippel-Lindau tumor suppressor protein to Elongin B and C. Science 1995;269:1444–1446.
36. Chen F, Slife L, Kishida T, et al: Genotype-phenotype correlation in von Hippel-Lindau disease: Identification of a mutation associated with VHL type 2A. J Med Genet 1996;33:716–717.
37. Ezzat S, Melmed S: Pituitary tumors in the elderly. *In* Morley JE, Korenman SG (eds): Endocrinology and

Metabolism in the Elderly. Boston, Blackwell Scientific, 1991, p 5869.
38. Mukai K: Pituitary adenomas: Immunocytochemical study of 150 tumors with clinicopathologic correlation. Cancer 1983;52:648–653.
39. Asa SL: The role of hypothalamic hormones in the pathogenesis of pituitary adenomas. Pathol Res Pract 1991;187:581–583.
40. Asa SL, Kovacs K, Stefaneanu L, et al: Pituitary adenomas in mice transgenic for growth hormone-releasing hormone. Endocrinology 1992;131:2083–2089.
41. Alexander JM, Biller BM, Bikkal H, et al: Clinically nonfunctioning pituitary tumors are monoclonal in origin. J Clin Invest 1990;86:336–340.
42. Herman V, Fagin J, Gonsky R, et al: Clonal origin of pituitary adenomas. J Clin Endocrinol Metab 1990; 71:1427–1433.
43. Vallar L, Spada A, Giannattasio G: Altered Gs and adenylate cyclase activity in human GH-secreting pituitary adenomas. Nature 1987;330:566–568.
44. Karga HJ, Alexander JM, Hedley-Whyte ET, et al: *Ras* mutations in human pituitary tumors. J Clin Endocrinol Metab 1992;74:914–919.
45. Pei L, Melmed S, Scheithauer B, et al: H-*ras* mutations in human pituitary carcinoma metastases. J Clin Endocrinol Metab 1994;78:842–846.
46. Cai WY, Alexander JM, Hedley-Whyte ET, et al: *ras* mutations in human prolactinomas and pituitary carcinomas. J Clin Endocrinol Metab 1994;78:89–93.
47. Alvaro V, Levy L, Dubray C, et al: Invasive human pituitary tumors express a point-mutated alpha-protein kinase-C. J Clin Endocrinol Metab 1993;77: 1125–1129.
48. Ezzat S, Zheng L, Smyth HS, Asa SL: The c-*erbB-2/neu* proto-oncogene in human pituitary tumours. Clin Endocrinol (Oxford) 1997;46:599–606.
49. Cryns VL, Alexander JM, Klibanski A, Arnold A: The retinoblastoma gene in human pituitary tumors. J Clin Endocrinol Metab 1993;77:644–646.
50. Zhu J, Leon SP, Beggs AH, et al: Human pituitary adenomas show no loss of heterozygosity at the retinoblastoma gene locus. J Clin Endocrinol Metab 1994;78: 922–927.
51. Sumi T, Stefaneanu L, Kovacs K, et al: Immunohistochemical study of p53 protein in human and animal pituitary tumors. Endocr Pathol 1993;4:9599.
52. Boggild MD, Jenkinson S, Pistorello M, et al: Molecular genetic studies of sporadic pituitary tumors. J Clin Endocrinol Metab 1994;78:387–392.
53. Dong Q, Debelenko LV, Chandrasekharappa SC, et al: Loss of heterozygosity at 11q13: Analysis of pituitary tumors, lung carcinoids, lipomas, and other uncommon tumors in subjects with familial multiple endocrine neoplasia type 1. J Clin Endocrinol Metab 1997;82: 1416–1420.
54. Bettio D, Rizzi N, Giardino D, et al: Cytogenetic study of pituitary adenomas. Cancer Genet Cytogenet 1997; 98:131–136.
55. Capra E, Rindi G, Santi G, et al: Chromosome abnormalities in a case of pituitary adenoma. Cancer Genet Cytogenet 1993;68:140–142.
56. Dietrich CU, Pandis N, Bjerre P, et al: Simple numerical chromosome aberrations in two pituitary adenomas. Cancer Genet Cytogenet 1993;69:118–121.
57. Rey JA, Bello MJ, de Campos JM, et al: A case of pituitary adenoma with 58 chromosomes. Cancer Genet Cytogenet 1986;23:171–174.
58. Rock JP, Babu VR, Drumheller T, Chason J: Cytogenetic findings in pituitary adenoma: Results of a pilot study. Surg Neurol 1993;40:224–229.
59. Daniely M, Aviram A, Adams EF, et al: Comparative genomic hybridization analysis of nonfunctioning pituitary tumors. J Clin Endocrinol Metab 1998;83: 1801–1805.
60. Metzger AK, Mohapatra G, Minn YA, et al: Multiple genetic aberrations including evidence of chromosome 11q13 rearrangement detected in pituitary adenomas by comparative genomic hybridization. J Neurosurg 1999; 90:306–314.
61. Bates AS, Farrell WE, Bicknell EJ, et al: Allelic deletion in pituitary adenomas reflects aggressive biological activity and has potential value as a prognostic marker. J Clin Endocrinol Metab 1997;82:818–824.
62. Clayton RN, Boggild M, Bates AS, et al: Tumour suppressor genes in the pathogenesis of human pituitary tumours. Horm Res 1997;47:185–193.
63. Woloschak M, Yu A, Post KD: Frequent inactivation of the *p16* gene in human pituitary tumors by gene methylation. Mol Carcinog 1997;19:221–224.
64. Barlier A, Pellegrini-Bouiller I, Caccavelli L, et al: Abnormal transduction mechanisms in pituitary adenomas. Horm Res 1997;47:227–234.
65. Clementi E, Malgaretti N, Meldolesi J, Taramelli R: A new constitutively activating mutation of the Gs protein alpha subunit-*gsp* oncogene is found in human pituitary tumours. Oncogene 1990;5:1059–1061.
66. Landis CA, Harsh G, Lyons J, et al: Clinical characteristics of acromegalic patients whose pituitary tumors contain mutant Gs protein. J Clin Endocrinol Metab 1990;71:1416–1420.
67. Gaiddon C, Mercken L, Bancroft C, Loeffler JP: Transcriptional effects in GH3 cells of Gs alpha mutants associated with human pituitary tumors: Stimulation of adenosine 3′,5′-monophosphate response element binding protein–mediated transcription and of prolactin and growth hormone promoter activity via protein kinase A. Endocrinology 1995;136:4331–4338.
68. Barlier A, Gunz G, Zamora AJ, et al: Prognostic and therapeutic consequences of Gs alpha mutations in somatotroph adenomas. J Clin Endocrinol Metab 1998;83: 1604–1610.
69. Tordjman K, Stern N, Ouaknine G, et al: Activating mutations of the Gs alpha-gene in nonfunctioning pituitary tumors. J Clin Endocrinol Metab 1993;77:765–769.
70. Harris PE: Gs protein mutations and the pathogenesis and function of pituitary tumors. Metabolism 1996; 45(8 Suppl 1):120–122.
71. Pei L, Melmed S, Scheithauer B, et al: Frequent loss of heterozygosity at the retinoblastoma susceptibility gene *(RB)* locus in aggressive pituitary tumors: Evidence for a chromosome 13 tumor suppressor gene other than *RB*. Cancer Res 1995;55:1613–1616.

72. Kawamoto H, Uozumi T, Kawamoto K, et al: Type IV collagenase activity and cavernous sinus invasion in human pituitary adenomas. Acta Neurochir (Wien) 1996;138:390–395.
73. Ikeda H, Yoshimoto T: The relationship between c-*myc* protein expression, the bromodeoxyuridine labeling index and the biological behavior of pituitary adenomas. Acta Neuropathol (Berl) 1992;83:361–364.
74. Blevins LSJ, Verity DK, Allen G: Aggressive pituitary tumors. Oncology (Huntington) 1998;12:1307–1312, 1315.
75. Buchfelder M, Fahlbusch R, Adams EF, et al: Proliferation parameters for pituitary adenomas. Acta Neurochir Suppl (Wien) 1996;65:18–21.
76. Daita G, Yonemasu Y: Dural invasion and proliferative potential of pituitary adenomas. Neurol Med Chir (Tokyo) 1996;36:211–214.
77. Ekramullah SM, Saitoh Y, Arita N, et al: The correlation of Ki-67 staining indices with tumour doubling times in regrowing non-functioning pituitary adenomas. Acta Neurochir (Wien) 1996;138:1449–1455.
78. Knosp E, Kitz K, Perneczky A: Proliferation activity in pituitary adenomas: Measurement by monoclonal antibody Ki-67. Neurosurgery 1989;25:927–930.
79. Kitz K, Knosp E, Koos WT, Korn A: Proliferation in pituitary adenomas: Measurement by MAb KI 67. Acta Neurochir Suppl (Wien) 1991;53:60–64.
80. Landolt AM, Shibata T, Kleihues P: Growth rate of human pituitary adenomas. J Neurosurg 1987;67: 803–806.
81. Chae YS, Flotte T, Hsu DW, et al: Flow cytometric DNA ploidy and cells phase fractions in recurrent human pituitary adenomas: A correlative study of flow cytometric analysis and the expression of proliferating cell nuclear antigen. Gen Diagn Pathol 1996;142: 89–95.
82. Fornas O, Mato ME, Viader M, et al: Flow cytometry analysis of pituitary adenomas. Horm Res 1996;46: 257–262.
83. Pegolo G, Buckwalter JG, Weiss MH, Hinton DR: Pituitary adenomas: Correlation of the cytologic appearance with biologic behavior. Acta Cytol 1995;39:887–892.
84. Croue A, Beldent V, Rousselet MC, et al: Contribution of immunohistochemistry, electron microscopy, and cell culture to the characterization of nonfunctioning pituitary adenomas: A study of 40 cases. Hum Pathol 1992; 23:1332–1339.
85. Thapar K, Scheithauer BW, Kovacs K, et al: p53 expression in pituitary adenomas and carcinomas: Correlation with invasiveness and tumor growth fractions. Neurosurgery 1996;38:763–770.
86. Pernicone PJ, Scheithauer BW, Sebo TJ, et al: Pituitary carcinoma: A clinicopathologic study of 15 cases. Cancer 1997;79:804–812.
87. Hinton DR, Hahn JA, Weiss MH, Couldwell WT: Loss of Rb expression in an ACTH-secreting pituitary carcinoma. Cancer Lett 1998;126:209–214.
88. Pearce SH, Trump D, Wooding C, et al: Loss of heterozygosity studies at the retinoblastoma and breast cancer susceptibility *(BRCA2)* loci in pituitary, parathyroid, pancreatic and carcinoid tumours. Clin Endocrinol (Oxford) 1996;45:195–200.
89. Kulig E, Jin L, Qian X, et al: Apoptosis in nontumorous and neoplastic human pituitaries: Expression of the bcl-2 family of proteins. Am J Pathol 1999;154:767–774.
90. Leblond-Francillard M, Picon A, Bertagna X, de Keyzer Y: High expression of the POU factor Brn3a in aggressive neuroendocrine tumors. J Clin Endocrinol Metab 1997; 82:89–94.
91. Fitzgibbons PL, Appley AJ, Turner RR, et al: Flow cytometric analysis of pituitary tumors: Correlation of nuclear antigen p105 and DNA content with clinical behavior. Cancer 1988;62:1556–1560.
92. Asa SL, Penz G, Kovacs K, Ezrin C: Prolactin cells in the human pituitary: A quantitative immunocytochemical analysis. Arch Pathol Lab Med 1982;106: 360–363.
93. Ezzat S, Asa SL, Stefaneanu L, et al: Somatotroph hyperplasia without pituitary adenoma associated with a long standing growth hormone releasing hormone–producing bronchial carcinoid. J Clin Endocrinol Metab 1994;78: 555–560.
94. McNicol AM: Patterns of corticotropic cells in the adult human pituitary in Cushing's disease. Diagn Histopathol 1981;4:335–341.
95. McKeever PE, Koppelman MC, Metcalf D, et al: Refractory Cushing's disease caused by multinodular ACTH-cell hyperplasia. J Neuropathol Exp Neurol 1982;41:490–499.
96. Kubota T, Hayashi M, Kabuto M, et al: Corticotroph cell hyperplasia in a patient with Addison disease: Case report. Surg Neurol 1992;37:441–447.
97. Fialkow PJ, Jackson CE, Block MA, Greenawald KA: Multicellular origin of parathyroid "adenomas." N Engl J Med 1977;297:696–698.
98. Arnold A, Brown MF, Urena P, et al: Monoclonality of parathyroid tumors in chronic renal failure and in primary parathyroid hyperplasia. J Clin Invest 1995;95: 2047–2053.
99. Shan L, Nakamura M, Nakamura Y, et al: Comparative analysis of clonality and pathology in primary and secondary hyperparathyroidism. Virchows Arch 1997;430: 247–251.
100. Tominaga Y, Kohara S, Namii Y, et al: Clonal analysis of nodular parathyroid hyperplasia in renal hyperparathyroidism. World J Surg 1996;20:744–750.
101. Friedman E, Sakaguchi K, Bale AE, et al: Clonality of parathyroid tumors in familial multiple endocrine neoplasia type 1. N Engl J Med 1989;321:213–218.
102. Yong JL, Vrga L, Warren BA: A study of parathyroid hyperplasia in chronic renal failure. Pathology 1994; 26:99–109.
103. McHenry CR, Lee K, Saadey J, et al: Parathyroid localization with technetium-99m-sestamibi: A prospective evaluation. J Am Coll Surg 1996;183:25–30.
104. Erickson LA, Jin L, Wollan P, et al: Parathyroid hyperplasia, adenomas, and carcinomas: Differential expression of p27Kip1 protein. Am J Surg Pathol 1999;23:288–295.
105. Noguchi S, Motomura K, Inaji H, et al: Clonal analysis of parathyroid adenomas by means of the polymerase chain reaction. Cancer Lett 1994;78:93–97.
106. Agarwal SK, Schrock E, Kester MB, et al: Comparative genomic hybridization analysis of human parathyroid tumors. Cancer Genet Cytogenet 1998;106:30–36.

107. Tahara H, Smith AP, Gas RD, et al: Genomic localization of novel candidate tumor suppressor gene loci in human parathyroid adenomas. Cancer Res 1996;56:599–605.
108. Palanisamy N, Imanishi Y, Rao PH, et al: Novel chromosomal abnormalities identified by comparative genomic hybridization in parathyroid adenomas. J Clin Endocrinol Metab 1998;83:1766–1770.
109. Hammami MM, al-Zahrani A, Butt A, et al: Primary hyperparathyroidism-associated polyostotic fibrous dysplasia: Absence of McCune-Albright syndrome mutations. J Endocrinol Invest 1997;20:552–558.
110. Arnold A, Kim HG, Gaz RD, et al: Molecular cloning and chromosomal mapping of DNA rearranged with the parathyroid hormone gene in a parathyroid adenoma. J Clin Invest 1989;83:2034–2040.
111. Rosenberg CL, Motokura T, Kronenberg HM, Arnold A: Coding sequence of the overexpressed transcript of the putative oncogene PRAD1/cyclin D1 in two primary human tumors. Oncogene 1993;8:519–521.
112. Farnebo F, Teh BT, Dotzenrath C, et al: Differential loss of heterozygosity in familial, sporadic, and uremic hyperparathyroidism. Hum Genet 1997;99:342–349.
113. Teh BT, Farnebo F, Twigg S, et al: Familial isolated hyperparathyroidism maps to the hyperparathyroidism-jaw tumor locus in 1q21-q32 in a subset of families. J Clin Endocrinol Metab 1998;83:2114–2120.
114. Pausova Z, Soliman E, Amizuka N, et al: Role of the *RET* proto-oncogene in sporadic hyperparathyroidism and in hyperparathyroidism of multiple endocrine neoplasia type 2. J Clin Endocrinol Metab 1996;81:2711–2718.
115. Komminoth P, Roth J, Muletta-Feurer S, et al: *RET* proto-oncogene point mutations in sporadic neuroendocrine tumors. J Clin Endocrinol Metab 1996;81:2041–2046.
116. Williams GH, Rooney S, Carss A, et al: Analysis of the *RET* proto-oncogene in sporadic parathyroid adenomas. J Pathol 1996;180:138–141.
117. Chaiwun B, Cote RJ, Taylor CR: Diffuse neuroendocrine and endocrine systems. *In* Taylor CR, Cote RJ (eds): Immunomicroscopy: A Diagnosic Tool for the Surgical Pathologist. Philadelphia, WB Saunders, 1994, pp 163–199.
118. Streeten EA, Weinstein LS, Norton JA, et al: Studies in a kindred with parathyroid carcinoma. J Clin Endocrinol Metab 1992;75:362–366.
119. Yoshimoto K, Endo H, Tsuyuguchi M, et al: Familial isolated primary hyperparathyroidism with parathyroid carcinomas: Clinical and molecular features. Clin Endocrinol (Oxford) 1998;48:67–72.
120. Jenkins PJ, Satta MA, Simmgen M, et al: Metastatic parathyroid carcinoma in the MEN2A syndrome. Clin Endocrinol (Oxf) 1997;47:747–751.
121. Subramaniam P, Wilkinson S, Shepherd JJ: Inactivation of retinoblastoma gene in malignant parathyroid growths: A candidate genetic trigger? Aust N Z J Surg 1995;65:714–716.
122. Cryns VL, Thor A, Xu HJ, et al: Loss of the retinoblastoma tumor-suppressor gene in parathyroid carcinoma. N Engl J Med 1994;330:757–761.
123. Cryns VL, Rubio MP, Thor AD, et al: p53 abnormalities in human parathyroid carcinoma. J Clin Endocrinol Metab 1994;78:1320–1324.
124. Harlow S, Roth SI, Bauer K, Marshall RB: Flow cytometric DNA analysis of normal and pathologic parathyroid glands. Mod Pathol 1991;4:310–315.
125. Obara T, Fujimoto Y, Hirayama A, et al: Flow cytometric DNA analysis of parathyroid tumors with special reference to its diagnostic and prognostic value in parathyroid carcinoma. Cancer 1990;65:1789–1793.
126. Howard S, Anderson C, Diels W, et al: Nuclear DNA density of parathyroid lesions. Pathol Res Pract 1992;188:497–499.
127. Bocsi J, Perner F, Szucs J, et al: DNA content of parathyroid tumors. Anticancer Res 1998;18:2901–2904.
128. Bowlby LS, DeBault LE, Abraham SR: Flow cytometric DNA analysis of parathyroid glands: Relationship between nuclear DNA and pathologic classifications. Am J Pathol 1987;128:338–344.
129. Abbona GC, Papotti M, Gasparri G, Bussolati G: Proliferative activity in parathyroid tumors as detected by Ki-67 immunostaining. Hum Pathol 1995;26:135–138.
130. Vargas MP, Vargas HI, Kleiner DE, Merino MJ: The role of prognostic markers (MiB-1, RB, and bcl-2) in the diagnosis of parathyroid tumors. Mod Pathol 1997;10:12–17.
131. Sadler GP, Morgan JM, Jasani B, et al: Epidermal growth factor receptor status in hyperparathyroidism: Immunocytochemical and in situ hybridization study. World J Surg 1996;20:736–742.
132. Chiovato L, Lapi P, Fiore E, et al: Thyroid autoimmunity and female gender. J Endocrinol Invest 1993;16:384–391.
133. Barbesino G, Tomer Y, Concepcion E, et al: Linkage analysis of candidate genes in autoimmune thyroid disease: 1. Selected immunoregulatory genes. International Consortium for the Genetics of Autoimmune Thyroid Disease. J Clin Endocrinol Metab 1998;83:1580–1584.
134. Hochberg Z: Subclinical Hashimoto's thyroiditis in gonadal dysgenesis. Isr J Med Sci 1980;16:847–848.
135. Kawai K, Kondo I, Terasaki T, Ogata E: A case of Turner's syndrome with hyperthyroidism. Endocrinol Jpn 1978;25:631–634.
136. Marcocci C, Bartalena L, Martino E, et al: Graves' disease and Turner's syndrome. J Endocrinol Invest 1980;3:429–431.
137. Tsuji S, Matsuoka Y, Suzuki Y, et al: Turner's syndrome associated with Hashimoto's thyroiditis and sarcoidosis: A case report. Intern Med 1992;31:131–133.
138. Tomer Y, Barbesino G, Greenberg DA, et al: A new Graves' disease–susceptibility locus maps to chromosome 20q11.2. International Consortium for the Genetics of Autoimmune Thyroid Disease. Am J Hum Genet 1998;63:1749–1756.
139. Conaway DH, Padgett GA, Bunton TE, et al: Clinical and histological features of primary progressive, familial thyroiditis in a colony of borzoi dogs. Vet Pathol 1985;22:439–446.
140. Phillips D, McLachlan S, Stephenson A, et al: Autosomal dominant transmission of autoantibodies to thyroglobulin and thyroid peroxidase. J Clin Endocrinol Metab 1990;70:742–746.

141. Ben-Ezra J, Wu A, Sheibani K: Hashimoto's thyroiditis lacks detectable clonal immunoglobulin and T cell receptor gene rearrangements. Hum Pathol 1988;19: 1444–1448.
142. Hsi ED, Singleton TP, Svoboda SM, et al: Characterization of the lymphoid infiltrate in Hashimoto thyroiditis by immunohistochemistry and polymerase chain reaction for immunoglobulin heavy chain gene rearrangement. Am J Clin Pathol 1998;110:327–333.
143. Matsuzuka F, Fukata S, Kuma K, et al: Gene rearrangement of immunoglobulin as a marker of thyroid lymphoma. World J Surg 1998;22:558–561.
144. Kaulfersch W, Baker JRJ, Burman KD, et al: Immunoglobulin and T cell antigen receptor gene arrangements indicate that the immune response in autoimmune thyroid disease is polyclonal. J Clin Endocrinol Metab 1988;66:958–963.
145. Demeure MJ, Doffek KM, Komorowski RA, Gorski J: Gip-2 codon 179 oncogene mutations: Absent in adrenal cortical tumors. World J Surg 1996;20:928–931.
146. Belge G, Thode B, Bullerdiek J, Bartnitzke S: Aberrations of chromosome 19: Do they characterize a subtype of benign thyroid adenomas? Cancer Genet Cytogenet 1992;60:23–26.
147. Cigudosa JC, Pedrosa GA, Otero GA, et al: Translocation (5;19)(q13;q13) in a multinodular thyroid goiter. Cancer Genet Cytogenet 1995;82:67–69.
148. Ferrer-Roca O, Perez-Gomez JA, Cigudosa JC, et al: Genetic heterogeneity of benign thyroid lesions: Static and flow cytometry, karyotyping and in situ hybridization analysis. Anal Cell Pathol 1998;16:101–110.
149. Roque L, Gomes P, Correia C, et al: Thyroid nodular hyperplasia: Chromosomal studies in 14 cases. Cancer Genet Cytogenet 1993;69:31–34.
150. Criado B, Barros A, Suijkerbuijk RF, et al: Detection of numerical alterations for chromosomes 7 and 12 in benign thyroid lesions by in situ hybridization: Histological implications. Am J Pathol 1995;147:136–144.
151. Hostetter AL, Hrafnkelsson J, Wingren SO, et al: A comparative study of DNA cytometry methods for benign and malignant thyroid tissue. Am J Clin Pathol 1988; 89:760–763.
152. Joensuu H, Klemi PJ, Eerola E: Diagnostic value of flow cytometric DNA determination combined with fine needle aspiration biopsy in thyroid tumors. Anal Quant Cytol Histol 1987;9:328–334.
153. Mizukami Y, Nonomura A, Michigishi T, et al: Flow cytometric DNA measurement in benign and malignant human thyroid tissues. Anticancer Res 1992;12: 2213–2217.
154. Chung DH, Kang GH, Kim WH, Ro JY: Clonal analysis of a solitary follicular nodule of the thyroid with the polymerase chain reaction method. Mod Pathol 1999;12: 265–271.
155. Kim H, Piao Z, Park C, et al: Clinical significance of clonality in thyroid nodules. Br J Surg 1998;85:1125–1128.
156. Namba H, Matsuo K, Fagin JA: Clonal composition of benign and malignant human thyroid tumors. J Clin Invest 1990;86:120–125.
157. Apel RL, Ezzat S, Bapat BV, et al: Clonality of thyroid nodules in sporadic goiter. Diagn Mol Pathol 1995;4: 113–121.
158. Harrer P, Broecker M, Zint A, et al: Thyroid nodules in recurrent multinodular goiters are predominantly polyclonal. J Endocrinol Invest 1998;21:380–385.
159. Couch RM, Hughes IA, DeSa DJ, et al: An autosomal dominant form of adolescent multinodular goiter. Am J Hum Genet 1986;39:811–816.
160. Bignell GR, Canzian F, Shayeghi M, et al: Familial nontoxic multinodular thyroid goiter locus maps to chromosome 14q but does not account for familial nonmedullary thyroid cancer. Am J Hum Genet 1997;61:1123–1130.
161. Baas F, Bikker H, van Ommen GJ, de Vijlder JJ: Unusual scarcity of restriction site polymorphism in the human thyroglobulin gene: A linkage study suggesting autosomal dominance of a defective thyroglobulin allele. Hum Genet 1984;67:301–305.
162. Ieiri T, Cochaux P, Targovnik HM, et al: A 3′ splice site mutation in the thyroglobulin gene responsible for congenital goiter with hypothyroidism. J Clin Invest 1991;88:1901–1905.
163. Targovnik HM, Medeiros-Neto G, Varela V, et al: A nonsense mutation causes human hereditary congenital goiter with preferential production of a 171-nucleotide-deleted thyroglobulin ribonucleic acid messenger. J Clin Endocrinol Metab 1993;77:210–215.
164. Targovnik HM, Vono J, Billerbeck AE, et al: A 138-nucleotide deletion in the thyroglobulin ribonucleic acid messenger in a congenital goiter with defective thyroglobulin synthesis. J Clin Endocrinol Metab 1995;80: 3356–3360.
165. Capella G, Matias-Guiu X, Ampudia X, et al: *Ras* oncogene mutations in thyroid tumors: Polymerase chain reaction-restriction-fragment-length polymorphism analysis from paraffin-embedded tissues. Diagn Mol Pathol 1996;5:45–52.
166. Namba H, Rubin SA, Fagin JA: Point mutations of *ras* oncogenes are an early event in thyroid tumorigenesis. Mol Endocrinol 1990;4:1474–1479.
167. Johnson TL, Lloyd RV, Thor A: Expression of *ras* oncogene p21 antigen in normal and proliferative thyroid tissues. Am J Pathol 1987;127:60–65.
168. Ezzat S, Zheng L, Kolenda J, et al: Prevalence of activating ras mutations in morphologically characterized thyroid nodules. Thyroid 1996;6:409–416.
169. Pasini B, Hofstra RM, Yin L, et al: The physical map of the human *RET* proto-oncogene. Oncogene 1995;11: 1737–1743.
170. Nakayama T, Ito M, Ohtsuru A, et al: Expression of the *ets*-1 proto-oncogene in human thyroid tumor. Mod Pathol 1999;12:61–68.
171. Oyama T, Ichimura E, Sano T, et al: c-*Met* expression of thyroid tissue with special reference to papillary carcinoma. Pathol Int 1998;48:763–768.
172. Davila RM, Bedrossian CW, Silverberg AB: Immunocytochemistry of the thyroid in surgical and cytologic specimens. Arch Pathol Lab Med 1988;112:51–56.
173. Dockhorn-Dworniczak B, Franke WW, Schroder S, et al: Patterns of expression of cytoskeletal proteins in human thyroid gland and thyroid carcinomas. Differentiation 1987;35:53–71.
174. Fucich LF, Freeman SM, Marrogi AJ: An immunohistochemical study of leu 7 and PCNA expression in thyroid neoplasms. Biotech Histochem 1996;71:298–303.

175. Hiasa Y, Nishioka H, Kitahori Y, et al: Immunohistochemical analysis of estrogen receptors in 313 paraffin section cases of human thyroid tissue. Oncology 1993;50:132–136.
176. van Hoeven KH, Kovatich AJ, Miettinen M: Immunocytochemical evaluation of HBME-1, CA 19-9, and CD-15 (Leu-M1) in fine-needle aspirates of thyroid nodules. Diagn Cytopathol 1998;18:93–97.
177. Bondeson L, Bengtsson A, Bondeson AG, et al: Chromosome studies in thyroid neoplasia. Cancer 1989;64: 680–685.
178. Teyssier JR, Liautaud-Roger F, Ferre D, et al: Chromosomal changes in thyroid tumors. Relation with DNA content, karyotypic features, and clinical data. Cancer Genet Cytogenet 1990;50:249–263.
179. Sozzi G, Bongarzone I, Miozzo M, et al: Cytogenetic and molecular genetic characterization of papillary thyroid carcinomas. Genes Chromosomes Cancer 1992;5: 212–218.
180. Antonini P, Linares G, Gaillard N, et al: Cytogenetic characterization of a new human papillary thyroid carcinoma permanent cell line (GLAG-66). Cancer Genet Cytogenet 1993;67:117–122.
181. Roque L, Castedo S, Gomes P, et al: Cytogenetic findings in 18 follicular thyroid adenomas. Cancer Genet Cytogenet 1993;67:1–6.
182. Belge G, Thode B, Bartnitzke S, Bullerdiek J: Cytogenetic biclonality corresponding to multiphasic differentiation in an atypical thyroid adenoma. Cancer Genet Cytogenet 1994;78:102–104.
183. Belge G, Roque L, Soares J, et al: Cytogenetic investigations of 340 thyroid hyperplasias and adenomas revealing correlations between cytogenetic findings and histology. Cancer Genet Cytogenet 1998;101: 42–48.
184. van den Berg E, Oosterhuis JW, de Jong B, et al: Cytogenetics of thyroid follicular adenomas. Cancer Genet Cytogenet 1990;44:217–222.
185. Taruscio D, Carcangiu ML, Ried T, Ward DC: Numerical chromosomal aberrations in thyroid tumors detected by double fluorescence in situ hybridization. Genes Chromosomes Cancer 1994;9:180–185.
186. Dal Cin P, Sneyers W, Aly MS, et al: Involvement of 19q13 in follicular thyroid adenoma. Cancer Genet Cytogenet 1992;60:99–101.
187. Bartnitzke S, Herrmann ME, Lobeck H, et al: Cytogenetic findings on eight follicular thyroid adenomas including one with a t(10;19). Cancer Genet Cytogenet 1989;39:65–68.
188. Herrmann MA, Hay ID, Bartelt DHJ, et al: Cytogenetics of six follicular thyroid adenomas including a case report of an oxyphil variant with t(8;14)(q13; q24.1). Cancer Genet Cytogenet 1991;56(2):231–235.
189. Belge G, Garcia E, de Jong P, et al: FISH analyses of a newly established thyroid tumor cell line showing a t(1;19)(p35 or p36.1;q13) reveal that the breakpoint lies between 19q13.3–13.4 and 19q13.4. Cytogenet Cell Genet 1995;69:220–222.
190. Hruban RH, Huvos AG, Traganos F, et al: Follicular neoplasms of the thyroid in men older than 50 years of age. A DNA flow cytometric study. Am J Clin Pathol 1990;94:527–532.
191. Joensuu H, Klemi P, Eerola E: DNA aneuploidy in follicular adenomas of the thyroid gland. Am J Pathol 1986;124:373–376.
192. van Thiel TP, van der Linden JC, Baak JP, et al: Reproducibility of flow cytometric assessment of follicular tumours of the thyroid. J Clin Pathol 1989;42:260–263.
193. Oyama T, Vickery ALJ, Preffer FI, Colvin RB: A comparative study of flow cytometry and histopathologic findings in thyroid follicular carcinomas and adenomas. Hum Pathol 1994;25:271–275.
194. Hemmer S, Wasenius VM, Knuutila S, et al: Comparison of benign and malignant follicular thyroid tumours by comparative genomic hybridization. Br J Cancer 1998; 78:1012–1017.
195. Marsh DJ, Zheng Z, Zedenius J, et al: Differential loss of heterozygosity in the region of the Cowden locus within 10q22-23 in follicular thyroid adenomas and carcinomas. Cancer Res 1997;57:500–503.
196. Marsh DJ, Dahia PL, Coulon V, et al: Allelic imbalance, including deletion of *PTEN/MMACI*, at the Cowden disease locus on 10q22-23, in hamartomas from patients with Cowden syndrome and germline *PTEN* mutation. Genes Chromosomes Cancer 1998;21:61–69.
197. Matsuo K, Tang SH, Fagin JA: Allelotype of human thyroid tumors: Loss of chromosome 11q13 sequences in follicular neoplasms. Mol Endocrinol 1991;5:1873–1879.
198. Zhang JS, Nelson M, McIver B, et al: Differential loss of heterozygosity at 7q31.2 in follicular and papillary thyroid tumors. Oncogene 1998;17:789–793.
199. Soares P, dos SN, Seruca R, et al: Benign and malignant thyroid lesions show instability at microsatellite loci. Eur J Cancer 1997;33:293–296.
200. Challeton C, Bounacer A, Du VJ, et al: Pattern of *ras* and *gsp* oncogene mutations in radiation-associated human thyroid tumors. Oncogene 1995;11:601–603.
201. Merkler DJ, Young SD: Recombinant type A rat 75-kDa alpha-amidating enzyme catalyzes the conversion of glycine-extended peptides to peptide amides via an alpha-hydroxyglycine intermediate. Arch Biochem Biophys 1991;289:192–196.
202. Horie H, Yokogoshi Y, Tsuyuguchi M, Saito S: Point mutations of ras and Gs alpha subunit genes in thyroid tumors. Jpn J Cancer Res 1995;86:737–742.
203. Monden T, Yamada M, Satoh T, et al: Analysis of the TSH receptor gene structure in various thyroid disorders: DNA from thyroid adenomas can have large insertions or deletions. Thyroid 1992;2:189–192.
204. O'Sullivan C, Barton CM, Staddon SL, et al: Activating point mutations of the *gsp* oncogene in human thyroid adenomas. Mol Carcinog 1991;4:345–349.
205. Murti KG, Kaur K, Goorha RM: Protein kinase C associates with intermediate filaments and stress fibers. Exp Cell Res 1992;202:36–44.
206. Parma J, Van Sande J, Swillens S, et al: Somatic mutations causing constitutive activity of the thyrotropin receptor are the major cause of hyperfunctioning thyroid adenomas: Identification of additional mutations activating both the cyclic adenosine 3′,5′-monophosphate and inositol phosphate-Ca^{2+} cascades. Mol Endocrinol 1995;9: 725–733.
207. Paschke R, Tonacchera M, Van Sande J, et al: Identification and functional characterization of two new somatic

mutations causing constitutive activation of the thyrotropin receptor in hyperfunctioning autonomous adenomas of the thyroid. J Clin Endocrinol Metab 1994;79: 1785–1789.

208. Russo D, Arturi F, Wicker R, et al: Genetic alterations in thyroid hyperfunctioning adenomas. J Clin Endocrinol Metab 1995;80:1347–1351.

209. Derwahl M, Manole D, Sobke A, Broecker M: Pathogenesis of toxic thyroid adenomas and nodules: Relevance of activating mutations in the TSH-receptor and Gs-alpha gene, the possible role of iodine deficiency and secondary and TSH-independent molecular mechanisms. Exp Clin Endocrinol Diabetes 1998; 106(Suppl 4):S6–S9.

210. Esapa C, Foster S, Johnson S, et al: G protein and thyrotropin receptor mutations in thyroid neoplasia. J Clin Endocrinol Metab 1997;82:493–496.

211. Ringel MD, Saji M, Schwindinger WF, et al: Absence of activating mutations of the genes encoding the alpha-subunits of G11 and Gq in thyroid neoplasia. J Clin Endocrinol Metab 1998;83:554–559.

212. Pinducciu C, Borgonovo G, Arezzo A, et al: Toxic thyroid adenoma: Absence of DNA mutations of the TSH receptor and Gs alpha. Eur J Endocrinol 1998;138:37–40.

213. Derwahl M: Molecular aspects of the pathogenesis of nodular goiters, thyroid nodules and adenomas. Exp Clin Endocrinol Diabetes 1996;104(Suppl 4):32–35.

214. Spambalg D, Sharifi N, Elisei R, et al: Structural studies of the thyrotropin receptor and Gs alpha in human thyroid cancers: Low prevalence of mutations predicts infrequent involvement in malignant transformation. J Clin Endocrinol Metab 1996;81:3898–3901.

215. Apple SK, Alzona MC, Jahromi SA, Grody WW: Can different thyroid tumor types be distinguished by polymerase chain reaction-based K-*ras* mutation detection? Mol Diagn 1998;3:143–147.

216. Karga H, Lee JK, Vickery ALJ, et al: *Ras* oncogene mutations in benign and malignant thyroid neoplasms. J Clin Endocrinol Metab 1991;73:832–836.

217. Bouras M, Bertholon J, Dutrieux-Berger N, et al: Variability of Ha-*ras* (codon 12) proto-oncogene mutations in diverse thyroid cancers. Eur J Endocrinol 1998;139: 209–216.

218. Lemoine NR, Mayall ES, Wyllie FS, et al: High frequency of *ras* oncogene activation in all stages of human thyroid tumorigenesis. Oncogene 1989;4:159–164.

219. Zou M, Shi Y, Farid NR: *p53* mutations in all stages of thyroid carcinomas. J Clin Endocrinol Metab 1993;77: 1054–1058.

220. Salvatore D, Celetti A, Fabien N, et al: Low frequency of *p53* mutations in human thyroid tumours: *p53* and *Ras* mutation in two out of fifty-six thyroid tumours. Eur J Endocrinol 1996;134:177–183.

221. Cheng AJ, Lin JD, Chang T, Wang TC: Telomerase activity in benign and malignant human thyroid tissues. Br J Cancer 1998;77:2177–2180.

222. Haugen BR, Nawaz S, Markham N, et al: Telomerase activity in benign and malignant thyroid tumors. Thyroid 1997;7:337–342.

223. Collin F, Salmon I, Rahier I, et al: Quantitative nuclear cell image analyses of thyroid tumors from archival material. Hum Pathol 1991;22:191–196.

224. Slowinska-Klencka D, Klencki M, Sporny S, Lewinski A: Karyometric analysis in the cytologic diagnosis of thyroid lesions. Anal Quant Cytol Histol 1997;19:507–513.

225. Crissman JD, Drozdowicz S, Johnson C, Kini SR: Fine needle aspiration diagnosis of hyperplastic and neoplastic follicular nodules of the thyroid: A morphometric study. Anal Quant Cytol Histol 1991;13:321–328.

226. Deshpande V, Kapila K, Sai KS, Verma K: Follicular neoplasms of the thyroid: Decision tree approach using morphologic and morphometric parameters. Acta Cytol 1997;41:369–376.

227. Salmon I, Gasperin P, Pasteels JL, et al: Relationship between histopathologic typing and morphonuclear assessments of 238 thyroid lesions: Digital cell image analysis performed on Feulgen-stained nuclei from formalin-fixed, paraffin-embedded materials. Am J Clin Pathol 1992;97:776–786.

228. Veneti S, Athanassiadou P, Kandaraki C, Kyrkou K: Evaluation of HMFG2 and thyroglobulin in the diagnosis of thyroid fine needle aspiration (FNA). Cytopathology 1997;8:13–19.

229. Ghali VS, Jimenez EJ, Garcia RL: Distribution of Leu-7 antigen (HNK-1) in thyroid tumors: Its usefulness as a diagnostic marker for follicular and papillary carcinomas. Hum Pathol 1992;23:21–25.

230. Czyz W, Joensuu H, Pylkkanen L, Klemi PJ: p53 protein, PCNA staining, and DNA content in follicular neoplasms of the thyroid gland. J Pathol 1994;174: 267–274.

231. Moore D, Ohene-Fianko D, Garcia B, Chakrabarti S: Apoptosis in thyroid neoplasms: Relationship with p53 and bcl-2 expression. Histopathology 1998;32:35–42.

232. van den Berg E, van Doormaal JJ, Oosterhuis JW, et al: Chromosomal aberrations in follicular thyroid carcinoma: Case report of a primary tumor and its metastasis. Cancer Genet Cytogenet 1991;54:215–222.

233. Jenkins RB, Hay ID, Herath JF, et al: Frequent occurrence of cytogenetic abnormalities in sporadic nonmedullary thyroid carcinoma. Cancer 1990;66:1213–1220.

234. Roque L, Clode A, Belge G, et al: Follicular thyroid carcinoma: Chromosome analysis of 19 cases. Genes Chromosomes Cancer 1998;21:250–255.

235. Roque L, Castedo S, Clode A, Soares J: Deletion of 3p25 → pter in a primary follicular thyroid carcinoma and its metastasis. Genes Chromosomes Cancer 1993;8: 199–203.

236. Herrmann MA, Hay ID, Bartelt DHJ, et al: Cytogenetic and molecular genetic studies of follicular and papillary thyroid cancers. J Clin Invest 1991;88:1596–1604.

237. Dahia PL, Marsh DJ, Zheng Z, et al: Somatic deletions and mutations in the Cowden disease gene, *PTEN*, in sporadic thyroid tumors. Cancer Res 1997;57: 4710–4713.

238. Tung WS, Shevlin DW, Kaleem Z, et al: Allelotype of follicular thyroid carcinomas reveals genetic instability consistent with frequent nondisjunctional chromosomal loss. Genes Chromosomes Cancer 1997;19:43–51.

239. Ward LS, Brenta G, Medvedovic M, Fagin JA: Studies of allelic loss in thyroid tumors reveal major differences in chromosomal instability between papillary and follicular carcinomas. J Clin Endocrinol Metab 1998;83: 525–530.

240. Bartolone L, Vermiglio F, Finocchiaro MD, et al: Thyroid follicular oncogenesis in iodine-deficient and iodine-sufficient areas: Search for alterations of the *ras*, *met* and *bFGF* oncogenes and of the *Rb* anti-oncogene. J Endocrinol Invest 1998;21:680–687.
241. Manenti G, Pilotti S, Re FC, et al: Selective activation of *ras* oncogenes in follicular and undifferentiated thyroid carcinomas. Eur J Cancer 1994;30A:987–993.
242. Namba H, Gutman RA, Matsuo K, et al: H-*ras* protooncogene mutations in human thyroid neoplasms. J Clin Endocrinol Metab 1990;71:223–229.
243. Dobashi Y, Sugimura H, Sakamoto A, et al: Stepwise participation of *p53* gene mutation during dedifferentiation of human thyroid carcinomas. Diagn Mol Pathol 1994;3:9–14.
244. Fagin JA, Matsuo K, Karmakar A, et al: High prevalence of mutations of the *p53* gene in poorly differentiated human thyroid carcinomas. J Clin Invest 1993;91:179–184.
245. Matias-Guiu X, Villanueva A, Cuatrecasas M, et al: p53 in a thyroid follicular carcinoma with foci of poorly differentiated and anaplastic carcinoma. Pathol Res Pract 1996; 192:1242–1249.
246. Sapi Z, Lukacs G, Sztan M, et al: Contribution of *p53* gene alterations to development of metastatic forms of follicular thyroid carcinoma. Diagn Mol Pathol 1995;4: 256–260.
247. Soares P, Cameselle-Teijeiro J, Sobrinho-Simoes M: Immunohistochemical detection of p53 in differentiated, poorly differentiated and undifferentiated carcinomas of the thyroid. Histopathology 1994;24:205–210.
248. Erickson LA, Jin L, Wollan PC, et al: Expression of p27kip1 and Ki-67 in benign and malignant thyroid tumors. Mod Pathol 1998;11:169–174.
249. Katoh R, Bray CE, Suzuki K, et al: Growth activity in hyperplastic and neoplastic human thyroid determined by an immunohistochemical staining procedure using monoclonal antibody MIB-1. Hum Pathol 1995;26: 139–146.
250. Shimizu T, Usuda N, Yamanda T, et al: Proliferative activity of human thyroid tumors evaluated by proliferating cell nuclear antigen/cyclin immunohistochemical studies. Cancer 1993;71:2807–2812.
251. Brabant G, Hoang-Vu C, Cetin Y, et al: E-cadherin: A differentiation marker in thyroid malignancies. Cancer Res 1993;53:4987–4993.
252. Dahlman T, Grimelius L, Wallin G, et al: Integrins in thyroid tissue: Upregulation of $alpha_2beta_1$ in anaplastic thyroid carcinoma. Eur J Endocrinol 1998;138:104–112.
253. Serini G, Trusolino L, Saggiorato E, et al: Changes in integrin and E-cadherin expression in neoplastic versus normal thyroid tissue. J Natl Cancer Inst 1996;88: 442–449.
254. Soares P, Berx G, van Roy F, Sobrinho-Simoes M: E-cadherin gene alterations are rare events in thyroid tumors. Int J Cancer 1997;70:32–38.
255. Christov K: Flow cytometric DNA measurements in human thyroid tumors. Virchows Arch B Cell Pathol Incl Mol Pathol 1986;51:255–263.
256. Jonasson JG, Hrafnkelsson J: Nuclear DNA analysis and prognosis in carcinoma of the thyroid gland: A nationwide study in Iceland on carcinomas diagnosed 1955–1990. Virchows Arch 1994;425:349–355.
257. Albores-Saavedra J, Nadji M, Civantos F, Morales AR: Thyroglobulin in carcinoma of the thyroid: An immunohistochemical study. Hum Pathol 1983;14: 62–66.
258. Beltrami CA, Barbatelli G, Criante P, et al: An immunohistochemical study in thyroid cancer. Appl Pathol 1987; 5:229–245.
259. Watanabe K, Koizumi N, Ozaki O, et al: Immunohistochemical studies on thyroid peroxidase and thyroglobulin in 13 human thyroid tumors and 7 Graves' goiters. Endocr J 1993;40:683–690.
260. Miettinen M, Kovatich AJ, Karkkainen P: Keratin subsets in papillary and follicular thyroid lesions: A paraffin section analysis with diagnostic implications. Virchows Arch 1997;431:407–413.
261. Yossie AdC, Longatto FA, Alves VA, et al: Lactoferrin in thyroid lesions: Immunoreactivity in fine needle aspiration biopsy samples. Acta Cytol 1996;40:408–413.
262. Schelfhout LJ, van Muijen GN, Fleuren GJ: Expression of keratin 19 distinguishes papillary thyroid carcinoma from follicular carcinomas and follicular thyroid adenoma. Am J Clin Pathol 1989;92:654–658.
263. Ostrowski ML, Brown RW, Wheeler TM, et al: Leu-7 immunoreactivity in cytologic specimens of thyroid lesions, with emphasis on follicular neoplasms. Diagn Cytopathol 1995;12:297–302.
264. Herrmann ME, Talpos GB, Mohamed AN, et al: Genetic markers in thyroid tumors. Surgery 1991;110: 941–947.
265. Segev DL, Saji M, Phillips GS, et al: Polymerase chain reaction–based microsatellite polymorphism analysis of follicular and Hürthle cell neoplasms of the thyroid. J Clin Endocrinol Metab 1998;83:2036–2042.
266. Zedenius J, Wallin G, Svensson A, et al: Allelotyping of follicular thyroid tumors. Hum Genet 1995;96:27–32.
267. Takiyama Y, Saji M, Clark DP, et al: Polymerase chain reaction–based microsatellite analysis of fine-needle aspirations from Hürthle cell neoplasms. Thyroid 1997; 7:853–857.
268. Kanthan R, Radhi JM: Immunohistochemical analysis of thyroid adenomas with Hürthle cells. Pathology 1998; 30:4–6.
269. Zedenius J, Larsson C, Wallin G, et al: Alterations of p53 and expression of WAF1/p21 in human thyroid tumors. Thyroid 1996;6:1–9.
270. Papotti M, Torchio B, Grassi L, et al: Poorly differentiated oxyphilic (Hürthle cell) carcinomas of the thyroid. Am J Surg Pathol 1996;20:686–694.
271. Schark C, Fulton N, Jacoby RF, et al: N-*ras* 61 oncogene mutations in Hürthle cell tumors. Surgery 1990; 108:994–999.
272. Masood S, Auguste LJ, Westerband A, et al: Differential oncogenic expression in thyroid follicular and Hürthle cell carcinomas. Am J Surg 1993;166:366–368.
273. Russo D, Wong MG, Costante G, et al: A Val 677 activating mutation of the thyrotropin receptor in a Hürthle cell thyroid carcinoma associated with thyrotoxicosis. Thyroid 1999;9:13–17.
274. Graff JR, Greenberg VE, Herman JG, et al: Distinct patterns of E-cadherin CpG island methylation in papillary, follicular, Hürthle's cell, and poorly differentiated human thyroid carcinoma. Cancer Res 1998;58: 2063–2066.

275. Campo E, Perez M, Charonis AA, et al: Patterns of basement membrane laminin distribution in nonneoplastic and neoplastic thyroid tissue. Mod Pathol 1992;5: 540–546.
276. Bronner MP, Clevenger CV, Edmonds PR, et al: Flow cytometric analysis of DNA content in Hürthle cell adenomas and carcinomas of the thyroid. Am J Clin Pathol 1988;89:764–769.
277. Camargo RS, Scafuri AG, de Tolosa EM, Ferreira EA: DNA image cytometric analysis of differentiated thyroid adenocarcinoma specimens. Am J Surg 1992;164: 640–645.
278. Zaccheroni V, Vacirca A, Lucci E, et al: An immunohistochemical study of progesterone receptor in thyroidal Hürthle cells tumors. J Exp Clin Cancer Res 1998;17: 291–298.
279. Johnson TL, Lloyd RV, Burney RE, Thompson NW: Hürthle cell thyroid tumors: An immunohistochemical study. Cancer 1987;59:107–112.
280. Roque L, Clode AL, Gomes P, et al: Cytogenetic findings in 31 papillary thyroid carcinomas. Genes Chromosomes Cancer 1995;13:157–162.
281. Herrmann ME, Mohamed A, Talpos G, Wolman SR: Cytogenetic study of a papillary thyroid carcinoma with a rearranged chromosome 10. Cancer Genet Cytogenet 1991;57:209–217.
282. Pierotti MA, Santoro M, Jenkins RB, et al: Characterization of an inversion on the long arm of chromosome 10 juxtaposing D10S170 and RET and creating the oncogenic sequence RET/PTC. Proc Natl Acad Sci U S A 1992;89:1616–1620.
283. Antonini P, Venuat AM, Caillou B, et al: Cytogenetic studies on 19 papillary thyroid carcinomas. Genes Chromosomes Cancer 1992;5:206–211.
284. Grieco M, Santoro M, Berlingieri MT, et al: PTC is a novel rearranged form of the *ret* proto-oncogene and is frequently detected in vivo in human thyroid papillary carcinomas. Cell 1990;60:557–563.
285. Bongarzone I, Pierotti MA, Monzini N, et al: High frequency of activation of tyrosine kinase oncogenes in human papillary thyroid carcinoma. Oncogene 1989;4: 1457–1462.
286. Santoro M, Carlomagno F, Hay ID, et al: *Ret* oncogene activation in human thyroid neoplasms is restricted to the papillary cancer subtype. J Clin Invest 1992;89: 1517–1522.
287. Tong Q, Li Y, Smanik PA, et al: Characterization of the promoter region and oligomerization domain of H4 (D10S170), a gene frequently rearranged with the *ret* proto-oncogene. Oncogene 1995;10:1781–1787.
288. Sozzi G, Bongarzone I, Miozzo M, et al: A t(10;17) translocation creates the *RET/PTC2* chimeric transforming sequence in papillary thyroid carcinoma. Genes Chromosomes Cancer 1994;9:244–250.
289. Santoro M, Dathan NA, Berlingieri MT, et al: Molecular characterization of *RET/PTC3:* A novel rearranged version of the *RET* proto-oncogene in a human thyroid papillary carcinoma. Oncogene 1994;9:509–516.
290. Klugbauer S, Lengfelder E, Demidchik EP, Rabes HM: A new form of *RET* rearrangement in thyroid carcinomas of children after the Chernobyl reactor accident. Oncogene 1996;13:1099–1102.
291. Minoletti F, Butti MG, Coronelli S, et al: The two genes generating RET/PTC3 are localized in chromosomal band 10q11.2. Genes Chromosomes Cancer 1994;11: 51–57.
292. Fugazzola L, Pierotti MA, Vigano E, et al: Molecular and biochemical analysis of *RET/PTC4,* a novel oncogenic rearrangement between *RET* and *ELE1* genes, in a post-Chernobyl papillary thyroid cancer. Oncogene 1996;13:1093–1097.
293. Klugbauer S, Demidchik EP, Lengfelder E, Rabes HM: Detection of a novel type of *RET* rearrangement *(PTC5)* in thyroid carcinomas after Chernobyl and analysis of the involved *RET*-fused gene *RFG5.* Cancer Res 1998; 58:198–203.
294. Bounacer A, Wicker R, Schlumberger M, et al: Oncogenic rearrangements of the *ret* proto-oncogene in thyroid tumors induced after exposure to ionizing radiation. Biochimie 1997;79:619–623.
295. Bounacer A, Wicker R, Caillou B, et al: High prevalence of activating *ret* proto-oncogene rearrangements in thyroid tumors from patients who had received external radiation. Oncogene 1997;15:1263–1273.
296. Fugazzola L, Pilotti S, Pinchera A, et al: Oncogenic rearrangements of the *RET* proto-oncogene in papillary thyroid carcinomas from children exposed to the Chernobyl nuclear accident. Cancer Res 1995;55: 5617–5620.
297. Greco A, Pierotti MA, Bongarzone I, et al: *TRK-T1* is a novel oncogene formed by the fusion of *TPR* and *TRK* genes in human papillary thyroid carcinomas. Oncogene 1992;7:237–242.
298. Sugg SL, Zheng L, Rosen IB, et al: *ret/PTC-1, -2,* and *-3* oncogene rearrangements in human thyroid carcinomas: Implications for metastatic potential? J Clin Endocrinol Metab 1996;81:3360–3365.
299. Bongarzone I, Vigneri P, Mariani L, et al: *RET/NTRK1* rearrangements in thyroid gland tumors of the papillary carcinoma family: Correlation with clinicopathological features. Clin Cancer Res 1998;4:223–228.
300. Zitzelsberger H, Lehmann L, Hieber L, et al: Cytogenetic changes in radiation-induced tumors of the thyroid. Cancer Res 1999;59:135–140.
301. Califano JA, Johns MM, Westra WH, et al: An allelotype of papillary thyroid cancer. Int J Cancer 1996; 69: 442–444.
302. Bird IM, Hanley NA, Word RA, et al: Human NCI-H295 adrenocortical carcinoma cells: A model for angiotensin-II-responsive aldosterone secretion. Endocrinology 1993;133:1555–1561.
303. Roth KA, Wilson DM, Eberwine J, et al: Acromegaly and pheochromocytoma: A multiple endocrine syndrome caused by a plurihormonal adrenal medullary tumor. J Clin Endocrinol Metab 1986;63:1421–1426.
304. Sargon MF, Hamdi CH, Demiryurek D, Dagdeviren A: Fine structure of the human coccygeal body: A light and electron microscopic study. Anat Anz 1998;180:11–14.
305. Akslen LA, Varhaug JE: Oncoproteins and tumor progression in papillary thyroid carcinoma: Presence of epidermal growth factor receptor, c-erbB-2 protein, estrogen receptor related protein, p21-ras protein, and proliferation indicators in relation to tumor recurrences and patient survival. Cancer 1995;76:1643–1654.

306. Omura K, Nagasato A, Kanehira E, et al: Retinoblastoma protein and proliferating-cell nuclear antigen expression as predictors of recurrence in well-differentiated papillary thyroid carcinoma. J Clin Oncol 1997;15:3458–3463.
307. Arber DA, Tamayo R, Weiss LM: Paraffin section detection of the c-*kit* gene product (CD117) in human tissues: Value in the diagnosis of mast cell disorders. Hum Pathol 1998;29:498–504.
308. Chhieng DC, Ross JS, McKenna BJ: CD44 immunostaining of thyroid fine-needle aspirates differentiates thyroid papillary carcinoma from other lesions with nuclear grooves and inclusions. Cancer 1997;81:157–162.
309. Figge J, del Rosario AD, Gerasimov G, et al: Preferential expression of the cell adhesion molecule CD44 in papillary thyroid carcinoma. Exp Mol Pathol 1994;61: 203–211.
310. Khan A, Baker SP, Patwardhan NA, Pullman JM: CD57 (Leu-7) expression is helpful in diagnosis of the follicular variant of papillary thyroid carcinoma. Virchows Arch 1998;432:427–432.
311. Miettinen M, Franssila K, Lehto VP, et al: Expression of intermediate filament proteins in thyroid gland and thyroid tumors. Lab Invest 1984;50:262–270.
312. Miettinen M, Karkkainen P: Differential reactivity of HBME-1 and CD15 antibodies in benign and malignant thyroid tumours: Preferential reactivity with malignant tumours. Virchows Arch 1996;429:213–219.
313. Nishimura R, Yokose T, Mukai K: S-100 protein is a differentiation marker in thyroid carcinoma of follicular cell origin: An immunohistochemical study. Pathol Int 1997;47:673–679.
314. Scappaticci S, Arrigoni G, Capra E, et al: Cytogenetics of multiple endocrine neoplasia syndromes: I. Two different, unique clonal chromosome changes in a medullary thyroid carcinoma and in a C-cell thyroid hyperplasia. Cancer Genet Cytogenet 1992;59:51–53.
315. Wurster-Hill DH, Pettengill OS, Noll WW, et al: Hypodiploid, pseudodiploid, and normal karyotypes prevail in cytogenetic studies of medullary carcinomas of the thyroid and metastatic tissues. Cancer Genet Cytogenet 1990;47:227–241.
316. Cooley LD, Elder FF, Knuth A, Gagel RF: Cytogenetic characterization of three human and three rat medullary thyroid carcinoma cell lines. Cancer Genet Cytogenet 1995;80:138–149.
317. Ekman ET, Bergholm U, Backdahl M, et al: Nuclear DNA content and survival in medullary thyroid carcinoma. Swedish Medullary Thyroid Cancer Study Group. Cancer 1990;65:511–517.
318. Narod SA, Sobol H, Nakamura Y, et al: Linkage analysis of hereditary thyroid carcinoma with and without pheochromocytoma. Hum Genet 1989;83:353–358.
319. Lairmore TC, Howe JR, Korte JA, et al: Familial medullary thyroid carcinoma and multiple endocrine neoplasia type 2B map to the same region of chromosome 10 as multiple endocrine neoplasia type 2A. Genomics 1991;9:181–192.
320. Ceccherini I, Pasini B, Pacini F, et al: Somatic in frame deletions not involving juxtamembranous cysteine residues strongly activate the *RET* proto-oncogene. Oncogene 1997;14:2609–2612.
321. Eng C, Mulligan LM, Smith DP, et al: Mutation of the *RET* protooncogene in sporadic medullary thyroid carcinoma. Genes Chromosomes Cancer 1995;12:209–212.
322. Alemi M, Lucas SD, Sallstrom JF, et al: A novel deletion in the *RET* proto-oncogene found in sporadic medullary thyroid carcinoma. Anticancer Res 1996;16: 2619–2622.
323. Alemi M, Lucas SD, Sallstrom JF, et al: A complex nine base pair deletion in RET exon 11 common in sporadic medullary thyroid carcinoma. Oncogene 1997;14: 2041–2045.
324. Eng C, Mulligan LM, Smith DP, et al: Low frequency of germline mutations in the *RET* proto-oncogene in patients with apparently sporadic medullary thyroid carcinoma. Clin Endocrinol (Oxford) 1995;43:123–127.
325. Fink M, Weinhusel A, Niederle B, Haas OA: Distinction between sporadic and hereditary medullary thyroid carcinoma (MTC) by mutation analysis of the RET proto-oncogene. Study Group Multiple Endocrine Neoplasia Austria (SMENA). Int J Cancer 1996; 69: 312–316.
326. Khosla S, Patel VM, Hay ID, et al: Loss of heterozygosity suggests multiple genetic alterations in pheochromocytomas and medullary thyroid carcinomas. J Clin Invest 1991;87:1691–1699.
327. Herfarth KK, Wick MR, Marshall HN, et al: Absence of *TP53* alterations in pheochromocytomas and medullary thyroid carcinomas. Genes Chromosomes Cancer 1997;20:24–29.
328. Moley JF, Brother MB, Wells SA, et al: Low frequency of *ras* gene mutations in neuroblastomas, pheochromocytomas, and medullary thyroid cancers. Cancer Res 1991;51:1596–1599.
329. Holm R, Nesland JM: Retinoblastoma and *p53* tumour suppressor gene protein expression in carcinomas of the thyroid gland. J Pathol 1994;172:267–272.
330. Gimm O, Marsh DJ, Andrew SD, et al: Germline dinucleotide mutation in codon 883 of the *RET* proto-oncogene in multiple endocrine neoplasia type 2B without codon 918 mutation. J Clin Endocrinol Metab 1997;82: 3902–3904.
331. Zedenius J, Larsson C, Bergholm U, et al: Mutations of codon 918 in the *RET* proto-oncogene correlate to poor prognosis in sporadic medullary thyroid carcinomas. J Clin Endocrinol Metab 1995;80:3088–3090.
332. Roncalli M, Viale G, Grimelius L, et al: Prognostic value of N-*myc* immunoreactivity in medullary thyroid carcinoma. Cancer 1994;74:134–141.
333. Schroder S, Schwarz W, Rehpenning W, et al: Leu-M1 immunoreactivity and prognosis in medullary carcinomas of the thyroid gland. J Cancer Res Clin Oncol 1988;114: 291–296.
334. Deftos LJ, Bone HG, Parthemore JG: Immunohistological studies of medullary thyroid carcinoma and C cell hyperplasia. J Clin Endocrinol Metab 1980;51: 857–862.
335. Grauer A, Raue F, Rix E, et al: Neuron-specific enolase in medullary thyroid carcinoma: Immunohistochemical demonstration, but no significance as serum tumor marker. J Cancer Res Clin Oncol 1987;113:599–602.
336. Harach HR, Wilander E, Grimelius L, et al: Chromogranin A immunoreactivity compared with argyrophilia, calcitonin immunoreactivity, and amyloid as tumour

markers in the histopathological diagnosis of medullary (C-cell) thyroid carcinoma. Pathol Res Pract 1992;188: 123–130.

337. Deftos LJ, Woloszczuk W, Krisch I, et al: Medullary thyroid carcinomas express chromogranin A and a novel neuroendocrine protein recognized by monoclonal antibody HISL-19. Am J Med 1988;85:780–784.
338. Kimura N, Sasano N, Yamada R, Satoh J: Immunohistochemical study of chromogranin in 100 cases of pheochromocytoma, carotid body tumour, medullary thyroid carcinoma and carcinoid tumour. Virchows Arch A Pathol Anat Histopathol 1988;413:33–38.
339. Schroder S, Dockhorn-Dworniczak B, Kastendieck H, et al: Intermediate-filament expression in thyroid gland carcinomas. Virchows Arch A Pathol Anat Histopathol 1986;409:751–766.
340. Dasovic-Knezevic M, Bormer O, Holm R, et al: Carcinoembryonic antigen in medullary thyroid carcinoma: An immunohistochemical study applying six novel monoclonal antibodies. Mod Pathol 1989;2:610–617.
341. Holm R, Sobrinho-Simoes M, Nesland JM, et al: Medullary thyroid carcinoma with thyroglobulin immunoreactivity: A special entity? Lab Invest 1987;57:258–268.
342. Antonaci A, Brierley J, Bacchi G, et al: Thyroid carcinoma. *In* Hermanek P, Gospodarowicz MK, Hensen DE, et al (eds): Prognostic Factors in Cancer. Berlin, Springer, 1995, pp 28–36.
343. Mark J, Ekedahl C, Dahlenfors R, Westermark B: Cytogenetical observations in five human anaplastic thyroid carcinomas. Hereditas 1987;107:163–174.
344. Roque L, Soares J, Castedo S: Cytogenetic and fluorescence in situ hybridization studies in a case of anaplastic thyroid carcinoma. Cancer Genet Cytogenet 1998;103: 7–10.
345. Ekman ET, Wallin G, Backdahl M, et al: Nuclear DNA content in anaplastic giant-cell thyroid carcinoma. Am J Clin Oncol 1989;12:442–446.
346. Klemi PJ, Joensuu H, Eerola E: DNA aneuploidy in anaplastic carcinoma of the thyroid gland. Am J Clin Pathol 1988;89:154–159.
347. Stringer BM, Rowson JM, Parkar MH, et al: Detection of the H-*RAS* oncogene in human thyroid anaplastic carcinomas. Experientia 1989;45:372–376.
348. Zou M, Shi Y, al-Sedairy S, et al: The expression of the *MDM2* gene, a p53 binding protein, in thyroid carcinogenesis. Cancer 1995;76:314–318.
349. Battista S, Martelli ML, Fedele M, et al: A mutated *p53* gene alters thyroid cell differentiation. Oncogene 1995; 11:2029–2037.
350. Donghi R, Longoni A, Pilotti S, et al: Gene *p53* mutations are restricted to poorly differentiated and undifferentiated carcinomas of the thyroid gland. J Clin Invest 1993;91:1753–1760.
351. Ito T, Seyama T, Mizuno T, et al: Unique association of *p53* mutations with undifferentiated but not with differentiated carcinomas of the thyroid gland. Cancer Res 1992;52:1369–1371.
352. Pierotti MA, Bongarzone I, Borello MG, et al: Cytogenetics and molecular genetics of carcinomas arising from thyroid epithelial follicular cells. Genes Chromosomes Cancer 1996;16:1–14.
353. Moretti F, Farsetti A, Soddu S, et al: p53 re-expression inhibits proliferation and restores differentiation of human thyroid anaplastic carcinoma cells. Oncogene 1997;14:729–740.
354. Tallini G, Santoro M, Helie M, et al: *RET/PTC* oncogene activation defines a subset of papillary thyroid carcinomas lacking evidence of progression to poorly differentiated or undifferentiated tumor phenotypes. Clin Cancer Res 1998;4:287–294.
355. Okubo T, Inokuma S, Takeda S, et al: Expression of *nm23-H1* gene product in thyroid, ovary, and breast cancers. Cell Biophys 1995;26:205–213.
356. Arai T, Yamashita T, Urano T, et al: Preferential reduction of *nm23-H1* gene product in metastatic tissues from papillary and follicular carcinomas of the thyroid. Mod Pathol 1995;8:252–256.
357. Zou M, Shi Y, al-Sedairy S, Farid NR: High levels of *Nm23* gene expression in advanced stage of thyroid carcinomas. Br J Cancer 1993;68:385–388.
358. Cerrato A, Fulciniti F, Avallone A, et al: Beta- and gamma-catenin expression in thyroid carcinomas. J Pathol 1998;185:267–272.
359. Aasland R, Lillehaug JR, Male R, et al: Expression of oncogenes in thyroid tumours: coexpression of c-*erbB2/-neu* and c-*erbB*. Br J Cancer 1988;57:358–363.
360. Zeki K, Spambalg D, Sharifi N, et al: Mutations of the adenomatous polyposis coli gene in sporadic thyroid neoplasms. J Clin Endocrinol Metab 1994;79:1317–1321.
361. Tung WS, Shevlin DW, Bartsch D, et al: Infrequent *CDKN2* mutation in human differentiated thyroid cancers. Mol Carcinog 1996;15:5–10.
362. Takano T, Matsuzuka F, Miyauchi A, et al: Restricted expression of oncofetal fibronectin mRNA in thyroid papillary and anaplastic carcinoma: An in situ hybridization study. Br J Cancer 1998;78:221–224.
363. Hashimoto T, Matsubara F, Mizukami Y, et al: Tumor markers and oncogene expression in thyroid cancer using biochemical and immunohistochemical studies. Endocrinol Jpn 1990;37:247–254.
364. Basolo F, Pollina L, Fontanini G, et al: Apoptosis and proliferation in thyroid carcinoma: Correlation with bcl-2 and p53 protein expression. Br J Cancer 1997;75:537–541.
365. Perros P, Palmer JM, Yeaman SJ, Kendall-Taylor P: Anti-mitochondrial antibodies in patients with Graves' disease may not signify primary biliary cirrhosis. Postgrad Med J 1994;70:17–18.
366. Hurlimann J, Gardiol D, Scazziga B: Immunohistology of anaplastic thyroid carcinoma: A study of 43 cases. Histopathology 1987;11:567–580.
367. Ordonez NG, el-Naggar AK, Hickey RC, Samaan NA: Anaplastic thyroid carcinoma: Immunocytochemical study of 32 cases. Am J Clin Pathol 1991;96:15–24.
368. Burt A, Goudie RB: Diagnosis of primary thyroid carcinoma by immunohistological demonstration of thyroglobulin. Histopathology 1979;3:279–286.
369. Carcangiu ML, Steeper T, Zampi G, Rosai J: Anaplastic thyroid carcinoma: A study of 70 cases. Am J Clin Pathol 1985;83:135–158.
370. Kashima K, Yokoyama S, Daa T, et al: Cytoplasmic biotin-like activity interferes with immunohistochemical analysis of thyroid lesions: A comparison of antigen retrieval methods. Mod Pathol 1997;10:515–519.

371. Wedell A: An update on the molecular genetics of congenital adrenal hyperplasia: Diagnostic and therapeutic aspects. J Pediatr Endocrinol Metab 1998;11:581–589.
372. Wedell A: Molecular genetics of congenital adrenal hyperplasia (21-hydroxylase deficiency): Implications for diagnosis, prognosis and treatment. Acta Paediatr 1998;87:159–164.
373. Lee HH, Chao HT, Ng HT, Choo KB: Direct molecular diagnosis of *CYP21* mutations in congenital adrenal hyperplasia. J Med Genet 1996;33:371–375.
374. Day DJ, Speiser PW, Schulze E, et al: Identification of non-amplifying *CYP21* genes when using PCR-based diagnosis of 21-hydroxylase deficiency in congenital adrenal hyperplasia (CAH) affected pedigrees. Hum Mol Genet 1996;5:2039–2048.
375. Rheaume E, Simard J, Morel Y, et al: Congenital adrenal hyperplasia due to point mutations in the type II 3 beta-hydroxysteroid dehydrogenase gene. Nat Genet 1992;1: 239–245.
376. Kagimoto K, Waterman MR, Kagimoto M, et al: Identification of a common molecular basis for combined 17 alpha-hydroxylase/17,20-lyase deficiency in two Mennonite families. Hum Genet 1989;82:285–286.
377. Geley S, Kapelari K, Johrer K, et al: *CYP11B1* mutations causing congenital adrenal hyperplasia due to 11 beta-hydroxylase deficiency. J Clin Endocrinol Metab 1996; 81:2896–2901.
378. Lin D, Sugawara T, Strauss JF, et al: Role of steroidogenic acute regulatory protein in adrenal and gonadal steroidogenesis. Science 1995;267:1828–1831.
379. Beuschlein F, Reincke M, Karl M, et al: Clonal composition of human adrenocortical neoplasms. Cancer Res 1994;54:4927–4932.
380. Boston BA, Mandel S, LaFranchi S, Bliziotes M: Activating mutation in the stimulatory guanine nucleotide-binding protein in an infant with Cushing's syndrome and nodular adrenal hyperplasia. J Clin Endocrinol Metab 1994;79:890–893.
381. Williamson EA, Johnson SJ, Foster S, et al: G protein gene mutations in patients with multiple endocrinopathies. J Clin Endocrinol Metab 1995;80:1702–1705.
382. Yamakita N, Murai T, Ito Y, et al: Adrenocorticotropin-independent macronodular adrenocortical hyperplasia associated with multiple colon adenomas/carcinomas which showed a point mutation in the APC gene. Intern Med 1997;36:536–542.
383. Hodge BO, Froesch TA: Familial Cushing's syndrome: Micronodular adrenocortical dysplasia. Arch Intern Med 1988;148:1133–1136.
384. Pascoe L, Jeunemaitre X, Lebrethon MC, et al: Glucocorticoid-suppressible hyperaldosteronism and adrenal tumors occurring in a single French pedigree. J Clin Invest 1995;96:2236–2246.
385. Bettio D, Rizzi N, Giardino D, et al: Translocation (7;17)(q22;p13) as a sole karyotypic change in an adrenal adenoma. Cancer Genet Cytogenet 1998;103:180–181.
386. Gordon RD, Stowasser M, Martin N, et al: Karyotypic abnormalities in benign adrenocortical tumors producing aldosterone. Cancer Genet Cytogenet 1993;68:78–81.
387. Kjellman M, Kallioniemi OP, Karhu R, et al: Genetic aberrations in adrenocortical tumors detected using comparative genomic hybridization correlate with tumor size and malignancy. Cancer Res 1996;56: 4219–4223.
388. Gicquel C, Bertagna X, Schneid H, et al: Rearrangements at the 11p15 locus and overexpression of insulin-like growth factor-II gene in sporadic adrenocortical tumors. J Clin Endocrinol Metab 1994;78:1444–1453.
389. Gortz B, Roth J, Speel EJ, et al: *MEN1* gene mutation analysis of sporadic adrenocortical lesions. Int J Cancer 1999;80:373–379.
390. Moul JW, Bishoff JT, Theune SM, Chang EH: Absent *ras* gene mutations in human adrenal cortical neoplasms and pheochromocytomas. J Urol 1993;149:1389–1394.
391. Reincke M, Karl M, Travis WH, et al: *p53* mutations in human adrenocortical neoplasms: Immunohistochemical and molecular studies. J Clin Endocrinol Metab 1994;78:790–794.
392. Reincke M, Wachenfeld C, Mora P, et al: *p53* mutations in adrenal tumors: Caucasian patients do not show the exon 4 "hot spot" found in Taiwan. J Clin Endocrinol Metab 1996;81:3636–3638.
393. Hough AJ, Hollifield JW, Page DL, Hartmann WH: Prognostic factors in adrenal cortical tumors: A mathematical analysis of clinical and morphologic data. Am J Clin Pathol 1979;72:390–399.
394. Vargas MP, Vargas HI, Kleiner DE, Merino MJ: Adrenocortical neoplasms: Role of prognostic markers MIB-1, P53, and RB. Am J Surg Pathol 1997;21:556–562.
395. Nakazumi H, Sasano H, Iino K, et al: Expression of cell cycle inhibitor p27 and Ki-67 in human adrenocortical neoplasms. Mod Pathol 1998;11:1165–1170.
396. Sasano H, Imatani A, Shizawa S, et al: Cell proliferation and apoptosis in normal and pathologic human adrenal. Mod Pathol 1995;8:11–17.
397. Cibas ES, Medeiros LJ, Weinberg DS, et al: Cellular DNA profiles of benign and malignant adrenocortical tumors. Am J Surg Pathol 1990;14:948–955.
398. Amberson JB, Vaughan EDJ, Gray GF, Naus GJ: Flow cytometric analysis of nuclear DNA from adrenocortical neoplasms: A retrospective study using paraffin-embedded tissue. Cancer 1987;59:2091–2095.
399. Haak HR, Cornelisse CJ, Hermans J, et al: Nuclear DNA content and morphological characteristics in the prognosis of adrenocortical carcinoma. Br J Cancer 1993;68: 151–155.
400. Lu X, Stallmach T, Gebbers JO: Image cytometric DNA analysis of adrenocortical neoplasms as a prognostic parameter: A clinico-pathologic study of 13 patients. Anal Cell Pathol 1996;12:1–11.
401. Remmelink M, Salmon I, Pasteels JL, et al: Nuclear DNA content, proliferation index and nuclear size determination in normal and tumoral adrenal tissues, pheochromocytomas and metastases. Acta Cytol 1995;39: 416–422.
402. Mertens F, Kullendorff CM, Moell C, et al: Complex karyotype in a childhood adrenocortical carcinoma. Cancer Genet Cytogenet 1998;105:190–192.
403. Marks JL, Wyandt HE, Beazley RM, et al: Cytogenetic studies of an adrenal cortical carcinoma. Cancer Genet Cytogenet 1992;61:96–98.
404. Limon J, Dal Cin P, Gaeta J, Sandberg AA: Translocation t(4;11)(q35;p13) in an adrenocortical carcinoma. Cancer Genet Cytogenet 1987;28:343–348.

405. Limon J, Dal Cin P, Kakati S, et al: Cytogenetic findings in a primary adrenocortical carcinoma. Cancer Genet Cytogenet 1987;26:271–277.
406. Birch JM, Hartley AL, Tricker KJ, et al: Prevalence and diversity of constitutional mutations in the *p53* gene among 21 Li-Fraumeni families. Cancer Res 1994;54: 1298–1304.
407. Ohgaki H, Kleihues P, Heitz PU: *p53* mutations in sporadic adrenocortical tumors. Int J Cancer 1993; 54:408–410.
408. Heppner C, Reincke M, Agarwal SK, et al: *MEN1* gene analysis in sporadic adrenocortical neoplasms. J Clin Endocrinol Metab 1999;84:216–219.
409. Fogt F, Vargas MP, Zhuang Z, Merino MJ: Utilization of molecular genetics in the differentiation between adrenal cortical adenomas and carcinomas. Hum Pathol 1998;29:518–521.
410. Yashiro T, Hara H, Fulton NC, et al: Point mutations of *ras* genes in human adrenal cortical tumors: Absence in adrenocortical hyperplasia. World J Surg 1994;18:455–460.
411. Hirano Y, Fujita K, Suzuki K, et al: Telomerase activity as an indicator of potentially malignant adrenal tumors. Cancer 1998;83:772–776.
412. Tartour E, Caillou B, Tenenbaum F, et al: Immunohistochemical study of adrenocortical carcinoma: Predictive value of the D11 monoclonal antibody. Cancer 1993;72: 3296–3303.
413. Bahr G, Gilbert F, Balaban G, Engler W: Homogeneously staining regions and double minutes in a human cell line: Chromatin organization and DNA content. J Natl Cancer Inst 1983;71:657–661.
414. Schwab M, Alitalo K, Klempnauer KH, et al: Amplified DNA with limited homology to *myc* cellular oncogene is shared by human neuroblastoma cell lines and a neuroblastoma tumour. Nature 1983;305:245–248.
415. Amler LC, Schurmann J, Schwab M: The *DDX1* gene maps within 400 kbp 5′ to *MYCN* and is frequently coamplified in human neuroblastoma. Genes Chromosomes Cancer 1996;15:134–137.
416. Brodeur GM, Seeger RC, Schwab M, et al: Amplification of N-*myc* sequences in primary human neuroblastomas: Correlation with advanced disease stage. Prog Clin Biol Res 1985;175:105–113.
417. Brodeur GM, Hayes FA, Green AA, et al: Consistent N-*myc* copy number in simultaneous or consecutive neuroblastoma samples from sixty individual patients. Cancer Res 1987;47:4248–4253.
418. Tsuda T, Obara M, Hirano H, et al: Analysis of N-*myc* amplification in relation to disease stage and histologic types in human neuroblastomas. Cancer 1987;60: 820–826.
419. Seeger RC, Brodeur GM, Sather H, et al: Association of multiple copies of the N-*myc* oncogene with rapid progression of neuroblastomas. N Engl J Med 1985;313: 1111–1116.
420. Noguchi M, Hirohashi S, Tsuda H, et al: Detection of amplified N-*myc* gene in neuroblastoma by in situ hybridization using the single-step silver enhancement method. Mod Pathol 1988;1:428–432.
421. Cohen PS, Seeger RC, Triche TJ, Israel MA: Detection of N-*myc* gene expression in neuroblastoma tumors by in situ hybridization. Am J Pathol 1988;131:391–397.
422. Grady-Leopardi EF, Schwab M, Ablin AR, Rosenau W: Detection of N-*myc* oncogene expression in human neuroblastoma by in situ hybridization and blot analysis: Relationship to clinical outcome. Cancer Res 1986;46: 3196–3199.
423. Nisen PD, Waber PG, Rich MA, et al: N-*myc* oncogene RNA expression in neuroblastoma. J Natl Cancer Inst 1988;80:1633–1637.
424. Fong CT, Dracopoli NC, White PS, et al: Loss of heterozygosity for the short arm of chromosome 1 in human neuroblastomas: Correlation with N-*myc* amplification. Proc Natl Acad Sci U S A 1989;86: 3753–3757.
425. Weith A, Martinsson T, Cziepluch C, et al: Neuroblastoma consensus deletion maps to 1p36.1–2. Genes Chromosomes Cancer 1989;1:159–166.
426. White PS, Maris JM, Sulman EP, et al: Molecular analysis of the region of distal 1p commonly deleted in neuroblastoma. Eur J Cancer 1997;33:1957–1961.
427. Caron H, Peter M, van Sluis P, et al: Evidence for two tumour suppressor loci on chromosomal bands 1p35–36 involved in neuroblastoma: One probably imprinted, another associated with N-*myc* amplification. Hum Mol Genet 1995;4:535–539.
428. Cheng JM, Hiemstra JL, Schneider SS, et al: Preferential amplification of the paternal allele in neuroblastomas with N-*myc* amplification. Prog Clin Biol Res 1994;385: 43–49.
429. Christiansen H, Lampert F: Tumour karyotype discriminates between good and bad prognostic outcome in neuroblastoma. Br J Cancer 1988;57:121–126.
430. Hayashi Y, Kanda N, Inaba T, et al: Cytogenetic findings and prognosis in neuroblastoma with emphasis on marker chromosome 1. Cancer 1989;63:126–132.
431. Caron H: Allelic loss of chromosome 1 and additional chromosome 17 material are both unfavourable prognostic markers in neuroblastoma. Med Pediatr Oncol 1995;24:215–221.
432. Brinkschmidt C, Christiansen H, Terpe HJ, et al: Comparative genomic hybridization (CGH) analysis of neuroblastomas—an important methodological approach in paediatric tumour pathology. J Pathol 1997; 181: 394–400.
433. Akeson R, Bernards R: N-*myc* down-regulates neural cell adhesion molecule expression in rat neuroblastoma. Mol Cell Biol 1990;10:2012–2016.
434. Lastowska M, Nacheva E, McGuckin A, et al: Comparative genomic hybridization study of primary neuroblastoma tumors. United Kingdom Children's Cancer Study Group. Genes Chromosomes Cancer 1997; 18: 162–169.
435. Vandesompele J, Van Roy N, Van Gele M, et al: Genetic heterogeneity of neuroblastoma studied by comparative genomic hybridization. Genes Chromosomes Cancer 1998;23:141–152.
436. Altura RA, Maris JM, Li H, et al: Novel regions of chromosomal loss in familial neuroblastoma by comparative genomic hybridization. Genes Chromosomes Cancer 1997;19:176–184.
437. Castresana JS, Bello MJ, Rey JA, et al: No *TP53* mutations in neuroblastomas detected by PCR-SSCP analysis. Genes Chromosomes Cancer 1994;10:136–138.

438. Goldman SC, Chen CY, Lansing TJ, et al: The p53 signal transduction pathway is intact in human neuroblastoma despite cytoplasmic localization. Am J Pathol 1996; 148:1381–1385.

439. Imamura J, Bartram CR, Berthold F, et al: Mutation of the *p53* gene in neuroblastoma and its relationship with N-*myc* amplification. Cancer Res 1993;53:4053–4058.

440. Vogan K, Bernstein M, Leclerc JM, et al: Absence of *p53* gene mutations in primary neuroblastomas. Cancer Res 1993;53:5269–5273.

441. Berg PE, Liu J, Yin J, et al: Microsatellite instability is infrequent in neuroblastoma. Cancer Epidemiol Biomarkers Prev 1995;4:907–909.

442. Oppedal BR, Storm-Mathisen I, Lie SO, Brandtzaeg P: Prognostic factors in neuroblastoma: Clinical, histopathologic, and immunohistochemical features and DNA ploidy in relation to prognosis. Cancer 1988;62: 772–780.

443. Taylor SR, Blatt J, Costantino JP, et al: Flow cytometric DNA analysis of neuroblastoma and ganglioneuroma: A 10-year retrospective study. Cancer 1988;62:749–754.

444. Gansler T, Chatten J, Varello M, et al: Flow cytometric DNA analysis of neuroblastoma: Correlation with histology and clinical outcome. Cancer 1986; 58: 2453–2458.

445. Christiansen H, Sahin K, Berthold F, et al: Comparison of DNA aneuploidy, chromosome 1 abnormalities, *MYCN* amplification and CD44 expression as prognostic factors in neuroblastoma. Eur J Cancer 1995; 31A: 541–544.

446. Brinkschmidt C, Poremba C, Christiansen H, et al: Comparative genomic hybridization and telomerase activity analysis identify two biologically different groups of 4s neuroblastomas. Br J Cancer 1998; 77: 2223–2229.

447. Hiyama E, Hiyama K, Ohtsu K, et al: Telomerase activity in neuroblastoma: Is it a prognostic indicator of clinical behaviour? Eur J Cancer 1997;33:1932–1936.

448. Castle VP, Heidelberger KP, Bromberg J, et al: Expression of the apoptosis-suppressing protein bcl-2 in neuroblastoma is associated with unfavorable histology and N-*myc* amplification. Am J Pathol 1993;143:1543–1550.

449. Krajewski S, Chatten J, Hanada M, Reed JC: Immunohistochemical analysis of the Bcl-2 oncoprotein in human neuroblastomas. Comparisons with tumor cell differentiation and N-Myc protein. Lab Invest 1995; 72:42–54.

450. Layfield LJ, Thompson JK, Dodge RK, Kerns BJ: Prognostic indicators for neuroblastoma: Stage, grade, DNA ploidy, MIB-1-proliferation index, p53, HER-2/neu and EGFr—a survival study. J Surg Oncol 1995;59:21–27.

451. Rudolph P, Lappe T, Hero B, et al: Prognostic significance of the proliferative activity in neuroblastoma. Am J Pathol 1997;150:133–145.

452. Thomas JO, Nijjar J, Turley H, et al: NB84: A new monoclonal antibody for the recognition of neuroblastoma in routinely processed material. J Pathol 1991; 163:69–75.

453. Miettinen M, Chatten J, Paetau A, Stevenson A: Monoclonal antibody NB84 in the differential diagnosis of neuroblastoma and other small round cell tumors. Am J Surg Pathol 1998;22:327–332.

454. Kiechle-Schwarz M, Neumann HP, Decker HJ, et al: Cytogenetic studies on three pheochromocytomas derived from patients with von Hippel-Lindau syndrome. Hum Genet 1989;82:127–130.

455. Okazaki M, Miya A, Tanaka N, et al: Allele loss on chromosome 10 and point mutation of *ras* oncogenes are infrequent in tumors of MEN 2A. Henry Ford Hosp Med J 1989;37:112–115.

456. Santoro M, Rosati R, Grieco M, et al: The *ret* proto-oncogene is consistently expressed in human pheochromocytomas and thyroid medullary carcinomas. Oncogene 1990;5:1595–1598.

457. Takaya K, Yoshimasa T, Arai H, et al: The RET proto-oncogene in sporadic pheochromocytomas. Intern Med 1996;35:449–452.

458. Beldjord C, Desclaux-Arramond F, Raffin-Sanson M, et al: The *RET* protooncogene in sporadic pheochromocytomas: Frequent MEN 2–like mutations and new molecular defects. J Clin Endocrinol Metab 1995; 80: 2063–2068.

459. Rodien P, Jeunemaitre X, Dumont C, et al: Genetic alterations of the RET proto-oncogene in familial and sporadic pheochromocytomas. Horm Res 1997; 47: 263–268.

460. Brauch H, Hoeppner W, Jahnig H, et al: Sporadic pheochromocytomas are rarely associated with germline mutations in the *vhl* tumor suppressor gene or the *ret* proto-oncogene. J Clin Endocrinol Metab 1997; 82: 4101–4104.

461. Moley JF, Wallin GK, Brother MB, et al: Oncogene and growth factor expression in MEN 2 and related tumors. Henry Ford Hosp Med J 1992;40:284–288.

462. Vargas MP, Zhuang Z, Wang C, et al: Loss of heterozygosity on the short arm of chromosomes 1 and 3 in sporadic pheochromocytoma and extra-adrenal paraganglioma. Hum Pathol 1997;28:411–415.

463. Shin E, Fujita S, Takami K, et al: Deletion mapping of chromosome 1p and 22q in pheochromocytoma. Jpn J Cancer Res 1993;84:402–408.

464. Yokogoshi Y, Yoshimoto K, Saito S: Loss of heterozygosity on chromosomes 1 and 11 in sporadic pheochromocytomas. Jpn J Cancer Res 1990;81:632–638.

465. Goto K, Ogo A, Yanase T, et al: Expression of c-*fos* and c-*myc* proto-oncogenes in human adrenal pheochromocytomas. J Clin Endocrinol Metab 1990;70:353–357.

466. Liu J, Voutilainen R, Kahri AI, Heikkila P: Expression patterns of the c-*myc* gene in adrenocortical tumors and pheochromocytomas. J Endocrinol 1997;152:175–181.

467. Kubota Y, Nakada T, Sasagawa I, et al: Elevated levels of telomerase activity in malignant pheochromocytoma. Cancer 1998;82:176–179.

468. Amberson JB, Vaughan EDJ, Gray GF, Naus GJ: Flow cytometric determination of nuclear DNA content in benign adrenal pheochromocytomas. Urology 1987;30: 102–104.

469. Hosaka Y, Rainwater LM, Grant CS, et al: Pheochromocytoma: Nuclear deoxyribonucleic acid patterns studied by flow cytometry. Surgery 1986;100:1003–1010.

470. Klein FA, Kay S, Ratliff JE, et al: Flow cytometric determinations of ploidy and proliferation patterns of adrenal neoplasms: An adjunct to histological classification. J Urol 1985;134:862–866.

471. Lai MK, Sun CF, Chen CS, et al: Deoxyribonucleic acid flow cytometric study in pheochromocytomas and its correlation with clinical parameters. Urology 1994;44: 185–188.
472. Pang LC, Tsao KC: Flow cytometric DNA analysis for the determination of malignant potential in adrenal and extra-adrenal pheochromocytomas or paragangliomas. Arch Pathol Lab Med 1993;117: 1142–1147.
473. Clarke MR, Weyant RJ, Watson CG, Carty SE: Prognostic markers in pheochromocytoma. Hum Pathol 1998;29:522–526.
474. Saeger W: Pathology of adrenal neoplasms. Minerva Endocrinol 1995;20:1–8.
475. DeBold CR, Menefee JK, Nicholson WE, Orth DN: Proopiomelanocortin gene is expressed in many normal human tissues and in tumors not associated with ectopic adrenocorticotropin syndrome. Mol Endocrinol 1988;2: 862–870.
476. Devilee P, van Schothorst EM, Bardoel AF, et al: Allelotype of head and neck paragangliomas: Allelic imbalance is confined to the long arm of chromosome 11, the site of the predisposing locus PGL. Genes Chromosomes Cancer 1994;11:71–78.
477. Mariman EC, van Beersum SE, Cremers CW, et al: Fine mapping of a putatively imprinted gene for familial nonchromaffin paragangliomas to chromosome 11q13.1: Evidence for genetic heterogeneity. Hum Genet 1995; 95:56–62.
478. Baysal BE, Farr JE, Rubinstein WS, et al: Fine mapping of an imprinted gene for familial nonchromaffin paragangliomas, on chromosome 11q23. Am J Hum Genet 1997;60:121–132.
479. Baysal BE, van Schothorst EM, Farr JE, et al: A high-resolution STS, EST, and gene-based physical map of the hereditary paraganglioma region on chromosome 11q23. Genomics 1997;44:214–221.
480. Carney JA: The triad of gastric epithelioid leiomyosarcoma, pulmonary chondroma, and functioning extra-adrenal paraganglioma: A five-year review. Medicine (Baltimore) 1983;62:159–169.
481. Carney JA: The triad of gastric epithelioid leiomyosarcoma, functioning extra-adrenal paraganglioma, and pulmonary chondroma. Cancer 1979;43:374–382.
482. Tisherman SE, Tisherman BG, Tisherman SA, et al: Three-decade investigation of familial pheochromocytoma: An allele of von Hippel-Lindau disease? Arch Intern Med 1993;153:2550–2556.
483. Blasius S, Brinkschmidt C, Poremba C, et al: Metastatic retroperitoneal paraganglioma in a 16-year-old girl: Case report, molecular pathological and cytogenetic findings. Pathol Res Pract 1998;194:439–444.
484. Achilles E, Padberg BC, Holl K, et al: Immunocytochemistry of paragangliomas--value of staining for S-100 protein and glial fibrillary acid protein in diagnosis and prognosis. Histopathology 1991;18:453–458.
485. Kliewer KE, Wen DR, Cancilla PA, Cochran AJ: Paragangliomas: Assessment of prognosis by histologic, immunohistochemical, and ultrastructural techniques. Hum Pathol 1989;20:29–39.
486. DeLellis RA, Tischler AS, Lee AK, et al: Leu-enkephalin-like immunoreactivity in proliferative lesions of the human adrenal medulla and extra-adrenal paraganglia. Am J Surg Pathol 1983;7:29–37.
487. Gee MS, Kliewer KE, Hinton DR: Nucleolar organizer regions in paragangliomas of the head and neck. Arch Otolaryngol Head Neck Surg 1992;118:380–383.
488. van der Mey AG, Cornelisse CJ, Hermans J, et al: DNA flow cytometry of hereditary and sporadic paragangliomas (glomus tumours). Br J Cancer 1991;63:298–302.
489. Chung DC, Smith AP, Louis DN, et al: A novel pancreatic endocrine tumor suppressor gene locus on chromosome 3p with clinical prognostic implications. J Clin Invest 1997;100:404–410.
490. Scappaticci S, Brandi ML, Capra E, et al: Cytogenetics of multiple endocrine neoplasia syndrome: II. Chromosome abnormalities in an insulinoma and a glucagonoma from two subjects with MEN1. Cancer Genet Cytogenet 1992;63:17–21.
491. Maraschio P, Pezzolo A, Brandi ML, et al: Cytogenetics of multiple endocrine neoplasia syndromes: III. Analysis of an insulinoma from a subject with MEN 1 by chromosome painting. Cancer Genet Cytogenet 1993;70: 68–70.
492. Larsson C, Skogseid B, Oberg K, et al: Multiple endocrine neoplasia type 1 gene maps to chromosome 11 and is lost in insulinoma. Nature 1988;332:85–87.
493. Debelenko LV, Zhuang Z, Emmert-Buck MR, et al: Allelic deletions on chromosome 11q13 in multiple endocrine neoplasia type 1–associated and sporadic gastrinomas and pancreatic endocrine tumors. Cancer Res 1997;57: 2238–2243.
494. Roncalli M, Springall DR, Varndell IM, et al: Oncoprotein immunoreactivity in human endocrine tumours. J Pathol 1991;163:117–127.
495. Pavelic K, Hrascan R, Kapitanovic S, et al: Multiple genetic alterations in malignant metastatic insulinomas. J Pathol 1995;177:395–400.
496. Pavelic K, Hrascan R, Kapitanovic S, et al: Molecular genetics of malignant insulinoma. Anticancer Res 1996; 16:1707–1717.
497. Nakamura T, Iwamura Y, Kaneko M, et al: Deletions and rearrangements of the retinoblastoma gene in hepatocellular carcinoma, insulinoma and some neurogenic tumors as found in a study of 121 tumors. Jpn J Clin Oncol 1991;21:325–329.
498. Iwamura Y, Futagawa T, Kaneko M, et al: Co-deletions of the retinoblastoma gene and Wilms' tumor gene and rearrangement of the Krev-1 gene in a human insulinoma. Jpn J Clin Oncol 1992;22:6–9.
499. Chung DC, Smith AP, Louis DN, et al: Analysis of the retinoblastoma tumour suppressor gene in pancreatic endocrine tumours. Clin Endocrinol (Oxford) 1997;47: 523–528.
500. Lloyd RV, Mervak T, Schmidt K, et al: Immunohistochemical detection of chromogranin and neuron-specific enolase in pancreatic endocrine neoplasms. Am J Surg Pathol 1984;8:607–614.
501. Bordi C, Pilato FP, D'Adda T: Comparative study of seven neuroendocrine markers in pancreatic endocrine tumours. Virchows Arch A Pathol Anat Histopathol 1988;413:387–398.
502. Graeme-Cook F, Nardi G, Compton CC: Immunocytochemical staining for human chorionic gonadotropin

subunits does not predict malignancy in insulinomas. Am J Clin Pathol 1990;93:273–276.

503. Bottger T, Seidl C, Seifert JK, et al: Value of quantitative DNA analysis in endocrine tumors of the pancreas. Oncology 1997;54:318–323.
504. Alanen KA, Joensuu H, Klemi PJ, et al: DNA ploidy in pancreatic neuroendocrine tumors. Am J Clin Pathol 1990;93:784–788.
505. Graeme-Cook F, Bell DA, Flotte TJ, et al: Aneuploidy in pancreatic insulinomas does not predict malignancy. Cancer 1990;66:2365–2368.
506. Herrmann ME, Rydstedt LL, Talpos GB, et al: Chromosomal aberrations in two sporadic gastrinomas. Cancer Genet Cytogenet 1993;67:44–49.
507. Sawicki MP, Wan YJ, Johnson CL, et al: Loss of heterozygosity on chromosome 11 in sporadic gastrinomas. Hum Genet 1992;89:445–449.
508. Bartsch D, Kopp I, Bergenfelz A, et al: *MEN1* gene mutations in 12 MEN1 families and their associated tumors. Eur J Endocrinol 1998;139:416–420.
509. Wang EH, Ebrahimi SA, Wu AY, et al: Mutation of the MENIN gene in sporadic pancreatic endocrine tumors. Cancer Res 1998;58:4417–4420.
510. Goebel SU, Vortmeyer AO, Zhuang Z, et al: Identical clonality of sporadic gastrinomas at multiple sites. Cancer Res 2000;60:60–63.
511. Evers BM, Rady PL, Sandoval K, et al: Gastrinomas demonstrate amplification of the *HER-2/neu* proto-oncogene. Ann Surg 1994;219:596–601.
512. Chaudhry A, Gobl A, Eriksson B, et al: Different splice variants of CD44 are expressed in gastrinomas but not in other subtypes of endocrine pancreatic tumors. Cancer Res 1994;54:981–986.
513. Creutzfeldt W, Arnold R, Creutzfeldt C, Track NS: Pathomorphologic, biochemical, and diagnostic aspects of gastrinomas (Zollinger-Ellison syndrome). Hum Pathol 1975;6:47–76.
514. Perkins PL, McLeod MK, Jin L, et al: Analysis of gastrinomas by immunohistochemistry and in situ hybridization histochemistry. Diagn Mol Pathol 1992; 1: 155–164.
515. Metz DC, Kuchnio M, Fraker DL, et al: Flow cytometry and Zollinger-Ellison syndrome: Relationship to clinical course. Gastroenterology 1993;105:799–813.
516. Goudswaard WB, Houthoff HJ, Koudstaal J, Zwierstra RP: Nesidioblastosis and endocrine hyperplasia of the pancreas: A secondary phenomenon. Hum Pathol 1986; 17:46–54.
517. Falkmer UG, Falkmer S: The value of cytometric DNA analysis as a prognostic tool in neuroendocrine neoplastic diseases. Pathol Res Pract 1995;191:281–303.
518. Heitz PU, Kasper M, Polak JM, Kloppel G: Pathology of the endocrine pancreas. J Histochem Cytochem 1979;27:1401–1402.
519. Dahms BB, Landing BH, Blaskovics M, Roe TF: Nesidioblastosis and other islet cell abnormalities in hyperinsulinemic hypoglycemia of childhood. Hum Pathol 1980;11:641–649.
520. Bani ST, Bani D, Biliotti G: The endocrine pancreas in patients with insulinomas: An immunocytochemical and ultrastructural study of the nontumoral tissue with morphometrical evaluations. Int J Pancreatol 1989; 5:11–28.
521. Glaser B, Phillip M, Carmi R, et al: Persistent hyperinsulinemic hypoglycemia of infancy ("nesidioblastosis"): Autosomal recessive inheritance in 7 pedigrees. Am J Med Genet 1990;37:511–515.
522. Glaser B, Chiu KC, Anker R, et al: Familial hyperinsulinism maps to chromosome 11p14-15.1, 30 cM centromeric to the insulin gene. Nat Genet 1994;7:185–188.
523. Glaser B, Chiu KC, Liu L, et al: Recombinant mapping of the familial hyperinsulinism gene to an 0.8 cM region on chromosome 11p15.1 and demonstration of a founder effect in Ashkenazi Jews. Hum Mol Genet 1995;4: 879–886.
524. Fantes JA, Oghene K, Boyle S, et al: A high-resolution integrated physical, cytogenetic, and genetic map of human chromosome 11: Distal p13 to proximal p15.1. Genomics 1995;25:447–461.
525. Thornton PS, Satin-Smith MS, Herold K, et al: Familial hyperinsulinism with apparent autosomal dominant inheritance: Clinical and genetic differences from the autosomal recessive variant. J Pediatr 1998;132:9–14.
526. Thomas PM, Cote GJ, Hallman DM, Mathew PM: Homozygosity mapping, to chromosome 11p, of the gene for familial persistent hyperinsulinemic hypoglycemia of infancy. Am J Hum Genet 1995;56:416–421.
527. de Lonlay P, Fournet JC, Rahier J, et al: Somatic deletion of the imprinted 11p15 region in sporadic persistent hyperinsulinemic hypoglycemia of infancy is specific of focal adenomatous hyperplasia and endorses partial pancreatectomy. J Clin Invest 1997;100:802–807.
528. Thomas PM, Cote GJ, Wohllk N, et al: Mutations in the sulfonylurea receptor gene in familial persistent hyperinsulinemic hypoglycemia of infancy. Science 1995;268: 426–429.
529. Thomas PM, Cote GJ, Wohllk N, et al: The molecular basis for familial persistent hyperinsulinemic hypoglycemia of infancy. Proc Assoc Am Physicians 1996;108: 14–19.
530. Nestorowicz A, Wilson BA, Schoor KP, et al: Mutations in the sulfonylurea receptor gene are associated with familial hyperinsulinism in Ashkenazi Jews. Hum Mol Genet 1996;5:1813–1822.
531. Thomas P, Ye Y, Lightner E: Mutation of the pancreatic islet inward rectifier Kir6.2 also leads to familial persistent hyperinsulinemic hypoglycemia of infancy. Hum Mol Genet 1996;5:1809–1812.

JEFFERY K. TAUBENBERGER
NADINE S. I. AGUILERA
SUSAN L. ABBONDANZO

14

Hematologic and Lymphoid System

Hematopathology is an ever-changing field in which adjunctive procedures have become integral to the processing and diagnosis of the pathologic tissue. Even before the specimen is processed, it is important to be aware of the assays and tests available to process the tissue correctly. The most frequent tests performed on hematopathologic specimens include flow cytometry, immunohistochemistry (both in frozen and paraffin-embedded tissue), molecular diagnostic techniques, including polymerase chain reaction (PCR) and Southern blot assays (both on fresh and paraffin-embedded tissue), cytogenetics, and in situ hybridization. Because many of the procedures that can now be performed on fixed tissue were at one time only performed on fresh or frozen tissue, the need to be fastidious about obtaining and storing fresh or frozen tissue until the diagnosis is rendered is often no longer necessary. Many of the assays once only used in frozen tissue immunohistochemistry or flow cytometry can now be performed on fixed embedded tissue. The same is true of most molecular diagnostic techniques.

The classification of lymphoid neoplasms has been burdened by a confusing complexity for the general pathologist, and even, if the truth be known, for the hematopathologist, given the competing classification systems that have been promulgated. Many pathologists view an ever-growing list of immunophenotypic and molecular tests available for the diagnosis of lymphoid neoplasms as adding to the confusion. The good news is that the hematoxylin and eosin stain is still the single most important diagnostic tool in hematopathology. Armed with a good differential from hematoxylin and eosin staining, the diagnosis often needs few supporting studies to arrive at the diagnosis. However, the advent of adjunctive techniques in immunophenotypic analysis and molecular diagnostics makes it possible to achieve an accurate diagnosis in most cases for which the histologic features of a given lesion are not classic.

The Revised European-American Classification for Lymphoid Neoplasms (REAL) was reported and has been used since 1994.[1] Since that time the World Health Organization (WHO) has attempted to update the REAL and add the few entities inadvertently left out of the original classification.[2*] The WHO classification also attempts to subdivide T-cell lymphomas more appropriately.[2] We will use the REAL in this chapter and make comments about the proposed WHO classification as necessary. The REAL and WHO classifications both cover three types of lymphoma: B-cell, T-cell and natural killer (NK)-cell, and Hodgkin's disease. Other lesions not covered by the REAL classification include post-transplant lymphoproliferative disorders (PT-LPDs) and immune deficiency–associated lymphoproliferative disorders.

Lymphoid neoplasms that present primarily as acute leukemias are covered superficially by the REAL and are not covered in this chapter. Acute leukemias are extremely complex and require cytogenetics or molecular diagnostic studies to be fully characterized. Primary bone marrow malignancies such as myelodysplasias are also not covered in this chapter. For further information about these entities, the reader is referred to recent reviews.[3–6]

The entities that are accepted by the REAL classification are listed in Table 14–1. The WHO has modified some of the names and the understanding of the underlying disease has changed in some cases since the REAL was adopted. We will endeavor to point out these changes when they occur. Before we begin our "trek" through the lymphoid neoplasms, in which characteristic immunophenotypic and molecular genetic changes will be highlighted, a short review of antigen receptor rearrangement and its significance for molecular diagnostics is presented. Assays designed to detect monoclonal rearrangements of the antigen receptor genes and chromosomal translocations are useful adjunct methods to support a diagnosis of lymphoma or leukemia. It must, however, be made clear that the results of these assays must be interpreted only in the context of all available clinicopathologic information.

*See revised classification system: Jaffe ES, Harris NL, Stein H, Vardiman JW (eds): Pathology and Genetics of Tumors of Haematopoietic and Lymphoid Tissues. Lyon, France, IARC Press, 2001.

TABLE 14–1

Disease Entities Accepted by the REAL Classification

B-Cell Neoplasms
I. Precursor B-Cell Neoplasms
  A. Precursor B-cell lymphoblastic leukemia/lymphoma
II. Peripheral B-Cell Neoplasms
  A. B-cell chronic lymphocytic leukemia/small lymphocytic lymphoma/prolymphocytic leukemia
  B. Lymphoplasmacytic lymphoma/immunocytoma
  C. Mantle cell lymphoma
  D. Follicle center lymphoma, follicular (grade I, II, III)
  E. Marginal zone B-cell lymphoma (extranodal and nodal)
  F. Splenic marginal zone lymphoma
  G. Hairy cell leukemia
  H. Plasmacytoma/plasma cell myeloma
  I. Diffuse large B-cell lymphoma
  J. Burkitt's lymphoma

T-Cell and NK-Cell Neoplasms
I. Precursor T-Cell Neoplasms (Includes NK Cell)
  A. Precursor T-lymphoblastic lymphoma/leukemia
II. Peripheral T-Cell Neoplasms
  A. T-cell chronic lymphocytic leukemia/prolymphocytic leukemia
  B. Large granular lymphocyte leukemia
    1. T-cell type
    2. NK-cell type
  C. Mycosis fungoides/Sézary syndrome
  D. Peripheral T-cell lymphoma
    1. γδ T-cell lymphoma
    2. Subcutaneous panniculitic T-cell lymphoma
  E. Angioimmunoblastic T-cell lymphoma
  F. Angiocentric lymphoma
  G. Intestinal T-cell lymphoma
  H. Adult T-cell lymphoma/leukemia
  I. Anaplastic large cell lymphoma $CD30^+$

Hodgkin's Disease
I. Lymphocyte Predominance
II. Nodular Sclerosis
III. Mixed Cellularity
IV. Lymphocyte Depletion
V. Lymphocyte-Rich Classic Hodgkin's Disease

ANTIGEN RECEPTOR GENES

Structure and Function

Mature B and T lymphocytes express antigen receptor glycoproteins (immunoglobulins and T-cell receptor [TCR] complexes, respectively), which are fundamental to the normal function of these cells. Each lymphocyte has a genetically and structurally unique antigen receptor derived by a remarkable process of somatic gene recombination.[7–9] These unique gene rearrangements are clonally expanded as a component of a normal polyclonal immune response and also serve as diagnostic markers of clonality in lymphoid malignancy. Identification of clonally rearranged antigen receptor genes is a key component of hematopathologic molecular diagnostics. This information is used primarily to support a diagnosis of malignancy and is often helpful in the assignment of lineage. Molecular diagnostic tools used for assessment are Southern blot and PCR.[10–12] A basic understanding of the underlying mechanism of antigen receptor gene rearrangement is essential for the interpretation of the tests used to assess them. A brief description of the normal processes is presented next.

The B-cell antigen receptor is encoded by the immunoglobulin genes. Both the immunoglobulin heavy chain and light chain (κ and λ) genes rearrange. Resulting immunoglobulins can be cell-surface bound or secreted and consist of a disulfide-bonded complex of two identical heavy chains and two identical light chains (either κ or λ). The TCR consists of a disulfide-bonded heteroduplex of either an α or a β chain or a heteroduplex of the TCR γ and δ chains. The antigen receptor genes are homologous members of the immunoglobulin superfamily whose structures are variations on a theme (Table 14–2). However, the basic mechanisms of their rearrangement are the same. For simplicity, the rearrangement of the immunoglobulin heavy chain will be used as a model.

The germline structure of the immunoglobulin heavy chain gene *(IgH)* is shown in Figure 14–1, line 1. It consists of 51 functional variable (V) region segments, 25 functional diversity (D), and 6 functional joining (J) region segments.[15] Early in B-cell development, one allele of the *IgH* gene is selected to undergo rearrangement to produce a functional antibody-encoding gene. The initial mechanism responsible for antigenic diversity is the rearrangement of VDJ segments by a process that induces double-strand breaks in the DNA and the deletion of large sections of intervening germline DNA. This is followed by DNA repair at the site of recombination. Starting with germline DNA, one IgH diversity (D) segment is fused to one joining (J) segment (see Fig. 14–1, line 2). If successful, this rearranged DJ segment is then fused with one variable (V) segment (see Fig. 14–1, line 3) to form a functional VDJ exon that encodes the variable antigen recognition site of the IgH protein (see Fig. 14–1, line 4).[7, 24, 25]

In germline configuration, V, D, and J segments are flanked with recombination signal sequences (RSS), which contain conserved heptamer and nonamer motifs separated by a 12- or 23-base pair (bp) spacer (Fig. 14–2*A*).[8] The sites of recombination are determined by the RSS, between one with a 12-bp spacer and one with a 23-bp spacer (12/23 rule), ensuring that V(D)J recombination occurs between two coding segments of different types (e.g., D and J segments) (see Fig. 14–2*B*).[25] The specificity of V(D)J rearrangement (including the 12/23 rule) and double-strand break is mediated by the coordinate expression of RAG1 and RAG2 proteins. Subsequent DNA repair steps overlap with other DNA repair mechanisms.[26–28]

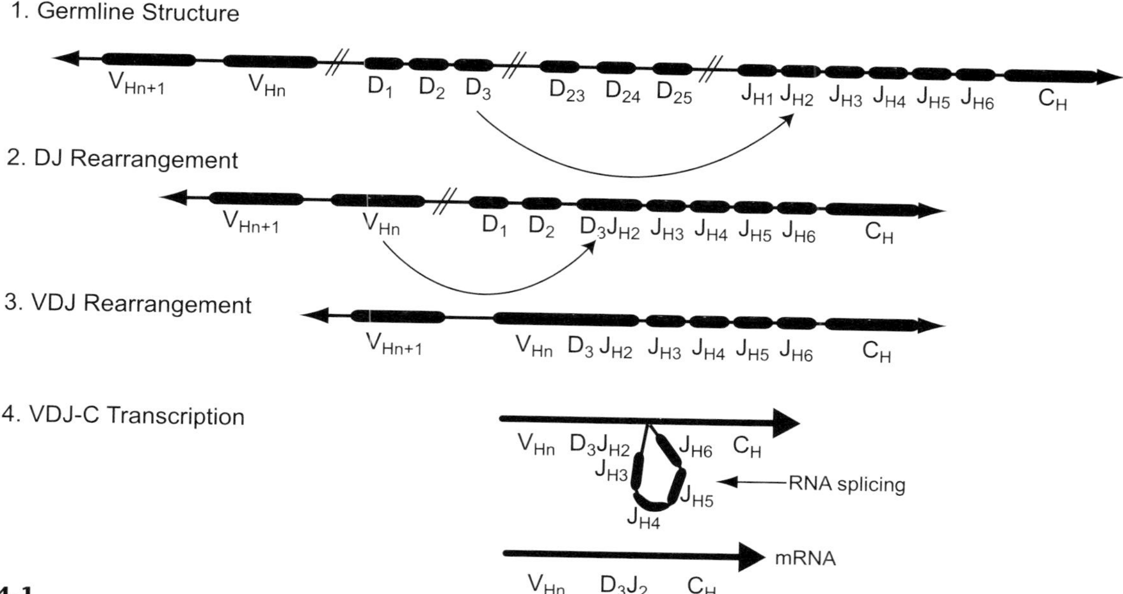

FIGURE 14–1
Schematic model of immunoglobulin heavy-chain (IgH) VDJ rearrangement. *Line 1* shows germline structure of IgH prior to the onset of rearrangement. As shown in Table 14–1, there are 51 functional V_H regions, 25 D_H, and 6 J_H segments available for rearrangement. *Arrow* shows random apposition of a D_H segment to a J_H segment, initiated by the expression of the RAG1/RAG2 complex. *Line 2* shows apposition of a random V_H segment to the successful D_HJ_H rearrangement to complete the VDJ rearrangement process, *line 3*. *Line 4* shows transcription of IgH mRNA. Note that the constant region exons are not involved in the rearrangement process, but spliced to form mature IgH mRNA before translation.

Recombinational diversity alone, although enormous, cannot account for the full range of diversity of the immunoglobulin repertoire. Nucleotide loss and random nucleotide addition (N nucleotides) between the D-J and V-DJ joints by the enzyme terminal deoxynucleotidyl transferase (TdT) add even more diversity. Other components of diversity include variable combinations between rearranged heavy- and light-chain genes to form the antigen recognition site of the mature immunoglobulin complex and somatic mutation of the germline sequences of the hypervariable complementarity-determining regions (CDRs) of the V regions.[13] The process of VDJ rearrangement of the heavy chain must lead to a functional (i.e., coding) section of the immunoglobulin heavy chain without frameshift or nonsense mutations. A successful IgH rearrangement induces subsequent rearrangement of a light chain allele and leads to suppression of rearrangement of the second IgH allele (a process termed *allelic exclusion*).[29, 30] B cells that fail to make a functional IgH VDJ rearrangement on the first allele can undergo a second IgH rearrangement on the second allele. Therefore, a single B-cell clone may bear two IgH rearrangements: a functional one coding for the expressed IgH and a nonfunctional rearrangement. Cells that fail to produce a functional IgH or light-chain rearrangement are eliminated through apoptotic processes.[7, 25]

The rearrangement of antigen receptor genes in lymphocyte development is hierarchical. In B cells, as just shown, IgH rearrangements occur developmentally before light-chain rearrangements. Therefore, assessment of IgH rearrangement status is the most useful molecular test in B-cell neoplasia, including precursor B-cell neoplasms. Allelic exclusion prevents a B cell from expressing antibodies with two different antigen receptor specificities. Light-chain rearrangement generally only begins after successful IgH rearrangement, and it in itself is ordered. The κ light chain rearranges preferentially, and only if both κ alleles fail to produce a functional rearrangement does the λ light chain rearrange.[7] T-cell rearrangement is also hierarchical and induces allelic exclusion. In the fetal and neonatal thymus, the TCR γ chain is often the first gene to rearrangement in T-cell development. This may lead to rearrangement of the TCR δ chain gene and development of a functional γδ TCR-bearing T cell. However, rearrangement of the γ gene in T-cell development postnatally usually leads to subsequent rearrangement of the TCR β chain. Successful β chain rearrangement induces α gene rearrangement to produce a functional αβ TCR-bearing T cell. Approximately 95% of mature T cells bear αβ TCR. Note here that an αβ TCR-positive T-cell clone may often have a TCR γ rearrangement without having expressed rearranged γ on the cell surface. Because the TCR δ locus is contained within the α locus, rearrangement of α eliminates δ (for that allele). Pairing rules also only allow expression of functional TCRαβ or TCRγδ dimers. Surface expression is linked to a complement of other proteins (CD3 and either CD4 or CD8) to produce a functional TCR complex.

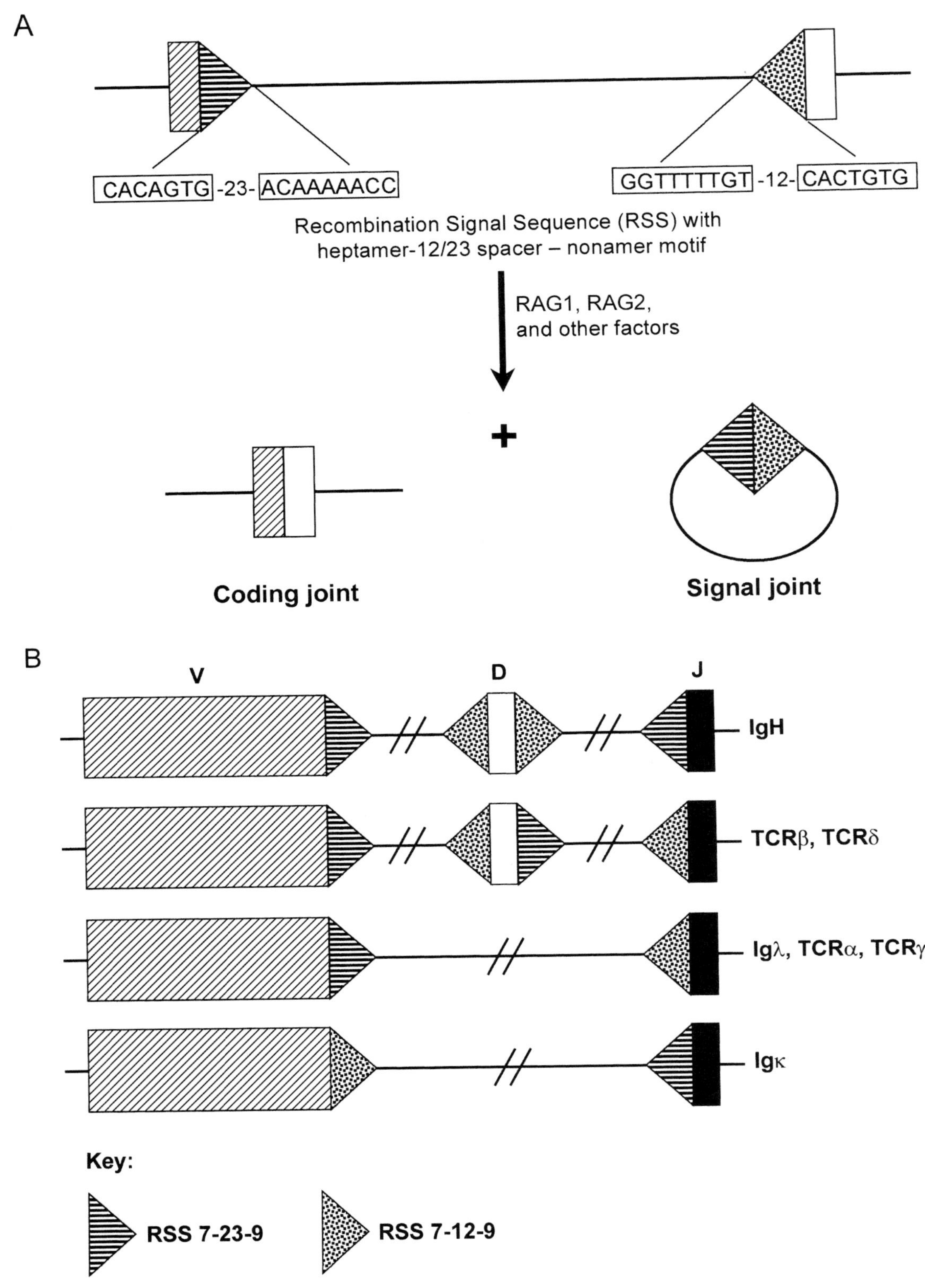

FIGURE 14–2
A, Structure of the coding and signal ends of the V(D)J segments. Recombination signal sequences (RSS) have a conserved heptamer-nonamer motif with either a 12-bp or 23-bp spacer. Rearrangement (as coordinated by expression of RAG1/RAG2 complex) forms a coding joint and an excised, circularized signal joint. The signal joint is lost with cell division. *B,* Structure of the antigen receptor genes in germline configuration showing RSS configuration. Only matched pairs of RSS with one 12-bp spacer RSS can rearrange with a complementary 23-bp spacer RSS. This ensures proper rearrangement of the V(D)J segments.

TABLE 14–2

Antigen Receptor Gene Structure

Immunoglobulin heavy-chain gene[7, 13–15]:

- *Location*: the long arm of chromosome 14, near the telomere at 14q32.
- *Organization*: 51 functional V_H segments, 25 functional D_H segments, and 6 functional J_H segments.
- On rearrangement, these are transcribed with one of the nine constant region C_H segments, resulting in the five different forms of the immunoglobulin heavy chain (C_μ, C_δ, C_γ, C_ϵ and C_α) by the mechanism of class switching. When coupled with a functionally rearranged light-chain protein (either κ or λ), these produce the five different antibody classes: IgM, IgD, IgG, IgE, and IgA, respectively.

Immunoglobulin light-chain genes:

κ[14, 15]:

- *Location*: short arm of chromosome 2, at 2p12
- *Organization:* 38 functional V_κ, 5 J_κ, and 1 constant region, C_κ

λ[14, 15]:

- *Location*: long arm of chromosome 22, at 22q11
- *Organization:* 31 functional V_λ, with 4 tandemly arranged J_λ-C_λ complexes

T-cell receptor genes: consist of a heterodimer (either TCR α/β or TCR γ/δ) associated on the T-cell surface with the invariant CD3 complex and either CD4 or CD8

β T-cell receptor[16]:

- *Location*: long arm of chromosome 7, at 7q34
- *Organization:* 46 functional V_β segments, with 2 tandem D_β-J_β-C_β complexes, each containing 1 D_β and 6 or 7 J_β segments

α T-cell receptor[17–19]:

- *Location*: long arm of chromosome 14, at 14q11
- *Organization:* ~42 V_α segments, with a single C_α (not yet completely mapped)

δ T-cell receptor[20,21]:

- *Location*: long arm of chromosome 14, at 14q11 *nested within* the α gene
- *Organization*: 4 V_δ segments, 2 D_δ, 3 J_δ and 1 C_δ segment; eliminated with productive α rearrangement

γ T-cell receptor[22, 23]:

- *Location*: short arm of chromosome 7, at 7p15
- *Organization:* 8 functional V_γ segments, with two tandem J_γ-C_γ segments, with 5 J_γ segments, and 2 C_γ segments

After successful rearrangement, immunoglobulin genes in mature B cells can undergo even further changes, in a process referred to as receptor editing. At least three mechanisms can occur: (1) IgH isotype switching, (2) somatic hypermutation, and (3) V-segment substitution by a second round of rearrangement:

1. Isotype or class switching allows a given IgH VDJ rearrangement to be transcribed to various heavy-chain classes, such as IgM, IgG, or IgA (see Table 14–2). Thus, a given B cell can produce different antibody classes, all bearing the identical idiotypic rearrangement.[31, 32]

2. Somatic V-region hypermutation involves the affinity maturation of an already rearranged antigen receptor gene by the introduction of point mutations, small insertions, and/or deletions. This process occurs in B cells in the germinal center or postgerminal center–derived B cells and is an antigen-dependent process.[33–36] The mechanisms are not yet fully elucidated but are linked to transcription of the gene.[37] Such receptor editing is rare in CD5⁺ B-cell derivatives such as mantle cell lymphoma and chronic lymphocytic leukemia.[7]

3. Antigen receptor genes can undergo a second round of rearrangement as a form of affinity maturation (receptor editing). This mechanism has been newly described and remarkably involves a RAG1/RAG2-dependent secondary rearrangement in the germinal center.[38–40] This mechanism has been observed for both immunoglobulin and TCR genes.

Analysis of Their Rearrangements

Classically, Southern blot assays have been used to assess clonality of the antigen receptor genes in lymphoid lesions. Although still considered the "gold standard" for such assessments, PCR-based assays have largely supplanted the Southern blot assays in diagnostic laboratories. A detailed account of Southern blot gene rearrangement assays can be found in the National Committee for Clinical Laboratory Standards (NCCLS) guidelines[12]; a summary is presented here. Southern blot assays take advantage of the changes in the germline structure of the antigen receptor gene with rearrangement. Restriction endonuclease sites in the germline structure of these genes have been carefully mapped. During V(D)J rearrangement, particular restriction sites will be deleted whereas novel restriction sites may be created. Cells with their antigen receptor genes in germline form will show a consistent pattern of the number and size of bands observed in a Southern blot (depending on the probe and restriction enzyme used). In a polyclonal population where each lymphocyte represents a unique clonal rearrangement (e.g., a normal lymph node), changes to the germline gene structure will not be consistent clone to clone, so no particular band will be visible on the blot. If a particular clonal population (e.g., a lymphoma) makes up a large enough percentage of the total cell population in the sample, a novel band differing in size from the germline band will be visible on the Southern blot, reflecting the clonally rearranged antigen receptor gene (Fig. 14–3). Thus, the proportion of the sample making up the clonal population is a critical feature of analysis.

Depending on the number of probes used (and the number of restriction digests employed with each probe), 50 to 100 μg of high-molecular-weight DNA will be needed for antigen receptor analysis by Southern blot.[12] This translates into about 500 mg of tissue or 2×10^8 nucleated cells. For the commonly used probes (J_H for immunoglobulin heavy chain, J_λ and J_κ for immunoglobulin light chain, J_β and C_β for TCR β), restriction with a minimum of three enzymes, *Eco*RI, *Bam*HI, and *Hin*dIII, is recommended. Care must be

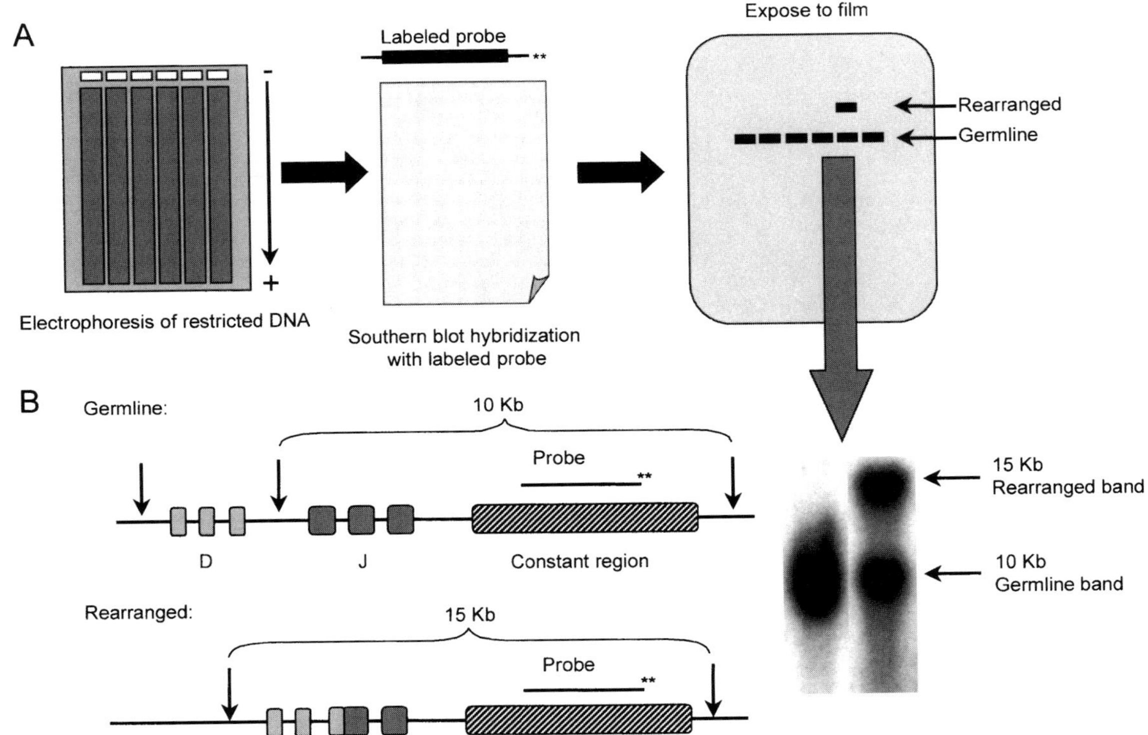

FIGURE 14–3
A, Diagram of Southern blot analysis for IgH gene rearrangement. Restriction-digested high-molecular-weight DNA is electrophoresed through an agarose gel, Southern blotted with labeled probe, and exposed to x-ray film. Rearranged band(s) appear as bands with a different molecular weight from the germline band. *B*, Diagram of the IgH region in germline configuration and after DJ rearrangement. Note the loss of a restriction site between the germline D and J segments in the rearranged allele. This changes the size of the restriction fragment hybridizing to the constant region probe.

exercised in the interpretation of a clonally rearranged allele. Ideally, lanes from two different restriction digests should show evidence of a clonal rearrangement. Verification of a band seen only with one enzyme may require use of a fourth restriction enzyme (commonly *Bgl*II). Interpretation should also take into consideration recognized test limitations including the proportion of clonal cells in a polyclonal background of lymphocytes. Sensitivity of gene rearrangement detection by genomic Southern blot is ideally at the 5% level. Partial or incomplete restriction enzyme digestion may yield spurious bands. Finally, a monoclonal gene rearrangement may also be detected in a non-neoplastic clonal proliferation.

PCR-based methodologies are rapidly becoming the standard of practice in molecular diagnostic laboratories to assess rearrangement status of the antigen receptor genes. Although PCR is known to be exquisitely sensitive, being able under ideal conditions to amplify a single target DNA molecule, this absolute sensitivity is not a relevant factor in PCR for immunoglobulin or TCR clonality studies. PCR-based methods, like Southern blot assays, also are dependent on the proportion of clonal cells in a polyclonal background. To understand this limitation with PCR, it is necessary to summarize how these methods work. Unlike Southern blotting, which relies on the differences between germline and dominantly rearranged alleles of the gene in question, diagnostic PCR-based assays only amplify rearranged antigen receptor gene alleles. PCR primers are designed to span portions of the rearranging gene, such as V-region and J-region primers. Rearrangement brings the primers close enough together that they can amplify the intervening target. In the germline state, the primers hybridize to sequences too far apart for routine amplification to occur. Therefore, PCR only assesses differences in *size* between uniquely *rearranged* alleles. Recall that TdT adds random numbers of random nucleotides between the V-D and D-J or V-J joints to increase overall repertoire diversity. PCR takes advantage of this phenomenon by assuming that different rearrangements will differ in size, by as little as a single base pair, over a certain range. Products are visualized after electrophoresis through a gel or capillary.[7, 41, 42] Polyclonal patterns appear either as a ladder of bands or a smear, depending on the sensitivity of resolution, whereas monoclonal rearrangements appear as a single band or a dominant band over a polyclonal ladder (Fig. 14–4). A sample protocol for IgH PCR is shown in SOP 14.1.

There are several caveats to the use of gene rearrangement assays in hematopathology. First, none of the assays provides 100% sensitivity—that is, there are lymphomas that will not show evidence of clonality by

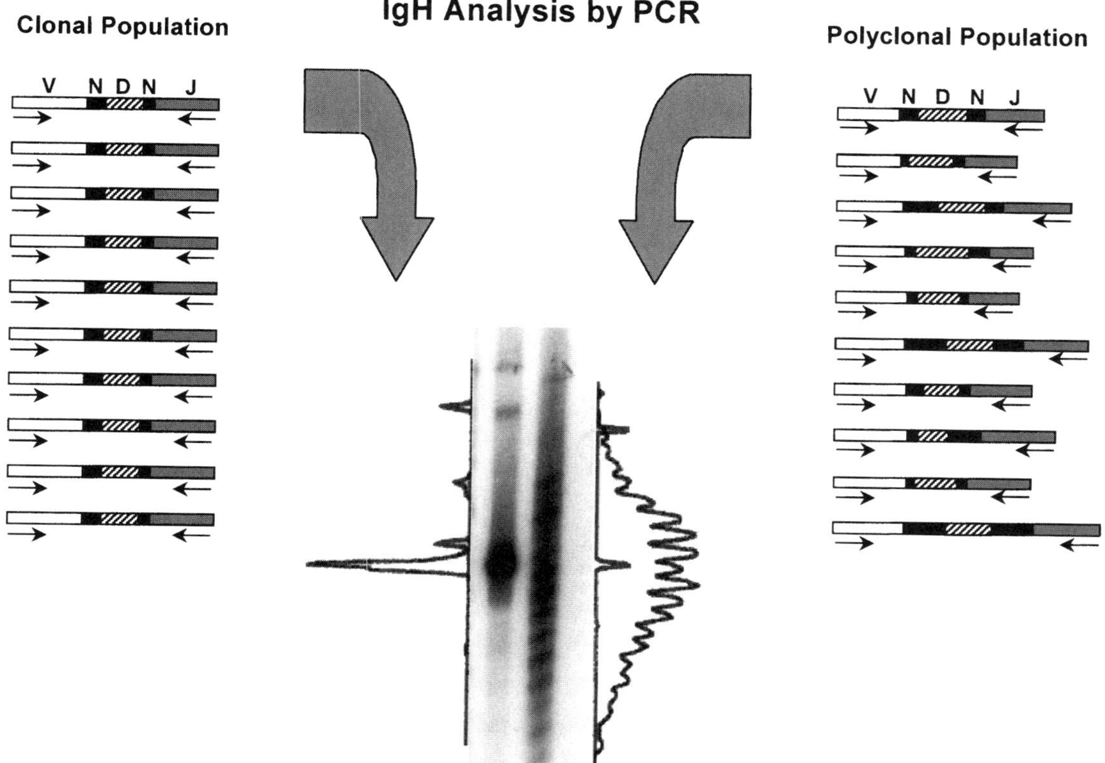

FIGURE 14–4
Analysis of IgH rearrangement by PCR (see Methods Box). Each VDJ rearrangement is unique in sequence and in size because of N-region addition and nucleotide loss during rearrangement. A polyclonal (reactive) population will consist of a ladder of VDJ products differing in size by three base pair intervals (*right side of figure*). A monoclonal rearrangement consists of only one rearrangement or a single dominant rearrangement over a polyclonal background (*left side of figure*).

certain assays, so one must be aware of false-negative results when interpreting the tests.[43] This can be caused by the proportion of the monoclonal population compared with the surrounding polyclonal background. For most methods, monoclonal B-cell populations less than 5% of the total B-cell pool in the sample will not be detected by either PCR or Southern blot. For focal lesions, microdissection of the suspect area may increase detection sensitivity. Other reasons for false-negative results include poor DNA quality or amount (both methods), incomplete restriction digestion (Southern blot), and somatic hypermutation of the rearranged antigen receptor gene such that poor primer binding occurs (PCR). Somatic hypermutation is a characteristic of germinal center–derived B-cell clones[38] and is known to decrease PCR detection sensitivity in follicle-center lymphomas and their derivatives.[7] The false-negative rate in PCR-based detection of IgH clonality in follicular lymphoma may be as high as 40% to 50%.[44]

Another caveat to the use of gene rearrangement assays is assignment of a lymphoma's lineage by analysis of antigen receptor genes. Lineage infidelity, or lineage promiscuity, in which a lymphocyte bears "inappropriate" rearrangements, is a well-known phenomenon in molecular pathology. Lineage infidelity is defined as a B-cell neoplasm that harbors rearrangements of TCR genes or as a T-cell neoplasm that shows immunoglobulin gene rearrangements.[7, 10, 42, 43, 45–48] Lineage infidelity is more common in neoplasms with precursor B-cell or T-cell phenotypes (e.g., lymphoblastic leukemias/lymphomas). In precursor B-cell leukemia/lymphoma, the majority of cases have undergone TCR γ V_γ-J_γ rearrangements and partial TCR δ rearrangements on at least one allele.[7] TCR β rearrangements are seen in 20% to 30% of cases.[7, 44] IgH rearrangements are seen in 15% to 30% of precursor T-lymphoblastic leukemia/lymphoma cases by Southern blot.[7, 44] The percentage of T-cell lymphoblastic leukemia cases showing IgH rearrangements by PCR is lower, suggesting that many of these tumors bear only partial D_H-J_H rearrangements not detected in routine IgH PCR assays.[7] Lineage infidelity is less common in neoplasms arising from more mature lymphocytes. Mature B-cell neoplasms show TCR rearrangements as assessed by Southern blot[44] or PCR[42] in 5% to 10% of cases, and mature T-cell neoplasms show IgH rearrangements in an even smaller percentage of cases.[42, 44]

CHROMOSOMAL ABNORMALITIES OF LYMPHOID NEOPLASMS

Cells from virtually all cases of lymphoma have clonal chromosomal abnormalities. Unlike most carcinomas, however, most non-Hodgkin's lymphomas have recurring, nonrandom cytogenetic abnormalities that correlate with clinical, histologic, and immunophenotypic parameters.[9, 49–51] Although classic cytogenetic analysis remains an important diagnostic technique, molecular cytogenetic analysis by Southern blot, PCR, or fluorescent in situ hybridization (FISH) allows the molecular pathologist to detect most such translocations.[11, 52, 53] Not only does detection of a specific translocation allow for initial diagnosis for many lymphoid neoplasms, but it also allows for prognostic information and minimal residual disease detection. Additionally, advances in molecular biology have made it possible to identify the underlying genetic mechanisms involved in many of these chromosomal rearrangements. At the chromosomal level, lymphomas often exhibit only single abnormalities (commonly reciprocal translocations). The occurrence of particular chromosomal translocations is highly associated with particular entities as defined in the REAL classification, suggesting that the mechanisms underlying these translocations are associated with lymphomagenesis. That microsatellite instability is rare in non-Hodgkin's lymphomas also suggests that these translocations occur by specific mechanisms rather than by generalized chromosomal instability or defects in DNA repair mechanisms.[49, 54]

There are two mechanisms by which translocations can result in altered gene function (which may play a significant role in transformation and lymphomagenesis): the deregulation of gene expression and the expression of a novel fusion protein. The first mechanism is the predominant one seen in lymphoma translocations and involves immunoglobulin genes in B-cell tumors and TCR genes in T-cell tumors. These translocations result in the overexpression or aberrant expression of a normal cellular gene by bringing it (by translocation) under the regulatory control of a constitutively expressed antigen receptor gene. Figure 14–5 shows a diagram of the t(14;18) translocation of follicular lymphoma. The second mechanism is the expression of a chimeric fusion product, in which coding portions of two different genes are brought together by translocation. This is the most common form seen in leukemia translocations. All the translocations identified in myeloid leukemias result in a fusion protein. In lymphomas, the one example of a fusion translocation is the NPM/ALK chimeric protein from the t(2;5)

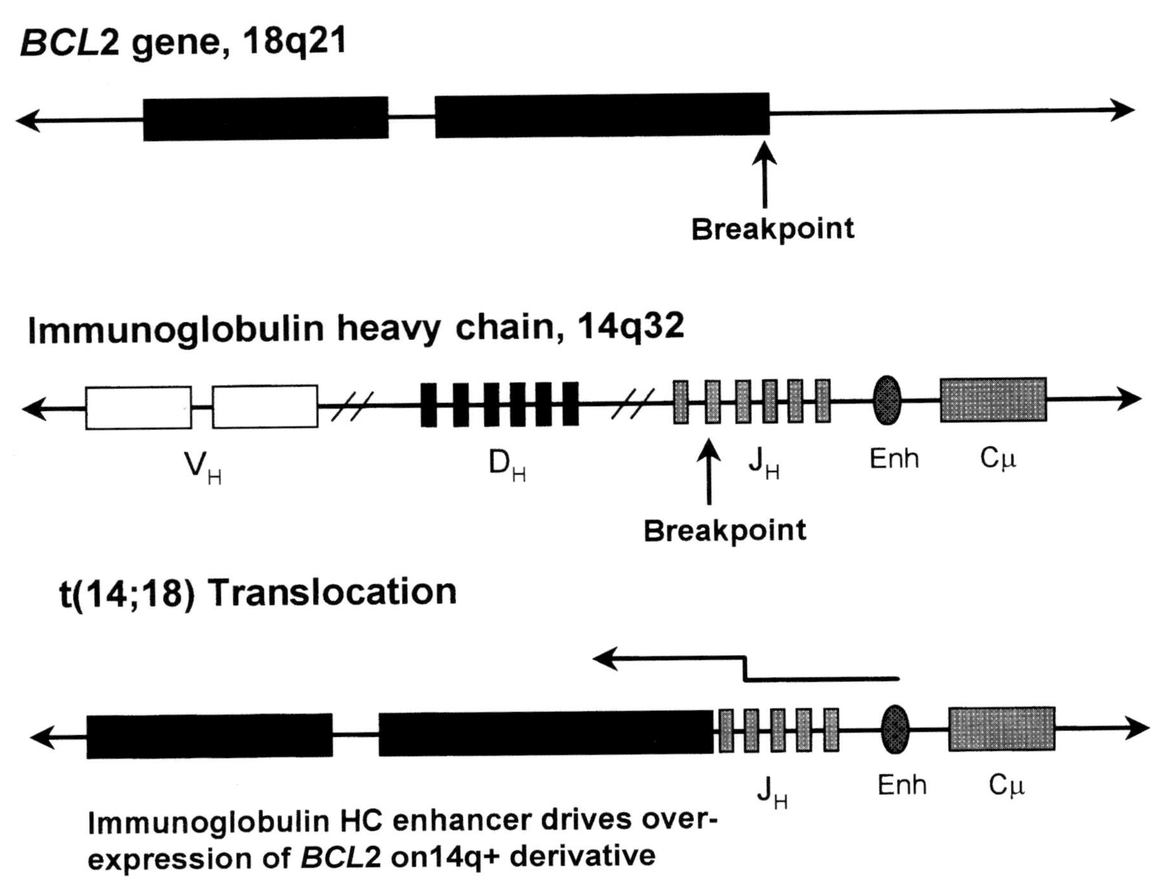

FIGURE 14–5
Diagram of the t(14;18)(q32;q21) IgH-*BCL2* translocation. The *BCL2* gene is translocated to the *IgH* gene at 14q32 and brought under the regulatory control of the IgH enhancer (Enh) located upstream of the IgH constant region.

translocation in anaplastic large cell lymphoma. Table 14–3 shows examples of common translocations in non-Hodgkin's lymphoma. Specific translocations as associated with particular lymphomas are described with the individual tumors in the next section.

Chromosomal translocations can be detected not only by classic cytogenetics but also by molecular genetic techniques including Southern blot, PCR (or reverse transcriptase [RT]-PCR), and FISH.[7, 44, 52] As stated earlier, molecular diagnostics assays do not eliminate the need for classic cytogenetic analyses but serve to complement them. Detection of specific chromosomal translocations in general is, however, very amenable to molecular genetic techniques. However, although molecular genetic translocation detection techniques only detect the specific changes assayed, cytogenetic screening allows for simultaneous detection of multiple chromosomal abnormalities (e.g., translocations, deletions, trisomy) not biased by assay choice.

Southern blot hybridization serves as an excellent method for detecting translocations. Like the assay for detection of antigen receptor gene rearrangement, the germline structure of the gene in question must first be mapped. Rearrangement through translocation deletes restriction enzyme sites, resulting in a different-sized product on a gel from the germline band. A caveat, however, is that this method does not generally allow assessment of a particular translocation partner, just evidence of disruption of the normal germline structure of a given gene. If a specific translocation is suspected, DNA probes specific to both partners in the translocation can be used. The detection of a non-germline band that hybridizes with both probes provides direct evidence for a particular translocation. Such a technique is cumbersome and is not generally performed. Southern blotting requires large amounts of high-molecular-weight DNA and thus is only applicable to fresh/frozen tissues.

Just as PCR is becoming the most common method to detect gene rearrangements, PCR for translocations in lymphoma diagnosis is quite common and easily performed. PCR can be performed from fixed tissue specimens and from small numbers of cells; thus, it is applicable for routinely processed specimens, microdissected specimens, and cytology samples. PCR can only be performed on translocations in which the breakpoints are tightly clustered and flanking sequences are known. Chromosomal translocations that have widely distributed breakpoint sites, such as *MYC* in t(8;14), or involve a gene that has numerous translocation partners, such as *BCL6* at 3q27, are not amenable to routine PCR analyses. For such translocations, Southern blotting is more practical. Fusion translocations (rare in lymphoma) in which a chimeric transcript is expressed can be assessed by RT-PCR. This technique is commonly used to detect the t(2;5)(p23;q35) *NPM-ALK* translocation in anaplastic large cell lymphoma.

FISH is a third molecular technique for translocation detection. It can be used with either interphase or metaphase preparations.[52] FISH assays are useful in detection of chromosomal translocations in which the breakpoints are widely dispersed, because typical FISH probes are much larger than probes used in Southern blot, often larger than 100 kb.[44] For example, FISH probes can detect virtually all the *MYC* 8q24 breakpoints in the t(8;14)(q24;q32) translocation in Burkitt's lymphoma, which span over 400 kb.[52] Just like Southern blot analysis, FISH assays that use a single probe can detect breakpoints within a chromosome that serve only as presumptive evidence for a specific translocation. To detect a specific chromosomal translocation with FISH, two probes labeled with different fluorescent dyes are needed, often by chromosome painting. Thus in the previous example, interphase probes for chromosomes 8 and 14 may be labeled red and green, respectively. Intact chromosomes

TABLE 14–3

Lymphoma Translocation Examples

Entity	Translocation	Genes Involved	Gene Function	Mechanism
Follicular lymphoma, DLBCL	t(14;18)(q32;q21)	*IgH, BCL2*	Antiapoptosis	Overexpression
Burkitt's lymphoma	t(8;14)(q24;q32)	*MYC, IgH*	Transcription factor	Overexpression
	t(2;8)(p12;q24)	*IgLκ, MYC*	Transcription factor	Overexpression
	t(8;22)(q24;q11)	*MYC, IgL λ*	Transcription factor	Overexpression
Mantle zone	t(11;14)(q13;q32)	*BCL1, IgH*	G1 cyclin	Overexpression
Lymphoplasmacytoid lymphoma	t(9;14)(p13;q32)	*PAX5, IgH*	Transcription factor	Overexpression
DLBCL	t(3;22)(q27;q11)	*BCL6, IgL λ*	Transcription factor	Overexpression
	t(3;14)(q27;q32)	*BCL6, IgH*	Transcription factor	Overexpression
T-lymphoblastic lymphoma/leukemia	t(10;14)(q24;q11)	*HOX11, TCR α/δ*	Transcription factor	Overexpression
	t(7;10)(q35;q24)	*TCR β, HOX11*	Transcription factor	Overexpression
Anaplastic large cell lymphoma	t(2;5)(p23;q35)	*ALK, NPM*	Tyrosine kinase (ALK)	Fusion protein

DLBCL, diffuse large B-cell lymphoma.

will be stained with one color probe only, while both probes will hybridize to the t(8;14), resulting in a blended yellow color.[52]

IMMUNOHISTOCHEMISTRY AND FLOW CYTOMETRY

The diagnostic utility of flow cytometry and immunohistochemistry has greatly expanded in the past decade. The number of antibody reagents for use in hematopathology, both for fresh and fixed tissue specimens, have grown exponentially. Very few fields of pathology have embraced these techniques to the extent of hematopathology. A list of commonly used antibodies in immunohistochemical analyses of lymphoid lesions is shown in Table 14–4. Because of limitations in use and interpretation of all immunohistochemical modalities, most hematopathologists advocate using a combined approach with morphology and molecular diagnostic techniques to arrive at a correct diagnosis. This strategy is reflected in the REAL classification. Techniques in immunohistochemistry and flow cytometry are found elsewhere in this book. For more information on the use of immunohistochemistry and flow cytometry in hematopathology, see the reviews in references 51–57.

FEATURES OF SPECIFIC LYMPHOMAS

B-Cell Neoplasms

The immunophenotypes of B-cell neoplasms are listed in Table 14–5. An immunohistochemical basis for clonality in a B-cell process is a κ to λ ratio greater than 5:1,

TABLE 14–4

Immunohistochemical Antibodies in Hematopathology

CD	Clone/Name	Use
CD1a	O10	Cortical thymocytes, Langerhans' cells, interdigitating reticulum cells
CD2		T cells, T-cell neoplasms
CD3	CLB-T3	T cells, T-cell neoplasms
CD4	IF6	T-helper cells, T cells, T-cell neoplasms
CD5	CD5	T cells, T-cell neoplasms, B-cell neoplasms
CD8	C8/144B	T-suppressor cells, T cells, T-cell neoplasms
CD10	CALLA	Germinal center cells, progenitor cells in bone marrow, lymphoblastic and follicular lymphoma
CD11c		Subset of B cells, subset of T cells, monocytes
CD15	Leu-M1	Granulocytes, Reed-Sternberg cells in classic Hodgkin's disease
CD20	L26	B cells (except premature and plasma cells), B-cell neoplasms, lymphocyte-predominant Hodgkin's disease
CD21		Follicular dendritic cells
CD22		B cells, B-cell precursors
CD30	Ki-1, Ber H2	Immunoblasts, plasma cells, Reed-Sternberg cells in classic Hodgkin's disease, anaplastic large-cell lymphoma
CD34	Qbend	Hematopoietic progenitor cells, vascular endothelial cells, granulocytic sarcoma
CD43	MT1	T cells, T-cell neoplasms, small cell B-cell lymphomas, natural killer cells, hematopoietic cells
CD45RB	LCA	Leukocytes, hematolymphoid neoplasms
CD45RO	UCHL-1	T cells, T-cell neoplasms, monocytes, some B-cell lymphomas
CD45RA	MT2	Paracortical T cell, mantle zone B cells, natural killer cells, follicular lymphoma
CD56		Large granular cytotoxic T cells, natural killer cells, and neoplasms
CD57		Large granular cytotoxic T cells, natural killer cells and neoplasms, lymphocytes surrounding neoplastic cells in lymphocyte-predominant Hodgkin's disease
CD68	KP-1	Macrophages, monocytes, myeloid precursors, histiocytic neoplasms, acute myeloid leukemia, and granular sarcoma
CD79a	Mb-1	B cells including plasma cells, B-cell and plasmacytic neoplasms, some lymphoblastic lymphomas
	Bcl-2	Protein overexpressed in follicular lymphomas associated with t(11;14)
β F1	8A3	T-cell β receptor
	κ/λ	Immunoglobulin light chain; restriction is indicative of a clonal B-cell process
	Cyclin-D1, bcl-1	Protein amplified in mantle cell lymphoma associated with t(11;14)
	Myeloperoxidase	Cytoplasmic granules in granulocytes and granulocytic neoplasms
	Lysozyme	Granulocytes, monocytes, macrophages, and corresponding neoplasms
TCRδ1	TCR1061	T-cell γδ receptor
	TdT	Cortical thymocytes, immature bone marrow lymphocytes, lymphoblastic lymphoma/leukemia
	TIA-1	Cytotoxic granules in T cells, natural killer cells, and neoplasms
	VS38C	Plasma cells and plasmacytoid lymphocytes
	ALK-1	Protein expressed in anaplastic large cell lymphoma associated with t(2;5)

which is the upper limit of normal, or less than 0.7:1, which is the lower limit of normal.[58]

PRECURSOR B-LYMPHOBLASTIC LEUKEMIA/LYMPHOMA

This entity presents uncommonly as a lymphoma and is equivalent to acute lymphoblastic leukemia. The presentation is similar to T-lymphoblastic lymphoma in tissue. Immunophenotype varies and bone marrow biopsy with flow cytometry and cytogenetic studies are the key to diagnosis and prognosis. Because of the numerous cytogenetic and immunophenotypic permutations described, this tumor is best covered in a text on acute leukemias[3–6] and is not covered here.

B-CELL CHRONIC LYMPHOCYTIC LEUKEMIA (B-CLL)/SMALL LYMPHOCYTIC LYMPHOMA (CLL/SLL), PROLYMPHOCYTIC LEUKEMIA (PLL)

SLL and CLL are thought to be the same disease with different presentations; one presents in lymph nodes (SLL), the other in the blood (CLL). Prolymphocytic leukemia was once thought to be the terminal transformation of CLL but is now believed to be a different disease and is recognized as such in the WHO classification. Our discussion concentrates on CLL/SLL.

Immunophenotype. The immunophenotype is (CD20, CD79a, CD5, CD23, CD43, BCL2)$^+$; (CD10, cyclin D1)$^-$.

Genotype. IgH and light chains are rearranged. Karyotypic abnormalities are seen in up to 50% in B-CLL and 70% in SLL.[59, 60] Abnormalities of 13q14, mainly deletions, are most common. Detection methods are classic cytogenetics, Southern blot, and FISH. By Southern blot, 13q14 deletions can be detected in 40% to 50% of B-CLL cases.[60, 61] These 13q deletions are clonal and present in more than 95% cells within the tumor, suggesting that this is an early event. Deletions at 13q14 are seen in a large percentage of other B-cell neoplasms, including mantle cell lymphoma (70%), B-lymphoblastic leukemia/lymphoma (>10%), and multiple myeloma, suggesting that a common genetic lesion at 13q14 functions as a "B-cell lymphoma" gene.[62] The deletions map 1.6 cM telomeric to the *RB1* gene,[63] and reports of deletions of *BRCA2* at 13q12.3 have been reported but not confirmed.[64] The gene(s) involved at 13q14 in these lymphomas have not been identified, and it is unknown whether the same genetic change is seen in the various B-cell lymphomas with these deletions.[62]

Other genetic abnormalities are also seen in these lesions: trisomy 12 is seen in about 15% of B-CLL. That it is rarely clonal, and that a varying percentage of cells carry the abnormality, suggest that trisomy 12 is a secondary genetic change occurring after transformation has taken place.[61] Deletions of 11q are seen in up to 20% of B-CLL and are associated with a poor

TABLE 14–5

Immunophenotype of B-Cell Neoplasms

CD	Pre B	CLL/SLL	LPL/I	MCL	FCL	MZL	SMZ*	HCL*	PC/M	DLCL	PTLD
CD20	−/+	+	+/−	+	+	+	+	+	−/+	+	+/−
CD22	+/−	+	+/−	+	+	+	+	+	−/+	+	+/−
CD79a	+/−	+	+	+	+	+	+	+	+/−	+	+
CD5	−	+	−/+	+	−	−	−/+	−	−	−/+	−
CD10	+/−	−	−	−	+	−	−/+	−	−	+/−	−
CD23	−	+/−	−	−	+/−	−	−/+	−	−	−	−
CD43	+	+/−	+/−	+/−	−	+/−	+/−	−	+	−/+	−/+
BCL2	−/+	+	+/−	+	+/−	+/−	+	+/−	+/−	+/−	−/+
BCL6	−	−	−	−	+	−	−	−	+/−	+/−	−
Cyclin D1	−	−	−	+	−	−	−	Rare	−	−	−
EMA	−	−	−/+	−	−	−	−	−	−	−	−/+
CD30	−	−	−/+	−	−	−	−	−	−/+	−/+	−/+
CD34	+/−	−	−	−	−	−	−	−	−	−	−
TdT	+	−	−	−	−	−	−	−	−	−	−
VS38	−	−	+/−	−	−	−	−	−	−/+	−/+	−/+
CD25	−	−	−	−	−	−	−/+	+	−	−	−
CD103	−	−	−	−	−	−	−	+	−	−	−
CD11C	−	−	−	−	−	−	−/+	+	−	−	−

*Best studied by flow cytometry.

Pre B, precursor B-cell neoplasm; CLL/SLL, chronic lymphocytic leukemia/small lymphocytic lymphoma; LPL/I, lymphoplasmacytic lymphoma/immunocytoma; MCL, mantle cell lymphoma; FCL, follicle center lymphoma; MZL, marginal zone lymphoma; SMZ, splenic marginal zone lymphoma; HCL, hairy cell leukemia; PC/M, plasmacytoma/myeloma; DLCL, diffuse large B-cell lymphoma; PTLD, post-transplant lymphoproliferative disorder.

prognosis.[65] The 17p deletion (*TP53*) is seen in more than 10% of CLL and is also a late-stage abnormality associated with a poor prognosis.[62] Deletions at 6q21-23 are seen in 25% of SLL, suggesting that SLL and CLL have a different pathogenesis.[62]

BCL2 is overexpressed in 85% of B-CLL cyclin D2 is also overexpressed in 85% of B-CLL, whereas MDM2 has been shown to be overexpressed in 50%.[66–68]

Because CLL/SLL is CD5 positive, it has been postulated that it is a tumor derived from naive pre–germinal center B cells, possibly arising in the follicular mantle zone.[69] Pre–germinal center B cells have not undergone antigenically induced somatic hypermutation (see earlier). However, studies have shown that the immunoglobulin heavy-chain genes of about half of CLL cases harbor somatic hypermutations, suggesting two subsets of tumors, the latter with a memory B-cell post–germinal center phenotype.[69] Interestingly, tumors with unmutated immunoglobulin V_H genes were associated with trisomy 12 whereas those cases with somatic hypermutations were associated with 13q14 abnormalities.[69] These two groups could also be divided by CD38 expression. CLL cases with unmutated immunoglobulin V_H genes had higher percentages of $CD38^+$ cells than those with somatic hypermutations.[70] Survival characteristics between the two groups are also markedly different. Those cases that display somatic hypermutations and show low percentages of CD38 expression have a much better prognosis.[69, 70] These data strongly support the concept that CLL can be divided into two distinct entities.[71]

LYMPHOPLASMACYTOID LYMPHOMA/ IMMUNOCYTOMA

This is an unusual and rare lymphoma, which in the REAL classification is equivalent to lymph node involvement of Waldenström's macroglobulinemia. The WHO classification modifies the name to "lymphoplasmacytic" lymphoma/immunocytoma, as was originally intended in the Kiel classification. The Kiel classification also recognized that this entity occurs independently from Waldenström's macroglobulinemia. This type of lymphoma may originate in the hilum of the lymph node (post–germinal center B-cell phenotype).[40]

Immunophenotype. The immunophenotype is $(CD20, CD79a,)^+$, $(CD43, BCL2)^{+/-}$, $(CD5, CD10)^-$.

Genotype. IgH and light chains are rearranged. A specific chromosomal translocation, t(9;14)(p13;q32), between the *PAX5* gene and *IgH* has been associated with lymphoplasmacytoid lymphoma in at least 50% of cases.[72–75] This nonfusion type translocation results in the dysregulation and overexpression of PAX5, known to be a crucial regulatory protein in normal B-cell differentiation.[76] The breakpoints involved in the translocation are scattered over a wide range, like the t(8;14) translocation in Burkitt's lymphoma, making PCR-based assays that span the translocation difficult. Therefore, detection of the translocation has been predominantly by classic cytogenetics or FISH. One article has been published that described a FISH technique that detects 80% of the translocations.[74]

MANTLE CELL LYMPHOMA

This tumor was not recognized in a classification scheme in the United States until the REAL classification.[77] Mantle cell lymphoma is the most aggressive of the small B-cell lymphomas. It has been referred to as centrocytic lymphoma in the Kiel classification, as diffuse small cleaved in the Working Formulation, and as intermediately differentiated lymphoma. This type of lymphoma is believed to originate in the inner mantle zone of the lymph node (pre–germinal center phenotype).[40]

Immunophenotype. The immunophenotype is $(CD20, CD79a, CD43, BCL2, CD5, cyclin D1)^+$, $(CD23, CD10)^-$.

Genotype. IgH and light chains are rearranged. Mantle cell lymphoma, like other $CD5^+$ B-cell lymphomas, rarely shows somatic hypermutation of the IgH. Therefore, PCR-based detection methods for clonality in mantle cell lymphoma show higher sensitivity than germinal center–derived B-cell neoplasms such as follicular lymphoma.[7, 78]

The characteristic translocation of mantle cell lymphoma is the nonfusion t(11;14)(q13;q32), which involves the *BCL1* gene translocated to IgH locus, leading to overexpression of the G_1 cyclin, cyclin D1 (CCND1 or PRAD1).[79, 80] Several different methods have been used to detect either the translocation or the overexpression of *BCL1*: classic cytogenetics, FISH, Southern blot, PCR, Northern blot, and RT-PCR for cyclin D1 messenger RNA (mRNA) detection and immunohistochemistry for cyclin D1 protein detection. To detect the translocation, FISH has proved the best technique, detecting mantle cell lymphoma in 95% to 100% of cases.[81, 82] The breakpoints are widely scattered on 11q13, but 70% to 80% are localized to a 1-kb DNA segment known as the major translocation cluster (MTC).[83] Within the MTC, the breakpoints cluster in an 80-bp region.[84] Breakpoints 3′ to the *BCL1* gene have also been described.[85] The breakpoints on 14q32 cluster in the 5′ area of one of the J_H segments. Because of the localization of these breakpoints, the translocation is amenable to PCR across the breakpoint, although breakpoints falling outside this cluster are not detected by PCR. It has been shown that in only 33% to 50% of mantle cell lymphomas can the translocation be detected by PCR.[78, 83, 86] Because of this low sensitivity of detection, PCR for t(11;14) cannot be recommended for routine clinical diagnosis.

An alternative approach for diagnosis is to detect overexpression of cyclin D1 mRNA (by Northern blot[87] or semiquantitative RT-PCR[78]) and cyclin D1 protein by immunohistochemistry.[78, 88] In the study by

Aguilera and associates,[78] 96% of mantle cell lymphoma cases were positive for cyclin D1 mRNA overexpression and 70% were positive for cyclin D1 immunohistochemistry. It must be noted, however, that simple detection by RT-PCR is inadequate to make a diagnosis of mantle cell lymphoma, because many other non-Hodgkin's lymphomas examined in this study expressed low levels of cyclin D1 mRNA. Therefore, a quantitative assay is needed to distinguish cyclin D1 levels compatible with mantle cell lymphoma from lower expression levels seen in other lymphoid malignancies.

The t(11;14) translocation is not specific for mantle cell lymphoma but has been reported in splenic lymphoma with villous lymphocytes (SLVL), prolymphocytic leukemia, hairy cell leukemia, and multiple myeloma.[89] It has been suggested, however, that the t(11;14)-positive SLVL cases may actually represent mantle cell lymphomas.[80] The t(11;14) in multiple myeloma has been shown to involve the switch region of IgH rather than the J_H region, suggesting a translocation later in B-cell development than with mantle cell lymphoma.[90] Interestingly, t(8;14) translocations of *MYC* to *IgH* in Burkitt's lymphoma also show breakpoints in J_H (endemic Burkitt's) and switch regions (sporadic Burkitt's), suggesting that translocation in this disease can also occur at different stages of B-cell differentiation (see later).

FOLLICLE CENTER LYMPHOMA

Follicle center lymphoma is a common lymphoma, derived from the germinal center of the follicle. The WHO has again changed the name back to follicular lymphoma.

Immunophenotype. The immunophenotype is $(CD20, CD19, CD10, BCL6)^+$; $(CD23, BCL2)^{+/-}$; $(CD43, CD5)^-$. Follicle center lymphomas are almost uniformly $CD43^-$.

Genotype. IgH and light chains are rearranged. The characteristic translocation t(14;18)(q32;q21) is seen in 70% to 95% of follicular lymphomas and 20% of diffuse large B-cell lymphomas (see later).[62, 91] The t(14;18) juxtaposes the *BCL2* gene on chromosome 18 to the *IgH* gene on chromosome 14, with the subsequent dysregulation and overexpression of BCL2 (see Fig. 14–5). The *BCL2* gene is thought to block programmed cell death, or apoptosis.[49, 92] It encodes a 26-kd protein that localizes to the mitochondrial outer membrane, smooth endoplasmic reticulum, and perinuclear membrane. Detection of the translocation has been reported by classic cytogenetics,[93] Southern blot,[94] FISH,[95, 96] conventional PCR,[97, 98] and 5′-exonuclease based real-time PCR.[99] Aberrant BCL2 protein detection can also be performed by immunohistochemistry with a detection rate of 90% of cases.[7]

The breakpoints on chromosome 18 are clustered primarily into two small regions. In 50% to 60%, the breakpoints span a 150-bp region in the 3′ untranslated region (3′ UTR) of the gene; this region has been called the major breakpoint region, or mbr. In 20% to 25% of cases, the breakpoints cluster in a region 20-kb downstream of the mbr, at the minor breakpoint cluster region, or mcr.[91, 93] In the remaining cases, the breakpoints are found either at 5′ or 3′ of the *BCL2* gene.[100] The breakpoints on 14q32 seem to cluster to the J_H segments of *IGH*, and it was thought that translocation was mediated by RSS-like sequences in *BCL2*, but recent studies suggest that the mechanism of translocation rearrangement is initially mediated by χ-like octamer sequences (prokaryotic activator of recombination) in *BCL2* and the D_H region of *IgH*.[101] Subsequent D_H-J_H rearrangement brings the translocated *BCL2* gene to the J_H region. Interestingly, χ-like sequences are found at sites of many nonfusion translocations involving antigen receptor genes, including *BCL1*, *BCL2*, *MYC*, *TCL1*, and *TCL2*,[101] suggesting a common mechanism for translocation pathogenesis.

Although breakpoint clustering makes PCR-based assays amenable to t(14;18) detection, single primer sets cannot detect both mbr and mcr breakpoints, and other nonclustered breakpoints cannot be detected. Overall detection sensitivity is 50% to 70% by PCR.[7] Boosting sensitivity of PCR by using nested primer sets has demonstrated t(14;18) translocations in follicular hyperplasia and other benign lesions.[102, 103] However, when using conventional PCR, t(14;18) was not detected in non-neoplastic lesions.[98] The significance of detecting the translocation in benign and hyperplastic tissues remains unknown. PCR has been used successfully for minimal residual disease detection and evaluation of autologous bone marrow transplantation.[104] Studies using 5′-exonuclease real-time PCR[99] or interphase FISH[96] show nearly 100% sensitivity of detection in follicular lymphoma.

Detection of IgH rearrangement by PCR-based clonality assays is hampered in follicular lymphoma by somatic hypermutation of V-region sequences as a consequence of germinal center–mediated receptor editing.[105] As a practical consequence, false-negative rates as high as 30% to 50% are common in conventional IgH PCR using only one V-region primer.[7, 11, 44]

MARGINAL ZONE B-CELL LYMPHOMA (MALT-TYPE)

The extranodal and nodal forms of marginal zone B-cell lymphoma have been accepted in the WHO classification. These lymphomas were at one time referred to as monocytoid B-cell lymphomas, but a recent study showed that marginal zone B cells and monocytoid B cells have different immunophenotypic properties and are distinct B-cell subtypes.[106]

Immunophenotype. Immunophenotypically this is a diagnosis of exclusion: $(CD20, CD79a)^+$; $(CD5, CD10, CD23, cyclin D1)^-$; $(CD43, CD11c, BCL2)^{+/-}$.

Genotype. IgH and light chains are rearranged. No single characteristic translocations are associated with marginal zone B-cell lymphomas, including no characteristic *BCL1*, *BCL2*, or *MYC* rearrangements. However, clonal chromosomal abnormalities have been reported in 74% of cases.[107] These include trisomy 3 (found in 58% of low-grade mucosa-associated lymphoid tissue [MALT] lymphomas,[108, 109]), trisomy 18 (29% of cases[107]), and rearrangements involving chromosome 1, with 1q21 rearrangements in 29% and 1p34 rearrangements in 19%. Translocation t(11;18) and rare cases with t(1;14) have also been reported.[108] These abnormalities have been detected by classic cytogenetics, FISH, and Southern blot. The t(1;14)(p22;q32) translocation involves a newly characterized gene at 1p22, *BCL10*, translocated to the IgH locus at 14q32.[110] Comparative genomic hybridization (CGH) analysis provides evidence of gains at 3q21-23 and 3q25-29, which correlates with the high incidence of trisomy 3, and suggests that gains at these sites might be particularly important with marginal zone lymphomas.[111] Indeed, a study has demonstrated *BCL6* translocations, t(3;14)(q27;q32), in 9% of MALT lymphomas.[112]

Marginal zone B-cell lymphomas are thought to arise from germinal center marginal zone B cells in spleen and equivalent cells in lymph node and extranodal lymphoid tissues.[113] As with follicular lymphoma, the IgH genes in marginal zone lymphomas demonstrate evidence of somatic hypermutation in over 90% of cases.[108] Consequently, false-negative results may be seen in these cases when assayed for IgH clonality by PCR. However, evidence of ongoing mutations by antigen selection was observed in only a minority of cases,[113] suggesting that marginal zone lymphomas may arise by malignant transformation of different subsets of normal marginal zone B cells (virgin, early, and late memory B cells) and that not all are driven by antigen selection.[108, 113, 114]

Extranodal marginal zone lymphomas (MALT type) provide further evidence of antigen stimulation (reflecting a post–germinal center B memory cell origin), with studies demonstrating not only somatic mutation but also intraclonal mutational variation, suggesting ongoing mutation.[115, 116] Extranodal MALT lymphomas are seen at many sites, including the gastrointestinal tract (especially stomach and intestine), salivary glands, respiratory tract (including lung, trachea, larynx, and pharynx), thyroid, ocular adnexa, thymus, liver, genitourinary tract, breast, skin, and dura.[108] Evidence of their relation to chronic antigenic stimulation is supplied by relation to infection: nodal marginal zone lymphoma is the most common lymphoma found in chronic hepatitis C virus infection,[117] and MALT lymphomas are commonly observed in chronically hepatitis C virus–infected individuals.[117–119] Other evidence linking extranodal MALT-type marginal zone B-cell lymphomas with chronic antigen stimulation comes from gastric lymphomas in *Helicobacter pylori* infection. Approximately 70% of cases of low-grade gastric MALT lymphoma regress after eradication of *H. pylori* with appropriate antibiotic therapy.[120] High-grade lesions, however, typically do not respond to antibiotic therapy. This corresponds to detecting *H. pylori* in 63% of low-grade and only 38% of high-grade gastric MALT lymphomas.[121] Strains of *H. pylori* containing the *cagA* gene may have a relation to tumorigenesis. A PCR-based study demonstrated the presence of this gene in 38% of low-grade and 77% of high-grade gastric MALT lesions.[122]

SPLENIC MARGINAL ZONE LYMPHOMA

This entity is fully accepted in the WHO classification. There is some debate as to the similarity of this lymphoma to the marginal zone B-cell lymphoma of the MALT type. Splenic lymphoma with villous lymphocytes (SLVL) is a low-grade B-cell lymphoma with splenomegaly and circulating villous lymphocytes. Although the splenic histology between SLVL and splenic marginal zone lymphoma (SMZL) is identical, the relationship between these two lesions is not clear.[123] The diagnosis of SLVL is made by the morphology of the circulating villous cells and their immunophenotype, which is distinct from chronic lymphocytic leukemia (CLL) and hairy cell leukemia (HCL).[63]

Immunophenotype. The immunophenotype is similar to that of marginal zone B cell of nodal and extranodal type. BCL2 immunoreactivity appears to be uniformly present. CD43 is negative.[124]

Genotype. Immunoglobulin gene rearrangements are present. Trisomy 3 has been reported in the majority of marginal zone B-cell lymphomas[108] but has been reported to be negative in SLVL. However, in a recent study it was shown that trisomy 3, although not detected by classic cytogenetic studies, is in fact present in 17% of cases of SLVL using FISH.[123] It was also detected in 36% of SMZL.[125] No t(14;18)(q32;q21) translocations were found in a study of 13 cases of SMZL.[124] The t(11;14) has been reported in rare cases, but its association with SMZL remains controversial. Another recent study failed to detect cyclin D1 mRNA (by Northern blot) or cyclin D1 protein by immunohistochemistry in SMZL.[126] No t(11;14)(q13;q32) translocations were detected in a study of 19 SMZL cases.[125] This study did, however, demonstrate clonal chromosomal abnormalities in 58% of cases. The most frequent abnormalities involved del(3) and del(7q). These findings support SMZL as a separate biologic entity from nonsplenic marginal zone B-cell lymphoma.

HAIRY CELL LEUKEMIA

This lymphoid neoplasms presents most often as leukemia, although it may present as a lymphomatous infiltrate.

Immunophenotype. The immunophenotype is (CD20, CD79a, CD19, CD11c [strong], CD25 [strong],

CD103, DBA44, TRAP, FMC7)$^+$; (CD5, CD10, CD23)$^-$; T-cell antigen negative. Coexpression of CD103 with pan–B-cell markers is highly suggestive of hairy cell leukemia.[127]

Genotype. IgH and light chains are rearranged. The t(11;14) translocation with corresponding overexpression of cyclin D1 is rarely present. However, overexpression of cyclin D1 as detected by Northern blot, Western blot, or immunohistochemistry is seen in 95% of cases.[128, 129] In these studies, totaling 40 cases, no 11q13 abnormalities were observed. A case report described a novel translocation, t(11;20)(q13;q11), in a hairy cell leukemia case.[130] These and other studies suggest that overexpression of cyclin D1 is quite common in hairy cell leukemia, but the mechanism of this overexpression is not generally dependent on the t(11;14)(q13;q32) translocation or other chromosomal abnormalities of 11q13 characteristic of mantle cell lymphoma.

PLASMACYTOMA/PLASMA CELL MYELOMA

Solitary extraosseous plasmacytomas are often found in the head and neck and constitute less than 5% of plasma cell neoplasms.[131] Because in this chapter we are not discussing bone marrow lesions, typical multiple myeloma will not be discussed here and the reader is referred to literature reviews.[132, 133] A solitary plasmacytoma is rare and more often is associated with a plasma cell myeloma. Plasma cells are cells of terminal B-cell differentiation and often lose expression of B-cell antigens as well as the leukocyte common antigen.

Immunophenotype. The immunophenotype is (CD79a, CD45RB, HLA-DR, epithelial membrane antigen, CD43, CD56, CD30)$^{+/-}$; (VS38 (CD38))$^+$.

Genotype. IgH and light chains are rearranged or deleted. The t(11;14) translocation is rarely present,[134] but like in other B-cell lymphomas, overexpression of cyclin D1 mRNA and protein has been reported. The study by Vasef and colleagues demonstrated cyclin D1 protein expression by immunohistochemistry in 26% of cases.[134]

DIFFUSE LARGE B-CELL LYMPHOMA

One of the most common types of lymphoma, representing 40% of B-cell non-Hodgkin's lymphoma,[135] this inclusive diagnosis includes several entities,[1, 135] some of which the WHO now consider unique tumors. These include mediastinal (thymic), intravascular, and primary effusion lymphomas.[2] The biologic heterogeneity of diffuse large B-cell lymphoma (DLBCL) is underscored by its striking heterogeneity of clinical presentation and response to therapy. As the biologic understanding of this lymphoma advances, it is likely that other separate diagnostic entities will be created.

Immunophenotype. The immunophenotype is (CD20, CD79a, CD22, CD19)$^+$, (CD45RB, CD5, CD10)$^{+/-}$. A study by Harada and co-workers[136] divided DLBCL into three groups by immunophenotypic profile. All three groups were cyclin D1 negative. Group 1 (17.5%) was CD5$^+$. Group 2 (30%) was CD5$^-$, CD10$^+$. Group 3 (52.5%) was CD5$^-$, CD10$^-$. This subgrouping was clinically and statistically significant, with CD5$^+$ cases (group 1) having the worst survival. Immunohistochemical detection of BCL2 was less frequent in group 2. This phenotype (CD5$^-$, CD10$^+$, BCL2$^-$) correlates to a normal germinal center phenotype. In this study, BCL6 protein was detected in 92% of cases, irrespective of grouping. In contrast, in a recent study only 71% of DLBCL cases (but 100% of follicular lymphoma cases) showed BCL6 protein expression.[137] BCL6 protein expression failed to correlate with 3q27 rearrangements (see later).

Genotype. IgH and light chains are rearranged. As expected by clinical and immunophenotypic heterogeneity, there are multiple patterns of genetic lesions in DLBCL, suggesting different mechanisms of molecular pathogenesis. Clonal genetic abnormalities are present in the majority of cases.[135] Common findings include rearrangement of the *BCL2* locus in 16% to 18.5%, rearrangement of the *BCL6* locus in 20% to 40%,[138, 139] and 6q abnormalities in 16%. *MYC* rearrangements are seen in rare cases. Rearrangements of *BCL6* were the sole genetic abnormality detected in 14% of cases.[135, 140, 141] A small percentage of cases possess a t(14;15)(q32;q11-13) translocation involving a newly described gene, *BCL8*, on chromosome 15 and the *IgH* locus at 14q32.[142]

BCL6, or *LAZ3*, is a proto-oncogene located in the 3q27 region and can be rearranged in association with different chromosomes, including but not limited to 14q32 (heavy chain) and 2p12 or 22q11 (light chains). Translocations are of the nonfusion type, with *BCL6* coding sequences linked downstream to heterologous regulatory regions, most commonly immunoglobulin genes. *BCL6* is normally expressed in germinal center B cells.[143] The protein functions as a zinc-finger transcriptional repressor essential for germinal center formation.[141, 144] In the study by Harada and colleagues,[136] 25% of cases had evidence of *BCL6* rearrangement by Southern blot. There may be a correlation to *BCL6* rearrangement and tumor location: 44% of extranodal cases showed *BCL6* rearrangement, whereas it is seen in only 20% of nodal DLBCL. BCL6 protein expression did not, however, correlate with 3q27 rearrangements. DLBCL cases without evidence of 3q27 abnormality were positive for BCL6 protein in 85% of cases. In contrast, 38% of cases with 3q27 rearrangements were BCL6 protein negative.[137]

Note: High-grade B-cell lymphoma, Burkitt-like, is also included in this diagnosis by most hematopathologists. This is supported by the fact that *MYC* is uncommon and *BCL2* is rearranged in about 30% of these lymphomas, as is the case in DLBCL. One study of high-grade B-cell lymphoma, Burkitt-like, identified three groups of patients[145]: those with a *MYC* translocation (28%), those with dual translocations of *MYC* and *BCL2* (33%), and those with other cytogenetic abnormalities (39%). The *MYC* group was younger and had a better clinical prognostic factor profile. A proportion of the dual translocation group had transformed from a previously diagnosed follicular lymphoma and presented with advanced stage with poorer prognostic features. However, all groups had poor survival.

BURKITT'S LYMPHOMA

Burkitt's lymphoma is one of the more extensively studied lymphomas. It has an extremely high cell proliferation rate. The origin of Burkitt's lymphoma is unknown, although it has been speculated to arise in the dark cap (or blastic area) of the germinal center. Two types of the lymphoma are recognized: endemic (African) Burkitt's lymphoma and sporadic Burkitt's lymphoma. Despite many similarities, there are numerous molecular genetic differences between them, suggesting different pathophysiologies.

Immunophenotype. The immunophenotype is $(\text{sIgM, CD19, CD20, CD22, CD79a, CD10, CD43})^{+}$; $(\text{CD5, CD23, TdT})^{-}$, $(\text{LMP})^{+/-}$.

Genotype. IgH and light chains are rearranged. Characteristic translocations involving *MYC* on 8q24 are seen in this lymphoma. The t(8:14)(q24;q32) is the most common (80%), placing the *MYC* gene under heterologous control of the IgH region. Translocation of *MYC* to the light chain loci—t(2:8) and t(8:22)—occurs in the remaining 20% of cases.[141] The diagnosis is made by classic cytogenetics, FISH, or Southern blot. PCR analysis of 8q24 translocations is hindered by the extensive breakpoint heterogeneity of up to 400 kb on either side of the *MYC* coding region.

MYC breakpoints tend to be 5′ of *MYC* in t(8;14), and 3′ of the coding region in *MYC* translocations involving the light chains t(2;8) and t(8;22). Sporadic Burkitt's lymphoma and a majority of acquired immunodeficiency syndrome (AIDS)–related Burkitt's lymphomas involve sequences within or immediately 5′ to *MYC* (<3 kb). Endemic (African) Burkitt's lymphoma cases have breakpoints on 8q24 at a distance greater than 100 kb 5′ to the *MYC* coding region. Breakpoints in the *IgH* locus are also heterogeneous, with translocations involving the J_H region in endemic Burkitt's lymphoma and the heavy-chain switch region in sporadic Burkitt's lymphoma.[141] These findings suggest that the translocation in endemic Burkitt's lymphoma occurs at an earlier stage of B-cell differentiation than does sporadic Burkitt's lymphoma. Because of this translocation heterogeneity, PCR cannot be used for conventional molecular diagnosis of the t(8;14). FISH is probably the most superior diagnostic method, and a recent method allows detection of a wide variety of 8q24 rearrangements including t(8;14), t(2;22), and t(8;22).[146]

Although these translocations are nonfusion-type translocations bringing a normal cellular proto-oncogene under heterologous control of one of the immunoglobulin genes, translocated *MYC* may also show mutations in the first exon/intron boundary corresponding to *MYC* regulatory regions, as well as mutations in exon 2, which contains phosphorylation and transactivation domains.[141] Thus, translocation of 8q24 in Burkitt's lymphoma leads to *MYC* deregulation by four known mechanisms: (1) constitutive activation by a heterologous promoter, (2) truncations within *MYC* that remove coding exons from the intragenic coding region, (3) mutations in *MYC* regulatory region that alter *MYC* responsiveness to factors regulating *MYC* expression, and (4) mutations in *MYC* that affect functional domains of the protein (transactivation potential or phosphorylation).

The role of EBV in Burkitt's pathophysiology remains unclear.[147–150] EBV is associated with 90% of endemic Burkitt's lymphoma and 30% to 40% of sporadic Burkitt's lymphoma.[150] Because EBV is a ubiquitous human pathogen, it alone cannot explain the narrow range of African Burkitt's lymphoma. Malaria has been suggested as a cofactor for the development of endemic Burkitt's lymphoma.[149] EBV has been shown to have oncogenic potential and can function to immortalize human B cells. Malaria may depress cytotoxic T-cell responses controlling polyclonal EBV-infected B-cell proliferations that may subsequently develop a *MYC* translocation. In EBV-positive Burkitt's lymphoma, the regulation of EBV genes remains puzzling. EBNA1 is expressed, but the other EBNAs and membrane antigens are usually absent.[147] It has been shown that EBNA2, EBNA3, and LMP1 are necessary to transform a normal B cell.[148] Either these proteins are not required for neoplastic transformation or they are down-regulated once transformation has occurred.

Like other germinal center–derived B-cell lymphomas, Burkitt's lymphomas show somatic mutations of immunoglobulin genes in both sporadic and endemic forms.[151] As such, false-negative results may be encountered when assessing *IgH* rearrangement in these lymphomas by PCR. In a study of the molecular heterogeneity in Burkitt's lymphoma, tumors from individual patients were found to have identical *MYC* translocations, identical *BCL6* status (wild-type or mutant), and the same productive *IgH* rearrangement. However, within each patient, intraclonal variation with respect to EBV, *TP53* mutations, and *MYC* mutations was observed. These findings suggest that *MYC* translocations and *BCL6* mutations are early events in the pathogenesis of Burkitt's lymphoma.[152]

T-Cell and NK-Cell Neoplasms

A short discussion is in order to explain the relationship between T cells and NK cells. T cells and NK cells are thought to derive from a common progenitor cell.[153, 154] At some point the progenitor cell is committed to become a T cell; this is thought to occur after the cell acquires a TCR. Before this occurs the cell can also become an NK cell. NK cells do not acquire TCRs and therefore do not undergo TCR rearrangements (Fig. 14–6).

Unlike B-cell lymphomas, in which the architecture is often the key to the diagnosis and cell type, T-cell lymphomas do not compartmentalize as readily and it is difficult to determine the cell type by morphology. However, some generalizations can be made: 95% of all T cells express the TCR αβ, with only 2% to 5% expressing the TCR γδ. Therefore, most T-cell lymphomas undergo rearrangement of TCR α and β (usually after rearrangement of TCR γ). Mature αβ-positive T cells express either the CD4 or CD8 antigen. The most common type of T-cell lymphoma is $CD4^+$. The γδ T cells usually do not express CD4 or CD8 (with the exception of a small $CD8^+$ subgroup). Because there is no definitive immunohistochemical marker of T-cell clonality (e.g., κ-to-λ ratio in B cells), the loss of T-cell antigens (aberrant phenotype) generally is indicative of malignancy in a T-cell lymphoma (Table 14–6). Therefore, clonality in T-cell neoplasia can only be established by assessment of the TCR rearrangement status. Most T-cell lesions are TCR αβ positive, but many also bear TCR γ rearrangements. Evidence of TCR γ clonality is thus not an indicator for a TCR γδ process. Southern blot assays still form the "gold standard" for assessing clonality,[12] but PCR-based assays for TCR γ and β especially are seeing more common use in molecular diagnostic laboratories, with results when used together approaching the sensitivity of Southern blot.[42] The advantage of PCR (as with *IgH* rearrangement) is the applicability to DNA extracted from tiny tissue specimens and fixed tissues.[42, 155] Southern blot or PCR for translocations associated with T-cell neoplasia can also be a useful adjunct to diagnosis.[7] Recently, using FISH probes derived from 14q11 (TCR α/δ) yeast artificial chromosomes (YAC) clones, detection of chromosomal abnormalities in T-cell lymphoproliferative disorders has been enhanced.[156] NK-cell neoplasms are extremely rare and occur in both an immature and mature form. Note that true NK cells and their malignant counterparts do not have TCR gene rearrangements.

PRECURSOR T-LYMPHOBLASTIC LYMPHOMA/LEUKEMIA

Precursor T-lymphoblastic lymphoma is predominantly a tissue disease with varying amounts of bone

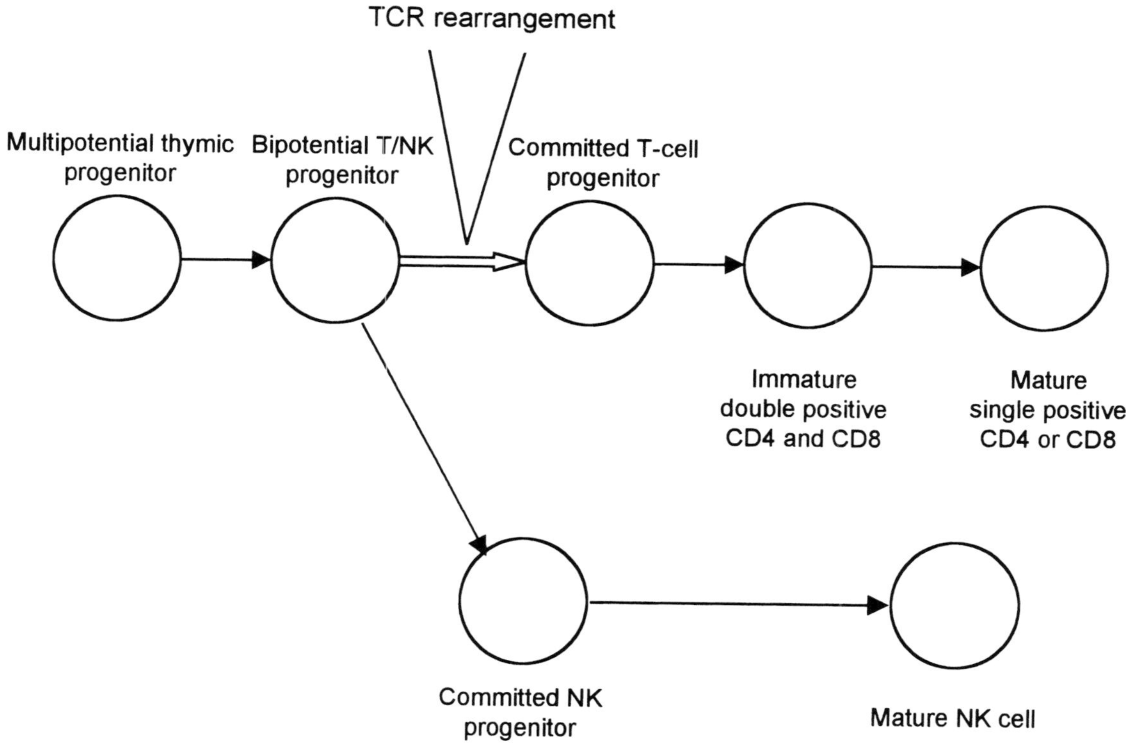

FIGURE 14–6
Simplified diagram of T-cell and NK-cell differentiation. During hematopoiesis a bipotential T/NK-precursor cell gives rise to both lineages. NK cells differentiate in their own pathway without undergoing TCR rearrangement. Thymocytes (T-cell precursors) develop in the thymus where they undergo hierarchical TCR rearrangement and coordinated expression of surface proteins. Immature thymocytes are $CD4^+$ $CD8^+$ "double positive" cells, while mature thymocytes and peripheral T cells are either $CD4^+$ $CD8^-$ (T_{helper} phenotype) or $CD4^-$ $CD8^+$ ($T_{cytotoxic}$ phenotype) "single-positive" cells.

TABLE 14–6

Immunophenotype of T-Cell Neoplasms*

CD	Pre-T LL/L	T-Pro L	T-LGL	NK-L	T/NK	MF/Sez	PTCL	AILD	ALCL	ATLL	Subcu pann	Hepato-splenic	Entero-pathy
CD1a	+/−	−	−	−	−	−	−	−	−	−	−	−	−
CD2	+/−	+	+	+	+	+	+	+	+/−	+	+	+	+
CD3	+	+	+	+	+	+	+	+	+/−	+	+	+	+
CD4	+/−	+	−	−	−	+	+	+	+/−	+	−	−	+/−
CD5	+/−	+	+/−	+/−	+/−	+	+	+	+/−	+	+	+	+
CD7	+	+	+/−	+/−	+/−	+	+	+	+/−	+	+	+	+
CD8	+/−	−	+	+/−	+/−	−/+	−/+	−	+/−	−	+	−	+/−
CD10	+/−	−	−	−	−	−	−	−	−	−	−	−	−
CD16	+/−	−	+	+/−	−	−	−	−	−	−	−	−	−
CD30	−	−	−	−	−	−	−/+	−	+	−	−	−	+/−
CD34	+	−	−	−	−	−	−	−	−	−	−	−	−
CD43	+	+	+/−	+/−	+/−	+	+	+	+	+	+	+	+
CD45RO	+	+	+/−	+/−	+/−	+	+	+	+/−	+	+	+	+
CD56	+/−	−	+/−	+	+	−	−	−	−	−	−	+/−	−
CD57	+/−	−	+	+/−	−/+	−	−	−	−	−	−	−	−
TIA-1	−	−	+	+	+	−	−/+	−	+	−	+	−	+/−
TdT	+	−	−	−	−	−	−	−	−	−	−	−	−
βF-1	+/−	+/−	+	−	−	+	+	+	+/−	+/−	+	−	+
TCR-γ/δ	+/−	−/+	−	−	−	−	−/+	−	+/−	−	−	+	−
EBV	−	−	−	+/−	+/−	−	−	+/−	−	−	−	−	−
CD103	−	−	−	−	−	−	−	−	−	−	−	−	+

*Aberrant phenotype (antigenic loss) is characteristic of T-cell neoplasms.

Pre-T LL/L precursor T-cell lymphoblastic lymphoma/leukemia; T-pro L, T-cell prolymphocytic leukemia; T-LGL, T-cell large granular lymphocytic leukemia; NK-L, natural killer cell leukemia; T/NK, extranodal natural killer/T-cell lymphoma; MF/Sez , mycosis fungoides/Sézary syndrome; PTCL, peripheral T-cell lymphoma, unspecified; AILD, angioimmunoblastic T-cell lymphoma; ALCL, anaplastic large cell lymphoma ($CD30^+$); ATLL, adult T-cell leukemia/lymphoma (HTLV-1^+); Subcu pann, subcutaneous panniculitis–like T-cell lymphoma; Hepatosplenic, hepatosplenic γ/δ T-cell lymphoma; Enteropathy, enteropathy-type intestinal T-cell lymphoma.

marrow involvement. The neoplasm is designated as a lymphoma or leukemia depending on the extent of bone marrow involvement (greater than 50% bone marrow involvement would be leukemia).

Immunophenotype. The immunophenotype is (CD7, CD3c, TdT, CD34, CD43, BCL2)$^+$; (CD2, CD5, CD1a, CD10 [CALLA])$^{+/-}$; it may be CD4 and CD8 double positive or negative.[157] CD57, CD16, or CD56 may be expressed. The expression of CD56 usually is seen on very aggressive disease.[158]

Genotype. Cells may express TCR γδ or TCR αβ or no TCR. *TCR* rearrangement is variable and *IgH* rearrangement can be seen (lineage infidelity). Variable cytogenetic abnormalities are reported in 60% of cases.[159] Of these, 18% of cases showed a 6q deletion, 17% a translocation involving a 14q11 breakpoint (*TCR* α/δ locus), and fewer cases showing 9p deletions, trisomy 8, and 11q23 and 14q32 translocations. The translocation t(10;14)(q24;q11) involving the *HOX11* *(TCL3)* gene deregulated by heterologous promoter control at the *TCR* α/δ locus is seen in 5% to 7% of tumors.[160] The translocation fuses *HOX11* to the *TCR* δ $J_{\delta 1}$ region. Rarely the t(7;10)(q35;q24) translocation places *HOX11* downstream of *TCR* β. However, one third of leukemic blast cells in precursor T-lymphoblastic leukemia overexpress *HOX11*[160] by mechanisms that remain unclear.

T-PROLYMPHOCYTIC LEUKEMIA

This type of T-cell neoplasm presents most often as an aggressive leukemia. Although it does not have the blastic appearance of an acute leukemia, there is a characteristic appearance of the cells. This neoplasm is seen more commonly in patients with ataxia-telangiectasia, a DNA repair disorder.[161] The WHO classification does not recognize a "chronic" form of this neoplasm as does the REAL classification (T-cell chronic lymphocytic leukemia/prolymphocytic leukemia). In most cases this T-cell neoplasm is highly aggressive.

Immunophenotype. T-prolymphocytic leukemia (T-PLL) is (CD7, CD2, CD3, CD5)$^+$, $CD25^-$. Most cases (65%) are $CD4^+$, $CD8^-$. The $CD8^+$, $CD4^-$ phenotype is seen in 13%, and the $CD4^-$ $CD8^-$ phenotype is seen in 21%.[161]

T-cell chronic lymphocytic leukemia/lymphoma (T-CLL) is predominantly $CD4^+$, but about 12% are $CD8^+$.[162] It may be difficult to distinguish T-CLL from the leukemic phase of peripheral T-cell lymphoma and some cases of Sézary syndrome. The terminology

"T-cell chronic lymphocytic leukemia/lymphoma" arose from its morphologic resemblance to B-CLL/SLL, but it is in fact a highly aggressive disease, clinically dissimilar to B-CLL/SLL.

Genotype. *TCR* rearrangements are present. Inv 14(q11;q32) or t(14;14)(q11;q32) is present in 60% to 75% of cases.[163, 164] The *TCL1* gene at 14q32 is involved in an inversion or translocation to the *TCR* α/δ locus at 14q11. TCL1 protein overexpression may inhibit apoptosis.[165] Detection of the inversion or translocation can be made by classic cytogenetics, Southern blot, or FISH.[156] TCL1 is normally expressed in pre–B cells and in $CD4^-$ $CD8^-$ thymocytes.[166] It has 40% identity (60% homology) to MTCP1,[166] a gene product cloned from a t(X;14)(q24;q11) translocation in a T-PLL from a patient with ataxia-telangiectasia.[167] These may represent members of a new class of oncogenes with currently unknown function.

Other common genetic abnormalities are listed: trisomy or multisomy for 8q resulting from i(8q) has been reported in 60% of cases.[164] Homozygous disruptions of *ATM* (the ataxia-telangiectasia gene) have been reported in the majority of T-PLL cases.[168] In this study of T-PLL in patients without ataxia-telangiectasia, deletions of 11q22-23 were observed in 63% of cases. In a follow-up study, mutations were detected in the second *ATM* allele in 6 of 6 cases examined, demonstrating biallelic loss of *ATM* by deletion and mutation. This suggests that *ATM* may serve as a tumor suppressor gene in T-PLL in patients without ataxia-telangiectasia.

T-CELL LARGE GRANULAR LYMPHOCYTIC LEUKEMIA (LGL)

The REAL classification includes both a T-cell form and an NK-cell form of the large granular lymphocytic leukemia. In the WHO classification the two forms are separate, which makes sense because they present as distinct clinical diseases. We follow the WHO classification in this discussion of LGL. Large granular lymphocytes in peripheral blood can be divided into two subsets: $CD3^+$ $CD8^+$ cytotoxic T cells and $CD3^-$ $CD56^+$ NK cells. The T-LGL counterpart makes up at least 80% of all LGL leukemias.[161, 169]

Immunophenotype. The immunophenotype is $(CD2, CD3, CD8, TIA1, TCR\alpha\beta, CD16)^+$; $(CD5, CD7, CD57, CD56)^{+/-}$; $(CD7, CD25)^-$. Less than 5% of cases are $CD4^+$.[161]

Genotype. TCR rearrangements are present.[170] In the vast majority of cases, the expressed TCR is αβ. Only 5% of cases show TCR γδ.[161] However, TCR $\alpha\beta^+$ cases may have TCR γ rearrangements.[170] It had been suggested that human T-cell lymphotrophic virus (HTLV) type I or II may have a role in LGL, but in a recent study none of 28 LGL cases examined demonstrated evidence of the virus by PCR.[171]

AGGRESSIVE NATURAL KILLER CELL LEUKEMIA

This diagnosis in the WHO classification is equivalent to the NK-cell LGL in the REAL classification.[161, 169]

Immunophenotype. The immunophenotype is $(CD2, CD3c, CD56, TIA1)^+$; $(CD3s, CD5, TCR\alpha\beta, TCR\gamma\delta, CD4)^-$; $(CD8, CD16, CD57)^{+/-}$.

Genotype. *TCR*s are not rearranged. No consistent cytogenetic abnormalities are reported. As earlier, retroviruses have been postulated to play a role in LGL. Interestingly, mice transgenic for the *tax* gene of HTLV-I develop NK-LGL.[172] However, no evidence of HTLV-I or II was seen by PCR in a series of LGLs examined.[171]

T/NATURAL KILLER CELL LYMPHOMA

This is equivalent to angiocentric lymphoma in the REAL classification. The WHO classification changed the name to reflect the fact that the cell of origin is the NK cell with rare examples of T-cell origin. This entity has also been called nasal-type T/NK-cell lymphoma and lethal midline granulomatosis. It occurs often in extranodal tissues.[173–178] In a study of 16 patients, 11 were nasal or nasopharyngeal in location.[175]

Immunophenotype. The immunophenotype is $(CD2, CD3c, CD56, EBV\ type\ 2, TIA1)^+$; $(CD4, CD8, CD5, CD7, CD16, CD57)^-$.

Genotype. *TCR*s are not rearranged.[175] While *TCR* is in germline, CD3 proteins may be expressed in the cytoplasm (surface $CD3^-$). No consistent cytogenetic abnormalities are reported. This tumor has a strong association with EBV, and in situ hybridization for EBV can be a useful adjunct to diagnosis.[178]

MYCOSIS FUNGOIDES/SÉZARY SYNDROME

The WHO[2] and the European Organization for Research and Treatment of Cancer (EORTC)[179] separate mycosis fungoides (MF) and Sézary syndrome for diagnosis. Sézary syndrome (SS) is thought to be the peripheralized form of mycosis fungoides, but the EORTC believes that the aggressive nature of SS as compared with MF warrants the separate classification.[179] The diagnosis relies on clinical presentation and history.[180] Mycosis fungoides should be distinguished from other non-Hodgkin's lymphomas that involve skin, such as peripheral T-cell lymphoma and adult T-cell leukemia/lymphoma (see later).

Immunophenotype. The immunophenotype is $(CD3, CD2, CD5, CD4, CD45RO)^+$; $(CD7)^{+/-}$; $(CD8, CD30)^-$. Most cases show a memory T-cell phenotype, $CD45RO^+$ $CD4^+$. Rare cases expressing a $CD3^+$ $CD4^-$ $CD8^+$ phenotype have been reported.[179] Loss of CD7 expression is seen in about two thirds of cases.[181] Sézary syndrome cells are $CD4^+$ $CD7^-$.[180]

Genotype. *TCR* is rearranged (both *TCR* αβ and *TCR* γ). Biphenotypic rearrangements of *TCR* and *IgH* have been reported.[181] Genetic abnormalities (translocations and deletions) reported most commonly involve chromosome 1 (*LCK* gene) and chromosome 6. The significance of these abnormalities in MF is unclear.[182] Sézary syndrome cells also have *TCR* rearrangements.

The role of various viruses in the pathogenesis of this tumor remains controversial, and the significance of the findings is unclear.[180, 183] HTLV-I sequences (*pol* and/or *tax*) have been demonstrated by PCR in more than 90% of cases. EBV is also associated with 100% of cases, and most cultures of peripheral blood leukocytes from MF/SS patients elaborate EBV. MF patients also have increased titers of EBV antibodies compared with controls.[161] Other viruses have been reported in these cases, including HTLV-II, human immunodeficiency virus (HIV), herpes simplex viruses types 1 and 2, and human herpesvirus type 6.[183] The significance of these findings to the pathogenesis of MF/SS remains unclear.

ANGIOIMMUNOBLASTIC T-CELL LYMPHOMA

This diagnosis includes what was once thought to be a premalignant T-cell process, angioimmunoblastic lymphadenopathy (AILD). This entity now is considered to be in the spectrum of low-grade to higher grade T-cell lymphoma.[184]

Immunophenotype. The immunophenotype is $(CD2, CD3, CD5, CD7)^+$; CD4 > CD8; loss of CD7 is common.

Genotype. *TCR*s are rearranged, with evidence in the literature for *TCR* β as well as *TCR* γ rearrangements.[185–187] Monoclonal *IgH* rearrangements have also been reported. In two studies for which *IgH* clonality was assessed, a total of 38 cases showed 11 cases with *IgH* rearrangements (29%), whereas *TCR* rearrangements were detected in 35 cases (92%).[185, 186] Only one case of the 38 showed a clonal IgH in the absence of detectable *TCR* rearrangement.[186] Other clonal cytogenetic abnormalities have also been reported in angioimmunoblastic T-cell lymphoma. These include trisomy 3 and trisomy 5, an additional X chromosome, and structural abnormalities of chromosome 1, especially at 1p31-32.[188] Chromosome 1 abnormalities and an additional X chromosome are highly significant clinically, associated with a poorer prognosis. Trisomy 3 had no impact on survival, and there was a trend for better prognosis with trisomy 5.[188]

Despite the numerous reports on the role of Epstein-Barr virus in AILD,[189, 190] it is not known whether the presence of EBV is associated with the immune defect that accompanies AILD or whether it plays an etiologic role.[184]

ANAPLASTIC LARGE CELL LYMPHOMA, $CD30^+$

Anaplastic large cell lymphoma (ALCL) is heterogeneous, both clinically and histologically. Thus, it may really represent more than one specific entity.[191] ALCL cases can be divided by histologic features, immunophenotype, or clinical features. Histologic variants include pleomorphic, monomorphic, small cell variant, and Hodgkin's disease–related forms. ALCL can be divided by immunophenotype into T-cell, B-cell, and null forms. Clinical variants include nodal, systemic, primary cutaneous, HIV-related, and secondary forms.[191] Note that in the REAL classification, this diagnosis includes the primary cutaneous form, whereas the WHO classification separates these forms into systemic ALCL and primary cutaneous ALCL.[2] It is important to distinguish the primary cutaneous form of ALCL from skin involvement by systemic ALCL for proper patient management,[191] because primary cutaneous ALCL has an excellent prognosis.[192, 193]

Immunophenotype. Sixty to 70% of cases show a T-cell phenotype, 10% to 20% have a B-cell phenotype, and 10% to 30% have a "null" phenotype in that they do not express either T- or B-cell markers.[191] Those having a B-cell phenotype are classified as DLBCL in the REAL classification (see B-cell lymphoma, earlier). ALCL has a distinctive translocation, t(2;5) (see later) that results in a fusion protein, NPM/ALK. Recently, antibodies against the fusion protein (p80) or the ALK domain of the fusion (ALK1) have become available for ALCL diagnosis.[194] A study by Nakamura and colleagues[195] found ALK expression in 64% of ALCL, but not in Hodgkin's disease. The ALK^+ cases form a homogeneous group, with a younger average age and more favorable clinical course than the ALK^- ALCL cases.[195, 196] Other general immunophenotypic markers are shown for systemic and cutaneous forms. Note that ALK1 is negative by immunohistochemistry and in situ hybridization in the primary cutaneous form of ALCL[197]:

- Systemic form: $(CD30, TIA1, ALK1[p80], \text{epithelial membrane antigen [EMA]})^+$; $(CD3, CD45RB, CD25, CD15, CD43, CD45RO)^{+/-}$.
- Cutaneous form: $(CD30, TIA1)^+$; $(ALK1, EMA)^-$; $(CD3, CD43, CD45RO, CD5, CD7)^{+/-}$.

In the small cell variant, while diffusely $CD30^+$, only scattered large pleomorphic cells may be seen. However, the t(2;5) translocation or *ALK* gene overexpression is seen in 76% of such cases, and 25% transform to typical ALCL, providing strong evidence for the relationship to ALCL.[191] B-cell lymphomas that have the t(2;5) or are $p80^+$ may have diffuse large B-cell lymphoma features ($CD30^{+/-}$ and EMA^-). Ten percent to 15% of ALCL express CD15. The distinction between ALCL and Hodgkin's disease may thus be difficult. A $t(2;5)^+$ or $ALK1^+$ tumor favors ALCL, as does expression of T-cell antigens, EMA, and CD45. Expression of CD15,

CD40, and EBV and lack of expression of CD45 and EMA favor Hodgkin's disease.[191]

Genotype. *TCR* gene rearrangements are detected in 50% to 60% of ALCL. However, *TCR* gene rearrangements are detected in 90% of ALCL of T-cell or null-cell phenotype.[198] Immunoglobulin heavy chain rearrangements are detected in B-cell ALCL. Sequence analysis of clonal *IgH* rearrangements in these cases finds evidence of somatic mutation, characteristic of germinal center or post–germinal center B cells.[199]

Recently, additional chromosomal translocations in ALCL, which produce fusion proteins involving the *ALK* gene, have been reported[199a]: an *ATIC-ALK* fusion formed by an inversion of chromosome 2, inv(2)(p23;q35); a *TFG-ALK* fusion formed by a t(2;3)(p23;q21) translocation; a TPM3-ALK fusion formed by a t(1;2)(q25;p23) translocation, and a CTLCL-ALK fusion formed by a t(2;22)(p23;q11) translocation. Like the *NPM-ALK* fusion described previously, all of these translocations contain a consistent *ALK* breakpoint near the transmembrane domain, allowing a fusion protein to be made containing the functional *ALK* kinase domain. *NPM* and the other fusion partner genes do not share sequence homology with each other, but they are all ubiquitously expressed genes that contain a dimerization motif which presumably allows constitutive activation of the ALK tyrosine kinase.[199a]

Overall, almost half of all ALCL cases carry the t(2;5), with an incidence significantly higher in pediatric ALCL (83%) versus adult ALCL (31%).[199a] Approximately 15–20% of ALCL that express ALK do not contain the t(2;5), suggesting that additional *ALK* fusion translocations will be found. Recently the category "ALK lymphoma" or "ALKoma" has emerged as a distinct pathological entity within the ALCL group.[199a, 199b] That ALK$^+$ ALCL patients experience significantly better survival than ALK$^-$ ALCL demonstrates the important prognostic and biologic implications of these observations.[199a]

The systemic form of ALCL has a characteristic translocation, t(2;5)(p23;q35), resulting in expression of a fusion transcript between the *NPM* gene at 5q35 and the *ALK* gene at 2p13.[200, 201] NPM is a constitutively expressed nuclear phosphoprotein, and ALK is a previously unknown tyrosine kinase not normally expressed in hematopoietic cells. The translocation brings the *ALK* gene under control of the *NPM* promoter.[191] The translocation has been detected by Southern blot, DNA PCR, or RT-PCR to detect the fusion transcript. Immunohistochemistry may be used to detect either the p80 fusion protein or the ALK domain (see earlier). By using these methods, evidence of ALK overexpression can be identified in 30% to 60% of ALCL.[191] FISH was used to identify cryptic translocations in ALK1$^+$ ALCL cases without cytogenetic evidence of t(2;5), which nonetheless resulted in ALK1 overexpression.[196] When the t(2;5) translocation was correlated to phenotype, 80% of monomorphic types, 75% of small cell variants, and 30% to 50% of pleomorphic types were positive.[191] The primary cutaneous form lacks the t(2;5)(p23;q35).

ADULT T-CELL LEUKEMIA/LYMPHOMA

This lymphoma is the result of T cells becoming infected with the HTLV-I virus, the first human malignancy to be associated with a retrovirus.[202] Cases of adult T-cell leukemia/lymphoma (ATLL) are strongly associated with areas of endemic HTLV-I circulation: southern Japan, West Africa, and the Caribbean.[203–205] Although the association of ATLL with HTLV-I is a distinct feature of the disease, the mechanism whereby HTLV-I infection leads to malignancy is still obscure. Unlike other acute transforming retroviruses, HTLV-I does not express any genes with direct oncogenic potential.[206]

Immunophenotype. The immunophenotype is (CD2, CD3, CD5, CD25$^+$); CD4 ≫ CD8.

Genotype. TCR gene rearrangements are observed. HTLV-I genomes are clonally integrated and can be detected by Southern blot or PCR.[195, 196, 207, 208] Viral integration does not occur at a specific site. Multiple integration sites (as detected by Southern blot) are associated with an aggressive clinical course.[209] A novel single-cell PCR assay has shown evidence of HTLV-I integration in both the cytologically abnormal and normal-appearing T cells in smears from patients with ATLL.[210] No distinctive chromosomal abnormalities have been reported[211]; however, 80% of the cases show aneuploidy. TCL1 overexpression is seen in all ATLL cases.[206] Fifteen percent to 20% of ATLL cases show *CDKN2 (P16INK4A)* gene alterations. This subset is associated with an aggressive clinical course.[212]

PERIPHERAL T-CELL LYMPHOMA, UNSPECIFIED

This diagnosis includes γδ T-cell lymphoma[213] and subcutaneous panniculitic T-cell lymphoma,[214] both of which are recognized as separate entities in the WHO classification.[161] These two lymphomas are extremely rare. γδ T-cell lymphomas are extranodal and have been described in hepatosplenic, cutaneous, intestinal, and thyroidal locations.[213]

Immunophenotype. The immunophenotype is (CD3, CD5, CD2)$^+$, CD8 > CD4, CD7$^{+/-}$; (loss of CD7 is common).

Genotype. *TCR* rearrangements are present. In a study of γδ T-cell lymphoma, 5 of 5 cases were positive for clonal *TCR* δ rearrangements by Southern blot.[213] In a study of 11 cases of subcutaneous panniculitic T-cell lymphoma, 8 of 10 cases showed evidence of clonal *TCR* β or δ rearrangement, whereas all expressed surface TCR (9 were TCR αβ$^+$ and 2 were TCR γδ$^+$).[214]

In hepatosplenic γδ T-cell lymphoma, FISH analyses have shown that isochromosome 7q and trisomy 8 are consistent genetic abnormalities.[215]

HEPATOSPLENIC γδ T-CELL LYMPHOMA

Most peripheral T-cell lymphomas are TCR α/β$^+$. However, TCR γ/δ$^+$ T-cell lymphomas are observed. Hepatosplenic γδ T-cell lymphoma is one such type. This type of lymphoma is extremely rare, affects young men, and is extremely aggressive.[216] Presentation usually includes marked hepatosplenomegaly in the absence of lymphadenopathy. It is usually disseminated at presentation.

Immunophenotype. The immunophenotype is (CD2, CD3, CD7, TCRδ1$^+$); (CD56, CD5)$^{+/-}$; (CD4, CD8, CD25)$^-$. CD8 may be expressed in some cases. In situ hybridization for EBV in this tumor is negative.[217]

Genotype. *TCR* γ rearrangements are observed, and *TCR* β rearrangements are variable. A distinctive chromosomal abnormality has been reported with this diagnosis (isochromosome 7q), often as the only observable cytogenetic abnormality.[217–220] Trisomy 8 has also been reported in a subset of cases.[215]

SUBCUTANEOUS PANNICULITIC T-CELL LYMPHOMA

This is a rare T-cell lymphoma with a morphology that is distinctive, although in the early stages it is difficult to diagnose. Genetic studies are extremely helpful in many cases. It generally presents as subcutaneous nodules.

Immunophenotype. The immunophenotype is (CD8, CD3, CD5, TIA1)$^+$; (CD56)$^-$.[216] The cells express a CD8$^+$ cytotoxic T-cell phenotype. Seventy-five percent of cases are TCR α/β$^+$ with βF1 positivity. The remaining 25% show a TCR γ/δ phenotype.

Genotype. *TCR* β, *TCR* γ, and/or *TCR* δ are rearranged in the majority of cases.[214, 221] EBV is negative by in situ hybridization.[214, 221]

ENTEROPATHY-TYPE INTESTINAL T-CELL LYMPHOMA

This extremely rare T-cell lymphoma occurs in adults with a history of gluten-sensitive enteropathy.[216, 222] Cases without such a history may still reveal villous atrophy or other pathologic changes in the small bowel. The small bowel frequently demonstrates ulcerations and perforations.[223] Cytologic features of the tumor may resemble ALCL, and 50% of cases express CD30.

Immunophenotype. The immunophenotype is (CD3, CD7, CD103[MLA])$^+$; (CD56, CD8, CD4, CD56, CD30)$^{+/-}$; EBV$^-$. EBV is typically negative in Western patients. Two thirds of cases are CD4$^-$ CD8$^-$, one third are CD8$^+$ CD4$^-$, and only rare cases are found to be CD4$^+$ CD8$^-$.[216, 224]

Genotype. *TCR* genes are rearranged. Most cases have *TCR* α/β rearrangements. Some cases may express *TCR* γ/δ.[216]

Hodgkin's Disease (Lymphoma)

In recent years, advances in molecular pathology have revolutionized our understanding of the nature of Hodgkin's disease. Although classic Hodgkin's disease (HD) and its histologic variants have long been recognized as distinct entities, only recently has the nature of the origin of Reed-Sternberg (RS) cells become known. Prior characterization of RS cells was hampered because these cells made up such a small percentage of the hematopoietic cells of the lesion. Classic RS cells and their histologic variants make up less than 1% of the total cell population in these lesions. However, microdissection of single RS cells and subsequent molecular analyses of these cells has conclusively demonstrated a monoclonal B-cell origin for nearly all cases of classic HD and lymphocyte-predominant Hodgkin's disease (LPHD).[225–230] Although these findings alone do not explain the pathophysiology of HD, this is the most significant advance in hematopathology in recent years. The WHO classification recognizes this incredible gain in knowledge by changing the name Hodgkin's disease to Hodgkin's lymphoma.[2] Molecular analyses have shown differences between classic HD and LPHD.

CLASSIC HODGKIN'S DISEASE: NODULAR SCLEROSIS, MIXED CELLULARITY, LYMPHOCYTE RICH, AND LYMPHOCYTE DEPLETION

These are the classic types of HD. The immunophenotype of the RS cell is similar in all these types.

Immunophenotype. The immunophenotype is (CD30, CD15)$^+$, (CD20, EMA, latent membrane protein for Epstein-Barr virus)$^{+/-}$; (CD45RB, CD3 [and other T-cell associated antigens])$^-$.

Genotype. Single-cell microdissection shows that the RS cells have clonal IgH rearrangements in 95% of cases.[226, 229, 230] Whether the minority of HD cases for which RS cells do not show clonal *IgH* rearrangements are T-cell derived is also currently unknown. The *IgH* genes from RS cells of a given case are clonal, arising from a single transformed B cell. In another study demonstrating that RS cells in classic HD are derived from germinal center B-cell precursors, two cases in which HD was associated with non-Hodgkin's lymphoma (NHL) in the same case were examined. Molecular analysis identified a common germinal center B-cell precursor but ruled out a linear progression from HD to NHL in each case. The sequence results of the *IgH* genes from the HD RS cells and NHL in each case suggest that the two lymphomas shared a common precursor but underwent separate transforming events.[231] In two patients with relapses of classic HD for which sequential biopsy specimens were available, the different specimens had identical clonotypic *IgH* rearrangements with identical somatic mutations, demonstrating the persistence and the dissemination of a clonal tumor cell population.[232]

Sequence analysis reveals that the *IgH* genes in RS cells have large numbers of somatic mutations, characteristic of a derivation from germinal center B cells. Furthermore, sequences of V regions show evidence of crippling mutations (e.g., in-frame stop codons in the coding sequence) in RS cells. This suggests that these mutations may prevent RS precursors from ongoing antigenic selection but that transformation events somehow allow escape from apoptosis.[229]

What the transforming event(s) is and how it leads to the complete histologic and clinical spectrum of HD is not yet known. Because normal germinal center B cells that are not antigen selected are signaled to undergo apoptosis, several studies have examined the role of BCL2 in RS cells. BCL2 expression was observed by immunohistochemistry in over 60% of RS cells in classic HD.[233] Whether RS cells possess t(14;18) translocations has remained controversial, but studies suggest that RS cells in a minority of cases do show t(14;18).[234, 235] In 40% of cases, 14q chromosomal abnormalities that were not limited to t(14;18) were observed.[236]

EBV has also been suggested to play a role in transformation of RS cells in classic HD.[237, 238] EBV has been localized in RS cells by Southern blot and DNA in situ hybridization for EBV genomic DNA,[237] by in situ hybridization for expression of EBER1 mRNA,[239] and by immunohistochemical analysis for LMP.[240] This study and others failed to demonstrate EBNA2 expression, suggesting a latency type II pattern of EBV gene expression in classic HD.[238, 241] Germinal center B cells can delay apoptosis by signaling through surface immunoglobulin (sIg) and/or through CD40. Because RS cells in classic HD have crippling mutations that do not allow IgH expression, an alternative mechanism for delaying apoptosis must exist. EBV infection and LMP1 expression may provide such an alternative pathway in which LMP1 might function like a constitutively active CD40 molecule.[238, 242]

The proportion of EBV-positive HD varies by type. Greater than 50% of mixed cellularity HD but only 10% to 50% of nodular sclerosis HD are EBV positive. As will be seen, lymphocyte-predominant HD has many differentiating features from the classic HD types, including EBV. This form of HD is EBV negative.[238]

LYMPHOCYTE-PREDOMINANT HD

Lymphocyte-predominant Hodgkin's disease (LPHD) makes up about 5% of total HD cases. Like their counterparts in classic HD, the lymphocytic and histiocytic (L&H) cell variants of RS cells in LPHD have also been shown conclusively to be B-cell–derived by molecular analyses.[225, 227] Even before such studies, however, the B-cell nature of L&H cells was supported by immunophenotypic studies.

Immunophenotype of L&H Cells. The immunophenotype is $(CD45RB, CD20, BCL6, J\text{-chain})^{+}$; $(CD3, BCL2, CD15, CD30)^{-}$; CD57 stains the background T cells and "rings" the L&H cells. Note that L&H cells are $CD45^{+}$ and $CD30^{-}$, $CD15^{-}$ as opposed to RS cells in classic HD. Strong nuclear BCL6 reactivity is observed in the majority of L&H cells in all LPHD cases but is only observed in a small percentage of RS cells in about 30% of classic HD.[243]

Genotype. Sequence analysis of *IgH* from L&H cells demonstrates a major clonal population at presentation. However, unlike RS cells in classic HD, the *IgH* gene rearrangements in L&H cells of LPHD often show evidence of intraclonal diversity, that is, sequence evidence of continued somatic mutation, such that 60% of LPHD cases show ongoing somatic mutation after transformation.[226, 227, 244–246] Most clones, however, lack the crippling mutations of classic HD that would prevent IgH translation. This intraclonal IgH sequence diversity by ongoing somatic mutation is similar to that seen in follicular lymphoma and marginal zone B-cell lymphoma, which are "classic" germinal center B-cell–derived tumors. Whether L&H cells in LPHD are subjected to continual antigenic selection pressure is unclear. In contrast, RS cells in classic HD undergo a transformation event early in their evolution, making cell survival independent of antigen-receptor signaling.[227] As with classic HD, evidence for a clonal relationship of LPHD to subsequent diffuse large B-cell lymphomas has also been obtained.[227, 247] TCR rearrangement in L&H cells has not been reported.

In developed nations, EBV has only been very infrequently associated with L&H cells,[227] but studies suggest that EBV does not play a role in LPHD.[238, 248] These studies found no evidence of EBV by in situ hybridization. Unlike classic HD, BCL2 expression (as assessed by immunohistochemistry) was also not observed in LPHD.[233, 248]

The immunophenotype and genotype of L&H cells suggest that their origin (or at least normal counterpart) is the centroblast, or proliferating germinal center B cell.[228, 245] Together these results suggest that the pathophysiology of LPHD is different from that of the classic types of HD.

Immunodeficiency-Associated Lymphoproliferative Disorders

Lymphoproliferative disorders, both reactive and neoplastic, occur in a variety of immunodeficiency states, including congenital, iatrogenic, and acquired.[249–251] Whereas the immunodeficiency states and their associated lymphoproliferative disorders are variable, they have some common features, often including B-cell derivation, extranodal localization, aggressive clinical course, and the frequent involvement of EBV.[249] Children with congenital immunodeficiencies, such as Wiscott-Aldrich syndrome, ataxia-telangiectasia, or combined variable immunodeficiency disorder have a significant risk of developing malignant lymphomas.[9, 252–254]

Post-transplant lymphoproliferative disorders (PT-LPD) are becoming more common as transplants become more widespread. The incidence varies depending on the type of transplant and adjuvant immunosuppressive therapy, but it may be as high as 10%.[255] Several schemes for diagnosing these neoplasms have been proposed. The most recent, by Knowles and colleagues,[249, 256] uses only three morphologic types. They include plasmacytic hyperplasia, polymorphic lymphoproliferative disorder, and non-Hodgkin's lymphoma or multiple myeloma. These three morphologic classifications are characterized by molecular changes indicative of the clinical behavior of the lymphoproliferation. Immunohistochemical studies are not as helpful as the molecular findings in many cases. The vast majority of these lymphoproliferative disorders are B cell derived, with only rare T-cell cases. Many of these cases are associated with EBV and may be associated with mutations in proto-oncogenes.

PT-LPD PLASMACYTIC HYPERPLASIA

These lesions usually present shortly after organ transplant but regress with discontinuation of the immunosuppressive drugs.

Immunophenotype. The immunophenotype for B cells is CD20$^+$; κ and λ are usually not monoclonal. B cells are EBV$^+$ by LMP immunohistochemistry or in situ hybridization for EBERs.

Genotype. These lesions are polyclonal mixtures of B cells and T cells and thus do not show evidence of clonal *IgH*, immunoglobulin light chain, or *TCR* gene rearrangements. Many cases show evidence of EBV, and Southern blot analysis can show infection to be polyclonal, oligoclonal, or monoclonal. Structural alterations in *BCL1*, *BCL2*, *MYC*, *HRAS*, *NRAS*, *KRAS*, and *TP53* are absent.[256]

PT-LPD POLYMORPHIC LYMPHOPROLIFERATIVE DISORDER

This category of PT-LPD contains the lesions "polymorphic B-cell hyperplasia" as described by Knowles and "polymorphic B-cell lymphoma" as described by Frizzera and associates.[257] They are often extranodal, and median interval from transplantation to presentation is less than 1 year.[249] The clinical course is variable, from regression after discontinuation of immunosuppressive therapy to an aggressive course.

Immunophenotype. The immunophenotype is CD20$^+$; κ and λ are often monoclonal or absent. B cells are EBV positive by LMP immunohistochemistry or in situ hybridization for EBERs.

Genotype. These lesions usually show monoclonal *IgH* rearrangements and also light chain rearrangements. They usually lack monoclonal *TCR* rearrangements. Most are EBV$^+$, and Southern blot analysis shows it often to be a clonal EBV infection. Structural alterations in *BCL1*, *BCL2*, *MYC*, *HRASS*, *KRAS*, *NRAS*, and *TP53* are absent. *BCL6* shows no rearrangement but may show mutations.[256]

PT-LPD NON-HODGKIN'S LYMPHOMA/MULTIPLE MYELOMA

Neoplasms of PT-LPD may have histologies like that of non-Hodgkin's lymphomas (NHL) and multiple myelomas occurring in nontransplant patients. Most of these are diffuse large B-cell lymphomas or multiple myelomas. These lymphomas can be both nodal or extranodal. These lymphoproliferations usually have a poor clinical outcome and usually do not regress after discontinuation of immunosuppressive therapy.

Immunophenotype. The immunophenotype is CD20$^+$; κ or λ is monoclonal. Cells are EBV$^+$ by LMP immunohistochemistry or in situ hybridization for EBERs.

Genotype. *IgH* and light chains are rearranged. Most are EBV positive, and Southern blot analysis shows it often to be a clonal EBV infection. These consistently show structural alterations of one or more proto-oncogenes and/or tumor suppressor genes most commonly involving the *RAS*, *MYC*, or *TP53* genes.[249, 256] *BCL6* gene mutations occur in 90% of post-transplant, NHL and multiple myelomas. *BCL6* mutations are correlated with shortened survival and lack of regression after reduction in immunosuppression[258]; thus, *BCL6* mutations serve as molecular markers for an aggressive clinical course.

HIV-Related Lymphomas

Non-Hodgkin's lymphoma is a common neoplasm associated with HIV infection.[259] The revised criteria for the diagnosis of AIDS include diffuse aggressive intermediate- or high-grade NHL in an HIV-infected individual.[260] AIDS-related lymphomas can be classified by their anatomic site of origin: systemic (includes both nodal and extranodal), representing 80% of cases; primary central nervous system (20%); and primary effusion lymphomas (<5%).[249, 261, 262] Almost all HIV-related NHL are B cell in phenotype and have diffuse aggressive features. Histologic types include Burkitt's lymphoma and diffuse large B-cell lymphoma (including Burkitt-like lymphoma). HIV sequences are not detected in the genomes of AIDS-related lymphomas, suggesting that HIV is not directly etiologic in malignant transformation of B cells.[249] Primary effusion lymphomas (body cavity lymphomas) are unusual lymphomas associated with human herpesvirus-8 (HHV-8) or Kaposi's sarcoma herpesvirus.[263, 264]

Immunophenotype. The immunophenotype is $(CD45RB, CD20)^{+/-}$, $(LMP1)^{+}$.

Genotype. *IgH* and light chains show monoclonal rearrangements, although rare cases have no rearrangement.[265] EBV is often clonal as assessed by Southern blot. EBV and *MYC* rearrangements are detected in over 80% of Burkitt's lymphoma cases and in less than 50% of other AIDS-related NHL.[249, 266] In contrast, *BCL6* rearrangements are frequently seen in diffuse large B-cell lymphomas but are not observed in Burkitt's lymphoma cases.[249] Primary CNS lymphomas are associated with EBV in 85% to 100% of cases.[267]

PRIMARY EFFUSION LYMPHOMA

This unusual lymphoma was first described in HIV-positive patients and has since been reported in patients who are not immune compromised. This lymphoma does not have the ability to form mass lesions in most cases and presents as a lymphomatous effusion.[263] Interestingly, HHV-8 has been detected not only in primary effusion lymphoma in HIV infection but also in a large proportion of multicentric Castleman's disease cases (particularly those associated with HIV). It has been also implicated in the pathogenesis of multiple myeloma, where it has been identified in the bone marrow stromal cells but not in the neoplastic plasma cell population itself.[263]

Immunophenotype. The immunophenotype is $(CD45RB, CD38, CD30, HLA\text{-}Dr, LMP1)^{+}$ $(CD20, CD19, CD22, \kappa, \lambda)^{-}$.

Genotype. *IgH* is clonally rearranged. These cases are consistently positive for HHV-8 (40 to 80 copies per cell)[263] and usually positive for EBV.[263, 268] Analysis for viral detection is performed by Southern blot or PCR. HHV-8 detection in primary effusion lymphoma is easily observed by Southern blot because of the high copy number. In contrast, in Kaposi's sarcoma, approximately one copy of HHV-8 is seen per cell.[263] Primary effusion lymphoma lacks *MYC* rearrangements and lacks mutations in *BCL2*, *BCL6*, *RAS*, and *TP53*.[249, 263]

REFERENCES

1. Harris NL, Jaffe ES, Stein H, et al: A revised European-American classification of lymphoid neoplasms: A proposal from the International Lymphoma Study Group [see comments]. Blood 1994;84:1361–1392.
2. Jaffe ES, Harris NL, Diebold J, Muller-Hermelink HK: World Health Organization classification of neoplastic diseases of the hematopoietic and lymphoid tissues: A progress report. Am J Clin Pathol 1999;111(Suppl 1): S8–S12.
3. Appelbaum FR: Molecular diagnosis and clinical decisions in adult acute leukemia. Semin Hematol 1999;36: 401–410.
4. Taylor CG, Stasi R, Bastianelli C, et al: Diagnosis and classification of the acute leukemias: Recent advances and controversial issues. Hematopathol Mol Hematol 1996;10:1–38.
5. Tefferi A: Pathogenetic mechanisms in chronic myeloproliferative disorders: Polycythemia vera, essential thrombocythemia, agnogenic myeloid metaplasia, and chronic myelogenous leukemia. Semin Hematol 1999;36(Suppl 2): 3–8.
6. Willman CL: Molecular evaluation of acute myeloid leukemias. Semin Hematol 1999;36:390–400.
7. Macintyre EA, Delabesse E: Molecular approaches to the diagnosis and evaluation of lymphoid malignancies. Semin Hematol 1999;36:373–389.
8. Roth DB: V(D)J recombination. *In* Herzenberg LA, Weir DM, Herzenberg LA (eds): Weir's Handbook of Experimental Immunology. Cambridge, MA, Blackwell Science, 1996.
9. Vanasse GJ, Concannon P, Willerford DM: Regulated genomic instability and neoplasia in the lymphoid lineage. Blood 1999;94:3997–4010.
10. Sklar J: Antigen receptor genes: Structure, function, and techniques for analysis of their rearrangements. *In* Knowles DM (ed): Neoplastic Hematopathology. Baltimore, Williams & Wilkins, 1992.
11. Bagg A, Kallakury BV: Molecular pathology of leukemia and lymphoma. Am J Clin Pathol 1999;112(Suppl 1):S76–S92.
12. O'Leary TJ, Brinza, L, Kant JA, et al: Immunoglobulin and T-cell receptor gene rearrangement assays: Approved guideline. National Committee for Clinical and Laboratory Standards, 1995;15:1–30.
13. Cook GP, Tomlinson IM: The human immunoglobulin VH repertoire. Immunol Today 1995;16:237–242.
14. Tomlinson IM, Cook GP, Walter G, et al: A complete map of the human immunoglobulin VH locus. Ann NY Acad Sci 1995;764:43–46.
15. Tomlinson I: V Base. MRC Centre for Protein Engineering, 1997, http://www.mrc-cpe.com.ac.uk.
16. Rowen L, Koop BF, Hood L: The complete 685-kilobase DNA sequence of the human beta T cell receptor locus. Science 1996;272:1755–1762.
17. Koop BF, Rowen L, Wang K, et al: The human T-cell receptor TCRAC/TCRDC (C alpha/C delta) region: Organization, sequence, and evolution of 97.6 kb of DNA. Genomics 1994;19:478–493.
18. Klein MH, Concannon P, Everett M, et al: Diversity and structure of human T-cell receptor alpha-chain variable region genes. Proc Natl Acad Sci U S A 1987;84: 6884–6888.
19. Arden B, Clark SP, Kabelitz D, Mak TW: Human T-cell receptor variable gene segment families. Immunogenetics 1995;42:455–500.
20. Takihara Y, Champagne E, Griesser H, et al: Sequence and organization of the human T cell delta chain gene. Eur J Immunol 1988;18:283–287.
21. Takihara Y, Tkachuk D, Michalopoulos E, et al: Sequence and organization of the diversity, joining, and constant

region genes of the human T-cell delta-chain locus. Proc Natl Acad Sci U S A 1988;85:6097–6101.

22. Lefranc MP, Rabbitts TH: The human T-cell receptor gamma (TRG) genes. Trends Biochem Sci 1989;14: 214–218.
23. Lefranc MP, Chuchana P, Dariavach P, et al: Molecular mapping of the human T cell receptor gamma (TRG) genes and linkage of the variable and constant regions. Eur J Immunol 1989;19:989–994.
24. Bogue M, Roth DB: Mechanism of V(D)J recombination. Curr Opin Immunol 1996;8:175–180.
25. Ramsden DA, van Gent DC, Gellert M: Specificity in V(D)J recombination: New lessons from biochemistry and genetics. Curr Opin Immunol 1997;9:114–120.
26. Agrawal A, Eastman QM, Schatz DG: Transposition mediated by RAG1 and RAG2 and its implications for the evolution of the immune system. Nature 1998;394: 744–751.
27. Grawunder U, West RB, Lieber MR: Antigen receptor gene rearrangement. Curr Opin Immunol 1998;10: 172–180.
28. Schatz DG: Transposition mediated by RAG1 and RAG2 and the evolution of the adaptive immune system. Immunol Res 1999;19:169–182.
29. Alt FW, Yancopoulos GD, Blackwell TK, et al: Ordered rearrangement of immunoglobulin heavy chain variable region segments. Embo J 1984;3:1209–1219.
30. Kitamura D, Rajewsky K: Targeted disruption of mu chain membrane exon causes loss of heavy-chain allelic exclusion. Nature 1992;356:154–156.
31. Stavnezer J: Antibody class switching. Adv Immunol 1996;61:79–146.
32. Stavnezer J: Immunoglobulin class switching. Curr Opin Immunol 1996;8:199–205.
33. Wiesendanger M, Scharff MD, Edelmann W: Somatic hypermutation, transcription, and DNA mismatch repair [comment]. Cell 1998;94:414–418.
34. Storb U: Progress in understanding the mechanism and consequences of somatic hypermutation. Immunol Rev 1998;162:5–11.
35. Goossens T, Klein U, Kuppers R: Frequent occurrence of deletions and duplications during somatic hypermutation: Implications for oncogene translocations and heavy chain disease. Proc Natl Acad Sci U S A 1998; 95:2463–2468.
36. Klein U, Goossens T, Fischer M, et al: Somatic hypermutation in normal and transformed human B cells. Immunol Rev 1998;162:261–280.
37. Storb U, Peters A, Klotz E, et al: Immunoglobulin transgenes as targets for somatic hypermutation. Int J Dev Biol 1998;42:977–982.
38. Kelsoe G: V(D)J hypermutation and receptor revision: Coloring outside the lines. Curr Opin Immunol 1999; 11:70–75.
39. Hertz M, Nemazee D: Receptor editing and commitment in B lymphocytes. Curr Opin Immunol 1998;10:208–213.
40. Küppers R, Klein U, Hansmann ML, Rajewsky K: Cellular origin of human B-cell lymphomas. N Engl J Med 1999;341:1520–1529.
41. Miller JE, Wilson SS, Jaye DL, Kronenberg M: An automated semiquantitative B and T cell clonality assay. Mol Diagn 1999;4:101–117.
42. Krafft AE, Taubenberger JK, Sheng ZM, et al: Enhanced sensitivity with a novel TCR gamma PCR assay for clonality studies in 569 formalin-fixed, paraffin-embedded (FFPE) cases. Mol Diagn 1999;4:119–133.
43. Rockman SP: Determination of clonality in patients who present with diagnostic dilemmas: A laboratory experience and review of the literature. Leukemia 1997;11: 852–862.
44. Medeiros LJ, Carr J: Overview of the role of molecular methods in the diagnosis of malignant lymphomas. Arch Pathol Lab Med 1999;123:1189–1207.
45. Alaibac M, Barbarossa G, Mori M, et al: Polymerase chain reaction analysis of T-cell receptor gamma gene rearrangements in cutaneous B-cell lymphomas. Oncol Rep 1998;5:409–411.
46. Papadopoulos KP, Bagg A, Bezwoda WR, Mendelow BV: The routine diagnostic utility of immunoglobulin and T-cell receptor gene rearrangements in lymphoproliferative disorders. Am J Clin Pathol 1989;91:633–638.
47. Pelicci PG, Knowles DM, Dalla Favera R: Lymphoid tumors displaying rearrangements of both immunoglobulin and T cell receptor genes. J Exp Med 1985;162: 1015–1024.
48. Hey MM, Feller AC, Kirchner T, et al: Genomic analysis of T-cell receptor and immunoglobulin antigen receptor genes and breakpoint cluster regions in gastrointestinal lymphomas. Hum Pathol 1990;21:1283–1287.
49. Ong ST, Le Beau MM: Chromosomal abnormalities and molecular genetics of non-Hodgkin's lymphoma. Semin Oncol 1998;25:447–460.
50. Mitelman F, Mertens F, Johansson B: A breakpoint map of recurrent chromosomal rearrangements in human neoplasia. Nat Genet 1997;15:417–474.
51. Fifth International Workshop on Chromosomes in Leukemia-Lymphoma. Correlation of chromosome abnormalities with histologic and immunologic characteristics in non-Hodgkin's lymphoma and adult T cell leukemia-lymphoma. Blood 1987;70:1554–1564.
52. Kluin PH, Schuuring E: FISH and related techniques in the diagnosis of lymphoma. Cancer Surv 1997;30:3–20.
53. Klein G: Immunoglobulin gene–associated chromosomal translocations in B-cell derived tumors. Curr Top Microbiol Immunol 1999;246:161–167.
54. Gamberi B, Gaidano G, Parsa N, et al: Microsatellite instability is rare in B-cell non-Hodgkin's lymphomas. Blood 1997;89:975–979.
55. Abbondanzo SL: Paraffin immunohistochemistry as an adjunct to hematopathology. Ann Diagn Pathol 1999; 3:318–327.
56. Chu PG, Chang KL, Arber DA, Weiss LM: Practical applications of immunohistochemistry in hematolymphoid neoplasms. Ann Diagn Pathol 1999;3:104–133.
57. Jennings CD, Foon KA: Recent advances in flow cytometry: Application to the diagnosis of hematologic malignancy. Blood 1997;90:2863–2892.
58. Westermann CD, Hurtubise PE, Linnemann CC, Swerdlow SH: Comparison of histologic nodal reactive patterns, cell suspension immunophenotypic data, and HIV status. Mod Pathol 1990;3:54–60.
59. Pangalis GA, Angelopoulou MK, Vassilakopoulos TP, et al: B-chronic lymphocytic leukemia, small lymphocytic lymphoma, and lymphoplasmacytic lymphoma, including

Waldenström's macroglobulinemia: A clinical, morphologic, and biologic spectrum of similar disorders. Semin Hematol 1999;36:104–114.
60. Reed JC: Molecular biology of chronic lymphocytic leukemia. Semin Oncol 1998;25:11–18.
61. Jabbar SA, Ganeshaguru K, Wickremasinghe RG, et al: Deletion of chromosome 13 (band q14) but not trisomy 12 is a clonal event in B-chronic lymphocytic leukaemia (CLL). Br J Haematol 1995;90:476–478.
62. Panayiotidis P, Kotsi P: Genetics of small lymphocyte disorders. Semin Hematol 1999;36:171–177.
63. Catovsky D, Matutes E: Splenic lymphoma with circulating villous lymphocytes/splenic marginal-zone lymphoma. Semin Hematol 1999;36:148–154.
64. Foroni L, Panayiotidis P, Hoffbrand AV: Lack of clonal *BCRA2* gene deletion on chromosome 13 in chronic lymphocytic leukaemia: An update of recent scientific reports [letter]. Br J Haematol 1998;100:800.
65. Dohner H, Stilgenbauer S, James MR, et al: 11q deletions identify a new subset of B-cell chronic lymphocytic leukemia characterized by extensive nodal involvement and inferior prognosis. Blood 1997;89:2516–2522.
66. Delmer A, Ajchenbaum-Cymbalista F, Tang R, et al: Overexpression of cyclin D2 in chronic B-cell malignancies. Blood 1995;85:2870–2876.
67. Hanada M, Delia D, Aiello A, et al: *bcl-2* gene hypomethylation and high-level expression in B-cell chronic lymphocytic leukemia. Blood 1993;82:1820–1828.
68. Watanabe T, Ichikawa A, Saito H, Hotta T: Overexpression of the *MDM2* oncogene in leukemia and lymphoma. Leuk Lymphoma 1996;21:391–397.
69. Hamblin TJ, Davis Z, Gardiner A, et al: Unmutated Ig V(H) genes are associated with a more aggressive form of chronic lymphocytic leukemia. Blood 1999;94: 1848–1854.
70. Damle RN, Wasil T, Fais F, et al: Ig V gene mutation status and CD38 expression as novel prognostic indicators in chronic lymphocytic leukemia. Blood 1999;94: 1840–1847.
71. Naylor M, Capra JD: Mutational status of Ig V(H) genes provides clinically valuable information in B-cell chronic lymphocytic leukemia. Blood 1999;94:1837–1839.
72. Offit K, Parsa NZ, Filippa D, et al: t(9;14) (p13;q32) denotes a subset of low-grade non-Hodgkin's lymphoma with plasmacytoid differentiation. Blood 1992;80: 2594–2599.
73. Iida S, Rao PH, Nallasivam P, et al: The t(9;14) (p13;q32) chromosomal translocation associated with lymphoplasmacytoid lymphoma involves the *PAX-5* gene. Blood 1996;88:4110–4117.
74. Iida S, Rao PH, Ueda R, et al: Chromosomal rearrangement of the *PAX-5* locus in lymphoplasmacytic lymphoma with t(9;14) (p13;q32). Leuk Lymphoma. 1999;34:25–33.
75. Amakawa R, Ohno H, Fukuhara S: t(9;14) (p13;q32) involving the *PAX-5*gene: A unique subtype of 14q32 translocation in B-cell non-Hodgkin's lymphoma. Int J Hematol 1999;69:65–69.
76. Baker SJ, Reddy EP: B cell differentiation: Role of E2A and Pax5/BSAP transcription factors. Oncogene 1995;11: 413–426.
77. Weisenburger DD, Armitage JO: Mantle cell lymphoma—an entity comes of age. Blood 1996;87:4483–4494.
78. Aguilera NS, Bijwaard KE, Duncan B, et al: Differential expression of cyclin D1 in mantle cell lymphoma and other non-Hodgkin's lymphomas. Am J Pathol 1998; 153:1969–1976.
79. Kurtin PJ: Mantle cell lymphoma. Adv Anat Pathol 1998;5:376–398.
80. Campo E, Raffeld M, Jaffe ES: Mantle-cell lymphoma. Semin Hematol 1999;36:115–27.
81. Li JY, Gaillard F, Moreau A, et al: Detection of translocation t(11;14) (q13;q32) in mantle cell lymphoma by fluorescence in situ hybridization. Am J Pathol 1999; 154:1449–1452.
82. Vaandrager JW, Schuuring E, Zwikstra E, et al: Direct visualization of dispersed 11q13 chromosomal translocations in mantle cell lymphoma by multicolor DNA fiber fluorescence in situ hybridization. Blood 1996;88: 1177–82.
83. Rimokh R, Berger F, Delsol G, et al: Detection of the chromosomal translocation t(11;14) by polymerase chain reaction in mantle cell lymphomas. Blood 1994;83(7): 1871–1875.
84. Pinyol M, Campo E, Nadal A, et al: Detection of the bcl-1 rearrangement at the major translocation cluster in frozen and paraffin-embedded tissues of mantle cell lymphomas by polymerase chain reaction. Am J Clin Pathol 1996;105:532–537.
85. de Boer CJ, Vaandrager JW, van Krieken JH, et al: Visualization of mono-allelic chromosomal aberrations 3′ and 5′ of the cyclin D1 gene in mantle cell lymphoma using DNA fiber fluorescence in situ hybridization. Oncogene 1997;15:1599–1603.
86. Lim LC, Segal GH, Wittwer CT: Detection of *bcl-1* gene rearrangement and B-cell clonality in mantle cell lymphoma using formalin-fixed, paraffin-embedded tissues. Am J Clin Pathol 1995;104:689–695.
87. de Boer CJ, van Krieken JH, Kluin-Nelemans HC, et al: Cyclin D1 messenger RNA overexpression as a marker for mantle cell lymphoma. Oncogene 1995;10:1833–1840.
88. Swerdlow SH, Yang WI, Zukerberg LR, et al: Expression of cyclin D1 protein in centrocytic/mantle cell lymphomas with and without rearrangement of the *BCL1*/cyclin D1 gene. Hum Pathol 1995;26:999–1004.
89. Jadayel D, Matutes E, Dyer MJ, et al: Splenic lymphoma with villous lymphocytes: Analysis of *BCL-1* rearrangements and expression of the cyclin D1 gene. Blood 1994;83:3664–3671.
90. Chesi M, Bergsagel PL, Brents LA, et al: Dysregulation of cyclin D1 by translocation into an IgH gamma switch region in two multiple myeloma cell lines. Blood 1996; 88:674–681.
91. Wang YL, Addya K, Edwards RH, et al: Novel bcl-2 breakpoints in patients with follicular lymphoma. Diagn Mol Pathol 1998;7:85–89.
92. Korsmeyer SJ: *BCL-2* gene family and the regulation of programmed cell death. Cancer Res 1999;59(Suppl 7): 1693s–1700s.
93. Medeiros LJ, Bagg A, Cossman J: Application of molecular genetics to the diagnosis of hematopoietic neoplasms. *In* Knowles DM (ed): Neoplastic Hematopathology. Baltimore, Williams & Wilkins, 1992.
94. Ladanyi M, Wang S: Detection of rearrangements of the BCL2 major breakpoint region in follicular lymphomas: Correlation of polymerase chain reaction results with Southern blot analysis. Diagn Mol Pathol 1992;1:31–35.

95. Rack KA, Salomon-Nguyen F, Radford-Weiss I, et al: FISH detection of chromosome 14q32/IgH translocations: Evaluation in follicular lymphoma. Br J Haematol 1998;103:495–504.
96. Vaandrager JW, Schuuring E, Raap T, et al: Interphase FISH detection of BCL2 rearrangement in follicular lymphoma using breakpoint-flanking probes. Genes Chromosomes Cancer 2000;27:85–94.
97. O'Leary TJ, Stetler-Stevenson M: Diagnosis of t(14;18) by polymerase chain reaction. The natural evolution of a laboratory test [editorial]. Arch Pathol Lab Med 1994;118:789–790.
98. Segal GH, Scott M, Jorgensen T, Braylan RC: Standard polymerase chain reaction analysis does not detect t(14;18) in reactive lymphoid hyperplasia. Arch Pathol Lab Med 1994;118:791–794.
99. Luthra R, McBride JA, Cabanillas F, and Sarris A: Novel 5′ exonuclease-based real-time PCR assay for the detection of t(14;18) (q32;q21) in patients with follicular lymphoma. Am J Pathol 1998;153(1):63–8.
100. Merup M, Spasokoukotskaja T, Einhorn S, et al: Bcl-2 rearrangements with breakpoints in both vcr and mbr in non-Hodgkin's lymphomas and chronic lymphocytic leukaemia. Br J Haematol 1996;92:647–652.
101. Wyatt RT, Rudders RA, Zelenetz A, et al: *BCL2* oncogene translocation is mediated by a chi-like consensus. J Exp Med 1992;175:1575–1588.
102. Aster JC, Kobayashi Y, Shiota M, et al: Detection of the t(14;18) at similar frequencies in hyperplastic lymphoid tissues from American and Japanese patients. Am J Pathol 1992;141:291–299.
103. Limpens J, Stad R, Vos C, et al: Lymphoma-associated translocation t(14;18) in blood B cells of normal individuals. Blood 1995;85:2528–2536.
104. Berinstein NL, Reis MD, Ngan BY, et al: Detection of occult lymphoma in the peripheral blood and bone marrow of patients with untreated early-stage and advanced-stage follicular lymphoma. J Clin Oncol 1993;11:1344–1352.
105. Storb U: The molecular basis of somatic hypermutation of immunoglobulin genes. Curr Opin Immunol 1996;8: 206–214.
106. Stein K, Hummel M, Korbjuhn P, et al: Monocytoid B cells are distinct from splenic marginal zone cells and commonly derive from unmutated naive B cells and less frequently from postgerminal center B cells by polyclonal transformation. Blood 1999;94:2800–2808.
107. Dierlamm J, Pittaluga S, Wlodarska I, et al: Marginal zone B-cell lymphomas of different sites share similar cytogenetic and morphologic features. Blood 1996;87: 299–307.
108. Nathwani BN, Drachenberg MR, Hernandez AM, et al: Nodal monocytoid B-cell lymphoma (nodal marginal-zone B-cell lymphoma). Semin Hematol 1999;36: 128–138.
109. Wotherspoon AC, Finn TM, Isaacson PG: Trisomy 3 in low-grade B-cell lymphomas of mucosa-associated lymphoid tissue. Blood 1995;85:2000–2004.
110. Willis TG, Jadayel DM, Du MQ, et al: Bcl10 is involved in t(1;14) (p22;q32) of MALT B cell lymphoma and mutated in multiple tumor types. Cell 1999;96:35–45.
111. Dierlamm J, Rosenberg C, Stul M, et al: Characteristic pattern of chromosomal gains and losses in marginal zone B cell lymphoma detected by comparative genomic hybridization. Leukemia 1997;11:747–758.
112. Dierlamm J, Pittaluga S, Stul M, et al: *BCL6* gene rearrangements also occur in marginal zone B-cell lymphoma. Br J Haematol 1997;98:719–725.
113. Tierens A, Delabie J, Pittaluga S, et al: Mutation analysis of the rearranged immunoglobulin heavy chain genes of marginal zone cell lymphomas indicates an origin from different marginal zone B lymphocyte subsets. Blood 1998;91:2381–2386.
114. Tierens A, Delabie J, Michiels L, et al: Marginal-zone B cells in the human lymph node and spleen show somatic hypermutations and display clonal expansion. Blood 1999;93:226–234.
115. Du M, Diss TC, Xu C, et al: Ongoing mutation in MALT lymphoma immunoglobulin gene suggests that antigen stimulation plays a role in the clonal expansion. Leukemia 1996;10:1190–1197.
116. Qin Y, Greiner A, Trunk MJ, et al: Somatic hypermutation in low-grade mucosa-associated lymphoid tissue-type B-cell lymphoma. Blood 1995;86:3528–3534.
117. Zuckerman E, Zuckerman T, Levine AM, et al: Hepatitis C virus infection in patients with B-cell non-Hodgkin lymphoma. Ann Intern Med 1997; 127:423–428.
118. Ascoli V, Lo Coco F, Artini M, et al: Extranodal lymphomas associated with hepatitis C virus infection. Am J Clin Pathol 1998;109:600–609.
119. Lai R, Weiss LM: Hepatitis C virus and non-Hodgkin's lymphoma [editorial; comment]. Am J Clin Pathol 1998; 109:508–510.
120. Isaacson PG: Mucosa-associated lymphoid tissue lymphoma. Semin Hematol 1999;36:139–147.
121. Bouzourene H, Haefliger T, Delacretaz F, Saraga E: The role of *Helicobacter pylori* in primary gastric MALT lymphoma. Histopathology 1999;34:118–123.
122. Peng H, Ranaldi R, Diss TC, et al: High frequency of $CagA^+$ *Helicobacter pylori* infection in high-grade gastric MALT B-cell lymphomas. J Pathol 1998;185:409–412.
123. Gruszka-Westwood AM, Matutes E, Coignet LJ, et al: The incidence of trisomy 3 in splenic lymphoma with villous lymphocytes: A study by FISH. Br J Haematol 1999;104:600–604.
124. Mollejo M, Menarguez J, Lloret E, et al: Splenic marginal zone lymphoma: A distinctive type of low-grade B-cell lymphoma: A clinicopathological study of 13 cases. Am J Surg Pathol 1995;19:1146–1157.
125. Sole F, Woessner S, Florensa L, et al: Frequent involvement of chromosomes 1, 3, 7, and 8 in splenic marginal zone B-cell lymphoma. Br J Haematol 1997;98:446–449.
126. Savilo E, Campo E, Mollejo M, et al: Absence of cyclin D1 protein expression in splenic marginal zone lymphoma. Mod Pathol 1998;11:601–606.
127. Tallman MS, Peterson LC, Hakimian D, et al: Treatment of hairy-cell leukemia: Current views. Semin Hematol 1999;36:155–163.
128. de Boer CJ, Kluin-Nelemans JC, Dreef E, et al: Involvement of the *CCND1* gene in hairy cell leukemia. Ann Oncol 1996;7:251–256.
129. Bosch F, Campo E, Jares P, et al: Increased expression of the *PRAD-1/CCND1* gene in hairy cell leukaemia. Br J Haematol 1995;91:1025–1030.

130. Ishida F, Kitano K, Ichikawa N, et al: Hairy cell leukemia with translocation (11;20)(q13;q11) and overexpression of cyclin D1. Leuk Res 1999;23:763–765.
131. Grogan TM, Spier CM: The B cell immunoproliferative disorders, including mutiple myeloma and amyloidosis. *In* Knowles DM (ed): Neoplastic Hematopathology. Baltimore, Williams & Wilkins, 1992.
132. Berenson JR: Etiology of multiple myeloma: What's new. Semin Oncol 1999;26(5 Suppl 13):2–9.
133. Anderson K: Advances in the biology of multiple myeloma: Therapeutic applications. Semin Oncol 1999; 26(Suppl 13):10–22.
134. Vasef MA, Medeiros LJ, Yospur LS, et al: Cyclin D1 protein in multiple myeloma and plasmacytoma: An immunohistochemical study using fixed, paraffin-embedded tissue sections. Mod Pathol 1997;10: 927–932.
135. Volpe G, Vitolo U, Carbone A, et al: Molecular heterogeneity of B-lineage diffuse large cell lymphoma. Genes Chromosomes Cancer 1996;16:21–30.
136. Harada S, Suzuki R, Uehira K, et al: Molecular and immunological dissection of diffuse large B cell lymphoma: $CD5^+$, and $CD5^-$ with $CD10^+$ groups may constitute clinically relevant subtypes. Leukemia 1999;13: 1441–1447.
137. Skinnider BF, Horsman DE, Dupuis B, Gascoyne RD: Bcl-6 and Bcl-2 protein expression in diffuse large B-cell lymphoma and follicular lymphoma: Correlation with 3q27 and 18q21 chromosomal abnormalities. Hum Pathol 1999;30:803–808.
138. Lo Coco F, Ye BH, Lista F, et al: Rearrangements of the *BCL6* gene in diffuse large cell non-Hodgkin's lymphoma. Blood 1994;83:1757–1759.
139. Pescarmona E, Lo Coco F, Pacchiarotti A, et al: Analysis of the *BCL-6* gene configuration in diffuse B-cell non-Hodgkin's lymphomas and Hodgkin's disease. J Pathol 1995;177:21–25.
140. Kramer MH, Hermans J, Wijburg E, et al: Clinical relevance of BCL2, BCL6, and MYC rearrangements in diffuse large B-cell lymphoma. Blood 1998;92:3152–3162.
141. Gaidano G, Pastore C, Volpe G: Molecular pathogenesis of non-Hodgkin lymphoma: A clinical perspective. Haematologica 1995;80:454–472.
142. Dyomin VG, Rao PH, Dalla-Favera R, Chaganti RSK: *BCL8*, a novel gene involved in translocations affecting band 15q11-13 in diffuse large-cell lymphoma. Proc Natl Acad Sci U S A 1997;94:5728–5732.
143. Cattoretti G, Chang CC, Cechova K, et al: BCL-6 protein is expressed in germinal-center B cells. Blood 1995; 86:45–53.
144. Ye BH, Cattoretti G, Shen Q, et al: The *BCL-6* proto-oncogene controls germinal-centre formation and Th2-type inflammation. Nat Genet 1997;16:161–170.
145. Macpherson N, Lesack D, Klasa R, et al: Small noncleaved, non-Burkitt's (Burkitt-like) lymphoma: Cytogenetics predict outcome and reflect clinical presentation. J Clin Oncol 1999;17:1558–1567.
146. Rack KA, Delabesse E, Radford-Weiss I, et al: Simultaneous detection of *MYC*, *BVR1*, and *PVT1* translocations in lymphoid malignancies by fluorescence in situ hybridization. Genes Chromosomes Cancer 1998;23: 220–226.
147. zur Hausen H: The role of Epstein Barr virus (EBV) in Burkitt's lymphomas. Jpn J Cancer Res 1998;89:inside cover.
148. Magrath IT, Jain V, Jaffe ES: Small noncleaved cell lymphoma. *In* Knowles DM (ed): Neoplastic Hematopathology. Baltimore, Williams & Wilkins, 1992.
149. de The G: The etiology of Burkitt's lymphoma and the history of the shaken dogmas. Blood Cells 1993;19: 667–673.
150. Klein G: Role of EBV and Ig/myc translocation in Burkitt lymphoma. Antibiot Chemother 1994;46: 110–116.
151. Ghia P, Nadler LM: Recent advances in lymphoma biology. Curr Opin Oncol 1997;9:403–412.
152. Gutierrez MI, Bhatia K, Cherney B, et al: Intraclonal molecular heterogeneity suggests a hierarchy of pathogenetic events in Burkitt's lymphoma. Ann Oncol 1997;8: 987–994.
153. Spits H, Blom B, Jaleco AC, et al: Early stages in the development of human T, natural killer and thymic dendritic cells. Immunol Rev 1998;165:75–86.
154. Spits H, Lanier LL, Phillips JH: Development of human T and natural killer cells. Blood 1995;85:2654–2670.
155. McCarthy KP, Sloane JP, Kabarowski JH, et al: A simplified method of detection of clonal rearrangements of the T-cell receptor-gamma chain gene. Diagn Mol Pathol 1992;1:173–179.
156. Rack KA, Cornelis F, Radford-Weiss I, et al: A chromosome 14q11/TCR alpha/delta specific yeast artificial chromosome improves the detection rate and characterization of chromosome abnormalities in T-lymphoproliferative disorders. Blood 1997;90:1233–1240.
157. Soslow RA, Bhargava V, Warnke RA: MIC2, TdT, bcl-2, and CD34 expression in paraffin-embedded high-grade lymphoma/acute lymphoblastic leukemia distinguishes between distinct clinicopathologic entities. Hum Pathol 1997;28:1158–1165.
158. Nakamura S, Koshikawa T, Yatabe Y, Suchi T: Lymphoblastic lymphoma expressing CD56 and TdT [letter; comment]. Am J Surg Pathol 1998;22:135–137.
159. Heerema NA, Sather HN, Sensel MG, et al: Frequency and clinical significance of cytogenetic abnormalities in pediatric T-lineage acute lymphoblastic leukemia: A report from the Children's Cancer Group. J Clin Oncol 1998;16:1270–1278.
160. Shimamoto T, Ohyashiki K, Toyama K, Takeshita K: Homeobox genes in hematopoiesis and leukemogenesis. Int J Hematol 1998;67:339–350.
161. Bartlett NL, Longo DL: T-small lymphocyte disorders. Semin Hematol 1999;36:164–170.
162. Hoyer JD, Ross CW, Li CY, et al: True T-cell chronic lymphocytic leukemia: A morphologic and immunophenotypic study of 25 cases. Blood 1995; 86:1163–1169.
163. Virgilio L, Narducci MG, Isobe M, et al: Identification of the *TCL1* gene involved in T-cell malignancies. Proc Natl Acad Sci U S A 1994;91:12530–12534.
164. Brito-Babapulle V, Pomfret M, Matutes E, Catovsky D: Cytogenetic studies on prolymphocytic leukemia: II. T cell prolymphocytic leukemia. Blood 1987;70:926–931.
165. Fu TB, Virgilio L, Narducci MG, et al: Characterization and localization of the *TCL-1* oncogene product. Cancer Res 1994;54:6297–6301.

166. Croce CM: Role of *TCL1* and *ALL1* in human leukemias and development. Cancer Res 1999;59(7 Suppl): 1778s–1783s.
167. Stern MH, Soulier J, Rosenzwajg M, et al: *MTCP-1:* A novel gene on the human chromosome Xq28 translocated to the T cell receptor alpha/delta locus in mature T cell proliferations. Oncogene 1993;8:2475–2483.
168. Stilgenbauer S, Schaffner C, Litterst A, et al: Biallelic mutations in the ATM gene in T-prolymphocytic leukemia. Nat Med 1997;3:1155–1159.
169. Loughran TP: Large granular lymphocytic leukemia: An overview. Hosp Pract (Off Ed) 1998;33:133–138.
170. Ryan DK, Alexander HD, Morris TC: Routine diagnosis of large granular lymphocytic leukaemia by Southern blot and polymerase chain reaction analysis of clonal T cell receptor gene rearrangement. Mol Pathol 1997;50:77–81.
171. Pawson R, Schulz TF, Matutes E, Catovsky D: The human T-cell lymphotropic viruses types I/II are not involved in T prolymphocytic leukemia and large granular lymphocytic leukemia. Leukemia 1997;11: 1305–1311.
172. Grossman WJ, Kimata JT, Wong FH, et al: Development of leukemia in mice transgenic for the *tax* gene of human T-cell leukemia virus type I. Proc Natl Acad Sci U S A 1995;92:1057–1061.
173. Ansai S, Maeda K, Yamakawa M, et al: CD56-positive (nasal-type T/NK cell) lymphoma arising on the skin: Report of two cases and review of the literature. J Cutan Pathol 1997;24:468–476.
174. Macon WR, Williams ME, Greer JP, et al: Natural killer-like T-cell lymphomas: Aggressive lymphomas of T-large granular lymphocytes. Blood 1996;87:1474–1483.
175. Emile JF, Boulland ML, Haioun C, et al: $CD5^-CD56^+$ T-cell receptor silent peripheral T-cell lymphomas are natural killer cell lymphomas. Blood 1996;87:1466–1473.
176. Hirakawa S, Kuyama M, Takahashi S, et al: Nasal and nasal-type natural killer/T-cell lymphoma. J Am Acad Dermatol 1999;40:268–272.
177. Yamashita Y, Tsuzuki T, Nakayama A, et al: A case of natural killer/T cell lymphoma of the subcutis resembling subcutaneous panniculitis-like T cell lymphoma. Pathol Int 1999;49:241–246.
178. Jaffe ES, Chan JK, Su IJ, et al: Report of the Workshop on Nasal and Related Extranodal Angiocentric T/Natural Killer Cell Lymphomas: Definitions, differential diagnosis, and epidemiology. Am J Surg Pathol 1996; 20:103–111.
179. Willemze R, Kerl H, Sterry W, et al: EORTC classification for primary cutaneous lymphomas: A proposal from the Cutaneous Lymphoma Study Group of the European Organization for Research and Treatment of Cancer. Blood 1997;90:354–371.
180. Kim YH, Hoppe RT: Mycosis fungoides and the Sézary syndrome. Semin Oncol 1999;26:276–289.
181. Barcos M: Mycosis fungoides: Diagnosis and pathogenesis. Am J Clin Pathol 1993;99:452–458.
182. Kuzel TM, Roenigk HH Jr, Rosen ST: Mycosis fungoides and the Sézary syndrome: A review of pathogenesis, diagnosis, and therapy. J Clin Oncol 1991;9:1298–1313.
183. Diamandidou E, Cohen PR, Kurzrock R: Mycosis fungoides and Sézary syndrome. Blood 1996;88:2385–2409.
184. Sallah S, Gagnon GA: Angioimmunoblastic lymphadenopathy with dysproteinemia: Emphasis on pathogenesis and treatment. Acta Haematol 1998;99:57–64.
185. Feller AC, Griesser H, Schilling CV, et al: Clonal gene rearrangement patterns correlate with immunophenotype and clinical parameters in patients with angioimmunoblastic lymphadenopathy. Am J Pathol 1988;133: 549–556.
186. Lorenzen J, Li G, Zhao-Hohn M, et al: Angioimmunoblastic lymphadenopathy type of T-cell lymphoma and angioimmunoblastic lymphadenopathy: A clinicopathological and molecular biological study of 13 Chinese patients using polymerase chain reaction and paraffin-embedded tissues. Virchows Arch 1994;424:593–600.
187. Araki A, Taniguchi M, Mikata A: T cell receptor V beta repertoires of angioimmunoblastic lymphadenopathy-like T cell lymphoma. Leuk Lymphoma 1994;16: 135–140.
188. Schlegelberger B, Zwingers T, Hohenadel K, et al: Significance of cytogenetic findings for the clinical outcome in patients with T-cell lymphoma of angioimmunoblastic lymphadenopathy type. J Clin Oncol 1996;14:593–599.
189. Anagnostopoulos I, Hummel M, Finn T, et al: Heterogeneous Epstein-Barr virus infection patterns in peripheral T-cell lymphoma of angioimmunoblastic lymphadenopathy type. Blood 1992;80:1804–1812.
190. Weiss LM, Jaffe ES, Liu XF, et al: Detection and localization of Epstein-Barr viral genomes in angioimmunoblastic lymphadenopathy and angioimmunoblastic lymphadenopathy-like lymphoma. Blood 1992;79: 1789–1795.
191. Kinney MC, Kadin ME: The pathologic and clinical spectrum of anaplastic large cell lymphoma and correlation with *ALK* gene dysregulation. Am J Clin Pathol 1999;111(Suppl 1):S56–S67.
192. Beljaards RC, Kaudewitz P, Berti E, et al: Primary cutaneous CD30-positive large cell lymphoma: Definition of a new type of cutaneous lymphoma with a favorable prognosis. A European Multicenter Study of 47 patients. Cancer 1993;71:2097–2104.
193. Tomaszewski MM, Lupton GP, Krishnan J, May DL: A comparison of clinical, morphological and immunohistochemical features of lymphomatoid papulosis and primary cutaneous CD30(Ki-1)-positive anaplastic large cell lymphoma. J Cutan Pathol 1995;22:310–318.
194. Shiota M, Fujimoto J, Takenaga M, et al: Diagnosis of t(2;5) (p23;q35)-associated Ki-1 lymphoma with immunohistochemistry. Blood 1994;84:3648–3652.
195. Nakamura S, Shiota M, Nakagawa A, et al: Anaplastic large cell lymphoma: A distinct molecular pathologic entity: A reappraisal with special reference to p80(NPM/ALK) expression. Am J Surg Pathol 1997; 21:1420–1432.
196. Pittaluga S, Wiodarska I, Pulford K, et al: The monoclonal antibody ALK1 identifies a distinct morphological subtype of anaplastic large cell lymphoma associated with 2p23/ALK rearrangements. Am J Pathol 1997;151: 343–351.
197. Herbst H, Sander C, Tronnier M, et al: Absence of anaplastic lymphoma kinase (ALK) and Epstein-Barr virus gene products in primary cutaneous anaplastic large cell lymphoma and lymphomatoid papulosis. Br J Dermatol 1997;137:680–686.

198. Foss HD, Anagnostopoulos I, Araujo I, et al: Anaplastic large-cell lymphomas of T-cell and null-cell phenotype express cytotoxic molecules. Blood 1996;88: 4005–4011.
199. Kuze T, Nakamura N, Hashimoto Y, Abe M: Most of CD30⁺ anaplastic large cell lymphoma of B cell type show a somatic mutation in the IgH V region genes. Leukemia 1998;12:753–757.
199a. Drexler HG, Gignac SM, von Wasielewski R, et al: Pathobiology of *NPM-ALK* and variant fusion genes in anaplastic large cell lymphoma and other lymphomas. Leukemia 2000;14:1533–1559.
199b. Benharroch D, Meguerian-Bedoyan Z, Lamant L, et al: ALK-positive lymphoma: A single disease with a broad spectrum of morphology. Blood 1998;91:2076–2084.
200. Kuefer MU, Look AT, Pulford K, et al: Retrovirus-mediated gene transfer of NPM-ALK causes lymphoid malignancy in mice. Blood 1997;90:2901–2910.
201. Morris SW, Kirstein MN, Valentine MB, et al: Fusion of a kinase gene, *ALK*, to a nucleolar protein gene, *NPM*, in non-Hodgkin's lymphoma [published erratum appears in Science 1995;267:316–317]. Science 1994; 263:1281–1284.
202. Blattner WA, Takatsuki K, Gallo RC: Human T-cell leukemia-lymphoma virus and adult T-cell leukemia. JAMA 1983;250:1074–1080.
203. Blattner WA, Kalyanaraman VS, Robert-Guroff M, et al: The human type-C retrovirus, HTLV, in blacks from the Caribbean region, and relationship to adult T-cell leukemia/lymphoma. Int J Cancer 1982;30: 257–264.
204. Hunsmann G, Schneider J, Schmitt J, Yamamoto N: Detection of serum antibodies to adult T-cell leukemia virus in non-human primates and in people from Africa. Int J Cancer 1983;32:329–332.
205. Uchiyama T, Yodoi J, Sagawa K, et al: Adult T-cell leukemia: Clinical and hematologic features of 16 cases. Blood 1977;50:481–492.
206. Narducci MG, Stoppacciaro A, Imada K, et al: TCL1 is overexpressed in patients affected by adult T-cell leukemias. Cancer Res 1997;57:5452–5456.
207. Jaffe ES, Blattner WA, Blayney DW, et al: The pathologic spectrum of adult T-cell leukemia/lymphoma in the United States: Human T-cell leukemia/lymphoma virus-associated lymphoid malignancies. Am J Surg Pathol 1984;8:263–275.
208. Franchini G: Molecular mechanisms of human T-cell leukemia/lymphotropic virus type I infection. Blood 1995;86:3619–3639.
209. Shimamoto Y, Kobayashi M, Miyamoto Y: Clinical implication of the integration patterns of human T-cell lymphotropic virus type I proviral DNA in adult T-cell leukemia/lymphoma. Leuk Lymphoma. 1996;20: 207–215.
210. Miyagi T, Murakami K, Sawada T, et al: A novel single cell PCR assay: Detection of human T lymphotropic virus type I DNA in lymphocytes of patients with adult T cell leukemia. Leukemia. 1998;12:1645–1650.
211. Verma RS, Macera MJ, Krishnamurthy M, et al: Chromosomal abnormalities in adult T-cell leukemia/lymphoma (ATL): A report of six cases with review of the literature. J Cancer Res Clin Oncol 1987;113: 192–196.
212. Uchida T, Kinoshita T, Murate T, et al: *CDKN2 (MTS1/p16INK4A)* gene alterations in adult T-cell leukemia/lymphoma. Leuk Lymphoma 1998;29:27–35.
213. Yamaguchi M, Ohno T, Nakamine H, et al: Gamma/delta T-cell lymphoma: A clinicopathologic study of 6 cases including extrahepatosplenic type. Int J Hematol 1999;69:186–195.
214. Salhany KE, Macon WR, Choi JK, et al: Subcutaneous panniculitis-like T-cell lymphoma: Clinicopathologic, immunophenotypic, and genotypic analysis of alpha/beta and gamma/delta subtypes. Am J Surg Pathol 1998;22:881–893.
215. Coventry S, Punnett HH, Tomczak EZ, et al: Consistency of isochromosome 7q and trisomy 8 in hepatosplenic gamma/delta T-cell lymphoma: Detection by fluorescence in situ hybridization of a splenic touch-preparation from a pediatric patient. Pediatr Dev Pathol 1999;2:478–483.
216. Jaffe ES, Krenacs L, Kumar S, et al: Extranodal peripheral T-cell and NK-cell neoplasms. Am J Clin Pathol 1999;111(Suppl 1):S46–S55.
217. Cooke CB, Krenacs L, Stetler-Stevenson M, et al: Hepatosplenic T-cell lymphoma: A distinct clinicopathologic entity of cytotoxic gamma/delta T-cell origin [see comments]. Blood 1996;88:4265–4274.
218. Wang CC, Tien HF, Lin MT, et al: Consistent presence of isochromosome 7q in hepatosplenic T gamma/delta lymphoma: A new cytogenetic-clinicopathologic entity. Genes Chromosomes Cancer 1995;12:161–164.
219. Alonsozana EL, Stamberg J, Kumar D, et al: Isochromosome 7q: The primary cytogenetic abnormality in hepatosplenic gamma/delta T cell lymphoma [letter]. Leukemia 1997;11:1367–1372.
220. Francois A, Lesesve JF, Stamatoullas A, et al: Hepatosplenic gamma/delta T-cell lymphoma: A report of two cases in immunocompromised patients, associated with isochromosome 7q. Am J Surg Pathol 1997;21:781–790.
221. Kumar S, Krenacs L, Medeiros J, et al: Subcutaneous panniculitic T-cell lymphoma is a tumor of cytotoxic T lymphocytes. Hum Pathol 1998;29:397–403.
222. Isaacson PG, O'Connor NT, Spencer J, et al: Malignant histiocytosis of the intestine: A T-cell lymphoma. Lancet 1985;2:688–691.
223. Chott A, Dragosics B, Radaszkiewicz T: Peripheral T-cell lymphomas of the intestine. Am J Pathol 1992;141: 1361–1371.
224. Chott A, Vesely M, Simonitsch I, et al: Classification of intestinal T-cell neoplasms and their differential diagnosis. Am J Clin Pathol 1999;111(1 Suppl 1):S68–S74.
225. Jaffe ES: Introduction: Hodgkin's lymphoma—pathology, pathogenesis, and treatment [editorial; comment]. Semin Hematol 1999;36:217–219.
226. Stein H, Hummel M: Cellular origin and clonality of classic Hodgkin's lymphoma: Immunophenotypic and molecular studies. Semin Hematol 1999;36:233–241.
227. Chan WC: Cellular origin of nodular lymphocyte-predominant Hodgkin's lymphoma: Immunophenotypic and molecular studies. Semin Hematol 1999;36: 242–252.
228. Harris NL: Hodgkin's disease: Classification and differential diagnosis. Mod Pathol 1999;12:159–175.
229. Kanzler H, Kuppers R, Hansmann ML, Rajewsky K: Hodgkin and Reed-Sternberg cells in Hodgkin's disease represent the outgrowth of a dominant tumor clone

derived from (crippled) germinal center B cells. J Exp Med 1996;184:1495–1505.

230. Küppers R, Rajewsky K, Zhao M, et al: Hodgkin disease: Hodgkin and Reed-Sternberg cells picked from histological sections show clonal immunoglobulin gene rearrangements and appear to be derived from B cells at various stages of development. Proc Natl Acad Sci U S A 1994; 91: 0962–10966.

231. Bräuninger A, Hansmann ML, Strickler JG, et al: Identification of common germinal-center B-cell precursors in two patients with both Hodgkin's disease and non-Hodgkin's lymphoma. N Engl J Med 1999;340:1239–1247.

232. Vockerodt M, Soares M, Kanzler H, et al: Detection of clonal Hodgkin and Reed-Sternberg cells with identical somatically mutated and rearranged VH genes in different biopsies in relapsed Hodgkin's disease. Blood 1998;92:2899–2907.

233. Smolewski P, Niewiadomska H, Blonski JZ, et al: Expression of proliferating cell nuclear antigen (PCNA) and p53, bcl-2 or C-erb B-2 proteins on Reed-Sternberg cells: Prognostic significance in Hodgkin's disease. Neoplasma 1998;45:140–147.

234. Reid AH, Cunningham RE, Frizzera G, O'Leary TJ: bcl-2 rearrangement in Hodgkin's disease: Results of polymerase chain reaction, flow cytometry, and sequencing on formalin-fixed, paraffin-embedded tissue. Am J Pathol 1993;142:395–402.

235. Gupta RK, Lister TA, Bodmer JG: The t(14;18) chromosomal translocation and Bcl-2 protein expression in Hodgkin's disease. Leukemia 1994;8:1337–1341.

236. Poppema S, Kaleta J, Hepperle B: Chromosomal abnormalities in patients with Hodgkin's disease: Evidence for frequent involvement of the 14q chromosomal region but infrequent bcl-2 gene rearrangement in Reed-Sternberg cells. J Natl Cancer Inst 1992;84: 1789–1793.

237. Weiss LM, Movahed LA, Warnke RA, Sklar J: Detection of Epstein-Barr viral genomes in Reed-Sternberg cells of Hodgkin's disease. N Engl J Med 1989;320:502–506.

238. Jarrett RF, MacKenzie J: Epstein-Barr virus and other candidate viruses in the pathogenesis of Hodgkin's disease. Semin Hematol 1999;36:260–269.

239. Wu TC, Mann RB, Charache P, et al: Detection of EBV gene expression in Reed-Sternberg cells of Hodgkin's disease. Int J Cancer 1990;46:801–804.

240. Pallesen G, Hamilton-Dutoit SJ, Rowe M, Young LS: Expression of Epstein-Barr virus latent gene products in tumour cells of Hodgkin's disease. Lancet 1991;337: 320–322.

241. Lyons SF, Liebowitz DN: The roles of human viruses in the pathogenesis of lymphoma. Semin Oncol 1998;25: 461–475.

242. Klein E, Teramoto N, Gogolak P, et al: LMP-1, the Epstein-Barr virus-encoded oncogene with a B cell activating mechanism similar to CD40. Immunol Lett 1999;68:147–154.

243. Falini B, Bigerna B, Pasqualucci L, et al: Distinctive expression pattern of the BCL-6 protein in nodular lymphocyte predominance Hodgkin's disease. Blood 1996; 87:465–471.

244. Ohno T, Stribley JA, Wu G, et al: Clonality in nodular lymphocyte-predominant Hodgkin's disease. N Engl J Med 1997;337:459–465.

245. Marafioti T, Hummel M, Anagnostopoulos I, et al: Origin of nodular lymphocyte-predominant Hodgkin's disease from a clonal expansion of highly mutated germinal-center B cells. N Engl J Med 1997;337:453–458.

246. Braeuninger A, Kuppers R, Strickler JG, et al: Hodgkin and Reed-Sternberg cells in lymphocyte predominant Hodgkin disease represent clonal populations of germinal center-derived tumor B cells [published erratum appears in Proc Natl Acad Sci U S A 1997;94:14211]. Proc Natl Acad Sci U S A. 1997;94:9337–9342.

247. Greiner TC, Gascoyne RD, Anderson ME, et al: Nodular lymphocyte-predominant Hodgkin's disease associated with large-cell lymphoma: Analysis of Ig gene rearrangements by V-J polymerase chain reaction. Blood 1996;88:657–666.

248. Alkan S, Ross CW, Hanson CA, Schnitzer B: Epstein-Barr virus and bcl-2 protein overexpression are not detected in the neoplastic cells of nodular lymphocyte predominance Hodgkin's disease. Mod Pathol 1995;8:544–547.

249. Knowles DM: Immunodeficiency-associated lymphoproliferative disorders. Mod Pathol 1999;12:200–217.

250. Harris NL, Ferry JA, Swerdlow SH: Posttransplant lymphoproliferative disorders: Summary of Society for Hematopathology Workshop. Semin Diagn Pathol 1997;14:8–14.

251. Swerdlow SH: Classification of the posttransplant lymphoproliferative disorders: From the past to the present. Semin Diagn Pathol 1997;14:2–7.

252. Perry GS, Spector BD, Schuman LM, et al: The Wiskott-Aldrich syndrome in the United States and Canada (1892–1979). J Pediatr 1980;97:72–78.

253. Morrell D, Cromartie E, Swift M: Mortality and cancer incidence in 263 patients with ataxia-telangiectasia. J Natl Cancer Inst 1986;77:89–92.

254. Cunningham-Rundles C, Siegal FP, Cunningham-Rundles S, Lieberman P: Incidence of cancer in 98 patients with common varied immunodeficiency. J Clin Immunol 1987;7:294–299.

255. Chadburn A, Chen JM, Hsu DT, et al: The morphologic and molecular genetic categories of posttransplantation lymphoproliferative disorders are clinically relevant. Cancer 1998;82:1978–1987.

256. Knowles DM, Cesarman E, Chadburn A, et al: Correlative morphologic and molecular genetic analysis demonstrates three distinct categories of posttransplantation lymphoproliferative disorders. Blood 1995;85:552–565.

257. Frizzera G, Hanto DW, Gajl-Peczalska KJ, et al: Polymorphic diffuse B-cell hyperplasias and lymphomas in renal transplant recipients. Cancer Res 1981;41: 4262–4279.

258. Cesarman E, Chadburn A, Liu YF, et al: *BCL-6* gene mutations in posttransplantation lymphoproliferative disorders predict response to therapy and clinical outcome. Blood 1998;92:2294–2302.

259. Beral V, Peterman T, Berkelman R, Jaffe H: AIDS-associated non-Hodgkin lymphoma. Lancet 1991;337: 805–809.

260. Centers for Disease Control: Revision of the CDC surveillance case definition for acquired immunodeficiency

syndrome. MMWR Morb Mortal Wkly Rep 1987; 36(Suppl):1S–5S.

261. Knowles DM: Etiology and pathogenesis of AIDS-related non-Hodgkin's lymphoma. Hematol Oncol Clin North Am 1996;10:1081–1109.

262. Knowles DM: Molecular pathology of acquired immunodeficiency syndrome-related non-Hodgkin's lymphoma. Semin Diagn Pathol 1997;14:67–82.

263. Cesarman E, Knowles DM: The role of Kaposi's sarcoma–associated herpesvirus (KSHV/HHV-8) in lymphoproliferative diseases. Semin Cancer Biol 1999;9: 165–174.

264. Chang Y, Cesarman E, Pessin MS, et al: Identification of herpesvirus-like DNA sequences in AIDS-associated Kaposi's sarcoma. Science 1994;266:1865–1869.

265. Nador RG, Cesarman E, Chadburn A, et al: Primary effusion lymphoma: A distinct clinicopathologic entity associated with the Kaposi's sarcoma–associated herpes virus. Blood 1996;88:645–656.

266. Subar M, Neri A, Inghirami G, et al: Frequent c-*myc* oncogene activation and infrequent presence of Epstein-Barr virus genome in AIDS-associated lymphoma. Blood 1988;72:667–671.

267. Said JW: Human immunodeficiency virus–related lymphoid proliferations. Semin Diagn Pathol 1997;14: 48–53.

268. Horenstein MG, Nador RG, Chadburn A, et al: Epstein-Barr virus latent gene expression in primary effusion lymphomas containing Kaposi's sarcoma–associated herpesvirus/human herpesvirus-8. Blood 1997;90:1186–1191.

CHAPTER 14 APPENDIX

SOP 14.1

IgH CLONALITY ASSAY:

DETECTION BY POLYACRYLAMIDE GEL ELECTROPHORESIS (PAGE) OR CAPILLARY ELECTROPHORESIS (CE)

ANALYSIS OF IgH PCR PRODUCT BY PAGE

Clonal populations of lymphocytes are detected by using polymerase chain reaction (PCR) with consensus primers for the V_H and J_H regions of the immunoglobulin heavy chain (*IgH*) gene. A single-round PCR procedure is used with hot start and ^{32}P-α-dATP incorporation. High-resolution polyacrylamide gel electrophoresis (PAGE) is used for PCR product detection. The expected size range for *IgH* gene rearrangements is between 105 and 120 base pairs. **Note: Handle all radioactivity behind a beta shield!**

PCR Conditions

The PCR reaction (50 μL final volume), containing 0.2, 1, or 5 μL of the DNA lysate, consists of:

1.25X PCR Buffer II (PE Applied Biosystems, Foster City, CA)
3.5 mmol/L $MgCl_2$
200 μmol dCTP, dGTP, and dTTP
20 μmol dATP
2 μCi ^{32}P-α-dATP (3000 Ci/mmol)
1.5 U AmpliTaq Gold DNA polymerase (PE Applied Biosystems, Foster City, CA)
100 nmol each primer:
IgH V_HFR3 5′-ACACGGC(C/T)(G/C)TGTATTACT GT-3′ (upstream)
IgH J_H 5′-ACCTGAGGAGACGGTGACC-3′ (downstream)
Molecular grade water to 50 μL

Samples are amplified in a PE GeneAmp 9600 or 9700 thermal cycler and cycled at the times and temperatures below:

Initial step:	10.5 min 95°C
40 cycles of:	1 min 94°C
	1 min 55°C
	1 min 72°C
Final step:	7 min 72°C

Samples are electrophoresed through a 6% denaturing PAGE gel (containing 6 mol/L urea), and the gel is dried and visualized by autoradiography.

Quality Control

Several types of positive and negative controls are run with each assay to ensure test performance. The placement of the controls within an assay is crucial to the detection of contamination at each step in the test system.

Positive Assay

The positive assay control is DNA from SUDHL-5 (a CLL cell line that contains a monoclonal *IgH* gene rearrangement).

Negative Assays

A negative control is used to control for each step in the test system: lysate preparation, reagent mix preparation, and carryover contamination from sample to sample in the assay setup procedure.

WATER CONTROL. A PCR reaction mix containing water as the sample tested is set up as first in the PCR run, before patient samples, to assess the purity of the assay reagents.

LYSATE CONTROL. A lysate (no DNA template) prepared in parallel with patient samples should give no detectable band, indicating that the tube was not contaminated with DNA during lysate preparation.

CONTAMINATION CONTROL AND AMPLIFICATION CONTROL-REACTIVE LYMPH NODE. A negative control lysate from a paraffin-embedded sample of a reactive lymph node is set up last in the PCR run, after the positive control. This reaction has two purposes.

1. It confirms the overall assay performance by demonstrating the amplification of a polyclonal pattern of *IgH* gene rearrangement.
2. It assesses the overall quality of the assay setup procedure in avoiding carryover contamination of a monoclonal band from a positive to an adjacent negative polyclonal sample.

Assay Controls

1. Run positive control and negative controls along with patient samples. Run 1 μL of positive control (SUDHL-5) lysate and negative controls along with patient samples.
2. Patient samples are tested at three concentrations: 1 μL of a 1:5 dilution of the sample lysate (0.2X), 1 μL of the undiluted lysate (1X), and 5 μL of the undiluted lysate (5X).

3. A tube with all reagents and 1 μL of lysate controls (an empty tube that was treated with the same reagents used during the preparation of the patient DNA extracts) serve as a negative control.
4. Five microliters of a water control, 1 μL of a lysate control, and 1 μL of a reactive lymph node serve as negative controls.

Reporting Results

A monoclonal *IgH* gene rearrangement appears as a dominant band of 105 to 120 bp. A positive result is reported as "A monoclonal band was detected." The monoclonal band must be observed in at least two of the three dilutions. If only a ladder of bands is observed, the result is reported as "No monoclonal band was detected." The assay for *IgH* rearrangement is indeterminate if there are no bands present or only one or two bands are observed, indicating the sample is poorly amplifiable. An alternate plausible explanation for the lack of bands in a sample is that the sample did not contain any B cells.

ANALYSIS OF IgH PCR PRODUCT ON ABI 310 GENETIC ANALYZER CAPILLARY ELECTROPHORESIS SYSTEM

Clonal populations of lymphocytes are detected by using PCR with the same consensus primers for the V_H and J_H regions of the *IgH* gene as reported earlier. A single round PCR procedure is used with hot start. High-resolution capillary electrophoresis (CE) is used for PCR product detection. The expected size range for *IgH* gene rearrangements is between 105 and 120 bp.

PCR Conditions

The PCR reaction (50 μL final volume), containing 0.2, 1, or 5 μL of the DNA lysate, consists of:

1.25X PCR Buffer II (PE Applied Biosystems, Foster City, CA)
3.5 mmol/L $MgCl_2$
0.2 mmol each dNTP
1.5 U AmpliTaq Gold DNA polymerase (PE Applied Biosystems, Foster City, CA)
100 nmol each primer
IgH V_HFR3 5′-ACACGGC(C/T)(G/C)TGTATTACT GT-3′ (upstream)
IgH J_H 5′-ACCTGAGGAGACGGTGACC-3′ (downstream)
Molecular grade water to 50 μL

Samples are amplified in a PE GeneAmp 9600 or 9700 thermal cycler and cycled at the times and temperatures below:

Initial step:	10.5 min 95°C
40 cycles of:	1 min 94°C
	1 min 55°C
	1 min 72°C
Final step:	7-min 72°C

One microliter of PCR product is diluted 1:10 in molecular grade-water (Sigma, St. Louis, MO) and mixed with 12 μL deionized formamide, pH 7 to 9 (Amresco, Inc., Solon, OH) and 0.5 μL GeneScan 500 [TAMRA] internal lane size standards. The samples are centrifuged and denatured for 5 minutes at 95°C and analyzed by capillary electrophoresis on the PE ABI Prism 310 Genetic Analyzer.

Quality Control

The same positive and negative assay controls need to be run with CE analysis of *IgH* gene rearrangement as described earlier.

Reporting Results

A monoclonal *IgH* gene rearrangement appears as a dominant peak of 105 to 120 bp. A positive result is reported as "A monoclonal band was detected." The monoclonal band must be observed in at least two of the three dilutions. If only a ladder of peaks is observed, the result is reported as "No monoclonal band was detected." The assay for *IgH* rearrangement is indeterminate if there are no peaks present or only one or two peaks are observed, indicating the sample is poorly amplifiable. An alternate plausible explanation for the lack of bands in a sample is that the sample did not contain any B cells.

REFERENCES

1. Abruzzo LV, Griffith LM, Nandedkar M, et al: Histologically discordant lymphomas with B-cell and T-cell components. Am J Clin Pathol 1997;108:316–323.
2. Krafft AE, Taubenberger JK, Sheng ZM, et al: Enhanced sensitivity with a novel TCR gamma PCR assay for clonality studies in 569 formalin-fixed, paraffin-embedded (FFPE) cases. Mol Diagn 1999;4:119–133.
3. Reed TJ, Reid A, Wallberg K, et al: Determination of B-cell clonality in paraffin-embedded lymph nodes using the polymerase chain reaction. Diagn Mol Pathol 1993;2:42–49.

TIMOTHY J. O'LEARY
DENNIS M. FRISMAN

15

Soft Tissue and Bones

Although tumors of the soft tissue and bone are relatively uncommon, they have been the subject of intense investigation in many laboratories. This interest has resulted, in part, from the fact that soft tissue tumors can often be grown in short-term cell culture and that subsequent cytogenetic studies frequently demonstrate the presence of chromosomal abnormalities that are present in a substantial fraction of tumors cultured. The presence of characteristic translocations or deletions, in turn, suggests genomic locations where positional cloning efforts may yield the identity of genes involved in the neoplastic process. In other cases, the identification of genetic abnormalities is facilitated by association with a genetic disease, such as von Recklinghausen's neurofibromatosis. Segregation analysis provides the target region for positional cloning efforts, and the specific genes involved in the neoplastic process are identified as a result.

In a large number of cases (Table 15–1), these efforts have demonstrated characteristic translocations that give rise to chimeric genes and fusion proteins. Although the mechanisms by which these chimeric genes exert their influence have only been partially elucidated, it has become possible to develop highly sensitive and specific molecular biologic tests based on fluorescent in situ hybridization (FISH) or reverse-transcriptase polymerase chain reaction (RT-PCR) techniques. In many cases, however, either the genetic changes have been too poorly elucidated to enable development of molecular laboratory methods, or the known changes generally consist of point mutations in a very large gene, resulting in economic limitations to routine molecular biologic analysis. In these cases, traditional morphologic and immunohistochemical (IHC) methods retain an undiminished role in diagnosis.

In this chapter, both the genetics of selected soft tissue and bone tumors and the role of ancillary methods in their diagnosis are explored. Where possible, the basic cytogenetic and molecular changes are outlined, along with the mechanisms by which the genetic abnormalities may give rise to a neoplastic process. The utility of molecular diagnostic methods, together with flow cytometry, image analysis, and immunohistochemistry, is then considered in the diagnosis and prognosis of each entity. Needless to say, much of the pertinent literature must be ignored, or go uncited. We hope, however, that the resulting text provides a context for understanding not only the role of molecular diagnosis but also for putting it in the context of earlier ancillary diagnostic techniques.

FIBROUS AND FIBROHISTIOCYTIC TUMORS

Intra-abdominal Desmoplastic Small Round Cell Tumor

Intra-abdominal desmoplastic small round cell tumor (IADSRCT) is a poorly differentiated aggressive intra-abdominal tumor that invariably demonstrates cytogenetic abnormalities of chromosomes 11p13 and 22q12, usually in the form of the reciprocal translocation t(11;22)(p13;q12).[1-3] This translocation results in fusion of the *EWS* (Ewing's sarcoma) and *WT1* (Wilms' tumor) genes to form a fusion gene that gives rise to a chimeric messenger RNA (mRNA).[4] The resulting protein is a potent transcriptional activator[5] that seems to increase expression of various autocrine and paracrine growth factors.[6] Flow cytometry of 11 cases showed nine tumors to be diploid, one tetraploid, and one aneuploid[7]; the relationship of ploidy to prognosis is unknown.

The t(11;22)(p13;q12) translocation may be detected in almost all cases of IADSRCT by RT-PCR techniques,[4, 8, 9] but the diagnosis may often be made in the absence of molecular data. These tumors typically demonstrate a distinctive IHC profile (Table 15–2) with reactivity for keratin, epithelial membrane antigen, neuron-specific enolase, and desmin.[1]

TABLE 15–1

Characteristic Translocations Found in Soft Tissue Tumors

Diagnosis	Translocation	Fusion Gene
Myxoid/round cell liposarcoma	t(12;16)(q13;p11) t(12;22)(q13;q12)	*FUS/DDIT3* *EWS/DDIT3*
Alveolar rhabdomyosarcoma	t(2;13)(q35;q14)	*PAX3/FOX01A* *PAX7/FOX01A*
Synovial sarcoma	t(X;18)(p11;q11)	*SSX1/SS18* *SSX2/SS18*
Ewing's sarcoma/primitive neuroectodermal tumor	t(11;22)(q24;q12) t(21;22)(q22;q12) t(2;22)(p22;p12) t(17;22)(q21;q12)	*EWS/FLI1* *EWS/ERG* *EWS/ETV1* *EWS/ETV4*
Desmoplastic intra-abdominal small round cell tumor	t(11;22)(p13;q12)	*EWS/WT1*
Clear cell sarcoma	t(12;22)(q13;q12)	*EWS/ATF1*
Extraskeletal myxoid chondrosarcoma	t(9;22)(q31;q12)	*EWS/NR4A3*

Solitary Fibrous Tumor

Solitary fibrous tumors are readily recognized in the pleura (fibrous mesothelioma) but may occur at virtually any site (where they easily may be misidentified). Although immunoreactivity for CD34 is well recognized,[10–12] this marker is not absolutely specific, because it is found in a small percentage of malignant fibrous histiocytomas and other tumors; the absence of reactivity for α_1-antitrypsin and α_1-antichymotrypsin is also useful in establishing the diagnosis from an IHC perspective (Table 15–3). Lack of CD34 reactivity, particularly when found in association with p53 accumulation, may be useful in identification of particularly aggressive tumors likely to result in recurrence and/or death.[13]

Cytogenetic and molecular biologic information regarding these tumors is very limited. Comparative genomic hybridization (CGH) studies have shown that large solitary fibrous tumors demonstrate greater cytogenetic abnormality than do small solitary fibrous tumors; these changes have included gains in 5q, 7, 8, 12, and 18 and losses in 13 and 20q.[14] Trisomy of chromosome 8 was seen in two cases, suggesting a relationship between solitary fibrous tumor and aggressive fibromatosis. Trisomy 21 has also been reported.[15] It is not clear whether either of these trisomies provides information predictive of outcome.

TABLE 15–2

Immunoreactivity of Selected/Markers in Intra-abdominal Desmoplastic Small Round Cell Tumor

Immunohistochemical Marker	Percentage of Cases Demonstrating Immunoreactivity
Keratin (pan)	93–100
Desmin	92–100
Epithelial membrane antigen	89–100
Neuron-specific enolase	52–77

Aggressive Fibromatosis (Desmoid Tumor)

Aggressive fibromatosis is a clonal proliferation of cytologically bland fibrocytes that can cause considerable morbidity.[16–18] Patterns of IHC reactivity that are useful in differentiation from solitary fibrous tumor are shown in Table 15–3. Trisomy 8 is frequently observed by FISH[19, 20]; it is not clear whether trisomy is an early event in these patients or whether it is acquired in the course of proliferation. Although trisomy 8 is only found in about 10% of patients with fibromatoses that do not recur after excision, it is observed in approximately 70% of patients whose tumors do recur.[21, 22] Trisomy 20 is also frequently observed in the same cells demonstrating trisomy 8.[20]

Desmoid tumors are seen in about 10% of individuals affected by the familial adenomatous polyposis syndrome and are associated with homozygous inactivation of the *APC* gene in these patients.[23] *APC* mutations have also been observed in sporadic desmoid tumors and are increased with an increase in β-catenin protein levels resulting from decreased protein degradation.[24] This is accompanied by estrogen or progesterone expression in two thirds of tumors and inappropriate expression of platelet-derived growth factor,[25] the level of which may be useful in predicting local aggressiveness.[26] Elastin synthesis is also increased[27]; telomerase expression is not observed.[28] An autosomal dominant pattern of desmoid tumor inheritance has also been seen in a few families affected by 3′ *APC* gene mutations[29, 30]; affected individuals do not demonstrate colonic polyposis.

Trisomy 8 is not associated with tumor size or proliferating cell nuclear antigen (PCNA) expression[22]; neither tumor size, PCNA immunohistochemistry, nor flow-cytometric S-phase fraction provides information useful for assessing recurrence risk. IHC stains generally contribute little to the clinical and morphologic diagnosis of this tumor. Thus, interphase cytogenetic identification of trisomy 8 is currently the only useful ancillary diagnostic technique for the pathologic diagnosis of aggressive fibromatosis.

Fibrosarcoma

Although fibrosarcoma was once frequently diagnosed in adults, the evolution of new diagnostic categories

TABLE 15–3

Immunoreactivity of Selected Immunohistochemical Markers in Solitary Fibrous Tumor and Aggressive Fibromatosis

Immunohistochemical Marker	Percentage of Solitary Fibrous Tumors Demonstrating Immunoreactivity	Percentage of Aggressive Fibromatoses Demonstrating Immunoreactivity
Factor 13A	100	0
α_1-Antitrypsin	0	79–100
CD34	88–96	0
α_1-Antichymotrypsin	0–13	62–98
Desmin	4–16	0
Vimentin	86–97	90–100
CAM 5.2	0–8	0
Epithelial membrane antigen	0–6	0

and techniques has caused it to become an uncommon diagnosis[31]; cases that were once diagnosed as fibrosarcoma are now frequently categorized as dermatofibrosarcoma protuberans, malignant fibrous histiocytoma, or monophasic synovial sarcoma. In part because criteria by which pathologists diagnose this tumor vary wildly, it is not possible to extract any meaningful information on the molecular biology of adult fibrosarcoma from the literature. Similarly, information on IHC reactions is "polluted." Clearly, these tumors may express actin and cytokeratins as well as vimentin and collagen type IV[32, 33]; desmin expression is rarely reported. IHC assessment of proliferation markers such as Ki-67, PCNA, p53, and BCL2 is not predictive of outcome, at least in the inflammatory variety of this tumor.[34] Fibrosarcomas tend to exhibit more proliferative activity than do fibromatoses, as assessed by both PCNA immunostaining and flow cytometry.[35] Furthermore, fibrosarcomas demonstrate aneuploidy detectable by flow cytometry in approximately one fourth of all cases; the prognostic value of this finding is uncertain.

Congenital fibrosarcoma is an often indolent tumor that may be identical to congenital mesonephric nephroma. Although trisomy 11 is the most frequently reported karyotypic abnormality in congenital fibrosarcoma,[20] trisomies of chromosomes 18, 17, and 20 are also reported, suggesting a strong relationship to the aggressive fibromatoses and to solitary fibrous tumors.[36, 37] A t(12;15)(p13;q25) translocation giving rise to a fusion between the *ETV6 (TEL)* gene and the *NTRK3* gene has also been reported in these patients and is not seen in adult fibrosarcomas or in fibromatoses.[38, 39]

Malignant Fibrous Histiocytoma

Malignant fibrous histiocytoma (MFH) is an often aggressive adult sarcoma. Although morphologic pattern remains the most useful criterion for diagnosis of MFH, IHC markers (Table 15–4) are sometimes helpful. The majority of cases demonstrate reactivity with α_1-antitrypsin and α_1-antichymotrypsin and are negative for desmin and actin. Nevertheless, desmin, actin, and even cytokeratin expression is sometimes observed,[40] so IHC assays must be interpreted with caution and careful consideration of both the clinical presentation and histomorphologic appearance.

Karyotypic analysis has revealed frequent rearrangements involving chromosomes 19p13, 11p11, 1q11, and 3p12; there is a tendency for tumors demonstrating 19p$^+$ markers to recur locally[41]; the extent of cytogenetic abnormality tends to correlate with histologic grade.[42] Surprisingly, these cytogenetic results do not correlate well with CGH studies, which do, however, suggest high-level amplifications in 4q12-21, 8p21-pter, 8q24.1-qter, 9q12-13, 12p11.2-pter, 12q12-15, and 15q 11.2-15.[43, 44] Chromosome 12q13-14 contains two oncogenes,

TABLE 15–4

Immunoreactivity of Selected Immunohistochemical Markers in Malignant Fibrous Histiocytoma

Immunohistochemical Marker	Percentage of Cases Demonstrating Immunoreactivity
Vimentin	93–99
α_1-Antichymotrypsin	67–79
α_1-Antitrypsin	64–79
Factor 13a	38–72
CD68	38–53
CD99	2–55
Epithelial membrane antigen	8–22
CAM 5.2	8–21
Lysozyme	4–21
Desmin	5–15
Actin	3–16
CD34	2–15
Myoglobin	0

SAS and *MDM2*, that are frequently amplified in MFH.[45] *SAS* amplification has been reported to be more characteristic of central tumors than those found in the arms and legs.[46] Amplification of *MDM2* is associated with the presence of ring chromosomes in karyotype preparations.[47] There is no relationship between *MDM2* amplification and survival, however.[48]

Mutation of the *TP53* gene and overaccumulation of the p53 protein are frequently observed in MFH.[48–55] Although IHC identification of p53 accumulation has not proven to be prognostically useful in multivariate analyses,[48, 49, 55, 56] there is some evidence that *TP53* gene mutation may be associated with shorter survival.[48]

Although p53 immunohistochemistry is clearly not useful in predicting outcome in patients with MFH, a variety of other IHC markers show promise in single studies. Increased urokinase-plasminogen activator levels appear to be associated with a worse prognosis[57]; expression of heat shock protein 27 (HSP-27)[58] and BCL2,[51] in contrast, appears to be associated with improved survival.

Perhaps not surprisingly, outcome in MFH has been associated with the extent of proliferative activity in a number of studies. High levels of the proliferation markers PCNA[59] and Ki-67[49, 55] appear to be associated with decreased survival, but the value added beyond histologic grading remains somewhat uncertain, largely because of the relatively small size of published investigations. Furthermore, although flow cytometric assessment of S-phase fraction has also proven to be useful in predicting outcome in MFH,[60] it is not clear whether flow cytometric assessment of proliferation provides information that is more useful, less useful, or independent of that provided by IHC assessment of proliferation markers. Finally, published investigations shed no light on whether morphometric measurements, which have also shown promise in a single study,[60] remain valuable if IHC information (which is considerably less expensive to obtain) is available.

Angiomatoid MFH is a variant that is typically characterized by somewhat less aggressive behavior than "typical" MFH. Most cases demonstrate diploid DNA histograms, but the presence of a diploid DNA distribution does not preclude recurrence.[61, 62] Unlike "typical" MFH, angiomatoid MFH frequently demonstrates desmin reactivity,[63] causing some authors to refer to the tumor as angiomatoid myosarcoma.[63, 64] Immunoreactivity for CD68, S-100, and factor 13A is seen in a minority of cases.[65]

In summary, diagnosis of MFH is best made on the basis of a histomorphologic impression formed, as necessary, through the use of IHC differentiation markers. Histologic grading may possibly be improved by IHC and flow cytometric assessment of proliferation, *TP53* mutation analysis, or image analysis; published studies remain too limited to recommend the routine use of any of these ancillary diagnostic methods.

LIPOMATOUS TUMORS

Lipomatous tumors are remarkable in that nearly all histologic categories demonstrate characteristic chromosomal alterations. Although one of these alterations, the t(12;16) translocation characteristic of myxoid/round cell liposarcoma, has been well-characterized, molecular testing strategies remain of limited use in routine diagnosis; likewise, IHC assessment has little use in the routine evaluation of lipomatous tumors. Nevertheless, cytogenetic and molecular studies have played an important role in forming our current understanding of the lipomatous tumors, providing a sound molecular basis for the belief that myxoid and round cell liposarcomas comprise one pathologic entity and that atypical lipoma and well-differentiated liposarcoma constitute another.

Lipoma

Diagnosis of "typical" well-differentiated lipomas from the subcutaneous tissue seldom presents diagnostic difficulty or need of ancillary diagnostic techniques. The identification of well-differentiated liposarcoma in deep tissues is primarily based on tumor size and location, and benefit from ancillary diagnostic methods has not been demonstrated in these tumors either. The diagnosis of spindle cell lipoma and pleomorphic lipomas may present challenges, however. Spindle cell lipomas tend to demonstrate strong reactivity for BCL2[66] and CD34[67]; these proteins are often expressed in other spindle cell tumors, such as dermatofibrosarcoma protuberans, emphasizing the need for panels of IHC assays in differential diagnosis of spindle cell tumors.

Cytogenetic analysis of typical lipomas usually demonstrate abnormalities of 12q13-14, either in the form of ring chromosomes or balanced rearrangements,[68] often involving chromosome 3. The breakpoints are common with those seen in uterine leiomyomas and pleomorphic adenomas in the salivary glands.[69] Although these breakpoints have been frequently related to the high-mobility protein gene *(HMGIC)*,[70] some map to locations more than 10 megabases away, suggesting involvement of several different genes in chromosome breakage in these tumors.[71] The chromosome 3 breakpoint has been mapped to 3q27-28, to a gene belonging to the LIM family[70]; the t(3;12) translocation is not specific for lipomas but is also seen in pulmonary chondroid hamartomas[72] and thus may relate to proliferation but not differentiation.

Atypical Lipoma/Well-Differentiated Liposarcoma

The histologic characteristics of atypical lipoma and well-differentiated liposarcoma are identical. Diagnostic distinction is generally based on location, with extremity neoplasms deemed "atypical lipoma" and central neoplasms called "well-differentiated liposarcoma," particularly when located in the retroperitoneum. Both are characterized cytogenetically by the presence of supernumerary ring chromosomes and, somewhat less frequently, by giant "marker" chromosomes[73–76] that result from high-level amplification of the *MDM2* gene.[47, 77] Neither *TP53* nor *RB1* gene mutations are seen in these tumors.[78] The presence of *FUS/DDIT3* fusion transcripts, characteristic of myxoid/round cell liposarcoma, has been reported in well-differentiated liposarcoma.[79]

Although the cytogenetic findings in these tumors are interesting, they are neither helpful in reaching a diagnosis nor useful in predicting ultimate outcome for the patient.

Myxoid/Round Cell Liposarcoma

A characteristic t(12;16)(q13;p11) translocation associated with myxoid liposarcoma[80–82] results from fusion of the *FUS(TLS)* gene on chromosome 16 and the *DDIT3(CHOP)* gene on chromosome 12, resulting in a chimeric FUS-DDIT3 message. Several different fusion transcripts have been sequenced. The FUS/DDIT3 fusion protein blocks adipocyte differentiation when expressed at a level comparable to that observed in human myxoid liposarcoma.[83] A second translocation, t(12;22), resulting from fusion between *DDIT3* and *EWS* has also been identified[84]; there seems to be no distinctive clinical difference between tumors demonstrating the two translocations. Although the distinctive translocations can be used diagnostically,[85, 86] they are not generally required to correctly characterize these tumors, and *FUS/DDIT3* fusion transcripts have been demonstrated in both pleomorphic liposarcoma and well-differentiated liposarcoma.[79]

The development of a defining molecular characteristic for liposarcomas enables development of more accurate IHC profiles than were previously possible. Virtually all cases demonstrate both vimentin and S-100 reactivity; desmin is observed in about half of the tumors.[81] Most round cell/myxoid liposarcomas also demonstrate CD36; CD34 is negative.

Pleomorphic Liposarcoma

The diagnosis of pleomorphic liposarcoma has become increasingly rare with the increasing tendency to diagnose malignant fibrous histiocytoma. There are no specific IHC, molecular biologic, or cytogenetic abnormalities characterizing this poorly studied group of tumors; *FUS/DDIT3* fusion transcripts, characteristic of round cell/myxoid liposarcoma, have been reported in nearly one third of pleomorphic liposarcomas.[79]

Lipoblastoma

Lipoblastomas are generally benign, often congenital, neoplasms present in infancy or childhood. Although neoplasms composed primarily of mature lipoblasts are readily diagnosed histologically, those with prominent myxoid stroma may be difficult to differentiate from myxoid liposarcoma; in these cases, assays capable of demonstrating the t(12;16) translocation may assist in diagnosis. Although lipoblastomas frequently demonstrate 8q11-q13 rearrangements,[20, 87, 88] the molecular nature of these translocations remains unknown, allowing their demonstration only by conventional cytogenetic studies.

Hibernoma

Hibernomas are tumors involving proliferation of brown fat that are readily diagnosed on histologic grounds alone. Cytogenetic changes are frequently observed in the 11q13 region,[20] but the underlying molecular abnormalities have not been elucidated.

SMOOTH MUSCLE TUMORS

The classification of "smooth muscle tumors" is undergoing revision as gastrointestinal tract tumors that had once been considered leiomyomas or leiomyosarcomas are increasingly referred to as "gastrointestinal stromal tumors." These tumors, which are significantly different from the smooth muscle tumors arising in the uterus and other sites, are considered separately. The diagnoses of both gastrointestinal stromal tumors and smooth muscle tumors arising in the soft tissues generally are based on classic histomorphologic criteria, but it is likely that these soon will be supplemented by molecular biologic tests.

Leiomyomas

The diagnosis of typical leiomyomas arising in the uterus provides a diagnostic challenge to neither clinician nor pathologist. Hence, consideration of cytogenetic, IHC, and molecular biologic data is with the objective of a better understanding of the pathogenesis of these benign yet debilitating tumors. The most striking cytogenetic finding in uterine leiomyomas is frequent translocation involving chromosomes 12 and 14 and deletion of the long arm of chromosome 7.[89–91] A subset of tumors demonstrates a characteristic translocation, t(12;14)(q14-15;q23-24).[89] The usual target gene on chromosome 12 for these translocations is the high-mobility group protein gene *HMGIC* (which contains a DNA-binding domain); the preferential translocation partner from chromosome 14 is the recombinational repair gene *RAD1B*,[92] although recombination with the mitochondrial aldehyde dehydrogenase gene has also been reported.[93] These cytogenetic changes have not been associated with oncogene amplification.[94]

In addition to the cytogenetic alterations just described, a variety of molecular biologic changes have been described in leiomyomas. Estrogen[95] and progesterone gene expression increase in comparison with normal myometrium. These changes are accompanied by estrogen-dependent modulation of HRAS, MYC, and EGF expression.[96, 97] Increased proliferation, as assessed by Ki-67 and PCNA, is observed in leiomyomas[98–100]; p53 immunoreactivity is not seen.[101]

Leiomyomas in other sites have not been so well characterized as those in the uterus. Both sporadic and Alport syndrome–associated diffuse esophageal leiomyomatosis has been associated with deletions in the *COL4A5/COL4A6* (collagen α5 and α6) gene cluster.[102] Diffuse leiomyomatosis in both lung[103] and peritoneum[104] has been associated with immunohistochemically detectable estrogen-receptor expression.

The multicentric smooth muscle tumors associated with the acquired immunodeficiency syndrome that arise in the bronchi,[105] adrenals,[106] meninges,[107] and other locations have been associated with the presence of replicating Epstein-Barr virus.[108, 109] This association suggests that some smooth muscle tumors can arise by means of interruption of apoptosis, a suggestion that is supported by the observation of abundant BCL2 expression in uterine leiomyomas.[110] Telomerase activity is not observed in uterine leiomyomas.[111]

The differentiation of bizarre leiomyomas from leiomyosarcomas is not always straightforward. The bizarre leiomyomas demonstrate karyotypic abnormalities that are considerably more complex than those associated with simple uterine leiomyomas.[112] Unfortunately, flow cytometric determinations of DNA aneuploidy and proliferation are insufficient to distinguish benign uterine smooth muscle tumors from leiomyosarcomas.[113, 114] Mitotic figure counting remains the preferred method by which to differentiate benign from malignant smooth muscle tumors in the uterus.

Leiomyosarcoma

The diagnosis of leiomyosarcoma is generally made by first establishing smooth muscle differentiation and then assessing the malignant potential by mitotic figure counting. Unfortunately, a number of tumors fall into "borderline" categories in which malignant potential cannot be predicted with certainty. In contrast to "ordinary" leiomyomas, leiomyosarcomas generally have very complex karyotypes. Such complex karyotypes are unfortunately also characteristic of bizarre leiomyomas, limiting the diagnostic use of cytogenetic analysis. Alterations in chromosome 1p are the most frequently reported cytogenetic abnormality; alterations involving the same regions of chromosomes 12 and 14 that are often involved in uterine leiomyomas are also observed.[91] CGH studies in soft tissue leiomyosarcomas demonstrate frequent losses in chromosomes 10q and 13q and frequent gains in chromosome 17p.[115] These complex chromosomal alterations are accompanied by aneuploidy that is frequently detectable by flow cytometry[113, 116] and an increased S-phase fraction that is an independent predictor of overall survival in multivariate analysis.[113, 117]

TABLE 15–5

Immunoreactivity of Selected Immunohistochemical Markers in Leiomyosarcoma

Immunohistochemical Marker	Percentage of Cases Demonstrating Immunoreactivity
Vimentin	86–95
Actin (HHF-35)	85–94
Actin (SM)	83–93
Desmin	59–71
CD68	30–47
AE1	6–37
α_1-Antichymotrypsin	10–28
CD99	9–29
CD34	11–24
S-100	6–17
CAM 5.2	0–21

Mutations of *TP53* occur in about 25% of leiomyosarcomas[118–120]; detection of mutation by molecular biologic methods does not correlate well with IHC staining for p53 protein. Although there is some evidence that *TP53* mutation detection may be prognostically useful,[121] most studies have been small and lacked follow-up. *HRAS* and *KRAS* mutations are observed only rarely[120, 122, 123] but may be associated with worse outcome.

Overexpression of the *MYC* oncogene is seen in about half of uterine leiomyosarcomas, a percentage similar to that seen in uterine leiomyomas.[124] Smooth muscle differentiation antigens are typically expressed in about 90% of cases (Table 15–5); a variety of other antigens not normally associated with smooth muscle differentiation may be seen in a minority of cases.

GASTROINTESTINAL STROMAL TUMORS

These tumors, now commonly called "GISTs," were for many years considered to be primary smooth muscle tumors arising in the gastrointestinal tract.[125–128] The histologic appearance can vary between that of well-differentiated smooth muscle and of an anaplastic tumor. Many, but not all, of these tumors demonstrate immunoreactivity for actin; desmin is seen only uncommonly.[129–131] Most tumors react with CD34; CD117 immunoreactivity is relatively specific for gastrointestinal stromal tumor[132] and suggests that these tumors are etiologically related to the interstitial cells of Cajal.[133] Nevertheless, CD117 has been reported to

TABLE 15–6

Spectrum of CD117 (KIT) Immunoreactivity

Diagnosis	Percentage of Cases Demonstrating Immunoreactivity
Gastrointestinal stromal tumor	78–96
Clear cell sarcoma	21–72
Malignant melanoma, metastatic	17–55
Hemangiopericytoma	0–45
Dermatofibrosarcoma protuberans	0–31
Malignant fibrous histiocytoma	0–15

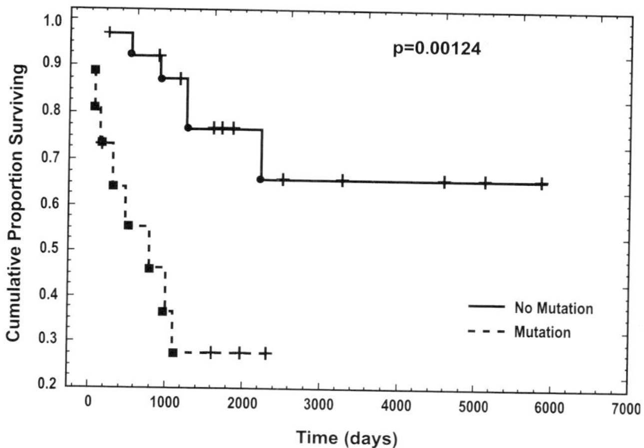

FIGURE 15–1
Survival as a function of *KIT* mutation, for patients with gastrointestinal stromal tumors. (From Ernst SI, Hubbs AE, Przygodzki RM, et al: *KIT* mutation portends poor prognosis in gastrointestinal stromal/smooth muscle tumors. Lab Invest 1998;78:1633–1636.)

react with a variety of other tumors (Table 15–6). The IHC profile of GIST is shown in Table 15–7.

Although tumor location,[134–136] size[127, 128, 137–139] and mitotic index[127, 128, 134] are all useful in predicting outcome, no histologic criterion reliably predicts malignant potential in all cases.[137] Although IHC assays for proliferation markers[140–142] and flow cytometry[137, 143–148] both improve outcome prediction somewhat, neither of these techniques, either alone or in combination with the other, allows determination of malignancy with certainty.

Recent investigations have demonstrated mutation of the *KIT* oncogene in some of these tumors.[149–151] The *KIT* gene codes for a transmembrane tyrosine kinase receptor; the deletion mutations that have been found in the *KIT* gene result in constitutive activation of this receptor.[150, 481, 482] On average, patients with tumors that demonstrate *KIT* mutations have a less favorable prognosis than those with tumors that do not demonstrate *KIT* mutations (Fig. 15–1),[149] but a significant number of patients have aggressive tumors that have no *KIT* gene abnormalities. This suggests that one or more other molecular alterations are important in the development of some GISTs and somewhat limits the diagnostic utility of *KIT* gene sequencing.

The constitutive activation of KIT that appears to be nearly ubiquitous in GIST provides a molecular target for therapeutic intervention. A small molecule tyrosine kinase inhibitor, imatinib mesylate (STI571, Gleevec) inhibits the tyrosine kinase activity of KIT[483–485]; its use as a chemotherapeutic agent in patients with disseminated GISTs is accompanied by a substantial clinical response rate and low toxicity.[486, 487] It seems likely that therapeutic agents directed against specific molecular targets will become increasingly important in the future.

TABLE 15–7

Immunoreactivity of Selected Markers in Gastrointestinal Stromal Tumors

Immunohistochemical Marker	Percentage of Cases Demonstrating Immunoreactivity
Vimentin	95–99
CD117	73–89
CD34	71–82
Actin (HHF-35)	52–63
Actin (SM)	38–49
Myosin (SM)	9–41
Desmin	14–21
S-100	6–10
Keratin (pan)	0–8
Chromogranin A	0–6
CD31	0
Glial fibrillary acidic protein	0
Neurofilament protein	0
Synaptophysin	0

TUMORS OF STRIATED MUSCLE

Rhabdomyoma

Little is known about the molecular biology of benign striated muscle tumors. A single karyotypic abnormality—reciprocal translocation involving chromosomes 15 and 17—has been reported in a single case.[152] Although allelic loss at chromosome 16p13.3 has been reported in a rhabdomyoma from a patient with tuberous sclerosis,[153] a relationship between chromosome 16 alterations and pathogenesis of sporadic rhabdomyomas has not been established.

Rhabdomyomas demonstrate diffuse reactivity for myoglobin, actin, desmin, and vimentin and do not demonstrate S-100 protein; this spectrum of reactivity is similar to that seen in normal cardiac muscle.[154] This finding, as well as the allelic loss seen at the site of the tuberous sclerosis complex, suggests that many or all rhabdomyomas represent hamartomas rather than true neoplasms.

Rhabdomyosarcoma

Although changes in diagnostic criteria have rendered the diagnosis of rhabdomyosarcoma uncommon in adults, striated muscle tumors account for a significant percentage of pediatric mesenchymal malignancies. Intensive research efforts have yielded considerable insight into the molecular pathogenesis of pediatric rhabdomyosarcoma, and molecular diagnosis is now an important technique in establishing the diagnosis of alveolar rhabdomyosarcoma.

EMBRYONAL RHABDOMYOSARCOMA

Cytogenetic studies of embryonal rhabdomyosarcoma have demonstrated complex patterns of chromosomal alteration. Extra copies of chromosomes 8, 11, and 12 are frequently observed by FISH, but the role of FISH in differential diagnosis and prognosis has not been established.[155, 156] Deletions on the short arm of chromosome 11, which is not observed in alveolar rhabdomyosarcoma, appears to be a reliable indicator of the embryonal form. CGH studies have demonstrated frequent gains on chromosomes 2, 7, 8, 12, and 13 and localized losses most frequently to chromosomes 1, 6, 9, 14, and 17.[488] These cytogenetic alterations correlate with the flow cytometric observation of aneuploidy in almost all embryonal rhabdomyosarcoma.[157, 158]

Loss of heterozygosity (LOH) studies point to the existence of one or more tumor suppressor genes on chromosome 11p15.5[159, 160]; there is some evidence that embryonal rhabdomyosarcoma is preferentially associated with functional loss of maternal alleles at this locus.[159, 161] Although it is likely that multiple genes near this locus are involved in the pathogenesis of embryonal rhabdomyosarcoma,[162] a specific tumor suppressor has yet to be identified.

There are several other molecular alterations that distinguish embryonal rhabdomyosarcoma from other tumors. Virtually all alveolar and embryonal rhabdomyosarcomas express mRNA for the acetylcholine receptor γ subunit; virtually all other tumors of children and adults express the ε subunit.[163] Studies using cDNA microarrays have demonstrated that gene expression profiles can readily distinguish this from other types of rhabdomyosarcoma.[489, 490]

Expression of MYOD1 is a distinguishing characteristic of rhabdomyosarcoma. Methylation of a 5-kb region upstream of the coding sequence is found in nearly all embryonal rhabdomyosarcomas and is only rarely observed in alveolar rhabdomyosarcomas.[164] Unfortunately, determination of DNA methylation patterns is sufficiently complex as to preclude its use as a routine diagnostic adjunct. IHC expression of most muscle differentiation antigens is sufficiently similar between embryonal rhabdomyosarcoma and other striated smooth muscle tumors as to render them useless in differential diagnosis. IHC identification of troponin T may be an exception, however; troponin T is identified in the majority of embryonal rhabdomyosarcomas but is not found in other histologic types of striated muscle tumor.[165]

ALVEOLAR RHABDOMYOSARCOMA

The diagnosis of "classic" alveolar rhabdomyosarcoma is, in theory, morphologically straightforward. Unfortunately, the frequent occurrence of solid variants that are readily confused with peripheral neuroectodermal tumor or neuroblastoma has made this an often difficult and/or erroneous diagnosis. Classic cytogenetic analysis demonstrates the presence of a t(2;13)(q37;q14) translocation in many cases.[166, 167] This translocation results from the fusion of the *PAX3* gene on chromosome 3 with the *FOXO1A (FKHR)* gene on chromosome 13.[168, 169] An alternative translocation, t(1;13)(p36;q14), results from fusion of the chromosome 1 *PAX7* gene with the *FOXO1A* gene.[170] The structure and expression of the products associated with the t(2;13)(q35;q14) translocation associated with alveolar rhabdomyosarcoma have been examined. The chromosome 13 *FOXO1A* gene is identified as a member of the forkhead domain family of transcription factors. The *PAX3* or the *PAX7* gene provides a DNA-binding domain to the fusion protein, presumably resulting in constitutive activation of *FOXO1A*. Although the translocation breakpoints are too variable to allow design of a robust direct PCR assay, RT-PCR assays are capable of detecting the fusion transcripts in the majority of cases.[171–173]

The *PAX3/FOXO1A* and *PAX7/FOXO1A* fusions give rise to distinct clinical phenotypes; the latter more often presents as a localized extremity lesion and is associated with a better prognosis (Fig. 15–2). FISH assays provide an alternative approach to identification of the translocation.[174–176]

Flow-cytometric measurements have demonstrated near-tetraploidy (1.80 to 2.60 times the DNA content of normal cells) in alveolar rhabdomysarcoma.[177] Image analysis is somewhat more sensitive than flow cytometry in detecting aneuploidy[178]; studies have given conflicting results on the relationship between tumor cell ploidy and clinical outcome.

Oncogene amplification is frequent in alveolar rhabdomyosarcomas. *MYCN* amplification occurs in approximately two thirds of cases and may be associated with a worse prognosis; it is not observed in embryonal rhabdomyosarcoma.[179–181] Amplification of *PAX3/FOXO1A* and *PAX7/FOXO1A* is also observed[182]; the prognostic significance is unclear. These may correspond to amplifications on chromosomes 1, 2, and 13 seen by CGH, which also demonstrates frequent amplification on chromosomes 12q13-15 and 8q13-21.[183]

Virtually all alveolar rhabdomyosarcomas express mRNA for the acetylcholine receptor γ subunit; virtually

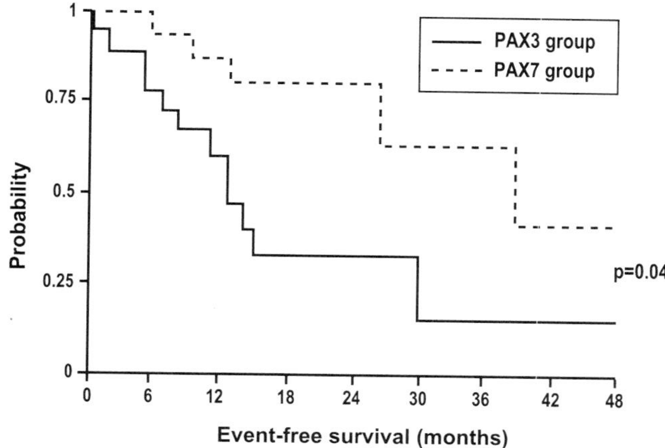

FIGURE 15–2
Kaplan-Meier curve for event-free survival of patients with *PAX3-FOXO1A* and *PAX7-FOXO1A* fusions. A significantly improved event-free survival was observed for patients with *PAX7-FOXO1A* fusion ($P = .04$). (From Kelly KM, Womer RB, Sorensen PH, et al: Common and variant gene fusions predict distinct clinical phenotypes in rhabdomyosarcoma. J Clin Oncol 1997;15:1831–1836.)

all non–striated-muscle tumors of children and adults demonstrate expression of the ε subunit instead.[163] Although IHC methods may be used to exploit this property in diagnosis, there does not appear to be an advantage over IHC testing for desmin[184, 185] and other muscle markers. If any three of the four markers—myosin, myoglobin, and the BB and MM isoenzymes of creatine kinase—can be identified immunohistochemically, striated muscle differentiation can be assumed.[186] Antibodies directed against skeletal muscle actin have also been produced and may possibly be useful in diagnosis.[187] Expression of nonskeletal markers should not necessarily deter one from the diagnosis of rhabdomyosarcoma (Table 15–8).[188]

TABLE 15–8
Immunoreactivity of Selected Markers in Rhabdomyosarcoma

Immunohistochemical Marker	Percentage of Cases Demonstrating Immunoreactivity
Actin (HHF-35)	94–100
Desmin	89–97
Vimentin	85–98
Myoglobin	2–72
CAM 5.2	21–53
α_1-Antichymotrypsin	20–53
Actin (SM)	23–49
CD99	13–25
CD68	3–31
S-100	0–13
CD45	0
Glial fibrillary acidic protein	0

PLEOMORPHIC RHABDOMYOSARCOMA

Pleomorphic rhabdomyosarcoma has become an increasingly uncommon diagnosis. Nevertheless, pleomorphic tumors in adults characterized by sarcomeres, Z-disks, and hexagonal myofilament arrays do exist and are properly placed in this category of tumors. Unfortunately, the apparent presence or absence of "cross striations" on light microscopy is not a reliable diagnostic criterion. IHC assessment of muscle antigens is helpful, because the majority of cases will demonstrate immunoreactivity for desmin, myoglobin, actin (HHF-35), and smooth-muscle actin.[189] Demonstration of immunoreactivity for MYOD1 may also be useful in establishing striated muscle differentiation in a pleomorphic sarcoma.[190]

TUMORS OF BLOOD VESSELS

Hemangiopericytoma

Approximately one fourth of hemangiopericytomas demonstrate cytogenetic abnormalities, in the form of inversions or translocations, at chromosome 12q13.[191, 192] Surprisingly, no chromosome copy number changes were seen in 11 hemangiopericytomas examined by CGH techniques.[14] However, *MDM2* amplification and overexpression have both been observed in the only hemangiopericytoma examined[193]; high levels of telomerase activity have also been observed in a single case.[194] Hemangiopericytomas do not demonstrate human herpesvirus 8 (HHV-8) sequences[195]; this may be used to differentiate fibrous hemangiopericytoma from Kaposi's sarcoma.

Only about 40 hemangiopericytomas have been studied by flow cytometry.[196, 197] Although DNA ploidy is not a useful indicator of biologic behavior, there is a trend toward more aggressive behavior in tumors with high S-phase fractions. A similar relationship exists between IHC proliferation markers (PCNA and Ki-67) and outcome.[198]

The reactivity of hemangiopericytoma and other vascular neoplasms with selected IHC differentiation markers is shown in Table 15–9. Histiopericytoma lacks IHC evidence of smooth muscle differentiation, thus differing from the normal pericyte.[199, 200]

Angiosarcoma

Angiosarcoma, an aggressive vascular neoplasm, has undergone limited cytogenetic investigation. Published karyotypes are often complex, and no characteristic rearrangements have been observed.[201–204] Recurrent changes include gains of 5pter-p11, 8p12-qter, and 20pter-q12 and losses of 7pter-p15, 22q13-qter, and -Y.[204] Flow cytometric assessments have found aneuploidy in 30% to

TABLE 15–9

Reactivity of Selected Markers in Vascular Neoplasms

	Percentage of Cells Demonstrating Immunoreactivity		
Immunohistochemical Marker	*Angiosarcoma*	*Hemangioendothelioma*	*Hemangiopericytoma*
Collagen IV	0–9	87–100	0–23
B72.3	36–78	0	–
Laminin	37–72	79–97	–
Vimentin	97–100	90–99	89–100
Factor XIIIA	–	100	62–93
CD99	–	–	45–78
Factor 8 RAG	70–83	–	0–12
CD31	69–85	78–92	0–8
CD34	80–100	76–100	49–70
Actin (SM)	8–29		0
CAM 5.2	24–55	0–15	–

80% of cases and have not demonstrated prognostic value.[197, 205] Most patients have high proliferative activity as assessed by IHC staining with MIB1; these patients have a poorer prognosis than those whose tumors demonstrate less MIB1 immunoreactivity.[206]

Between 20% and 50% of angiosarcomas demonstrate IHC accumulation of p53 or *TP53* mutations, but there is no evidence to suggest that these patients have an outcome different than those whose tumors demonstrate wild-type p53.[206–208] About half of the angiosarcomas demonstrate increased MDM2 reactivity.[208] Although HHV-8 sequences have been observed by several workers using nested PCR techniques, they have not been detected by simple PCR assays.[209] This suggests that HHV-8 is not involved in the pathogenesis of angiosarcoma and that simple PCR assays for HHV-8 may be useful in eliminating angiosarcoma from the differential diagnosis of soft tissue vascular tumors.

The reactivity of angiosarcomas and other vascular neoplasms with some IHC differentiation markers is shown in Table 15–9. Differentiation of angiosarcomas from other vascular neoplasms can generally be made using morphologic appearance supplemented by a panel of IHC markers.

Kaposi's Sarcoma

Kaposi's sarcoma (KS) is a monoclonal vascular proliferation found predominantly in immunosuppressed patients.[210–212] A previously unknown, actively transcribed herpesvirus, HHV-8, was discovered in Kaposi's sarcoma cells from human immunodeficiency virus (HIV)-infected patients using representational difference analysis.[213] This virus infects both endothelial cells and typical KS spindle cells and is also found in non–HIV-related KS.[214–216] Viral sequences can be found in the serum well before the appearance of KS lesions[217–219]; in one case there is evidence of a 40-year latency.[220] Viral sequences can be identified in semen[217] and saliva,[221] as well as in the KS lesions themselves. In contrast to other herpesviruses, in which transmission occurs in childhood and adolescence, transmission of HHV-8 appears to be limited to adults.[222]

Two small transcripts account for most HHV-8–encoded RNA in KS.[223] One of these transcripts accumulates in the nucleus; the other is a small BCL2 homologue that inhibits apoptosis.[224, 225] IHC stains almost invariably demonstrate strong reaction of KS cells with antibodies derived against BCL2,[226] suggesting that this protein is up-regulated in KS cells.[227] Abundant expression of RAS P21 may also be observed immunohistochemically.[227] The KS K1 open reading frame has demonstrated transforming potential, although it has yet to be directly implicated in the initiation and/or maintenance of KS.[228] In addition, HHV-8 encodes a cyclin that is expressed during latent infection, phosphorylating the retinoblastoma tumor suppressor protein and possibly playing a role in cell immortalization.[229, 230] Although IHC expression of p53 is seen in up to half of KS lesions, there is no convincing evidence favoring a role for p53 in the pathogenesis of this neoplasm.[231–234] Mutations of *TP53* have not been reported.

Only limited cytogenetic analysis of KS has been performed. Losses of chromosomes 14, 21, 22, and X have been observed,[203, 235] as have nonrandom translocations and deletions, accompanied by LOH, at 3p14-ter.[235] Flow cytometric studies show early-stage KS to have a diploid DNA distribution, whereas later lesions demonstrate aneuploidy or tetraploidy[205] and an increasing percentage of S-plus G_2M-phase cells.[236] This latter finding contrasts to IHC observations based on Ki-67 staining, which suggest no relationship between stage and proliferative activity in KS.[237] Interestingly, most patients whose KS lesions develop subsequent to steroid treatment show aneuploid flow histograms, in contrast to the diploid pattern shown by most tumors appearing in HIV-infected patients.[238]

Although most KS lesions may be diagnosed easily by consideration of morphologic and clinical features, early lesions may be difficult to differentiate from hemangiomas and later lesions may sometimes be hard to differentiate from angiosarcoma or spindle cell hemangioendothelioma. The IHC identification of type IV collagen, which is present in early KS lesions, may assist in diagnosis,[239] as may the identification of HHV-8 sequences, which are found in KS but not in either angiosarcoma or hemangioendothelioma.[240, 241]

Hemangioma

Relatively little is known about the genetic and molecular alterations underlying this class of readily diagnosed benign vascular lesions. Cytogenetic analysis of a cavernous hemangioma with transition to angiosarcoma demonstrated trisomy 5 and loss of the Y chromosome as the sole cytogenetic abnormalities.[242] Flow cytometric investigations have demonstrated hemangiomas to be uniformly diploid. An unusual epithelioid hemangioma-like lesion found in immunosuppressed patients has been associated with IHC localization of the cat-scratch disease bacillus.[243]

Cherry hemangiomas demonstrate capillaries with perivascular hyalinized sheaths. These have been demonstrated immunohistochemically to show increased staining for type VI collagen.[244]

SYNOVIAL SARCOMA

The diagnosis of synovial sarcoma, a tumor of adolescents and young adults, has been complicated by the fact that its appearance as a monophasic, spindle cell neoplasm is at least as frequent as its appearance in the traditional "biphasic" form. Following the original identification of the characteristic t(X;18) by traditional karyotypic analysis,[245] a large number of reports established that this translocation can be identified in 90% or more of the tumors diagnosed as synovial sarcoma on histologic grounds.[246–252] The translocation results in fusion of the chromosome 18 *SS18(SYT)* gene to either the Xp11.2 *SSX1* gene or *SSX2* gene, resulting in a hybrid gene that gives rise to either of two distinct fusion proteins, depending on which X chromosome gene is involved.[253, 254] The fusion protein is localized in the nucleus.[255, 256] The *SSX2* gene codes for a tumor antigen HOM-MEL-40, which is expressed by about half of malignant melanomas and a variety of other tumors; it is not expressed in normal tissues other than testis.[257, 258] The *SSX1/SSX2* portion of the fusion transcript contains a transcriptional repressor domain, whereas the *SS18* portion contains transcriptional activator sequences.[259] Although the details of how this gives rise to neoplastic transformation are unknown, synovial sarcoma almost invariably demonstrates BCL2 overexpression, suggesting the possibility that the fusion protein in some way disrupts the apoptosis pathway in this tumor.[49, 260] It also appears that there is a relationship between the nature of the fusion protein and both histology and long-term outcome in patients with synovial sarcoma; biphasic tumors typically demonstrate *SS18/SSX1* transcripts, whereas those with monophasic tumors demonstrate *SS18/SSX2* transcripts and a worse outcome (Figs. 15–3 and 15–4).[261] There is also a suggestion that *TP53* mutation may contribute to progression/metastasis in synovial sarcoma, but further study is required.[262] Although *MYC* amplification has been reported in synovial sarcoma,[263] the role of oncogene amplification in the pathogenesis and prognosis of this tumor has not received much attention.

CGH studies have demonstrated a variety of other aberrations in synovial sarcoma, including high-level amplifications and recurrent deletions at 8p12-qter and 21q21-qter.[264] Cytogenetic changes were more complex in monophasic than biphasic tumors.

IHC observation of high levels of proliferation using Ki-67 (MIB1) or PCNA staining is associated with a worse prognosis in patients with synovial sarcoma.[49, 265–267]

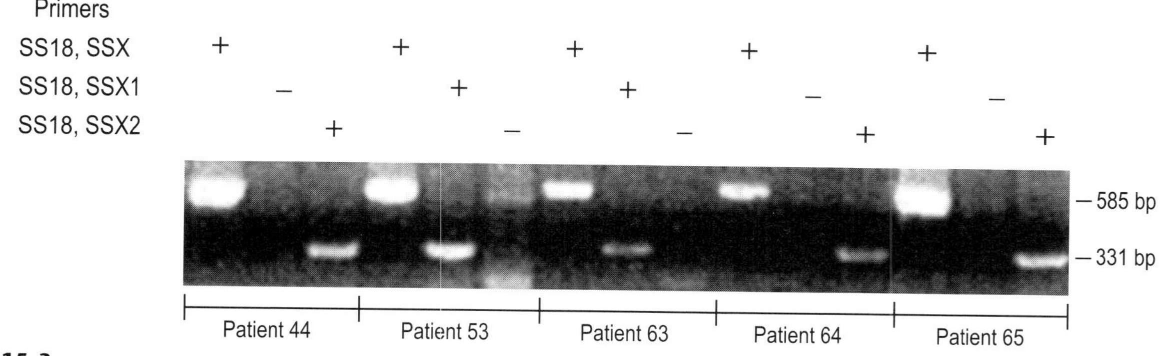

FIGURE 15–3
Analysis of *SS18-SSX* fusion transcripts in synovial sarcoma. Tumors from patients 53 and 63 contain the *SS18-SSX1* fusion transcript, whereas those from patients 44, 64, and 65 contain the *SS18-SSX2* fusion transcript. (From Kawai A, Woodruff J, Healey JH, et al: *SYT-SSX* gene fusion as a determinant of morphology and prognosis in synovial sarcoma. N Engl J Med 1998;338:153–160.)

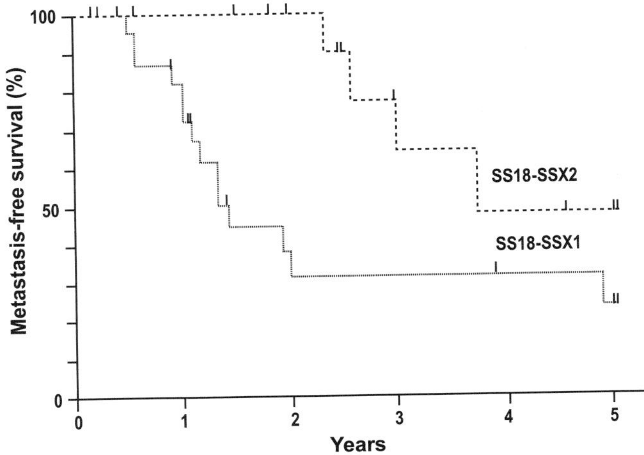

FIGURE 15–4
Metastasis-free survival in patients with localized tumors. Metastasis-free survival was significantly longer among those with the *SS18-SSX2* fusion transcript than those with *SS18-SSX1* (P =.03 by multivariate analysis). (From Kawai A, Woodruff J, Healey JH, et al: *SYT-SSX* gene fusion as a determinant of morphology and prognosis in synovial sarcoma. N Engl J Med 1998;338:153–160.)

Patients whose tumors demonstrate a diploid DNA histogram have a significantly better survival than those with aneuploid DNA histograms,[266] but there is no relationship between S-phase fraction and outcome.[266, 268, 269] Furthermore, multivariate analysis shows that determination of tumor ploidy does not provide information beyond that provided by IHC staining.[267]

The t(X;18) translocation can be identified by FISH in the interphase nuclei isolated from formalin-fixed, paraffin-embedded synovial sarcomas in about 90% of cases.[86, 270–273] RT-PCR assays provide an alternative approach, but RNA degradation appears to reduce the sensitivity to approximately 80%.[274–276] Furthermore, although molecular testing is useful in some cases to establish the diagnosis of synovial sarcoma, it is usually not necessary. Identification of high levels of vimentin and BCL2 staining in a cytologic malignant spindle cell proliferation is strongly suggestive of the diagnosis; a profile of the immunoreactivity of syncovial sarcoma for selected antigens is shown in Table 15–10.

PERIPHERAL NERVE SHEATH TUMORS

Schwannoma

Schwannomas are tumors of the cranial, spinal, and peripheral nerve sheaths composed of Schwann cells. These tumors may show local invasion but do not metastasize; nevertheless, they may demonstrate substantial nuclear pleomorphism. The most common cytogenetic abnormality is loss of chromosome 22, which is found in more than half the cases[277, 278]; CGH does not reveal other consistent chromosomal anomalies.[279] This cytogenetic abnormality is accompanied by inactivation of the *NF2* gene at chromosome 22q12,[280, 281] with resulting formation of a truncated form of a protein known as merlin or schwannomin.[282, 283] This molecular abnormality is found both in tumors from patients suffering from type 2 neurofibromatosis and in sporadic schwannomas[284]; the loss of merlin expression is universal in this tumor type and is found before the "tumorlet" stage of development.[285, 286] This protein is a member of a family of structural proteins that link cytoskeletal elements with the cell membrane; the mechanism by which its disruption gives rise to neoplasia has not been completely elucidated but may be related to the elevation of basal proliferation, aberrant membrane ruffling, and presence of fiber disorganization observed in

TABLE 15–10
Immunoreactivity of Selected Markers in Synovial Sarcoma

Immunohistochemical Marker	Percentage of Cases Demonstrating Immunoreactivity
Vimentin	100
BCL2	91–100
Keratin (pan)	69–83
Epithelial membrane antigen	65–79
CAM 5.2	41–79
CD99	30–58
Carcinoembryonic antigen (polyclonal)	9–36
Actin (SM)	1–24
CD68	1–21
S-100	0–11
α_1-Antichymotrypsin	0–13
CD31	0
CD34	0
Desmin	0

Schwann cells.[287–289] In patients with neurofibromatosis, protein-truncating mutations result in a more severe clinical presentation than mutations resulting in only a single amino acid change.[288] Whether the nature of *NF2* mutation affects the propensity to develop a malignant phenotype or the morphologic appearance of the schwannoma is unknown.

Telomerase activity is not observed in schwannomas.[290] IHC (Ki-67 and PCNA) and flow cytometric investigations have demonstrated no relationship between proliferation rate or ploidy and recurrence in cellular schwannoma.[291] Mutations of the *TP53* gene are not seen in schwannoma[292, 293]; although some authors have suggested that IHC identification of p53 is associated with recurrence and malignant transformation, others have not found such an association.[291]

Some IHC staining characteristics of schwannomas are outlined in Table 15–11. As with all mesenchymal tumors, cytokeratin expression is occasionally observed.[294] Unlike peripheral neurofibromas, schwannomas do not react with antibodies directed against factor 13a; this may assist in differential diagnosis.[295]

Neurofibroma

Although neurofibromas are most frequently found in patients with type 1 neurofibromatosis (von Recklinghausen's disease), an autosomal dominant disease characterized by the presence of café-au-lait spots and multiple neurofibromas, they may also occur sporadically. Plexiform and dermal neurofibromas are rarely observed in patients lacking stigmata of neurofibromatosis, and plexiform neurofibromas have a high propensity for malignant transformation.

Almost all studies on the molecular biology of neurofibroma have been performed on lesions taken from patients with neurofibromatosis. Neurofibromas are monoclonal proliferations that may, apparently, evolve into multiple subclones on occasion.[296–298] They demonstrate no characteristic cytogenetic abnormalities; linkage studies were required to identify the chromosome 17q11.2 gene *(NF1)* coding for a 280-kd RAS/GTPase-activating protein, neurofibromin, which is mutated or absent in patients with neurofibromatosis and presumably in sporadic neurofibromas.[299–302] Mutation or loss of both copies of this gene, leading to constitutive activation of the P21/RAS signal transduction pathway, is apparently required for neurofibromas to form.[303–305]

Approximately half of all cases of type 1 neurofibromatosis result from new mutations, which usually occur in the paternally derived allele.[306, 307] This may reflect a tendency for methylated CpG dinucleotides within the *NF1* gene to undergo C→T transition mutations.[306] Development of new *NF1* mutations may also be facilitated by germ-line mutations in the DNA mismatch repair gene *MLH1* associated with hereditary nonpolyposis colorectal cancer.[308]

Although IHC accumulation of p53 has been observed in neurofibromas,[309] chromosome 17p loss of heterozygosity has not been observed.[310] It seems unlikely, therefore, that *TP53* gene alterations are important in the pathogenesis of neurofibroma, although there is evidence that *TP53* mutation may play a role in malignant transformation to neurofibrosarcoma.

The diagnosis of neurofibroma is based primarily on histologic pattern. S-100 is nearly always identified immunohistochemically.

TABLE 15–11

Immunoreactivity of Selected Markers in Schwannoma

Immunohistochemical Marker	Percentage of Cases Demonstrating Immunoreactivity
S-100	100
Vimentin	100
CD34	23–48
Epithelial membrane antigen	13–58
Glial fibrillary acidic protein	21–45
Neurofilament protein	8–30

Malignant Peripheral Nerve Sheath Tumors

Malignant peripheral nerve sheath tumor (MPNST, neurofibrosarcoma, malignant schwannoma) arises most frequently in the setting of type 1 neurofibromatosis, but about one third of the time it appears de novo in soft tissue. Cytogenetic analysis has typically revealed complex karyotypes characterized by the frequent presence of chromosome 17 abnormalities and the somewhat less frequent occurrence of chromosome 22 aberrations,[311, 312] but characteristic abnormalities have not been identified. CGH studies of both sporadic MPNST and MPNST arising in the setting of type 1 neurofibromatosis have demonstrated an increase in copy number of 17q24-qter in tumors arising in neurofibromatosis patients, but not in patients with sporadic MPNST.[313] Loss of 13q sequences in the region 13q14-q21 was found in both sporadic tumors and in tumors arising in patients with neurofibromatosis. Although these findings suggest different pathogenesis for MPNST in patients with and without neurofibromatosis, at least one study has found substantial down-regulation of NF1 expression in a sporadic MPNST, suggesting that neurofibromin protein defects are common to both the sporadic and neurofibromatosis-associated neoplasms.[314, 315] Loss of the RAS/GTPase-activating activity of neurofibromin is, in turn, expected to cause constitutive activation of the P21/RAS signal transduction pathway,[305, 316–320] with a variety of consequences, including activation of KIT (a tyrosine kinase receptor)[321] and increased production of platelet-derived growth factor receptors.[322]

Although constitutive activation of RAS signaling pathways appears to be common to both neurofibromas and MPNSTs, molecular alterations beyond those found in NF1 must be invoked to explain malignant transformation. A variety of molecular alterations have been found in MPNSTs that are not observed in neurofibromas. Some MPNSTs demonstrate a higher expression of both hepatocyte growth factor and its receptor, the *MET* proto-oncogene product, than do benign neurofibromas.[323] Amplification and overexpression of the *MDM2* gene has been observed in three of six MPNSTs examined.[193] Homozygous deletions of the putative tumor-suppressor gene *CDKN2A*, which encodes an inhibitor of CDK4, were found in two of eight MPNSTs, suggesting that aberration of the cyclin pathway may play a role in malignant transformation of some or all of these tumors.[324] There is also strong evidence for an involvement of *TP53* in the development of some, but not all, MPNSTs, because mutation of this tumor suppressor has been found in a few cases.[310]

The IHC characteristics of MPNST are illustrated in Table 15–12. Most MPNSTs can be expected to demonstrate either S-100 protein, myelin basic protein (MBP), or Leu-7, and about a third demonstrate all three antigens.[325] The interpretation of IHC results is complicated by frequent reports of reactivity for both muscle and fibrohistiocytic markers. Immunoreactivity for muscle markers in MPNST is generally quite focal, in contrast to the diffuse presentation in tumors of muscle origin. S-100 staining is also typically weaker and more diffuse than in neurofibroma. Careful consideration of the clinical setting and detailed examination to determine evolution from benign nerve sheath elements facilitates the diagnosis.

TABLE 15–12

Immunoreactivity of Selected Markers in Malignant Peripheral Nerve Sheath Tumors

Immunohistochemical Marker	Percentage of Cases Demonstrating Immunoreactivity
Vimentin	70–90
S-100	56–71
CD57	33–73
CD68	25–56
Neuron-specific enolase	25–55
α_1-Antichymotrypsin	11–47
BCL2	11–44
Epithelial membrane antigen	7–33
Actin (HHF-35)	8–27
Keratin (pan)	4–24
Desmin	0–22
CD34	1–17
Neurofilament protein	0–13
Actin (SM)	0
CD31	0
Glial fibrillary acidic protein	0
HMB-45	0

Ewing's Sarcoma/Primitive Neuroectodermal Tumor

Although Ewing's sarcoma (ES) and primitive neuroectodermal tumor (PNET) were once considered distinct neoplasms, molecular characterization has shown them to be a single entity that may appear in almost completely undifferentiated (ES) or better differentiated (PNET) forms. Cytogenetic analysis reveals a characteristic t(11; 22)(q24;q12) translocation, or a variant involving either 11q24 or 22q12, in over 90% of cases.[326–331] This t(11;22) translocation results in the fusion of the chromosome 22 gene *EWS* with the chromosome 11 gene *FLI1*, leading to the synthesis of a chimeric transcript,[332, 333] which produces a fusion protein localizing in the nucleus. Alternative t(7;22), t(21;22) translocations give rise to fusion of *EWS* with the *ETV1*,[334–338] *ERG*,[334–338] and *ETV4* *(E1A-F)*[339] genes, respectively.[334, 335, 337, 338] Each of these translocations replaces the RNA-binding domain of EWS with a DNA-binding domain from the fusion partner. Thus, the chimeric protein has the properties of a transcription factor, with the transcriptional activation domain contributed by EWS and the DNA-binding domain contributed by the fusion partner. These fusion proteins are highly potent transcriptional activators for the target gene of FLI1, and presumably of other EWS fusion partners.[340, 341] The structure of the *EWS/FLI1* fusion transcript is predictive of prognosis (Fig. 15–5).

CGH studies have suggested additional cytogenetic changes in ES/PNET.[342–344] Gains at 1q, 4p, 5p, 5q, 7q, 8p, 8q, 9p, 12p, 12q, and 17q (including high-level amplifications on 1q, 2p24, and 8q24), together with losses at 17p, have been observed.[342, 343] These results suggest the possibility of *MYC* gene amplification.

A variety of molecular alterations have been reported in a minority of ES/PNET. Amplification of *MYC*, *FLG*, *SPRR3*, *MDM2*, and *CDK4* have been reported,[344–347] usually in association with advanced disease. Although most Ewing's sarcomas are diploid by flow cytometry, both aneuploid and tetraploid tumors have been reported.[348] Loss of the CDK4 inhibitor CDKN2A has been seen in about one third of ES/PNET; post-transcriptional *CDKN2A* inactivation has also been observed, and *CDKN2A* abnormalities appear to be among the most frequent secondary molecular aberration in ES/PNET.[349] LOH at 11p15 and 17p13 is each seen in one third to one half of cases.[347, 350] Mutations

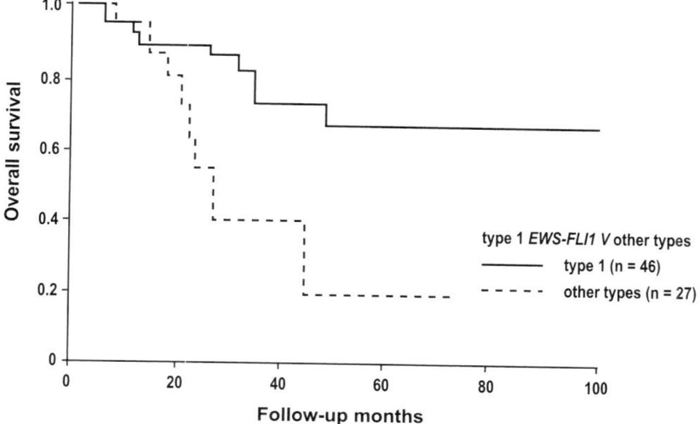

FIGURE 15–5
Kaplan-Meier survival plots for all patients regardless of stage with tumors that contain type 1 *EWS-FLI1* fusions versus all other types (multivariate $P = .014$). (From de Alava E, Kawai A, Healey JH, et al: *EWS-FLI1* fusion transcript structure is an independent determinant of prognosis in Ewing's sarcoma. J Clin Oncol 1998;16:1248–1255.)

of *TP53* are seen in a small subset of tumors, generally also in association with advanced stage disease.[349, 351] Although patients with *MYC* amplification appear to have a poor prognosis, the relationship of other molecular abnormalities (other than formation of fusion genes) to outcome is unclear.

Diagnosis of ES/PNET is greatly facilitated by the availability of FISH[86, 352–355] and RT-PCR[8, 172, 356–358] assays, both of which can readily be carried out in formalin-fixed, paraffin-embedded tissue (see SOP 15.1). In frozen tissue, the sensitivity of the RT-PCR assay is approximately 99%, substantially higher than that for classic cytogenetics (39%) or FISH (75%).[8] Differentiation from other small round cell tumors is also facilitated by IHC analysis; the IHC profile of ES is shown in Table 15–13. Although CD99 was originally thought to be a marker specific for ES/PNET, it has since been found in a wide variety of tumors and must therefore be used as part of a diagnostic panel rather than a "stand alone" immunoassay.

NEOPLASMS OF UNCERTAIN HISTOGENESIS

Clear Cell Sarcoma

Clear cell sarcoma of tendons and aponeuroses (CCS) has also been called "malignant melanoma of soft parts," because both melanin and differentiation antigens associated with melanoma are occasionally observed. A characteristic t(12;22)(q13;q12) translocation (which is not observed in malignant melanoma) has been described in a number of cases[359–363]; this translocation results in fusion of EWS, a chromosome 22q12 DNA-binding protein with the bZIP domain of ATF1, a cyclic adenosine monophosphate (AMP)–dependent transcriptional activating factor coded by a gene on chromosome 12q13. The resulting fusion protein binds only weakly to DNA but can serve as a constitutive transcriptional activator for some promoters[364, 365] while repressing other promoters that contain ATF1-binding sites[366] and blocking cyclic AMP–induced transcription.[367] The net result is deregulation of transcription and proliferation in the tumor.

Clear cell sarcoma generally demonstrates IHC reactivity for vimentin together with focal staining for S-100, neuron-specific enolase, and HMB-45.[368, 369] Synaptophysin and Leu-7 are occasionally identified, but cytokeratin, epithelial membrane antigen, carcinoembryonic antigen, desmin, muscle-specific actin, and leukocyte common antigen are absent.[369]

TABLE 15–13
Immunoreactivity of Selected Markers in Ewing's Sarcoma

Immunohistochemical Marker	Percentage of Cases Demonstrating Immunoreactivity
CD99	92–96
Vimentin	77–91
Neuron-specific enolase	32–50
β_2-Microglobulin	17–55
Neurofilament protein	18–51
CD57	15–38
NB 84	12–33
S-100	9–29
CD68	0–19
Actin (HHF-35)	0–8
AE1/AE3	0–9
Keratin (pan)	0–6
Desmin	0–2
Actin (SM)	0
CD15	0
CD45	0
Epithelial membrane antigen	0
Factor VIII RAG	0
Synaptophysin	0

Myxoma

Although they are most frequently associated with the cardiac atrium, myxomas may also present in the soft tissues and other sites. Although most cases are sporadic, some atrial myxomas occur in association with pigmented micronodular adrenal disease and abnormal skin pigmentation (Carney's complex). Linkage analysis has mapped the gene for this complex to 2p16[370]; whether a gene in this location is associated with sporadic myxomas is unknown. No specific mutations or gene amplifications have been identified in these tumors.

The diagnosis of myxoma occasionally requires IHC assays to differentiate it from unrelated myxoid lesions. Myxomas are generally vimentin-positive[371] and S-100 negative.[372] In addition, they may express epithelial markers (keratin, carcinoembryonic antigen, epithelial membrane antigen), neuroendocrine markers (neuron-specific enolase, synaptophysin), histiocytic markers (α_1-antitrypsin, α_1-antichymotrypsin), and smooth muscle actin.[371, 373–375]

Approximately 20% of myxomas show tumor aneuploidy by flow cytometry, and an equal fraction demonstrates an elevated S-phase fraction. Although the significance of increased S-phase fraction is somewhat uncertain,[376, 377] the finding of a tetraploid DNA histogram is a strong predictor of recurrence.[378] The IHC assessment of proliferation using PCNA or Ki-67 staining has not been shown to have clinical utility.

Alveolar Soft Part Sarcoma

Alveolar soft part sarcoma is an uncommon mesenchymal tumor occurring primarily in children and young adults. IHC evidence of muscle differentiation includes the presence of both actin and desmin,[379] but there is no evidence of MYOD1 or myogenin expression.[380] Electron microscopic studies do not demonstrate myofilaments.[379]

CGH studies show little case-to-case consistency, and copy number changes are observed in a minority of cases.[381] Gains are occasionally observed in 1q, 8q, 12q, and 16p.

Rhabdoid Tumor

Rhabdoid tumors are neoplasms that typically present in the kidneys but that may also develop in the soft tissue in nearly any site. Rhabdoid tumors arising in the soft tissues are usually aggressively malignant. A variety of karyotypic abnormalities have been reported, including isochromosome 12p in a malignant rhabdoid tumor,[382] t(11;22)(p15.5;q11.23) translocation,[383] inversion in 1p15,[384] and abnormalities at 22q11.2.[385] Gene mapping studies have defined multiple candidate loci for a suppressor gene within chromosome 11p15[386] and suggest that the *KCNQ1 (KVLQT1)* gene,[387] *STIM1 (GOK)* gene,[388] or both may be involved. The abnormalities in chromosome 22q11.2 have failed to yield a candidate suppressor gene.[389]

IHC stains demonstrate vimentin in over 90% of cases and cytokeratin and epithelial membrane antigen in about 60%.[390, 391] More than half the cases contain demonstrable CD99 and synaptophysin, whereas none demonstrates myoglobin or desmin.[390] Thus, rhabdoid tumor shares many features with neuroectodermal tumors such as Ewing's sarcoma.

Extraskeletal Myxoid Chondrosarcoma

Extraskeletal myxoid chondrosarcoma (EMC) is a clinically and pathologically distinct low-grade sarcoma that usually arises in the muscle and is characterized (in about 75% of cases) by the specific chromosomal translocation t(9;22)(q22-31;q12).[392–398] Although the EMCs are superficially similar to myxoid chondrosarcomas that occur in the bones, they generally occur in a somewhat older age group, demonstrate more aggressive behavior, and show significant ultrastructural differences. Furthermore, evidence of t(9;22) is generally lacking in skeletal myxoid chondrosarcomas.[399]

FISH studies demonstrate that the fusion gene from chromosome 22q12 is *EWS*.[395] *EWS* is fused to a chromosome 9q22 gene designated as *NR4A3 (CHN, TEC)*, a member of the steroid/thyroid receptor gene superfamily that has a zinc finger DNA-binding domain and that localizes to the nucleus.[394, 400] This fusion gene codes a transcript that contains the amino-terminal transactivation domain of EWS linked to the entire NR4A3 protein.[401] Interestingly, EMC demonstrates immunoreactivity for CD99, most often associated with Ewing's sarcoma, in approximately 20% of cases.[402]

Chordoma

Chordomas are slow-growing malignancies that typically appear in the sacrococcygeal region and that have been supposed to arise from fetal notochord remnants. A variety of cytogenetic abnormalities have been reported[403, 404] but provide little clue to its pathogenesis. Telomerase activity has been observed in one of two tumors examined.[404] Flow cytometric analyses show frequent aneuploidy.[405, 406] Although Ki-67 and p53 expression has been examined immunohistochemically,[406] the relationships between high levels of expression and either outcome or pathogenesis is unclear and neither these ancillary diagnostic techniques nor flow cytometry shows obvious clinical utility.

TABLE 15–14

Immunoreactivity of Selected Markers in Chordoma

Immunohistochemical Marker	Percentage of Cases Demonstrating Immunoreactivity
AE1/AE3	100
CAM 5.2	100
Cytokeratin 19	100
HBME-1	100
Vimentin	100
Epithelial membrane antigen	91–98
Neuron-specific enolase	89–99
S-100	84–93
Carcinoembryonic antigen (polyclonal)	31–53
HMB-45	15–54
CD57	20–44
Glial fibrillary acidic protein	13–41
Synaptophysin	0–19
Desmin	0–8
Chromogranin	0

Chordomas demonstrate a wide variety of mesenchymal and epithelial differentiation antigens; the IHC staining characteristics of this tumor are depicted in Table 15–14.

BENIGN PROLIFERATIVE DISORDERS

Proliferative Myositis

Proliferative myositis is a benign pseudosarcomatous lesion of uncertain etiology. IHC stains generally demonstrate actin and smooth muscle actin, but only rarely desmin[407] and never myoglobin or the MM isoenzyme of creatine kinase.[408] Origin from pericytes,[407] myofibroblasts,[409] and fibroblasts[408] has been suggested.

Little has been learned about the cytogenetics or molecular biology of this proliferative disorder. Trisomy 2 has been described in cultured cells,[410] as has the t(6;14)(q23;q32) translocation.[411]

Nodular Fasciitis

Nodular fasciitis is a benign pseudosarcomatous lesion that may occasionally be confused with malignant fibrous histiocytoma.[412, 413] The characteristic IHC profile (strong staining for smooth muscle and muscle-specific actin, vimentin, and the histiocytic marker CD68) should, when assisted by a clinical history of extremely rapid growth, preclude misdiagnosis. IHC stains for PCNA typically show numerous strongly positive cells[35]; stains for BCL2 are negative,[66, 414] and p53 staining is only rarely observed.[52]

TUMORS OF BONE

Chondroma

Rearrangement of chromosome 12q13 is the most frequently reported cytogenetic abnormality in chondroma[415, 416]; the molecular abnormalities underlying this finding have not yet been characterized. Morphometric assessment may occasionally be useful in differentiating chondroma from low-grade chondrosarcoma.[417]

Osteochondroma

Osteochondromas (osteocartilaginous exostoses) typically develop near the metaphyses of long bones. Although most are sporadic and solitary, multiple lesions occur in the Langer-Giedion syndrome and in the multiple hereditary exostosis syndrome, both of which exhibit autosomal dominant transmission. Cytogenetic studies reveal the most frequent chromosomal alterations in both sporadic osteochondromas and Langer-Giedion osteochondromas to be loss or rearrangement of 8q24.1,[418] although DNA copy number changes have not been observed by CGH.[419] The chromosomal alterations at 8q24.1 correspond to the locus of the *EXT1* gene; chromosomal microdeletions at this site are responsible for the hereditary exostosis syndrome and apparently for many sporadic osteochrondromas as well. A second gene found at 11p11-12, *EXT2*, may be implicated in a second subset of osteochondromas, both sporadic and hereditary.[418, 420, 421]

Chondrosarcoma

Chondrosarcoma typically displays an extremely complex karyotype. Abnormalities at 6q13-21 appear to be associated with locally aggressive behavior in cartilage tumors, but the genetic basis of this behavior is unknown.[422] CGH studies generally demonstrate gains of whole chromosomes or whole chromosome arms, most frequently at 20q and 17p. High-level amplifications occur in less than 20% of cases; localized losses are equally rare, occurring at 6cen-q22 and 9p.[423] The relationship between CGH changes observed on chromosome 6q and clinical behavior has not been established but might be expected to be similar to those found through classic cytogenetic techniques. Interestingly, chromosome 9p is involved in the translocation of extraskeletal myxoid chondrosarcoma, although this translocation is not seen in "garden variety" chondrosarcoma. After pedigree studies linked the familial osteochondroma syndrome to the *EXT1* and *EXT2* genes,[424] it was shown that chondrosarcoma frequently also exhibits LOH at these gene loci[425] and also demonstrates

10q abnormalities that do not correlate with grade or prognosis in two thirds of cases.[426] LOH in the region of *TP53* on 17p is found in 25% of cases overall, and in 80% of high-grade chondrosarcomas.[427] LOH is accompanied by *TP53* gene mutations; the presence of *TP53* gene mutation is correlated with high tumor grade and indicative of aggressive behavior in long-term follow-up studies.[427–430] LOH also is found near the retinoblastoma gene locus (13q) in 36% of chondrosarcomas and again is more common in high-grade tumors.[427]

Amplification of the *MYC* and *CDK4* genes has been observed in chondrosarcoma, but the clinical significance has not been determined.[431, 432]

IHC assessment of p53 accumulation reveals that overexpression, like mutation, is associated with high-grade lesions, increased cellular proliferation, and a worse prognosis.[428–430, 433–436] IHC evidence of increased proliferative activity by PCNA or Ki-67 assessment is also associated with adverse outcome[434, 435, 437]; multivariate analysis suggests that assessment of the Ki-67 (MIB1) index has independent prognostic significance and that assessment of IHC accumulation of p53 conveys no additional prognostic information.[434]

Flow cytometry and image analysis of high-grade chondrosarcoma demonstrates aneuploid DNA histograms, in keeping with the complex karyotypes observed in these tumors[433, 438–440]; well-differentiated components of these tumors display aneuploid histograms, however.[433] Diploid chondrosarcomas tend to be of low histologic grade and not recur[438]; whether DNA histogram assessment provides prognostic information beyond that given by tumor grade and/or IHC assessment of proliferation fraction is unknown.

Although the diagnosis of chondrosarcoma is usually made on radiologic and morphologic grounds, IHC assays (Table 15–15) may occasionally help with the diagnosis of a dedifferentiated tumor.

TABLE 15–15

Immunoreactivity of Selected Markers in Chondrosarcoma

Immunohistochemical Marker	Percentage of Cases Demonstrating Immunoreactivity
Vimentin	95–100
HBME-1	93–100
S-100	90–99
CAM 5.2	0–15
Epithelial membrane antigen	0–6
AE1/AE3	0
Carcinoembryonic antigen	0
Desmin	0

Giant Cell Tumor

Giant cell tumor, which constitutes about 1 in 20 primary bone tumors, is generally benign but may be locally very destructive. The most common cytogenetic finding is random telomeric fusion, with most frequent involvement of 11p, 13p, 15p, 18p, 19p, and 21p.[441–443] Telomerase activity is found in most or all giant cell tumors[444]; tumors showing the greatest telomere reduction are those most likely to demonstrate telomeric fusion.[445] The factors that promote telomere fusion in giant cell tumor, but not other tumors with high telomerase activity, are unknown. Clonal structural karyotypic abnormalities are relatively uncommon and most frequently involve 11p15 and fusions of chromosomes 14p or 15p with chromosome 21p.[442] Most tumors that behave benignly demonstrate no chromosomal abnormalities, whereas chromosomal abnormalities are found in 90% of those tumors that are locally aggressive, recurrent, or metastatic.[441]

Although alterations in *MYCN*, *MYC*, and *FOS* oncogenes have been detected in giant cell tumors, the relationship of these changes to pathogenesis or prognosis is unclear.[446] IHC accumulation of p53 has been observed in slightly more than 10% of cases and may be associated with a worse prognosis.[447] Microsatellite instability does not appear to play a role in the pathogenesis of giant cell tumors.[448] DNA flow cytometry has no demonstrated value in the assessment of giant cell tumors.[449]

Osteosarcoma

The most common malignant tumors of bone are found in both children and adults. Cytogenetic analysis typically reveals complex karyotypic features, although relatively normal karyotypes may also be observed.[450, 451] Although no specific chromosomal aberrations have been described, losses of chromosome 3, 10, 13, and 15 are frequently described.[452] Chromosome 13 losses, which occur in half of cases, may be associated with inactivation of the 13q14 retinoblastoma *(RB1)* gene, alterations of which are frequent in osteosarcoma.[453–456] Patients whose tumors demonstrate structural abnormalities at the *RB1* locus appear to have a worse prognosis than those that do not.[457]

The mechanism by which RB1 suppresses tumor formation has only partially been elucidated. There appears to be a role for the protein in suppression of apoptosis,[458] as well as in suppression of tumor cell invasion.[459] The most important and well-elucidated role, however, appears to be as a phosphorylated nuclear DNA-binding protein acting as part of a cell-cycle control pathway that includes the gene product CDKN2A, and CDK4.[460] Inactivation of *RB1* by mutation, deletion, methylation, or viral sequestration results in inactivation of the $G_1 \rightarrow S$ phase cell cycle checkpoint, with resulting unchecked cell cycling that is linked to changes in the phosphorylation and dephosphorylation of RB1.[461, 462] Mutational inactivation of the *CDKN2A* gene product is frequently observed in osteosarcomas that lack *RB1* alterations.[460] Abnormalities of *CDKN2A* or *RB1* appear to be present in virtually all osteosarcomas. Both *RB1* and *CDKN2A* abnormalities are generally accompanied by amplification of the *CDK4* gene, which seems to occur in association with (and possibly as a result of) compensatory overexpression.[432, 460, 461] Amplifications have also been observed in *MYC*, *CHOP*, *RAF1*, *GLI*, and *MDM2*[431, 463–467] but do not appear to have great clinical significance. *CDK4* mutations have not been detected in osteosarcoma, suggesting the possibility that mutations at this locus are fatal to the cell.

The *TP53* gene codes for a binding protein that blocks progression of cells through the cell cycle late in the G_1 phase of cell replication, before the G_1/S checkpoint and may also be involved in regulation at the G_2/M checkpoint. Thus, cells that lack functional p53 do not exhibit G_1 arrest. Modulation of p53 activity affects a number of other regulatory proteins, including MDM2, cyclin G_1, BAX, and CDKN1A. Point mutations or deletions of the *TP53* gene are found in about 20% of osteosarcomas,[436, 468–473] including tumors with features of low-grade malignancy.[474] IHC accumulation of p53 is associated with neither higher proliferative rate in osteosarcomas[466] nor outcome.[475] Thus, the significance of p53 alterations in the pathogenesis of osteosarcoma remains obscure.

IHC assessment of proliferation demonstrates strong correlation between adverse outcome and overexpression of cyclin A,[476] cyclin D1,[476] or Ki-67.[437] These findings correlate with histologic grade, however, and probably do not have independent prognostic significance. Flow and image cytometry commonly reveal aneuploid DNA histograms (in keeping with the karyotypic complexity of osteosarcoma) that correlate well with the degree of histologic differentiation and provide no prognostic information beyond that obtained by histologic examination.[477] Most osteosarcomas show no telomerase activity.[478]

Diagnosis of osteosarcoma is based primarily on consideration of morphologic and radiologic findings and seldom requires immunocytochemical assistance. Selected IHC characteristics are shown in Table 15–16. Osteonectin, although commonly observed in osteosarcoma, is of little practical diagnostic value because it is found frequently in a wide variety of other tumors, including spindle cell carcinoma and soft tissue sarcomas.

TABLE 15–16

Immunoreactivity of Selected Markers in Osteosarcoma

Immunohistochemical Marker	Percentage of Cases Demonstrating Immunoreactivity
Vimentin	100
Osteonectin	83–100
α_1-Antichymotrypsin	61–97
α_1-Antitrypsin	54–100
Actin (SM)	37–67
CD99	21–49
Epithelial membrane antigen	22–46
S-100	20–44
Desmin	2–20
Keratin (pan)	0–8
CAM 5.2	0

PAROSTEAL OSTEOSARCOMA

Parosteal (juxtacortical) osteosarcoma is an osteosarcoma variant with a characteristic clinical/radiologic presentation, diploid DNA histogram,[477] and a relatively good prognosis. These tumors are characterized cytogenetically by the presence of a supernumerary ring chromosome, often as the sole anomaly.[451, 479] CGH demonstrates gains in 12q13-15 in nearly every tumor.[479] These gains are strongly correlated with the presence of ring chromosomes, which have been shown by chromosome painting to consist entirely of chromosome 12 material. These changes are accompanied by amplification of the *CDK4*, *MDM2*, and *SAS* genes, which are in turn overexpressed.[480] The relationship between these findings and the relative indolence of parosteal osteosarcoma is unknown, and other characteristic molecular abnormalities have not been identified.

REFERENCES

1. Gerald WL, Miller HK, Battifora H, et al: Intra-abdominal desmoplastic small round-cell tumor: Report of 19 cases of a distinctive type of high-grade polyphenotypic malignancy affecting young individuals [see comments]. Am J Surg Pathol 1991;15:499–513.
2. Biegel JA, Conard K, Brooks JJ: Translocation (11;22)(p13;q12): Primary change in intra-abdominal desmoplastic small round cell tumor. Genes Chromosomes Cancer 1993;7:119–121.
3. Rodriguez E, Sreekantaiah C, Gerald W, et al: A recurring translocation, t(11;22)(p13;q11.2), characterizes intra-abdominal desmoplastic small round-cell tumors. Cancer Genet Cytogenet 1993;69:17–21.
4. Ladanyi M, Gerald W: Fusion of the *EWS* and *WT1* genes in the desmoplastic small round cell tumor. Cancer Res 1994;54:2837–2840.
5. Benjamin LE, Fredericks WJ, Barr FG, Rauscher FJ: Fusion of the *EWS1* and *WT1* genes as a result of the t(11;22)(p13;q12) translocation in desmoplastic small round cell tumors. Med Pediatr Oncol 1996;27:434–439.

6. Froberg K, Brown RE, Gaylord H, Manivel C: Intra-abdominal desmoplastic small round cell tumor: Immunohistochemical evidence for up-regulation of autocrine and paracrine growth factors. Ann Clin Lab Sci 1998; 28:386–393.
7. Ordonez NG, el-Naggar AK, Ro JY, et al: Intra-abdominal desmoplastic small cell tumor: A light microscopic, immunocytochemical, ultrastructural, and flow cytometric study [see comments]. Hum Pathol 1993;24:850–865.
8. Barr FG, Chatten J, D'Cruz CM, et al: Molecular assays for chromosomal translocations in the diagnosis of pediatric soft tissue sarcomas. JAMA 1995;273:553–557.
9. de Alava E, Ladanyi M, Rosai J, Gerald WL: Detection of chimeric transcripts in desmoplastic small round cell tumor and related developmental tumors by reverse transcriptase polymerase chain reaction: A specific diagnostic assay. Am J Pathol 1995;147:1584–1591.
10. Ali SZ, Hoon V, Hoda S, et al: Solitary fibrous tumor: A cytologic-histologic study with clinical, radiologic, and immunohistochemical correlations. Cancer 1997;81: 116–121.
11. Khalifa MA, Montgomery EA, Azumi N, et al: Solitary fibrous tumors: A series of lesions, some in unusual sites. South Med J 1997;90:793–799.
12. van de Rijn M, Lombard CM, Rouse RV: Expression of CD34 by solitary fibrous tumors of the pleura, mediastinum, and lung [see comments]. Am J Surg Pathol 1994; 18:814–820.
13. Yokoi T, Tsuzuki T, Yatabe Y, et al: Solitary fibrous tumour: Significance of p53 and CD34 immunoreactivity in its malignant transformation. Histopathology 1998;32: 423–432.
14. Miettinen MM, el-Rifai W, Sarlomo-Rikala M, et al: Tumor size-related DNA copy number changes occur in solitary fibrous tumors but not in hemangiopericytomas. Mod Pathol 1997;10:1194–1200.
15. Dal Cin P, Sciot R, Fletcher CD, et al: Trisomy 21 in solitary fibrous tumor. Cancer Genet Cytogenet 1996; 86:58–60.
16. Alman BA, Pajerski ME, Diaz-Cano S, et al: Aggressive fibromatosis (desmoid tumor) is a monoclonal disorder. Diagn Mol Pathol 1997;6:98-101.
17. Lucas DR, Shroyer KR, McCarthy PJ, et al: Desmoid tumor is a clonal cellular proliferation: PCR amplification of HUMARA for analysis of patterns of X-chromosome inactivation. Am J Surg Pathol 1997;21:306–311.
18. Li M, Cordon-Cardo C, Gerald WL, Rosai J: Desmoid fibromatosis is a clonal process. Hum Pathol 1996;27: 939–943.
19. Dal Cin P, Sciot R, Aly MS, et al: Some desmoid tumors are characterized by trisomy 8. Genes Chromosomes Cancer 1994;10:131–135.
20. Dei TA, Dal Cin P: The role of cytogenetics in the classification of soft tissue tumours. Virchows Arch 1997;431: 83–94.
21. Fletcher JA, Naeem R, Xiao S, Corson JM: Chromosome aberrations in desmoid tumors: Trisomy 8 may be a predictor of recurrence [see comments]. Cancer Genet Cytogenet 1995;79:139–143.
22. Kouho H, Aoki T, Hisaoka M, Hashimoto H: Clinicopathological and interphase cytogenetic analysis of desmoid tumours. Histopathology 1997;31:336–341.
23. de Silva DC, Wright MF, Stevenson DA, et al: Cranial desmoid tumor associated with homozygous inactivation of the adenomatous polyposis coli gene in a 2-year-old girl with familial adenomatous polyposis. Cancer 1996; 77:972–976.
24. Alman BA, Li C, Pajerski ME, et al: Increased beta-catenin protein and somatic APC mutations in sporadic aggressive fibromatoses (desmoid tumors). Am J Pathol 1997;151:329–334.
25. Alman BA, Goldberg MJ, Naber SP, et al: Aggressive fibromatosis. J Pediatr Orthop 1992;12:1–10.
26. Alman BA, Naber SP, Terek RM, et al: Platelet-derived growth factor in fibrous musculoskeletal disorders: A study of pathologic tissue sections and in vitro primary cell cultures. J Orthop Res 1995;13:67–77.
27. Naito Y, Ohori K, Tanaka M, et al: Collagen and elastin synthesis by desmoid tumor in vitro. Pathol Int 1998;48:603–610.
28. Scates DK, Clark SK, Phillips RK, Venitt S: Lack of telomerase in desmoids occurring sporadically and in association with familial adenomatous polyposis. Br J Surg 1998;85:965–969.
29. Eccles DM, van der Luijt R, Breukel C, et al: Hereditary desmoid disease due to a frameshift mutation at codon 1924 of the *APC* gene [see comments]. Am J Hum Genet 1996;59:1193–1201.
30. Scott RJ, Froggatt NJ, Trembath RC, et al: Familial infiltrative fibromatosis (desmoid tumours) (MIM135290) caused by a recurrent 3′ *APC* gene mutation. Hum Mol Genet 1996;5:1921–1924.
31. Frankenthaler R, Ayala AG, Hartwick RW, Goepfert H: Fibrosarcoma of the head and neck. Laryngoscope 1990; 100:799–802.
32. Madhavan M, Krishnan KB: Cell marker studies in undifferentiated soft tissue sarcoma. Indian J Pathol Microbiol 1991;34:99–103.
33. Meis JM, Enzinger FM: Inflammatory fibrosarcoma of the mesentery and retroperitoneum: A tumor closely simulating inflammatory pseudotumor. Am J Surg Pathol 1991;15:1146–1156.
34. Meis-Kindblom JM, Kjellstrom C, Kindblom LG: Inflammatory fibrosarcoma: Update, reappraisal, and perspective on its place in the spectrum of inflammatory myofibroblastic tumors. Semin Diagn Pathol 1998;15: 133–143.
35. Oshiro Y, Fukuda T, Tsuneyoshi M: Fibrosarcoma versus fibromatoses and cellular nodular fasciitis: A comparative study of their proliferative activity using proliferating cell nuclear antigen, DNA flow cytometry, and p53. Am J Surg Pathol 1994;18:712–719.
36. Miettinen MM, el-Rifai W, Sarlomo-Rikala M, et al: Tumor size–related DNA copy number changes occur in solitary fibrous tumors but not in hemangiopericytomas. Mod Pathol 1997;10:1194–1200.
37. Schofield DE, Fletcher JA, Grier HE, Yunis EJ: Fibrosarcoma in infants and children: Application of new techniques. Am J Surg Pathol 1994;18:14–24.
38. Knezevich SR, McFadden DE, Tao W, et al: A novel *ETV6-NTRK3* gene fusion in congenital fibrosarcoma. Nat Genet 1998;18:184–187.
39. Knezevich SR, Garnett MJ, Pysher TJ, et al: *ETV6-NTRK3* gene fusions and trisomy 11 establish a histogenetic link

between mesoblastic nephroma and congenital fibrosarcoma. Cancer Res 1998;58:5046–5048.

40. Miettinen M: Antibody specific to muscle actins in the diagnosis and classification of soft tissue tumors. Am J Pathol 1988;130:205–215.
41. Mandahl N, Heim S, Willen H, et al: Characteristic karyotypic anomalies identify subtypes of malignant fibrous histiocytoma. Genes Chromosomes Cancer 1989; 1:9–14.
42. Mertens F, Fletcher CD, Dal Cin P, et al: Cytogenetic analysis of 46 pleomorphic soft tissue sarcomas and correlation with morphologic and clinical features: A report of the CHAMP Study Group. Chromosomes and Morphology. Genes Chromosomes Cancer 1998;22:16–25.
43. Sakabe T, Shinomiya T, Mori T, et al: Identification of a novel gene, *MASL1*, within an amplicon at 8p23.1 detected in malignant fibrous histiocytomas by comparative genomic hybridization. Cancer Res 1999;59:511–515.
44. Hinze R, Schagdarsurengin U, Taubert H, et al: Assessment of genomic imbalances in malignant fibrous histiocytomas by comparative genomic hybridization. Int J Mol Med 1999;3:75–79.
45. Jankowski SA, Mitchell DS, Smith SH, et al: *SAS*, a gene amplified in human sarcomas, encodes a new member of the transmembrane 4 superfamily of proteins. Oncogene 1994;9:1205–1211.
46. Smith SH, Weiss SW, Jankowski SA, et al: *SAS* amplification in soft tissue sarcomas. Cancer Res 1992;52: 3746–3749.
47. Nilbert M, Rydholm A, Willen H, et al: *MDM2* gene amplification correlates with ring chromosome in soft tissue tumors. Genes Chromosomes Cancer 1994;9: 261–265.
48. Reid AH, Tsai MM, Venzon DJ, et al: *MDM2* amplification, *P53* mutation, and accumulation of the P53 gene product in malignant fibrous histiocytoma. Diagn Mol Pathol 1996;5:65–73.
49. Jensen V, Sorensen FB, Bentzen SM, et al: Proliferative activity (MIB-1 index) is an independent prognostic parameter in patients with high-grade soft tissue sarcomas of subtypes other than malignant fibrous histiocytomas: A retrospective immunohistological study including 216 soft tissue sarcomas. Histopathology 1998;32:536–546.
50. Leach FS, Tokino T, Meltzer P, et al: *p53* Mutation and *MDM2* amplification in human soft tissue sarcomas. Cancer Res 1993;53(10 Suppl):2231–2234.
51. Nakanishi H, Ohsawa M, Naka N, et al: Immunohistochemical detection of bcl-2 and p53 proteins and apoptosis in soft tissue sarcoma: Their correlations with prognosis. Oncology 1997;54:238–244.
52. Soini Y, Vahakangas K, Nuorva K, et al: p53 immunohistochemistry in malignant fibrous histiocytomas and other mesenchymal tumours. J Pathol 1992;168:29–33.
53. Szadowska A, Olborski B, Harezga-Bal B, Debiec-Rychter M: Immunohistochemical status of p53, mdm2 and Ki-67 in malignant fibrous histiocytoma. Pol J Pathol 1998;49:15–21.
54. Taubert H, Wurl P, Meye A, et al: Molecular and immunohistochemical *p53* status in liposarcoma and malignant fibrous histiocytoma: Identification of seven new mutations for soft tissue sarcomas. Cancer 1995; 76:1187–1196.
55. Yang P, Hirose T, Hasegawa T, et al: Prognostic implication of the p53 protein and Ki-67 antigen immunohistochemistry in malignant fibrous histiocytoma. Cancer 1995;76:618–625.
56. Stefanou DG, Nonni AV, Agnantis NJ, et al: p53/MDM-2 immunohistochemical expression correlated with proliferative activity in different subtypes of human sarcomas: A ten-year follow-up study. Anticancer Res 1998; 18:4673–4681.
57. Choong PF, Ferno M, Akerman M, et al: Urokinase-plasminogen-activator levels and prognosis in 69 soft-tissue sarcomas. Int J Cancer 1996;69:268–272.
58. Tetu B, Lacasse B, Bouchard HL, et al: Prognostic influence of HSP-27 expression in malignant fibrous histiocytoma: A clinicopathological and immunohistochemical study. Cancer Res 1992;52:2325–2328.
59. Dreinhofer KE, Akerman M, Willen H, et al: Proliferating cell nuclear antigen (PCNA) in high-grade malignant fibrous histiocytoma: Prognostic value in 48 patients. Int J Cancer 1994;59:379–382.
60. Becker RLJ, Venzon D, Lack EE, et al: Cytometry and morphometry of malignant fibrous histiocytoma of the extremities: Prediction of metastasis and mortality. Am J Surg Pathol 1991;15:957–964.
61. Pettinato G, Manivel JC, De Rosa G, et al: Angiomatoid malignant fibrous histiocytoma: Cytologic, immunohistochemical, ultrastructural, and flow cytometric study of 20 cases. Mod Pathol 1990;3:479–487.
62. el-Naggar AK, Ro JY, Ayala AG, et al: Angiomatoid malignant fibrous histiocytoma: Flow cytometric DNA analysis of six cases. J Surg Oncol 1989;40:201–204.
63. Fletcher CD: Angiomatoid "malignant fibrous histiocytoma": An immunohistochemical study indicative of myoid differentiation. Hum Pathol 1991;22:563–568.
64. Granter SR, Badizadegan K, Fletcher CD: Myofibromatosis in adults, glomangiopericytoma, and myopericytoma: A spectrum of tumors showing perivascular myoid differentiation. Am J Surg Pathol 1998;22:513–525.
65. Rosenberg AE, O'Connell JX, Dickersin GR, Bhan AK: Expression of epithelial markers in malignant fibrous histiocytoma of the musculoskeletal system: An immunohistochemical and electron microscopic study. Hum Pathol 1993;24:284–293.
66. Suster S, Fisher C, Moran CA: Expression of bcl-2 oncoprotein in benign and malignant spindle cell tumors of soft tissue, skin, serosal surfaces, and gastrointestinal tract. Am J Surg Pathol 1998;22:863–872.
67. Templeton SF, Solomon ARJ: Spindle cell lipoma is strongly CD34 positive: An immunohistochemical study. J Cutan Pathol 1996;23:546–550.
68. Mandahl N, Heim S, Johansson B, et al: Lipomas have characteristic structural chromosomal rearrangements of 12q13-q14. Int J Cancer 1987;39:685–688.
69. Wanschura S, Kazmierczak B, Schoenmakers E, et al: Regional fine mapping of the multiple-aberration region involved in uterine leiomyoma, lipoma, and pleomorphic adenoma of the salivary gland to 12q15 [see comments]. Genes Chromosomes Cancer 1995;14:68–70.
70. Petit MR, Mols R, Schoenmakers EF, et al: LPP, the preferred fusion partner gene of HMGIC in lipomas, is a novel member of the LIM protein gene family. Genomics 1996;36:118–129.

71. Merscher S, Marondel I, Pedeutour F, et al: Identification of new translocation breakpoints at 12q13 in lipomas. Genomics 1997;46:70–77.
72. Rogalla P, Kazmierczak B, Meyer-Bolte K, et al: The t(3;12)(q27;q14-q15) with underlying HMGIC-LPP fusion is not determining an adipocytic phenotype. Genes Chromosomes Cancer 1998;22:100–104.
73. Iwasaki H, Ohjimi Y, Ishiguro M, et al: Supernumerary ring chromosomes and nuclear blebs in some low-grade malignant soft tissue tumours: Atypical lipomatous tumours and dermatofibrosarcoma protuberans. Virchows Arch 1998;432:521–528.
74. Mandahl N, Akerman M, Aman P, et al: Duplication of chromosome segment 12q15-24 is associated with atypical lipomatous tumors: A report of the CHAMP collaborative study group. CHromosomes And MorPhology. Int J Cancer 1996;67:632–635.
75. Tallini G, Dal Cin P, Rhoden KJ, et al: Expression of HMGI-C and HMGI(Y) in ordinary lipoma and atypical lipomatous tumors: Immunohistochemical reactivity correlates with karyotypic alterations. Am J Pathol 1997; 151:37–43.
76. Dal Cin P, Kools P, Sciot R, et al: Cytogenetic and fluorescence in situ hybridization investigation of ring chromosomes characterizing a specific pathologic subgroup of adipose tissue tumors. Cancer Genet Cytogenet 1993;68: 85–90.
77. Nilbert M, Rydholm A, Mitelman F, et al: Characterization of the 12q13-15 amplicon in soft tissue tumors. Cancer Genet Cytogenet 1995;83:32–36.
78. Schneider-Stock R, Walter H, Radig K, et al: *MDM2* amplification and loss of heterozygosity at *Rb* and *p53* genes: No simultaneous alterations in the oncogenesis of liposarcomas. J Cancer Res Clin Oncol 1998;124:532–540.
79. Willeke F, Ridder R, Mechtersheimer G, et al: Analysis of FUS-CHOP fusion transcripts in different types of soft tissue liposarcoma and their diagnostic implications. Clin Cancer Res 1998;4:1779–1784.
80. Forus A, Kools PF, Schoenmakers EF, et al: A long range restriction map spanning the myxoid liposarcoma breakpoint in the q13-14 region of human chromosome 12. Hum Genet 1994;94:259–264.
81. Gibas Z, Miettinen M, Limon J, et al: Cytogenetic and immunohistochemical profile of myxoid liposarcoma. Am J Clin Pathol 1995;103:20–26.
82. Tallini G, Akerman M, Dal Cin P, et al: Combined morphologic and karyotypic study of 28 myxoid liposarcomas: Implications for a revised morphologic typing (a report from the CHAMP Group). Am J Surg Pathol 1996;20:1047–1055.
83. Adelmant G, Gilbert JD, Freytag SO: Human translocation liposarcoma-CCAAT/enhancer binding protein (C/EBP) homologous protein (TLS-CHOP) oncoprotein prevents adipocyte differentiation by directly interfering with C/EBPbeta function. J Biol Chem 1998;273: 15574–15581.
84. Dal Cin P, Sciot R, Panagopoulos I, et al: Additional evidence of a variant translocation t(12;22) with EWS/CHOP fusion in myxoid liposarcoma: Clinicopathological features. J Pathol 1997;182:437–441.
85. Hisaoka M, Tsuji S, Morimitsu Y, et al: Detection of TLS/FUS-CHOP fusion transcripts in myxoid and round cell liposarcomas by nested reverse transcription-polymerase chain reaction using archival paraffin-embedded tissues. Diagn Mol Pathol 1998;7:96–101.
86. Yoshida H, Nagao K, Ito H, et al: Chromosomal translocations in human soft tissue sarcomas by interphase fluorescence in situ hybridization. Pathol Int 1997;47: 222–229.
87. Dal Cin P, Sciot R, De Wever I, et al: New discriminative chromosomal marker in adipose tissue tumors: The chromosome 8q11-q13 region in lipoblastoma. Cancer Genet Cytogenet 1994;78:232–235.
88. Fletcher CD, Akerman M, Dal Cin P, et al: Correlation between clinicopathological features and karyotype in lipomatous tumors: A report of 178 cases from the Chromosomes and Morphology (CHAMP) Collaborative Study Group. Am J Pathol 1996;148:623–630.
89. Heim S, Nilbert M, Vanni R, et al: A specific translocation, t(12;14)(q14-15;q23-24), characterizes a subgroup of uterine leiomyomas. Cancer Genet Cytogenet 1988; 32:13–17.
90. Karaiskos C, Pandis N, Bardi G, et al: Cytogenetic findings in uterine epithelioid leiomyomas. Cancer Genet Cytogenet 1995;80:103–106.
91. Nibert M, Heim S: Uterine leiomyoma cytogenetics. Genes Chromosomes Cancer 1990;2:3–13.
92. Schoenmakers EF, Huysmans C, Van de Ven WJ: Allelic knockout of novel splice variants of human recombination repair gene RAD51B in t(12;14) uterine leiomyomas. Cancer Res 1999;59:19–23.
93. Kazmierczak B, Hennig Y, Wanschura S, et al: Description of a novel fusion transcript between HMGI-C, a gene encoding for a member of the high mobility group proteins, and the mitochondrial aldehyde dehydrogenase gene. Cancer Res 1995;55:6038–6039.
94. Arheden K, Nilbert M, Heim S, et al: No amplification or rearrangement of *INT1*, *GLI*, or *COL2A1* in uterine leiomyomas with t(12;14)(q14-15;q23-24). Cancer Genet Cytogenet 1989;39:195–201.
95. Brandon DD, Erickson TE, Keenan EJ, et al: Estrogen receptor gene expression in human uterine leiomyomata. J Clin Endocrinol Metab 1995;80:1876–1881.
96. Harrison-Woolrych ML, Charnock-Jones DS, Smith SK: Quantification of messenger ribonucleic acid for epidermal growth factor in human myometrium and leiomyomata using reverse transcriptase polymerase chain reaction. J Clin Endocrinol Metab 1994;78: 1179–1184.
97. Fujimoto J, Hori M, Ichigo S, et al: Tissue differences in the expression of mRNAs of Ha-ras, c-myc, fos and jun in human uterine endometrium, myometrium and leiomyoma under the influence of estrogen/progesterone. Tumour Biol 1994;15:311–317.
98. Shimomura Y, Matsuo H, Samoto T, Maruo T: Up-regulation by progesterone of proliferating cell nuclear antigen and epidermal growth factor expression in human uterine leiomyoma. J Clin Endocrinol Metab 1998;83: 2192–2198.
99. Kawaguchi K, Fujii S, Konishi I, et al: Immunohistochemical analysis of oestrogen receptors, progesterone receptors and Ki-67 in leiomyoma and myometrium during the menstrual cycle and pregnancy. Virchows Arch A Pathol Anat Histopathol 1991;419:309–315.

100. Zhai YL, Kobayashi Y, Mori A, et al: Expression of steroid receptors, Ki-67, and p53 in uterine leiomyosarcomas. Int J Gynecol Pathol 1999;18:20–28.
101. Niemann TH, Raab SS, Lenel JC, et al: p53 protein overexpression in smooth muscle tumors of the uterus. Hum Pathol 1995;26:375–379.
102. Ueki Y, Naito I, Oohashi T, et al: Topoisomerase I and II consensus sequences in a 17-kb deletion junction of the *COL4A5* and *COL4A6* genes and immunohistochemical analysis of esophageal leiomyomatosis associated with Alport syndrome. Am J Hum Genet 1998; 62:253–261.
103. Gal AA, Brooks JS, Pietra GG: Leiomyomatous neoplasms of the lung: A clinical, histologic, and immunohistochemical study [see comments]. Mod Pathol 1989; 2:209–216.
104. Due W, Pickartz H: Immunohistologic detection of estrogen and progesterone receptors in disseminated peritoneal leiomyomatosis. Int J Gynecol Pathol 1989; 8:46–53.
105. Bluhm JM, Yi ES, Diaz G, et al: Multicentric endobronchial smooth muscle tumors associated with the Epstein-Barr virus in an adult patient with the acquired immunodeficiency syndrome: A case report. Cancer 1997;80:1910–1913.
106. Jimenez-Heffernan JA, Hardisson D, Palacios J, et al: Adrenal gland leiomyoma in a child with acquired immunodeficiency syndrome. Pediatr Pathol Lab Med 1995;15:923–929.
107. Kleinschmidt-DeMasters BK, Mierau GW, Sze CI, et al: Unusual dural and skull-based mesenchymal neoplasms: A report of four cases. Hum Pathol 1998;29: 240–245.
108. McClain KL, Leach CT, Jenson HB, et al: Association of Epstein-Barr virus with leiomyosarcomas in children with AIDS [see comments]. N Engl J Med 1995;332: 12–18.
109. Jenson HB, Leach CT, McClain KL, et al: Benign and malignant smooth muscle tumors containing Epstein-Barr virus in children with AIDS. Leuk Lymphoma 1997;27:303–314.
110. Matsuo H, Maruo T, Samoto T: Increased expression of Bcl-2 protein in human uterine leiomyoma and its up-regulation by progesterone. J Clin Endocrinol Metab 1997;82:293–299.
111. Zheng PS, Iwasaka T, Yamasaki F, et al: Telomerase activity in gynecologic tumors. Gynecol Oncol 1997; 64:171–175.
112. Nilbert M, Heim S, Mandahl N, et al: Complex karyotypic anomalies in a bizarre leiomyoma of the uterus. Genes Chromosomes Cancer 1989;1:131–134.
113. Peters WA, Howard DR, Andersen WA, Figge DC: Deoxyribonucleic acid analysis by flow cytometry of uterine leiomyosarcomas and smooth muscle tumors of uncertain malignant potential. Am J Obstet Gynecol 1992;166:1646–1653.
114. Tsushima K, Stanhope CR, Gaffey TA, Lieber MM: Uterine leiomyosarcomas and benign smooth muscle tumors: Usefulness of nuclear DNA patterns studied by flow cytometry. Mayo Clin Proc 1988;63:248–255.
115. el-Rifai W, Sarlomo-Rikala M, Knuutila S, Miettinen M: DNA copy number changes in development and progression in leiomyosarcomas of soft tissues. Am J Pathol 1998;153:985–990.
116. Nordal RR, Kristensen GB, Kaern J, et al: The prognostic significance of stage, tumor size, cellular atypia and DNA ploidy in uterine leiomyosarcoma. Acta Oncol 1995;34:797–802.
117. Blom R, Guerrieri C, Stal O, et al: Leiomyosarcoma of the uterus: A clinicopathologic, DNA flow cytometric, p53, and mdm-2 analysis of 49 cases. Gynecol Oncol 1998;68:54–61.
118. de Vos S, Wilczynski SP, Fleischhacker M, Koeffler P: p53 alterations in uterine leiomyosarcomas versus leiomyomas. Gynecol Oncol 1994;54:205–208.
119. Dei TA, Maestro R, Doglioni C, et al: Tumor suppressor genes and related molecules in leiomyosarcoma. Am J Pathol 1996;148:1037–1045.
120. Hall KL, Teneriello MG, Taylor RR, et al: Analysis of Ki-*ras*, *p53*, and *MDM2* genes in uterine leiomyomas and leiomyosarcomas. Gynecol Oncol 1997;65:330–335.
121. Konomoto T, Fukuda T, Hayashi K, et al: Leiomyosarcoma in soft tissue: Examination of p53 status and cell proliferating factors in different locations. Hum Pathol 1998;29:74–81.
122. Hill MA, Gong C, Casey TJ, et al: Detection of K-*ras* mutations in resected primary leiomyosarcoma. Cancer Epidemiol Biomarkers Prev 1997;6:1095–1100.
123. Wilke W, Maillet M, Robinson R: H-*ras*-1 point mutations in soft tissue sarcomas. Mod Pathol 1993;6:129–132.
124. Jeffers MD, Richmond JA, Macaulay EM: Overexpression of the c-*myc* proto-oncogene occurs frequently in uterine sarcomas. Mod Pathol 1995;8:701–704.
125. Appelman HD, Helwig EB: Sarcomas of the stomach. Am J Clin Pathol 1977;67:2–10.
126. Appelman HD: Smooth muscle tumors of the gastrointestinal tract. What we know now that Stout didn't know. Am J Surg Pathol 1986;10 (Suppl 1):83–99.
127. Appleman HD, Helwig EB: Gastric epithelioid leiomyoma and leiomyosarcoma (leiomyoblastoma). Cancer 1976;38:708–728.
128. Ranchod M, Kempson RL: Smooth muscle tumors of the gastrointestinal tract and retroperitoneum: A pathologic analysis of 100 cases. Cancer 1977;39:255–262.
129. Erlandson RA, Klimstra DS, Woodruff JM: Subclassification of gastrointestinal stromal tumors based on evaluation by electron microscopy and immunohistochemistry [see comments]. Ultrastruct Pathol 1996;20:373–393.
130. Hurlimann J, Gardiol D: Gastrointestinal stromal tumours: An immunohistochemical study of 165 cases. Histopathology 1991;19:311–320.
131. Ma CK, Amin MB, Kintanar E, et al: Immunohistologic characterization of gastrointestinal stromal tumors: A study of 82 cases compared with 11 cases of leiomyomas. Mod Pathol 1993;6:139–144.
132. Sarlomo-Rikala M, Kovatich AJ, Barusevicius A, Miettinen M: CD117: A sensitive marker for gastrointestinal stromal tumors that is more specific than CD34. Mod Pathol 1998;11:728–734.
133. Kindblom LG, Remotti HE, Aldenborg F, Meis-Kindblom JM: Gastrointestinal pacemaker cell tumor (GIPACT): Gastrointestinal stromal tumors show phenotypic characteristics of the interstitial cells of Cajal. Am J Pathol 1998;152:1259–1269.

134. Emory TS, Sobin LH, Lukes L, et al: Prognosis of gastrointestinal smooth-muscle (stromal) tumors: Dependence on anatomic site. Am J Surg Pathol 1999;23:82–87.
135. Goldblum JR, Appelman HD: Stromal tumors of the duodenum: A histologic and immunohistochemical study of 20 cases. Am J Surg Pathol 1995;19:71–80.
136. Tworek JA, Appelman HD, Singleton TP, Greenson JK: Stromal tumors of the jejunum and ileum. Mod Pathol 1997;10:200–209.
137. Cunningham RE, Federspiel BH, McCarthy WF, et al: Predicting prognosis of gastrointestinal smooth muscle tumors: Role of clinical and histologic evaluation, flow cytometry, and image cytometry. Am J Surg Pathol 1993;17:588–594.
138. Roy M, Sommers SC: Metastatic potential of gastric leiomyosarcoma. Pathol Res Pract 1989;185:874–877.
139. Milanezi MF, Schmitt F: Pseudosarcomatous myofibroblastic proliferation of the spermatic cord (proliferative funiculitis) [letter]. Histopathology 1997;31: 387–388.
140. Emory TS, Derringer GA, Sobin LH, O'Leary TJ: Ki-67 (MIB-1) immunohistochemistry as a prognostic factor in gastrointestinal smooth-muscle tumors. J Surg Pathol 1997;2:239–242.
141. Franquemont DW, Frierson HF Jr: Proliferating cell nuclear antigen immunoreactivity and prognosis of gastrointestinal stromal tumors. Mod Pathol 1995;8: 473–477.
142. Sbaschnig RJ, Cunningham RE, Sobin LH, O'Leary TJ: Proliferating-cell nuclear antigen immunocytochemistry in the evaluation of gastrointestinal smooth-muscle tumors. Mod Pathol 1994;7:780–783.
143. Cooper PN, Quirke P, Hardy GJ, Dixon MF: A flow cytometric, clinical, and histological study of stromal neoplasms of the gastrointestinal tract. Am J Surg Pathol 1992;16:163–170.
144. el-Naggar AK, Ro JY, McLemore D, et al: Gastrointestinal stromal tumors: DNA flow-cytometric study of 58 patients with at least five years of follow-up. Mod Pathol 1989;2:511–515.
145. Kiyabu MT, Bishop PC, Parker JW, et al: Smooth muscle tumors of the gastrointestinal tract: Flow cytometric quantitation of DNA and nuclear antigen content and correlation with histologic grade. Am J Surg Pathol 1988;12:954–960.
146. Lerma E, Lee SJ, Tugues D, et al: Ploidy of 36 stromal tumors of the gastrointestinal tract: A comparative study with flow cytometry and image analysis. Anal Quant Cytol Histol 1994;16:435–440.
147. Shimamoto T, Haruma K, Sumii K, et al: Flow cytometric DNA analysis of gastric smooth muscle tumors. Cancer 1992;70:2031–2034.
148. Tsushima K, Rainwater LM, Goellner JR, et al: Leiomyosarcomas and benign smooth muscle tumors of the stomach: Nuclear DNA patterns studied by flow cytometry. Mayo Clin Proc 1987;62:275–280.
149. Ernst SI, Hubbs AE, Przygodzki RM, et al: *KIT* mutation portends poor prognosis in gastrointestinal stromal/ smooth muscle tumors. Lab Invest 1998;78:1633–1636.
150. Hirota S, Isozaki K, Moriyama Y, et al: Gain-of-function mutations of c-*kit* in human gastrointestinal stromal tumors. Science 1998;279:577–580.
151. Lasota J, Jasinski M, Sarlomo-Rikala M, Miettinen M: Mutations in exon 11 of c-*Kit* occur preferentially in malignant versus benign gastrointestinal stromal tumors and do not occur in leiomyomas or leiomyosarcomas. Am J Pathol 1999;154:53–60.
152. Gibas Z, Miettinen M: Recurrent parapharyngeal rhabdomyoma: Evidence of neoplastic nature of the tumor from cytogenetic study. Am J Surg Pathol 1992;16: 721–728.
153. Green AJ, Smith M, Yates JR: Loss of heterozygosity on chromosome 16p13.3 in hamartomas from tuberous sclerosis patients. Nat Genet 1994;6:193–196.
154. Burke AP, Virmani R: Cardiac rhabdomyoma: A clinicopathologic study. Mod Pathol 1991;4:70–74.
155. Afify A, Mark HF: Trisomy 8 in embryonal rhabdomyosarcoma detected by fluorescence in situ hybridization. Cancer Genet Cytogenet 1999;108:127–132.
156. Lee W, Han K, Harris CP, Meisner LF: Detection of aneuploidy and possible deletion in paraffin-embedded rhabdomyosarcoma cells with FISH. Cancer Genet Cytogenet 1993;68:99-103.
157. Boyle ETJ, Reiman HM, Kramer SA, et al: Embryonal rhabdomyosarcoma of bladder and prostate: Nuclear DNA patterns studied by flow cytometry. J Urol 1988; 140:1119–1121.
158. Kowal-Vern A, Gonzalez-Crussi F, Turner J, et al: Flow and image cytometric DNA analysis in rhabdomyosarcoma. Cancer Res 1990;50:6023–6027.
159. Casola S, Pedone PV, Cavazzana AO, et al: Expression and parental imprinting of the *H19* gene in human rhabdomyosarcoma [published erratum appears in Oncogene 1997;15:875]. Oncogene 1997;14:1503–1510.
160. Samuel DP, Tsokos M, DeBaun MR: Hemihypertrophy and a poorly differentiated embryonal rhabdomyosarcoma of the pelvis. Med Pediatr Oncol 1999; 32:38–43.
161. Chung WY, Yuan L, Feng L, et al: Chromosome 11p15.5 regional imprinting: Comparative analysis of *KIP2* and *H19* in human tissues and Wilms' tumors. Hum Mol Genet 1996;5:1101–1108.
162. Loh WEJ, Scrable HJ, Livanos E, et al: Human chromosome 11 contains two different growth suppressor genes for embryonal rhabdomyosarcoma. Proc Natl Acad Sci U S A 1992;89:1755–1759.
163. Gattenloehner S, Vincent A, Leuschner I, et al: The fetal form of the acetylcholine receptor distinguishes rhabdomyosarcomas from other childhood tumors. Am J Pathol 1998;152:437–444.
164. Chen B, Dias P, Jenkins JJ, et al: Methylation alterations of the MyoD1 upstream region are predictive of subclassification of human rhabdomyosarcomas. Am J Pathol 1998;152:1071–1079.
165. Dodd S, Malone M, McCulloch W: Rhabdomyosarcoma in children: A histological and immunohistochemical study of 59 cases. J Pathol 1989; 158:13–18.
166. Douglass EC, Valentine M, Etcubanas E, et al: A specific chromosomal abnormality in rhabdomyosarcoma [published erratum appears in Cytogenet Cell Genet 1988;47:232]. Cytogenet Cell Genet 1987;45:148–155.
167. Wang-Wuu S, Soukup S, Ballard E, et al: Chromosomal analysis of sixteen human rhabdomyosarcomas. Cancer Res 1988;48:983–987.

168. Barr FG, Nauta LE, Hollows JC: Structural analysis of *PAX3* genomic rearrangements in alveolar rhabdomyosarcoma. Cancer Genet Cytogenet 1998;102:32–39.
169. Galili N, Davis RJ, Fredericks WJ, et al: Fusion of a fork head domain gene to *PAX3* in the solid tumour alveolar rhabdomyosarcoma [published erratum appears in Nat Genet 1994;6:214]. Nat Genet 1993;5: 230–235.
170. Weber-Hall S, McManus A, Anderson J, et al: Novel formation and amplification of the *PAX7-FKHR* fusion gene in a case of alveolar rhabdomyosarcoma. Genes Chromosomes Cancer 1996;17:7–13.
171. Chen BF, Chen ML, Liang DC, et al: Detection of PAX3-FKHR and PAX7-FKHR fusion transcripts in rhabdomyosarcoma by reverse transcriptase-polymerase chain reaction using paraffin-embedded tissue. Chung Hua I Hsueh Tsa Chih (Taipei) 1999;62:86–91.
172. Downing JR, Khandekar A, Shurtleff SA, et al: Multiplex RT-PCR assay for the differential diagnosis of alveolar rhabdomyosarcoma and Ewing's sarcoma. Am J Pathol 1995;146:626–634.
173. Reichmuth C, Markus MA, Hillemanns M, et al: The diagnostic potential of the chromosome translocation t(2;13) in rhabdomyosarcoma: A PCR study of fresh-frozen and paraffin-embedded tumour samples. J Pathol 1996;180:50–57.
174. Biegel JA, Nycum LM, Valentine V, et al: Detection of the t(2;13)(q35;q14) and *PAX3-FKHR* fusion in alveolar rhabdomyosarcoma by fluorescence in situ hybridization. Genes Chromosomes Cancer 1995;12:186–192.
175. McManus AP, O'Reilly MA, Jones KP, et al: Interphase fluorescence in situ hybridization detection of t(2;13) (q35;q14) in alveolar rhabdomyosarcoma—a diagnostic tool in minimally invasive biopsies. J Pathol 1996;178: 410–414.
176. Sozzi G, Minoletti F, Miozzo M, et al: Relevance of cytogenetic and fluorescent in situ hybridization analyses in the clinical assessment of soft tissue sarcoma. Hum Pathol 1997;28:134–142.
177. Shapiro DN, Parham DM, Douglass EC, et al: Relationship of tumor-cell ploidy to histologic subtype and treatment outcome in children and adolescents with unresectable rhabdomyosarcoma [published erratum appears in J Clin Oncol 1991;9:893]. J Clin Oncol 1991;9: 159–166.
178. Kilpatrick SE, Teot LA, Geisinger KR, et al: Relationship of DNA ploidy to histology and prognosis in rhabdomyosarcoma: Comparison of flow cytometry and image analysis. Cancer 1994;74:3227–3233.
179. Dias P, Kumar P, Marsden HB, et al: N-*myc* gene is amplified in alveolar rhabdomyosarcomas (RMS) but not in embryonal RMS. Int J Cancer 1990;45:593–596.
180. Driman D, Thorner PS, Greenberg ML, et al: *MYCN* gene amplification in rhabdomyosarcoma. Cancer 1994; 73:2231–2237.
181. Hachitanda Y, Toyoshima S, Akazawa K, Tsuneyoshi M: N-*myc* gene amplification in rhabdomyosarcoma detected by fluorescence in situ hybridization: Its correlation with histologic features. Mod Pathol 1998;11: 1222–1227.
182. Barr FG, Nauta LE, Davis RJ, et al: In vivo amplification of the *PAX3-FKHR* and *PAX7-FKHR* fusion genes in alveolar rhabdomyosarcoma. Hum Mol Genet 1996; 5:15–21.
183. Weber-Hall S, Anderson J, McManus A, et al: Gains, losses, and amplification of genomic material in rhabdomyosarcoma analyzed by comparative genomic hybridization. Cancer Res 1996;56:3220–3224.
184. Miettinen M, Lehto VP, Badley RA, Virtanen I: Alveolar rhabdomyosarcoma: Demonstration of the muscle type of intermediate filament protein, desmin, as a diagnostic aid. Am J Pathol 1982;108:246–251.
185. Seidal T, Kindblom LG, Angervall L: Myoglobin, desmin and vimentin in ultrastructurally proven rhabdomyomas and rhabdomyosarcomas: An immunohistochemical study utilizing a series of monoclonal and polyclonal antibodies. Appl Pathol 1987;5:201–219.
186. Tsokos M, Howard R, Costa J: Immunohistochemical study of alveolar and embryonal rhabdomyosarcoma. Lab Invest 1983;48:148–155.
187. de Jong AS, Kessel-van Vark M, Albus-Lutter CE, et al: Skeletal muscle actin as tumor marker in the diagnosis of rhabdomyosarcoma in childhood. Am J Surg Pathol 1985;9:467–474.
188. Miettinen M, Rapola J: Immunohistochemical spectrum of rhabdomyosarcoma and rhabdomyosarcoma-like tumors: Expression of cytokeratin and the 68-kD neurofilament protein. Am J Surg Pathol 1989;13:120–132.
189. Gaffney EF, Dervan PA, Fletcher CD: Pleomorphic rhabdomyosarcoma in adulthood: Analysis of 11 cases with definition of diagnostic criteria. Am J Surg Pathol 1993;17:601–609.
190. Wesche WA, Fletcher CD, Dias P, et al: Immunohistochemistry of MyoD1 in adult pleomorphic soft tissue sarcomas. Am J Surg Pathol 1995;19:261–269.
191. Henn W, Wullich B, Thonnes M, et al: Recurrent t(12;19)(q13;q13.3) in intracranial and extracranial hemangiopericytoma. Cancer Genet Cytogenet 1993; 71:151–154.
192. Mandahl N, Orndal C, Heim S, et al: Aberrations of chromosome segment 12q13-15 characterize a subgroup of hemangiopericytomas. Cancer 1993; 71:3009–3013.
193. Florenes VA, Maelandsmo GM, Forus A, et al: *MDM2* gene amplification and transcript levels in human sarcomas: Relationship to *TP53* gene status [see comments]. J Natl Cancer Inst 1994;86:1297–1302.
194. Aue G, Muralidhar B, Schwartz HS, Butler MG: Telomerase activity in skeletal sarcomas. Ann Surg Oncol 1998;5:627–634.
195. McDonagh DP, Liu J, Gaffey MJ, et al: Detection of Kaposi's sarcoma-associated herpesvirus-like DNA sequence in angiosarcoma. Am J Pathol 1996;149: 1363–1368.
196. Finn WG, Goolsby CL, Rao MS: DNA flow cytometric analysis of hemangiopericytoma. Am J Clin Pathol 1994; 101:181–185.
197. Fukunaga M, Shimoda T, Nikaido T, et al: Soft tissue vascular tumors: A flow cytometric DNA analysis. Cancer 1993;71:2233–2241.
198. Middleton LP, Duray PH, Merino MJ: The histological spectrum of hemangiopericytoma: Application of immunohistochemical analysis including proliferative markers to facilitate diagnosis and predict prognosis. Hum Pathol 1998;29:636–640.

199. Porter PL, Bigler SA, McNutt M, Gown AM: The immunophenotype of hemangiopericytomas and glomus tumors, with special reference to muscle protein expression: An immunohistochemical study and review of the literature. Mod Pathol 1991;4:46–52.
200. Schurch W, Skalli O, Lagace R, et al: Intermediate filament proteins and actin isoforms as markers for soft-tissue tumor differentiation and origin: III. Hemangio pericytomas and glomus tumors. Am J Pathol 1990; 136:771–786.
201. Cerilli LA, Huffman HT, Anand A: Primary renal angiosarcoma: A case report with immunohistochemical, ultrastructural, and cytogenetic features and review of the literature. Arch Pathol Lab Med 1998;122:929–935.
202. Gil-Benso R, Lopez-Gines C, Soriano P, et al: Cytogenetic study of angiosarcoma of the breast. Genes Chromosomes Cancer 1994;10:210–212.
203. Kindblom LG, Stenman G, Angervall L: Morphological and cytogenetic studies of angiosarcoma in Stewart-Treves syndrome. Virchows Arch A Pathol Anat Histopathol 1991;419:439–445.
204. Schuborg C, Mertens F, Rydholm A, et al: Cytogenetic analysis of four angiosarcomas from deep and superficial soft tissue. Cancer Genet Cytogenet 1998;100:52–56.
205. Dictor M, Ferno M, Baldetorp B: Flow cytometric DNA content in Kaposi's sarcoma by histologic stage: Comparison with angiosarcoma. Anal Quant Cytol Histol 1991;13:201–208.
206. Meis-Kindblom JM, Kindblom LG: Angiosarcoma of soft tissue: A study of 80 cases. Am J Surg Pathol 1998;22:683–697.
207. Naka N, Tomita Y, Nakanishi H, et al: Mutations of *p53* tumor-suppressor gene in angiosarcoma. Int J Cancer 1997;71:952–955.
208. Zietz C, Rossle M, Haas C, et al: MDM-2 oncoprotein overexpression, *p53* gene mutation, and VEGF up-regulation in angiosarcomas. Am J Pathol 1998;153: 1425–1433.
209. Lasota J, Miettinen M: Absence of Kaposi's sarcoma-associated virus (human herpesvirus-8) sequences in angiosarcoma. Virchows Arch 1999;434:51–56.
210. Delabesse E, Oksenhendler E, Lebbe C, et al: Molecular analysis of clonality in Kaposi's sarcoma. J Clin Pathol 1997;50:664–668.
211. Rabkin CS, Bedi G, Musaba E, et al: AIDS-related Kaposi's sarcoma is a clonal neoplasm. Clin Cancer Res 1995;1:257–260.
212. Rabkin CS, Janz S, Lash A, et al: Monoclonal origin of multicentric Kaposi's sarcoma lesions [see comments]. N Engl J Med 1997;336:988–993.
213. Chang Y, Cesarman E, Pessin MS, et al: Identification of herpesvirus-like DNA sequences in AIDS-associated Kaposi's sarcoma [see comments]. Science 1994;266: 1865–1869.
214. Boshoff C, Schulz TF, Kennedy MM, et al: Kaposi's sarcoma–associatfed herpesvirus infects endothelial and spindle cells. Nat Med 1995;1:1274–1278.
215. Rady PL, Yen A, Martin RW, et al: Herpesvirus-like DNA sequences in classic Kaposi's sarcomas. J Med Virol 1995;47:179–183.
216. Alkan S, Karcher DS, Ortiz A, et al: Human herpesvirus-8/Kaposi's sarcoma-associated herpesvirus in organ transplant patients with immunosuppression. Br J Haematol 1997;96:412–414.
217. Monini P, de Lellis L, Fabris M, et al: Kaposi's sarcoma–associated herpesvirus DNA sequences in prostate tissue and human semen [see comments]. N Engl J Med 1996;334:1168–1172.
218. Verbeek W, Frankel M, Miles S, et al: Seroprevalence of HHV-8 antibodies in HIV-positive homosexual men without Kaposi's sarcoma and their clinical follow-up. Am J Clin Pathol 1998;109:778–783.
219. Moore PS, Kingsley LA, Holmberg SD, et al: Kaposi's sarcoma–associated herpesvirus infection prior to onset of Kaposi's sarcoma. AIDS 1996; 10:175–180.
220. Kowalzick L, Hoffmann I, Neipel F, et al: Detection of HHV-8 DNA in a German patient with classical Kaposi's sarcoma may allow an estimation of the incubation period. Eur J Dermatol 1998;8:432–434.
221. Vieira J, Huang ML, Koelle DM, Corey L: Transmissible Kaposi's sarcoma–associated herpesvirus (human herpesvirus 8) in saliva of men with a history of Kaposi's sarcoma. J Virol 1997;71:7083–7087.
222. Blauvelt A, Sei S, Cook PM, et al: Human herpesvirus 8 infection occurs following adolescence in the United States. J Infect Dis 1997;176:771–774.
223. Zhong W, Wang H, Herndier B, Ganem D: Restricted expression of Kaposi sarcoma–associated herpesvirus (human herpesvirus 8) genes in Kaposi sarcoma. Proc Natl Acad Sci U S A 1996;93:6641–6646.
224. Cheng EH, Nicholas J, Bellows DS, et al: A Bcl-2 homolog encoded by Kaposi sarcoma–associated virus, human herpesvirus 8, inhibits apoptosis but does not heterodimerize with Bax or Bak. Proc Natl Acad Sci U S A 1997;94:690–694.
225. Sarid R, Sato T, Bohenzky RA, et al: Kaposi's sarcoma–associated herpesvirus encodes a functional bcl-2 homologue. Nat Med 1997;3:293–298.
226. Dada MA, Chetty R, Biddolph SC, et al: The immunoexpression of bcl-2 and p53 in Kaposi's sarcoma. Histopathology 1996;29:159–163.
227. Simonart T, Degraef C, Noel JC, et al: Overexpression of Bcl-2 in Kaposi's sarcoma–derived cells. J Invest Dermatol 1998;111:349–353.
228. Lee H, Veazey R, Williams K, et al: Deregulation of cell growth by the *K1* gene of Kaposi's sarcoma–associated herpesvirus. Nat Med 1998;4:435–440.
229. Horenstein MG, Cesarman E, Wang X, et al: Cyclin D1 and retinoblastoma protein expression in Kaposi's sarcoma. J Cutan Pathol 1997;24:585–589.
230. Sarid R, Wiezorek JS, Moore PS, Chang Y: Characterization and cell cycle regulation of the major Kaposi's sarcoma–associated herpesvirus (human herpesvirus 8) latent genes and their promoter. J Virol 1999;73: 1438–1446.
231. Bergman R, Ramon M, Kilim S, et al: An immunohistochemical study of p53 protein expression in classical Kaposi's sarcoma [see comments]. Am J Dermatopathol 1996;18:367–370.
232. Kennedy MM, O'Leary JJ, Oates JL, et al: Human herpes virus 8 (HHV-8) in Kaposi's sarcoma: Lack of association with Bcl-2 and p53 protein expression. Mol Pathol 1998;51:155–159.

233. Li JJ, Huang YQ, Cockerell CJ, et al: Expression and mutation of the tumor suppressor gene *p53* in AIDS-associated Kaposi's sarcoma [see comments]. Am J Dermatopathol 1997;19:373–378.
234. Pillay P, Chetty R, Reddy R: Bcl-2 and p53 immunoprofile in Kaposi's sarcoma. Pathol Oncol Res 1999;5:17–20.
235. Popescu NC, Zimonjic DB, Leventon-Kriss S, et al: Deletion and translocation involving chromosome 3 (p14) in two tumorigenic Kaposi's sarcoma cell lines. J Natl Cancer Inst 1996;88:450–455.
236. Bisceglia M, Bosman C, Quirke P: A histologic and flow cytometric study of Kaposi's sarcoma. Cancer 1992;69:793–798.
237. De Thier F, Simonart T, Hermans P, et al: Early- and late-stage Kaposi's sarcoma lesions exhibit similar proliferation fraction [in process citation]. Am J Dermatopathol 1999;21:25–27.
238. Reizis Z, Trattner A, Katzenelson V, et al: Flow cytometric DNA analysis of classic and steroid-induced Kaposi's sarcoma [see comments]. Br J Dermatol 1995;132:548–550.
239. Penneys NS, Bernstein H, Leonardi C: Confirmation of early Kaposi's sarcoma by polyclonal antibody to type IV collagen. J Am Acad Dermatol 1988;19:447–450.
240. Hisaoka M, Hashimoto H, Iwamasa T: Diagnostic implication of Kaposi's sarcoma–associated herpesvirus with special reference to the distinction between spindle cell hemangioendothelioma and Kaposi's sarcoma. Arch Pathol Lab Med 1998;122:72–76.
241. Jin YT, Tsai ST, Yan JJ, et al: Detection of Kaposi's sarcoma–associated herpesvirus-like DNA sequence in vascular lesions: A reliable diagnostic marker for Kaposi's sarcoma. Am J Clin Pathol 1996;105:360–363.
242. Mandahl N, Jin YS, Heim S, et al: Trisomy 5 and loss of the Y chromosome as the sole cytogenetic anomalies in a cavernous hemangioma/angiosarcoma. Genes Chromosomes Cancer 1990;1:315–316.
243. LeBoit PE, Berger TG, Egbert BM, et al: Epithelioid haemangioma-like vascular proliferation in AIDS: Manifestation of cat scratch disease bacillus infection? Lancet 1988;1:960–963.
244. Tamm E, Jungkunz W, Marsch WC, Lutjen-Drecoll E: Increase in types IV and VI collagen in cherry haemangiomas. Arch Dermatol Res 1992;284:275–282.
245. Limon J, Dal Cin P, Sandberg AA: Translocations involving the X chromosome in solid tumors: Presentation of two sarcomas with t(X;18)(q13;p11). Cancer Genet Cytogenet 1986;23:87–91.
246. Turc-Carel C, Dal Cin P, Limon J, et al: Involvement of chromosome X in primary cytogenetic change in human neoplasia: Nonrandom translocation in synovial sarcoma. Proc Natl Acad Sci U S A 1987; 84:1981–1985.
247. Limon J, Mrozek K, Mandahl N, et al: Cytogenetics of synovial sarcoma: Presentation of ten new cases and review of the literature. Genes Chromosomes Cancer 1991;3:338–345.
248. Knight JC, Reeves BR, Kearney L, et al: Localization of the synovial sarcoma t(X;18)(p11.2;q11.2) breakpoint by fluorescence in situ hybridization. Hum Mol Genet 1992;1:633–637.
249. Dal Cin P, Rao U, Jani-Sait S, et al: Chromosomes in the diagnosis of soft tissue tumors: I. Synovial sarcoma. Mod Pathol 1992;5:357–362.
250. Karakousis CP, Dal Cin P, Turc-Carel C, et al: Chromosomal changes in soft-tissue sarcomas: A new diagnostic parameter. Arch Surg 1987;122:1257–1260.
251. Nojima T, Wang YS, Abe S, et al: Morphological and cytogenetic studies of a human synovial sarcoma xenotransplanted into nude mice. Acta Pathol Jpn 1990;40:486–493.
252. Reeves BR, Smith S, Fisher C, et al: Characterization of the translocation between chromosomes X and 18 in human synovial sarcomas. Oncogene 1989;4:373–378.
253. Clark J, Rocques PJ, Crew AJ, et al: Identification of novel genes, *SYT* and *SSX*, involved in the t(X;18)(p11.2;q11.2) translocation found in human synovial sarcoma. Nat Genet 1994;7:502–508.
254. Crew AJ, Clark J, Fisher C, et al: Fusion of *SYT* to two genes, *SSX1* and *SSX2*, encoding proteins with homology to the Kruppel-associated box in human synovial sarcoma. EMBO J 1995;14:2333–2340.
255. dos Santos NR, de Bruijn DR, Balemans M, et al: Nuclear localization of SYT, SSX and the synovial sarcoma-associated SYT-SSX fusion proteins. Hum Mol Genet 1997;6:1549–1558.
256. Brett D, Whitehouse S, Antonson P, et al: The SYT protein involved in the t(X;18) synovial sarcoma translocation is a transcriptional activator localised in nuclear bodies. Hum Mol Genet 1997;6:1559–1564.
257. Tureci O, Sahin U, Schobert I, et al: The *SSX-2* gene, which is involved in the t(X;18) translocation of synovial sarcomas, codes for the human tumor antigen HOM-MEL-40. Cancer Res 1996;56:4766–4772.
258. Gure AO, Tureci O, Sahin U, et al: SSX: A multigene family with several members transcribed in normal testis and human cancer. Int J Cancer 1997;72:965–971.
259. Thaete C, Brett D, Monaghan P, et al: Functional domains of the SYT and SYT-SSX synovial sarcoma translocation proteins and co-localization with the SNF protein BRM in the nucleus. Hum Mol Genet 1999;8:585–591.
260. Hirakawa N, Naka T, Yamamoto I, et al: Overexpression of bcl-2 protein in synovial sarcoma: A comparative study of other soft tissue spindle cell sarcomas and an additional analysis by fluorescence in situ hybridization. Hum Pathol 1996;27:1060–1065.
261. Kawai A, Woodruff J, Healey JH, et al: *SYT-SSX* gene fusion as a determinant of morphology and prognosis in synovial sarcoma [see comments]. N Engl J Med 1998;338:153–160.
262. Pollock RE, Lang A, Luo J, et al: Soft tissue sarcoma metastasis from clonal expansion of p53 mutated tumor cells. Oncogene 1996;12:2035–2039.
263. Barrios C, Castresana JS, Ruiz J, Kreicbergs A: Amplification of the c-*myc* proto-oncogene in soft tissue sarcomas. Oncology 1994;51:13–17.
264. Szymanska J, Serra M, Skytting B, et al: Genetic imbalances in 67 synovial sarcomas evaluated by comparative genomic hybridization [in process citation]. Genes Chromosomes Cancer 1998;23:213–219.
265. Lopes JM, Bjerkehagen B, Holm R, et al: Proliferative activity of synovial sarcoma: An immunohistochemical

evaluation of Ki-67 labeling indices of 52 primary and recurrent tumors. Ultrastruct Pathol 1995;19:101–106.
266. Lopes JM, Hannisdal E, Bjerkehagen B, et al: Synovial sarcoma: Evaluation of prognosis with emphasis on the study of DNA ploidy and proliferation (PCNA and Ki-67) markers. Anal Cell Pathol 1998;16:45–62.
267. Oda Y, Hashimoto H, Takeshita S, Tsuneyoshi M: The prognostic value of immunohistochemical staining for proliferating cell nuclear antigen in synovial sarcoma. Cancer 1993;72:478–485.
268. el-Naggar AK, Ayala AG, Abdul-Karim FW, et al: Synovial sarcoma: A DNA flow cytometric study. Cancer 1990;65:2295–2300.
269. Mune T, Yasuda K, Ishii M, et al: Tetany due to hypomagnesemia induced by cisplatin and doxorubicin treatment for synovial sarcoma. Intern Med 1993;32:434–437.
270. Lee W, Han K, Harris CP, et al: Use of FISH to detect chromosomal translocations and deletions: Analysis of chromosome rearrangement in synovial sarcoma cells from paraffin-embedded specimens. Am J Pathol 1993;143:15–19.
271. Nagao K, Ito H, Yoshida H: Chromosomal translocation t(X;18) in human synovial sarcomas analyzed by fluorescence in situ hybridization using paraffin-embedded tissue. Am J Pathol 1996;148:601–609.
272. Yang P, Hirose T, Hasegawa T, et al: Dual-colour fluorescence in situ hybridization analysis of synovial sarcoma. J Pathol 1998;184:7–13.
273. Zilmer M, Harris CP, Steiner DS, Meisner LF: Use of nonbreakpoint DNA probes to detect the t(X;18) in interphase cells from synovial sarcoma: Implications for detection of diagnostic tumor translocations. Am J Pathol 1998;152:1171–1177.
274. Fligman I, Lonardo F, Jhanwar SC, et al: Molecular diagnosis of synovial sarcoma and characterization of a variant SYT-SSX2 fusion transcript. Am J Pathol 1995;147:1592–1599.
275. Lasota J, Jasinski M, Debiec-Rychter M, et al: Detection of the SYT-SSX fusion transcripts in formaldehyde-fixed, paraffin-embedded tissue: A reverse transcription polymerase chain reaction amplification assay useful in the diagnosis of synovial sarcoma. Mod Pathol 1998; 11:626–633.
276. Willeke F, Mechtersheimer G, Schwarzbach M, et al: Detection of SYT-SSX1/2 fusion transcripts by reverse transcriptase-polymerase chain reaction (RT-PCR) is a valuable diagnostic tool in synovial sarcoma. Eur J Cancer 1998;34:2087–2093.
277. Stenman G, Kindblom LG, Johansson M, Angervall L: Clonal chromosome abnormalities and in vitro growth characteristics of classical and cellular schwannomas. Cancer Genet Cytogenet 1991;57:121–131.
278. Bello MJ, de Campos JM, Kusak ME, et al: Clonal chromosome aberrations in neurinomas. Genes Chromosomes Cancer 1993;6:206–211.
279. Sarlomo-Rikala M, el-Rifai W, Lahtinen T, et al: Different patterns of DNA copy number changes in gastrointestinal stromal tumors, leiomyomas, and schwannomas. Hum Pathol 1998;29:476–481.
280. Bijlsma EK, Merel P, Bosch DA, et al: Analysis of mutations in the SCH gene in schwannomas. Genes Chromosomes Cancer 1994;11:7–14.
281. Twist EC, Ruttledge MH, Rousseau M, et al: The neurofibromatosis type 2 gene is inactivated in schwannomas. Hum Mol Genet 1994;3:147–151.
282. Gusella JF, Ramesh V, MacCollin M, Jacoby LB: Neurofibromatosis 2:Loss of merlin's protective spell. Curr Opin Genet Dev 1996;6:87–92.
283. Gutmann DH, Giordano MJ, Fishback AS, Guha A: Loss of merlin expression in sporadic meningiomas, ependymomas and schwannomas. Neurology 1997; 49: 267–270.
284. Leone PE, Bello MJ, Mendiola M, et al: Allelic status of 1p, 14q, and 22q and *NF2* gene mutations in sporadic schwannomas. Int J Mol Med 1998;1:889–892.
285. Stemmer-Rachamimov AO, Xu L, Gonzalez-Agosti C, et al: Universal absence of merlin, but not other ERM family members, in schwannomas. Am J Pathol 1997; 151:1649–1654.
286. Stemmer-Rachamimov AO, Ino Y, Lim ZY, et al: Loss of the *NF2* gene and merlin occur by the tumorlet stage of schwannoma development in neurofibromatosis 2. J Neuropathol Exp Neurol 1998;57:1164–1167.
287. Gutmann DH, Sherman L, Seftor L, et al: Increased expression of the *NF2* tumor suppressor gene product, merlin, impairs cell motility, adhesion and spreading. Hum Mol Genet 1999;8:267–275.
288. Ruttledge MH, Andermann AA, Phelan CM, et al: Type of mutation in the neurofibromatosis type 2 gene *(NF2)* frequently determines severity of disease. Am J Hum Genet 1996;59:331–342.
289. Pelton PD, Sherman LS, Rizvi TA, et al: Ruffling membrane, stress fiber, cell spreading and proliferation abnormalities in human schwannoma cells. Oncogene 1998;17:2195–2209.
290. Hiraga S, Ohnishi T, Izumoto S, et al: Telomerase activity and alterations in telomere length in human brain tumors. Cancer Res. 1998;58:2117–2125.
291. Casadei GP, Scheithauer BW, Hirose T, et al: Cellular schwannoma: A clinicopathologic, DNA flow cytometric, and proliferation marker study of 70 patients. Cancer 1995;75:1109–1119.
292. Nozaki M, Tada M, Matsumoto R, et al: Rare occurrence of inactivating *p53* gene mutations in primary non-astrocytic tumors of the central nervous system: Reappraisal by yeast functional assay. Acta Neuropathol (Berl) 1998;95:291–296.
293. Ohgaki H, Eibl RH, Schwab M, et al: Mutations of the *p53* tumor suppressor gene in neoplasms of the human nervous system. Mol Carcinog 1993;8:74–80.
294. Gray MH, Rosenberg AE, Dickersin GR, Bhan AK: Glial fibrillary acidic protein and keratin expression by benign and malignant nerve sheath tumors. Hum Pathol 1989;20:1089–1096.
295. Gray MH, Smoller BR, McNutt NS, Hsu A: Immunohistochemical demonstration of factor XIIIa expression in neurofibromas: A practical means of differentiating these tumors from neurotized melanocytic nevi and schwannomas [see comments]. Arch Dermatol 1990;126:472–476.
296. Daschner K, Assum G, Eisenbarth I, et al: Clonal origin of tumor cells in a plexiform neurofibroma with LOH in NF1 intron 38 and in dermal neurofibromas without LOH of the *NF1* gene. Biochem Biophys Res Commun 1997;234:346–350.

297. Skuse GR, Kosciolek BA, Rowley PT: The neurofibroma in von Recklinghausen neurofibromatosis has a unicellular origin. Am J Hum Genet 1991;49:600–607.
298. Rey JA, Bello MJ, de Campos JM, et al: Cytogenetic clones in a recurrent neurofibroma. Cancer Genet Cytogenet 1987;26:157–163.
299. Cawthon RM, O'Connell P, Buchberg AM, et al: Identification and characterization of transcripts from the neurofibromatosis 1 region: The sequence and genomic structure of EVI2 and mapping of other transcripts. Genomics 1990;7:555–565.
300. Cawthon RM, Weiss R, Xu GF, et al: A major segment of the neurofibromatosis type 1 gene: cDNA sequence, genomic structure, and point mutations [published erratum appears in Cell 1990;62:following 608]. Cell 1990; 62:193–201.
301. Viskochil D, Buchberg AM, Xu G, et al: Deletions and a translocation interrupt a cloned gene at the neurofibromatosis type 1 locus. Cell 1990;62:187–192.
302. Wallace MR, Marchuk DA, Andersen LB, et al: Type 1 neurofibromatosis gene: Identification of a large transcript disrupted in three NF1 patients [published erratum appears in Science 1990;250:1749]. Science 1990; 249:181–186.
303. Sawada S, Florell S, Purandare SM, et al: Identification of *NF1* mutations in both alleles of a dermal neurofibroma. Nat Genet 1996;14:110–112.
304. Serra E, Puig S, Otero D, et al: Confirmation of a double-hit model for the *NF1* gene in benign neurofibromas. Am J Hum Genet 1997;61:512–519.
305. Cowley GS, Murthy AE, Parry DM, et al: Genetic variation in the 3′ untranslated region of the neurofibromatosis 1 gene: Application to unequal allelic expression. Somat Cell Mol Genet 1998;24:107–119.
306. Rodenhiser DI, Coulter-Mackie MB, Singh SM: Evidence of DNA methylation in the neurofibromatosis type 1 *(NF1)* gene region of 17q11.2. Hum Mol Genet 1993;2:439–444.
307. Elyakim S, Lerer I, Zlotogora J, et al: Neurofibromatosis type I (NFI) in Israeli families: Linkage analysis as a diagnostic tool. Am J Med Genet 1994;53:325–334.
308. Ricciardone MD, Ozcelik T, Cevher B, et al: Human MLH1 deficiency predisposes to hematological malignancy and neurofibromatosis type 1. Cancer Res 1999; 59:290–293.
309. Halling KC, Scheithauer BW, Halling AC, et al: p53 expression in neurofibroma and malignant peripheral nerve sheath tumor: An immunohistochemical study of sporadic and NF1-associated tumors [see comments]. Am J Clin Pathol 1996;106:282–288.
310. Menon AG, Anderson KM, Riccardi VM, et al: Chromosome 17p deletions and *p53* gene mutations associated with the formation of malignant neurofibrosarcomas in von Recklinghausen neurofibromatosis. Proc Natl Acad Sci U S A 1990;87:5435–5439.
311. Jhanwar SC, Chen Q, Li FP, et al: Cytogenetic analysis of soft tissue sarcomas: Recurrent chromosome abnormalities in malignant peripheral nerve sheath tumors (MPNST). Cancer Genet Cytogenet 1994;78:138–144.
312. Mertens F, Rydholm A, Bauer HF, et al: Cytogenetic findings in malignant peripheral nerve sheath tumors. Int J Cancer 1995;61:793–798.
313. Lothe RA, Karhu R, Mandahl N, et al: Gain of 17q24-qter detected by comparative genomic hybridization in malignant tumors from patients with von Recklinghausen's neurofibromatosis. Cancer Res 1996;56:4778–4781.
314. Takahashi K, Suzuki H, Hatori M, et al: Reduced expression of neurofibromin in the soft tissue tumours obtained from patients with neurofibromatosis type I. Clin Sci (Colch) 1995;88:581–585.
315. Gutmann DH, Silos-Santiago I, Geist RT, et al: Lack of NF1 expression in a sporadic schwannoma from a patient without neurofibromatosis. J Neurooncol 1995;25: 103–111.
316. Tang Y, Marwaha S, Rutkowski JL, et al: A role for Pak protein kinases in Schwann cell transformation. Proc Natl Acad Sci U S A 1998;95:5139–5144.
317. Yan N, Ricca C, Fletcher J, et al: Farnesyltransferase inhibitors block the neurofibromatosis type I (NF1) malignant phenotype. Cancer Res 1995;55:3569–3575.
318. Basu TN, Gutmann DH, Fletcher JA, et al: Aberrant regulation of ras proteins in malignant tumour cells from type 1 neurofibromatosis patients [see comments]. Nature 1992;356:713–715.
319. DeClue JE, Papageorge AG, Fletcher JA, et al: Abnormal regulation of mammalian p21ras contributes to malignant tumor growth in von Recklinghausen (type 1) neurofibromatosis. Cell 1992;69:265–273.
320. Guha A, Lau N, Huvar I, et al: Ras-GTP levels are elevated in human NF1 peripheral nerve tumors. Oncogene 1996;12:507–513.
321. Badache A, Muja N, De Vries GH: Expression of Kit in neurofibromin-deficient human Schwann cells: Role in Schwann cell hyperplasia associated with type 1 neurofibromatosis. Oncogene 1998;17:795–800.
322. Badache A, De Vries GH: Neurofibrosarcoma-derived Schwann cells overexpress platelet-derived growth factor (PDGF) receptors and are induced to proliferate by PDGF BB. J Cell Physiol 1998;177:334–342.
323. Rao UN, Surti U, Hoffner L, Yaw K: Cytogenetic and histologic correlation of peripheral nerve sheath tumors of soft tissue. Cancer Genet Cytogenet 1996;88:17–25.
324. Maelandsmo GM, Berner JM, Florenes VA, et al: Homozygous deletion frequency and expression levels of the *CDKN2* gene in human sarcomas—relationship to amplification and mRNA levels of CDK4 and CCND1. Br J Cancer 1995;72:393–398.
325. Wick MR, Swanson PE, Scheithauer BW, Manivel JC: Malignant peripheral nerve sheath tumor: An immunohistochemical study of 62 cases. Am J Clin Pathol 1987;87:425–433.
326. Aurias A, Rimbaut C, Buffe D, et al: Translocation involving chromosome 22 in Ewing's sarcoma: A cytogenetic study of four fresh tumors. Cancer Genet Cytogenet 1984;12:21–25.
327. Casorzo L, Fessia L, Sapino A, et al: Extraskeletal Ewing's tumor with translocation t(11;22) in a patient with Down syndrome. Cancer Genet Cytogenet 1989; 37:79–84.
328. Douglass EC, Valentine M, Green AA, et al: t(11;22) and other chromosomal rearrangements in Ewing's sarcoma. J Natl Cancer Inst 1986;77:1211–1215.
329. Turc-Carel C, Philip I, Berger MP, et al: Chromosome study of Ewing's sarcoma (ES) cell lines: Consistency of

a reciprocal translocation t(11;22)(q24;q12). Cancer Genet Cytogenet 1984;12(1):1–19.

330. Turc-Carel C, Aurias A, Mugneret F, et al: Chromosomes in Ewing's sarcoma: I. An evaluation of 85 cases of remarkable consistency of t(11;22)(q24;q12). Cancer Genet Cytogenet 1988;32:229–238.
331. Whang-Peng J, Triche TJ, Knutsen T, et al: Cytogenetic characterization of selected small round cell tumors of childhood. Cancer Genet Cytogenet 1986;21:185–208.
332. Delattre O, Zucman J, Plougastel B, et al: Gene fusion with an ETS DNA-binding domain caused by chromosome translocation in human tumours.
333. Zucman J, Delattre O, Desmaze C, et al: Cloning and characterization of the Ewing's sarcoma and peripheral neuroepithelioma t(11;22) translocation breakpoints. Genes Chromosomes Cancer 1992;5:271–277.
334. Desmaze C, Brizard F, Turc-Carel C, et al: Multiple chromosomal mechanisms generate an *EWS/FLI1* or an *EWS/ERG* fusion gene in Ewing tumors. Cancer Genet Cytogenet 1997;97:12–19.
335. Hibshoosh H, Lattes R: Immunohistochemical and molecular genetic approaches to soft tissue tumor diagnosis: A primer. Semin Oncol 1997;24:515–525.
336. Kaneko Y, Kobayashi H, Handa M, et al: EWS-ERG fusion transcript produced by chromosomal insertion in a Ewing sarcoma. Genes Chromosomes Cancer 1997; 18:228–231.
337. Ladanyi M: The emerging molecular genetics of sarcoma translocations. Diagn Mol Pathol 1995;4:162–173.
338. Peter M, Couturier J, Pacquement H, et al: A new member of the ETS family fused to EWS in Ewing tumors. Oncogene 1997;14:1159–1164.
339. Urano F, Umezawa A, Hong W, et al: A novel chimera gene between EWS and E1A-F, encoding the adenovirus E1A enhancer-binding protein, in extraosseous Ewing's sarcoma. Biochem Biophys Res Commun 1996;219:608–612.
340. May WA, Lessnick SL, Braun BS, et al: The Ewing's sarcoma *EWS/FLI-1* fusion gene encodes a more potent transcriptional activator and is a more powerful transforming gene than *FLI-1*. Mol Cell Biol 1993;13: 7393–7398.
341. Lessnick SL, Braun BS, Denny CT, May WA: Multiple domains mediate transformation by the Ewing's sarcoma *EWS/FLI-1* fusion gene. Oncogene 1995;10:423–431.
342. Schutz BR, Scheurlen W, Krauss J, et al: Mapping of chromosomal gains and losses in primitive neuroectodermal tumors by comparative genomic hybridization. Genes Chromosomes Cancer 1996;16:196–203.
343. Knuutila S, Armengol G, Bjorkqvist AM, et al: Comparative genomic hybridization study on pooled DNAs from tumors of one clinical-pathological entity. Cancer Genet Cytogenet 1998;100:25–30.
344. Armengol G, Tarkkanen M, Virolainen M, et al: Recurrent gains of 1q, 8 and 12 in the Ewing family of tumours by comparative genomic hybridization. Br J Cancer 1997;75:1403–1409.
345. Ladanyi M, Lewis R, Jhanwar SC, et al: *MDM2* and *CDK4* gene amplification in Ewing's sarcoma. J Pathol 1995;175:211–217.
346. Kovar H, Auinger A, Jug G, et al: Narrow spectrum of infrequent *p53* mutations and absence of *MDM2* amplification in Ewing tumours. Oncogene 1993;8: 2683–2690.
347. Scheurlen WG, Schwabe GC, Joos S, et al: Molecular analysis of childhood primitive neuroectodermal tumors defines markers associated with poor outcome. J Clin Oncol 1998;16:2478–2485.
348. Kowal-Vern A, Walloch J, Chou P, et al: Flow and image cytometric DNA analysis in Ewing's sarcoma. Mod Pathol 1992;5:56–60.
349. Kovar H, Jug G, Aryee DN, et al: Among genes involved in the RB dependent cell cycle regulatory cascade, the *p16* tumor suppressor gene is frequently lost in the Ewing family of tumors. Oncogene 1997;15:2225–2232.
350. Fults D, Petronio J, Noblett BD, Pedone CA: Chromosome 11p15 deletions in human malignant astrocytomas and primitive neuroectodermal tumors. Genomics 1992;14:799–801.
351. Komuro H, Hayashi Y, Kawamura M, et al: Mutations of the *p53* gene are involved in Ewing's sarcomas but not in neuroblastomas. Cancer Res 1993;53:5284–5288.
352. Kumar S, Pack S, Kumar D, et al: Detection of EWS-FLI-1 fusion in Ewing's sarcoma/peripheral primitive neuroectodermal tumor by fluorescence in situ hybridization using formalin-fixed paraffin-embedded tissue [in process citation]. Hum Pathol 1999;30:324–330.
353. McManus AP, Gusterson BA, Pinkerton CR, Shipley JM: Diagnosis of Ewing's sarcoma and related tumours by detection of chromosome 22q12 translocations using fluorescence in situ hybridization on tumour touch imprints. J Pathol 1995;176:137–142.
354. Nagao K, Ito H, Yoshida H, et al: Chromosomal rearrangement t(11;22) in extraskeletal Ewing's sarcoma and primitive neuroectodermal tumour analysed by fluorescence in situ hybridization using paraffin-embedded tissue. J Pathol 1997;181:62–66.
355. Shipley JM, Jones TA, Patel K, et al: Ordering of probes surrounding the Ewing's sarcoma breakpoint on chromosome 22 using fluorescent in situ hybridization to interphase nuclei. Cytogenet Cell Genet 1993;64:233–239.
356. Barr FG, Xiong QB, Kelly K: A consensus polymerase chain reaction–oligonucleotide hybridization approach for the detection of chromosomal translocations in pediatric bone and soft tissue sarcomas. Am J Clin Pathol 1995;104:627–633.
357. Dockhorn-Dworniczak B, Schafer KL, Dantcheva R, et al: Diagnostic value of the molecular genetic detection of the t(11;22) translocation in Ewing's tumours. Virchows Arch 1994;425:107–112.
358. Downing JR, Head DR, Parham DM, et al: Detection of the (11;22) (q24;q12) translocation of Ewing's sarcoma and peripheral neuroectodermal tumor by reverse transcription polymerase chain reaction. Am J Pathol 1993; 143:1294–1300.
359. Bridge JA, Borek DA, Neff JR, Huntrakoon M: Chromosomal abnormalities in clear cell sarcoma: Implications for histogenesis. Am J Clin Pathol 1990;93:26–31.
360. Limon J, Debiec-Rychter M, Nedoszytko B, et al: Aberrations of chromosome 22 and polysomy of chromosome 8 as non-random changes in clear cell sarcoma. Cancer Genet Cytogenet 1994;72:141–145.
361. Mrozek K, Karakousis CP, Perez-Mesa C, Bloomfield CD: Translocation t(12;22)(q13; q12.2-12.3) in a clear

cell sarcoma of tendons and aponeuroses. Genes Chromosomes Cancer 1993;6:249–252.

362. Peulve P, Michot C, Vannier JP, et al: Clear cell sarcoma with t(12;22)(q13-14;q12) [see comments]. Genes Chromosomes Cancer 1991;3:400–402.

363. Reeves BR, Fletcher CD, Gusterson BA: Translocation t(12;22)(q13;q13) is a nonrandom rearrangement in clear cell sarcoma. Cancer Genet Cytogenet 1992;64: 101–103.

364. Pan S, Ming KY, Dunn TA, et al: The EWS/ATF1 fusion protein contains a dispersed activation domain that functions directly. Oncogene 1998;16:1625–1631.

365. Fujimura Y, Ohno T, Siddique H, et al: The *EWS-ATF-1* gene involved in malignant melanoma of soft parts with t(12;22) chromosome translocation encodes a constitutive transcriptional activator. Oncogene 1996;12: 159–167.

366. Brown AD, Lopez-Terrada D, Denny C, Lee KA: Promoters containing ATF-binding sites are de-regulated in cells that express the EWS/ATF1 oncogene. Oncogene 1995;10:1749–1756.

367. Li KK, Lee KA: MMSP tumor cells expressing the EWS/ATF1 oncogene do not support cAMP-inducible transcription. Oncogene 1998;16:1325–1331.

368. Mechtersheimer G, Tilgen W, Klar E, Moller P: Clear cell sarcoma of tendons and aponeuroses: Case presentation with special reference to immunohistochemical findings. Hum Pathol 1989;20:914–917.

369. Swanson PE, Wick MR: Clear cell sarcoma: An immunohistochemical analysis of six cases and comparison with other epithelioid neoplasms of soft tissue. Arch Pathol Lab Med 1989;113:55–60.

370. Stratakis CA, Carney JA, Lin JP, et al: Carney complex, a familial multiple neoplasia and lentiginosis syndrome: Analysis of 11 kindreds and linkage to the short arm of chromosome 2. J Clin Invest 1996;97:699–705.

371. Curschellas E, Toia D, Borner M, et al: Cardiac myxomas: Immunohistochemical study of benign and malignant variants. Virchows Arch A Pathol Anat Histopathol 1991;418:485–491.

372. Hashimoto H, Tsuneyoshi M, Daimaru Y, et al: Intramuscular myxoma: A clinicopathologic, immunohistochemical, and electron microscopic study. Cancer 1986; 58:740–747.

373. Goldman BI, Frydman C, Harpaz N, et al: Glandular cardiac myxomas: Histologic, immunohistochemical, and ultrastructural evidence of epithelial differentiation. Cancer 1987;59:1767–1775.

374. Krikler DM, Rode J, Davies MJ, et al: Atrial myxoma: A tumour in search of its origins. Br Heart J 1992;67: 89–91.

375. Landon G, Ordonez NG, Guarda LA: Cardiac myxomas: An immunohistochemical study using endothelial, histiocytic, and smooth-muscle cell markers. Arch Pathol Lab Med 1986;110:116–120.

376. Kotylo PK, Kennedy JE, Waller BF, Sample RB: DNA analysis of atrial myxomas. Chest 1991; 99:1203–1207.

377. Seidman JD, Berman JJ, Hitchcock CL, et al: DNA analysis of cardiac myxomas: Flow cytometry and image analysis. Hum Pathol 1991;22:494–500.

378. McCarthy PM, Schaff HV, Winkler HZ, et al: Deoxyribonucleic acid ploidy pattern of cardiac myxomas: Another predictor of biologically unusual myxomas. J Thorac Cardiovasc Surg 1989;98:1083–1086.

379. Miettinen M, Ekfors T: Alveolar soft part sarcoma: Immunohistochemical evidence for muscle cell differentiation [see comments]. Am J Clin Pathol 1990;93: 32–38.

380. Wang NP, Bacchi CE, Jiang JJ, et al: Does alveolar soft-part sarcoma exhibit skeletal muscle differentiation? An immunocytochemical and biochemical study of myogenic regulatory protein expression. Mod Pathol 1996; 9:496–506.

381. Kiuru-Kuhlefelt S, el-Rifai W, Sarlomo-Rikala M, et al: DNA copy number changes in alveolar soft part sarcoma: A comparative genomic hybridization study. Mod Pathol 1998;11:227–231.

382. Comtesse PP, Simons A, Siepman A, et al: Isochromosome (12p) and peritriploidy in a highly malignant extrarenal rhabdoid tumor [in process citation]. Cancer Genet Cytogenet 1999;109:175–177.

383. Besnard-Guerin C, Cavenee W, Newsham I: The t(11;22) (p15.5;q11.23) in a retroperitoneal rhabdoid tumor also includes a regional deletion distal to *CRYBB2* on 22q. Genes Chromosomes Cancer 1995;13:145–150.

384. Kaiserling E, Ruck P, Handgretinger R, et al: Immunohistochemical and cytogenetic findings in malignant rhabdoid tumor. Gen Diagn Pathol 1996;141:327–337.

385. Ota S, Crabbe DC, Tran TN, et al: Malignant rhabdoid tumor: A study with two established cell lines. Cancer 1993;71:2862–2872.

386. Hoovers JM, Kalikin LM, Johnson LA, et al: Multiple genetic loci within 11p15 defined by Beckwith-Wiedemann syndrome rearrangement breakpoints and subchromosomal transferable fragments. Proc Natl Acad Sci U S A 1995;92:12456–12460.

387. Reid LH, Davies C, Cooper PR, et al: A 1-Mb physical map and PAC contig of the imprinted domain in 11p15.5 that contains *TAPA1* and the *BWSCR1/WT2* region. Genomics 1997;43:366–375.

388. Sabbioni S, Barbanti-Brodano G, Croce CM, Negrini M: *GOK:* A gene at 11p15 involved in rhabdomyosarcoma and rhabdoid tumor development. Cancer Res 1997;57:4493–4497.

389. Mori T, Fukuda Y, Kuroda H, et al: Cloning and characterization of a novel Rab-family gene, *Rab36*, within the region at 22q11.2 that is homozygously deleted in malignant rhabdoid tumors. Biochem Biophys Res Commun 1999;254:594–600.

390. Fanburg-Smith JC, Hengge M, Hengge UR, et al: Extrarenal rhabdoid tumors of soft tissue: A clinicopathologic and immunohistochemical study of 18 cases. Ann Diagn Pathol 1998;2:351–362.

391. Kodet R, Newton WAJ, Sachs N, et al: Rhabdoid tumors of soft tissues: A clinicopathologic study of 26 cases enrolled on the Intergroup Rhabdomyosarcoma Study. Hum Pathol 1991;22:674–684.

392. Hinrichs SH, Jaramillo MA, Gumerlock PH, et al: Myxoid chondrosarcoma with a translocation involving chromosomes 9 and 22. Cancer Genet Cytogenet 1985;14: 219–226.

393. Turc-Carel C, Dal Cin P, Rao U, et al: Recurrent breakpoints at 9q31 and 22q12.2 in extraskeletal myxoid chondrosarcoma. Cancer Genet Cytogenet 1988;30:145–150.

394. Clark J, Benjamin H, Gill S, et al: Fusion of the *EWS* gene to *CHN*, a member of the steroid/thyroid receptor gene superfamily, in a human myxoid chondrosarcoma. Oncogene 1996;12:229–235.
395. Gill S, McManus AP, Crew AJ, et al: Fusion of the *EWS* gene to a DNA segment from 9q22-31 in a human myxoid chondrosarcoma. Genes Chromosomes Cancer 1995; 12:307–310.
396. Kilpatrick SE, Inwards CY, Fletcher CD, et al: Myxoid chondrosarcoma (chordoid sarcoma) of bone: A report of two cases and review of the literature. Cancer 1997;79:1903–1910.
397. Sciot R, Dal Cin P, Fletcher C, et al: t(9;22)(q22-31; q11-12) is a consistent marker of extraskeletal myxoid chondrosarcoma: Evaluation of three cases. Mod Pathol 1995;8:765–768.
398. Tarkkanen M, Wiklund T, Virolainen M, et al: Dedifferentiated chondrosarcoma with t(9;22)(q34;q11-12). Genes Chromosomes Cancer 1994;9:136–140.
399. Antonescu CR, Argani P, Erlandson RA, et al: Skeletal and extraskeletal myxoid chondrosarcoma: A comparative clinicopathologic, ultrastructural, and molecular study. Cancer 1998;83:1504–1521.
400. Brody RI, Ueda T, Hamelin A, et al: Molecular analysis of the fusion of EWS to an orphan nuclear receptor gene in extraskeletal myxoid chondrosarcoma. Am J Pathol 1997;150:1049–1058.
401. Labelle Y, Zucman J, Stenman G, et al: Oncogenic conversion of a novel orphan nuclear receptor by chromosome translocation. Hum Mol Genet 1995;4:2219–2226.
402. Devaney K, Abbondanzo SL, Shekitka KM, et al: MIC2 detection in tumors of bone and adjacent soft tissues. Clin Orthop 1995;310:176–187.
403. Bridge JA, Pickering D, Neff JR: Cytogenetic and molecular cytogenetic analysis of sacral chordoma. Cancer Genet Cytogenet 1994;75:23–25.
404. Butler MG, Dahir GA, Hedges LK, et al: Cytogenetic, telomere, and telomerase studies in five surgically managed lumbosacral chordomas. Cancer Genet Cytogenet 1995;85:51–57.
405. Hruban RH, Traganos F, Reuter VE, Huvos AG: Chordomas with malignant spindle cell components: A DNA flow cytometric and immunohistochemical study with histogenetic implications. Am J Pathol 1990;137:435–447.
406. Naka T, Fukuda T, Chuman H, et al: Proliferative activities in conventional chordoma: A clinicopathologic, DNA flow cytometric, and immunohistochemical analysis of 17 specimens with special reference to anaplastic chordoma showing a diffuse proliferation and nuclear atypia. Hum Pathol 1996;27:381–388.
407. el-Jabbour JN, Bennett MH, Burke MM, et al: Proliferative myositis: An immunohistochemical and ultrastructural study. Am J Surg Pathol 1991;15:654–659.
408. Ushigome S, Takakuwa T, Takagi M, et al: Proliferative myositis and fasciitis: Report of five cases with an ultrastructural and immunohistochemical study. Acta Pathol Jpn 1986;36:963–971.
409. Navas-Palacios JJ: The fibromatoses: An ultrastructural study of 31 cases. Pathol Res Pract 1983;176:158–175.
410. Ohjimi Y, Iwasaki H, Ishiguro M, et al: Trisomy 2 found in proliferative myositis cultured cell [letter]. Cancer Genet Cytogenet 1994;76:157.
411. McComb EN, Neff JR, Johansson SL, et al: Chromosomal anomalies in a case of proliferative myositis. Cancer Genet Cytogenet 1997;98:142–144.
412. Chung EB, Enzinger FM: Proliferative fasciitis. Cancer 1975;36:1450–1458.
413. Montgomery EA, Meis JM: Nodular fasciitis: Its morphologic spectrum and immunohistochemical profile. Am J Surg Pathol 1991;15:942–948.
414. Miettinen M, Sarlomo-Rikala M, Kovatich AJ: Cell-type- and tumour-type-related patterns of bcl-2 reactivity in mesenchymal cells and soft tissue tumours. Virchows Arch 1998;433:255–260.
415. Bridge JA, Bhatia PS, Anderson JR, Neff JR: Biologic and clinical significance of cytogenetic and molecular cytogenetic abnormalities in benign and malignant cartilaginous lesions. Cancer Genet Cytogenet 1993;69: 79–90.
416. Mertens F, Jonsson K, Willen H, et al: Chromosome rearrangements in synovial chondromatous lesions. Br J Cancer 1996;74:251–254.
417. Bohm G, Salzer-Kuntschik M, Lintner F: Morphometric analysis of cartilaginous tumors. Pathol Res Pract 1992;188:570–575.
418. Bridge JA, Nelson M, Orndal C, et al: Clonal karyotypic abnormalities of the hereditary multiple exostoses chromosomal loci 8q24.1 (EXT1) and 11p11-12 (EXT2) in patients with sporadic and hereditary osteochondromas. Cancer 1998;82:1657–1663.
419. Larramendy ML, Valle J, Tarkkanen M, et al: No DNA copy number changes in osteochondromas: A comparative genomic hybridization study. Cancer Genet Cytogenet 1997;97:76–78.
420. Wuyts W, Van Hul W, Hendrickx J, et al: Identification and characterization of a novel member of the *EXT* gene family, EXTL2. Eur J Hum Genet 1997;5:382–389.
421. Wuyts W, Van Hul W, De Boulle K, et al: Mutations in the *EXT1* and *EXT2* genes in hereditary multiple exostoses. Am J Hum Genet 1998;62:346–354.
422. Sawyer JR, Swanson CM, Lukacs JL, et al: Evidence of an association between 6q13-21 chromosome aberrations and locally aggressive behavior in patients with cartilage tumors. Cancer 1998;82:474–483.
423. Larramendy ML, Tarkkanen M, Valle J, et al: Gains, losses, and amplifications of DNA sequences evaluated by comparative genomic hybridization in chondrosarcomas. Am J Pathol 1997;150:685–691.
424. Hecht JT, Hogue D, Strong LC, et al: Hereditary multiple exostosis and chondrosarcoma: Linkage to chromosome II and loss of heterozygosity for EXT-linked markers on chromosomes 11 and 8. Am J Hum Genet 1995;56:1125–1131.
425. Hecht JT, Hogue D, Wang Y, et al: Hereditary multiple exostoses (EXT): Mutational studies of familial EXT1 cases and EXT-associated malignancies. Am J Hum Genet 1997;60:80–86.
426. Raskind WH, Conrad EU, Matsushita M: Frequent loss of heterozygosity for markers on chromosome arm 10q in chondrosarcomas. Genes Chromosomes Cancer 1996;16:138–143.
427. Yamaguchi T, Toguchida J, Wadayama B, et al: Loss of heterozygosity and tumor suppressor gene mutations in chondrosarcomas. Anticancer Res 1996;16:2009–2015.

428. Dobashi Y, Sugimura H, Sato A, et al: Possible association of p53 overexpression and mutation with high-grade chondrosarcoma. Diagn Mol Pathol 1993;2:257–263.
429. Oshiro Y, Chaturvedi V, Hayden D, et al: Altered p53 is associated with aggressive behavior of chondrosarcoma: A long term follow-up study. Cancer 1998;83:2324–2334.
430. Terek RM, Healey JH, Garin-Chesa P, et al: *p53* mutations in chondrosarcoma. Diagn Mol Pathol 1998;7:51–56.
431. Barrios C, Castresana JS, Ruiz J, Kreicbergs A: Amplification of c-*myc* oncogene and absence of c-Ha-*ras* point mutation in human bone sarcoma. J Orthop Res 1993;11:556–563.
432. Kanoe H, Nakayama T, Murakami H, et al: Amplification of the *CDK4* gene in sarcomas: Tumor specificity and relationship with the *RB* gene mutation. Anticancer Res 1998;18:2317–2321.
433. Coughlan B, Feliz A, Ishida T, et al: p53 expression and DNA ploidy of cartilage lesions. Hum Pathol 1995;26:620–624.
434. Nawa G, Ueda T, Mori S, et al: Prognostic significance of Ki67 (MIB1) proliferation index and p53 overexpression in chondrosarcomas. Int J Cancer 1996;69:86–91.
435. Simms WW, Ordonez NG, Johnston D, et al: p53 expression in dedifferentiated chondrosarcoma. Cancer 1995;76:223–227.
436. Wadayama B, Toguchida J, Yamaguchi T, et al: p53 expression and its relationship to DNA alterations in bone and soft tissue sarcomas. Br J Cancer 1993;68:1134–1139.
437. Scotlandi K, Serra M, Manara MC, et al: Clinical relevance of Ki-67 expression in bone tumors. Cancer 1995;75:806–814.
438. Helio H, Karaharju E, Bohling T, et al: Chondrosarcoma of bone: A clinical and DNA flow cytometric study. Eur J Surg Oncol 1995;21:408–413.
439. Kreicbergs A, Silvfersward C, Tribukait B: Flow DNA analysis of primary bone tumors: Relationship between cellular DNA content and histopathologic classification. Cancer 1984;53:129–136.
440. Mankin HJ, Connor JF, Schiller AL, et al: Grading of bone tumors by analysis of nuclear DNA content using flow cytometry. J Bone Joint Surg [Am] 1985;67:404–413.
441. Bridge JA, Neff JR, Bhatia PS, et al: Cytogenetic findings and biologic behavior of giant cell tumors of bone. Cancer 1990;65:2697–2703.
442. Bridge JA, Neff JR, Mouron BJ: Giant cell tumor of bone: Chromosomal analysis of 48 specimens and review of the literature. Cancer Genet Cytogenet 1992;58:2–13.
443. McComb EN, Johansson SL, Neff JR, et al: Chromosomal anomalies exclusive of telomeric associations in giant cell tumor of bone. Cancer Genet Cytogenet 1996;88:163–166.
444. Schwartz HS, Juliao SF, Sciadini MF, et al: Telomerase activity and oncogenesis in giant cell tumor of bone. Cancer 1995;75:1094–1099.
445. Schwartz HS, Dahir GA, Butler MG: Telomere reduction in giant cell tumor of bone and with aging. Cancer Genet Cytogenet 1993;71:132–138.
446. Pompetti F, Rizzo P, Simon RM, et al: Oncogene alterations in primary, recurrent, and metastatic human bone tumors. J Cell Biochem 1996;63:37–50.
447. Masui F, Ushigome S, Fujii K: Giant cell tumor of bone: A clinicopathologic study of prognostic factors. Pathol Int 1998;48:723–729.
448. Scheiner M, Hedges L, Schwartz HS, Butler MG: Lack of microsatellite instability in giant cell tumor of bone. Cancer Genet Cytogenet 1996;88:35–38.
449. Sara AS, Ayala AG, el-Naggar A, et al: Giant cell tumor of bone: A clinicopathologic and DNA flow cytometric analysis. Cancer 1990;66:2186–2190.
450. Hoogerwerf WA, Hawkins AL, Perlman EJ, Griffin CA: Chromosome analysis of nine osteosarcomas. Genes Chromosomes Cancer 1994;9:88–92.
451. Mertens F, Mandahl N, Orndal C, et al: Cytogenetic findings in 33 osteosarcomas. Int J Cancer 1993;55:44–50.
452. Shimizu N, Goseki T, Yamaguchi M, et al: In vitro cellular aging stimulates interleukin-1 beta production in stretched human periodontal-ligament–derived cells. J Dent Res 1997;76:1367–1375.
453. Araki N, Uchida A, Kimura T, et al: Involvement of the retinoblastoma gene in primary osteosarcomas and other bone and soft-tissue tumors. Clin Orthop 1991;270:271–277.
454. Belchis DA, Meece CA, Benko FA, et al: Loss of heterozygosity and microsatellite instability at the retinoblastoma locus in osteosarcomas. Diagn Mol Pathol 1996;5:214–219.
455. Wunder JS, Czitrom AA, Kandel R, Andrulis IL: Analysis of alterations in the retinoblastoma gene and tumor grade in bone and soft-tissue sarcomas. J Natl Cancer Inst 1991;83:194–200.
456. Yamaguchi T, Toguchida J, Yamamuro T, et al: Allelotype analysis in osteosarcomas: Frequent allele loss on 3q, 13q, 17p, and 18q. Cancer Res 1992;52:2419–2423.
457. Feugeas O, Guriec N, Babin-Boilletot A, et al: Loss of heterozygosity of the *RB* gene is a poor prognostic factor in patients with osteosarcoma [published erratum appears in J Clin Oncol 1996;14:2411]. J Clin Oncol 1996;14:467–472.
458. Haas-Kogan DA, Kogan SC, Levi D, et al: Inhibition of apoptosis by the retinoblastoma gene product. EMBO J 1995;14:461–472.
459. Li J, Hu SX, Perng GS, et al: Expression of the retinoblastoma *(RB)* tumor suppressor gene inhibits tumor cell invasion in vitro. Oncogene 1996;13:2379–2386.
460. Nielsen GP, Burns KL, Rosenberg AE, Louis DN: *CDKN2A* gene deletions and loss of p16 expression occur in osteosarcomas that lack RB alterations. Am J Pathol 1998;153:159–163.
461. Benassi MS, Molendini L, Gamberi G, et al: Altered G1 phase regulation in osteosarcoma. Int J Cancer 1997;74:518–522.
462. Wei G, Lonardo F, Ueda T, et al: *CDK4* gene amplification in osteosarcoma: Reciprocal relationship with *INK4A* gene alterations and mapping of 12q13 amplicons. Int J Cancer 1999;80:199–204.
463. Forus A, Florenes VA, Maelandsmo GM, et al: The protooncogene *CHOP/GADD153*, involved in growth arrest and DNA damage response, is amplified in a sub-

set of human sarcomas. Cancer Genet Cytogenet 1994; 78:165–171.

464. Ikeda S, Sumii H, Akiyama K, et al: Amplification of both c-*myc* and c-*raf*-1 oncogenes in a human osteosarcoma. Jpn J Cancer Res 1989;80:6–9.

465. Ladanyi M, Cha C, Lewis R, et al: *MDM2* gene amplification in metastatic osteosarcoma. Cancer Res 1993; 53:16–18.

466. Lonardo F, Ueda T, Huvos AG, et al: p53 and MDM2 alterations in osteosarcomas: Correlation with clinicopathologic features and proliferative rate. Cancer 1997; 79:1541–1547.

467. Khatib ZA, Matsushime H, Valentine M, et al: Coamplification of the *CDK4* gene with *MDM2* and *GLI* in human sarcomas. Cancer Res 1993;53:5535–5541.

468. Miller CW, Aslo A, Won A, et al: Alterations of the *p53*, *Rb* and *MDM2* genes in osteosarcoma. J Cancer Res Clin Oncol 1996;122:559–565.

469. Patino-Garcia A, Sierrasesumaga L: Analysis of the *p16INK4* and *TP53* tumor suppressor genes in bone sarcoma pediatric patients. Cancer Genet Cytogenet 1997; 98:50–55.

470. Radig K, Schneider-Stock R, Oda Y, et al: Mutation spectrum of *p53* gene in highly malignant human osteosarcomas. Gen Diagn Pathol 1996;142:25–32.

471. Scholz RB, Kabisch H, Weber B, et al: Studies of the *RB1*gene and the *p53* gene in human osteosarcomas [see comments]. Pediatr Hematol Oncol 1992;9:125–137.

472. Smith-Sorensen B, Gebhardt MC, Kloen P, et al: Screening for *TP53* mutations in osteosarcomas using constant denaturant gel electrophoresis (CDGE). Hum Mutat 1993;2:274–285.

473. Yokoyama R, Schneider-Stock R, Radig K, et al: Clinicopathologic implications of *MDM2*, *p53* and K-*ras* gene alterations in osteosarcomas: *MDM2* amplification and *p53* mutations found in progressive tumors. Pathol Res Pract 1998;194:615–621.

474. Radig K, Schneider-Stock R, Haeckel C, et al: *p53* gene mutations in osteosarcomas of low-grade malignancy. Hum Pathol 1998;29:1310–1316.

475. Serra M, Maurici D, Scotlandi K, et al: Relationship between P-glycoprotein expression and p53 status in high-grade osteosarcoma. Int J Oncol 1999;14:301–307.

476. Molendini L, Benassi MS, Magagnoli G, et al: Prognostic significance of cyclin expression in human osteosarcoma. Int J Oncol 1998;12:1007–1011.

477. Bauer HC: DNA cytometry of osteosarcoma. Acta Orthop Scand Suppl 1988;228:1–39.

478. Aue G, Muralidhar B, Schwartz HS, Butler MG: Telomerase activity in skeletal sarcomas [in process citation]. Ann Surg Oncol 1998;5:627–634.

479. Szymanska J, Mandahl N, Mertens F, et al: Ring chromosomes in parosteal osteosarcoma contain sequences from 12q13-15: A combined cytogenetic and comparative genomic hybridization study. Genes Chromosomes Cancer 1996;16:31–34.

480. Wunder JS, Eppert K, Burrow SR, et al: Co-amplification and overexpression of CDK4, SAS and MDM2 occurs frequently in human parosteal osteosarcomas. Oncogene 1999;18:783–788[ED51].

481. Berman J, O'Leary TJ: Gastrointestinal stromal tumor workshop. Human Pathology 2001;32:578–582.

482. Rubin BP, Singer S, Tsao C, et al: KIT activation is a ubiquitous feature of gastrointestinal stromal tumors. Cancer Res 2001;61:8118–8121.

483. Demetri GD: Targeting *c-kit* mutations in Solid Tumors: Scientific Rationale and Novel Therapeutic Options. Seminars in Oncol 2001;28:19–26.

484. Heinrich MC, Blanke CD, Druker BJ, Corless CL: Inhibition of KIT tyrosine kinase activity: a novel molecular approach to the treatment of KIT-positive malignancies. J Clin Oncol 2002;20:1692–1703.

485. Tuveson DA, Willis NA, Jacks T, et al: ST1571 inactivation of the gastrointestinal stromal tumor c-kit oncoprotein: biological and clinical implications. Oncogene 2001;20:5054–5058.

486. Joensuu H, Roberts PJ, Sarlomo-Rikala M. Effect of the tyrosine kinase inhibitor ST1571 in a patient with a metastatic gastrointestinal stromal tumor. N Engl J Med 2001;344:1052–1056.

487. vanOosterom AT, Judson I, Verweij J et al: Safety and efficacy of imatinib (ST1571) in metastatic gastrointestinal stromal tumors: a phase I study. Lancet 2001;358: 1421–1423.

488. Bridge JA, Liu J, Weibolt V, et al: Novel genomic imbalances in embryonal rhabdomyosarcoma revealed by comparative genomic hybridization and fluorescence in situ hybridization: an intergroup rhabdomyosarcoma study. Genes Chromosomes Cancer 2000;27:337–344.

489. Triche TJ, Schofield D, Buckley J: DNA microarrays in pediatric cancer. Cancer J 2001;7:2–15. Review.

490. Pandita A, Zielenska M, Thorner P, et al: Application of comparative genomic hybridization, spectral karyotyping, and microarray analysis in the identification of subtype-specific patterns of genomic changes in rhabdomyosarcoma. Neoplasia 1999;1:262–275.

CHAPTER 15 APPENDIX

SOP 15.1*

t(11;22): *EWS/FLI1* TRANSLOCATION RT-PCR/SOUTHERN BLOT PROCEDURE

PRINCIPLE

The t(11;22)(q24;q12) translocation, also known as *EWS/FLI1*, occurs in approximately 85% of Ewing's sarcoma and greater than 90% of peripheral primitative neuroectodermal tumors (pPNET). This translocation results in the production of a chimeric gene between a novel putative RNA-binding gene, *EWS* at 22q12 and *FLI1*, a member of the *ETS* family of transcription factors located at 11q24. The translocation occurs at variable breakpoints along both chromosomes 11 (*FLI1* exons 4–9) and 22 (*EWS* exons 7–10) and results in the formation of up to 12 currently identified fusion types. The most common (~60%), type 1, results from the fusion of exon 7/6 *(EWS/FLI1)*; type 2 (~25%)—exon 7/5; type 3—exon 10/6; type 4—exon 7+10/6; type 5—exon 10/5; type 6—exon 7/8; type 7—exon 9/4; type X, and so on. The various *EWS/FLI1* type fusions can be determined by synthesizing the corresponding complementary DNA with reverse transcriptase and amplifying it with PCR by using multiple primers flanking the translocation function. The base-pair size of the resulting products can be used to determine the fusion type. The A673 (type 1), RD-ES and SK-ES-1 (type 2), and Tc-135 (type 3) cell lines are used as controls.

SPECIMEN (see SOP 1)

REAGENTS, SUPPLIES, AND EQUIPMENT

ALWAYS WEAR GLOVES WHEN HANDLING REAGENTS. FOLLOW PROCEDURES FOR AVOIDING CONTAMINATION OF PCR REACTIONS!! (See SOP 2.)

The primers and a probe for the t(11;22) *EWS/FLI1* are adapted from published sequences. t(11;22) EWS/FLI1 primers and all PCR reagents, except $MgCl_2$ are stored in the DNA freezer in the PCR setup room. $MgCl_2$ is stored in the RNA refrigerator in the PCR setup area. RNA extracts and t(11;22) *EWS/FLI1* positive controls are kept in the −70°C freezer in the hallway. Probes for t(11;22) *EWS/FLI1* are kept in the freezer in the post-PCR room. Aliquots of reagents and controls are stored in microcentrifuge tubes (1.5 and 0.5 mL). Do not put unused aliquots back in tubes or containers. Throw them away!

The usual source of a reagent is indicated in brackets [ ]: Fisher [FI], PerkinElmer [PE], Promega [PR], etc. Homemade reagents are abbreviated [MDL], and the lot number in use has been quality control tested.

Cutting Blocks (see SOP 3)

Preparation of RNA Lysates (see SOP 5)

Polymerase Chain Reaction (PCR)

REAGENTS

[DEPC] Molecular-grade water [RG/SIGMA]
PCR buffer II (10X) [PE]
DTT (0.1 mol/L) [BRL]
Random primers [BRL] diluted 0.5 μg/μL with DEPC-molecular-grade water
dNTP 2.5 mmol/L each [PR] [MDL]
DMSO [SI]

1. To prepare, first make a 10-mmol/L solution from a 100-mmol/L stock (1:10 dilution) of each dNTP (dATP, dCTP, dGTP, and dTTP) as follows. To four microcentrifuge tubes, add 900 μL of water, and then add 100 μL of dNTP (100 mmol/L). Mix well.
2. Next, mix equal volumes of each 10 mmol/L solution to make each dNTP 2.5 mmol/L in the final mix.
3. Aliquot and label tubes. Store in DNA freezer.

Taq polymerase (5 U/μL) [PE]
$MgCl_2$ (25 mmol/L) [PE]

PRIMERS

EWS/FLI1 primers are stored in the freezer in a working dilution of 15 μmol/L. β_2-Microglobulin primers (BM3/BM5) are stored at a working dilution of 15 μmol/L.

EWS 1S
5′-TCC TAC AGC CAA GCT CCA AGT C-3′ (temp. = 55°C)
EWS 3S
5′-GAG AGC GAG GTG GCT TCA AT- 3′ (temp. = 53.4°C)
EWS 4S
5′-GAG AAC CGG AGC ATG AGT GG-3′ (temp. = 54.4°C)
FLI1 2AS
5′-GCT GGT CGG GCC CAG GAT CT-3′ (temp. = 62°C)
FLI1 3AS
5′-ACT CAA TCG TGA GGA TTG GTC G-3′ (temp. = 55.5°C)
FLI1 4AS
5′-GCA CTT CCG TGT TGT AGA GG-3′ (temp. = 51°C)

* SOP 15.1 written by Karen Bijwaard, MS, Department of Cellular Pathology and Genetics, Armed Forces Institute of Pathology, Rockville, Maryland.

Fusion Type Frequency, Location, Primer and Probe Information

Type	Frequency (%)	EWS exon	FLI1	5′ Primer	Exon Location	3′ Primer	Exon Location	Est. Prod (bp)	Probe	Exon Location
1	60–70	7	6	EWS 1S	7	FLI1 2AS	8	214	EWSP1	EWS 7
2	20–25	7	5	EWS 1S	7	FLI1 3AS	5	114	EWSP1	EWS 7
3	4–5	10	6	EWS 3S	9	FLI1 2AS	8	218	EWSP3	EWS 10
4	2–3	10*	6	EWS 1S	7	FLI1 2AS	8	247	EWSP1	EWS 7
5	4	10	5	EWS 3S	9	FLI1 3AS	5	123	EWSP3	EWS 10
6	2	7	8	EWS 1S	7	FLI1 2AS	8	87	EWSP1	EWS 7
7	2	9	4	EWS 5S	8	FLI1 4AS	5	169	EWS3S	EWS 9
?	1–2	9	7	EWS 5S	8	FLI1 2AS	8	135	EWS3S	EWS 9

* EWS exon 7 is fused to EWS exon 10 (exons 8 and 9 are spliced out).

Primer combinations to be used are as follows:

EWS/FLI1 Primer and Probe Groupings

	EWS/FLI1 Groupings			
	A	*B*	*C*	*D (β_2-Microglobulin)*
Primers 5′	EWS 1S	EWS 3S	EWS 5S	BM5
3′	FLI1 2AS	FLI1 2AS	FLI1 2AS	BM3
	FLI1 3AS	FLI1 3AS	FLI1 4AS	
Probe	EWS P1	EWS P3	EWS 3S	BMP1

EWS/FLI1 and β_2 Microglobulin Product Sizes

Group A	Size (bp)	Group B	Size (bp)	Group C	Size (bp)	Group D	Size (bp)
Type		Type		Type		β_2-Microglobulin	158
1	214	3	218	7	169/410		
2	114/358	5	123/256	?	135		
3	472						
4	247						
6	87						

Make 40 μL of complementary DNA. Setup for reactions to include A, B, and D. If A and B are negative, a setup for C should be performed with remaining 10 μL of complementary DNA.

Master Mix

REVERSE TRANSCRIPTASE (RT) SARCOMA MASTER MIX

Final reaction volume is 40 μL with 4 μL and 20 μL of sample (corresponding to 1 μL and 5 μL per assay).

4 μL	10X PCR Buffer II
2.4 μL	25 mmol/L $MgCl_2$ (1.5 mmol/L final concentration)
4 μL	0.1 mol/L DTT
2 μL	2.5 mmol/L dNTP
0.6 μL	RNase inhibitor
4 μL	DEPC-dH_2O
17 μL	

Note: 2 μL × N random primers (0.5 μg/μL) and 1 μL × N MMLV-RT (1.8 U/reaction) is added to the RT Sarcoma Master Mix before use.

PCR-RNA SARCOMA MASTER MIX

The volumes to make 40 μL of reaction mixture are as follows:

	Each EWS/FLI1 Mix	β_2-Microglobulin Mix
10× PCR Buffer II	5 μL	5 μL
25 mmol/L $MgCl_2$ (1.5 mmol/L final)	3 μL	3 μL
2.5 mmol/L dNTP	4 μL	4 μL
DEPC-dH_2O	17.5 μL	24.3 μL
	29.5 μL	36.3 μL

Refer to previous table: 2.5 μL × N of each respective EWS and FLI1 primer (10 μmol/L each) and 2.5 μL × N DMSO are added to groups A, B, and C. 1.6 μL × N (15 μmol/L each) and 6.8 μL × N DEPC-dH_2O are added to the β_2-Microglobulin Mix. Add 0.5 μL × N of Taq polymerase to each PCR-RNA Sarcoma Master Mix. Then 10 μL of complementary DNA is added to the PCR-RNA Sarcoma Master Mix for each fusion reaction and the β_2-microglobulin amplification control.

Supplies and Equipment

Microcentrifuge tubes (1.5 mL, 0.5 mL and 0.2 mL)
Aerosol-resistant pipette tips (ART tips)
Disposable gloves
Extra-fine-point permanent marker and racks
Pipettes
Microcentrifuge (reserved for pre-PCR use only)
PerkinElmer Thermal Cycler GeneAmp 9700
Vortexer

Agarose Gel Electrophoresis (see SOP 6)

All reagents except agarose are in the post-PCR room. Agarose is in the pre-PCR room. Use 2.5% agarose.

Chemiluminescence: Southern Blotting of PCR Products (see SOP 9)

Chemiluminescence: End-Labeling Oligonucleotide Probes (see SOP 7)

t(11;22) EWS/FLI1 Probes [BRL/IDT]

Oligonucleotide probes are stored in the post-PCR room freezer in a working dilution of 15 μmol/L (15 pmol/μL).
EWSP1
5′-TAG CTG CTG CTC TGT TGG C-3′
EWSP3
5′-CCA TGG ATG AAG GAC CAG AT-3′
EWS 3S
5′-GAG AGC GAG GTG GCT TCA AT-3′

Chemiluminescence: Hybridization and Washing Southern Blots (see SOP 12)

Prewarm first wash buffer (0.1X SSC/0.1%SDS) to 42°C before washing.

EXPOSING AND DEVELOPING FILM (SEE SOP 11)

QUALITY CONTROL

Several types of positive and negative controls are run with each assay to ensure test performance. The placement of the controls within an assay is crucial to the detection of contamination at each step in the test system.

Positive Assay Control

This also serves as a sensitivity control. The t(11;22) EWS/FLI1 positive control is a lysate from paraffin-embedded cell lines RDES (T2), SK-ES-1(T2), A673 (T1), and TC-135 (T1). See table in "Primers" for product sizes. T2 = type 2

Negative Assay Controls

A negative control is used to control for each step in the test system: lysate preparation, reagent mix preparation, and carryover contamination from sample to sample in the assay setup procedure.

WATER CONTROL. A PCR reaction mix containing water as the sample tested is set up as the first sample in the PCR run, before patient samples, to assess the purity of the assay reagents.

LYSATE CONTROL. A control lysate (no RNA template) prepared in parallel with patient samples but with no tissue specimen should give no detectable band, indicating that the reagents used in lysate preparation were not contaminated.

CONTAMINATION CONTROL. A negative control PCR reaction containing water as the sample tested is also set up last in the PCR run, after the positive control. This reaction assesses the overall quality of the assay setup procedure in avoiding carryover contamination from a positive to an adjacent negative sample.

AMPLIFICATION CONTROL. Paraffin-embedded tissues may contain inhibitors of RT-PCR or fixatives that severely compromise nucleic acid integrity. A control gene must be tested for each sample to assess whether amplifiable nucleic acid is present in the sample.

Positive controls are tested at one concentration: 0.6 to 1 μL of the stock (new vials should be tested before use).

A water control (equiv. to 5 μL water/combination) and lysate controls (1μL equiv./combination) (an empty tube that was treated with the same reagents used during the preparation of the patient DNA extracts) serve as negative controls.

Patient samples are tested at two concentrations: 1 μL of the undiluted lysate (1X) and 5 μL of the undiluted lysate (5X).

The current master mix lot, containing all reaction components except RNA, MMLV, or Taq polymerase and random primers, is prepared and tested in advance with positive and negative controls.

PROCEDURE

FOLLOW PROCEDURES FOR AVOIDING CONTAMINATION OF PCR REACTIONS!! (See SOP 2)

Cutting Blocks (see SOP 3)

Preparation of RNA Lysates (see SOP 5)

RT-Polymerase Chain Reaction (RT-PCR)

Use PerkinElmer Thermal Cycler GeneAmp 9700.

1. Determine the number of samples to be assayed (two dilutions of each patient extract, two water controls, at least one lysate control, and one positive control for each group [if available]). Prepare enough reagents for two additional assays (two plus the number of samples and controls = N). Remove the appropriate number of master mix aliquots for the setup. Aliquots of master mix are sufficient for approximately nine samples. Record the master mix lot numbers on the worksheet. The RT Sarcoma Master Mix is aliquoted for 17 μL per sample, and the RNA PCR Sarcoma Master Mix is aliquoted for 29.5 μL per sample. Calculate the amount of RT Sarcoma Master Mix needed by multiplying

N × 17. Calculate the amount of RNA-PCR Sarcoma Master Mix by N × 29.5.

2. Number the side of each microamp tube, consecutively. Record the assay number, identity of each sample, and dilution on the worksheet (i.e., MDL#, Control, 1X, 5X).

3. Add 2 μL × N Random Primers (0.5 μg/μL) and 1 μL × N MMLV to 17 × N of the RT Sarcoma Master mix (2 + 1 + 17 = 20). Tap tube gently to mix.

4. Add 20 μL DEPC-dH_2O to the water control and 16 μL DEPC-dH_2O to each tube that corresponds to 1X of extract. Add 18 to 19.4 μL DEPC-dH_2O to the tubes containing the positive controls (No. 7 below).

5. Add 20 μL of the master mix to each tube. Close caps.

6. Add 4 μL and 20 μL of undiluted sample extract to each tube designated for 1X and 5X, respectively. The final volume of the RT reaction is 40 μL.

7. Add 0.6 to 2 μL of each positive control (the optimum amount of each positive control should be determined empirically before the control being put into use and DEPC-dH_2O volume to be adjusted accordingly).

8. Add 20 μL DEPC-dH_2O to the remaining water control (negative).

9. Place in PerkinElmer Thermal Cycler GeneAmp 9700 and incubate 1 hour at 37°C, 5 minutes at 95°C, and finally at 4°C.

10. Remove tubes from thermal cycler. Label three additional tubes for each tube from the previous steps, using the same numbers but designate #A, #B, #D. (A = group A; B = group B; D = β_2-microglobulin).

11. Add 29.7 × N of RNA PCR Sarcoma Master Mix to 1.5-mL Eppendorf tubes labeled A, B, and D. To tubes A and B, add 2.5 μL × N of each primer and DMSO to each tube (see earlier table). To tube D, add 1.6 μL × N of BM3 and BM5 each, and 6.8 μL × N DEPC-dH_2O. Add 0.5 μL × N of Taq polymerase to each tube.

12. Aliquot 40 μL RNA PCR Sarcoma Master Mix for group A into each of the group A tubes. Repeat for group B and D. Add 10 μL of the 40 μL complementary DNA to its respective tube (A, B, D). Cap tubes. Reserve the remaining 10 μL of complementary DNA in the RNA refrigerator for future amplification for group C, if necessary. Label rack with assay and setup date.

13. Place tube in PerkinElmer Thermal Cycler GeneAmp 9700 and cycle using the times and temperatures below:

Initial step:	5 min 94°C
40 cycles of:	1 min 94°C
	1 min 60°C
	1 min 72°C
Final step:	7 min 72°C
Soak:	4°C

14. Place samples in refrigerator in post-PCR room.

Agarose Gel Electrophoresis (see SOP 6)

All reagents are in the post-PCR room. The PCR products are resolved on 2.5% agarose (2% LMP, 0.5% agarose) in 1X TBE.

Chemiluminescence: Southern Blotting (see SOP 9)

Chemiluminescence: End-Labeling Oligonucleotide Probes (see SOP 7)

Chemiluminescence: Hybridization and Washing Southern Blots (see SOP 10)

Prewarm first wash buffer (0.1X SSC/0.1%SDS) to 42°C before washing.

Exposing and Developing Film (see SOP 11)

REPORTING RESULTS

A positive result for the t(11;22)(q24;q12) translocation is reported if a positive signal is seen in the patient sample, provided all the appropriate controls are working. If not, repeat the assay.

If there is a positive signal for the β_2-microglobulin gene and a negative signal for the t(11;22)(q24;q12) translocation, the t(11;22)(q24;q12) result is reported as negative.

If there is a negative signal for the β_2-microglobulin gene and a negative signal for the t(11;22)(q24;q12) translocation, the t(11;22)(q24;q12) result is reported as indeterminate.

REFERENCES

Delattre O, Zucman J, Plougastel B, et al: Gene fusion with an ETS DNA-binding domain caused by chromosome translocation in human tumours. Nature 1992;359:163–165.

Downing JR, Head DR, Parham DM, et al: Detection of the (11;22)(q24;q12) translocation of Ewing's sarcoma and peripheral neuroectodermal tumor by reverse transcription polymerase chain reaction. Am J Pathol 1993;143: 1294–1300.

Ida K, Kobayashi S, Taki T, et al: EWS-FLI-1 and EWS-ERG chimeric mRNAs in Ewing's sarcoma and primitive neuroectodermal tumor. Int J Cancer 1995;63:500–504.

Ladanyi M: The emerging molecular genetics of sarcoma translocations. Diagn Mol Pathol 1995;4:162–173.

Plougastel B, Zucman J, Peter M, et al: Genomic structure of the *EWS* gene and its relationship to EWSR1, a site of tumor-associated chromosome translocation. Genomics 1993;18:609–615.

Sorensen PHB, Liu XF, Delattre O, et al: Reverse transcriptase PCR amplification of EWS/FLI-1 fusion transcripts as a diagnostic test for peripheral primitive neuroectodermal tumors of childhood. Diagn Mol Pathol 1993;2:147–157.

TIMOTHY J. O'LEARY

16

Skin

EPITHELIAL TUMORS

Basal Cell Carcinoma

Basal cell carcinoma (BCC) is the most common malignant neoplasm. The distinctive histologic and clinical presentation renders unnecessary the use of ancillary diagnostic methods in all but a vanishingly small number of cases. Nevertheless, BCC is interesting from a molecular biologic perspective, both because it provides insight into the role of DNA damage repair in neoplasia and because the rare occurrence of metastatic disease provides an exceptional opportunity to separately consider factors influencing tumor proliferation and metastatic potential.

Gorlin's (basal cell nevus) syndrome, an autosomal dominant disease characterized by the appearance of multiple BCCs beginning in childhood, provides a "natural experiment" by which to attempt an understanding of molecular alterations in BCC. Linkage analysis suggests that the genetic defect in Gorlin's syndrome occurs in the region of 9q22,[1–3] through mutation of the *PTCH* (patched) gene.[4–7] Most mutations result in protein truncation, and there is no obvious genotype/phenotype correlation in patients with Gorlin's syndrome.[8]

Most sporadic BCCs demonstrate loss of heterozygosity (LOH) on chromosome 9q22.[9–14] Karyotypic studies also demonstrate frequent 9q22 structural rearrangements.[15, 16] In spite of the strong association between sun exposure and the development of BCC, no relationship between 9q22 LOH and sun exposure has been seen.[9] LOH is associated with mutation of the *PTCH* gene, which codes a transmembrane protein homologous to a *Drosophila*,[17] and is in turn associated with very high levels of PTCH expression.[18, 19] In contrast to the germline mutations of Gorlin's syndrome, which are most frequently frameshift type, missense mutations in highly conserved alleles are often identified in sporadic BCC.[20, 21]

The mechanism by which *PTCH* mutation gives rise to BCC is not understood. Patients with Gorlin's syndrome demonstrate a significant level of spontaneous chromatid and chromosome rearrangements, accompanied by cell cycle lengthening; these findings suggest that *PTCH* mutation gives rise to chromosome instability and that the protein may have a role in DNA repair.[22]

A number of other molecular abnormalities have been reported in BCC. Although one study has reported that about 3% of BCC patients demonstrate LOH at the *HRAS* locus,[23] other studies have suggested that *HRAS* mutations are rare in BCC[24, 25]; *KRAS* mutations have also been reported in a minority of patients.[26] It seems likely that *RAS* gene mutations are not involved in the pathogenesis of BCC but that they serve as a general indicator of sun exposure and genetic damage from ultraviolet radiation.

Although BCC frequently demonstrates p53 by immunohistochemical (IHC) methods, mutation is seen in a minority of cases.[27–29] Mutations of *TP53* are more frequent in patients who develop tumors later in life than in those presenting before age 40[30]; most frequently only a single allele is mutated, in contrast to other tumors that frequently demonstrate *TP53* mutations.[31] IHC staining for p53 may have prognostic significance, because some workers report p53 reactivity to be more common in lesions that recur or metastasize than in those that do not[28]; other workers have failed to confirm this observation.[32] Because a very small proportion of BCCs metastasize, however, it is likely that the vast majority of p53-positive BCCs will remain localized.

IHC studies of cellular proliferation show wide variations in the levels of Ki-67 (MIB1) reactivity. Although the average growth fraction differs somewhat depending on the histologic variant, there is great overlap across tumor types.[33, 34] Some workers have reported that tumors demonstrating high levels of Ki-67 (MIB1) immunoreactivity are more likely to recur than those with lower levels of immunoreactivity[32]; similar results have been reported for proliferating cell nuclear antigen (PCNA) immunohistochemistry.[35] Cytometric studies demonstrate that BCCs demonstrating partial or diffuse growth patterns are more likely to be aneuploid than those with circumscribed growth patterns.[36] Taken together with other findings in BCC, this result suggests that multiple genetic abnormalities, in addition to those related to PTCH function, are probably involved in the pathogenesis of many or most BCCs.

Although the diagnosis of BCC and its differentiation from skin appendage tumors with which it is frequently confused is seldom aided by IHC assessment, the IHC staining characteristics have not been extensively studied. Most are cytokeratin and BCL2 positive; stains for glandular differentiation are negative, and S-100 immunoreactivity is not observed.

Keratoacanthoma

Keratoacanthoma is a benign and usually self-healing squamous proliferation that bears a resemblance to squamous cell carcinoma (SCC). Some investigators believe that keratoacanthoma is biologically and clinically indistinguishable from well-differentiated SCC.[37] Other investigators have observed differences in IHC staining patterns of keratoacanthoma and SCC that would suggest definite biologic distinctions.[38] A single karyotype has been reported for keratoacanthoma; the reported clonal changes were very complex.[39] DNA cytometry reveals near-diploid aneuploidy in most keratoacanthomas but severe aneuploidy in only a small percentage.[40, 41]

The genetic alterations contributing to the development of keratoacanthomas are not well established. Although most investigators have not identified human papillomaviruses within keratoacanthomas,[42, 43] others have reported detecting a wide variety of papillomavirus types by polymerase chain reaction (PCR).[44] Keratoacanthomas are relatively common in individuals with certain familial mismatch repair gene abnormalities (Muir-Torre syndrome),[45] and microsatellite instability is generally observed in the keratoacanthomas from these patients.[46] In contrast, microsatellite instability is rare in patients with isolated, sporadic keratoacanthomas.[47, 48] A second syndrome associated with multiple self-healing keratoacanthomas, Ferguson-Smith syndrome, has been linked to a locus on 9q22-31 at or near the site of the *PTCH* gene,[49] which is frequently mutated in BCCs. To date, *PTCH* mutations have not been reported, however, and LOH at 9q22-31 is infrequent in sporadic keratocanthomas.[50]

Keratoacanthomas frequently demonstrate IHC staining for p53,[51–54] but mutations are rarely detected by sequencing.[29, 55] IHC staining is not useful in differentiating keratoacanthomas from SCC.[52, 56] Activating *RAS* mutations have been reported but appear to be uncommon[25, 57] and are not clearly related to pathogenesis.

IHC staining for PCNA shows that the fraction of proliferating cells is higher in proliferating keratoacanthomas than in regressing keratoacanthomas and that it overlaps that of well-differentiated SCC.[58] Similar overlap is seen when Ki-67 (MIB1) expression is assessed.[59] The pattern of PCNA and Ki-67 staining differs somewhat between keratoacanthomas and SCC, with the former demonstrating a more "peripheral" pattern of staining.[60–62] Nevertheless, IHC assays of cell proliferation have limited use in distinguishing between these histologically similar lesions.

Squamous Cell Carcinoma

Squamous cell carcinoma of the skin is an aggressive tumor that is frequently associated with radiation or other skin damage. Although many cases arise in the setting of preexisting actinic keratoses or Bowen's disease (carcinoma in situ), neither is a requisite precondition for pathogenesis of SCC. Cytogenetic studies of SCC originating in the skin do not reveal consistent clonal karyotypic abnormalities.[63–72] In situ hybridization and comparative genomic hybridization studies are sparse and unrewarding.[73]

LOH studies have demonstrated frequent loss on 9p, 9q, 13q, 17p, 17q, and 3p.[13, 74–76] One of the areas frequently displaying LOH, chromosome 9q22.3, is the site of the *PTCH* gene, which is frequently mutated in BCC. Sequence analysis has, however, failed to demonstrate mutation of *PTCH* in any of 14 SCCs examined.[74] A nearby gene, *ZNF189*, which codes for a zinc-finger protein, is likewise not mutated in these tumors.[77]

Ultraviolet light, which is thought to be the major cause of human skin cancer, readily causes mutation of the *TP53* tumor suppressor gene. Such mutations are found in more than half of actinic keratoses, Bowen's disease, and SCC.[78–80] In addition, large patches of morphologically normal skin with *TP53* mutations are a frequent finding in humans; such patches may be up to 100,000 times more frequent than dysplasia and are not conclusively premalignant.[80] Mutations of the *TP53* gene are uncommon in arsenic-related skin cancers, however.[81]

Mutations of the *CDKN2A* gene, which encodes two proteins involved in cell cycle regulation, have also been reported in approximately 15% of SCC.[82]

The flat warts of epidermodysplasia verruciformis frequently transform to SCC. HPV 17 has been detected in epidermodysplasia verruciformis by PCR.[83] HPV-related sequences are also frequently detected in both actinic keratoses and SCCs of patients immunosuppressed as a result of organ transplantation[84, 85] or human immunodeficiency virus (HIV) infection.[86] A large number of HPV subtypes have been implicated. HPV (particularly HPV-16) has also been found in the lesions of bowenoid papulosis and SCC of the vulva, even in the absence of immunosuppression.[87, 88] HPV is also seen in SCC originating in the finger[88]; it seems unlikely that HPV is playing an important role in the pathogenesis of these tumors.[42] Studies have yielded contradictory reports regarding the roles of Epstein-Barr virus (EBV) and human herpesvirus type 8 in squamous skin lesions of immunosuppressed patients.[89–92] Herpes simplex virus has been detected in SCC.[93]

Investigations of the role of *RAS* genes in development of squamous carcinoma have been highly variable, with some investigators reporting only rare activating mutations[24, 94] and others claiming that these mutations may be found in up to 90% of cases.[23]

Merkel Cell Carcinoma

Merkel cell carcinoma is an uncommon neuroendocrine tumor arising from the skin and skin appendages. Most tumors are characterized by multiple chromosomal abnormalities; almost all karyotypes have demonstrated chromosome 1 derangement, ranging from trisomy to deletions.[95–103] Although classic karyotyping has not revealed characteristic recurrent cytogenetic abnormalities, deletions and translocations involving chromosome 1p36 have several times been reported as the major cytogenetic abnormalities[95, 99]; LOH at chromosome 1p36 is frequently observed by microsatellite analysis.[104–107] Other regions in which cytogenetic changes are frequently observed, both by karyotypic analysis and comparative genomic hybridization, are 3p, 13q, 5p, 8q, and 19,[99, 104] but considerable case-to-case variation is observed.[108] Microsatellite studies demonstrate that, as for 1p36, allelic deletions of 13q[109] and 3p[107] are common. Trisomies of chromosomes 1, 11, and 18 have also been seen by chromosome-specific in situ hybridization.[110]

Merkel cell carcinomas frequently demonstrate IHC staining for p53 protein[111]; studies attempting to relate p53 expression to prognosis have yielded conflicting results.[111, 112] Mutation of the *TP53* gene has not been reported.[113] There is apparently no relationship between expression of PCNA or Ki-67 (MIB1) and outcome.[112, 114]

The IHC characteristics of Merkel cell carcinoma are outlined in Table 16–1. This tumor is most easily distinguished from lymphoma or melanoma by IHC staining for keratin[115]; CK20 staining can be used further to distinguish Merkel cell carcinoma from small cell carcinomas originating in the lung and elsewhere.[116, 117]

MESENCHYMAL TUMORS

Atypical Fibroxanthoma

Although some authors consider atypical fibroxanthoma (AFX) to be nothing more than an extremely superficial form of malignant fibrous histiocytoma (MFH),[118] there is little cytogenetic or molecular biologic evidence to support this claim. Although AgNOR counts are similar,[119] the IHC profiles of AFX and MFH differ significantly (Table 16–2), with AFX significantly more likely to express actin and S-100. This suggests significant biologic differences between the two tumors.

Most cases of AFX demonstrate IHC reactivity for p53[120, 121]; these cases demonstrate mutations with a pattern suggestive of ultraviolet radiation–induced mutagenesis.[120] The frequency of p53 mutation (approximately 70% of cases) in AFX is much higher than that in MFH (approximately 15% of cases).[122] Reports differ on the frequency of tumor aneuploidy.[123, 124] There is, as yet, no reliable method for predicting which of these tumors will develop metastases.

TABLE 16–1

Immunohistochemical Characteristics of Merkel Cell Carcinoma

Antigen	Percentage of Cases Demonstrating Immunoreactivity
Keratin (pan)	92–100
CK 20	92–100
CAM 5.2	80–98
Epithelial membrane antigen	73–95
Neuron-specific enolase	70–88
Chromogranin A	46–74
Neurofilament protein	30–70
Gastrin-releasing peptide (bombesin)	14–56
Synaptophysin	19–48
Somatostatin	16–49
Calcitonin	1–24
Vimentin	0–12
CD45	0
HMB-45	0
S-100	0
Serotonin	0

TABLE 16–2

Reactivity of Selected Immunohistochemical Markers in Malignant Fibrous Histiocytoma (MFH), Atypical Fibroxanthoma (AFX), and Dermatofibrosarcoma Protuberans (DFSP)

Antigen	Percentage of MFHs Positive	Percentage of AFXs Positive	Percentage of DFSPs Positive
α_1-Antitrypsin	64–79	49–79	0
α_1-Antichymotrypsin	67–79	48–80	0–15
Actin (HHF-35)	3–16	32–56	47–68
Actin (SM)	1–15	22–48	28–48
CD34	2–15	8–42	73–85
CD68	38–53	40–70	2–20
S-100	0–4	6–20	0–3
Vimentin	93–99	100	100

Dermatofibroma

Little is known about the pathogenesis of dermatofibroma (DF). Neither cytogenetic nor comparative genomic hybridization studies have been performed; whether this tumor represents a monoclonal proliferation has not been established. High levels of *PDGFB* messenger RNA are found,[125] suggesting a possible relationship to dermatofibrosarcoma protuberans (DFSP), in which this gene is often deregulated. IHC staining for p53 is seen seldom, if ever.[121, 126, 127] Although the proliferation rate determined by Ki-67 (MIB1) staining is low,[128, 129] high levels of PCNA staining are observed.[130]

Differentiation of DF from DFSP is usually straightforward, both morphologically and immunohistochemically (Table 16–3).

Dermatofibrosarcoma Protuberans

Dermatofibrosarcoma protuberans (DFSP) is a monoclonal[131] spindle cell proliferation of intermediate malignant potential. Although a number of chromosomal abnormalities have been reported,[132–141] the t(17;22)(q22;q13) translocation[134, 135, 142] and the presence of supernumerary ring chromosomes containing material from 17q22 and 22q13 are the most common findings.[135, 136, 143] This material is made up of amplified *COL1A1* and *PDGFB* sequences[135]; the gene fusion appears to result in deletion of *PDGF* exon 1, with resulting constitutive activation.[144–146] Interestingly, translocations and ring chromosomes seldom occur in combination, suggesting that both events accomplish the same biologic result.

Although IHC evidence of p53 accumulation is seen in almost all DFSPs,[121, 126] this is apparently not accompanied by mutation[147] and is not correlated with the proliferation rate.[126] One small study suggests that IHC staining for p53 is possibly associated with more aggressive behavior.[147] Studies comparing the proliferation rates of DFSP and DF have reached contradictory conclusions.[126, 128, 129]

The antigenic profiles of DF and DFSP differ substantially (see Table 16–3), although IHC characterization is seldom required to make a diagnosis of DF. The more common problem of differentiating DFSP from AFX and MFH may also be assisted by IHC methods, because, unlike AFX and MFH, DFSP seldom reacts with antibodies directed against α_1-antitrypsin or α_1-antichymotrypsin (see Table 16–2).

Mycosis Fungoides

A wide variety of T-cell lymphomas affect the skin, including mycosis fungoides (MF), its leukemic variant

TABLE 16–3

Immunohistochemical Profile Differences Between Dermatofibroma (DF) and Dermatofibrosarcoma Protuberans (DFSP)

Antigen	Percentage of DF Cases Positive	Percentage of DFSP Cases Positive
α_1-Antichymotrypsin	23–49	67–79
Actin (SM)	63–88	28–48
CD34	5–16	73–85
CD68	43–91	2–20

the Sézary syndrome, lymphomatoid papulosis, CD30+ large cell lymphoma, and adult T-cell leukemia/lymphoma. MF is a neoplasm of middle age that typically has a fatal 4- to 5-year clinical course. Cytogenetic abnormalities of chromosome 14q have been reported for many years[148] and are most frequently identified at 14q32,[149] but a wide variety of other cytogenetic abnormalities have also been reported.[150, 151] Although these cytogenetic abnormalities may provide important clues to disease pathogenesis, they have not been followed up.

Although IHC staining for p53 is rarely observed in early cases of MF, it is frequently seen in tumors that have undergone large cell transformation[152]; mutation of *TP53* is not necessarily observed[152] but has nevertheless been reported in approximately 25% of patients.[153] Ki-67 (MIB1) immunoreactivity tends to increase as MF progresses[154] but also appears to be useful in predicting prognosis of patients with limited disease.[155]

Although Epstein-Barr virus has been found in MF cells, the virus is nonreplicating and does not appear to have a role in pathogenesis.[156, 157] A retrovirus, human T-cell lymphotrophic virus-I (HTLV-I) has occasionally been identified in MF cells[158] Even though some studies suggest that the vast majority of patients do not harbor this virus,[159–161] others find it in almost all cases.[162–164] The wide variation in reported results suggests methodologic difficulties in the identification of HTLV-I sequences and militates against the use of assays of HTLV-I in the diagnosis of cutaneous leukemia/lymphoma.

T-cell proliferations, including MF, are characterized by rearrangement of the T-cell receptor genes.[165] Identification of T-cell β or γ chain rearrangement by Southern blotting or PCR is a diagnostically useful way to establish the identity of a monoclonal T-cell proliferation[166]; most laboratories have found PCR assays for the T-cell γ chain rearrangement to be most easily incorporated into routine clinical practice.[167, 168] Although Southern blot tests detect a higher proportion of potential rearrangements, the small number of cells present in many skin biopsy specimens often results in an insufficient quantity of recoverable DNA for Southern blotting. Limited cellularity may also cause difficulties in interpreting PCR results, however, because the appearance of a "clonal band" based on amplification of cellular DNA from four or five cells may mislead one into inferring malignancy when none is present.[169] Detection of a monoclonal T-cell population in morphologically uninvolved lymph nodes suggests a poor prognosis.[170]

IHC assays typically demonstrate the pan–T-cell antigens CD2, CD3, and CD5 but often fail to show CD7. Most cases show the mature helper T-cell phenotype, CD4+/CD8−.[165] CD15 (Leu-M1) positivity is often associated with tumor progression.[171]

MALIGNANT MELANOMA

Malignant melanoma is a common cancer. The lifetime risk for melanoma of a resident of the United States is approximately 1 in 90; this incidence has increased 20-fold in the past 70 years.[172] Clearly, damage by solar ultraviolet radiation is the major etiologic factor. Absorption of this radiation in the upper epidermis by melanin pigment provides significant protection to dark-skinned individuals. In addition, the observation of "melanoma families" (in particular, those afflicted with the dysplastic nevus syndrome) indicates a strong hereditary component that has proven useful in the search for the genetic alterations causing this highly aggressive cancer.

Karyotypic analysis demonstrates frequent clonal abnormalities in chromosomes 1p, 6q, 7, and 9p, with less frequent abnormalities on chromosomes 2, 3, 10, and 11.[173] Karyotypes of congenital and common nevi seldom demonstrate karyotypic abnormalities[174, 175]; those of dysplastic nevi are most commonly normal but may show a variety of cytogenetic alterations.[174, 175] In contrast, karyotypes of malignant melanoma are virtually all abnormal.[174] Losses of chromosome 9p represent the only common alteration found in dysplastic nevi and malignant melanomas, suggesting strongly the involvement of chromosome 9p (particularly 9pter-p22) in the pathogenesis of dysplastic nevus syndrome–associated melanoma.[174, 176] Linkage studies also point to chromosome 9p as the site of a dysplastic nevus syndrome gene,[177, 178] and LOH studies demonstrate 9p21 LOH in over 85% of malignant melanomas[179] and in nearly as many dysplastic nevi.[180] Comparative genomic hybridization reveals changes in a similar proportion of cases.[181] These alterations are frequently associated with frameshift mutations in the cell-cycle regulating *CDKN2A* gene (*p16, INK4)*, a part of the retinoblastoma gene pathway.[182, 183] Although this potentially provides a substrate for molecular diagnosis of dysplastic nevus syndrome, the clinical characteristics are sufficiently unique to suggest that such a test would find little practical utility for most families. There is a relatively low incidence of *CDKN2A* mutation in sporadic melanoma, however, even when 9p21 LOH is demonstrated,[184] and many familial melanomas do not demonstrate *CDKN2A* mutations,[185] further limiting the clinical use of such a test. Retinoblastoma gene activity and CDK4 function are also lost in malignant melanoma, albeit in a much smaller fraction of tumors lose CDKN2A function.[186, 187] Nevertheless, the aggregate effect is that nearly 100% of melanoma cell lines demonstrate alterations of *CDKN2A*, *CDKN2B*, or one of their downstream targets.[188] These changes are all typically associated with overexpression of *CCND1*[189] and confirm the importance of the retinoblastoma/cyclase pathway in the pathogenesis of malignant melanoma.

Rearrangements of chromosome 1, in most cases involving 1p12-22, are found in most cases of advanced melanoma but less commonly identified in early melanoma.[173, 190, 191] Deletions of 1p36 are also common, and linkage analysis suggests involvement of 1p36 in at least some dysplastic nevus syndrome families.[192] Deletions of 1p36 are found in a large number of advanced cancers with varying histogenesis, but the specific molecular alterations are as yet not well defined. In melanomas, however, loss of heterozygosity in this region appears to be associated only with nodular melanoma, rather than with superficial spreading disease.[193] A metastasis suppressor gene called *KISS1*, loss of which may be associated with dissemination of malignant melanoma, has been mapped to 1p32.[194, 195]

Chromosome 6 rearrangements are found in about half of all melanomas[173, 190, 196, 197]; deletions of 6q and amplifications of 6p are each identified in about one fourth of cases by comparative genomic hybridization.[181] LOH studies show 6q loss to occur most frequently in the 6q22-27 region,[198] but specific gene mutations of this region have not been characterized.

An increase in chromosome 7 copy number is seen in about half of melanomas,[173, 181, 199, 200] particularly late in the clinical course. Nevertheless, the clinical significance of this finding is unknown. In addition to chromosome duplication, gene amplifications of chromosomes 4q12, 5p13-pter, 7q33-qter, 8q12-13, 11q13-14, and 17q25 have been observed by comparative genomic hybridization[181] and increases in chromosome 20q copy number have been observed by fluorescent in situ hybridization.[201] *MYCN* amplification has also been reported in two patients.[202]

Flow and image cytometric analysis of malignant melanoma are complex. Aneuploidy is detected by image cytometry in nearly 80% of fresh melanoma specimens but in fewer than half of formalin-fixed, paraffin-embedded tumors.[203] Image cytometry, in turn, is clearly superior to flow cytometry for detection of aneuploidy.[204] Tumor aneuploidy appears to be associated with metastasis[205] and with high proliferation rates.[206] The use of cytometric measurements in predicting long-term survival is complicated by the fact that both aneuploidy[207] and S-phase fractions appear to be associated with response to some therapeutic regimens.[208] Further investigation is required.

Expression and mutation of the *TP53* gene in malignant melanoma has been the subject of numerous investigations, yielding results that often conflict with one another. The p53 protein can be identified in about half of all malignant melanomas and appears to be more common in those with a nodular configuration than in those of the superficial spreading variety.[209–211] Results vary substantially from laboratory to laboratory, however, with some laboratories reporting that as few as 5% of all primary melanomas demonstrate p53 immunoreactivity[212] and others reporting immunoreactivity in up to 85% of cases.[213] There appears to be little or no association between p53 immunoreactivity and *TP53* gene mutation in melanoma,[209, 214] and *TP53* mutation is rarely observed in melanoma biopsy specimens.[209, 215] Although some investigators have suggested that IHC staining for p53 is prognostically useful in early melanoma,[211, 216, 217] other investigators have not only failed to find an association between clinical utility and poor outcome[205, 218, 219] but even found an association between p53 immunoreactivity and favorable prognosis.[220] These large discrepancies, together with the substantial interlaboratory variation in this assay, militate against the clinical use of p53 immunohistochemistry in assessment of melanoma prognosis.

Activating mutations of *RAS* proto-oncogenes occur in approximately 10% of malignant melanomas. These mutations, which usually are found in nodular melanomas rather than those of superficial spreading type, generally occur in codon 61 of *NRAS*.[173, 221, 222] Mutations of *KRAS* and *HRAS* are uncommon.[222, 223]

The protein product of the *KIT* proto-oncogene is a tyrosine kinase receptor that, when mutated, serves as a constitutively activated dominant oncogene in mast cell and gastrointestinal stromal tumors. In contrast, KIT expression is down-regulated in malignant melanoma,[224, 225] apparently allowing melanoma to escape stem cell factor–induced apoptosis.[226] Loss of KIT expression apparently results from loss of a transcription factor, AP-2.[227] Neither the frequency nor mechanism of AP-2 loss has yet been determined.

The clinical utility of IHC assessment of cellular proliferation markers (PCNA and Ki-67/MIB1) has been extensively investigated.[228, 229] These studies suggest that high levels of MIB1 immunoreactivity are associated with metastatic dissemination in malignant melanomas measuring more than 1.5 mm in thickness,[217, 230, 231] but not in thin melanomas.[232] PCNA immunostaining appears to be of little prognostic value. Some studies find an association between high PCNA index and metastasis[233]; others suggest that high levels of PCNA staining are associated with an improved prognosis.[231, 234] Perhaps not surprisingly, most authors conclude that PCNA immunohistochemistry has little prognostic utility in malignant melanoma.[228, 235, 236]

Although immunohistochemistry is of limited prognostic utility in malignant melanoma, it is the mainstay of diagnosis when this disease appears, as it so frequently does, as metastatic disease of unknown primary tumor. The IHC profile of malignant melanoma is shown in Tables 16–4 and 16–5 (which highlights characteristics of desmoplastic malignant melanoma). The usual absence of HMB-45 staining in desmoplastic malignant melanoma should be noted, as should the frequent staining with polyclonal antibodies directed against carcinoembyronic antigen, because both of these characteristics frequently cause unnecessary diagnostic confusion.

INHERITED DISEASES OF SKIN

There are an extremely large number of inherited diseases of the skin, skin appendages, and subcutaneous

TABLE 16–4

Immunoreactivity of Selected Immunohistochemical Markers in Malignant Melanoma

Antigen	Percentage of Cases Demonstrating Immunoreactivity
CD146	100
S-100	94–99
Myosin	91–100
Vimentin	93–99
Tubulin	84–100
HMB-45	86–92
Melan-A	79–93
CD68	68–82
Neuron-specific enolase	63–82
CD117	57–74
α_1-Antichymotrypsin	43–82
α_1-Antitrypsin	39–75
Actin (SM)	33–59
Carcinoembryonic antigen (polyclonal)	25–56
CD99	1–13
Epithelial membrane antigen	0–13
Keratin (pan)	0–5
CD31	0
CD34	0
CD45	0
Carcinoembryonic antigen (monoclonal)	0
Factor VIII–related antigen	0

tissue. In this section I briefly discuss the clinical and molecular biologic features of a few of these diseases, chosen because they illustrate the wide range of mutational events that can give rise to histologically and clinically similar inherited disorders.

Cutis Laxa

Cutis laxa is a disease in which marked laxity of the skin is present. An X-linked form that is associated by a characteristic facies, skeletal abnormalities, and structural abnormalities of the genitourinary tract has been described,[237] as has an autosomal dominant form that may occur with or without pulmonary and cardiovascular compromise.[238, 239] The histopathologic features of fragmented and branched elastin fibrils are similar to those of normal cutaneous aging.[240, 241] In the autosomal dominant form, this is accompanied by reduced elastin gene expression[242] and secondary structure abnormalities that result from frameshift mutations in the elastin gene.[239, 243] In the X-linked form, it appears as a mutation in a copper-transporting adenosine triphosphatase.[243, 244] Although only a few of these mutations have been characterized, it appears that they may occur in any of several exons. Thus, molecular testing will require sequence analysis and is likely to be more useful for genetic counseling than initial diagnosis.

TABLE 16–5

Immunoreactivity of Selected Immunohistochemical Markers in Desmoplastic Malignant Melanoma

Antigen	Percentage of Cases Demonstrating Immunoreactivity
Neuron-specific enolase	100
S-100	92–100
Vimentin	64–100
CD63	28–72
HMB-45	4–20

Epidermolysis Bullosa Simplex

Epidermolysis bullosa simplex (EBS) is a form of epidermolysis bullosa in which blistering is entirely intradermal. A variety of subtypes have been proposed, based on the distribution of lesions and histologic and electron microscopic findings. Mutations of the keratin 5 gene *(KRT5)*[245–250] or the keratin 14 gene *(KRT14)*[245, 246, 251–253] appear to cause all of the various subtypes (Weber-Cockayne, Kobner, Dowling-Meara); missense mutation in the same codon can give rise to all three subtypes, suggesting that the specific nature of each mutation must be considered when weighing its likely clinical importance.[254]

Generalized Atrophic Benign Epidermolysis Bullosa

This is an adult-onset, nonlethal, inherited subepidermal blistering disease in which structural abnormalities are found in the hemidesmosome-anchoring filament complexes.[255, 256] Both autosomal dominant and autosomal recessive inheritance have been reported; associated abnormalities include hypoplasia and pitting of the dental enamel.[257] Frameshift mutation of any of several loci in the gene for type XVII collagen, *COL17A1/BPAG2*, apparently gives rise to both structural changes and reduced gene expression, resulting in disrupted junctional stability.[255, 257–260]

Epidermolysis Bullosa Letalis (Herlitz-Pearson Type Epidermolysis Bullosa)

Epidermolysis bullosa letalis is a disorder of the perinatal period in which the appearance of bullous lesions is often followed by sloughing of skin, loss of protein, and infection. It appears that this disorder may be caused by disruption in any of the three laminin 5 (nicein, kalinin) polypeptides—α_3 (coded by *LAMA3*),[261, 262] β_3 (coded by *LAMB3*).[261, 263, 264] and γ_2 (coded by *LAMC2*).[261, 265, 266] Thirty percent to 40% of all mutations occur at a single mutational hot spot in the *LAMB3* gene[261, 264]; the relatively small number of regions in which mutations are identified has facilitated prenatal molecular testing.[267–269] IHC analysis of laminin 5 subunits is not useful in predicting the chain affected by mutation.[270]

A variant of epidermolysis bullosa letalis in which pyloric atresia also occurs has been associated with defective integrin $\alpha6\beta4$ expression.[271]

Ehlers-Danlos syndrome

Ehlers-Danlos syndrome (EDS) is a constellation of inherited connective tissue diseases characterized by fragile, bruisable skin, joint laxity, and frequent premature rupture of fetal membranes. A large variety of clinical manifestations have been reported, and at least 10 clinical "types" have been described on the basis of varying clinical and biochemical features. Differing molecular abnormalities giving rise to defective collagen assembly have been described for each type.[272]

CLASSIC TYPE (TYPES 1 AND 2)

Skin hyperextensibility with widened atrophic scars and joint hypermobility characterize the autosomal dominant "classic type" of EDS. Traditionally, the term *type 1* was reserved for those patients with severe manifestations and *type 2* for those with a less severe form. DNA sequence analysis has shown this distinction to be suspect, but the occurrence of serious internal complications, including rupture of the large vessels, diverticulosis, and rupture of the bowel, make an assessment of the global severity of disease useful clinically. Linkage analysis demonstrates a strong association between clinical disease and the *COL5A1* gene,[273–275] and mutations in both *COL5A1* and in *COL5A2* have been found in patients with classic EDS.[276–281]

VASCULAR TYPE (TYPE 4)

Type 4 EDS is an autosomal dominant disorder characterized by extremely thin skin through which blood vessels are readily visualized and vascular fragility that leads to extensive bruising even after minor trauma.[282, 283] This increased vascular fragility leads to an increased predisposition to spontaneous rupture of the aorta; ruptures of cerebral vessels intestinal and uterine rupture are also reported.[284] Unlike other forms of EDS, joint hypermobility is typically confined to the fingers and the skin is not particularly hyperextensible.

Mutations occur in a gene coding for type 3 collagen (*COL3A1*),[285–292] with reduction of type 3 collagen caused by effects on secretion and fibrillogenesis.[293, 294] The spectrum of mutations appears to be limited, and denaturing gradient gel electrophoresis of PCR products has been used as a molecular diagnostic test.[290]

KYPHOSCOLIOSIS TYPE (TYPE 6)

Type 6 EDS is characterized by severe infantile muscular hypotonia, kyphoscoliosis from an early age, and scleral fragility, together with the usual EDS features of recurrent joint dislocations and stretchable skin. This form has been associated with lysyl hydroxylase deficiency,[295] and the clinical diagnosis is typically confirmed by identification of an insufficiency of hydroxylysine on analysis of hydrolyzed dermis.[296] Enzymatic insufficiency results from mutations in the *PLOD* gene on chromosome 1p36.3.[297–303] Although about one fifth of EDS families show a duplication of seven exons in the *PLOD*,[302] a variety of mutation types has been reported. Thus, sequence analysis is most useful not for diagnosis but rather for genetic counseling purposes.[304]

ARTHROCHALASIA TYPE (TYPE 7B)

This form of EDS is characterized by congenital dislocation of the hip, together with the usual skin manifestations, severe joint hypermobility, mild bone loss, short stature, and a small mandible. This form of EDS is autosomal dominant; many cases appear to result from new mutations, which result in deletion of exon 6 of the *COL1A1* or *COL1A2* genes.[305–308] This exon codes the N-telopeptide cleavage side of the procollagen chains, and its deletion inhibits conversion of procollagen to collagen. The restricted range of mutations enables straightforward molecular diagnosis.

DERMATOSPARAXIS TYPE (TYPE 7C)

Patients with this autosomal recessive form of EDS have striking fragility of their soft, doughy, and redundant skin (which resembles that of cutis laxa) and substantial bruising. Blue sclerae, umbilical hernia, and failure to normally mineralize the cranial vault are also characteristic. Electron microscopy demonstrates not an absence of collagen bundles but rather a loose and disorganized fibril meshwork.[309–311] Although the precise genetic defects have not been characterized, there is evidence that the enzyme that cleaves the amino-terminal propeptides from the pro-α1(I) and pro-α2(I) chains of type I procollagen molecules is defective.[311]

REFERENCES

1. Farndon PA, Del Mastro RG, Evans DG, Kilpatrick MW: Location of gene for Gorlin syndrome. Lancet 1992;339:581–582.
2. Wicking C, Berkman J, Wainwright B, Chenevix-Trench G: Fine genetic mapping of the gene for nevoid basal cell carcinoma syndrome. Genomics 1994;22:505–511.
3. Farndon PA, Morris DJ, Hardy C, et al: Analysis of 133 meioses places the genes for nevoid basal cell carcinoma (Gorlin) syndrome and Fanconi anemia group C in a 2.6-cM interval and contributes to the fine map of 9q22.3. Genomics 1994;23:486–489.
4. Johnson RL, Rothman AL, Xie J, et al: Human homolog of patched, a candidate gene for the basal cell nevus syndrome. Science 1996;272:1668–1671.
5. Wicking C, Bale AE: Molecular basis of the nevoid basal cell carcinoma syndrome. Curr Opin Pediatr 1997;9:630–635.
6. Wicking C, Gillies S, Smyth I, et al: De novo mutations of the Patched gene in nevoid basal cell carcinoma syndrome help to define the clinical phenotype. Am J Med Genet 1997;73:304–307.
7. Wicking C, Shanley S, Smyth I, et al: Most germ-line mutations in the nevoid basal cell carcinoma syndrome lead to a premature termination of the PATCHED protein, and no genotype-phenotype correlations are evident. Am J Hum Genet 1997;60:21–26.
8. Bale AE: The nevoid basal cell carcinoma syndrome: Genetics and mechanism of carcinogenesis. Cancer Invest 1997;15:180–186.
9. Gailani MR, Leffell DJ, Ziegler A, et al: Relationship between sunlight exposure and a key genetic alteration in basal cell carcinoma. J Natl Cancer Inst 1996;88:349–354.
10. Holmberg E, Rozell BL, Toftgard R: Differential allele loss on chromosome 9q22.3 in human non-melanoma skin cancer. Br J Cancer 1996;74:246–250.
11. Konishi K, Yamanishi K, Ishizaki K, et al: Analysis of *p53* gene mutations and loss of heterozygosity for loci on chromosome 9q in basal cell carcinoma. Cancer Lett 1994;79:67–72.
12. Quinn AG, Sikkink S, Rees JL: Delineation of two distinct deleted regions on chromosome 9 in human non-melanoma skin cancers. Genes Chromosomes Cancer 1994;11:222–225.
13. Quinn AG, Sikkink S, Rees JL: Basal cell carcinomas and squamous cell carcinomas of human skin show distinct patterns of chromosome loss. Cancer Res 1994;54:4756–4759.
14. Shanley SM, Dawkins H, Wainwright BJ, et al: Fine deletion mapping on the long arm of chromosome 9 in sporadic and familial basal cell carcinomas. Hum Mol Genet 1995;4:129–133.
15. Jin Y, Mertens F, Persson B, et al: Nonrandom numerical chromosome abnormalities in basal cell carcinomas. Cancer Genet Cytogenet 1998;103:35–42.
16. Jin Y, Merterns F, Persson B, et al: The reciprocal translocation t(9;16)(q22;p13) is a primary chromosome abnormality in basal cell carcinomas. Cancer Res 1997;57:404–406.
17. Hahn H, Wicking C, Zaphiropoulous PG, et al: Mutations of the human homolog of *Drosophila* patched in the nevoid basal cell carcinoma syndrome. Cell 1996;85:841–851.
18. Gailani MR, Stahle-Backdahl M, Leffell DJ, et al: The role of the human homologue of *Drosophila* patched in sporadic basal cell carcinomas. Nat Genet 1996;14:78–81.
19. Nagano T, Bito T, Kallassy M, et al: Overexpression of the human homologue of *Drosophila* patched *(PTCH)* in skin tumours: Specificity for basal cell carcinoma. Br J Dermatol 1999;140:287–290.
20. Unden AB, Holmberg E, Lundh-Rozell B, et al: Mutations in the human homologue of *Drosophila* patched (*PTCH*) in basal cell carcinomas and the Gorlin syndrome: Different in vivo mechanisms of *PTCH* inactivation. Cancer Res 1996;56:4562–4565.
21. Wolter M, Reifenberger J, Sommer C, et al: Mutations in the human homologue of the *Drosophila* segment polarity gene patched (PTCH) in sporadic basal cell carcinomas of the skin and primitive neuroectodermal tumors of the central nervous system. Cancer Res 1997;57:2581–2585.
22. Shafei-Benaissa E, Savage JR, Babin P, et al: The naevoid basal-cell carcinoma syndrome (Gorlin syndrome) is a chromosomal instability syndrome. Mutat Res 1998;397:287–292.
23. Ananthaswamy HN, Applegate LA, Goldberg LH, Bales ES: Deletion of the c-Ha-*ras*-1 allele in human skin cancers. Mol Carcinog 1989;2:298–301.
24. Campbell C, Quinn AG, Rees JL: Codon 12 Harvey-*ras* mutations are rare events in non-melanoma human skin cancer. Br J Dermatol 1993;128:111–114.
25. Lieu FM, Yamanishi K, Konishi K, et al: Low incidence of Ha-*ras* oncogene mutations in human epidermal tumors. Cancer Lett 1991;59:231–235.
26. van der Schroeff JG, Evers LM, Boot AJ, Bos JL: *Ras* oncogene mutations in basal cell carcinomas and squamous cell carcinomas of human skin. J Invest Dermatol 1990;94:423–425.

27. Campbell C, Quinn AG, Angus B, Rees JL: The relation between *p53* mutation and p53 immunostaining in non-melanoma skin cancer. Br J Dermatol 1993;129:235–241.
28. De Rosa G, Staibano S, Barra E, et al: p53 protein in aggressive and non-aggressive basal cell carcinoma. J Cutan Pathol 1993;20:429–434.
29. Kubo Y, Urano Y, Yoshimoto K, et al: *p53* gene mutations in human skin cancers and precancerous lesions: Comparison with immunohistochemical analysis. J Invest Dermatol 1994;102:440–444.
30. D'Errico M, Calcagnile AS, Corona R, et al: *p53* mutations and chromosome instability in basal cell carcinomas developed at an early or late age. Cancer Res 1997;57:747–752.
31. van der Riet P, Karp D, Farmer E, et al: Progression of basal cell carcinoma through loss of chromosome 9q and inactivation of a single p53 allele. Cancer Res 1994;54: 25–27.
32. Healy E, Angus B, Lawrence CM, Rees JL: Prognostic value of Ki67 antigen expression in basal cell carcinomas. Br J Dermatol 1995;133:737–741.
33. Barrett TL, Smith KJ, Hodge JJ, et al: Immunohistochemical nuclear staining for p53, PCNA, and Ki-67 in different histologic variants of basal cell carcinoma. J Am Acad Dermatol 1997;37:430–437.
34. Baum HP, Meurer I, Unteregger G: Ki-67 antigen expression and growth pattern of basal cell carcinomas. Arch Dermatol Res 1993;285:291–295.
35. Toth DP, Guenther LC, Shum DT: Proliferating cell nuclear antigen (PCNA); prognostic value in the clinical recurrence of primary basal cell carcinoma. J Dermatol Sci 1996;11:36–40.
36. Herzberg AJ, Garcia JA, Kerns BJ, et al: DNA ploidy of basal cell carcinoma determined by image cytometry of fresh smears. J Cutan Pathol 1993;20:216–222.
37. Beham A, Regauer S, Soyer HP, Beham-Schmid C: Keratoacanthoma: A clinically distinct variant of well-differentiated squamous cell carcinoma. Adv Anat Pathol 1998;5:269–280.
38. Ho T, Horn T, Finzi E: Transforming growth factor alpha expression helps to distinguish keratoacanthomas from squamous cell carcinomas. Arch Dermatol 1991; 127:1167–1171.
39. Mertens F, Heim S, Mandahl N, et al: Clonal chromosome aberrations in a keratoacanthoma and a basal cell papilloma. Cancer Genet Cytogenet 1989;39:227–232.
40. Pilch H, Weiss J, Heubner C, Heine M: Differential diagnosis of keratoacanthomas and squamous cell carcinomas: Diagnostic value of DNA image cytometry and p53 expression. J Cutan Pathol 1994;21:507–513.
41. Seidman JD, Berman JJ, Moore GW, Yetter RA: Multiparameter DNA flow cytometry of keratoacanthoma. Anal Quant Cytol Histol 1992;14:113–119.
42. Kawashima M, Favre M, Obalek S, et al: Premalignant lesions and cancers of the skin in the general population: Evaluation of the role of human papillomaviruses. J Invest Dermatol 1990;95:537–542.
43. Lu S, Syrjanen SL, Havu VK, Syrjanen S: Known HPV types have no association with keratoacanthomas. Arch Dermatol Res 1996;288:129–132.
44. Hsi ED, Svoboda-Newman SM, Stern RA, et al: Detection of human papillomavirus DNA in keratoacanthomas by polymerase chain reaction. Am J Dermatopathol 1997;19:10–15.
45. Esche C, Kruse R, Lamberti C, et al: Muir-Torre syndrome: Clinical features and molecular genetic analysis. Br J Dermatol 1997;136:913–917.
46. Honchel R, Halling KC, Schaid DJ, et al: Microsatellite instability in Muir-Torre syndrome. Cancer Res 1994; 54:1159–1163.
47. Langenbach N, Kroiss MM, Ruschoff J, et al: Assessment of microsatellite instability and loss of heterozygosity in sporadic keratoacanthomas. Arch Dermatol Res 1999;291:1–5.
48. Peris K, Magrini F, Keller G, et al: Analysis of microsatellite instability and loss of heterozygosity in keratoacanthoma. Arch Dermatol Res 1997;289:185–188.
49. Richards FM, Goudie DR, Cooper WN, et al: Mapping the multiple self-healing squamous epithelioma (MSSE) gene and investigation of xeroderma pigmentosum group A (XPA) and PATCHED (PTCH) as candidate genes. Hum Genet 1997;101:316–322.
50. Waring AJ, Takata M, Rehman I, Rees JL: Loss of heterozygosity analysis of keratoacanthoma reveals multiple differences from cutaneous squamous cell carcinoma. Br J Cancer 1996;73:649–653.
51. Borkowski A, Bennett WP, Jones RT, et al: Quantitative image analysis of p53 protein accumulation in keratoacanthomas. Am J Dermatopathol 1995;17:335–338.
52. Cain CT, Niemann TH, Argenyi ZB: Keratoacanthoma versus squamous cell carcinoma: An immunohistochemical reappraisal of p53 protein and proliferating cell nuclear antigen expression in keratoacanthoma-like tumors. Am J Dermatopathol 1995;17:324–331.
53. Kerschmann RL, McCalmont TH, LeBoit PE: p53 oncoprotein expression and proliferation index in keratoacanthoma and squamous cell carcinoma. Arch Dermatol 1994;130:181–186.
54. Lee YS, Teh M: p53 expression in pseudoepitheliomatous hyperplasia, keratoacanthoma, and squamous cell carcinoma of skin. Cancer 1994;73:2317–2323.
55. Perez MI, Robins P, Biria S, et al: P53 oncoprotein expression and gene mutations in some keratoacanthomas. Arch Dermatol 1997;133:189–193.
56. Stephenson TJ, Royds J, Silcocks PB, Bleehen SS: Mutant p53 oncogene expression in keratoacanthoma and squamous cell carcinoma. Br J Dermatol 1992; 127:566–570.
57. Corominas M, Kamino H, Leon J, Pellicer A: Oncogene activation in human benign tumors of the skin (keratoacanthomas): Is *HRAS* involved in differentiation as well as proliferation? Proc Natl Acad Sci USA 1989;86: 6372–6376.
58. Li J, Lee YS: Proliferating cell nuclear antigen (PCNA) expression in pseudoepitheliomatous hyperplasia, keratoacanthoma and squamous cell carcinoma of the skin. Ann Acad Med Singapore 1996;25:526–530.
59. Matsuta M, Kimura S, Kosegawa G, Kon S: Immunohistochemical detection of Ki-67 in epithelial skin tumors in formalin-fixed paraffin-embedded tissue sections using a new monoclonal antibody (MIB-1). J Dermatol 1996;23:147–152.
60. Royds JA, Stephenson TJ, Silcocks PB, Bleehen SS: Proliferating cell nuclear antigen immunostaining in

keratoacanthoma and squamous cell carcinoma of the skin. Pathologica 1994;86:612–616.

61. Skalova A, Michal M: Patterns of cell proliferation in actinic keratoacanthomas and squamous cell carcinomas of the skin: Immunohistochemical study using the MIB 1 antibody in formalin-fixed paraffin sections. Am J Dermatopathol 1995;17:332–334.

62. Sagol O, Kurtoglu B, Ozer E, Pabuccuoglu U: Stereological estimation of mean nuclear volume and staining pattern of Ki-67 antigen in keratoacanthomas and squamous cell carcinomas. Gen Diagn Pathol 1998;143: 305–309.

63. Atkin NB, Baker MC, Petkovic I: Squamous cell carcinoma of the skin with an unusual marker chromosome. Cytobios 1988;54:161–166.

64. Atkin NB, Fox MF: Possibly identical marker chromosome der(16)t(?13;16)(?q13or14;q22) in a squamous cell carcinoma of the skin and larynx. Cancer Genet Cytogenet 1992;58:198–200.

65. Boukamp P, Tilgen W, Dzarlieva RT, et al: Phenotypic and genotypic characteristics of a cell line from a squamous cell carcinoma of human skin. J Natl Cancer Inst 1982;68:415–427.

66. Heim S, Jin Y, Mandahl N, et al: Multiple unrelated clonal chromosome abnormalities in an in situ squamous cell carcinoma of the skin. Cancer Genet Cytogenet 1988;36:149–153.

67. Heim S, Caron M, Jin Y, et al: Genetic convergence during serial in vitro passage of a polyclonal squamous cell carcinoma. Cytogenet Cell Genet 1989;52:133–135.

68. Heim S, Mertens F, Jin YS, et al: Diverse chromosome abnormalities in squamous cell carcinomas of the skin. Cancer Genet Cytogenet 1989;39:69–76.

69. MacHino H, Miki Y, Teramoto T, et al: Cytogenetic studies in a patient with porokeratosis of Mibelli, multiple cancers and a forme fruste of Werner's syndrome. Br J Dermatol 1984;111:579–586.

70. Swanson GP, Dobin SM, Arber JM, et al: Chromosome 11 abnormalities in Bowen disease of the vulva. Cancer Genet Cytogenet 1997;93:109–114.

71. Worsham MJ, Carey TE, Benninger MS, et al: Clonal cytogenetic evolution in a squamous cell carcinoma of the skin from a xeroderma pigmentosum patient. Genes Chromosomes Cancer 1993;7:158–164.

72. Zaslav AL, Stamberg J, Steinberg BM, et al: Cytogenetic analysis of head and neck carcinomas. Cancer Genet Cytogenet 1991;56:181–187.

73. Dobler M, Schuh J, Kiesewetter F, et al: Deletion monitoring in skin tumors by interphase-FISH using band-specific DNA probes. Int J Oncol 1999;14: 571–576.

74. Eklund LK, Lindstrom E, Unden AB, et al: Mutation analysis of the human homologue of *Drosophila* patched and the xeroderma pigmentosum complementation group A genes in squamous cell carcinomas of the skin. Mol Carcinog 1998;21:87–92.

75. Quinn AG, Campbell C, Healy E, Rees JL: Chromosome 9 allele loss occurs in both basal and squamous cell carcinomas of the skin. J Invest Dermatol 1994; 102:300–303.

76. Zaphiropoulos PG, Soderkvist P, Hedblad MA, Toftgard R: Genetic instability of microsatellite markers in region q22.3-q31 of chromosome 9 in skin squamous cell carcinomas. Biochem Biophys Res Commun 1994;201:1495–1501.

77. Odeberg J, Rosok O, Gudmundsson GH, et al: Cloning and characterization of *ZNF189*, a novel human Kruppel-like zinc finger gene localized to chromosome 9q22-q31. Genomics 1998;50:213–221.

78. Brash DE, Rudolph JA, Simon JA, et al: A role for sunlight in skin cancer: UV-induced *p53* mutations in squamous cell carcinoma. Proc Natl Acad Sci USA 1991;88: 10124–10128.

79. Brash DE, Ziegler A, Jonason AS, et al: Sunlight and sunburn in human skin cancer: *p53*, apoptosis, and tumor promotion. J Invest Dermatol Symp Proc 1996;1:136–142.

80. Ren ZP, Ahmadian A, Ponten F, et al: Benign clonal keratinocyte patches with *p53* mutations show no genetic link to synchronous squamous cell precancer or cancer in human skin. Am J Pathol 1997;150:1791–1803.

81. Castren K, Ranki A, Welsh JA, Vahakangas KH: Infrequent *p53* mutations in arsenic-related skin lesions. Oncol Res 1998;10:475–482.

82. Kubo Y, Urano Y, Matsumoto K, et al: Mutations of the INK4a locus in squamous cell carcinomas of human skin. Biochem Biophys Res Commun 1997;232:38–41.

83. Yutsudo M, Shimakage T, Hakura A: Human papillomavirus type 17 DNA in skin carcinoma tissue of a patient with epidermodysplasia verruciformis. Virology 1985;144:295–298.

84. Bens G, Wieland U, Hofmann A, et al: Detection of new human papillomavirus sequences in skin lesions of a renal transplant recipient and characterization of one complete genome related to epidermodysplasia verruciformis-associated types. J Gen Virol 1998;79:779–787.

85. Euvrard S, Chardonnet Y, Pouteil-Noble C, et al: Association of skin malignancies with various and multiple carcinogenic and noncarcinogenic human papillomaviruses in renal transplant recipients. Cancer 1993;72: 2198–2206.

86. Cuesta KH, Palazzo JP, Mittal KR: Detection of human papillomavirus in verrucous carcinoma from HIV-seropositive patients. J Cutan Pathol 1998;25:165–170.

87. Bergeron C, Naghashfar Z, Canaan C, et al: Human papillomavirus type 16 in intraepithelial neoplasia (bowenoid papulosis) and coexistent invasive carcinoma of the vulva. Int J Gynecol Pathol 1987;6:1–11.

88. Eliezri YD, Silverstein SJ, Nuovo GJ: Occurrence of human papillomavirus type 16 DNA in cutaneous squamous and basal cell neoplasms. J Am Acad Dermatol 1990;23:836–842.

89. Nishimoto S, Inagi R, Yamanishi K, et al: Prevalence of human herpesvirus-8 in skin lesions. Br J Dermatol 1997;137:179–184.

90. Huston BM, Maia DM: Absence of latent Epstein-Barr virus in cutaneous squamoproliferative lesions after solid organ transplantation. Mod Pathol 1997;10:1188–1193.

91. Kohler S, Kamel OW, Chang PP, Smoller BR: Absence of human herpesvirus 8 and Epstein-Barr virus genome sequences in cutaneous epithelial neoplasms arising in immunosuppressed organ-transplant patients. J Cutan Pathol 1997;24:559–563.

92. Ternesten-Bratel A, Kjellstrom C, Ricksten A: Specific expression of Epstein-Barr virus in cutaneous squamous

cell carcinomas from heart transplant recipients. Transplantation 1998;66:1524–1529.
93. Claudy AL, Chignol MC, Chardonnet Y: Detection of herpes simplex virus DNA in a cutaneous squamous cell carcinoma by in situ hybridization. Arch Dermatol Res 1989;281:333–335.
94. Arrighi F: Parapsoriasiforme lichen planus. Bull Soc Fr Dermatol Syphiligr 1968;75:619–620.
95. Gibas Z, Weil S, Chen ST, McCue PA: Deletion of chromosome arm 1p in a Merkel cell carcinoma (MCC). Genes Chromosomes Cancer 1994;9:216–220.
96. Koduru PR, Dicostanzo DP, Jhanwar SC: Nonrandom cytogenetic changes characterize Merkel cell carcinoma. Dis Markers 1989;7:153–161.
97. Kusyk CJ, Romsdahl MM: Cytogenetic study of a Merkel cell carcinoma. Cancer Genet Cytogenet 1986; 20:311–316.
98. Larsimont D, Verhest A: Chromosome 6 trisomy as sole anomaly in a primary Merkel cell carcinoma. Virchows Arch 1996;428:305–309.
99. Leonard JH, Leonard P, Kearsley JH: Chromosomes 1, 11, and 13 are frequently involved in karyotypic abnormalities in metastatic Merkel cell carcinoma. Cancer Genet Cytogenet 1993;67:65–70.
100. Perlman EJ, Lumadue JA, Hawkins AL, et al: Primary cutaneous neuroendocrine tumors: Diagnostic use of cytogenetic and MIC2 analysis. Cancer Genet Cytogenet 1995;82:30–34.
101. Sandbrink F, Muller L, Fiebig HH, Kovacs G: Short communication: Deletion 7q, trisomy 6 and 11 in a case of Merkel-cell carcinoma. Cancer Genet Cytogenet 1988;33:305–309.
102. Tope WD, Sangueza OP: Merkel cell carcinoma: Histopathology, immunohistochemistry, and cytogenetic analysis. J Dermatol Surg Oncol 1994;20:648–652.
103. Vazquez-Mazariego Y, Vallcorba I, Ferro MT, et al: Cytogenetic study of neuroendocrine carcinoma of Merkel cells. Cancer Genet Cytogenet 1996;92:79–81.
104. Van Gele M, Van Roy N, Ronan SG, et al: Molecular analysis of 1p36 breakpoints in two Merkel cell carcinomas. Genes Chromosomes Cancer 1998;23:67–71.
105. Vortmeyer AO, Merino MJ, Boni R, et al: Genetic changes associated with primary Merkel cell carcinoma. Am J Clin Pathol 1998;109:565–570.
106. Harnett PR, Kearsley JH, Hayward NK, et al: Loss of allelic heterozygosity on distal chromosome 1p in Merkel cell carcinoma: A marker of neural crest origins? Cancer Genet Cytogenet 1991;54:109–113.
107. Leonard JH, Williams G, Walters MK, et al: Deletion mapping of the short arm of chromosome 3 in Merkel cell carcinoma. Genes Chromosomes Cancer 1996; 15:102–107.
108. Harle M, Arens N, Moll I, et al: Comparative genomic hybridization (CGH) discloses chromosomal and subchromosomal copy number changes in Merkel cell carcinomas. J Cutan Pathol 1996;23:391–397.
109. Leonard JH, Hayard N: Loss of heterozygosity of chromosome 13 in Merkel cell carcinoma. Genes Chromosomes Cancer 1997;20:93–97.
110. Amo-Takyi BK, Tietze L, Tory K, et al: Diagnostic relevance of chromosomal in-situ hybridization in Merkel cell carcinoma: Targeted interphase cytogenetic tumour analyses. Histopathology 1999;34:163–169.
111. Kennedy MM, Blessing K, King G, Kerr KM: Expression of bcl-2 and p53 in Merkel cell carcinoma: An immunohistochemical study. Am J Dermatopathol 1996;18:273–277.
112. Carson HJ, Reddy V, Taxy JB: Proliferation markers and prognosis in Merkel cell carcinoma. J Cutan Pathol 1998;25:16–19.
113. Schmid M, Janssen K, Dockhorn-Dworniczak B, et al: p53 abnormalities are rare events in neuroendocrine (Merkel cell) carcinoma of the skin: An immunohistochemical and SSCP analysis. Virchows Arch 1997; 430:233–237.
114. Parrado C, Bjornhagen V, Eusebi V, et al: Prognosticating tools in primary neuroendocrine (Merkel-cell) carcinomas of the skin: Histopathological subdivision, DNA cytometry, cell proliferation analyses (Ki-67 immunoreactivity) and NCAM immunohistochemistry: A clinicopathological study in 25 patients. Pathol Res Pract 1998;194:11–23.
115. Battifora H, Silva EG: The use of antikeratin antibodies in the immunohistochemical distinction between neuroendocrine (Merkel cell) carcinoma of the skin, lymphoma, and oat cell carcinoma. Cancer 1986;58:1040–1046.
116. Chan JK, Suster S, Wenig BM, et al: Cytokeratin 20 immunoreactivity distinguishes Merkel cell (primary cutaneous neuroendocrine) carcinomas and salivary gland small cell carcinomas from small cell carcinomas of various sites. Am J Surg Pathol 1997;21:226–234.
117. Miettinen M: Keratin 20: Immunohistochemical marker for gastrointestinal, urothelial, and Merkel cell carcinomas. Mod Pathol 1995;8:384–388.
118. Fish FS: Soft tissue sarcomas in dermatology. Dermatol Surg 1996;22:268–273.
119. Merot Y, Durgniat AC, Frenk E: Nucleolar organizer regions in fibrohistiocytic tumors of the skin. J Cutan Pathol 1990;17:122–126.
120. Dei TA, Maestro R, Doglioni C, et al: Ultraviolet-induced *p53* mutations in atypical fibroxanthoma. Am J Pathol 1994;145:11–17.
121. Lee CS, Chou ST: p53 protein immunoreactivity in fibrohistiocytic tumors of the skin. Pathology 1998;30: 272–275.
122. Reid AH, Tsai MM, Venzon DJ, et al: *MDM2* amplification, *P53* mutation, and accumulation of the *P53* gene product in malignant fibrous histiocytoma. Diagn Mol Pathol 1996;5:65–73.
123. Michie BA, Reid RP, Fallowfield ME: Aneuploidy in atypical fibroxanthoma: DNA content quantification of 10 cases by image analysis. J Cutan Pathol 1994;21: 404–407.
124. Breathnach AS: Development and differentiation of dermal cells in man. J Invest Dermatol 1978;71:2–8.
125. Smits A, Funa K, Vassbotn FS, et al: Expression of platelet-derived growth factor and its receptors in proliferative disorders of fibroblastic origin. Am J Pathol 1992;140:639–648.
126. Diaz-Cascajo C, Bastida-Inarrea J, Borrego L, Carretero-Hernandez G: Comparison of p53 expression in dermatofibrosarcoma protuberans and dermatofibroma: Lack of correlation with proliferation rate. J Cutan Pathol 1995;22:304–309.
127. Haerslev T, Rossen K, Hou-Jensen K, Jacobsen GK: Immunohistochemical detection of p53 in epidermal

proliferations overlying dermatofibromas. Acta Derm Venereol 1995;75:187–189.

128. Ooe M, Nogita T, Kawashima M: Comparative study of Ki-67 immunostaining and nuclear DNA content in histiofibrous tumors. J Dermatol 1992;19:12–18.

129. Hsi ED, Nickoloff BJ: Dermatofibroma and dermatofibrosarcoma protuberans: An immunohistochemical study reveals distinctive antigenic profiles. J Dermatol Sci 1996;11:1–9.

130. Li DF, Iwasaki H, Kikuchi M, et al: Dermatofibroma: Superficial fibrous proliferation with reactive histiocytes: A multiple immunostaining analysis. Cancer 1994;74: 66–73.

131. Allan AE, Tsou HC, Harrington A, et al: Clonal origin of dermatofibrosarcoma protuberans. J Invest Dermatol 1993;100:99–102.

132. Craver RD, Correa H, Kao Y, Van Brunt T: Dermatofibrosarcoma protuberans with 46,XY,t(X;7) abnormality in a child. Cancer Genet Cytogenet 1995;80:75–77.

133. Iwasaki H, Ohjimi Y, Ishiguro M, et al: Supernumerary ring chromosomes and nuclear blebs in some low-grade malignant soft tissue tumours: Atypical lipomatous tumours and dermatofibrosarcoma protuberans. Virchows Arch 1998;432:521–528.

134. Dei TA, Dal Cin P: The role of cytogenetics in the classification of soft tissue tumours. Virchows Arch 1997; 431:83–94.

135. Gisselsson D, Hoglund M, O'Brien KP, et al: A case of dermatofibrosarcoma protuberans with a ring chromosome 5 and a rearranged chromosome 22 containing amplified COL1A1 and PDGFB sequences. Cancer Lett 1998;133:129–134.

136. Minoletti F, Miozzo M, Pedeutour F, et al: Involvement of chromosomes 17 and 22 in dermatofibrosarcoma protuberans. Genes Chromosomes Cancer 1995;13:62–65.

137. Orndal C, Mandahl N, Rydholm A, et al: Supernumerary ring chromosomes in five bone and soft tissue tumors of low or borderline malignancy. Cancer Genet Cytogenet 1992;60:170–175.

138. Pedeutour F, Simon MP, Minoletti F, et al: Ring 22 chromosomes in dermatofibrosarcoma protuberans are low-level amplifiers of chromosome 17 and 22 sequences. Cancer Res 1995;55:2400–2403.

139. Pedeutour F, Lacour JP, Perrin C, et al: Another case of t(17;22) (q22;q13) in an infantile dermatofibrosarcoma protuberans. Cancer Genet Cytogenet 1996;89:175–176.

140. Sonobe H, Furihata M, Iwata J, et al: Dermatofibrosarcoma protuberans harboring t(9;22)(q32;q12.2). Cancer Genet Cytogenet 1999;110:14–18.

141. Stephenson CF, Berger CS, Leong SP, et al: Ring chromosome in a dermatofibrosarcoma protuberans. Cancer Genet Cytogenet 1992;58:52–54.

142. Pedeutour F, Simon MP, Minoletti F, et al: Translocation, t(17;22)(q22;q13), in dermatofibrosarcoma protuberans: A new tumor-associated chromosome rearrangement. Cytogenet Cell Genet 1996;72:171–174.

143. Pedeutour F, Coindre JM, Sozzi G, et al: Supernumerary ring chromosomes containing chromosome 17 sequences: A specific feature of dermatofibrosarcoma protuberans? Cancer Genet Cytogenet 1994;76:1–9.

144. Greco A, Fusetti L, Villa R, et al: Transforming activity of the chimeric sequence formed by the fusion of collagen gene *COL1A1* and the platelet-derived growth factor b-chain gene in dermatofibrosarcoma protuberans. Oncogene 1998;17:1313–1319.

145. O'Brien KP, Seroussi E, Dal Cin P, et al: Various regions within the alpha-helical domain of the *COL1A1* gene are fused to the second exon of the *PDGFB* gene in dermatofibrosarcomas and giant-cell fibroblastomas. Genes Chromosomes Cancer 1998;23:187–193.

146. Simon MP, Pedeutour F, Sirvent N, et al: Deregulation of the platelet-derived growth factor B-chain gene via fusion with collagen gene *COL1A1* in dermatofibrosarcoma protuberans and giant-cell fibroblastoma. Nat Genet 1997;15:95–98.

147. Hisaoka M, Okamoto S, Morimitsu Y, et al: Dermatofibrosarcoma protuberans with fibrosarcomatous areas: Molecular abnormalities of the p53 pathway in fibrosarcomatous transformation of dermatofibrosarcoma protuberans. Virchows Arch 1998;433:323–329.

148. Fukuhara S, Rowley JD, Variakojis D: Banding studies of chromosomes in a patient with mycosis fungoides. Cancer 1978;42:2262–2268.

149. Fukuhara S, Rowley JD: Chromosome 14 translocations in non-Burkitt lymphomas. Int J Cancer 1978;22:14–21.

150. Thangavelu M, Finn WG, Yelavarthi KK, et al: Recurring structural chromosome abnormalities in peripheral blood lymphocytes of patients with mycosis fungoides/ Sézary syndrome. Blood 1997;89:3371–3377.

151. van Vloten WA, Pet EA, Geraedts JP: Chromosome studies in mycosis fungoides. Br J Dermatol 1980; 102:507–513.

152. Strohl RA: The role of total skin electron beam radiation therapy in the management of mycosis fungoides. Dermatol Nurs 1994;6:191–194, 196, 220.

153. McGregor JM, Crook T, Fraser-Andrews EA, et al: Spectrum of *p53* gene mutations suggests a possible role for ultraviolet radiation in the pathogenesis of advanced cutaneous lymphomas. J Invest Dermatol 1999;112:317–321.

154. Dummer R, Michie SA, Kell D, et al: Expression of bcl-2 protein and Ki-67 nuclear proliferation antigen in benign and malignant cutaneous T-cell infiltrates. J Cutan Pathol 1995;22:11–17.

155. Kristensen M, Illum D, Sogaard H, et al: Mycosis fungoides: A review of the clinical picture, treatment and course in 107 patients. Ugeskr Laeger 1990;152: 1371–1375.

156. Anagnostopoulos I, Hummel M, Kaudewitz P, et al: Low incidence of Epstein-Barr virus presence in primary cutaneous T-cell lymphoproliferations. Br J Dermatol 1996;134:276–281.

157. Chan AC, Ho JW, Chiang AK, Srivastava G: Phenotypic and cytotoxic characteristics of peripheral T-cell and NK-cell lymphomas in relation to Epstein-Barr virus association. Histopathology 1999;34:16–24.

158. Detmar M, Pauli G, Anagnostopoulos I, et al: A case of classical mycosis fungoides associated with human T-cell lymphotropic virus type I. Br J Dermatol 1991; 124:198–202.

159. Fujihara K, Goldman B, Oseroff AR, et al: HTLV-associated diseases: Human retroviral infection and cutaneous T-cell lymphomas. Immunol Invest 1997;26: 231–242.

160. Bazarbachi A, Soriano V, Pawson R, et al: Mycosis fungoides and Sézary syndrome are not associated with HTLV-I infection: An international study. Br J Haematol 1997;98:927–933.
161. Wood GS, Schaffer JM, Boni R, et al: No evidence of HTLV-I proviral integration in lymphoproliferative disorders associated with cutaneous T-cell lymphoma. Am J Pathol 1997;150:667–673.
162. Pancake BA, Zucker-Franklin D, Coutavas EE: The cutaneous T cell lymphoma, mycosis fungoides, is a human T cell lymphotropic virus-associated disease: A study of 50 patients. J Clin Invest 1995;95:547–554.
163. Khan ZM, Sebenik M, Zucker-Franklin D: Localization of human T-cell lymphotropic virus-1 tax proviral sequences in skin biopsies of patients with mycosis fungoides by in situ polymerase chain reaction. J Invest Dermatol 1996;106:667–672.
164. Manca N, Piacentini E, Gelmi M, et al: Persistence of human T cell lymphotropic virus type 1 (HTLV-1) sequences in peripheral blood mononuclear cells from patients with mycosis fungoides. J Exp Med 1994; 180:1973–1978.
165. Knowles DM: Immunophenotypic and antigen receptor gene rearrangement analysis in T cell neoplasia. Am J Pathol 1989;134:761–785.
166. Liebmann RD, Anderson B, McCarthy KP, Chow JW: The polymerase chain reaction in the diagnosis of early mycosis fungoides. J Pathol 1997;182:282–287.
167. Ashton-Key M, Diss TC, Du MQ, et al: The value of the polymerase chain reaction in the diagnosis of cutaneous T-cell infiltrates. Am J Surg Pathol 1997;21: 743–747.
168. Curco N, Servitje O, Llucia M, et al: Genotypic analysis of cutaneous T-cell lymphoma: A comparative study of Southern blot analysis with polymerase chain reaction amplification of the T-cell receptor-gamma gene. Br J Dermatol 1997;137:673–679.
169. Wood GS, Tung RM, Haeffner AC, et al: Detection of clonal T-cell receptor gamma gene rearrangements in early mycosis fungoides/Sézary syndrome by polymerase chain reaction and denaturing gradient gel electrophoresis (PCR/DGGE). J Invest Dermatol 1994;103:34–41.
170. Kern DE, Kidd PG, Moe R, et al: Analysis of T-cell receptor gene rearrangement in lymph nodes of patients with mycosis fungoides. Prognostic implications. Arch Dermatol 1998;134:158–164.
171. Wieczorek R, Suhrland M, Ramsay D, et al: Leu-M1 antigen expression in advanced (tumor) stage mycosis fungoides. Am J Clin Pathol 1986;86:25–32.
172. Kamb A, Herlyn M: Malignant melanoma. *In* Vogelstein B, Kinzler KW (eds): The Genetic Basis of Human Cancer. New York, McGraw-Hill, 1998, pp 507–518.
173. Worsham MJ, Nathanson SD, Lee M, et al. Cytogenetic biomarkers in skin cancer. *In* Wolman SR, Sell S (eds): Human Cytogenetic Cancer Markers. Totawa, NJ, Humana, 1997, pp 289–317.
174. Cowan JM, Halaban R, Francke U: Cytogenetic analysis of melanocytes from premalignant nevi and melanomas. J Natl Cancer Inst 1988;80:1159–1164.
175. Balaban GB, Herlyn M, Clark WHJ, Nowell PC: Karyotypic evolution in human malignant melanoma. Cancer Genet Cytogenet 1986;19:113–122.
176. Cowan JM, Francke U: Cytogenetic analysis in melanoma and nevi. Cancer Treat Res 1991;54:3–16.
177. Bergman W, Gruis NA, Sandkuijl LA, Frants RR: Genetics of seven Dutch familial atypical multiple mole–melanoma syndrome families: A review of linkage results including chromosomes 1 and 9. J Invest Dermatol 1994;103(Suppl 5):122S–125S.
178. Goldstein AM, Dracopoli NC, Engelstein M, et al: Linkage of cutaneous malignant melanoma/dysplastic nevi to chromosome 9p, and evidence for genetic heterogeneity. Am J Hum Genet 1994;54:489–496.
179. Fountain JW, Karayiorgou M, Ernstoff MS, et al: Homozygous deletions within human chromosome band 9p21 in melanoma. Proc Natl Acad Sci USA 1992;89:10557–10561.
180. Park WS, Vortmeyer AO, Pack S, et al: Allelic deletion at chromosome 9p21(p16) and 17p13(p53) in microdissected sporadic dysplastic nevus. Hum Pathol 1998;29: 127–130.
181. Bastian BC, LeBoit PE, Hamm H, et al: Chromosomal gains and losses in primary cutaneous melanomas detected by comparative genomic hybridization. Cancer Res 1998;58:2170–2175.
182. Puig S, Ruiz A, Lazaro C, et al: Chromosome 9p deletions in cutaneous malignant melanoma tumors: The minimal deleted region involves markers outside the p16 (CDKN2) gene. Am J Hum Genet 1995;57: 395–402.
183. Puig S, Ruiz A, Castel T, et al: Inherited susceptibility to several cancers but absence of linkage between dysplastic nevus syndrome and *CDKN2A* in a melanoma family with a mutation in the *CDKN2A* (P16INK4A) gene. Hum Genet 1997;101:359–364.
184. Healy E, Sikkink S, Rees JL: Infrequent mutation of *p16INK4* in sporadic melanoma. J Invest Dermatol 1996;107:318–321.
185. Kamb A, Shattuck-Eidens D, Eeles R, et al: Analysis of the *p16* gene (CDKN2) as a candidate for the chromosome 9p melanoma susceptibility locus. Nat Genet 1994;8:23–26.
186. Bartkova J, Lukas J, Guldberg P, et al: The p16-cyclin D/Cdk4-pRb pathway as a functional unit frequently altered in melanoma pathogenesis. Cancer Res 1996;56:5475–5483.
187. Tsao H, Benoit E, Sober AJ, et al: Novel mutations in the *p16/CDKN2A* binding region of the cyclin-dependent kinase-4 gene. Cancer Res 1998;58:109–113.
188. Walker GJ, Flores JF, Glendening JM, et al: Virtually 100% of melanoma cell lines harbor alterations at the DNA level within *CDKN2A*, *CDKN2B*, or one of their downstream targets. Genes Chromosomes Cancer 1998;22:157–163.
189. Maelandsmo GM, Florenes VA, Hovig E, et al: Involvement of the pRb/p16/cdk4/cyclin D1 pathway in the tumorigenesis of sporadic malignant melanomas. Br J Cancer 1996;73:909–916.
190. Balaban G, Herlyn M, Guerry D, et al: Cytogenetics of human malignant melanoma and premalignant lesions. Cancer Genet Cytogenet 1984;11:429–439.
191. Dracopoli NC, Harnett P, Bale SJ, et al: Loss of alleles from the distal short arm of chromosome 1 occurs late in melanoma tumor progression. Proc Natl Acad Sci USA 1989;86:4614–4618.

192. Goldstein AM, Goldin LR, Dracopoli NC, et al: Two-locus linkage analysis of cutaneous malignant melanoma/dysplastic nevi. Am J Hum Genet 1996;58:1050–1056.
193. Poetsch M, Woenckhaus C, Dittberner T, et al: Differences in chromosomal aberrations between nodular and superficial spreading malignant melanoma detected by interphase cytogenetics. Lab Invest 1998;78:883–888.
194. Lee JH, Miele ME, Hicks DJ, et al: *KiSS-1*, a novel human malignant melanoma metastasis-suppressor gene. J Natl Cancer Inst 1996;88:1731–1737.
195. West A, Vojta PJ, Welch DR, Weissman BE: Chromosome localization and genomic structure of the KiSS-1 metastasis suppressor gene (KISS1). Genomics 1998;54:145–148.
196. Cowan JM, Halaban R, Lane AT, Francke U: The involvement of 6p in melanoma. Cancer Genet Cytogenet 1986;20:255–261.
197. Thompson FH, Emerson J, Olson S, et al: Cytogenetics of 158 patients with regional or disseminated melanoma: Subset analysis of near-diploid and simple karyotypes. Cancer Genet Cytogenet 1995;83:93–104.
198. Millikin D, Meese E, Vogelstein B, et al: Loss of heterozygosity for loci on the long arm of chromosome 6 in human malignant melanoma. Cancer Res 1991;51:5449–5453.
199. D'Alessandro I, Zitzelsberger H, Hutzler P, et al: Numerical aberrations of chromosome 7 detected in 15-micron paraffin-embedded tissue sections of primary cutaneous melanomas by fluorescence in situ hybridization and confocal laser scanning microscopy. J Cutan Pathol 1997;24:70–75.
200. Matsuta M, Imamura Y, Sasaki K, Kon S: Detection of numerical chromosomal aberrations in malignant melanomas using fluorescence in situ hybridization. J Cutan Pathol 1997;24:201–205.
201. Barks JH, Thompson FH, Taetle R, et al: Increased chromosome 20 copy number detected by fluorescence in situ hybridization (FISH) in malignant melanoma. Genes Chromosomes Cancer 1997;19:278–285.
202. Bauer J, Sokol L, Stribrna J, et al: Amplification of N-*myc* oncogene in human melanoma cells. Neoplasma 1990;37:233–238.
203. Herzberg AJ, Kerns BJ, Borowitz MJ, et al: DNA ploidy of malignant melanoma determined by image cytometry of fresh frozen and paraffin-embedded tissue. J Cutan Pathol 1991;18:440–448.
204. Klapperstuck T, Wohlrab W: DNA image cytometry on sections as compared with image cytometry on smears and flow cytometry in melanoma. Cytometry 1996;25:82–89.
205. Reddy VB, Gattuso P, Aranha G, Carson HJ: Cell proliferation markers in predicting metastases in malignant melanoma. J Cutan Pathol 1995;22:248–251.
206. Steinbeck ZG, Heselmeyer KM, Gerlach B, et al: Diagnostic impact of nuclear DNA content and proliferative activity in benign and malignant melanocytic lesions. Melanoma Res 1996;6:37–43.
207. Hahka-Kemppinen M, Muhonen T, Nordling S, Pyrhonen S: DNA flow cytometry and the outcome of chemoimmunotherapy in metastatic melanoma. Melanoma Res 1997;7:329–334.
208. Karlsson M, Jungnelius U, Aamdal S, et al: Correlation of DNA ploidy and S-phase fraction with chemotherapeutic response and survival in a randomized study of disseminated malignant melanoma. Int J Cancer 1996;65:1–5.
209. Albino AP, Vidal MJ, McNutt NS, et al: Mutation and expression of the *p53* gene in human malignant melanoma. Melanoma Res 1994;4:35–45.
210. Barnhill RL, Castresana JS, Rubio MP, et al: p53 expression in cutaneous malignant melanoma: An immunohistochemical study of 87 cases of primary, recurrent, and metastatic melanoma. Mod Pathol 1994;7:533–535.
211. Lee CS, Pirdas A, Lee MW: p53 in cutaneous melanoma: Immunoreactivity and correlation with prognosis. Australas J Dermatol 1995;36:192–195.
212. Lassam NJ, From L, Kahn HJ: Overexpression of p53 is a late event in the development of malignant melanoma. Cancer Res 1993;53(10 Suppl):2235–2238.
213. Stretch JR, Gatter KC, Ralfkiaer E, et al: Expression of mutant *p53* in melanoma. Cancer Res 1991;51:5976–5979.
214. Akslen LA, Monstad SE, Larsen B, et al: Frequent mutations of the *p53* gene in cutaneous melanoma of the nodular type. Int J Cancer 1998;79:91–95.
215. Poremba C, Yandell DW, Metze D, et al: Immunohistochemical detection of p53 in melanomas with rare *p53* gene mutations is associated with mdm-2 overexpression. Oncol Res 1995;7:331–339.
216. McGregor JM, Yu CC, Dublin EA, et al: p53 immunoreactivity in human malignant melanoma and dysplastic naevi. Br J Dermatol 1993;128:606–611.
217. Vogt T, Zipperer KH, Vogt A, et al: p53-protein and Ki-67-antigen expression are both reliable biomarkers of prognosis in thick stage I nodular melanomas of the skin. Histopathology 1997;30:57–63.
218. Weiss J, Heine M, Korner B, et al: Expression of p53 protein in malignant melanoma: Clinicopathological and prognostic implications. Br J Dermatol 1995;133:23–31.
219. Straume O, Akslen LA: Alterations and prognostic significance of p16 and p53 protein expression in subgroups of cutaneous melanoma. Int J Cancer 1997;74:535–539.
220. Florenes VA, Holm R, Fodstad O: Accumulation of p53 protein in human malignant melanoma: Relationship to clinical outcome. Melanoma Res 1995;5:183–187.
221. Albino AP, Fountain JW: Molecular genetics of human malignant melanoma. Cancer Treat Res 1993;65:201–255.
222. Jafari M, Papp T, Kirchner S, et al: Analysis of *ras* mutations in human melanocytic lesions: Activation of the *ras* gene seems to be associated with the nodular type of human malignant melanoma. J Cancer Res Clin Oncol 1995;121:23–30.
223. Albino AP, Nanus DM, Davis ML, McNutt NS: Lack of evidence of Ki-*ras* codon 12 mutations in melanocytic lesions. J Cutan Pathol 1991;18:273–278.
224. Natali PG, Nicotra MR, Winkler AB, et al: Progression of human cutaneous melanoma is associated with loss of expression of c-*kit* proto-oncogene receptor. Int J Cancer 1992;52:197–201.

225. Funasaka Y, Boulton T, Cobb M, et al: c-*Kit*-kinase induces a cascade of protein tyrosine phosphorylation in normal human melanocytes in response to mast cell growth factor and stimulates mitogen-activated protein kinase but is down-regulated in melanomas. Mol Biol Cell 1992;3:197–209.
226. Huang S, Luca M, Gutman M, et al: Enforced c-*KIT* expression renders highly metastatic human melanoma cells susceptible to stem cell factor–induced apoptosis and inhibits their tumorigenic and metastatic potential. Oncogene 1996;13:2339–2347.
227. Huang S, Jean D, Luca M, et al: Loss of AP-2 results in downregulation of c-*KIT* and enhancement of melanoma tumorigenicity and metastasis. EMBO J 1998;17: 4358–4369.
228. Bjornhagen V, Mansson-Brahme E, Lindholm J, et al: Morphometric, DNA and PCNA in thin malignant melanomas. Med Oncol Tumor Pharmacother 1993; 10:87–94.
229. Bjornhagen V, Bonfoco E, Brahme EM, et al: Morphometric, DNA, and proliferating cell nuclear antigen measurements in benign melanocytic lesions and cutaneous malignant melanoma. Am J Dermatopathol 1994;16:615–623.
230. Boni R, Doguoglu A, Burg G, et al: MIB-1 immunoreactivity correlates with metastatic dissemination in primary thick cutaneous melanoma. J Am Acad Dermatol 1996;35:416–418.
231. Niezabitowski A, Czajecki K, Rys J, et al: Prognostic evaluation of cutaneous malignant melanoma: A clinicopathologic and immunohistochemical study. J Surg Oncol 1999;70:150–160.
232. Sparrow LE, English DR, Taran JM, Heenan PJ: Prognostic significance of MIB-1 proliferative activity in thin melanomas and immunohistochemical analysis of MIB-1 proliferative activity in melanocytic tumors. Am J Dermatopathol 1998;20:12–16.
233. Kanoko M, Ueda M, Ichihashi M: PCNA expression and nucleolar organizer regions in malignant melanoma and nevus cell nevus. Kobe J Med Sci 1994;40:107–123.
234. Evans AT, Blessing K, Orrell JM, Grant A: Mitotic indices, anti-PCNA immunostaining, and AgNORs in thick cutaneous melanomas displaying paradoxical behaviour. J Pathol 1992;168:15–22.
235. Woosley JT, Dietrich DR: Prognostic significance of PCNA grade in malignant melanoma. J Cutan Pathol 1993;20:498–503.
236. Girod SC, Groth W, Junk M, Gerlach KL: p53 and PCNA expression in malignant melanomas of the head and neck. Pigment Cell Res 1994;7:354–357.
237. Byers PH, Siegel RC, Holbrook KA, et al: X-linked cutis laxa: Defective cross-link formation in collagen due to decreased lysyl oxidase activity. N Engl J Med 1980;303:61–65.
238. Damkier A, Brandrup F, Starklint H: Cutis laxa: Autosomal dominant inheritance in five generations. Clin Genet 1991;39:321–329.
239. Zhang MC, He L, Giro M, et al: Cutis laxa arising from frameshift mutations in exon 30 of the elastin gene (ELN). J Biol Chem 1999;274:981–986.
240. Fazio MJ, Olsen DR, Uitto JJ: Skin aging: Lessons from cutis laxa and elastoderma. Cutis 1989;43:437–444.
241. Holbrook KA, Byers PH: Structural abnormalities in the dermal collagen and elastic matrix from the skin of patients with inherited connective tissue disorders. J Invest Dermatol 1982;79(Suppl 1):7s–16s.
242. Olsen DR, Fazio MJ, Shamban AT, et al: Cutis laxa: Reduced elastin gene expression in skin fibroblast cultures as determined by hybridizations with a homologous cDNA and an exon 1–specific oligonucleotide. J Biol Chem 1988;263:6465–6467.
243. Kaler SG, Gallo LK, Proud VK, et al: Occipital horn syndrome and a mild Menkes phenotype associated with splice site mutations at the MNK locus. Nat Genet 1994;8:195–202.
244. Das S, Levinson B, Vulpe C, et al: Similar splicing mutations of the Menkes/mottled copper-transporting ATPase gene in occipital horn syndrome and the blotchy mouse. Am J Hum Genet 1995;56:570–576.
245. Chan YM, Yu QC, Fine JD, Fuchs E: The genetic basis of Weber-Cockayne epidermolysis bullosa simplex. Proc Natl Acad Sci USA 1993;90:7414–7418.
246. Bonifas JM, Rothman AL, Epstein EHJ: Epidermolysis bullosa simplex: Evidence in two families for keratin gene abnormalities. Science 1991;254:1202–1205.
247. Dong W, Ryynanen M, Uitto J: Identification of a leucine-to-proline mutation in the keratin 5 gene in a family with the generalized Kobner type of epidermolysis bullosa simplex. Hum Mutat 1993;2:94–102.
248. Ehrlich P, Sybert VP, Spencer A, Stephens K: A common keratin 5 gene mutation in epidermolysis bullosa simplex–Weber-Cockayne. J Invest Dermatol 1995; 104:877–879.
249. Galligan P, Listwan P, Siller GM, Rothnagel JA: A novel mutation in the L12 domain of keratin 5 in the Kobner variant of epidermolysis bullosa simplex. J Invest Dermatol 1998;111:524–527.
250. Muller FB, Kuster W, Bruckner-Tuderman L, et al: Novel K5 and K14 mutations in German patients with the Weber-Cockayne variant of epidermolysis bullosa simplex. J Invest Dermatol 1998;111:900–902.
251. Chan YM, Cheng J, Gedde-Dahl TJ, et al: Genetic analysis of a severe case of Dowling-Meara epidermolysis bullosa simplex. J Invest Dermatol 1996;106:327–334.
252. Chen H, Bonifas JM, Matsumura K, et al: Keratin 14 gene mutations in patients with epidermolysis bullosa simplex. J Invest Dermatol 1995;105:629–632.
253. Hachisuka H, Morita M, Karashima T, Sasai Y: Keratin 14 gene point mutation in the Kobner and Dowling-Meara types of epidermolysis bullosa simplex as detected by the PASA method. Arch Dermatol Res 1995;287: 142–145.
254. Shemanko CS, Mellerio JE, Tidman MJ, et al: Severe palmo-plantar hyperkeratosis in Dowling-Meara epidermolysis bullosa simplex caused by a mutation in the keratin 14 gene (*KRT14*). J Invest Dermatol 1998; 111:893–895.
255. McGrath JA, Gatalica B, Christiano AM, et al: Mutations in the 180-kD bullous pemphigoid antigen (BPAG2), a hemidesmosomal transmembrane collagen (COL17A1), in generalized atrophic benign epidermolysis bullosa. Nat Genet 1995;11:83–86.
256. Shimizu H: New insights into the immunoultrastructural organization of cutaneous basement membrane zone molecules. Exp Dermatol 1998;7:303–313.

257. McGrath JA, Gatalica B, Li K, et al: Compound heterozygosity for a dominant glycine substitution and a recessive internal duplication mutation in the type XVII collagen gene results in junctional epidermolysis bullosa and abnormal dentition. Am J Pathol 1996;148:1787–1796.
258. Chavanas S, Gache Y, Tadini G, et al: A homozygous in-frame deletion in the collagenous domain of bullous pemphigoid antigen BP180 (type XVII collagen) causes generalized atrophic benign epidermolysis bullosa. J Invest Dermatol 1997;109:74–78.
259. Darling TN, McGrath JA, Yee C, et al: Premature termination codons are present on both alleles of the bullous pemphigoid antigen 2/type XVII collagen gene in five Austrian families with generalized atrophic benign epidermolysis bullosa. J Invest Dermatol 1997;108:463–468.
260. Pohla-Gubo G, Lazarova Z, Giudice GJ, et al: Diminished expression of the extracellular domain of bullous pemphigoid antigen 2 (BPAG2) in the epidermal basement membrane of patients with generalized atrophic benign epidermolysis bullosa. Exp Dermatol 1995;4:199–206.
261. Ashton GH, Mellerio JE, Dunnill MG, et al: A recurrent laminin 5 mutation in British patients with lethal (Herlitz) junctional epidermolysis bullosa: Evidence for a mutational hotspot rather than propagation of an ancestral allele. Br J Dermatol 1997;136:674–677.
262. Kivirikko S, McGrath JA, Baudoin C, et al: A homozygous nonsense mutation in the alpha 3 chain gene of laminin 5 (LAMA3) in lethal (Herlitz) junctional epidermolysis bullosa. Hum Mol Genet 1995;4:959–962.
263. Pulkkinen L, Cserhalmi-Friedman PB, Tang M, et al: Molecular analysis of the human laminin alpha-3a chain gene (LAMA3a): A strategy for mutation identification and DNA-based prenatal diagnosis in Herlitz junctional epidermolysis bullosa. Lab Invest 1998;78:1067–1076.
264. Kivirikko S, McGrath JA, Pulkkinen L, et al: Mutational hotspots in the *LAMB3* gene in the lethal (Herlitz) type of junctional epidermolysis bullosa. Hum Mol Genet 1996;5:231–237.
265. Aberdam D, Galliano MF, Vailly J, et al: Herlitz's junctional epidermolysis bullosa is linked to mutations in the gene (*LAMC2*) for the gamma 2 subunit of nicein/kalinin (LAMININ-5). Nat Genet 1994;6:299–304.
266. Airenne T, Haakana H, Sainio K, et al: Structure of the human laminin gamma 2 chain gene (*LAMC2*): Alternative splicing with different tissue distribution of two transcripts. Genomics 1996;32:54–64.
267. Christiano AM, Pulkkinen L, McGrath JA, Uitto J: Mutation-based prenatal diagnosis of Herlitz junctional epidermolysis bullosa. Prenat Diagn 1997;17:343–354.
268. Marinkovich MP, Meneguzzi G, Burgeson RE, et al: Prenatal diagnosis of Herlitz junctional epidermolysis bullosa by amniocentesis. Prenat Diagn 1995;15:1027–1034.
269. McGrath JA, Kivirikko S, Ciatti S, et al: A homozygous nonsense mutation in the alpha 3 chain gene of laminin 5 *(LAMA3)* in Herlitz junctional epidermolysis bullosa: Prenatal exclusion in a fetus at risk. Genomics 1995;29:282–284.
270. McMillan JR, McGrath JA, Pulkkinen L, et al: Immunohistochemical analysis of the skin in junctional epidermolysis bullosa using laminin 5 chain specific antibodies is of limited value in predicting the underlying gene mutation. Br J Dermatol 1997;136:817–822.
271. Brown TA, Gil SG, Sybert VP, et al: Defective integrin alpha 6 beta 4 expression in the skin of patients with junctional epidermolysis bullosa and pyloric atresia. J Invest Dermatol 1996;107:384–391.
272. Beighton P, De Paepe A, Steinmann B, et al: Ehlers-Danlos syndromes: Revised nosology, Villefranche, 1997. Ehlers-Danlos National Foundation (USA) and Ehlers-Danlos Support Group (UK). Am J Med Genet 1998;77:31–37.
273. Burrows NP, Nicholls AC, Yates JR, et al: The gene encoding collagen alpha 1(V) (*COL5A1*) is linked to mixed Ehlers-Danlos syndrome type I/II. J Invest Dermatol 1996;106:1273–1276.
274. Burrows NP, Nicholls AC, Yates JR, et al: Genetic linkage to the collagen alpha 1 (V) gene (*COL5A1*) in two British Ehlers-Danlos syndrome families with variable type I and II phenotypes. Clin Exp Dermatol 1997;22:174–176.
275. Loughlin J, Irven C, Hardwick LJ, et al: Linkage of the gene that encodes the alpha 1 chain of type V collagen (COL5A1) to type II Ehlers-Danlos syndrome (EDS II). Hum Mol Genet 1995;4:1649–1651.
276. Burrows NP, Nicholls AC, Richards AJ, et al: A point mutation in an intronic branch site results in aberrant splicing of *COL5A1* in Ehlers-Danlos syndrome type II in two British families. Am J Hum Genet 1998;63:390–398.
277. De Paepe A, Nuytinck L, Hausser I, et al: Mutations in the *COL5A1* gene are causal in the Ehlers-Danlos syndromes I and II. Am J Hum Genet 1997;60:547–554.
278. Nicholls AC, Oliver JE, McCarron S, et al: An exon skipping mutation of a type V collagen gene (*COL5A1*) in Ehlers-Danlos syndrome. J Med Genet 1996;33:940–946.
279. Richards AJ, Martin S, Nicholls AC, et al: A single base mutation in *COL5A2* causes Ehlers-Danlos syndrome type II. J Med Genet 1998;35:846–848.
280. Toriello HV, Glover TW, Takahara K, et al: A translocation interrupts the *COL5A1* gene in a patient with Ehlers-Danlos syndrome and hypomelanosis of Ito. Nat Genet 1996;13:361–365.
281. Wenstrup RJ, Langland GT, Willing MC, et al: A splice-junction mutation in the region of *COL5A1* that codes for the carboxyl propeptide of pro alpha 1(V) chains results in the gravis form of the Ehlers-Danlos syndrome (type I). Hum Mol Genet 1996;5:1733–1736.
282. Pope FM, Nicholls AC, Jones PM, et al: EDS IV (acrogeria): New autosomal dominant and recessive types. J R Soc Med 1980;73:180–186.
283. Superti-Furga A, Saesseli B, Steinmann B, Bollinger A: Microangiopathy in Ehlers-Danlos syndrome type IV. Int J Microcirc Clin Exp 1992;11:241–247.
284. North KN, Whiteman DA, Pepin MG, Byers PH: Cerebrovascular complications in Ehlers-Danlos syndrome type IV. Ann Neurol 1995;38:960–964.

285. Superti-Furga A, Gugler E, Gitzelmann R, Steinmann B: Ehlers-Danlos syndrome type IV: A multi-exon deletion in one of the two COL3A1 alleles affecting structure, stability, and processing of type III procollagen. J Biol Chem 1988;263:6226–6232.
286. Ades LC, Waltham RD, Chiodo AA, Bateman JF: Myocardial infarction resulting from coronary artery dissection in an adolescent with Ehlers-Danlos syndrome type IV due to a type III collagen mutation. Br Heart J 1995;74:112–116.
287. Benchellal ZA, Huten N, Danquechin DE, et al: Abdominal emergencies in type IV Ehlers-Danlos syndrome. Gastroenterol Clin Biol 1998;22:343–345.
288. Chiodo AA, Sillence DO, Cole WG, Bateman JF: Abnormal type III collagen produced by an exon-17-skipping mutation of the *COL3A1* gene in Ehlers-Danlos syndrome type IV is not incorporated into the extracellular matrix. Biochem J 1995;311:939–943.
289. Gilchrist D, Schwarze U, Shields K, et al: Large kindred with Ehlers-Danlos syndrome type IV due to a point mutation (G571S) in the *COL3A1* gene of type III procollagen: Low risk of pregnancy complications and unexpected longevity in some affected relatives. Am J Med Genet 1999;82:305–311.
290. Johnson PH, Richards AJ, Lloyd JC, et al: Efficient strategy for the detection of mutations in acrogeric Ehlers-Danlos syndrome type IV. Hum Mutat 1995; 6:336–342.
291. Kontusaari S, Tromp G, Kuivaniemi H, et al: Inheritance of an RNA splicing mutation (G^+ 1 IVS20) in the type III procollagen gene (*COL3A1*) in a family having aortic aneurysms and easy bruisability: Phenotypic overlap between familial arterial aneurysms and Ehlers-Danlos syndrome type IV. Am J Hum Genet 1990;47:112–120.
292. Kuivaniemi H, Tromp G, Bergfeld WF, et al: Ehlers-Danlos syndrome type IV: A single base substitution of the last nucleotide of exon 34 in *COL3A1* leads to exon skipping. J Invest Dermatol 1995;105:352–356.
293. Smith LT, Schwarze U, Goldstein J, Byers PH: Mutations in the *COL3A1* gene result in the Ehlers-Danlos syndrome type IV and alterations in the size and distribution of the major collagen fibrils of the dermis. J Invest Dermatol 1997;108:241–247.
294. Superti-Furga A, Steinmann B: Impaired secretion of type III procollagen in Ehlers-Danlos syndrome type IV fibroblasts: Correction of the defect by incubation at reduced temperature and demonstration of subtle alterations in the triple-helical region of the molecule. Biochem Biophys Res Commun 1988;150:140–147.
295. Wenstrup RJ, Murad S, Pinnell SR: Ehlers-Danlos syndrome type VI: Clinical manifestations of collagen lysyl hydroxylase deficiency. J Pediatr 1989;115:405–409.
296. Steinmann B, Eyre DR, Shao P: Urinary pyridinoline cross-links in Ehlers-Danlos syndrome type VI. Am J Hum Genet 1995;57:1505–1508.
297. Brinckmann J, Acil Y, Feshchenko S, et al: Ehlers-Danlos syndrome type VI: Lysyl hydroxylase deficiency due to a novel point mutation (W612C). Arch Dermatol Res 1998;290:181–186.
298. Ha VT, Marshall MK, Elsas LJ, et al: A patient with Ehlers-Danlos syndrome type VI is a compound heterozygote for mutations in the lysyl hydroxylase gene. J Clin Invest 1994;93:1716–1721.
299. Hautala T, Byers MG, Eddy RL, et al: Cloning of human lysyl hydroxylase: Complete cDNA-derived amino acid sequence and assignment of the gene (*PLOD*) to chromosome 1p36.3-p36.2. Genomics 1992; 13:62–69.
300. Hyland J, Ala-Kokko L, Royce P, et al: A homozygous stop codon in the lysyl hydroxylase gene in two siblings with Ehlers-Danlos syndrome type VI. Nat Genet 1992;2:228–231.
301. Pousi B, Hautala T, Hyland JC, et al: A compound heterozygote patient with Ehlers-Danlos syndrome type VI has a deletion in one allele and a splicing defect in the other allele of the lysyl hydroxylase gene. Hum Mutat 1998;11:55–61.
302. Yeowell HN, Walker LC, Murad S, Pinnell SR: A common duplication in the lysyl hydroxylase gene of patients with Ehlers-Danlos syndrome type VI results in preferential stimulation of lysyl hydroxylase activity and mRNA by hydralazine. Arch Biochem Biophys 1997;347:126–131.
303. Yeowell HN, Walker LC: Ehlers-Danlos syndrome type VI results from a nonsense mutation and a splice site–mediated exon-skipping mutation in the lysyl hydroxylase gene. Proc Assoc Am Physicians 1997;109: 383–396.
304. Yeowell HN, Walker LC: Prenatal exclusion of Ehlers-Danlos syndrome type VI by mutational analysis. Proc Assoc Am Physicians 1999;111:57–62.
305. Chiodo AA, Hockey A, Cole WG: A base substitution at the splice acceptor site of intron 5 of the *COL1A2* gene activates a cryptic splice site within exon 6 and generates abnormal type I procollagen in a patient with Ehlers-Danlos syndrome type VII. J Biol Chem 1992;267:6361–6369.
306. Carr AJ, Chiodo AA, Hilton JM, et al: The clinical features of Ehlers-Danlos syndrome type VIIB resulting from a base substitution at the splice acceptor site of intron 5 of the *COL1A2* gene. J Med Genet 1994;31: 306–311.
307. Giunta C, Superti-Furga A, Spranger S, et al: Ehlers-Danlos syndrome type VII: Clinical features and molecular defects. J Bone Joint Surg Am 1999;81:225–238.
308. Lehmann HW, Mundlos S, Winterpacht A, et al: Ehlers-Danlos syndrome type VII: Phenotype and genotype. Arch Dermatol Res 1994;286:425–428.
309. Wertelecki W, Smith LT, Byers P: Initial observations of human dermatosparaxis: Ehlers-Danlos syndrome type VIIC. J Pediatr 1992;121:558–64.
310. Pierard GE, Hermanns-Le T, Arrese-Estrada J, et al: Structure of the dermis in type VIIC Ehlers-Danlos syndrome. Am J Dermatopathol 1993;15:127–132.
311. Smith LT, Wertelecki W, Milstone LM, et al: Human dermatosparaxis: A form of Ehlers-Danlos syndrome that results from failure to remove the amino-terminal propeptide of type I procollagen. Am J Hum Genet 1992;51:235–244.

TIMOTHY J. O'LEARY

17

Cytopathology

The Food and Drug Administration's approval of image-based automated cell analysis systems for interpretation of Papanicolaou (Pap) smears was a public proclamation of a quieter revolution that has been slowly occurring in cytology over many years. Although morphologic examination remains the mainstay of the cytotechnologist and cytopathologist, it is often no longer the "gold standard" on which final cytomorphologic diagnosis is based. Rather, image analysis systems may suggest that it is prudent to rescreen an apparently normal cervical smear, immunocytochemical assays may suggest that adenocarcinoma metastatic to the pleura was not appreciated on cytomorphologic examination, or a polymerase chain reaction (PCR)–based assay may suggest the optimal diagnostic intervention after a morphologic diagnosis of "atypical squamous cells of undetermined significance" (ASCUS).

Thousands of papers have now appeared that describe the uses or misuses of one or more of these ancillary diagnostic techniques. The very profusion of papers has frequently confused me as much as guided me; I am sure the same is true for others. To improve "publishability," authors often put the "most optimistic spin possible" on experimental results, even when prudent examination of the data suggests that an assay is of little clinical utility in everyday practice. Further confusion is caused by the fact that authors tend to be advocates for the techniques by which they make their academic careers. Biases, not always obvious, may creep into experimental results and conclusions. Seldom are the relative advantages and disadvantages of one technique compared with another.

This chapter is an attempt to put into perspective the clinical utility of immunocytochemical, molecular biologic, flow cytometric, and image analysis techniques in the current practice of diagnostic cytopathology and that which we may expect to see in the next few years. This perspective is based on some a priori biases based on the fact that, in my experience, immunocytochemical assays are the least expensive and most readily disseminated of the four types of approaches considered here, followed by molecular biologic assays, flow cytometric assays, and image analysis systems. There are some strong individual exceptions to this apparent bias, because, in my opinion, a widely distributed and highly regulated image analysis system, such as PAPNET or AutoPap, is more likely to be successfully adopted in a new laboratory than is any "home brew" immunocytochemical test. No doubt, this chapter retains unstated biases; furthermore, many excellent papers, both primary and review, that served as background are not cited. I hope that, in spite of these deficiencies, the resulting work will prove of some practical value in deciding when the use of immunocytochemical, molecular diagnostic, or cytometric techniques is appropriate.

EXFOLIATIVE CYTOLOGY

Papanicolaou Smears

FLOW CYTOMETRY

Perhaps because increased nucleus/cytoplasm ratio is both readily detectable by flow cytometry and one of the more important visual assessments in gynecologic cytopathology, many of the earliest investigations of diagnostic applications of flow cytometry focused on gynecologic samples.[1–8] Cervical swabs were collected in 50% ethanol and dissociated by mechanical agitation. Cells were then stained using propidium iodide (PI) and fluorescein isothiocyanate (FITC) to quantitate nucleic acids and cellular protein, respectively. Increases in the nucleus/cytoplasm (N/C) ratio thus resulted in an increased ratio of red (PI) to green (FITC) fluorescence. As few as 1% abnormal cells could be detected in experimental systems consisting of cultured mouse squamous cell carcinoma cells mixed with normal pooled gynecologic systems. Unfortunately, these promising results were not matched by equal performance on "natural" cytologic specimens, in which misclassification rates of approximately 20% were typical.

Using acridine orange staining and a slit scan system for Pap smear prescreening[9, 10] allows Pap staining to be performed after flow cytometry.[9] The prescreening system has a false-negative rate of approximately 3% and a false-positive rate of approximately 18% and classifies all specimens containing 0.1% or more abnormal cells as abnormal. Although this represents a significant improvement over previous flow cytometric results, it appears nevertheless only slightly more accurate than image-based automated prescreening systems.

Besides the high misclassification rates, the relative difficulty in preparing specimens for flow cytometric analysis significantly hindered the development of flow cytometry as a potential cervical cancer screening technique. It seems likely that adaptation of the ThinPrep technique will allow simple preparation of specimens for flow cytometry. Addition of antigen analysis[11] or nucleic acid hybridization[12, 13] techniques, together with methods that facilitate the detection of very rare abnormal cells,[14] might allow flow cytometry to complement automated image analysis in cervical cytodiagnosis.

IMAGE ANALYSIS

Several commercially available image analysis systems have proven their ability to effectively identify squamous intraepithelial lesions (SILs) in prescreening, rescreening, or primary screening modes.[15–26] One of these systems, PAPNET, uses a neural network algorithm to identify the most abnormal fields on a slide.[27] Images of these fields are presented to a cytotechnologist or cytopathologist, together with coordinates to help locate the field on the original microscope slide, for final interpretation. Another system, AutoPAP, identifies slides that have either a very low likelihood of harboring abnormal cells or an increased likelihood. The former need not be screened by the cytotechnologist; the latter are identified for double screening. Field-of-view locations can be provided to the cytotechnologist to assist in screening.[23]

Most of the studies on these systems demonstrate that they decrease the number of false-negative smears. They may also assist in differentiating low-grade SIL from high-grade SIL.[23a] Their cost-effectiveness has been called into question, because the objective of reducing the number of cases of cervical carcinoma can be achieved not only through computer-assisted techniques but also through manual rescreening of cervical smears and by obtaining smears from women who do not regularly get them.[28]

IMMUNOCYTOCHEMISTRY

Immunocytochemistry has little place in interpretation of Pap smears. Immunocytochemical methods have been used to assess *Chlamydia trachomatis* infection but detect only a small fraction of culture-positive patients.[29] Herpes simplex may be identified by immunocytochemical staining of Pap smears, with a sensitivity that appears to be the same as that of culture.[30, 31] Human papillomavirus (HPV) can sometimes be immunocytochemically identified in Pap smears, but the staining is generally weak and found in only a tiny subset of smears in which HPV can be identified by molecular diagnostic methods.

MOLECULAR DIAGNOSIS

Some of the greatest interest and uncertainty in the area of cervical pathology concerns the use of HPV testing as either an alternative or adjunct to the Pap smear. Although it has been clear for many years that HPV is etiologic in most cervical cancers of young women, it has been equally clear that many cases of HPV infection are transient and do not give rise to malignancy or its precursor lesions.[32] Demonstration of HPV in a woman's genital tract does not, therefore, equate to a need for treatment, although persistence of "high-risk" HPV types (HPV 16, 18, 31, 33, 35, 39, 45, 51, 52, 56, 68, and others) is strongly correlated with progression of cytologic and histologic abnormalities in young women.[33] In postmenopausal women the role of HPV is less clear.[34] To complicate matters further, a number of distinct laboratory methods have been used to detect HPV—Southern blot, dot blot, in situ hybridization (including fluorescent in situ hybridization [FISH]), PCR, and hybrid-capture assay. A fourth, in situ PCR, is useful in the research setting but currently too complex for routine diagnostic use.

Although in situ hybridization allows visualization of HPV-infected cells, the conditions necessary for the assay are harsh, and multiple samples are often required. For this reason, it is no longer in widespread use as a laboratory test in studies of clinical utility. The most commonly used approaches, the MY09/MY11 L1 consensus primer PCR-based test and the hybrid capture method, do not give equivalent results. The PCR test is clearly more sensitive and detects a greater range of HPV types. The sensitivity of the hybrid capture method is significantly higher for women with concurrent SILs than for women with normal cytologic findings.[35] Although the hybrid-capture assay is slightly less expensive and challenging technically, neither is difficult for the routine molecular diagnostic laboratory.

HPV testing need not be restricted to cervical smears; PCR tests for HPV detect the presence of viral sequences in about 90% of women with cytologic or histologic evidence of SILs or carcinoma (as well as in a large percentage of women without cytologic evidence of preneoplastic disease).[36] Home cervicovaginal lavage has also been proposed for collecting samples for HPV analysis.[37, 38] For these reasons, conclusions drawn about the utility of HPV testing must take into account not only population demographics[39–46] but also the specific types of sample, assay method, and clinical implications of a positive result.

Although data do not currently suggest that HPV testing replace the Pap smear as a screening test, there are data that suggest that HPV testing may be used to guide screening strategy.[46a] For example, large investigations have shown that progression to high-grade SIL is rare in women who are HPV negative at the time of cytologic screening.[47] Thus, it may be possible to increase the interval between Pap smears for women who do not harbor evidence of high-risk HPV subtypes. It may further be possible to improve the treatment of women whose smears are given a diagnosis of ASCUS. If women with a diagnosis of ASCUS are referred to colposcopy only if high-risk HPV is identified, far fewer women are unnecessarily subjected to this procedure and few cases of high-grade SIL will be missed.[48, 49] HPV testing may also be useful in interpretation of cellular atypia in postmenopausal women; the rate of HPV infection in biopsy-proven SIL is as high as for younger women, although few cases of cytologic atypia are associated with SIL.[50]

The telomerase repeat amplification protocol (TRAP) has also been proposed as an ancillary diagnostic technique for cervicovaginal cytology.[51, 52] Telomerase activity is seen in about half of SILs; occasionally, high telomerase activity has been associated with biopsy-proven SIL in the absence of cytomorphologic abnormalities in the smear.[51] However, because telomerase activity is frequently seen in histologically normal epithelium,[52] neither the sensitivity nor the specificity of this assay is appropriate to a cost-effective screening test.

Gastrointestinal Brushings

FLOW CYTOMETRY AND IMAGE ANALYSIS

Flow cytometry of gastrointestinal brushings has not proven useful. Significant increases in nuclear DNA are observed in patients with ulceration or inflammation of the gastric mucosa; attempts to use this as a criterion for malignant change yields an unacceptable false-positive rate.[53] Similarly, use of flow cytometry as an adjunct to cytomorphology for diagnosis of ampullary brushings gives only a slight increase in sensitivity at the cost of a serious loss in specificity.[54]

The PAPNET system, a neural net-based interactive computerized cell analysis system, has been used to examine cells from 138 esophageal smears. Abnormal cells were identified in all 35 patients with cancer, including one case of esophageal carcinoma in situ not previously recognized on either the smear or biopsy.[55] This suggests that the algorithms developed for cervical cancer screening may also be applicable to other exfoliated specimens.

IMMUNOCYTOCHEMISTRY

Accumulation of p53 protein is seen in esophageal brushings of patients with Barrett's esophagus[56] and in endobiliary brush specimens of biliary tract cancer patients[56a]; the results correlate well with immunocytochemical assays on corresponding biopsy specimens. Because there was a strong correlation between immunocytochemical and cytomorphologic findings, however, it does not appear that there is any additional diagnostic information to be gained from this immunocytochemical test.

As elsewhere, immunocytochemical assessment is useful in the characterization of unusual metastatic neoplasms.[57, 58]

MOLECULAR DIAGNOSIS

KRAS codon 12 mutations have been identified in brush specimens from approximately 40% of adenomas and carcinomas from the ampulla of Vater; thus, PCR for *KRAS* mutation may provide a tool for early identification of neoplasm but not for distinction between benign and malignant processes.[59]

The stools of colorectal cancer patients whose tumors contain *KRAS* mutations usually have detectable *RAS* mutations in DNA purified from the stool.[60, 61] This PCR-based test is likely to be both less sensitive and less cost effective than stool guaiac testing as a screening method but might be useful for detecting early recurrences.

A PCR-based telomerase assay has been investigated for detection of gastrointestinal cancers. About one third of patients with oral cancer or squamous carcinomas of the head and neck demonstrate telomerase activity in oral rinses.[62] There is no evidence that telomerase testing adds to findings of a careful physical examination. Telomerase activity is also detected in colonic washings of about two thirds of patients with colon cancer but not those with inflammatory bowel disease.[63] This suggests that telomerase activity may be a marker for colon carcinoma; this assay, too, seems likely to be less cost effective than stool guaiac testing.

Sputum, Bronchial Brushings, and Bronchoalveolar Lavage Fluid

FLOW CYTOMETRY AND IMAGE ANALYSIS

Flow cytometry has been used to enrich the population of malignant cells from sputum but has since found little diagnostic application,[64, 65] in spite of the availability of immunocytochemical markers to facilitate cell identification through multicolor cytometry. Deinlein and coworkers[66] examined bronchial washings from 73 patients with bronchogenic carcinoma, pneumonia, or no pulmonary disease by flow cytometry, comparing the flow cytometry results with cytologic and histologic findings. Using aneuploidy or high S fraction as evidence of malignancy, the flow cytometry results showed sensitivity and specificity for detection of cancer similar to that of visual cytologic examination. Like results were obtained by Fuhr and associates,[21] who found that adding flow cytometry to visual cytologic examination increased diagnostic sensitivity to 86%, with a specificity of 96%.[67]

Little recent attention has been given to image analysis methods, although early studies showed great promise.[68–70] A retrospective study of the PAPNET automated image analysis system suggests possible utility in screening or rescreening of sputum samples.[71] In addition, a retrospective study has suggested that it may be possible for image analysis systems to detect carcinomas in specimens that do not demonstrate currently accepted cytomorphologic criteria of malignancy.[72]

IMMUNOCYTOCHEMISTRY

Because cytomorphologic characteristics are generally sufficient for diagnosis and classification of the vast majority of lung tumors, immunocytochemical analysis is rarely performed on sputum, brushings, or bronchoalveolar fluid. Cytomorphologic identification of bronchoalveolar carcinoma is sometimes difficult, however, and p53 accumulation is seen immunocytochemically in about two thirds of bronchoalveolar carcinomas.[73] Although this may prove to be diagnostically useful, further validation is required. Thyroid transcription factor 1 (TTF1) staining may assist in differentiating primary from metastatic disease.[73a]

MOLECULAR DIAGNOSIS

KRAS and *TP53* mutations occur frequently in lung cancer, and even rare mutated cells are easily detected in carefully designed PCR assays. Approximately 60% of patients with non–small cell lung cancer demonstrate a normal *KRAS* allele by PCR. Because about 10% of patients without cancer carry this mutation, the diagnostic utility of *KRAS* mutation detection seems limited.[74] Mutations in *TP53* are less frequently encountered in patients without cancer, however, and in 80% of cases, a clonal population of mutated cells can be found in sputum before clinical diagnosis.[75] Although mutation-specific assays for *TP53* mutation are impractical as a screening tool, "enriched single-strand conformational polymorphism (E-SSCP)" permits detection of rare alleles with unknown mutations and also appears to be capable of detecting malignant cells months before the clinical appearance of disease.[76] An alternative approach, interphase FISH, is capable of detecting highly aneuploid cells in bronchial brushings that do not have cytomorphologic characteristics of malignancy.[77] Thus, molecular diagnosis shows promise of future use in pulmonary cytology.

FLUIDS

Cerebrospinal Fluid

Although most cerebrospinal fluid (CSF) examinations fail to yield a diagnosis, infectious organisms (particularly *Cryptococcus*), metastatic neoplasms, leukemias, and lymphomas are frequently identified.[78] The use of ancillary diagnostic methods has considerably increased the range of diagnoses that can be made and the speed with which accurate and specific diagnoses are reported.

FLOW AND IMAGE CYTOMETRY

Although CSF is often too acellular for flow cytometric evaluation, both surface marker and DNA flow cytometry are sometimes useful adjuncts to visual cytologic assessment of the CSF. Although flow cytometric tumor aneuploidy/elevated S-phase fraction only identifies approximately 70% of cytologically positive cases, it also identifies many cytologically negative cases in which laboratory or radiographic evidence of meningeal involvement is later found.[79] The combination of nucleic acid and cell surface marker flow cytometry is probably as sensitive as conventional cytology in identifying central nervous system (CNS) involvement by leukemia or lymphoma,[80] and the combination of cytologic examination and multicolor flow cytometry for cell surface markers is about 40% more sensitive than morphologic examination alone.[81, 81a]

An image cytometric study suggests that an abnormal DNA distribution should not be used as the sole criterion of malignancy, because there is significant overlap between the histograms generated by neoplastic processes and those resulting from viral (but not bacterial) infections.[82]

IMMUNOCYTOCHEMISTRY

Several studies have demonstrated that immunocytochemical assessment of epithelial membrane antigen (EMA) and carcinoembryonic antigen (CEA) increases the sensitivity of cytologic examination for leptomeningeal metastases by between 9% and 40%.[83–85] Immunocytochemical characterization of lymphoid cell populations is useful for distinguishing reactive processes from malignant lymphoma, as well as for characterization of lymphoid malignancies.[86]

Distinction among metastatic carcinoma, lymphoma, leukemia, and primary brain tumors is facilitated by use of an antibody panel consisting of antibodies directed against multiple glial fibrillary acidic protein subtypes, a pan-neuroectodermal antibody (UJ13A), B72.3, which recognizes a common tumor glycoprotein, and a panleukocyte antibody (2D1).[87]

MOLECULAR DIAGNOSIS

FISH may increase the sensitivity of cytologic examination by allowing detection of numerical chromosomal abnormalities but data are very sparse.[88] Use of in situ hybridization techniques to establish the diagnosis of virus infections, particularly herpes encephalitis,[89] has largely been replaced by PCR-based methods,[90–92] which enable improved outcomes and reduced use of acyclovir as compared with empirical decision making.[93]

PCR-based assays can also be used to diagnose a wide variety of other CNS infections.[94–111] Kits are available for performing many of these assays.

PCR-based immunoglobulin and T-cell receptor gene rearrangement assays are rapid and sensitive tests for the presence of leukemia or lymphoma in the CSF,[112–116] as are assays directed against specific chromosomal translocations.[117] These assays may provide a definitive diagnosis when cytomorphologic examination is inconclusive.[116] Similarly, PCR assays for patient-specific gene alterations, such as *TP53* mutation or *ERBB2* amplification, can provide a highly sensitive method by which to detect CNS metastases.[118, 119]

The majority of human neoplasms, including those of the CNS, express telomerase, which is not expressed in most adult benign tissue. As a result, assessment of telomerase activity may be a useful adjunct to CSF cytodiagnosis.[120]

Effusions

FLOW CYTOMETRY

Effusions are excellent substrates for flow cytometric evaluation, because little or no disaggregation is required for their analysis. The sensitivity of aneuploidy for diagnosis of malignancy has averaged about 70%, with a false-positive rate of 1% to 3% in various studies.[67, 121–128] Lima and colleagues[129] have suggested that the diagnostic utility depends on the type of effusion and have suggested a greater utility when the differential diagnosis includes lymphoma.

More favorable results may be obtained when immunocytochemical labeling of cells allows further selection of a cell subset for ploidy analysis. Croonen and coworkers[130] investigated 106 pleural and peritoneal effusions using anticytokeratin antibody to label epithelial cells with propidium iodide for DNA staining. This enabled easier identification of DNA aneuploidy when the fluid contained many lymphocytes. Joseph and associates have similarly noted greater utility for multiparameter flow cytometry than for single-parameter measurements.[131]

Taken together, the studies to date suggest that single-parameter flow cytometry usually has little clinical utility, although it may help in the diagnosis of some cytologically equivocal cases. Multiparameter flow cytometry may prove to be more useful but must compete with image cytometry[127] for a place as a diagnostic adjunct to visual examination.

IMAGE ANALYSIS

Image analysis methods are sometimes helpful in distinguishing benign from malignant effusions. Marchevsky and colleagues implemented an algorithm that correctly classified nearly 90% of pleural effusions, based on cell structural characteristics,[132] but the method is not readily implemented on other image analysis systems. DNA aneuploidy is also helpful in making this distinction, but, because it is observed in only about half of malignant effusions, is rather insensitive.[133, 134] The sensitivity for identification of mesothelioma, however, is about 70%.[135]

IMMUNOCYTOCHEMISTRY

Immunocytochemistry can be quite helpful in the identification of adenocarcinoma and mesothelioma in serous effusions. For distinguishing metastatic adenocarcinoma from mesothelial proliferations, most authors suggest a panel of antibodies, including anti-CEA and anti-EMA.[136–138] Antibodies B72.3[137, 139] and BER-EP4[140] are also excellent markers for glandular differentiation. Leu-M1 is highly specific for the presence of glandular cells. Tissue fragments or cell clusters that react with the Leu-M1 antibody are invariably of glandular differentiation, but only about half of glandular neoplasms demonstrate this antigen. EMA, on the other hand, is found in both glandular cells and many mesotheliomas but very rarely in reactive mesothelial proliferations; calretinin is found in mesothelial cells but not adenocarcinoma.[140a]

Several other markers may assist in the diagnosis of effusions. Diagnosis of metastatic malignant melanoma is assisted by HMB-45 and S-100. MART-1 may stain melanomas that do not express either of these antigens.[141] ERBB2 staining appears to be restricted to adenocarcinomas and is most likely to be found in breast or ovarian cancer, although other adenocarcinomas may also show ERBB2 overexpression.[142] MOC31,[143] the OV632 antibody, appears to react predominantly with ovarian carcinoma and malignant mesothelioma, but experience is limited.[136] Fibronectin reacts with reactive mesothelial cells but apparently not with adenocarcinomas.[138] Its utility in identifying malignant mesothelial cells in effusions is uncertain. Diagnosis of lymphoid effusions is facilitated by the identification of cells monomorphically expressing antigens reflecting either B- or T-cell lineage. Antibodies to CD45RO (UCHL-1) and CD20 (L26) are particularly useful; antibodies to immunoglobulin molecules are frequently noncontributory in effusions.

Although some authors have reported that p53 reactivity is not seen in benign effusions,[144] this has not been my experience. The presence of cells reactive for p53 in an effusion should raise one's index of suspicion for malignancy[145] but should only be used in combination with cytomorphologic features to reach a diagnosis of malignancy. Similarly, large numbers of cells demonstrating proliferating cell nuclear antigen (PCNA) reactivity are a frequent feature of malignancy but may also be seen in benign conditions.[146]

MOLECULAR DIAGNOSIS

Point mutations in *KRAS* are frequent in ascites from patients with pancreatic carcinoma; PCR assays may detect these mutations in cytomorphologically unremarkable specimens, suggesting that such tests may be a useful diagnostic adjunct in patients with this and other tumors that frequently show *KRAS* mutation.[147] In situ hybridization for albumin messenger RNA (mRNA) may assist in the diagnosis of hepatocellular carcinoma,[148] and PCR-based identification of specific translocations may assist in the diagnosis of tumors exhibiting these translocations. In each case, however, either good morphologic or clinical evidence to suggest the tumor type is necessary for the assay to be cost effective.

Telomerase mRNA is detectable in about 90% of effusions with definite cytomorphologic or histologic evidence of malignancy and 5% to 10% of nonmalignant effusions.[149, 150] Use of telomerase as a diagnostic adjunct may be appropriate in cases in which the increase in sensitivity offsets the decreased specificity of the combined cytomorphologic/telomerase assay test system.

Immunoglobulin heavy chain and T-cell receptor rearrangement assays are of great help in establishing the diagnosis of body cavity lymphoma, particularly when it is well differentiated.[151] In addition, identification of human herpesvirus type 8 (HHV8) may assist in the identification of primary effusion lymphoma.[151a]

FISH may be used to detect numeric chromosomal abnormalities in effusions with greater efficiency than either flow cytometry or image analysis techniques. Fish analysis may improve the sensitivity for detection of metastatic breast,[152, 153] pancreatic,[154] and other cancers.[155, 156] Aneuploidy appears to be extremely rare in benign effusions, so the addition of FISH analysis to cytomorphologic examination is expected to increase the sensitivity without significantly degrading specificity.

SYNOPSIS

Although flow- and image-based ploidy analysis are occasionally useful in the diagnosis of effusions, both are quite laborious. In most cases, immunocytochemical assays are sufficient to resolve diagnostic questions. Neither is likely to be as sensitive for the detection of an aneuploid population as FISH. For these reasons, cytometry should probably be reserved for the analysis of lymphoid effusions. Although molecular diagnostics show great promise, only those assays that distinguish among lymphoid cell populations are frequently helpful at present. In specific cases, a diagnosis may be aided by an assay for a tumor-specific translocation. The use of FISH to improve sensitivity is very promising, because it appears not to significantly degrade sensitivity. Nevertheless, FISH assays are fairly laborious and time consuming; work is needed to define those situations in which addition of FISH analysis to immunocytochemical testing provides diagnostic benefit. The telomerase assays appear to be less promising. Although they undoubtedly yield an increased sensitivity, they often do so at the cost of significantly reduced specificity.

Immunocytochemical assays remain the diagnostic adjuncts of choice for most diagnostic dilemmas arising from examination of effusions.

Urine and Urinary Tract Washings

FLOW CYTOMETRY

Although urine specimens are generally too poorly preserved to permit flow cytometric analysis, there is abundant evidence that cytometric methods improve accuracy of urinary tract cytodiagnosis from washings.[157–164] Flow cytometric findings typically agree with both cytologic and cystoscopic findings, but identification of aneuploid populations by flow cytometry may antedate the development of cystoscopically visible tumors by as much as a year.[162] Nevertheless, flow cytometry does not replace conventional cytologic examination; conventional cytologic examination is more sensitive than is flow cytometry analysis, largely owing to greater efficacy in identification of abnormalities in treated invasive cancers.[159, 164, 165] Instead, the two techniques are complementary. One significant advantage of flow cytometry is that it may frequently (50% to 70% of the time) identify abnormalities in low-grade bladder carcinomas[162, 166–168]; this is particularly useful in bladder washings, because "instrumentation artifact" frequently mimics the changes associated with low-grade carcinoma, in turn giving rise to frequent equivocal diagnoses in bladder wash specimens demonstrating changes typical for low-grade transitional cell carcinoma. Flow cytometry most frequently misses ulcerated invasive tumors that are generally straightforward cytologic diagnoses.[168]

Interpretation of urinary tract cytology is often more difficult during and after surgery, chemotherapy, and/-or treatment with bacille Calmette-Guérin (BCG). Although some authors suggest that flow cytometry is the best method for monitoring for recurrent tumors during treatment,[169] others reach differing conclusions, depending on the nature of the chemotherapy and the precise flow cytometric techniques.[170, 171] Both conventional examination and flow cytometry are negative in many tumor recurrences after BCG therapy[172] or chemotherapy.[157] Thus, interpretation of flow cytometry results after therapy requires close attention to the clinical situation.[173, 174] The lowest flow cytometry sensitivity and specificity are in patients treated by intravesicle chemotherapy; the highest are in those treated by surgery without additional therapy. Information about timing is as important as information about treatment history. Although flow cytometry examination misses many cystoscopically positive early recurrences when BCG treatment has been used, a negative flow cytometry at 6 months predicts treatment response as effectively as cystoscopic examination.[175]

The use of multiparameter flow cytometry may further improve the interpretation of urinary tract cytology specimens, particularly after chemotherapy or BCG therapy. For example, flow cytometry quantification of a urothelial antigen, Om5, and nuclear DNA has been used to assess response to intravesical BCG for carcinoma in situ.[161] Five of 9 patients with persistent Om5 positive cells after therapy had recurrent tumor by biopsy; 2 others had positive cytology. In contrast, none of the 4 without antigen-positive cells after therapy had clinical evidence of tumor. Another approach to multiparameter flow cytometry is the use of cytokeratin staining to separate epithelial from nonepithelial cell populations. This enables selective examination of urothelial cells and improved identification of aneuploid tumor cells.[176] Yet a third approach involves the use of the Tn antigen, which has been associated with bladder tumor prognosis, in a two-parameter assay with DNA ploidy.[177] Although multiparameter assessment may increase detection of high-grade tumors by flow cytometry, the lack of additional reports after these initial successes is not encouraging.

IMAGE ANALYSIS

Studies on the clinical utility of image cytometry as an adjunct to cytomorphologic examination of urine and urinary tract washings closely parallel those of flow cytometry. Quantitation of nuclear fluorescence from specimens dyed with DNA-intercalating dyes detects both low- and high-grade tumors earlier and with greater specificity than does cytomorphologic examination alone[178, 179] and may detect aneuploidy in cases where it was missed by flow cytometry.[180–182] This has led to claims of a combined sensitivity for image analysis and cytomorphologic examination from 85% to 100%.[183, 184] Some authors suggest that abnormal DNA ploidy by image analysis increases the detection of cancer only in patients demonstrating urothelial atypia and that ancillary diagnostic techniques can be avoided in patients with obvious malignancy or normal cytomorphologic examinations,[181] but this does not reflect the prevailing consensus. Cytomorphologic examination clearly detects cases missed by image cytometry and should not be omitted.[185]

The use of neural network for automated urine cytology holds great promise. Early results suggest that neural network analysis of cytomorphologic parameters correctly classifies approximately 97% of urinary cytology specimens,[185–188] even with Giemsa-stained specimens.

Although image analysis methods have not been tested as broadly in various clinical settings, it seems likely that their utility suffers from many of the same advantages and disadvantages as flow cytometry when applied to the same clinical situation.

IMMUNOCYTOCHEMISTRY

The clinical utility of immunocytochemical assays in urinary tract cytology has received surprisingly little attention. Immunocytochemical detection of p53 can be used to increase the sensitivity of the cytologic examination, but only at the cost of a reduction in specificity.[189] Similar results are found for the use of Lewis X, M244, and 19A211 antigens.[190]

MOLECULAR DIAGNOSIS

About 60% of bladder cancers have *TP53* mutations, which can be detected in the urine sediment.[191] Mutation-specific PCR may be useful as a marker of recurrence in patients whose tumors demonstrate mutations.

Telomerase mRNA is detected in the voided urine of about 80% of patients with bladder cancer and may be found in patients without cytomorphologic abnormalities.[192] Although telomerase mRNA is most frequently observed in tumors, it provides the greater increase in sensitivity in detection of low-grade tumors.[193, 194] Telomerase mRNA is detectable in about 5% of patients without bladder cancer[192] and is frequently found in patients with bladder inflammation.[195, 196] This limitation may be overcome by the use of quantitative assays, however.[197]

The specificity of the telomerase assay is between 80% and 100%, depending on the patient population and assay method[197, 198]; this is probably slightly lower than the specificity for cytomorphologic examination. The sensitivity of telomerase assay is 70% to 80%,[197, 198] compared with 40% to 50% for morphologic examination. Telomerase assay thus appears to be a very promising adjunct to urinary cytology, provided the assessment is performed via mRNA reverse transcriptase (RT)–PCR rather than telomerase repeat assay.[196]

A new FISH method, UroVysion (Vysis, Downers Grove, IL), has recently been approved for monitoring bladder cancer recurrence. This assay relies on the fact that deletions in chromosome 9p21, together with polysomy of chromosomes 3, 7, and 17, are common in transitional cell carcinoma. Data suggest that addition of the FISH assay to cytologic examination improves the sensitivity for detecting bladder cancer by about 20%.[196a,b]

FINE-NEEDLE ASPIRATION

Fine-needle aspiration (FNA) biopsy is well established as a definitive diagnostic method for many lesions. Nevertheless, a few FNAs from all sites remain diagnostically difficult, in spite of the well-characterized morphology of many common lesions. Although many articles reporting flow cytometry results suggest diagnostic utility in at least a fraction of cases, analysis of the literature suggests a low diagnostic yield, except when immunophenotypic analysis is used to help characterize lymphoid proliferations.

Thyroid

FLOW CYTOMETRY

DNA flow cytometry does not allow unambiguous diagnosis in any of the differential diagnoses currently not resolvable by aspiration cytology, such as follicular carcinoma versus follicular adenoma.[199] Similarly, identification of a monoclonal cell population by flow cytometry fails to differentiate Hashimoto's thyroiditis from malignant lymphoma.[200] Thus, flow cytometry has little use in thyroid aspiration cytology at this time.

IMAGE ANALYSIS

Although many articles have appeared regarding the use of image analysis in the classification of thyroid FNAs, the potential applicability for the technique in the routine laboratory is limited not only by the heterogeneity of results reported but also by the fact of the limited standardization of the image analysis equipment on which these results are based. The most optimistic results suggest that neural network classification of nuclear size, shape, and texture results in 98% correct diagnosis of malignancy in patients with a wide variety of benign and malignant thyroid disorders.[201] Although, this compares very favorably with visual cytomorphologic assessment, other investigations have found significant overlap in nuclear characteristics among subsets of thyroid FNAs,[202] and these promising results have not been replicated by an independent group. Thus, though image analysis shows more promise than flow cytometry as an adjunctive method for thyroid FNA, it is as yet unproved.

IMMUNOCYTOCHEMISTRY

Immunocytochemical evaluation of thyroid FNAs is nearly identical to that employed for surgical specimens. Undifferentiated neoplasms may be characterized by a panel of antibodies including anticytokeratin, anti-CD45 (LCA), and vimentin and further characterized if appropriate. Thyrocalcitonin is helpful in confirming a diagnosis of medullary carcinoma, but the differentiation among medullary, papillary, and follicular carcinomas can generally be made on the basis of cytomorphologic criteria. Cytokeratin 19 staining may sometimes prove helpful in differentiating papillary carcinomas from follicular neoplasms.[202a]

Immunocytochemical demonstration of lactoferrin is reported not to be seen in goiter, to be seen infrequently in adenoma, and to be commonly present in carcinoma.[203] Similarly, thyroid peroxidase has been proposed as an adjunct to establish a diagnosis of follicular carcinoma.[204] Although the sensitivity for identification of malignancy has been reported as 98%, the specificity is only 83% and the method relies on the use of a complex scoring system to ascertain staining.[205] Similarly, the carbohydrate-binding protein galectin-3 and the CD44 cell adhesion molecule are both commonly expressed in papillary and follicular carcinomas, but only rarely in adenomas.[204, 206] Given the limited experience with these antibodies and the likelihood that the surgical approach will not be affected by a specific diagnosis, none of these immunocytochemical tools can yet be considered other than investigational.

MOLECULAR DIAGNOSIS

PCR assays have demonstrated that the immunoglobulin heavy chain is not rearranged in Hashimoto's thyroiditis,[207] although rearrangement is readily identified in mucosa-associated lymphoid tissue (MALT) lymphoma of the thyroid.[208] In situ hybridization to determine light-chain restriction is also useful for establishing the presence of a monoclonal population in thyroid lymphoma[209] but is technically somewhat more cumbersome than immunoglobulin heavy-chain PCR. Both techniques are more useful than immunocytochemical assessment for the evaluation of monoclonality.

Mutation of the *RET* proto-oncogene is typical of medullary carcinoma. By comparing the sequence of the *RET* oncogene in a neck mass with that of peripheral blood, it has been possible to preoperatively differentiate between sporadic medullary carcinoma and multiple endocrine neoplasia, thus eliminating the need to search for other neoplasms.[210]

Telomerase activity is high in many malignancies but usually absent in normal adult tissue. High telomerase activity, as determined by the TRAP assay, has been shown in thyroid tumors demonstrating capsular or vascular invasion as well as in thyroid tissue demonstrating inflammatory changes. Telomerase activity has not been demonstrated in benign tumors but is also absent in a significant number of malignancies. Therefore, telomerase assays, whether performed by TRAP or by RT-PCR for telomerase mRNA, are unlikely to be an important diagnostic adjunct in thyroid FNA. Several other molecular biologic approaches demonstrate more promise for the identification of malignant changes in thyroid FNA. For example, mutation of the *RAS* oncogene has been identified in malignant, but not benign, thyroid FNAs.[211] Expression of oncofetal fibronectin mRNA (by RT-PCR) has been demonstrated in anaplastic and papillary carcinoma of the thyroid and demonstrates a sensitivity and specificity for diagnosis of these malignancies of 96.9 and 100%, respectively.[212] Similarly, overexpression of the *MUC1* gene has been associated with papillary carcinoma.[213]

With the exception of immunoglobulin gene rearrangement/restriction assays, the molecular methods discussed previously will not be ripe for clinical use until they have been evaluated in both a larger spectrum of disease and a larger number of laboratories.

Head and Neck

There is relatively little published information regarding the use of ancillary diagnostic methods on samples from FNAs of the head and neck. Flow cytometric assessment of cell surface markers may be useful in the diagnosis and characterization of extranodal lymphomas of the head and neck. Assessment of nuclear DNA content is probably of less value. Although some studies have suggested a relationship between aneuploidy or tumor proliferation rate (as assessed by the S-phase fraction),[214] others have found no such correlation.[215] Because interlaboratory variability is high for both flow cytometric and image analytic nuclear DNA measurements, it is prudent to determine the predictive value of these techniques on a laboratory-by-laboratory basis.

IMMUNOCYTOCHEMISTRY

With the exception of the rare instance in which they are required for characterization of an undifferentiated malignant neoplasm, immunocytochemical techniques are seldom useful in the characterization of head and neck neoplasms. In large part this reflects the limited spectrum of disease seen in this site. In children, however, the differentiation of various small, round, blue cell neoplasms may benefit from the use of the Ewing's sarcoma/peripheral neuroepithelial tumor marker CD99,[216] as well as from muscle- and lymphocyte-specific immunocytochemical assays.

MOLECULAR DIAGNOSIS

The role of molecular diagnosis in head and neck FNA is very limited. Although papillomavirus genomes may be demonstrated in some head and neck tumors by either in situ hybridization or PCR, their identification does not contribute clinically significant information to the diagnosis. Either in situ hybridization or PCR may be useful to identify Epstein-Barr virus (EBV), confirming an FNA diagnosis of undifferentiated nasopharyngal carcinoma; EBV genome is generally not identified by either method in other benign or malignant conditions.[217, 218]

As in other sites, immunoglobulin heavy-chain and T-cell receptor rearrangement analysis may prove helpful in establishing both a diagnosis and lineage for lymphoma and leukemia. In children, PCR-based assays for the t(11;22) (*EWS/FLI1*, Ewing's sarcoma)[219] and t(2;13)/t(1;13) (*PAX3-FOXO1A/PAX7-FOXO1A* alveolar rhabdomyosarcoma) gene fusions[220, 221] are often useful in differentiating among undifferentiated small cell tumors. Both sets of assays should be performed, because occasionally patients may demonstrate a tumor with molecular characteristics of both Ewing's sarcoma and rhabdomyosarcoma.[222] Detection of the myoD1 transcript may also be useful in establishing muscle differentiation.[223]

Salivary Gland

Patient history and clinical examination of the salivary glands, particularly the parotid gland, are highly accurate predictors of morphology and behavior.[224] Cytomorphologic examination further increases the accuracy of assessment, to the point where ancillary diagnostic techniques must provide truly spectacular results to be useful. Unfortunately, this is seldom the case.

FLOW CYTOMETRY AND IMAGE ANALYSIS

Although aneuploidy and increased S-phase fraction are more likely to be seen in malignant than benign salivary gland tumors, adjunctive use of flow cytometry or image analysis provides at most a marginal increase in diagnostic accuracy.[225] For this reason, the use of flow cytometry is best limited to assessment of lymphoid neoplasm cell surface markers.

IMMUNOCYTOCHEMISTRY

The differential diagnosis of salivary gland neoplasms is usually quite limited and resolved on the basis of cytomorphologic characteristics alone. Occasionally, the identification of a pleomorphic adenoma may be assisted by immunocytochemical demonstration of glial fibrillary acid protein, which appears to be unique to this neoplasm.[226–228]

Both salivary glands and their neoplasms occasionally show cross-reactivity for prostate-specific antigen (PSA). This may occasionally cause confusion between salivary gland neoplasm and metastatic prostate cancer.[229]

MOLECULAR DIAGNOSIS

Although PCR assays for immunoglobulin heavy-chain rearrangement are useful adjuncts for the diagnosis of salivary gland MALT lymphomas,[230] monoclonal bands are occasionally seen in benign conditions, such as myoepithelial sialadenitis,[231] and must be interpreted with caution. In situ hybridization studies for κ chain restriction must be interpreted with the same caution.[209]

A number of infectious diseases may give rise to masses and cysts in the salivary glands; the etiology is often not obvious either clinically or by visual examination of the aspirate. Use of PCR methods may be useful in the identification of atypical mycobacterial infections,[232] human immunodeficiency virus infection,[233] and other infectious causes.

Skin

FNA is rarely performed for the initial diagnosis of primary skin lesions; so the applications of ancillary diagnostic techniques to FNA samples has generally been dictated by clinical characteristics associated with one or more of the many tumors. For metastatic tumors, the role of adjunctive diagnostic techniques is similar to that encountered in lymph node metastases and is discussed in that section of this chapter. Several primary skin diseases have frequently been assessed by FNA, however, including leukemia/lymphoma, Merkel cell carcinoma, and disseminated histiocytosis.

IMMUNOCYTOCHEMISTRY

Cytologic diagnosis of Merkel cell carcinoma is facilitated by the observation of neuron-specific enolase (NSE), EMA, and S-100 staining to complement the observation of pseudorosettes of small cells with inconspicuous cytoplasm, finely granular chromatin, and multiple small nucleoli.[234] Dotlike cytokeratin staining, although highly characteristic of Merkel cell carcinoma, is seen in only about half of cases and depends on the particular anticytokeratin antibody employed.[235]

The diagnosis of peripheral T-cell lymphoma is aided by the observation of monomorphic staining for CD45-RO (UCHL-1). Nevertheless, the number of lymphoid cells observed is often small, and this finding should not be used alone to make a diagnosis of malignancy.

MOLECULAR DIAGNOSIS

PCR assays for T-cell γ receptor gene rearrangement are very useful in establishing a diagnosis of a peripheral T-cell neoplasm, such as mycosis fungoides, in skin FNA specimens.

Liver

The major diagnostic challenge for liver FNA is the differentiation of metastatic neoplasm, cholangiocarcinoma, hepatocellular carcinoma, and benign hepatic proliferative processes, including cirrhosis and adenoma. About 80% of malignant lesions may be diagnosed on clinical and cytomorphologic grounds, and ancillary diagnostic methods (predominantly immunocytochemistry) can resolve many of the remainder.[236]

FLOW AND IMAGE CYTOMETRY

Flow[237, 238] and image[239, 240] cytometry of liver FNA samples may be used to determine the ploidy of hepatocellular neoplasms and thus predict prognosis. Nevertheless, such studies are rarely pivotal in achieving a correct diagnosis[237] and are probably not cost effective in most cases.

IMMUNOCYTOCHEMISTRY

The diagnostic dilemma for which immunocytochemistry of liver FNA samples is most commonly employed is the differentiation of hepatocellular carcinoma, cholangiocarcinoma, and carcinoma metastatic from pancreas or colon (Table 17–1). In general, the distinction between hepatocellular carcinoma and carcinoma metastatic from the pancreas or colon is straightforward both cytomorphologically and immunocytochemically. In contrast, the distinction between cholangiocarcinoma and metastatic carcinoma is seldom made from aspirated material on either a morphologic or immunocytochemical basis. The distinction between cholangiocarcinoma and hepatocellular carcinoma is complicated by the existence of tumors demonstrating both forms of differentiation.

In addition to the assays shown in Table 17–1, the combination of CD34 and factor VIII has been suggested to

TABLE 17–1

Immunocytochemical Reactivity Patterns of Selected Abdominal Tumors

	Percent Positive			
Antigen	*Hepatocellular Carcinoma*	*Cholangiocarcinoma*	*Pancreatic Carcinoma*	*Colon Carcinoma*
α-Fetoprotein	52–66	3–20	0	6
Factor 13A	88–98	0	Unknown	Unknown
CK 19	9–16	92–99	100	70–97
AE1/3	10–29 (weak)	100 (strong)	100 (strong)	100 (strong)
CK 7	13–23	96–100	68–94	10–23
Carcinoembryonic antigen (polyclonal)	52–68	78–100	54–86	78–91
Vimentin	3–10	12–65	0	0–6

facilitate diagnosis of hepatocellular carcinoma, as neither antigen is typically expressed in metastatic tumor or non-neoplastic liver lesions.[241] Canalicular staining with CEA may also assist in the diagnosis.[242–244]

Differentiation of hepatocellular carcinoma and benign proliferative lesions in the liver can sometimes be difficult. Immunoreactivity for p53 is seen in hepatocellular carcinoma but not in regenerative nodules, adenoma, or focal nodular hyperplasia.[245] Unfortunately, p53 expression is only seldom seen in the well-differentiated hepatocellular carcinomas that are most likely to be a source of diagnostic confusion. PCNA reactivity is also higher in even well-differentiated hepatocellular carcinomas than in regenerative nodules, but the spectrum of reactivity in focal nodular hyperplasia and adenoma has not been defined.[246]

MOLECULAR DIAGNOSIS

Although albumin is expressed only in the liver, its uptake in nonhepatic cells limits the use of immunocytochemical assays for the diagnosis of hepatocellular carcinoma. In situ hybridization for albumin gene RNA overcomes this artifact and has demonstrated a sensitivity of 95% and specificity of 100% for diagnosis of hepatocellular lineage in aspirates[247, 248]; RT-PCR assays might be expected to achieve similar results. Molecular detection of albumin gene expression may thus prove useful in cases where cytomorphology and immunocytochemistry are insufficient to establish lineage of a hepatic aspirate with certainty.

Molecular assays for infectious disease are frequently useful in examining liver FNA specimens. PCR and RT-PCR assays reliably establish the diagnosis of hepatitis B and C, as well as a large variety of other infectious organisms that may be found in the liver.

Pancreas

FNA of the pancreas is generally performed to confirm a clinical diagnosis of pancreatic adenocarcinoma or islet cell tumor, permitting more informed treatment planning. Cytomorphologic examination alone is generally adequate to confirm either diagnosis if adequate tissue is obtained, but inadequate aspirates are frequently obtained from this site. As a result, both immunocytochemical and molecular biologic approaches to increasing the sensitivity of pancreatic FNA have been proposed.

IMMUNOCYTOCHEMISTRY

The monoclonal antibody B72.3 has been used to increase the sensitivity of cytologic examination of pancreatic aspirates.[249] In contrast to initial reports,[139] however, staining of benign cells is not uncommon, and this assay must be used with caution. Immunocytochemical demonstration of p53 has also been proposed for increasing the sensitivity of pancreatic FNA[250]; this is a promising technique, but it is currently limited by both the paucity of practical experience with this application as well as the broad range of reactivity of commercially available anti-p53 antibodies.

Immunocytochemical analysis is occasionally useful in distinguishing pancreatic adenocarcinoma from undifferentiated islet cell tumors. Synaptophysin is almost always expressed in islet cell tumors and chromogranin in about 60%; neither is seen in typical pancreatic adenocarcinoma. Islet cell tumors may be further characterized by more specific polypeptide markers such as gastrin and insulin.[251]

MOLECULAR DIAGNOSIS

Most pancreatic adenocarcinomas demonstrate mutation of the *KRAS* oncogene at codon 12. The use of PCR-based assays that detect this mutation in cytologic material demonstrates the mutation in about 80% of pancreatic adenocarcinomas and may thus increase the sensitivity of the FNA procedure.[252]

Adrenal Gland

FNA of the adrenal gland is performed most commonly for metastatic disease (lung and malignant melanoma are the most common metastatic tumors) but may also demonstrate adrenocortical carcinoma, myelolipoma, pheochromocytoma,[253] or neuroblastoma.[254] Each of the three primary adrenal tumors is treated by resection; thus, only immunocytochemistry is commonly employed as an ancillary diagnostic technique for adrenal FNA. Typical immunocytochemical profiles for the adrenal tumors, together with those of renal cell carcinoma and hepatocellular carcinoma, which often enter into the differential diagnosis of abdominal FNA specimens, are shown in Table 17–2. Neuroblastoma manifests itself in a younger age group than most of these neoplasms (although adrenal cortical carcinoma is not uncommon in older children) and is characterized by scanty cytoplasm, pseudorosettes, and multinucleated ganglion cells. These cytologic features are distinctive and seldom confused with those of other tumors commonly encountered in this site and age group. NSE is usually positive, and cytokeratin markers are generally negative.[255]

Kidney

Although FNA of the kidney may reveal lymphoma, metastatic neoplasm, or transitional cell carcinoma, it is most frequently performed in adults to establish a diagnosis of renal cell carcinoma. Although this diagnosis is frequently straightforward, the heterogeneous morphology of renal cell carcinoma sometimes results in uncertainty regarding differentiation and even malignancy.

TABLE 17–2

Immunoreactivity of Selected Abdominal Tumors

Antibody	Percentage of Cases Demonstrating Immunoreactivity			
	Adrenal Carcinoma	*Pheochromocytoma*	*Hepatocellular Carcinoma*	*Renal Cell Carcinoma*
AE1	0–9		27–43	50–78
AE1/3	0		10–29	80–93
CAM5.2	0–9		79–90	26–53
Carcinoembryonic antigen (CEA) (polyclonal)	0–87		52–68	0–26
Chromogranin A		90–100		0
CK 7			13–23	28–68
CK 19	0–9		9–16	38–70
Cytokeratin (pan)	5–22	9–27	100	83–94
D11	67–96	0		
Epithelial membrane antigen (EMA)	0–6	0	24–43	88–97
S-100	0	0		83–94
Vimentin	48–78	28–52	3–10	50–68

FLOW CYTOMETRY AND IMAGE ANALYSIS

Several studies have considered the utility of flow and image cytometry of renal cell carcinoma FNA samples.[256, 257] FNA material is insufficient to allow reliable identification of small aneuploid populations,[257] limiting the utility of FNA-based flow and image cytometry. There does appear to be some benefit from flow cytometric analysis of lymphocyte subpopulations within renal FNAs in the characterization of acute rejection, but experience is very limited.[258, 259]

IMMUNOCYTOCHEMISTRY

The most common application of immunocytochemistry to the evaluation of renal FNAs is to distinguish between undifferentiated transitional cell carcinoma of the renal pelvis and renal cell carcinoma. A panel consisting of cytokeratin 7, cytokeratin 20, and vimentin is useful in these unusual cases (Table 17–3). Actin may be useful in confirmation of a diagnosis of angiomyolipoma[260] or leiomyosarcoma.[261] The use of a renal cell carcinoma–specific antibody in the assessment of FNA material has been reported. The antibody appears to be useful in differentiating renal cell carcinoma from oncocytoma.[262]

MOLECULAR DIAGNOSIS

Diagnosis of cytomegalovirus in renal transplant recipients by in situ hybridization of FNA aspirates has been reported[263] but may not provide benefits that offset the increased price by comparison to immunocytochemistry. In situ hybridization or PCR-based assays may also be useful in characterizing EBV-stimulated lymphoproliferative disorders in these patients.

Immunoglobulin heavy-chain PCR of kidney FNA aspirates has proven to be useful in the characterization of post-transplant lymphoproliferative disorders,[258] and T-cell receptor PCR may be useful in the diagnosis of post-transplant leukemias.[264]

Prostate

FLOW CYTOMETRY AND IMAGE ANALYSIS

Flow cytometric investigations of prostate FNA aspirates have found that aneuploidy is specific for carcinoma and detected in 39% of cases; benign hyperplasia cases are diploid.[265] The incidence of aneuploidy

TABLE 17–3

Immunocytochemical Assays Distinguishing Transitional Cell Carcinoma from Renal Cell Carcinoma

Antigen	Percentage of Cases Demonstrating Immunoreactivity	
	Renal Cell Carcinoma	*Transitional Cell Carcinoma*
CK 7	28–68	100
CK 20	0–8	68–90
Vimentin	50–68	0

increases with the degree of dedifferentiation,[265, 266] reaching almost 95% in very poorly differentiated tumors, but the modal DNA value and cytologic grade are of prognostic value even in low-stage, low-grade untreated prostate cancer.[267] Image cytometry likewise provides prognostic information,[268] but the clinical utility of the prognostic information from both flow cytometry and image analysis remains unproved.

IMMUNOCYTOCHEMISTRY AND MOLECULAR DIAGNOSIS

Although immunocytochemical assessment of desmin and actin are occasionally useful in confirming this histogenesis of prostatic rhabdomyosarcoma,[269] there are few other applications for which these assays show clinical use for FNA.

FISH has been used to assess gene and chromosome copy numbers in prostate cancer.[270–272] Data suggest that FISH provides a better assessment of aneuploidy in prostate cancer than does flow cytometry.[272]

Breast

FLOW CYTOMETRY

In contrast to other sites, for which work relating flow cytometry and FNA has focused on the contribution of flow cytometry to diagnosis, studies on the breast have, for the most part, focused on the use of flow cytometry as a prognostic marker. Hundreds of studies have been published, with often conflicting results, making assessment of the cost-effectiveness of this technique difficult.

FNA may be used to obtain both ploidy and S-phase fraction information, and the flow cytometry data thus obtained have prognostic significance.[273] In 80% of cases, flow cytometry results from FNA material are qualitatively similar to those obtained from surgical biopsy specimens.[273] Although 99% of aneuploid specimens represent carcinomas, most of these cancers are identifiable by light microscopy and FNA appears to add little to the diagnostic yield, particularly because almost half of all carcinomas are diploid.[274–278] Flow cytometry of FNA specimens may occasionally prove useful in diagnosis of uncommon tumors, however. Corkill and colleagues[279] have suggested, for example, that identification of an aneuploid population may help in correct identification of intracystic papillary carcinoma.

Comparison of flow cytometry with image cytometric analysis strongly suggests that the latter provides a more sensitive method for identifying small aneuploid populations than does the former, in spite of the higher coefficients of variation associated with image cytometry.[274] Determination S-phase fraction is difficult using image cytometry, however. Immunocytochemical assessment of proliferation with Ki-67 (MIB1) is an alternative to determining S-phase fraction by flow cytometry. Although Ki-67 index and S-phase fraction are strongly correlated in breast FNA,[280] the Ki-67 index provides as much prognostic information at lower cost.[281]

Preoperative chemotherapy is increasingly employed in the treatment of breast cancer. Flow cytometric assessment of sequential FNA specimens provides a useful tool for following the effects of treatment,[282] but flow cytometric determination of S-phase fraction provides no information regarding the likelihood of response to treatment.[283]

Flow cytometric assessment of multidrug resistance *ABCB1 (MDR1)* gene expression may also be helpful in predicting potential drug resistance in the adjuvant chemotherapy setting.[284]

Flow cytometric assessment of breast FNA aspirates is an expensive procedure. It provides little or no information regarding likely responses to nonsurgical treatment. The limited benefits must be considered in light of the substantial costs when considering its use.

IMAGE ANALYSIS

Image analysis has been advocated as an alternative to manual scoring methods for the immunocytochemical quantitation of estrogen and progesterone receptor content.[285] The added benefit has been disputed, and use of these instruments seems to reflect the personality of the potential user more than the data provided. Like flow cytometry, image analysis of FNA specimens can be used to predict survival curves for breast cancer patients.[286] However, tumor grade predicted by image cytometry strongly correlates with that obtained by visual grading and flow cytometry and is more laborious than either of the latter methods.[287, 288]

Although the role of currently available image analysis techniques in the interpretation of breast FNA aspirates is severely limited by both cost and labor, newer, completely automated approaches to image cytometry promise to make these methods more cost effective.[289] Furthermore, the development of improved mathematical models for interpretation of cytometric results can be expected to make the methods more useful; algorithms have been developed that have a high degree of accuracy in diagnosing breast FNA specimens.[289] These algorithms use nuclear morphometric features derived from breast aspirates to predict time to recurrence more accurately than microscopic examination of lymph nodes,[290] and accurately diagnose aspirates that have received an inconclusive diagnosis based on cytomorphologic examination. One may therefore expect the development of automated systems that more nearly resemble the stand-alone machines being employed in cervical cancer screening.

IMMUNOCYTOCHEMISTRY

Immunocytochemical assays are occasionally helpful in the characterization of tumors metastatic to the breast,[291] and rare breast tumors,[292–295] but are only rarely used to assist in the diagnosis of "garden variety" breast carcinoma. Contrary to early reports,[139] immunocytochemical assessment of "tumor antigens" is of limited assistance in reaching a malignant diagnosis. Occasionally, immunocytochemical assessment of actin expression can assist in identifying myoepithelial cells[296] and thus clarify a morphologically confusing smear but, in general, cytomorphologic features provide the most reliable indicators of malignancy.

Accumulation of the *TP53* gene product is reliably determined by FNA[297, 298] but is only observed in 20% to 30% of invasive breast carcinomas. Similarly, the Ki-67 proliferation index[299] and PCNA index[297] can be obtained from FNA specimens, and ERBB2 overexpression can be assessed.[300, 301] Although p53 accumulation, increased Ki-67 proliferation index, and ERBB2 overexpression are all associated with adverse prognosis in breast cancer, their use in achieving a correct diagnosis has not been assessed in large studies, and they should not be considered "magic bullets" to assist with diagnosis.

Immunocytochemical loss of integrin expression in FNA specimens has been shown to predict nodal status[302]; it is not clear whether this will result in clinical utility for the assay.

Immunocytochemical assessment of estrogen and progesterone receptor status on FNA material is straightforward, correlates well with receptor quantitation performed in other ways,[303, 304, 304a] and can be used to predict response to tamoxifen.[299] Although immunocytochemical determination of ERBB2 overexpression can be used to select patients for treatment with the anti-ERBB2 monoclonal antibody Herceptin, this application has not been validated for specimens obtained by FNA.

MOLECULAR DIAGNOSIS

FISH is a reliable method for detecting amplification of the *ERBB2* oncogene[305] and is more readily performed on FNA aspirates than on biopsy specimens. In some laboratories, competitive PCR provides an alternative method for assessing *ERBB2* amplification,[306–308] and both immunocytochemistry and in situ hybridization[309] can provide assessments of gene overexpression in FNA specimens. The clinical use of these various approaches to *ERBB2* assessment has not been directly compared in FNA samples, nor validated for the selection of adjuvant chemotherapy.

In situ hybridization has also been used to detect numeric chromosome aberrations in breast aspirates.[152, 307, 310–315]

In general, it appears that numeric chromosome aberrations are not observed in benign tumors and that, when seen, they are strongly indicative of malignancy.[152, 311, 313] The degree to which this may assist in achieving correct cytopathologic diagnoses is not yet evident, however.

RT-PCR methods can be used to determine overexpression of the multidrug resistance gene *ABCB1* in breast aspirates.[284, 316, 317] The clinical use is uncertain, however, because ABCB1 overexpression does not reliably predict development of chemotherapy resistance.[317] Similarly, PCR followed by single-strand conformational polymorphism (SSCP), denaturing gradient gel electrophoresis (DGGE), or direct sequencing can be used to identify *TP53* mutations in breast aspirates.[284, 298, 318] As with immunocytochemical detection of p53 accumulation, however, the diagnostic utility of these techniques is unclear. Breast cancers harboring *TP53* mutations generally show abundant cytomorphologic characteristics of malignancy.

Lung

FLOW CYTOMETRY

FNA of lung, although not as commonly performed as FNA of breast and thyroid, is frequently useful in differentiating neoplastic from non-neoplastic pulmonary nodules. Diagnostic difficulties may occasionally arise because reparative/proliferative responses can have atypia simulating malignancy. Unfortunately, most investigations have focused not on resolving the diagnostic dilemmas but on measurement of cell proliferation kinetics.[319,320] These studies have shown unequivocally that lung FNA specimens may be used to determine ploidy and that the presence of an aneuploid population indicates malignancy with a false-positive rate of 1% to 2% and a false-negative rate of approximately 25%. The high false-negative rate appears to result from frequent near-diploid aneuploidy. Specimens are generally insufficient for routine cell cycle analysis,[319] but a more refined analysis can be obtained by dual-parameter flow cytometry.[320] In this technique, S-phase cells are labeled with 5-bromodeoxyuridine (BrdU), which can, in turn, be detected using a monoclonal antibody directed against BrdU. Although investigated on bronchial brushings, the techniques described should be equally applicable to FNA.

IMMUNOCYTOCHEMISTRY

In general, cytomorphologic criteria are sufficient to diagnose most lung aspirates. Occasionally, immunocytochemical staining with NSE, synaptophysin, chromogranin, or bombesin is helpful in making a diagnosis of small cell carcinoma, carcinoid, or large cell neuroendocrine carcinoma but usually these stains are unnecessary. Similarly, immunocytochemical demonstration of TAG72, CEA, Leu-M1, Ber-EP4, or other glandular markers is occasionally helpful in reaching a diagnosis of adenocarcinoma.

MOLECULAR DIAGNOSIS

PCR detection of HPV DNA in lung aspirates has been used to identify metastatic cervical cancer.[321]

Soft Tissue

FLOW CYTOMETRY AND IMAGE ANALYSIS

There is at most a limited role for these technologies in the assessment of soft tissue FNA material. Identification of an aneuploid population by flow cytometry may occasionally prompt reconsideration of an initially benign diagnosis,[322] but DNA flow cytometry of aspirates from this site is seldom informative. Flow cytometric characterization of cell surface markers from leukemias and lymphomas presenting in the soft tissue may contribute to the clinical management, however.[323]

Image analysis is unfortunately of little assistance in resolving the sometimes difficult differential diagnosis of proliferative myositis, fasciitis, and sarcoma, because both the pseudosarcomatous and malignant neoplasms often have similar DNA histograms.[324]

IMMUNOCYTOCHEMISTRY

The immunocytochemical characterization of soft tissue tumors is outlined in Chapter 5. Because classification and grading of soft tissue tumors are in many cases more dependent on morphology than antigen expression, one often is left with a somewhat imprecise cytologic diagnosis. Nevertheless, exclusion of spindle cell carcinoma and malignant melanoma, both of which frequently mimic sarcoma, is readily effected by a combination of cytokeratin, S-100, vimentin, and HMB-45. The use of antibodies against desmin and the various classes of actins may be of further assistance in some cases[325]; the markers for fibrohistiocytic differentiation are of little help.

The diagnosis of Ewing's sarcoma/primitive neuroepithelial tumor is facilitated by use of the MIC2 antibody,[216] but molecular diagnostics are generally more useful than immunocytochemical assays for specific diagnosis of soft tissue tumors.

MOLECULAR BIOLOGY

Many of the soft tissue tumors demonstrate specific translocations that allow unambiguous molecular diagnoses. Those that have been investigated in the context of FNA are shown in Table 17–4. Tumors demonstrating more than one translocation and biphenotypic differentiation have been observed.[222]

Lymph Node

The cytologic diagnosis of malignant lymphoma is rightfully regarded with suspicion by hematopathologists. The morphologic similarity between reactive and malignant lymphoid cells is striking, and monomorphic, cytologically abnormal lymphoid proliferations are seen in a variety of non-neoplastic processes. Nevertheless, the increasing importance of newer diagnostic methods in hematopathology has resulted in assays and diagnostic algorithms that enable correct diagnosis and classification of a large number of lymphoid neoplasms on the basis of FNA.[326, 327, 327a] Furthermore, aspiration of lymph nodes is an effective way to inexpensively document metastases and is often used to ascertain the tissue of origin when the primary site is unknown.[328]

Optimal use of the ancillary diagnostic methods below requires that lymphoma be considered at the time of initial aspiration, so that tissue may be used in a fresh or frozen state. Although some of the techniques below, such as PCR, work reasonably well on tissue that has been fixed on a slide or preserved in a cell block, none is as useful after fixation, and some, such

TABLE 17–4
Selected Tumor-Specific Translocations

Neoplasm	Chromosomal Translocation	Gene Fusion	Reference
Alveolar rhabdomyosarcoma	t(2;13) t(1;13)	*PAX3/FOXO1A* *PAX7/FOXO1A*	222
Ewing's sarcoma/primitive neuroectodermal tumor	t(11;22)	*EWS/FLI1*	219, 338
Synovial sarcoma	t(X;18)	*SSX1/SS18* *SSX2/SS18*	339

as flow cytometry for cell surface markers, are not applicable to fixed tissue.

FLOW CYTOMETRY AND IMAGE ANALYSIS

Flow cytometry is useful in the interpretation of lymph node aspirates, particularly when cell surface marker analysis is performed. Use of light-chain flow cytometry alone is sufficient to establish the diagnosis of lymphoma and/or its clinical stage approximately one third of the time.[329] Aneuploidy is observed in approximately 40% of high-grade lymphomas but virtually never in low-grade tumors; thus, aneuploidy cannot be used to distinguish low-grade lymphoma from benign processes. Addition of cell cycle analysis improves the diagnostic yield, however, such that about 80% of all lymphomas may be diagnosed using either aneuploidy or high S-phase as a diagnostic criterion[330]; addition of flow cytometry results to morphologic analysis appears to improve diagnostic accuracy. The combination of immunophenotypic and DNA flow cytometry further improves the diagnostic yield.[331, 332]

Although image analysis techniques yield ploidy and S-phase fraction results comparable to those obtained by flow cytometry,[333] there have been few applications to lymph node aspirates. It appears that the DNA distribution information obtained from these techniques can assist in reaching a diagnosis when flow cytometric information cannot be obtained.[334, 335]

IMMUNOCYTOCHEMISTRY

Most lymph node aspirates are performed to diagnose metastatic disease. When the patient has a known primary tumor, cytomorphologic examination alone is usually sufficient to confirm the presence of metastasis. Occasionally, however, the cytologic characteristics of the metastasis differ substantially from those of the primary tumor, or the aspirate has been obtained from a patient without a known primary tumor. Sometimes the features are those of a lymphoid malignancy rather than of a carcinoma. In these cases, the cytomorphologic features alone are seldom sufficient to determine the site of primary. Immunocytochemical assays, together with patient age, gender, and the location of the lymph node, can substantially focus the search for a primary in many of these cases.

The assessment of the unknown tumor generally proceeds through a series of panels of increasing specificity; depending on morphologic characteristics of the aspirate and the clinical situation, some of these panels may be modified or deleted. After this general assessment, which usually includes CD45 (LCA) for hematologic tumors, S-100 for malignant melanoma, a pancytokeratin for carcinomas, and vimentin as both a control and sarcoma marker, more specific panels based on specific intermediate filaments, surface markers, and secretory products are employed.

A large number of specific antigens and their utility are considered in Chapter 2. Although none of the antigens is absolutely specific for a particular tumor, some of them come pretty close. These are outlined in Table 17–5.

Immunocytochemical assessment of hematopoietic neoplasms is absolutely essential for complete classification and is often helpful in making the initial diagnosis. The identification of a monomorphic population of lymphocytes uniformly staining for either a B-cell (such as CD20 [L26]) or a T-cell marker (e.g., CD45RO [UCHL-1]) assists in making the diagnosis of lymphoma. Unfortunately, many cases present a mixed-cell population due to infiltration of uninvolved lymph nodes by malignant cells. Immunocytochemical markers for immunoglobulin chains are seldom of assistance unless they are performed on freshly prepared tissues. Most lymphomas express these genes at too low a level to detect by standard immunoperoxidase techniques on cell block material. Suspicion for follicular lymphoma may be assisted by strong staining for BCL2; suspicion for Hodgkin's disease may be increased by strong Leu-M1 and CD30 (BerH2) staining in a CD45 (LCA)-negative specimen, but the diagnosis still requires the identification of classic Reed-Sternberg cells. Mantle cell lymphoma is suggested by CD5 positivity, expression of one or more pan–B-cell markers, and immunoglobulin light-chain restriction.[336] Expression of the Ki-1 antigen can assist in the diagnosis of anaplastic large cell lymphoma.[337]

MOLECULAR DIAGNOSIS

Molecular diagnosis has strong roots in diagnostic hematopathology and is often critical to the successful diagnosis of lymphoma-containing FNA aspirates. PCR assays for immunoglobulin and T-cell receptor gene rearrangements, although expensive, are often highly informative. PCR-based assays for immunoglobulin

TABLE 17–5

Selected Tumor-Specific Antigens

HMB45	Malignant melanoma Chordoma
α-Fetoprotein	Hepatocellular carcinoma Cholanglocarcinoma
CD99 MIC2	Ewing's sarcoma Primitive neuorectodermal tumor
Calcitonin	Medullary carcinoma of thyroid
Thyroglobulin	Papillary carcinoma of thyroid Follicular carcinoma of thyroid
Prostate-specific antigen	Adenocarcinoma of prostate
Insulin	Islet cell tumor of pancreas
Gastrin	Gastrinoma of pancreas, duodenum, or stomach
TTF1	Carcinoma of lung

heavy-chain rearrangement are capable of detecting monoclonal populations of B cells constituting 5% to 25% of the total cell population. In the absence of an immunodeficiency syndrome or severe infectious process, the observation of a monoclonal heavy-chain rearrangement is almost tantamount to a diagnosis of malignancy. Furthermore, immunoglobulin heavy-chain rearrangement seldom displays lineage fidelity, allowing one to conclude that the lymphoma is of B-cell type. The observation of T-cell receptor β or γ chain rearrangement is a similar very strong sign of malignancy. Nevertheless, PCR-based assays for T-cell receptor gene rearrangements demonstrate lineage infidelity in about 10% of cases. Thus, more care must be taken in assigning lineage on the basis of this assay.

Follicular lymphoma may be quite difficult to distinguish from reactive hyperplasia in lymph node aspirates. Unfortunately, many PCR-based assays for immunoglobulin heavy-chain rearrangement do not reliably identified follicular lymphoma. The diagnosis of follicular lymphoma in FNA specimens is thus best assisted by the use of an immunocytochemical assay for BCL2 protein or detection of the *BCL2* rearrangement by PCR. If the latter approach is chosen, it is important to use a PCR assay that has not had its sensitivity boosted through the use of nesting or similar techniques. Nested, heminested, and otherwise enhanced assays for the *BCL2* rearrangement frequently identify a population of reactive cells that do not demonstrate malignant potential, so care must be taken in interpreting the results of these assays.

There are a few other lymphomas in which the demonstration of a particular translocation is straightforward and informative. Observation of the t(8;14) translocation by Southern blotting in Burkitt's lymphoma is useful in reaching a diagnosis. Identification of the t(2;5) translocation can enable the diagnosis of anaplastic large cell lymphoma, and identification of t(11;14) can facilitate a diagnosis of mantle cell lymphoma. Unfortunately, currently available PCR assays identify these translocations in only a minority of diagnosed cases.

CONCLUSIONS

Flow cytometry is a useful adjunct to cytologic examination in several settings. When properly interpreted, it can contribute greatly to the interpretation of bladder washings and is routinely performed for this purpose in many centers. It is also quite useful for the assessment of lymphoid lesions, whether they originate from FNA, CSF, or other sources. Optimal use of flow cytometry is frequently achieved only when more than one parameter is assessed; simultaneous use of cell differentiation markers and nuclear DNA quantitation is often significantly more useful than either alone. Improvement in image cytometric techniques may significantly limit the development of flow cytometry in cytology. Multiparameter measurements may also be accomplished with imaging techniques, which allow the further advantage of visual identification of cells with equivocal morphologic changes. The development of artificial intelligence methods for use with imaging technology has also significantly exceeded that associated with flow cytometry. Furthermore, several commercially available instruments designed to assist with Pap smear interpretation appear to be useful for other cytodiagnostic problems as well. Hence, with the exception of characterizing lymphoid cell surface markers, there are currently few applications in which flow cytometry is a useful, cost-effective adjunctive method.

The development and commercialization of image analysis systems can be expected to dramatically change the way cytology is practiced. As the "diagnostic abilities" of these machines improve and the cost of use decreases, cytotechnologist screening of Pap smears may disappear. Automated interpretation of FNA aspirates may be expected to follow, changing the role of the diagnostic cytopathologist.

Immunocytochemical methods are clearly today's most important adjunctive diagnostic techniques. They are inexpensive, effective, applicable to a wide range of diagnostic problems, and available in nearly every laboratory. Although assessment of ploidy by immunocytochemical methods is not possible, proliferation rates may be estimated by counting the number of tumor cell nuclei staining with antibodies directed against Ki-67 and other proliferation antigens. In addition, immunocytochemical methods can reliably identify cells that are not "where they should belong," such as glandular cells in a pleural fluid specimen. Many new immunocytochemical assays have resulted from advances in the molecular biologic understanding of disease, making the use of more complicated molecular diagnostic techniques unnecessary. Furthermore, automated interpretation of immunocytochemical assays is often quite straightforward.

With few exceptions, the role of molecular diagnosis in cytodiagnosis is still being defined. Clearly, molecular diagnostic methods are useful in the diagnosis of lymphoid and pediatric neoplasms for which well-characterized rearrangements and translocations have been recognized. FISH-based detection of aneuploidy is a potentially powerful and sensitive technique that may significantly increase the sensitivity of cytologic examination for a wide variety of tumors. Use of the more powerful amplification-based technologies, such as PCR-based mutation detection, is still limited to a few tumors and genes for which the variety of possible sequence abnormalities is severely limited. Assessment of telomerase expression appears to be a very sensitive indicator or the presence of malignant cells but is less specific than cytomorphology. Nevertheless, with the introduction of increasingly fast and powerful technologies for finding multiple aberrant gene expression patterns, molecular biologic techniques will certainly complement, and may even replace, both immunocytochemical and image analysis methods in the next decade.

REFERENCES

1. Bentley SA, Smith EM, Habbersett MC, Herman CJ: A pattern classification system for automated cervical cytologic screening based on flow microfluorometric analysis. Anal Quant Cytol 1979;1:61–66.
2. Fowlkes BJ, Herman CJ, Cassidy M: Flow microfluorometric system for screening gynecologic cytology specimens using propidium iodide-fluorescein isothiocyanate. J Histochem Cytochem 1976;24:322–331.
3. Habbersett MC, Shapiro M, Bunnag B, et al: Quantitative analysis of flow microfluorometric data for screening gynecologic cytology specimens. J Histochem Cytochem 1979;27:536–544.
4. Linden WA, Ochlich K, Baisch H, et al: Flow cytometric prescreening of cervical smears. J Histochem Cytochem 1979;27:529–535.
5. O'Leary TJ, O'Leary DP, Habbersett MC, Herman CJ: Classification of gynecologic flow cytometry data: A comparison of methods. Anal Quant Cytol 1981; 3:135–142.
6. Sprenger E, Rossner R, Otto C, et al: The mathematical evaluation of flow-through cytophotometric data in processing cervical cytology. Beitr Pathol 1974;153:289–296.
7. Sprenger E, Sandritter W, Naujoks H, et al: Routine use of flow-through photometric prescreening in the detection of cervical carcinoma. Acta Cytol 1977;21:435–440.
8. Titley I, Tee DE, Driver M, et al: Can flow cytometry reduce the workload for cervical screening? The results of a series of 622 specimens. Cytopathology 1991;2: 193–203.
9. Berkan TK, Reeder JE, Lopez PAJ, et al: A protocol for Papanicolaou staining of cytologic specimens following flow analysis. Cytometry 1986;7:101–103.
10. Wheeless LL, Patten SF, Berkan TK, et al: Multidimensional slit-scan prescreening system: Preliminary results of a single-blind clinical study. Cytometry 1984;5:1–8.
11. Suehiro Y, Kato H, Nagai M, Torigoe T: Flow cytometric analysis of tumor antigen TA-4 in cervical cytologic specimens. Cancer 1986;57:1380–1384.
12. Perticarari S, Presani G, Michelutti A, et al: Flow cytometric analysis of DNA content in cervical lesions. Pathol Res Pract 1989;185:686–688.
13. Siadat-Pajouh M, Periasamy A, Ayscue AH, et al: Detection of human papillomavirus type 16/18 DNA in cervicovaginal cells by fluorescence based in situ hybridization and automated image cytometry. Cytometry 1994;15: 245–257.
14. Gross HJ, Verwer B, Houck D, Recktenwald D: Detection of rare cells at a frequency of one per million by flow cytometry. Cytometry 1993;14:519–526.
15. Mitchell H, Medley G: Detection of laboratory false negative smears by the PAPNET cytologic screening system. Acta Cytol 1998;42:265–270.
16. Rosenthal DL, Acosta D, Peters RK: Computer-assisted rescreening of clinically important false negative cervical smears using the PAPNET Testing System. Acta Cytol 1996;40:120–126.
17. Sherman ME, Mango LJ, Kelly D, et al: PAPNET analysis of reportedly negative smears preceding the diagnosis of a high-grade squamous intraepithelial lesion or carcinoma. Mod Pathol 1994;7:578–581.
18. Sherman ME, Schiffman M, Herrero R, et al: Performance of a semiautomated Papanicolaou smear screening system: Results of a population-based study conducted in Guanacaste, Costa Rica. Cancer 1998;84: 273–280.
19. Solomon HM, Frist S: PAPNET testing for HSILs. The few cell/small cell challenge. Acta Cytol 1998;42: 253–259.
20. Slagel DD, Zaleski S, Cohen MB: Efficacy of automated cervical cytology screening. Diagn Cytopathol 1995;13: 26–30.
21. Colgan TJ, Patten SFJ, Lee JS: A clinical trial of the AutoPap 300 QC system for quality control of cervicovaginal cytology in the clinical laboratory. Acta Cytol 1995;39:1191–1198.
22. Colgan TJ, Bon N, Lee JS, Patten SFJ: AutoPap 300 QC system scoring of cervical smears without "epithelial cell abnormalities." Acta Cytol 1997;41:45–49.
23. Lee JS, Kuan L, Oh S, et al: A feasibility study of the AutoPap system location-guided screening. Acta Cytol 1998;42:221–226.

23a. Bollman R, Bollman M, Henson DE, Bodo M: DNA cytometry confirms the utility of the Bethesda system for classification of Pap smears. Cancer Cytopathol 2001;93:222–228.

24. Patten SFJ, Lee JS, Wilbur DC, et al: The AutoPap 300 QC System multicenter clinical trials for use in quality control rescreening of cervical smears: II. Prospective and archival sensitivity studies. Cancer 1997;81: 343–347.
25. Patten SFJ, Lee JS, Wilbur DC, et al: The AutoPap 300 QC System multicenter clinical trials for use in quality control rescreening of cervical smears: I. A prospective intended use study. Cancer 1997;81:337–342.
26. Wilbur DC, Bonfiglio TA, Rutkowski MA, et al: Sensitivity of the AutoPap 300 QC System for cervical cytologic abnormalities. Biopsy data confirmation. Acta Cytol 1996;40:127–132.
27. Mango LJ: Computer-assisted cervical cancer screening using neural networks. Cancer Lett 1994;77:155–162.
28. O'Leary TJ, Tellado M, Buckner SB, et al: PAPNET-assisted rescreening of cervical smears: Cost and accuracy compared with a 100% manual rescreening strategy. JAMA 1998;279:235–237.
29. Waters SA, Sterrett GF: Intracytoplasmic vacuoles in cervical smears: Relationship to chlamydial inclusions—morphology, mucin histochemistry, and immunocytochemistry. Diagn Cytopathol 1991;7:252–260.
30. Marsella RC, Buckner SB, Bratthauer GL, et al: Identification of genital herpes simplex virus infection by immunoperoxidase staining: Comparison with culture results and cytology. Appl Immunohistochem 1995; 3:184–189.
31. Kobayashi TK: Comparison of immunocytochemistry and in situ hybridization in the cytodiagnosis of genital herpetic infection. Diagn Cytopathol 1992;8:53–60.

32. Ho GY, Bierman R, Beardsley L, et al: Natural history of cervicovaginal papillomavirus infection in young women. N Engl J Med 1998;338:423–428.
33. Remmink AJ, Walboomers JM, Helmerhorst TJ, et al: The presence of persistent high-risk HPV genotypes in dysplastic cervical lesions is associated with progressive disease: Natural history up to 36 months. Int J Cancer 1995;61:306–311.
34. Gerbaldo D, Cristoforoni P, Leone M, et al: The incidental finding of abnormal cervical histology in postmenopausal patients. Maturitas 1995;21:115–120.
35. Cope JU, Hildesheim A, Schiffman MH, et al: Comparison of the hybrid capture tube test and PCR for detection of human papillomavirus DNA in cervical specimens. J Clin Microbiol 1997;35:2262–2265.
36. Vossler JL, Forbes BA, Adelson MD: Evaluation of the polymerase chain reaction for the detection of human papillomavirus from urine. J Med Virol 1995;45: 354–360.
37. Morrison EA, Goldberg GL, Hagan RJ, et al: Self-administered home cervicovaginal lavage: A novel tool for the clinical-epidemiologic investigation of genital human papillomavirus infections. Am J Obstet Gynecol 1992; 167:104–107.
38. Burk RD, Kadish AS, Calderin S, Romney SL: Human papillomavirus infection of the cervix detected by cervicovaginal lavage and molecular hybridization: Correlation with biopsy results and Papanicolaou smear. Am J Obstet Gynecol 1986;154:982–989.
39. Borg AJ, Medley G, Garland SM: Polymerase chain reaction: A sensitive indicator of the prevalence of human papillomavirus DNA in a population with sexually transmitted disease. Acta Cytol 1995;39:654–658.
40. Engels H, Nyongo A, Temmerman M, et al: Cervical cancer screening and detection of genital HPV-infection and chlamydial infection by PCR in different groups of Kenyan women. Ann Soc Belg Med Trop 1992; 72:53–62.
41. Hagmar B, Kalantari M, Skyldberg B, et al: Human papillomavirus in cell samples from Stockholm Gynecologic Health Screening. Acta Cytol 1995;39:741–745.
42. Johnson TL, Joseph CL, Caison-Sorey TJ, et al: Prevalence of HPV 16 and 18 DNA sequences in CIN III lesions of adults and adolescents. Diagn Cytopathol 1994;10:276–283.
43. Kjaer SK, van den Brule AJ, Bock JE, et al: Determinants for genital human papillomavirus (HPV) infection in 1000 randomly chosen young Danish women with normal Pap smear: Are there different risk profiles for oncogenic and nononcogenic HPV types? Cancer Epidemiol Biomarkers Prev 1997;6: 799–805.
44. Rymark P, Forslund O, Hansson BG, Lindholm K: Genital HPV infection not a local but a regional infection: Experience from a female teenage group. Genitourin Med 1993;69:18–22.
45. ter Meulen J, Eberhardt HC, Luande J, et al: Human papillomavirus (HPV) infection, HIV infection and cervical cancer in Tanzania, east Africa. Int J Cancer 1992; 51:515–521.
46. van Doornum GJ, Van den Hoek JA, Van Ameijden EJ, et al: Cervical HPV infection among HIV-infected prostitutes addicted to hard drugs. J Med Virol 1993; 41:185–190.
46a. Harrington CS: Does HPV testing have a role in primary cervical screening? Cytopathol 2001;12:71–74.
47. Rozendaal L, Walboomers JM, van der Linden JC, et al: PCR-based high-risk HPV test in cervical cancer screening gives objective risk assessment of women with cytomorphologically normal cervical smears. Int J Cancer 1996;68:766–769.
48. Cox JT, Lorincz AT, Schiffman MH, et al: Human papillomavirus testing by hybrid capture appears to be useful in triaging women with a cytologic diagnosis of atypical squamous cells of undetermined significance. Am J Obstet Gynecol 1995;172:946–954.
49. Cox JT, Schiffman MH, Winzelberg AJ, Patterson JM: An evaluation of human papillomavirus testing as part of referral to colposcopy clinics. Obstet Gynecol 1992; 80:389–395.
50. Symmans F, Mechanic L, MacConnell P, et al: Correlation of cervical cytology and human papillomavirus DNA detection in postmenopausal women. Int J Gynecol Pathol 1992;11:204–209.
51. Kyo S, Takakura M, Ishikawa H, et al: Application of telomerase assay for the screening of cervical lesions. Cancer Res 1997;57:1863–1867.
52. Yashima K, Ashfaq R, Nowak J, et al: Telomerase activity and expression of its RNA component in cervical lesions. Cancer 1998;82:1319–1327.
53. Sprenger E, Witte S: The diagnostic significance of flow cytometric nuclear DNA measurement in gastroscopic diagnosis of the stomach. Pathol Res Pract 1980;169: 269–275.
54. Ryan ME, Baldauf MC: Comparison of flow cytometry for DNA content and brush cytology for detection of malignancy in pancreaticobiliary strictures. Gastrointest Endosc 1994;40:133–139.
55. Koss LG, Morgenstern N, Tahir-Kheli N, et al: Evaluation of esophageal cytology using a neural net–based interactive scanning system (the PAPNET system): Its possible role in screening for esophageal and gastric carcinoma. Am J Clin Pathol 1998;109:549–557.
56. Tsai TT, Bongiorno PF, Orringer MB, Beer DG: Detection of p53 nuclear protein accumulation in brushings and biopsies of Barrett's esophagus. Cancer Detect Prev 1997;21:326–331.
56a. Steward CJR, Burke GM: Value of p53 immunostaining in pancreatico-biliary brush cytology specimens. Diag Cytopathol 2000;23:308–313.
57. Shidham VB, Weiss JP, Quinn TJ, Grotkowski CE: Fine needle aspiration cytology of gastric solitary fibrous tumor: A case report. Acta Cytol 1998;42:1159–1166.
58. Gorczyca W, Woyke S: Endoscopic brushing cytology of primary gastric choriocarcinoma: A case report. Acta Cytol 1992;36:551–554.
59. Chung CH, Wilentz RE, Polak MM, et al: Clinical significance of K-*ras* oncogene activation in ampullary neoplasms. J Clin Pathol 1996;49:460–464.
60. Sidransky D, Tokino T, Hamilton SR, et al: Identification of *ras* oncogene mutations in the stool of patients with curable colorectal tumors. Science 1992;256: 102–105.

61. Nollau P, Jung R, Neumaier M, Wagener C: Tumour diagnosis by PCR-based detection of tumour cells. Scand J Clin Lab Invest Suppl 1995;221:116–121.
62. Califano J, Ahrendt SA, Meininger G, et al: Detection of telomerase activity in oral rinses from head and neck squamous cell carcinoma patients. Cancer Res 1996; 56:5720–5722.
63. Yoshida K, Sugino T, Goodison S, et al: Detection of telomerase activity in exfoliated cancer cells in colonic luminal washings and its related clinical implications. Br J Cancer 1997;75:548–553.
64. Frost JK, Tyrer HW, Pressman NJ, et al: Automatic cell identification and enrichment in lung cancer: I. Light scatter and fluorescence parameters. J Histochem Cytochem 1979;27:545–551.
65. Tyrer HW, Pressman NJ, Albright CD, Frost JK: Automatic cell identification and enrichment in lung cancer: V. Adenocarcinoma and large cell undifferentiated carcinoma. Cytometry 1985;6:37–46.
66. Deinlein E, Sander U, Greiner C, Hornstein OP: Diagnostic significance of flow cytometric DNA analysis applied for the detection of cancer cells in bronchial washing fluid. Anal Quant Cytol Histol 1988;10:360–364.
67. Fuhr JE, Kattine AA, Sullivan TA, Nelson HSJ: Flow cytometric analysis of pulmonary fluids and cells for the detection of malignancies. Am J Pathol 1992;141: 211–215.
68. Greenberg SD, Smith S, Swank PR, et al: Visual cell profiles for quantitation of premalignant cells in sputum: A preliminary report. Acta Cytol 1982; 26:809–813.
69. Kimzey SL, Greenberg SD, Baky AA, Winkler DG: Cell atypia profiles for bronchial epithelial cells: Mathematical evaluation of sputum cellular atypia in squamous cell carcinogenesis of the lung. Anal Quant Cytol 1980;2: 186–194.
70. Tockman MS, Gupta PK, Pressman NJ, Mulshine JL: Cytometric validation of immunocytochemical observations in developing lung cancer. Diagn Cytopathol 1993;9:615–622.
71. Hoda RS, Saccomanno G, Schreiber K, et al: Automated sputum screening with PAPNET system: A study of 122 cases. Hum Pathol 1996;27:656–659.
72. Payne PW, Sebo TJ, Doudkine A, et al: Sputum screening by quantitative microscopy: A reexamination of a portion of the National Cancer Institute Cooperative Early Lung Cancer Study. Mayo Clin Proc 1997; 72:697–704.
73. Saleh HA, Haapaniemi J, Khatib G, Sakr W: Bronchioloalveolar carcinoma: Diagnostic pitfalls and immunocytochemical contribution. Diagn Cytopathol 1998;18: 301–306.
73a. Chhieng DC, Cangiarella JF, Zakowski MF, et al; Use of thyroid transcription factor 1, PE-10 and cytokeratins 7 and 20 in discriminating between primary lung carcinomas and metastatic lesions in fine-needle aspiration biopsy specimens. Cancer Cytopathol 2001;93:330–336.
74. Yakubovskaya MS, Spiegelman V, Luo FC, et al: High frequency of K-*ras* mutations in normal appearing lung tissues and sputum of patients with lung cancer. Int J Cancer 1995;63:810–814.
75. Mao L, Hruban RH, Boyle JO, et al: Detection of oncogene mutations in sputum precedes diagnosis of lung cancer. Cancer Res 1994;54:1634–1637.
76. Marchetti A, Buttitta F, Carnicelli V, et al: A highly sensitive method for the detection of unknown mutations: Application to the molecular diagnosis of lung cancer in sputum samples. Diagn Mol Pathol 1997;6:185–191.
77. Schenk T, Ackermann J, Brunner C, et al: Detection of chromosomal aneuploidy by interphase fluorescence in situ hybridization in bronchoscopically gained cells from lung cancer patients. Chest 1997;111:1691–1696.
78. Prayson RA, Fischler DF: Cerebrospinal fluid cytology: An 11-year experience with 5951 specimens. Arch Pathol Lab Med 1998;122:47–51.
79. Cibas ES, Malkin MG, Posner JB, Melamed MR: Detection of DNA abnormalities by flow cytometry in cells from cerebrospinal fluid. Am J Clin Pathol 1987; 88: 570–577.
80. Redner A, Melamed MR, Andreeff M: Detection of central nervous system relapse in acute leukemia by multiparameter flow cytometry of DNA, RNA, and CALLA. Ann N Y Acad Sci 1986;468:241–255.
81. Finn WG, Peterson LC, James C, Goolsby CL: Enhanced detection of malignant lymphoma in cerebrospinal fluid by multiparameter flow cytometry. Am J Clin Pathol 1998;110:341–346.
81a. French CA, Dorfman DM, Shaheen G, Cibas ES: Diagnosing lymphoproliferative disorders involving the cerebrospinal fluid: Increased sensitivity using flow cytometric analysis. Diagn Cytopathol 2000;23: 369–374.
82. Biesterfeld S, Bernhard B, Bamborschke S, Bocking A: DNA single cell cytometry in lymphocytic pleocytosis of the cerebrospinal fluid. Acta Neuropathol (Berl) 1993;86:428–432.
83. Boogerd W, Vroom TM, van Heerde P, et al: CSF cytology versus immunocytochemistry in meningeal carcinomatosis. J Neurol Neurosurg Psychiatry 1988; 51:142–145.
84. Jorda M, Ganjei-Azar P, Nadji M: Cytologic characteristics of meningeal carcinomatosis: Increased diagnostic accuracy using carcinoembryonic antigen and epithelial membrane antigen immunocytochemistry. Arch Neurol 1998;55:181–184.
85. Oschmann P, Kaps M, Volker J, Dorndorf W: Meningeal carcinomatosis: CSF cytology, immunocytochemistry and biochemical tumor markers. Acta Neurol Scand 1994;89:395–399.
86. Tani E, Costa I, Svedmyr E, Skoog L: Diagnosis of lymphoma, leukemia, and metastatic tumor involvement of the cerebrospinal fluid by cytology and immunocytochemistry. Diagn Cytopathol 1995;12:14–22.
87. Vick WW, Wikstrand CJ, Bullard DE, et al: The use of a panel of monoclonal antibodies in the evaluation of cytologic specimens from the central nervous system. Acta Cytol 1987;31:815–824.
88. van Oostenbrugge RJ, Hopman AH, Arends JW, et al: The value of interphase cytogenetics in cytology for the diagnosis of leptomeningeal metastases. Neurology 1998;51:906–908.
89. Bamborschke S, Porr A, Huber M, Heiss WD: Demonstration of herpes simplex virus DNA in CSF cells by in

situ hybridization for early diagnosis of herpes encephalitis. J Neurol 1990;237:73–76.

90. Cinque P, Vago L, Marenzi R, et al: Herpes simplex virus infections of the central nervous system in human immunodeficiency virus–infected patients: Clinical management by polymerase chain reaction assay of cerebrospinal fluid. Clin Infect Dis 1998;27:303–309.
91. Klapper PE, Cleator GM, Dennett C, Lewis AG: Diagnosis of herpes encephalitis via Southern blotting of cerebrospinal fluid DNA amplified by polymerase chain reaction. J Med Virol 1990;32:261–264.
92. Puchhammer-Stockl E, Popow-Kraupp T, Heinz FX, et al: Establishment of PCR for the early diagnosis of herpes simplex encephalitis. J Med Virol 1990;32:77–82.
93. Tebas P, Nease RF, Storch GA: Use of the polymerase chain reaction in the diagnosis of herpes simplex encephalitis: A decision analysis model. Am J Med 1998; 105:287–295.
94. Arribas JR, Clifford DB, Fichtenbaum CJ, et al: Detection of Epstein-Barr virus DNA in cerebrospinal fluid for diagnosis of AIDS-related central nervous system lymphoma. J Clin Microbiol 1995;33:1580–1583.
95. Brink NS, Sharvell Y, Howard MR, et al: Detection of Epstein-Barr virus and Kaposi's sarcoma–associated herpesvirus DNA in CSF from persons infected with HIV who had neurological disease. J Neurol Neurosurg Psychiatry 1998;65:191–195.
96. Cherian T, Lalitha MK, Manoharan A, et al: PCR-enzyme immunoassay for detection of *Streptococcus pneumoniae* DNA in cerebrospinal fluid samples from patients with culture-negative meningitis. J Clin Microbiol 1998;36:3605–3608.
97. Cinque P, Vago L, Dahl H, et al: Polymerase chain reaction on cerebrospinal fluid for diagnosis of virus-associated opportunistic diseases of the central nervous system in HIV-infected patients. AIDS 1996;10: 951–958.
98. De Luca A, Antinori A, Cingolani A, et al: Evaluation of cerebrospinal fluid EBV-DNA and IL-10 as markers for in vivo diagnosis of AIDS-related primary central nervous system lymphoma [published erratum appears in Br J Haematol 1995;91:1035]. Br J Haematol 1995;90: 844–849.
99. Ehrnst A: The clinical relevance of different laboratory tests in CMV diagnosis. Scand J Infect Dis Suppl 1996;100:64–71.
100. Fujimoto S, Kobayashi M, Uemura O, et al: PCR on cerebrospinal fluid to show influenza-associated acute encephalopathy or encephalitis. Lancet 1998;352:873–875.
101. Hammarin AL, Bogdanovic G, Svedhem V, et al: Analysis of PCR as a tool for detection of JC virus DNA in cerebrospinal fluid for diagnosis of progressive multifocal leukoencephalopathy. J Clin Microbiol 1996;34: 2929–2932.
102. Hosoya M, Honzumi K, Sato M, et al: Application of PCR for various neurotropic viruses on the diagnosis of viral meningitis. J Clin Virol 1998;11:117–124.
103. Kirchhoff LV: Use of a PCR assay for diagnosing African trypanosomiasis of the CNS: A case report. Cent Afr J Med 1998;44:134–136.
104. Novati R, Castagna A, Morsica G, et al: Polymerase chain reaction for *Toxoplasma gondii* DNA in the cerebrospinal fluid of AIDS patients with focal brain lesions. AIDS 1994;8:1691–1694.
105. Rappelli P, Are R, Casu G, et al: Development of a nested PCR for detection of *Cryptococcus neoformans* in cerebrospinal fluid. J Clin Microbiol 1998;36:3438–3440.
106. Reischl U, Lehn N, Wolf H, Naumann L: Clinical evaluation of the automated COBAS AMPLICOR MTB assay for testing respiratory and nonrespiratory specimens. J Clin Microbiol 1998;36:2853–2860.
107. Schmitz FJ, Steiert M, Hofmann B, et al: Detection of staphylococcal genes directly from cerebrospinal and peritoneal fluid samples using a multiplex polymerase chain reaction. Eur J Clin Microbiol Infect Dis 1998; 17:272–274.
108. Studahl M, Bergstrom T, Hagberg L: Acute viral encephalitis in adults—a prospective study. Scand J Infect Dis 1998;30:215–220.
109. Taggart EW, Byington CL, Hillyard DR, et al: Enhancement of the AMPLICOR enterovirus PCR test with a coprecipitant. J Clin Microbiol 1998;36: 3408–3409.
110. Weber T, Frye S, Bodemer M, et al: Clinical implications of nucleic acid amplification methods for the diagnosis of viral infections of the nervous system. J Neurovirol 1996; 2:175–190.
111. Weinberg A, Spiers D, Cai GY, et al: Evaluation of a commercial PCR kit for diagnosis of cytomegalovirus infection of the central nervous system. J Clin Microbiol 1998;36:3382–3384.
112. Januszkiewicz DA, Nowak JS: Molecular evidence for central nervous system involvement in children with newly diagnosed acute lymphoblastic leukemia. Hematol Oncol 1995;13:201–206.
113. van Dongen JJ, Breit TM, Adriaansen HJ, et al: Detection of minimal residual disease in acute leukemia by immunological marker analysis and polymerase chain reaction. Leukemia 1992;6(Suppl 1):47–59.
114. Garicochea B, Cliquet MG, Melo N, et al: Leptomeningeal involvement in chronic lymphocytic leukemia identified by polymerase chain reaction in stored slides: A case report. Mod Pathol 1997;10:500–503.
115. Galoin S, Daste G, Apoil PA, et al: Polymerase chain reaction on cerebrospinal fluid cells in the detection of leptomeningeal involvement by B-cell lymphoma and leukaemia: A novel strategy and its implications. Br J Haematol 1997;99:122–130.
116. Rhodes CH, Glantz MJ, Glantz L, et al: A comparison of polymerase chain reaction examination of cerebrospinal fluid and conventional cytology in the diagnosis of lymphomatous meningitis. Cancer 1996;77:543–548.
117. Harigae H, Kobayashi M, Mihara A, Watanabe N: Detection of minimal residual disease in cerebrospinal fluid of a patient with acute myelogenous leukemia with t(16;21)(p11;q22) translocation by reverse transcriptase-polymerase chain reaction. Tohoku J Exp Med 1997;183:297–302.
118. Rhodes CH, Honsinger C, Sorenson GD: Detection of tumor-derived DNA in cerebrospinal fluid. J Neuropathol Exp Neurol 1994;53:364–368.
119. Rhodes CH, Honsinger C, Sorenson GD: PCR-detection of tumor-derived p53 DNA in cerebrospinal fluid. Am J Clin Pathol 1995;103:404–408.

120. Kleinschmidt-DeMasters BK, Evans LC, Bitter MA, et al: Part II. Telomerase expression in cerebrospinal fluid specimens as an adjunct to cytologic diagnosis. J Neurol Sci 1998;161:124–134.
121. Crosby JH, Allsbrook WCJ, Pantazis CG, et al: Cytology and DNA flow cytometry of peritoneal washings in gynecologic patients. Mod Pathol 1992;5:153–157.
122. Finn CB, Ward K, Luesley DM, et al: Qualitative and quantitative analysis of peritoneal fluids from women with gynecologic diseases: Comparison of cytology and flow cytometry for the detection of malignancy in lavage and ascitic fluids. Anal Quant Cytol Histol 1991;13:182–186.
123. Hedley DW, Philips J, Rugg CA, Taylor IW: Measurement of cellular DNA content as an adjunct to diagnostic cytology in malignant effusions. Eur J Cancer Clin Oncol 1984;20:749–752.
124. Hostmark J, Vigander T, Skaarland E: Characterization of pleural effusions by flow-cytometric DNA analysis. Eur J Respir Dis 1985;66:315–319.
125. Jones MA, Hitchcox S, D'Ascanio P, et al: Flow cytometric DNA analysis versus cytology in the evaluation of peritoneal fluids. Gynecol Oncol 1991;43:226–232.
126. Katz RL, Johnson TS, Williamson KD: Comparison of cytologic and acridine-orange flow-cytometric detection of malignant cells in human body cavity fluids. Anal Quant Cytol Histol 1985;7:227–235.
127. Rijken A, Dekker A, Taylor S, et al: Diagnostic value of DNA analysis in effusions by flow cytometry and image analysis. A prospective study on 102 patients as compared with cytologic examination. Am J Clin Pathol 1991;95:6–12.
128. Zarbo RJ: Flow cytometric DNA analysis of effusions: A new test seeking validation [editorial; comment]. Am J Clin Pathol 1991;95:2–4.
129. Lima CE, Mizushima Y, Masuda S, Kitagawa M: Comparison of DNA flow cytometric analysis of body cavity fluids with conventional cytology. In Vivo 1994; 8:359–362.
130. Croonen AM, van der Valk P, Herman CJ, Lindeman J: Cytology, immunopathology and flow cytometry in the diagnosis of pleural and peritoneal effusions. Lab Invest 1988;58:725–732.
131. Joseph MG, Banerjee D, Harris P, et al: Multiparameter flow cytometric DNA analysis of effusions: A prospective study of 36 cases compared with routine cytology and immunohistochemistry. Mod Pathol 1995;8:686–693.
132. Marchevsky AM, Hauptman E, Gil J, Watson C: Computerized interactive morphometry as an aid in the diagnosis of pleural effusions. Acta Cytol 1987;31:131–136.
133. Banks ER, Jennings CD, Jacobs S, Davey DD: Comparative assessment of DNA analysis in effusions by image analysis and flow cytometry. Diagn Cytopathol 1994; 10:62–66.
134. el-Habashi AH, Freeman SM, el-Morsi B, et al: DNA ploidy and proliferating cell nuclear antigen image analysis of peritoneal and pleural effusions: A possible diagnostic role. Acta Cytol 1997;41:636–648.
135. Motherby H, Marcy T, Hecker M, et al: Static DNA cytometry as a diagnostic aid in effusion cytology: I. DNA aneuploidy for identification and differentiation of primary and secondary tumors of the serous membranes. Anal Quant Cytol Histol 1998;20:153–161.
136. Delahaye M, Hoogsteden HC, van der Kwast TH: Immunocytochemistry of malignant mesothelioma: OV632 as a marker of malignant mesothelioma. J Pathol 1991;165:137–143.
137. Frisman DM, McCarthy WF, Schleiff P, et al: Immunocytochemistry in the differential diagnosis of effusions: Use of logistic regression to select a panel of antibodies to distinguish adenocarcinomas from mesothelial proliferations. Mod Pathol 1993;6:179–184.
138. Lee JS, Nam JH, Lee MC, et al: Immunohistochemical panel for distinguishing between carcinoma and reactive mesothelial cells in serious effusions. Acta Cytol 1996; 40:631–636.
139. Johnston WW, Szpak CA, Thor A, et al: Applications of immunocytochemistry to clinical cytology [published erratum appears in Cancer Invest 1991;9:243–245]. Cancer Invest 1987;5:593–611.
140. Eyden BP, Banik S, Harris M: Malignant epithelial mesothelioma of the peritoneum: Observations on a problem case. Ultrastruct Pathol 1996;20:337–344.
140a. Kitazume H, Kitamura K, Mukai K, et al: Cytologic differential diagnosis among reactive mesothelial cells, malignant mesothelioma and adenocarcinoma: Utility of combined E-cadherin and calretinin immunostaining. Cancer Cytopathol 2000;90:55–60.
141. Beaty MW, Fetsch P, Wilder AM, et al: Effusion cytology of malignant melanoma: A morphologic and immunocytochemical analysis including application of the MART-1 antibody. Cancer 1997;81:57–63.
142. Ascoli V, Scalzo CC, Nardi F: C-*erbB*-2 oncoprotein immunostaining in serous effusions. Cytopathology 1993;4:207–218.
143. Chen LM, Lazcano O, Katzmann JA, et al: The role of conventional cytology, immunocytochemistry, and flow cytometric DNA ploidy in the evaluation of body cavity fluids: A prospective study of 52 patients. Am J Clin Pathol 1998;109:712–721.
144. Lee JS, Lee MC, Park CS, Juhng SW: Diagnostic value of p53 protein and flow cytometric DNA analysis in the study of serous effusions. Acta Cytol 1997;41:1719–1725.
145. Mullick SS, Green LK, Ramzy I, et al: p53 gene product in pleural effusions: Practical use in distinguishing benign from malignant cells. Acta Cytol 1996;40: 855–860.
146. el-Habashi AH, Freeman SM, el-Morsi B, et al: p53 and PCNA coexpression of 81 pleural and peritoneal effusion specimens: An immunohistochemical study. Pathol Res Pract 1996;192:834–839.
147. Yamashita K, Kuba T, Shinoda H, et al: Detection of K-*ras* point mutations in the supernatants of peritoneal and pleural effusions for diagnosis complementary to cytologic examination. Am J Clin Pathol 1998;109:704–711.
148. Stephen MR, Oien K, Ferrier RK, Burnett RA: Effusion cytology of hepatocellular carcinoma with in situ hybridisation for human albumin. J Clin Pathol 1997;50: 442–444.
149. Hiyama K, Hiyama E, Ishioka S, et al: Telomerase activity in small-cell and non–small-cell lung cancers. J Natl Cancer Inst 1995;87:895–902.
150. Yang CT, Lee MH, Lan RS, Chen JK: Telomerase activity in pleural effusions: Diagnostic significance. J Clin Oncol 1998;16:567–573.

151. Alkan S, Lehman C, Sarago C, et al: Polymerase chain reaction detection of immunoglobulin gene rearrangement and bcl-2 translocation in archival glass slides of cytologic material. Diagn Mol Pathol 1995;4:25–31.
151a. Gessain A, Briere J, Angelin-Duclos C, et al: Human herpesvirus γ (Kaposi's sarcoma herpes virus) and malignant lymphoproliferations in France: A molecular study of 250 cases including two AIDS-associated body cavity based lymphoma. Leukemia 1997;11:226–272.
152. Roka S, Fiegl M, Zojer N, et al: Aneuploidy of chromosome 8 as detected by interphase fluorescence in situ hybridization is a recurrent finding in primary and metastatic breast cancer. Breast Cancer Res Treat 1998;48:125–133.
153. Zojer N, Fiegl M, Angerler J, et al: Interphase fluorescence in situ hybridization improves the detection of malignant cells in effusions from breast cancer patients. Br J Cancer 1997;75:403–407.
154. Zojer N, Fiegl M, Mullauer L, et al: Chromosomal imbalances in primary and metastatic pancreatic carcinoma as detected by interphase cytogenetics: Basic findings and clinical aspects. Br J Cancer 1998;77: 1337–1342.
155. Larramendy ML, Bjorkqvist AM, Tammilehto L, et al: Absence of trisomy 7 in nonneoplastic human ascitic and pleural fluid cells: An interphase cytogenetic study. Cancer Genet Cytogenet 1994;78:78–81.
156. Johnson TM, Kuffel DG, Dewald GW: Detection of hyperdiploid malignant cells in pleural effusions with chromosome-specific probes and fluorescence in situ hybridization. Mayo Clin Proc 1996;71:643–648.
157. Hermansen DK, Reuter VE, Whitmore WFJ, et al: Flow cytometry and cytology as response indicators to M-VAC (methotrexate, vinblastine, doxorubicin and cisplatin). J Urol 1988;140:1394–1396.
158. Pritchett TR, Kanzler AW, Nichols PW, et al: A simple and practical technic for detecting cancer cells in urine and urinary bladder washings by flow cytometry. Am J Clin Pathol 1985;84:191–196.
159. Dean PJ, Murphy WM: Importance of urinary cytology and future role of flow cytometry. Urology 1985;26(4 Suppl):11–15.
160. Devonec M, Darzynkiewicz Z, Kostyrka-Claps ML, et al: Flow cytometry of low stage bladder tumors: Correlation with cytologic and cystoscopic diagnosis. Cancer 1982;49:109–118.
161. Huffman JL, Fradet Y, Cordon-Cardo C, et al: Effect of intravesical bacillus Calmette-Guérin on detection of a urothelial differentiation antigen in exfoliated cells of carcinoma in situ of the human urinary bladder. Cancer Res 1985;45:5201–5204.
162. Klein FA, Whitmore WFJ, Herr HW, Melamed MR: Flow cytometry followup of patients with low stage bladder tumors. J Urol 1982;128:88–92.
163. Melamed MR: Flow cytometry of the urinary bladder. Urol Clin North Am 1984;11:599–608.
164. Murphy WM: Urinary cytology in diagnostic pathology. Diagn Cytopathol 1985;1:173–175.
165. Murphy WM, Emerson LD, Chandler RW, et al: Flow cytometry versus urinary cytology in the evaluation of patients with bladder cancer. J Urol 1986;136:815–819.
166. Badalament RA, Kimmel M, Gay H, et al: The sensitivity of flow cytometry compared with conventional cytology in the detection of superficial bladder carcinoma. Cancer 1987;59:2078–2085.
167. Jitsukawa S, Tachibana M, Nakazono M, et al: Flow cytometry based on heterogeneity index score compared with urine cytology to evaluate their diagnostic efficacy in bladder tumor. Urology 1987;29:218–222.
168. Klein FA, White FK: Flow cytometry deoxyribonucleic acid determinations and cytology of bladder washings: Practical experience. J Urol 1988;139:275–278.
169. Adolphs HD, Schwabe HW, Helpap B, Volz C: Cytomorphological and histological studies on the urothelium during and after chemoimmune prophylaxis. Urol Res 1984;12:129–133.
170. Schwabe HW, Adolphs HD, Hartlapp J: Flow-cytophotometric studies on urine sediments of patients treated with anti-cancer drugs. Urol Res 1983;11:159–162.
171. Gregoire M, Fradet Y, Meyer F, et al: Diagnostic accuracy of urinary cytology, and deoxyribonucleic acid flow cytometry and cytology on bladder washings during followup for bladder tumors. J Urol 1997;157:1660–1664.
172. Badalament RA, Gay H, Whitmore WFJ, et al: Monitoring intravesical bacillus Calmette-Guérin treatment of superficial bladder carcinoma by serial flow cytometry. Cancer 1986;58:2751–2757.
173. Badalament RA, Fair WR, Whitmore WFJ, Melamed MR: The relative value of cytometry and cytology in the management of bladder cancer: The Memorial Sloan-Kettering Cancer Center experience. Semin Urol 1988;6:22–30.
174. Tetu B, Katz RL, Kalter SP, et al: Acridine-orange flow cytometry of urinary bladder washings for the detection of transitional cell carcinoma of the bladder: The influence of prior local therapy. Cancer 1987;60:1815–1822.
175. Bretton PR, Herr HW, Kimmel M, et al: Flow cytometry as a predictor of response and progression in patients with superficial bladder cancer treated with bacillus Calmette-Guérin. J Urol 1989;141:1332–1336.
176. Liedl T: Flow cytometric DNA/cytokeratin analysis of bladder lavage: Methodical aspects and clinical implications. Urol Int 1995;54:22–47.
177. Pinnock CB, Roxby DJ, Ross JM, et al: Ploidy and Tn-antigen expression in the detection of transitional cell neoplasia in non–tumour-bearing patients. Br J Urol 1995;75:461–469.
178. Hemstreet GP, West SS, Cook MS: Improved nuclear fluorescence screening technique. J Occup Med 1986; 28:1004–1010.
179. Koss LG, Eppich EM, Melder KH, Wersto R: DNA cytophotometry of voided urine sediment: Comparison with results of cytologic diagnosis and image analysis. Anal Quant Cytol Histol 1987;9:398–404.
180. Koss LG, Wersto RP, Simmons DA, et al: Predictive value of DNA measurements in bladder washings: Comparison of flow cytometry, image cytophotometry, and cytology in patients with a past history of urothelial tumors. Cancer 1989;64:916–924.
181. Slaton JW, Dinney CP, Veltri RW, et al: Deoxyribonucleic acid ploidy enhances the cytological prediction of recurrent transitional cell carcinoma of the bladder. J Urol 1997;158:806–811.

182. Van der Poel HG, Boon ME, van Stratum P, et al: Conventional bladder wash cytology performed by four experts versus quantitative image analysis. Mod Pathol 1997;10:976–982.
183. de la Roza GL, Hopkovitz A, Caraway NP, et al: DNA image analysis of urinary cytology: Prediction of recurrent transitional cell carcinoma. Mod Pathol 1996;9: 571–578.
184. Mora LB, Nicosia SV, Pow-Sang JM, et al: Ancillary techniques in the followup of transitional cell carcinoma: A comparison of cytology, histology and deoxyribonucleic acid image analysis cytometry in 91 patients. J Urol 1996;156:49–54.
185. Richman AM, Mayne ST, Jekel JF, Albertsen P: Image analysis combined with visual cytology in the early detection of recurrent bladder carcinoma. Cancer 1998;82: 1738–1748.
186. Pantazopoulos D, Karakitsos P, Pouliakis A, et al: Static cytometry and neural networks in the discrimination of lower urinary system lesions. Urology 1998;51:946–950.
187. Pantazopoulos D, Karakitsos P, Iokim-Liossi A, et al: Back propagation neural network in the discrimination of benign from malignant lower urinary tract lesions. J Urol 1998;159:1619–1623.
188. Pantazopoulos D, Karakitsos P, Iokim-Liossi A, et al: Comparing neural networks in the discrimination of benign from malignant lower urinary tract lesions. Br J Urol 1998;81:574–579.
189. Righi E, Rossi G, Ferrari G, et al: Does p53 immunostaining improve diagnostic accuracy in urine cytology? Diagn Cytopathol 1997;17:436–439.
190. Sagerman PM, Saigo PE, Sheinfeld J, et al: Enhanced detection of bladder cancer in urine cytology with Lewis X, M344 and 19A211 antigens. Acta Cytol 1994; 38:517–523.
191. Sidransky D, Von Eschenbach A, Tsai YC, et al: Identification of p53 gene mutations in bladder cancers and urine samples. Science 1991;252:706–709.
192. Ito H, Kyo S, Kanaya T, et al: Detection of human telomerase reverse transcriptase messenger RNA in voided urine samples as a useful diagnostic tool for bladder cancer. Clin Cancer Res 1998; 4:2807–2810.
193. Kinoshita H, Ogawa O, Kakehi Y, et al: Detection of telomerase activity in exfoliated cells in urine from patients with bladder cancer. J Natl Cancer Inst 1997; 89:724–730.
194. Lee DH, Yang SC, Hong SJ, et al: Telomerase: A potential marker of bladder transitional cell carcinoma in bladder washes. Clin Cancer Res 1998;4:535–538.
195. Mayfield MP, Shah T, Flannigan GM, et al: Telomerase activity in malignant and benign bladder conditions. Int J Mol Med 1998;1:835–840.
196. Muller M, Krause H, Heicappell R, et al: Comparison of human telomerase RNA and telomerase activity in urine for diagnosis of bladder cancer. Clin Cancer Res 1998; 4:1949–1954.
196a. Halling KC, King W, Sokolova IA, et al: A comparison of cytology and fluorescence in situ hybridization for the detection of urothelial carcinoma. J Urology 2000;164:1768–1775.
196b. Bubedorf L, Grilli B, Sauter G, et al: Multiprobe FISH for enhanced detection of bladder cancer in voided urine specimens and bladder washings. Am J Clin Pathol 2001;116:79–86.
197. Yokota K, Kanda K, Inoue Y, et al: Semi-quantitative analysis of telomerase activity in exfoliated human urothelial cells and bladder transitional cell carcinoma. Br J Urol 1998;82:727–732.
198. Landman J, Chang Y, Kavaler E, et al: Sensitivity and specificity of NMP-22, telomerase, and BTA in the detection of human bladder cancer. Urology 1998;52: 398–402.
199. Joensuu H, Klemi PJ, Eerola E: Diagnostic value of flow cytometric DNA determination combined with fine needle aspiration biopsy in thyroid tumors. Anal Quant Cytol Histol 1987;9:328–334.
200. Matsubayashi S, Tamai H, Morita T, et al: Hashimoto's thyroiditis manifesting monoclonal lymphocytic infiltration. Clin Exp Immunol 1990;79:170–174.
201. Karakitsos P, Cochand-Priollet B, Guillausseau PJ, Pouliakis A: Potential of the back propagation neural network in the morphologic examination of thyroid lesions. Anal Quant Cytol Histol 1996;18:494–500.
202. Slowinska-Klencka D, Klencki M, Sporny S, Lewinski A: Karyometric analysis in the cytologic diagnosis of thyroid lesions. Anal Quant Cytol Histol 1997;19:507–513.
202a. Nasser SM, Pitman MB, Pilch BZ, Faquin WC: Fine-needle aspiration biopsy of papillary thyroid carcinoma: Diagnostic utility of cytokeratin 19 immunostaining. Cancer Cytopathol 2000;90:307–311.
203. Yossie AdC, Longatto FA, Alves VA, et al: Lactoferrin in thyroid lesions: Immunoreactivity in fine needle aspiration biopsy samples. Acta Cytol 1996;40:408–413.
204. Orlandi F, Saggiorato E, Pivano G, et al: Galectin-3 is a presurgical marker of human thyroid carcinoma. Cancer Res 1998;58:3015–3020.
205. Faroux MJ, Theobald S, Pluot M, et al: Evaluation of the monoclonal antibody antithyroperoxidase MoAb47 in the diagnostic decision of cold thyroid nodules by fine-needle aspiration. Pathol Res Pract 1997;193:705–712.
206. Ross JS, del Rosario AD, Sanderson B, Bui HX: Selective expression of CD44 cell-adhesion molecule in thyroid papillary carcinoma fine-needle aspirates. Diagn Cytopathol 1996;14:287–291.
207. Hsi ED, Singleton TP, Svoboda SM, et al: Characterization of the lymphoid infiltrate in Hashimoto thyroiditis by immunohistochemistry and polymerase chain reaction for immunoglobulin heavy chain gene rearrangement. Am J Clin Pathol 1998;110:327–333.
208. Lovchik J, Lane MA, Clark DP: Polymerase chain reaction–based detection of B-cell clonality in the fine needle aspiration biopsy of a thyroid mucosa-associated lymphoid tissue (MALT) lymphoma. Hum Pathol 1997;28:989–992.
209. Stewart CJ, Farquharson MA, Kerr T, McCorriston J: Immunoglobulin light chain mRNA detected by in situ hybridisation in diagnostic fine needle aspiration cytology specimens. J Clin Pathol 1996;49:749–754.
210. Russo D, Arturi F, Chiefari E, et al: A case of metastatic medullary thyroid carcinoma: Early identification before surgery of an *RET* proto-oncogene somatic mutation in fine-needle aspirate specimens. J Clin Endocrinol Metab 1997;82:3378–3382.

211. Sciacchitano S, Paliotta DS, Nardi F, et al: PCR amplification and analysis of *ras* oncogenes from thyroid cytologic smears. Diagn Mol Pathol 1994;3:114–121.
212. Takano T, Miyauchi A, Yokozawa T, et al: Accurate and objective preoperative diagnosis of thyroid papillary carcinomas by reverse transcription-PCR detection of oncofetal fibronectin messenger RNA in fine-needle aspiration biopsies. Cancer Res 1998;58:4913–4917.
213. Weiss M, Baruch A, Keydar I, Wreschner DH: Preoperative diagnosis of thyroid papillary carcinoma by reverse transcriptase polymerase chain reaction of the *MUC1* gene. Int J Cancer 1996;66:55–59.
214. Strong EW, Kasdorf H, Henk JM: Squamous cell carcinoma of the head and neck. *In* Hermanek MK, Gospodarowicz MK, Henson DE, et al (eds): Prognostic Factors in Cancer. Heidelberg, Springer-Verlag, 1996, pp 12–22.
215. Pekkola-Heino K, Joensuu H, Klemi P, Grenman R: Relation of DNA ploidy and proliferation rate to radiation sensitivity in squamous carcinoma cell lines. Arch Otolaryngol Head Neck Surg 1994;120:750–754.
216. Collins BT, Cramer HM, Frain BE, Davis MM: Fine-needle aspiration biopsy of metastatic Ewing's sarcoma with MIC2 (CD99) immunocytochemistry. Diagn Cytopathol 1998;19:382–384.
217. Pacchioni D, Negro F, Valente G, Bussolati G: Epstein-Barr virus detection by in situ hybridization in fine-needle aspiration biopsies. Diagn Mol Pathol 1994;3: 100–104.
218. Feinmesser R, Miyazaki I, Cheung R, et al: Diagnosis of nasopharyngeal carcinoma by DNA amplification of tissue obtained by fine-needle aspiration. N Engl J Med 1992;326:17–21.
219. Schlott T, Nagel H, Ruschenburg I, et al: Reverse transcriptase polymerase chain reaction for detecting Ewing's sarcoma in archival fine needle aspiration biopsies. Acta Cytol 1997;41:795–801.
220. Kelly KM, Womer RB, Sorensen PH, et al: Common and variant gene fusions predict distinct clinical phenotypes in rhabdomyosarcoma. J Clin Oncol 1997;15: 1831–1836.
221. Anderson J, Renshaw J, McManus A, et al: Amplification of the t(2;13) and t(1;13) translocations of alveolar rhabdomyosarcoma in small formalin-fixed biopsies using a modified reverse transcriptase polymerase chain reaction. Am J Pathol 1997;150:477–482.
222. de Alava E, Lozano MD, Sola I, et al: Molecular features in a biphenotypic small cell sarcoma with neuroectodermal and muscle differentiation. Hum Pathol 1998;29: 181–184.
223. Frascella E, Rosolen A: Detection of the MyoD1 transcript in rhabdomyosarcoma cell lines and tumor samples by reverse transcription polymerase chain reaction. Am J Pathol 1998;152:577–583.
224. Phillips DE, Jones AS: Reliability of clinical examination in the diagnosis of parotid tumours. J R Coll Surg Edinb 1994;39:100–102.
225. Takashima S, Takayama F, Wang Q, et al: Parotid gland lesions: Diagnosis of malignancy with MRI and flow cytometric DNA analysis and cytology in fine-needle aspiration biopsy. Head Neck 1999;21:43–51.
226. Domagala W, Halczy-Kowalik L, Weber K, Osborn M: Coexpression of glial fibrillary acid protein, keratin and vimentin: A unique feature useful in the diagnosis of pleomorphic adenoma of the salivary gland in fine needle aspiration biopsy smears. Acta Cytol 1988;32: 403–408.
227. Gupta RK, Naran S, Dowle C, Simpson JS: Coexpression of vimentin, cytokeratin and S-100 in monomorphic adenoma of salivary gland; value of marker studies in the differential diagnosis of salivary gland tumours. Cytopathology 1992;3:303–309.
228. Ostrzega N, Cheng L, Layfield L: Glial fibrillary acid protein immunoreactivity in fine-needle aspiration of salivary gland lesions: A useful adjunct for the differential diagnosis of salivary gland neoplasms. Diagn Cytopathol 1989;5:145–149.
229. Holmes GF, Eisele DW, Rosenthal D, Westra WH: PSA immunoreactivity in a parotid oncocytoma: A diagnostic pitfall in discriminating primary parotid neoplasms from metastatic prostate cancer. Diagn Cytopathol 1998;19: 221–225.
230. Stewart CJ, Jackson R, Farquharson M, Richmond J: Fine-needle aspiration cytology of extranodal lymphoma. Diagn Cytopathol 1998;19:260–266.
231. Ruschenburg I, Korabiowska M, Schlott T, et al: The value of PCR technique in fine needle aspiration biopsy of salivary gland for diagnosis of low-grade B-cell lymphoma. Int J Mol Med 1998;2:339–341.
232. Cox HJ, Brightwell AP, Riordan T: Non-tuberculous mycobacterial infections presenting as salivary gland masses in children: Investigation and conservative management. J Laryngol Otol 1995;109:525–530.
233. Sperling NM, Lin PT, Lucente FE: Cystic parotid masses in HIV infection. Head Neck 1990;12:337–341.
234. Collins BT, Elmberger PG, Tani EM, et al: Fine-needle aspiration of Merkel cell carcinoma of the skin with cytomorphology and immunocytochemical correlation. Diagn Cytopathol 1998;18:251–257.
235. Pettinato G, De Chiara A, Insabato L, et al: Neuroendocrine (Merkel cell) tumor of the skin: Fine-needle aspiration cytology, histology, electron microscopy and immunohistochemistry of 12 cases. Appl Pathol 1988; 6:17–27.
236. Pisharodi LR, Lavoie R, Bedrossian CW: Differential diagnostic dilemmas in malignant fine-needle aspirates of liver: A practical approach to final diagnosis. Diagn Cytopathol 1995;12:364–370.
237. Fuhr JE, Kattine AA, Nelson HSJ: Flow cytometry of liver fine needle aspirates. J Surg Oncol 1994;56:153–158.
238. Cottier M, Jouffre C, Maubon I, et al: Prospective flow cytometric DNA analysis of hepatocellular carcinoma specimens collected by ultrasound-guided fine needle aspiration. Cancer 1994;74:599–605.
239. Zeppa P, Benincasa G, Troncone G, et al: Retrospective evaluation of DNA ploidy of hepatocarcinoma on cytologic samples. Diagn Cytopathol 1998;19:323–329.
240. Sampatanukul P, Mikuz G, Israsena S, et al: Cytomorphologic and DNA cytometric features of hepatocellular carcinoma in fine needle aspirates. Acta Cytol 1997;41: 435–442.

241. Gottschalk-Sabag S, Ron N, Glick T: Use of CD34 and factor VIII to diagnose hepatocellular carcinoma on fine needle aspirates. Acta Cytol 1998;42:691–696.
242. Johnson DE, Powers CN, Rupp G, Frable WJ: Immunocytochemical staining of fine-needle aspiration biopsies of the liver as a diagnostic tool for hepatocellular carcinoma. Mod Pathol 1992;5:117–123.
243. Rebello PM, Koelma IA, Kumar D: Fine needle aspiration of focal liver lesions. Cytopathology 1994;5:359–368.
244. Rishi M, Kovatich A, Ehya H: Utility of polyclonal and monoclonal antibodies against carcinoembryonic antigen in hepatic fine-needle aspirates. Diagn Cytopathol 1994;11:358–361.
245. Ojanguren I, Ariza A, Castella EM, et al: p53 immunoreactivity in hepatocellular adenoma, focal nodular hyperplasia, cirrhosis and hepatocellular carcinoma. Histopathology 1995;26:63–68.
246. Ojanguren I, Ariza A, Llatjos M, et al: Proliferating cell nuclear antigen expression in normal, regenerative, and neoplastic liver: A fine-needle aspiration cytology and biopsy study. Hum Pathol 1993;24:905–908.
247. Papotti M, Pacchioni D, Negro F, et al: Albumin gene expression in liver tumors: Diagnostic interest in fine needle aspiration biopsies. Mod Pathol 1994;7:271–275.
248. Salomao DR, Lloyd RV, Goellner JR: Hepatocellular carcinoma: Needle biopsy findings in 74 cases. Diagn Cytopathol 1997;16:8–13.
249. Ness MJ, Pour PM, Tempero MA, Linder J: Immunohistochemistry with monoclonal antibody B72.3 as an adjunct in the cytologic diagnosis of pancreatic carcinoma. Mod Pathol 1988;1:279–283.
250. Iwao T, Tsuchida A, Hanada K, et al: Immunocytochemical detection of p53 protein as an adjunct in cytologic diagnosis from pancreatic duct brushings in mucin-producing tumors of the pancreas. Cancer 1997;81:163–171.
251. al-Kaisi N, Weaver MG, Abdul-Karim FW, Siegler E: Fine needle aspiration cytology of neuroendocrine tumors of the pancreas: A cytologic, immunocytochemical and electron microscopic study. Acta Cytol 1992;36: 655–660.
252. Evans DB, Frazier ML, Charnsangavej C, et al: Molecular diagnosis of exocrine pancreatic cancer using a percutaneous technique. Ann Surg Oncol 1996;3:241–246.
253. Wadih GE, Nance KV, Silverman JF: Fine-needle aspiration cytology of the adrenal gland: Fifty biopsies in 48 patients. Arch Pathol Lab Med 1992;116:841–846.
254. Frostad B, Tani E, Kogner P, et al: The clinical use of fine needle aspiration cytology for diagnosis and management of children with neuroblastic tumours. Eur J Cancer 1998;34:529–536.
255. Silverman JF, Dabbs DJ, Ganick DJ, et al: Fine needle aspiration cytology of neuroblastoma, including peripheral neuroectodermal tumor, with immunocytochemical and ultrastructural confirmation. Acta Cytol 1988;32: 367–376.
256. Cajulis RS, Katz RL, Dekmezian R, et al: Fine needle aspiration biopsy of renal cell carcinoma: Cytologic parameters and their concordance with histology and flow cytometric data. Acta Cytol 1993;37:367–372.
257. Ljungberg B, Stenling R, Roos G: Flow cytometric DNA analysis of renal-cell carcinoma: A study of fine needle aspiration biopsies in comparison with multiple surgical samples. Anal Quant Cytol Histol 1987;9:505–508.
258. Collins BT, Ramos RR, Grosso LE: Combined fine needle aspiration biopsy and immunophenotypic and genotypic approach to posttransplantation lymphoproliferative disorders. Acta Cytol 1998;42:869–874.
259. Oliveira JG, Ramos JP, Xavier P, et al: Analysis of fine-needle aspiration biopsies by flow cytometry in kidney transplant patients. Transplantation 1997;64:97–102.
260. Wadih GE, Raab SS, Silverman JF: Fine needle aspiration cytology of renal and retroperitoneal angiomyolipoma: Report of two cases with cytologic findings and clinicopathologic pitfalls in diagnosis. Acta Cytol 1995; 39:945–950.
261. Chow LT, Chan SK, Chow WH: Fine needle aspiration cytodiagnosis of leiomyosarcoma of the renal pelvis: A case report with immunohistochemical study. Acta Cytol 1994;38:759–763.
262. Scharfe T, Yokoyama M, Alken P, et al: Immunoperoxidase staining of fine-needle aspiration biopsies of renal cell carcinoma using tumor-specific monoclonal antibody. Eur Urol 1987;13:331–333.
263. Murer L, Zacchello G, Basso G, et al: Early and rapid diagnosis of CMV infection by nonradioactive in situ hybridization in pediatric kidney transplant recipients. Nephron 1992;60:25–29.
264. Levendoglu-Tugal O, Weiss R, Ozkaynak MF, et al: T-cell acute lymphoblastic leukemia after renal transplantation in childhood. J Pediatr Hematol Oncol 1998;20: 548–551.
265. Paz-Bouza JI, Orfao A, Abad M, et al: Transrectal fine needle aspiration biopsy of the prostate combining cytomorphologic, DNA ploidy status and cell cycle distribution studies. Pathol Res Pract 1994;190:682–689.
266. Tribukait B, Esposti PL, Ronstrom L: Tumour ploidy for characterization of prostatic carcinoma: Flow-cytofluorometric DNA studies using aspiration biopsy material. Scand J Urol Nephrol Suppl 1980;55:59–64.
267. Adolfsson J, Ronstrom L, Hedlund PO, et al: The prognostic value of modal deoxyribonucleic acid in low grade, low stage untreated prostate cancer. J Urol 1990;144:1404–1406.
268. Azua J, Romeo P, Valle J, Azua JJ: DNA quantification as a prognostic factor in prostatic adenocarcinoma. Anal Quant Cytol Histol 1996;18:330–336.
269. Moroz K, Crespo P, de las M: Fine needle aspiration of prostatic rhabdomyosarcoma: A case report demonstrating the value of DNA ploidy. Acta Cytol 1995;39: 785–790.
270. Xiao S, Renshaw A, Cibas ES, et al: Novel fluorescence in situ hybridization approaches in solid tumors: Characterization of frozen specimens, touch preparations, and cytological preparations. Am J Pathol 1995; 147:896–904.
271. Qian J, Jenkins RB, Bostwick DG: Determination of gene and chromosome dosage in prostatic intraepithelial neoplasia and carcinoma. Anal Quant Cytol Histol 1998; 20:373–380.
272. Wang RY, Troncoso P, Palmer JL, et al: Trisomy 7 by dual-color fluorescence in situ hybridization: A potential biological marker for prostate cancer progression. Clin Cancer Res 1996;2:1553–1558.

273. Lykkesfeldt AE, Balslev I, Christensen IJ, et al: DNA ploidy and S-phase fraction in primary breast carcinomas in relation to prognostic factors and survival for premenopausal patients at high risk for recurrent disease. Acta Oncol 1988;27:749–756.
274. Cornelisse CJ, van Driel-Kulker AM: DNA image cytometry on machine-selected breast cancer cells and a comparison between flow cytometry and scanning cytophotometry. Cytometry 1985;6:471–477.
275. Levack PA, Mullen P, Anderson TJ, et al: DNA analysis of breast tumour fine needle aspirates using flow cytometry. Br J Cancer 1987;56:643–646.
276. Martelli G, Daidone MG, Mastore M, et al: Combined analysis of ploidy and cell kinetics on fine-needle aspirates from breast tumors. Cancer 1993;71:2522–2527.
277. Palmer JO, McDivitt RW, Stone KR, et al: Flow cytometric analysis of breast needle aspirates. Cancer 1988; 62:2387–2391.
278. Remvikos Y, Magdelenat H, Zajdela A: DNA flow cytometry applied to fine needle sampling of human breast cancer. Cancer 1988;61:1629–1634.
279. Corkill ME, Sneige N, Fanning T, el-Naggar A: Fine-needle aspiration cytology and flow cytometry of intracystic papillary carcinoma of breast. Am J Clin Pathol 1990;94:673–680.
280. Bozzetti C, Nizzoli R, Camisa R, et al: Comparison between Ki-67 index and S-phase fraction on fine-needle aspiration samples from breast carcinoma. Cancer 1997;81:287–292.
281. Ellis PA, Makris A, Burton SA, et al: Comparison of MIB-1 proliferation index with S-phase fraction in human breast carcinomas. Br J Cancer 1996;73:640–643.
282. Briffod M, Spyratos F, Hacene K, et al: Evaluation of breast carcinoma chemosensitivity by flow cytometric DNA analysis and computer-assisted image analysis. Cytometry 1992;13:250–258.
283. Makris A, Powles TJ, Dowsett M, et al: Prediction of response to neoadjuvant chemoendocrine therapy in primary breast carcinomas. Clin Cancer Res 1997;3: 593–600.
284. Chevillard S, Lebeau J, Pouillart P, et al: Biological and clinical significance of concurrent *p53* gene alterations, *MDR1* gene expression, and S-phase fraction analyses in breast cancer patients treated with primary chemotherapy or radiotherapy. Clin Cancer Res 1997;3: 2471–2478.
285. Auger M, Katz RL, Johnston DA, et al: Quantitation of immunocytochemical estrogen and progesterone receptor content in fine needle aspirates of breast carcinoma using the SAMBA 4000 image analysis system. Anal Quant Cytol Histol 1993;15:274–280.
286. Charpin C, Andrac L, Habib MC, et al: Immunodetection in fine-needle aspirates and multiparametric (SAMBA) image analysis: Receptors (monoclonal antiestrogen and antiprogesterone) and growth fraction (monoclonal Ki67) evaluation in breast carcinomas. Cancer 1989;63:863–872.
287. Davey DD, Banks ER, Jennings D, Powell DE: Comparison of nuclear grade and DNA cytometry in breast carcinoma aspirates to histologic grade in excised cancers. Am J Clin Pathol 1993;99:708–713.
288. Spyratos F, Briffod M: DNA ploidy and S-phase fraction by image and flow cytometry in breast cancer fine-needle cytopunctures. Mod Pathol 1997;10:556–563.
289. Wolberg WH, Street WN, Mangasarian OL: Image analysis and machine learning applied to breast cancer diagnosis and prognosis. Anal Quant Cytol Histol 1995;17:77–87.
290. Wolberg WH, Street WN, Mangasarian OL: Computer-derived nuclear features compared with axillary lymph node status for breast carcinoma prognosis. Cancer 1997;81:172–179.
291. Silverman JF, Feldman PS, Covell JL, Frable WJ: Fine needle aspiration cytology of neoplasms metastatic to the breast. Acta Cytol 1987;31:291–300.
292. Silverman JF, McLeod DL, Park HK: Fine-needle aspiration cytology of hematopoietic lesions from multiple sites. Diagn Cytopathol 1990;6:252–257.
293. Silverman JF, Geisinger KR, Park HK, et al: Fine-needle aspiration cytology of granulocytic sarcoma and myeloid metaplasia. Diagn Cytopathol 1990;6:106–111.
294. Silverman JF, Berns LA, Holbrook CT, et al: Fine needle aspiration cytology of primitive neuroectodermal tumors: A report of these cases. Acta Cytol 1992;36: 541–550.
295. Gorczyca W, Olszewski W, Tuziak T, et al: Fine needle aspiration cytology of rare malignant tumors of the breast. Acta Cytol 1992;36:918–926.
296. Masood S, Lu L, Assaf-Munasifi M, McCaulley K: Application of immunostaining for muscle specific actin in detection of myoepithelial cells in breast fine-needle aspirates. Diagn Cytopathol 1995;13:71–74.
297. Alexiev BA: Localization of p53 and proliferating cell nuclear antigen in fine-needle aspirates of benign and primary malignant tumors of the human breast: An immunocytochemical study using supersensitive monoclonal antibodies and the biotin-streptavidin-amplified method. Diagn Cytopathol 1996;15:277–281.
298. Lavarino C, Corletto V, Mezzelani A, et al: Detection of *TP53* mutation, loss of heterozygosity and DNA content in fine-needle aspirates of breast carcinoma. Br J Cancer 1998;77:125–130.
299. Makris A, Powles TJ, Allred DC, et al: Changes in hormone receptors and proliferation markers in tamoxifen treated breast cancer patients and the relationship with response. Breast Cancer Res Treat 1998;48:11–20.
300. Jorda M, Ganjei P, Nadji M: Retrospective c-*erbB*-2 immunostaining in aspiration cytology of breast cancer. Diagn Cytopathol 1994;11:262–265.
301. Sinha SK, Singh UR, Bhatia A: C-*erb* B2 oncoprotein expression: Correlation with the Ki-67 labeling index and AgNOR counts in breast carcinoma on fine needle aspiration cytology. Acta Cytol 1996;40:1217–1220.
302. Gui GP, Wells CA, Yeomans P, et al: Integrin expression in breast cancer cytology: A novel predictor of axillary metastasis. Eur J Surg Oncol 1996;22:254–258.
303. Cuthbert A, Herbert A, Coddington R, et al: Demonstration of oestrogen receptor in symptomatic breast carcinoma, using fine needle aspiration cytology. Cytopathology 1990;1:339–347.
304. Keshgegian AA, Inverso K, Kline TS: Determination of estrogen receptor by monoclonal antireceptor antibody in aspiration biopsy cytology from breast carcinoma. Am J Clin Pathol 1988;89:24–29.

304a. Tajford S, Bøhler PJ, Risberg B, Torlakovic E: Estrogen and progesterone hormone receptor status in breast carcinoma: Comparison of immunocytochemistry and immunohistochemistry. Diagn Cytopathol 2002;26:137–141.

305. Sauter G, Feichter G, Torhorst J, et al: Fluorescence in situ hybridization for detecting erbB-2 amplification in breast tumor fine needle aspiration biopsies. Acta Cytol 1996;40:164–173.

306. Li BD, Harlow SP, Budnick RM, et al: Detection of *HER-2/neu* oncogene amplification in flow cytometry-sorted breast ductal cells by competitive polymerase chain reaction. Cancer 1994;73:2771–2778.

307. Deng G, Yu M, Chen LC, et al: Amplifications of oncogene erbB-2 and chromosome 20q in breast cancer determined by differentially competitive polymerase chain reaction. Breast Cancer Res Treat 1996;40:271–281.

308. Medl M, Sevelda P, Czerwenka K, et al: DNA amplification of *HER-2/neu* and *INT-2* oncogenes in epithelial ovarian cancer. Gynecol Oncol 1995;59:321–326.

309. Soini Y, Mannermaa A, Winqvist R, et al: Application of fine-needle aspiration to the demonstration of ERBB2 and MYC expression by in situ hybridization in breast carcinoma. J Histochem Cytochem 1994;42:795–803.

310. Cajulis RS, Kotliar S, Haines GK, et al: Comparative study of interphase cytogenetics, flow cytometric analysis, and nuclear grade of fine-needle aspirates of breast carcinoma. Diagn Cytopathol 1994;11:151–158.

311. Ichikawa D, Hashimoto N, Hoshima M, et al: Analysis of numerical aberrations of specific chromosomes by fluorescent in situ hybridization as a diagnostic tool in breast cancer. Cancer 1996;77:2064–2069.

312. Patterson AH, McManus DT, Maxwell P: Detection of chromosomal numerical abnormalities in clinical breast tumour fine-needle aspirations by fluorescence in situ hybridisation (FISH): Refinement of a method. Br J Biomed Sci 1998;55:2–7.

313. Tsuda H, Takarabe T, Shimamura K, Hirohashi S: Detection of alterations in chromosomes 16 and 1 by fluorescence in situ hybridization in breast tumors cytologically or histologically equivocal for malignancy. Pathobiology 1998;66:268–273.

314. Schmitt FC, Soares R, Leitao D: Detection of numerical chromosome 17 abnormalities in fine-needle aspirates of breast cancer using a novel in situ hybridization signal amplification method. Diagn Cytopathol 1998; 19:141–146.

315. Truong K, Guilly MN, Gerbault-Seureau M, et al: Quantitative FISH by image cytometry for the detection of chromosome 1 imbalances in breast cancer: A novel approach analyzing chromosome rearrangements within interphase nuclei. Lab Invest 1998;78:1607–1613.

316. Beck J, Bohnet B, Brugger D, et al: Multiple gene expression analysis reveals distinct differences between G2 and G3 stage breast cancers, and correlations of PKC eta with MDR1, MRP and LRP gene expression. Br J Cancer 1998;77:87–91.

317. Wang CS, LaRue H, Fortin A, et al: mdr1 mRNA expression by RT-PCR in patients with primary breast cancer submitted to neoadjuvant therapy. Breast Cancer Res Treat 1997;45:63–74.

318. Sato T, Yuyama Y, Watabe K, et al: Detection of *p53* gene mutations in fine-needle aspiration biopsied breast cancer specimens: Correlations with nuclear p53 accumulations and tumor DNA aneuploidy patterns. Cancer Lett 1997;115:47–55.

319. Bunn PAJ, Carney DN, Gazdar AF, et al: Diagnostic and biological implications of flow cytometric DNA content analysis in lung cancer. Cancer Res 1983;43: 5026–5032.

320. ten Velde GP, Schutte B, Reijnders MM, et al: Cytokinetic analysis of lung cancer by bromodeoxyuridine labeling of cytology specimens. Cytometry 1989;10: 807–810.

321. Shibata D, Cosgrove M, Arnheim N, et al: Detection of human papillomavirus DNA in fine-needle aspirations of metastatic squamous-cell carcinoma of the uterine cervix using the polymerase chain reaction. Diagn Cytopathol 1989;5:40–43.

322. Bodensteiner D, Reidinger D, Rosenfeld C, et al: Flow cytometry of needle aspirates from bone and soft tissue tumors. South Med J 1991;84:1451–1454.

323. Wakely PEJ, Kornstein MJ: Aspiration cytopathology of lymphoblastic lymphoma and leukemia: The MCV experience. Pediatr Pathol Lab Med 1996;16:243–252.

324. Lundgren L, Kindblom LG, Willems J, et al: Proliferative myositis and fasciitis: A light and electron microscopic, cytologic, DNA-cytometric and immunohistochemical study. APMIS 1992;100:437–448.

325. Szadowska A, Lasota J, Mirecka B, Giryn I: Immunohistochemistry in the differential diagnosis of tumours of possible myogenic origin. Patol Pol 1991;42:10–16.

326. Steel BL, Schwartz MR, Ramzy I: Fine needle aspiration biopsy in the diagnosis of lymphadenopathy in 1,103 patients: Role, limitations and analysis of diagnostic pitfalls. Acta Cytol 1995;39:76–81.

327. Stewart CJ, Duncan JA, Farquharson M, Richmond J: Fine needle aspiration cytology diagnosis of malignant lymphoma and reactive lymphoid hyperplasia. J Clin Pathol 1998;51:197–203.

327a. Young NA, Al-Saleem T: Diagnosis of lymphoma by fine-needle aspiration cytology using the revised European-American classification of lymphoid neoplasms. Cancer Cytopathol 1999;87:325–345.

328. Pilotti S, Di Palma S, Alasio L, et al: Diagnostic assessment of enlarged superficial lymph nodes by fine needle aspiration. Acta Cytol 1993;37:853–866.

329. Johnson A, Akerman M, Cavallin-Stahl E: Flow cytometric detection of B-clonal excess in fine needle aspirates for enhanced diagnostic accuracy in non-Hodgkin's lymphoma in adults. Histopathology 1987; 11:581–590.

330. Joensuu H, Klemi PJ, Eerola E: Diagnostic value of DNA flow cytometry combined with fine needle aspiration biopsy in lymphomas. J Pathol 1988;154:237–245.

331. Hanson CA, Schnitzer B: Flow cytometric analysis of cytologic specimens in hematological disease. J Clin Lab Anal 1989;3:2–7.

332. Katz RL, Gritsman A, Cabanillas F, et al: Fine-needle aspiration cytology of peripheral T-cell lymphoma: A cytologic, immunologic, and cytometric study. Am J Clin Pathol 1989;91:120–131.

333. Wojcik EM, Katz RL, Johnston DA, et al: Comparative analysis of DNA ploidy and proliferative index in fine

needle aspirates of non-Hodgkin's lymphomas by image analysis and flow cytometry. Anal Quant Cytol Histol 1993;15:151–157.
334. Ruschenburg L, Misselwitz W, Korabiowska M, Droese M: Comparison of the DNA content in low and high grade non-Hodgkin lymphomas. Anticancer Res 1998; 18:1617–1620.
335. Ruschenburg I, Peters D, Korabiowska M, Droese M: Comparative cytophotometric analysis of reactive lymphoid hyperplasia and low malignant non-Hodgkin lymphoma. Anticancer Res 1998;18:1613–1616.
336. Gagneten D, Hijazi YM, Jaffe ES, Solomon D: Mantle cell lymphoma: A cytopathological and immunocytochemical study. Diagn Cytopathol 1996;14:32–37.
337. Tani E, Lowhagen T, Nasiell K, et al: Fine needle aspiration cytology and immunocytochemistry of large cell lymphomas expressing the Ki-1 antigen. Acta Cytol 1989;33:359–362.
338. Bakhos R, Andrey J, Bhoopalam N, et al: Fine-needle aspiration cytology of extraskeletal Ewing's sarcoma. Diagn Cytopathol 1998;18:137–140.
339. Kilpatrick SE, Ward WG, Chauvenet AR, Pettenati MJ: The role of fine-needle aspiration biopsy in the initial diagnosis of pediatric bone and soft tissue tumors: An institutional experience. Mod Pathol 1998;11:923–928.

APPENDIX

APPENDIX

This appendix consists of procedures that have been used in the molecular diagnostics laboratory at the Armed Forces Institute of Pathology and that have been referred to in procedures included in the body of this book. Many parts of this procedure manual (such as those pertaining to operation and maintenance of equipment) are not included, and others may have been updated. Although these procedures reflect clinical practice, most must be adapted to each individual laboratory situation before implementation, and "tweaking" of procedures is often required to make them work in a new laboratory environment.

The references to specific vendors and manufacturers should not be interpreted as an endorsement of these products. Other products may work as well or better; it is prudent to consider the appropriate sources of reagents and equipment on the basis of the individual circumstances of each laboratory.

SOP 1*

PROCEDURES TO PREVENT SPECIMEN LOSS, ALTERATION, OR CONTAMINATION

PRINCIPLE

SPECIMEN COLLECTION. Anatomic pathology samples, primarily formalin fixed and embedded in paraffin blocks, are obtained from patients in both civilian and military medical facilities.

SPECIMEN HANDLING. Each block is received in a labeled box or plastic bag to prevent sample mixup or contamination. Each sample (block or unstained slides) should be accompanied by

- Consultation request form
- Case folder
- Stained slides

Of these, only the block (or slides) and consultation request form are required.

*SOPs 1 through 13 written by Amy E. Kraftt, PhD, and SOPs 14 through 20 by Robert E. Cunningham, MS, both from the Department of Cellular Pathology and Genetics, Armed Forces Institute of Pathology, Rockville, Maryland.

ACCESSIONING. On receiving a specimen for consultation, determine the acceptability of the case according to criteria for rejection of unacceptable specimens. If the case is accepted, enter all pertinent clerical and medical information into the Consult Log Book. Assign each case a unique tracking number (an MDL number). Label the request form in the upper right-hand corner with the MDL number. Label the box or bag containing the paraffin blocks with the MDL number.

PREVENTION OF SPECIMEN LOSS AND ALTERATION. Store paraffin block or slide specimens in the cabinets in the tissue processing area. Storage of other types of specimens for research purposes only will be determined on a case-by-case basis after discussion with the MDL laboratory director.

RETURN OF SPECIMENS TO CONTRIBUTOR. Return all remaining specimens together with the typed case report. It is permissible to return case material to a contributor (generally a staff pathologist) before the assays have been completed if material for analysis has been obtained. However, if specimens are released from the laboratory before a report is issued, note that "specimen has been returned to contributor" on the request form and in the section of the Consult Log Book designated "Early Return of Cases."

PREVENTION OF SPECIMEN CONTAMINATION. Use disposable microtome blades for cutting paraffin blocks and **replace the blade each time a new block is cut.** Use plugged aerosol-resistant pipette tips (ART) for all liquid transfers used in the handling of specimens, including lysate preparation and setup of assays. Wear gloves when handling specimens at all times. Perform all pre-PCR procedures (cutting sections, preparation of lysate, and reaction setup) in the designated areas of the MDL. See SOP 2.

SPECIMEN IDENTIFICATION THROUGHOUT EACH STAGE OF THE ASSAY. Before a block is cut, check the case identifier on the block with the accompanying folder to verify its relation to the case in reference. Label two microcentrifuge tubes using an extra-fine-tip permanent marker with the MDL number **before** the block is cut. Label a round 1/2″ Avery Label 05053 with initials, date cut, and MDL number. Place label on cap of both tubes. Write MDL number on side of tube. Cut sections and place in tubes. Use one tube for lysate preparation. The date of lysate preparation is added to the side of each tube at that time. The DNA lysate or RNA extract is stored at −20°C in the DNA freezer or RNA freezer, respectively, in the PCR setup room while the sample is being analyzed. *DNA samples are moved to the −70°C freezer for long-term storage at quarterly intervals* (Jan 1, Apr 1, Jul 1, Oct 1). *RNA samples are moved to the −70°C free-*

zer for long-term storage after sample analysis. Save the second tube at room temperature in the consult boxes located in the cabinet in the PCR setup area. All specimens are saved for a minimum of 5 years.

ASSAY SETUP. Label assay tubes consecutively. Keep tubes in numerical order throughout all setup procedures. Identify the specimen associated with each assay tube on the data sheet with the MDL number or control. Verify that the MDL number on the tube and data sheet match for all assay setup procedures.

GELS AND AUTORADIOGRAMS. Identify the location of each specimen loaded on each lane of every gel on the appropriate data sheet in the assay notebook. Enter this information in the ENTER GEL RECORD form in the laboratory PC. Identify the location of gel lanes on Southern blots by horizontal dashes drawn in black ink. Identify lanes on autoradiograms by alignment with marked blots. Label each lane on the autoradiogram with specific identifiers, including the MDL number, dilution tested, and other identifiers as necessary (e.g., block number). Lanes containing molecular weight markers (lane 1) and control samples should be clearly labeled as such.

Complete autoradiograms are tagged by placing a label in the top right-hand corner. The tag indicates the technologist's initials, the date developed, and the gel number corresponding to record of data entered in the GEL RECORD form. The laboratory director's final review of the data is indicated by an initial on this tag.

REFERENCE

These procedures were developed within the MDL.

SOP 2

PROCEDURES FOR PHYSICAL CONTAINMENT TO MINIMIZE FALSE-POSITIVE RESULTS

PRINCIPLE

The polymerase chain reaction (PCR) procedure is a powerful tool for identifying DNA sequences that may be present in very small quantities. The method involves repeated synthesis of a particular region of DNA from sequence-specific primers by a heat-stable DNA polymerase. With the use of in vitro amplification, millions of copies of a specific DNA sequence can be generated. This makes it theoretically possible to analyze DNA sequences from a single cell or to detect specific sequences present in only one cell among thousands that do not harbor the sequence. This procedure is very sensitive, and great care must be taken to avoid contamination and false-positive results.

PROCEDURES TO MINIMIZE FALSE-POSITIVE RESULTS

General Considerations

Because PCR is so sensitive, molecular contamination of a sample reaction with as little as one molecule of target DNA or previously amplified DNA may lead to a spurious positive signal. To avoid this carryover problem, fastidious laboratory practice must be employed. This includes following rigorous procedures to keep the PCR laboratory equipment, supplies, and surroundings physically clean at all times.

The most common source of contamination of samples, a series of samples, or reagents is from previously amplified product, but it may result from introduction of nucleic acids from any source. A simple but effective procedure to minimize contamination is to ***discard all pipette tips and all microcentrifuge tubes into zip-locked bags.*** These sealed bags are then disposed of in laboratory waste containers. This eliminates leakage of products or spillage of tube contents that could subsequently aerosolize PCR products throughout the laboratory.

The laboratory is physically divided into pre-PCR, PCR setup, and post-PCR areas to separate the functions involved with sample preparation, reagent preparation, PCR assay setup, and analysis of PCR products. Steps are taken to avoid sample-to-sample spillover and contamination of the sample or reagent during or after amplification. The flow of amplified product is one way out of the PCR setup area to the post-PCR area for analysis. Any racks used to carry products must be thoroughly soaked in 10% bleach to inactivate DNA before reentering the pre-PCR and PCR setup area.

The **pre-PCR** area contains the microtome for cutting paraffin sections and the balance for weighing out chemicals used within the entire laboratory. The reagents stored in this room for sample preparation are Hemo-De and Ethanol. These solvents are used to thoroughly clean the microtome between samples. The supplies used in this area are gauze pads, cotton-tipped applicator sticks, disposable razor blades, and 1.5 mL microcentrifuge tubes for collecting the paraffin sections for PCR.

The **PCR setup** room is the space where PCR assays are set up and contains dedicated supplies, reagents, and equipment for *PCR SETUP ONLY.* GLOVES must be worn in this room at all times and **must be changed whenever entering the PCR setup room.** Fingertips of gloves are wiped on a bleach-soaked towel between patient samples during PCR setup procedures. The refrigerators and freezers in the PCR setup room are used for storage of PCR reagents and patient samples. A chemical hood is used for solvent extractions for RNA preparation and for adding radioactive dATP to phosphorus 32 (^{32}P) incorporation assays. The PCR thermal cyclers are also located in the PCR setup area. Most supplies entering this area are sterile and/or disposable.

Supplies that are stored in this area include:

Aerosol-resistant tips (ART) for pipettors: Only ART tips are used in the PCR laboratory to prevent contamination of pipettors. The pipettors in the PCR setup room are dedicated to use only in that area.

Tubes—microcentrifuge (0.5 mL and 1.5 mL): Handling is kept to a minimum. GLOVES must be worn at all times. Multicolor, nonsterile microcentrifuge tubes are purchased and dispensed into plastic-covered bins for daily use. Instead of putting hands into bins, pour tubes onto clean towels.

Tubes—sterile conical (15 mL and 50 mL)

Disposable sterile plugged pipettes (1 mL, 5 mL, 10 mL): Pipettes are manipulated with an electric Pipet-Aid (Drummond), which has a filtered nosepiece. Filters are replaced if fluid is aspirated into nosepiece. MOUTH PIPETTING IS PROHIBITED!!

REAGENTS

All reagents used in the pre-PCR or PCR setup area must be commercially obtained or prepared in the PCR setup room on a "clean day" using dedicated pipettors, ART tips, and disposable pipettes and tubes. A "clean day" is usually Monday, after the regular weekly cleaning with bleach and before work has begun on the case materials. All buffers and solutions used for PCR are aliquotted into tubes labeled with lot number and expiration date and are quality control tested before use.

ONLY ONE LOT OF A PARTICULAR REAGENT IS USED AT ANY TIME. ALL ALIQUOTS ARE DISPOSED OF AFTER USE. The following reagents are kept in the PCR setup area as a physical containment procedure to minimize contamination:

Hemo-De, ethanol, isopropanol, phenol:chloroform: isoamyl alcohol: These reagents are dispensed into sterile conical tubes for daily use only.
Sodium acetate, glycogen, proteinase K, DNA and RNA extraction buffers: Aliquots of these reagents are disposed of after a single use.
PCR reagents
dNTPs: Three dNTP formulas are used in the PCR laboratory (dNTP, Mix II, Mix III) and are described in the appropriate SOPs
Buffers (for reverse transcriptase and PCR)
$MgCl_2$
Oligonucleotide primers
Water—HPLC-grade water: Bottled HPLC-grade water used for PCR is purchased from Fisher. Upon opening, a bottle of water is aliquotted into 50-mL sterile conical centrifuge tubes and frozen at −20° C. When needed, a 50-mL aliquot is thawed and dispensed into 1.5-mL centrifuge tubes and stored at −20° C. Each aliquot is disposed of after single use.

The reagents for each assay are stored in kits. Assay kits contain pre-made and pre-tested master mixes. Master mix aliquots are discarded after use.

UNDER NO CIRCUMSTANCES SHOULD AMPLIFIED DNA BE BROUGHT INTO THE PCR SETUP ROOM—this includes storage of products, blots, or gels containing products, centrifugation of product, or incubation of product-enzyme mixtures in water baths.

The post-PCR area is used for analyzing PCR products by denaturing polyacrylamide and agarose gel electrophoresis.

THE REFRIGERATOR/FREEZER IS POSTED FOR RADIOACTIVE STORAGE. Unlabeled oligonucleotide probes are stored in the post-PCR freezer. Probes labeled with radioactive γATP in this area are stored in Lucite boxes in the freezer. Radioactively labeled PCR products are stored in Lucite boxes in the refrigerator. The post-PCR area contains the hybridization ovens for incubating ^{32}P-labeled probes with Southern blots. The refrigerators are used for storing PCR products and the reagents for product analysis.

LABORATORY DECONTAMINATION

Nondisposable Plasticware

Nondisposable plasticware, such as tube racks, must be soaked in 10% bleach before reuse in the laboratory.

Equipment

On Friday, bench tops, equipment, the fume hood, and floors should be cleaned with 10% bleach. The schedule for regularly cleaning specific areas is initialed on completion. The counter is wiped with 10% bleach and covered with fresh bench paper before every assay is set up in the PCR setup room. Bench paper is changed weekly in the post-PCR room.

REFERENCE

Kwok S: Procedures to minimize PCR-product carry-over. *In* Innis M, Gelfand D, Sninsky J, White T (eds): PCR Protocols. New York: Academic Press; 1990:142–145.

SOP 3

CUTTING BLOCKS

PRINCIPLE

Tissue sections for PCR are cut with a microtome fitted with a disposable blade. Before cutting a sample, the microtome is thoroughly cleansed with Hemo-De soaked gauze to remove any residual paraffin. The Hemo-De is removed by wiping thoroughly with ethanol. Usually, six 6-μm sections are cut for both DNA and RNA extracts. For small tissue samples, cut more sections.

REAGENTS

Hemo-De [Fisher]
Absolute ethanol

SUPPLIES AND EQUIPMENT

Disposable gloves
Gauze
Applicator sticks
Extra-fine-tip permanent markers
Microcentrifuge tubes
Disposable razor blades
Microtome

QUALITY CONTROL

1. Duplicate samples of each paraffin block are collected in two microcentrifuge tubes when sufficient sample is available. One is used for extraction. The other sample is stored at room temperature.
2. See SOP 1, Procedures to Prevent Specimen Loss, Alteration, or Contamination.
3. Visually inspect microtome and pre-PCR area for cleanliness.

PROCEDURE

1. Clean microtome with Hemo-De soaked gauze. Then wipe microtome with ethanol-soaked gauze. Let air dry before proceeding.
2. Set the section thickness selector at 6 μm.
3. Position the block in the microtome. Be certain that the block clears the blade holder.
4. Adjust the block to be parallel to the blade holder with the block holder screws.
5. Insert a disposable razor blade in the blade holder.

6. Rough cut the block by repeatedly advancing the block and taking a slice. Stop when the entire surface of the tissue is exposed ("facing the block").
7. After "facing the block," take six sections for each tube. Use more sections for small tissue samples.

How To Cut a Paraffin Block for Slides

a. Prepare heated water baths: 40°C for normal tissue, 37°C for brain tissue.
b. Dull blade finish by very lightly moving a xylene-soaked gauze pad across the blade edge.
c. Trim block on all sides to remove excess paraffin.
d. Notch all four corners of the paraffin block—this will aid in separating the sections.
e. Face off the block.
f. Use a wetted paintbrush to gently pull and lift the paraffin sections. DO NOT touch blade edge with the paintbrush.
g. Place the sections in a water bath at room temperature to determine if the entire face of the tissue is being sectioned. If so, proceed to step #7. If not, continue facing off the block.
h. Use newspaper to clear any residual paraffin from the surface of the water bath.
i. Chill the block on the microtome with a Kim-wipe soaked with cold water.
j. After soaking block, retract the stage slightly before cutting, owing to the expansion of the block.
k. Begin sectioning by using the paintbrush to lift the first tissue section. Hold the first paraffin section with your fingers. This section will be discarded.
l. To separate slices, use forceps and gently press at the edge of the section when it is in the room temperature water bath. If slices do not separate, use a glass slide on its edge and a pick to gently separate sections.
m. Transfer the sections from the room temperature water bath to the heated water bath using a non-treated slide. If the section is upside down, it will appear glossy. Do not use this section.
n. Leave the tissue in the heated bath long enough to remove wrinkles.
o. Pick up the section with a glass slide placed at a sharp angle.
p. Place the slide on its edge to allow slide to dry.

8. Use an applicator stick to push sections into labeled microcentrifuge tubes. Samples are collected in duplicate when possible.
9. Remove and dispose of blade in sharps container.

DISPOSAL OF TISSUES

DNA lysates and RNA extracts are prepared from formalin-fixed and unfixed tissue specimens, which are capable of transmitting serious disease. Universal precautions are used to handle all reagents and supplies that come into contact with specimens on the microtome stage where the blocks are cut and during tissue deparaffinization and protease digestion. All samples and reagents and supplies that are potentially contaminated with tissue samples are disposed of in biohazardous waste bags or sharps containers after use. Nondisposable supplies and equipment are decontaminated with 10% bleach after use. Each sample is considered infectious through preparation of the DNA lysate or RNA extract. The wastes generated in the PCR setup room are considered noninfectious.

REFERENCE

Reid AH: Polymerase chain reaction. *In* Mikel UV (ed): AFIP Advanced Laboratory Methods in Histology and Pathology. Washington, DC, AFIP, 1994, pp 81–83.

SOP 4

PREPARATION OF DNA LYSATES FROM PARAFFIN-EMBEDDED TISSUE

PRINCIPLE

Tissue is routinely received fixed and embedded in paraffin. To render DNA accessible to PCR, tissue sections are first deparaffinized with Hemo-De. The tissue is then washed in ethanol to remove residual Hemo-De. Cells are lysed in nonionic detergent buffer containing proteinase K. The proteinase is heat inactivated. The cell debris is precipitated by centrifugation. The DNA lysate is stored at −20°C.

REAGENTS

All reagents are in the pre-PCR setup room.
Hemo-De [Fisher] (500 mL, room temperature): Hemo-De is a biodegradable xylene substitute.
Absolute ethanol (pint, room temperature): Ethanol (more than one pint) is stored in the flammable cabinet.
Nonionic digestion buffer (NIB) [MDL]: Components: 50 mmol/L KCl, 10 mmol/L TRIS Cl (pH 8), 0.1 mmol/L EDTA, 0.5% Tween 20.
To make 50 mL:

45.75 mL	HPLC-grade water
2.5 mL	1 mol/L KCl
0.5 mL	1 mol/L TRIS, pH 8
1.0 mL	5 mmol/L EDTA
0.25 mL	Tween 20

Aliquot 1 mL into 1.5-mL tubes, label appropriately, and store in DNA freezer. Immediately before use, thaw proteinase K (20 mg/mL) [*source varies] and NIB aliquot. Add 6 μL proteinase K/1 mL NIB.

SUPPLIES AND EQUIPMENT

Microcentrifuge tubes (1.5 mL and 0.5 mL)
Aerosol-resistant pipette tips (ART tips)
Disposable gloves
Extra-fine-tip permanent marker and racks
Sterile conical tubes (15 mL and 50 mL)
Pipetters
Vortexer
Microcentrifuge
Oven (55°C)
Heating block (95°C)
Water bath (55°C)

QUALITY CONTROL

1. Check expiration dates on all reagents.
2. Inspect reagents for abnormal color, precipitate, or turbidity. If there is a problem, discard.
3. Be sure that tubes are labeled correctly. A round label with initials, date cut, and MDL number is on the cap

of the tube. The MDL number is also on the side of tube.

4. Label side of tube with date of lysate preparation.

PROCEDURE

Before starting extraction procedure, wipe work surface with 10% bleach. Place clean bench paper on counter. Organize tubes to be extracted in numerical order. Place an empty tube before the first tube and label as a lysate control.

1. Decant a sufficient amount of Hemo-De and ethanol from stock bottles into labeled sterile 15-mL conical tubes.
2. Add 800 μL of Hemo-De to tube containing two 6-μm sections of tissue. Vortex at full speed (setting 8) for 5 seconds. Add 400 μL of ethanol. Vortex at full speed for 5 seconds. Centrifuge at full speed (14,000 rpm) for 5 minutes.
3. Decant the liquid carefully and add 800 μL of ethanol. Vortex at full speed for 5 seconds. Centrifuge at full speed for 5 minutes. Decant the liquid.
4. Dry pellet in 55°C oven for approximately 5 minutes. Do not overdry.
5. Remove NIB buffer and proteinase K stock from freezer and thaw at room temperature. Tap proteinase K to mix. Vortex NIB buffer to mix. *Add 6μL proteinase K to 1 mL NIB buffer* and invert to mix.
6. Add NIB buffer (100 μL) to cell pellet and vortex a few seconds at slow speed (setting 2-3). Place in 55°C water bath for 2 hours.
7. Inactivate proteinase K by heating at 95°C for 5 minutes.
8. Centrifuge tube at full speed for 5 minutes to pellet cell debris.
9. Label side of tube with date of lysate preparation.
10. Store DNA lysate at −20°C in Consult box in numerical order. DNA samples are moved to the −70°C freezer for long-term storage at quarterly intervals (Jan 1, Apr 1, Jul 1, Oct 1).

DISPOSAL OF TISSUES

DNA lysates and RNA extracts are prepared from formalin-fixed and unfixed tissue specimens, which are capable of transmitting serious disease. Universal precautions are used to handle all reagents and supplies that come into contact with specimens on the microtome stage where the blocks are cut and during tissue deparaffinization and protease digestion. All samples and reagents and supplies that are potentially contaminated with tissue samples are disposed of in biohazardous waste bags or sharps containers after use. Nondisposable supplies and equipment are decontaminated with 10% bleach after use. Each sample is considered infectious through preparation of the DNA lysate or RNA extract. The wastes generated in the PCR setup room are considered noninfectious.

REFERENCE

Reid AH: Polymerase chain reaction. *In* Mikel UV (ed): AFIP Advanced Laboratory Methods in Histology and Pathology. Washington, DC, AFIP, 1994, pp 81–83.

SOP 5

PREPARATION OF RNA EXTRACTS

PRINCIPLE

Tissue is routinely received fixed and embedded in paraffin. To render RNA accessible to PCR, six tissue sections are first deparaffinized with Hemo-De. The tissue is then washed in ethanol to remove residual Hemo-De. Cells are lysed in buffer containing SDS, which also inhibits endogenous RNases. After proteinase K digestion, the lysate is extracted with phenol: chloroform:isoamyl alcohol twice, is isopropanol precipitated in the presence of glycogen, and is washed with ethanol. The pellet is resuspended in water, and the extract is stored at −70°C.

REAGENTS

All reagents are in the pre-PCR setup room. A set of reagents and supplies dedicated to RNA work are located in the cabinets above the right half of the work counter. The RNA freezer is below the right half of the counter.

Hemo-De [Fisher] (500 mL, room temperature): Hemo-De is a biodegradable xylene substitute.

Absolute ethanol (pint, room temperature): Ethanol (more than one pint) is stored in the flammable cabinet.

Extraction buffer [MDL]: Final concentration:20 mmol/L TRIS-HCL pH 7.6, 20 mmol/L EDTA, 1% SDS, 0.5 mg/mL proteinase K.

To make 100 mL:

2 mL	1 mol/L TRIS, pH 7.6
4 mL	0.5 mol/L EDTA
10 mL	10% SDS
84 mL	HPLC-grade water

Extraction buffer is stored in 1.8-mL aliquots at room temperature without proteinase K. Before use, proteinase K stocks are thawed and 45 μL of proteinase K stock (20 mg/mL) is added to 1.8 mL of extraction buffer.

80% ethanol is stored in 50-mL aliquots in the RNA cabinet. Absolute ethanol is stored in the flammable cabinet.

Isopropanol: One-liter bottles are stored in the flammable cabinet.

Phenol:chloroform:isoamyl alcohol (25:24:1) (PC) [BRL]: Aliquots are stored in the RNA refrigerator in 15-mL conical tubes.

Ethanol, isopropanol, and PC are decanted from stock bottles into 15-mL conical tubes before use. They are all hazardous substances and must be handled with caution and disposed of properly in labeled bottles under the hood.

3M Sodium acetate: Stored at room temperature in the RNA cabinet.

Glycogen: Stored in aliquots in the −20°C RNA freezer.

HPLC-grade water: Stored in −20°C RNA freezer.

Glycogen, sodium acetate, and water are stored in aliquots in microcentrifuge tubes and are disposed of after a single use.

SUPPLIES AND EQUIPMENT

Microcentrifuge tubes (1.5 mL)
Aerosol-resistant pipette tips (ART tips)
Disposable gloves
Extra-fine-tip permanent marker and racks

Sterile conical tubes (15 mL)
Pipetters
Vortexer
Microcentrifuge
Oven (55°C)
Water bath (55°C)
Spectrophotometer (Pharmacia-GeneQuant) to measure dilutions in 100 μL total volume.

QUALITY CONTROL

1. Check expiration dates on all reagents.
2. Inspect reagents for abnormal color, precipitate, or turbidity. If there is a problem, discard.
3. Be sure that tubes are labeled correctly. A round label with initials, date cut, and MDL number is on the cap of the tube. The MDL number is also on the side of tube.
4. Label side of tube with date of lysate preparation with extra-fine-point permanent marker.

PROCEDURE

1. Before starting lysate procedure, place clean bench paper on counter.
2. Decant a sufficient amount (at least 1 mL per specimen) of Hemo-De and ethanol from stock bottles into labeled sterile 15-mL conical tubes.
3. Add 800 μL of Hemo-De to tube containing six 6-μm sections of tissue. Vortex at full speed (setting 8) for 5 seconds. Add 400 μL of ethanol. Vortex at full speed for 5 seconds. Centrifuge at full speed (14,000 rpm) for 5 minutes.
4. Decant the liquid carefully and add 800 μL of ethanol. Vortex at full speed for 5 seconds. Centrifuge at full speed for 5 minutes. Decant the liquid.
5. Dry pellet in 55°C oven for approximately 5 minutes. Do not overdry.
6. Determine total amount of extraction buffer needed (600 μL/sample). Remove proteinase K stock from freezer and thaw at room temperature. Tap proteinase K to mix. Vortex extraction buffer to mix. Add 45 μL proteinase K to 1.8 mL extraction buffer and mix by tapping.
7. Add extraction buffer (600 μL) to cell pellet and vortex a few seconds at slow speed (setting 2-3). Place in 55°C water bath for 4 hours. Overnight incubation appears to give equal yields of RNA.
8. Purify nucleic acids with two phenol/chloroform (PC) extractions. Add an equal volume of PC (600 μL) to microcentrifuge tube and vortex vigorously. Centrifuge at full speed for 5 minutes. Remove upper aqueous layer to clean tube and repeat extraction with an equal volume of PC.
9. Add 1/10th volume of sodium acetate stock (3 mol/L) to give final concentration of 0.3 mol/L (60 μL to 600 μL) and 20 μg glycogen (1 μL). Mix well before adding 0.6 vol of isopropanol (396 μL isopropanol to 660 μL aqueous solution) and leave on ice for at least 5 minutes.
10. Collect precipitate by centrifugation at full speed for 5 minutes.
11. Wash pellet with 0.5 mL 80% ethanol; centrifuge at full speed for 5 minutes. Decant ethanol and repeat wash.
12. After second wash, decant ethanol and blot tube on clean Kim-wipe before rehydrating pellet in 25 μL of water.
13. OPTIONAL: Make a 1:50 dilution of RNA extract and measure the absorbance (OD) at 260 nm. Calculate the concentration using an OD 260 = 1.0 as equivalent to 40 μg/mL. Use 0.5 μg and 1 μg of A260 material in assay.
14. Store concentrated RNA extracts at −20°C in the RNA freezer in the PCR setup room while the sample is being analyzed. Samples are moved to the −70°C freezer after sample analysis for long-term storage.

LIMITATIONS

Procedure may not always yield RNA of adequate quality for amplification.

DISPOSAL OF TISSUES

DNA lysates and RNA extracts are prepared from formalin-fixed and unfixed tissue specimens, which are capable of transmitting serious disease. Universal precautions are used to handle all reagents and supplies that come into contact with specimens on the microtome stage where the blocks are cut and during tissue deparaffinization and protease digestion. All samples and reagents and supplies that are potentially contaminated with tissue samples are disposed of in biohazardous waste bags or sharps containers after use. Nondisposable supplies and equipment are decontaminated with 10% bleach after use. Each sample is considered infectious through preparation of the DNA lysate or RNA extract. The wastes generated in the PCR setup room are considered noninfectious.

REFERENCE

Krafft A, et al: Postmortem diagnosis of morbillivirus infection in bottlenose dolphins (Tursiops truncatus) in the Atlantic and Gulf of Mexico epizootics by polymerase chain reaction-based assay. J Wildl Dis 1995;31:410–415.

SOP 6

AGAROSE GEL ELECTROPHORESIS

PRINCIPLE

The standard method for DNA analysis is agarose gel electrophoresis. DNA is negatively charged and will migrate toward the anode at neutral pH. DNA molecules will separate by size because large molecules migrate more slowly than small molecules. PCR products amplified from formalin-fixed, paraffin-embedded tissues are typically 100 to 400 base pairs and are separated efficiently on 2.5% agarose in a TRIS-Borate-EDTA (TBE) running buffer. The detection limit of agarose gel electrophoresis followed by ethidium bromide staining is about 2 ng DNA.

REAGENTS

Agarose is in the cabinet in the pre-PCR area and TBE is in the post-PCR room. PCR products are analyzed by agarose gel electrophoresis in the post-PCR room.

TBE buffer (1X) [BRL] or [MDL] (room temperature): 1X TBE = 90 mmol/L TRIS-HCl pH 8.3, 90 mmol/L Borate, 2 mmol/L EDTA. To make: Dilute 5X or 10X stock to 1X in distilled water.

Loading dye (10X) [MDL] (Refrigerator): 35% glycerol, 0.25% bromophenol blue (BPB). To make:

25 mg BPB
3.5 mL glycerol
6.5 mL water

Digoxigenin-labeled molecular weight markers: Preparation of agarose molecular weight markers for nonisotopic Southern detection.

Reagent	Source	Catalog #	Volume
DNA MWM XIII (50 bp)—unlabeled	Boehringer Mannheim	1 721 925	40 μL
DNA MWM XI (100 bp)—digoxigenin-labeled	Boehringer Mannheim	1465 422	20 μL
Agarose gel loading dye	MDL	N/A	10 μL
1X TBE	BRL or MDL	N/A	130 μL

Storage: −20°C (post-PCR room)

ϕX174 RF DNA/Hae III Frag (molecular weight ladder) [BRL]: See SOP 8.

Radioactive ^{32}P-labeled ladder (freezer)

Low melting point agarose (room temperature): 2.0 g LMP agarose [Fisher] or [FMC]/0.5 g agarose [BRL] in 100 mL 1X TBE

Ethidium bromide EtBr (10 mg/mL in water): Refrigerate in foil-covered bottle. This fluorescent dye will enable visualization of the DNA under ultraviolet light. Stain gels with 0.5 μg/mL EtBr in running buffer. WARNING: ETHIDIUM BROMIDE IS A MUTAGEN. WEAR GLOVES AT ALL TIMES AND HANDLE WITH EXTREME CARE. BUFFERS CONTAINING ETHIDIUM BROMIDE MUST BE TREATED WITH ACTIVATED CHARCOAL FOR 1 HOUR BEFORE FILTERING. THE FILTRATE CAN BE POURED DOWN THE SINK.THE CHARCOAL IS DISPOSED OF IN HAZARDOUS WASTE CONTAINERS. Solid EtBr waste (gels) is disposed of in radioactive waste because gels have a radioactive molecular weight ladder on them.

SUPPLIES AND EQUIPMENT

Aerosol-resistant pipette tips (ART tips)
Parafilm
Latex gloves
Oven gloves for handling beakers containing hot agarose solutions
Beaker for melting agarose
Plastic wrap for covering beaker
Ultraviolet (UV) light–protective goggles
Polaroid 667 Film pack
Microwave oven
Direct current power source [PH LKB-EPS 500/400]
Horizontal gel electrophoresis apparatus [BRL 11.14], electric cables
Transilluminator [IBI]
Polaroid camera
Rotator
Balance

QUALITY CONTROL

1. Test wells for leaks before loading samples. Load 2 μL loading buffer per well. Let stand 2 minutes. Do not use wells that leak.
2. Identify the location of each specimen loaded on each lane of every gel in the appropriate data sheet in the assay notebook (top or bottom, lane 1–28).
3. Label photograph to identify assay, date, and lanes containing samples.

PROCEDURE

1. To prepare 2.5% LMP/agarose: Weigh out 2.0 g LMP agarose and 0.5 g agarose per 100 mL of 1X TBE buffer. Place in a beaker.
2. Add 1X TBE buffer, swirl gently to mix, and cover with plastic wrap. Microwave the solution until the agarose is dissolved (3 to 5 minutes). WEAR OVEN GLOVES when handling hot beaker.
3. Let the agarose solution cool to about 55°C.
4. Pour the solution into a gel mold, insert a well-former (comb), and allow the gel to harden (the gel turns opaque in about 15 minutes).
5. After pouring, wait a minimum of 30 minutes (but no longer than 2 hours). Place the gel in the electrophoresis apparatus and flood it with TBE buffer. Remove the well-former after carefully loosening each well by placing a narrow spatula between teeth of well-former and gel itself.
6. Note which samples are to be run in which wells. Always run the molecular weight markers in lane 1 and/or lane 15 (far left). Radioactive labeled markers are used to aid in aligning gel lanes and fragment sizes on film after autoradiography. RADIOACTIVE MATERIALS MUST BE HANDLED WITH GLOVES BEHIND BETA SHIELDS AND DISPOSED OF IN RADIOACTIVE WASTE.
7. Count the number of samples including a molecular weight marker for each row on the gel. Pipette 2 μL of dye solution per sample at well-spaced intervals onto a piece of parafilm to mix each sample before loading into well.
8. Add 20 μL of each PCR product to a spot with 2 μL of dye solution on the piece of parafilm. Mix by pipetting up and down and add 20 μL of the sample to a well on the gel. Save the leftover product in the refrigerator in case it is necessary to reconfirm blot results. Add 3 to 5 μL of labeled molecular weight marker to 2 μL of dye solution. Mix well and add to appropriate lanes on gel.
9. Connect the electrophoresis apparatus to the DC power source and electrophorese at 150 V until the bromophenol dye is near the bottom of the gel (about 1 hour).
10. Wearing gloves, carefully remove the gel from the electrophoresis rig and place in a plastic dish for staining. Add EtBr (0.5 μg/mL of running buffer) and rock on rotator for 15 minutes.
11. Place it on the transilluminator and photograph it with the Polaroid camera. When using the transilluminator, UV-protective goggles must be worn. The camera must be loaded with Type 667 film and equipped with a red filter. Photograph for 1/4 second, remove the film from the camera, and wait 30 seconds before peeling the backing from the film. If the picture is overexposed, try a shorter exposure.

PROCEDURE NOTES

WARNING: Ethidium bromide is mutagenic and UV light is harmful to the eyes. Gloves must be worn at all times when handling the concentrated ethidium bromide solution and the ethidium bromide–containing gel.

NOTE: When using electrophoresis units other than BRL 11.14, always load molecular weight ladder in the far left lane and sequentially number lanes from left to right.

Gels and buffers are RADIOACTIVE if a ^{32}P-labeled molecular weight ladder is used and must be handled taking precautions to minimize exposure to radiation.

Rinse agarose gel rig with tap water after use and dry before storing.

REFERENCE

Maniatis T, Fritsch EF, Sambrook J: Molecular Cloning: A Laboratory Manual. Cold Spring Harbor, NY, Cold Spring Harbor Laboratory, 1982.

SOP 7

END-LABELING OF OLIGONUCLEOTIDES (RADIOLABELING)

PRINCIPLE

Oligonucleotides (usually 10 to 50 bases) are too short to label by random priming. However, oligonucleotides can be labeled at the 5′-end with ^{32}P in a reaction utilizing [γ-^{32}P]-ATP and phage T4 polynucleotide kinase. The reaction relies on the fact that kinase will transfer the gamma phosphate of ATP to the unphosphorylated 5′ end of the oligonucleotide.

REAGENTS

REAGENTS are in −20°C freezer in post-PCR room.
Forward Kinase buffer (5X) [BRL]
T4 Polynucleotide kinase [BRL]
[γ-P-32]ATP (10 μCi/μL) [Amersham] in beta-shielded box

SUPPLIES AND EQUIPMENT

Microcentrifuge tubes (1.5 mL)
Gloves
Pipettors and pipette tips
Oncor safety station
Microcentrifuge
Water bath set at 37°C
Heat block set at 95°C
Vortexer

QUALITY CONTROL

1. Check reference date on γ-^{32}P-ATP source. The probe is used within 2 weeks of the reference date on the source. Label probe tube with lot number and expiration date (reference date plus 14 days).
2. Check solutions visually for signs of deterioration. Reagents must be clear and colorless and free of precipitate. If not, discard.
3. New lots of kinase are checked functionally by the demonstration that a probe labeled with the new lot produced a readily detectable signal on a Southern blot containing target sequence.

PROCEDURE

1. Work in the Oncor workstation. Put on two pairs of gloves and mix the following in a 1.5-mL microcentrifuge tube:
   1 μL of oligonucleotide (15 pmol/μL)
   5 μL of 5X forward kinase buffer
   1 μL of T4 kinase (20 U/μL)
   3 μL of [γ-32P]ATP (10 μCi/μL)
   15 μL of water
   Centrifuge for a few seconds to collect reagents at bottom of tube.
2. Incubate at 37°C for 45 minutes in water bath.
3. Incubate at 95°C for 5 minutes in heat block to inactivate kinase.
4. Add 175 μL of water, vortex the mix at full speed for 5 seconds, and store the labeled oligonucleotide in the shielded probe box in the −20°C freezer. Discard after 2 weeks from the reference date on the γ-^{32}P-ATP stock in zip-lock bag in radiation waste.

PROCEDURE NOTES

Always wear gloves when working with radioactivity. Wear a radiation badge, finger ring, and laboratory coat at all times while handling radioactive material. Work in the Oncor safety station or behind the Plexiglas shield, and always use special spill-absorbent paper. Place all radioactive wastes in the proper waste containers. After the procedure, monitor the work area with a Geiger counter and record in "Isotope User Survey Log." Decontaminate any radioactive spills or other contaminated areas/equipment. Record usage in Radioisotope Stock Record.

REFERENCE

Maniatis T, Fritsch EF, Sambrook J: Molecular Cloning: A Laboratory Manual. Cold Spring Harbor, NY, Cold Spring Harbor Laboratory, 1982.

SOP 8

END-LABELING OF MOLECULAR WEIGHT LADDER

PRINCIPLE

The PhiX174 DNA HaeIII cut ladder can be end-labeled with ^{32}P using the exchange reaction of T4 polynucleotide kinase and [γ-^{32}P]-ATP.

REAGENTS

Reagents are in −20°C freezer in post-PCR room.
PhiX174 DNA HaeIII cut ladder [BRL] (500 ng/μL)
Exchange kinase buffer (5X) [BRL]
T4 Polynucleotide kinase [BRL]
[γ-P-32]ATP (10 μCi/μL) [Amersham] in beta-shielded box
Redivue is stored in the refrigerator.

SUPPLIES AND EQUIPMENT

Microcentrifuge tubes (1.5 mL)
Gloves
Pipettors and pipette tips
Oncor safety station
Microcentrifuge
Water bath set at 37°C
Heat block set at 95°C
Vortexer

QUALITY CONTROL

1. Check reference date on γ-^{32}P-ATP. Use only within 2 weeks of the reference date. Label ladder tube with lot number and expiration date (reference date plus 14 days).
2. Check solutions visually for signs of deterioration. Reagents must be clear and colorless and free of precipitate. If not, discard.

PROCEDURE

1. Work in the Oncor safety station. Put on two pairs of gloves and mix the following in a 1.5-mL microcentrifuge tube:
   3.6 μL of molecular weight ladder (1.8 μg)
   5 μL of 5X exchange kinase buffer
   1 μL of T4 kinase (20 U/μL)
   3 μL of [γ-32P]ATP (10 μCi/μL)
   15 μL of HPLC-grade water
   Centrifuge for a few seconds to collect reagents at bottom of tube.
2. Incubate at 37°C for 45 minutes in water bath.
3. Incubate at 95°C for 5 minutes in heat block to inactivate kinase.
4. Add 175 μL of water, vortex the mix at full speed for 5 seconds, and store the labeled oligonucleotide in the shielded probe box in the −20°C freezer. Discard after 2 weeks.

PROCEDURE NOTES

Always wear gloves when working with radioactivity. Wear a radiation badge, finger ring, and laboratory coat at all times while handling radioactive material. Work in the Oncor safety station or behind the Plexiglas shield and always use special spill-absorbent paper. Place all radioactive wastes in the proper waste containers. After the procedure, monitor the work area with a Geiger counter and record in "Isotope User Survey Log." Decontaminate any radioactive spills or other contaminated areas/equipment. Record usage in Radioisotope Stock Record.

REFERENCE

Maniatis T, Fritsch EF, Sambrook J: Molecular Cloning: A Laboratory Manual. Cold Spring Harbor, NY, Cold Spring Harbor Laboratory, 1982.

SOP 9

SOUTHERN BLOTTING OF PCR PRODUCTS

PRINCIPLE

A Southern blot is a solid phase membrane to which separated DNA, transferred from a gel after electrophoresis, is bound so that it can be hybridized with a labeled nucleic acid probe. In this procedure, the separated double-stranded DNA is denatured in alkali solution. Single-stranded DNA is transferred by capillary action from the agarose to the nylon membrane (Southern blotted) overnight, followed by hybridization with a labeled probe to obtain a sensitivity in the 0.2-pg range.

REAGENTS

Reagents are in the post-PCR room.
Denaturation solution (0.5 M NaOH, 0.6 M NaCl) [MDL]

SUPPLIES AND EQUIPMENT

Nylon membrane filter (Sure Blot Hybridization Membrane) [Intergen]
Blotting pads [BRL]
Saran wrap
Glass plate (about 8 × 8 inches)
Weight (2 to 4 lb)
Gloves
Oven set at 77°C to 83°C
Rocker apparatus

QUALITY CONTROL

1. Denaturation solution should be clear and colorless.
2. Membranes should be uniformly white and intact (free of tears).
3. Blots should be free of bubbles.

PROCEDURE

1. Put on gloves. Take an electrophoresed agarose gel and soak 3 gel volumes of denaturation solution in a plastic dish for 30 minutes with gentle rocking on a rocker apparatus.
2. Place a glass plate on the counter. Place a stack of blotting paper (10 pieces) on top of the glass plate. Soak a piece of blotting paper and a piece of nylon membrane filter in denaturation solution. Place the wet blotting paper, then the filter, and then the gel on top of the dry blotting towels.
3. Immediately place plastic wrap on top of the gel and carefully remove air bubbles from between the gel and filter.
4. Place a glass plate on top of the stack and cover with a 2- to 4-lb weight (e.g., a large catalog).

5. Leave the stack undisturbed for 12 to 16 hours. During this time the liquid in the gel will be drawn through the filter into the blotting pads, carrying the DNA with it. The single-stranded DNA, however, will bind to the filter. After blotting, mark the filter with a pencil showing the date, gel number, and well position of lanes.
6. Remove the filter and dry it in an oven at 77°C to 83°C for 30 minutes. For chemiluminescent detection, dry for 60 minutes. Save the filter in the filter storage box.

PROCEDURE NOTES

It is very important to make sure that no bubbles are present between the gel and filter in step 3 because bubbles prevent the transfer of DNA. If the gel contains radioactive marker fragments, it must be disposed of in the radioactive waste.

REFERENCE

Maniatis T, Fritsch EF, Sambrook J: Molecular Cloning: A Laboratory Manual. Cold Spring Harbor, NY, Cold Spring Harbor Laboratory, 1982.

SOP 10

HYBRIDIZATION AND WASHING OF SOUTHERN BLOTS (RADIOLABELED)

PRINCIPLE

During the Southern blotting procedure, single-stranded DNA is transferred from an agarose gel to a filter membrane where it is bound. To visualize specific DNA sequences, the membrane is incubated with a radioactive probe that hybridizes specifically to complementary DNA. Washing the blot removes nonspecific material, and the specifically bound probe can be visualized by autoradiography.

REAGENTS

10X SSC (room temperature): To make: 20X SSC/liter = 175.3 g NaCl + 88.2 g NaCitrate, pH 7
Hybrisol I Intergen (room temperature): Prewarm in 55°C water bath and mix thoroughly
Wash solution (room temperature): 0.1X SSC, 0.1% SDS (15 mmol/L NaCl, 1.5 mmol/L NaCitrate, pH 7, 0.1% SDS). To make:
5 mL 20X SSC
10 mL 10% SDS
Dilute to 1000 mL

SUPPLIES AND EQUIPMENT

Pencil to mark lanes
Hybridization bottles
15-mL conical centrifuge tube to store probe
Beta shields and Plexiglas rack boxes
Blotting paper
Hybridization incubator
Film cassette
Kodak X-OMAT AR film
−70°C freezer

QUALITY CONTROL

Positive controls are run at two dilutions. One level is near the lowest detection limit of that assay using stringent hybridization conditions. Both control levels are kept low to minimize the chance of carryover from a strong positive control to a negative sample.

PROCEDURE

1. Put on gloves. Briefly wet blot in 10X SSC.
2. With forceps, roll blot and place inside a hybridization bottle. Try to remove air bubbles.
3. Add 5 mL prewarmed Hybrisol I to bottle to block membrane.
   Incubate at 42°C for 30 minutes to an hour, rotating.
4. Pour used Hybrisol I down the sink. Add 5 mL Hybrisol I and add 100 μL of specific ^{32}P-labeled probe.
5. Incubate the blot of PCR products with probe for a minimum of 4 hours at 42°C, rotating.
6. After hybridization, put on gloves, remove probe, and save in a 15-mL disposable tube in the beta-shielded storage box in the −20°C freezer [the probe can be reused once]. Label tube with lot number and expiration date of labeled probe. Probe expires 14 days later. Place in radioactive liquid waste if it is to be discarded.
7. Wash the blot three times for 5 minutes each at 42°C in wash solution (not prewarmed), rotating.
8. Blot filters gently with blotting paper to remove excess moisture. Place damp filter between two layers of Saran wrap or in a document protector.
9. Place the blot in a film cassette with intensifying screens and a piece of Kodak X-OMAT AR film. Place the cassette in the −70°C freezer or at room temperature for 2 to 24 hours. If the signals are weak, put on a second film for 24 to 48 hours.

PROCEDURE NOTES

Perform all manipulations in an area of the laboratory set aside for work with radioactive material. Personnel must wear gloves, a laboratory coat, and a film badge. Monitor the work area with a Geiger counter after the procedure. Place all contaminated materials in the radioactive waste cans. Decontaminate any equipment or work area.

To clean hybridization bottles, remove O-ring from cap assembly and rinse. Dry before reassembling cap assembly.

REFERENCE

Maniatis T, Fritsch EF, Sambrook J: Molecular Cloning: A Laboratory Manual. Cold Spring Harbor, NY, Cold Spring Harbor Laboratory, 1982.

SOP 11

EXPOSING AND DEVELOPING FILMS

PRINCIPLE

The radioactive label incorporated into nucleic acid molecules is detected by exposure to photographic film in a process known as autoradiography.

MATERIALS

Plastic wrap
Film cassette
XAR-2 film
Film processing equipment

QUALITY CONTROL

Each autoradiogram is examined for adequate clarity and resolution.

PROCEDURES

To Expose Film

1. Wrap blot in plastic wrap.
2. Place inside cassette.
3. Put cassette at room temperature or at −70°C, depending on the specific requirements of the assay. In general, all ^{32}P incorporation assay blot films must be exposed at −70°C, because the blots are not dried.

To Use the X-Omat Film Processer

1. Turn on flow of water by turning the faucet counterclockwise.
2. Turn on processor with the toggle switch on the left side.
3. Replace cover if removed.
4. If instrument has been on but no film has been processed for awhile, press the black button near the toggle switch to cycle chemicals.
5. If machine has been idle, start a blank film through by placing on the flat entry side and gently pushing toward the machine. The film will automatically be drawn into the instrument.
6. When ready to develop, turn off the overhead lights and turn on the safe light. Open the cassette, remove the film, and insert into machine as above. **DO NOT PUT BLOT IN FILM PROCESSER.**
7. When the beep sounds, the lights may be turned back on.
8. Label autoradiogram by superimposing over lanes of blot. Label each lane with the MDL number, dilution tested, and other identifiers as necessary.

PROCEDURE NOTES

The contract calls for chemical replenishment once per month. If the levels in the tanks become low, chemicals may be added directly. Make sure DEVELOPER and FIXER go in the respective tanks. Call contractor if there is instrument malfunction. Report problems to the supervisor.

SOP 12

HYBRIDIZATION AND WASHING OF SOUTHERN BLOTS

(CHEMILUMINESCENT DETECTION)

PRINCIPLE

During the Southern blotting procedure, single-stranded DNA is transferred from an agarose gel to a filter membrane, where it is bound. To visualize specific DNA sequences, the membrane is incubated with a DIG-labeled probe that hybridizes specifically to complementary DNA. Washing the membrane removes nonspecific material, and the specifically bound probe can be visualized by exposing film to the membrane after chemiluminescent detection.

MATERIALS

Preparation of Solutions for Southern Hybridization

10X SSC [MDL] for wetting membranes is stored at room temperature in the post-PCR area. A blue tray is filled with 10X SSC for pre-wetting of membranes. To make 10X SSC, dilute 20X SSC [Sigma] with an equal volume of deionized water.
(1) DIG Easy Hyb [Boehringer Mannheim] for Southern prehybridization and probe hybridization is a light-sensitive reagent and is stored at room temperature in a foil-wrapped bottle in the pre-PCR area. Need 10 mL/blot.
(2) Southern hybridization wash solution [MDL] for washing is stored in a carboy at room temperature. 0.1X SSC, 0.1% SDS (15 mmol/L NaCl, 1.5 mmol/L NaCitrate, pH 7, 0.1% SDS). To make 1 liter: 5 mL 20X SSC, 10 mL 10% SDS, dilute to 1000 mL.

Preparation of Solutions and Buffers for Detection

The DIG Wash and Block Buffer Set are purchased from Boehringer Mannheim {BM} and stored at room temperature when unopened. Bring all REFRIGERATED or FROZEN reagents and solutions to room temperature before use (i.e., frozen 10X blocking solution, Dig 1X wash buffer, and 1X maleic acid buffer). Maleic acid buffer, blocking solution, and antibody solution are made in the following volumes:

(3) Maleic acid buffer, 1X (Buffer 1) 1X = 0.1 mol/L maleic acid, 0.15 mol/L NaCl, pH 7.5. Dilute maleic acid buffer, 10X concentration {BM solution 2} to 1X with dH_2O.
(4) Blocking solution, 1X (Buffer 1 + blocking solution): Add blocking solution to Buffer 1 as follows: Dilute blocking solution, 10X concentration (stored as aliquots at −20°C) to 1X with Buffer 1 in 50-mL tube. Need 10 mL/blot. MAKE FRESH.
(5) Antibody solution (1X blocking solution + Antidig antibody): Anti-digoxigenin-alkaline phosphatase Fab fragments (Antidig antibody) is stored at 4°C. Centrifuge 2 minutes before making dilution to force particulate to bottom of tube and avoid black spots on film. Dilute Antidig antibody 1:10,000 with blocking solution from step 4 (e.g., add 0.5 μL of antibody to 5 mL of blocking solution).
(6) Washing buffer (Buffer 1 + Tween 20) 4°C
Dilute washing buffer, 10X concentration {BM solution 1} to 1X with dH_2O. To make own washing buffer, add 0.3% (w/v) Tween 20 to Buffer 1.
(7) Detection buffer 4°C:1X = 0.1 mol/L NaCl, 0.1 mol/L TRIS-HCl, pH 9.5: Dilute detection buffer, 10X concentration {BM solution 4} to 1X with dH_2O. MAKE FRESH.
(8) CDP-Star [BM] 4°C: Dilute 1:100 with detection buffer. MAKE FRESH.

SUPPLIES AND EQUIPMENT

Pencil to mark lanes on membrane
Roller bottles
15-mL conical centrifuge tubes

50-mL conical centrifuge tubes
Gloves
Pipettor and tips
Pipet-Aid and pipettes
Document protector and tape
Clear plastic box for detection
Hybridization incubator
Autoradiography cassettes and Kodak X-OMAT AR film

QUALITY CONTROL

Positive controls are run at two dilutions. One level is near the lowest detection limit of that assay using stringent hybridization conditions. Both control levels are kept low to minimize the chance of carryover from a strong positive control to a negative sample.

PROCEDURE

1. Wear gloves throughout the entire procedure. Prewarm hybridization oven to 42°C. Prewarm water bath to 37°C. Bring all reagents to room temperature.
   a. Determine the volume of DIG Easy Hyb and decant amount necessary for pre-hybridization to 50-mL conical tube. For pre-hybridization, allow 5 mL DIG Easy Hyb solution for blots in small and medium roller bottles, or 10 mL DIG Easy Hyb solution for blots in long roller bottles. *Prewarm* in 37°C water bath and mix thoroughly.
   b. For probe hybridization, label one 15-mL conical tube per probe and add same volumes of DIG Easy Hyb solution used for pre-hybridization (5 or 10 mL of DIG Easy Hyb) to 1-mL conical tube. Add digoxigenin-labeled probe to 15-mL conical tube, vortex, and prewarm at 37°C. (Stock probe concentration is 4.5 pmol/μL; therefore, add 1.1 μL probe to 5 mL DIG Easy Hyb in 15-mL conical tube.)
2. Remove blot from oven and cut if necessary. Wet in 10X SSC.
3. With forceps, roll each blot and place inside a roller hybridization bottle, being careful to not scratch the membrane.
4. Add 5 mL *prewarmed* DIG Easy Hyb from 1a to roller hybridization bottle to block membrane. Incubate at 42°C for a minimum of 30 minutes (30 to 60 minutes) while rotating.
5. Discard used DIG Easy Hyb in the sink. Add *prewarmed* probe from 1b: 5 mL fresh DIG Easy Hyb containing 1 pmol/μL of specific digoxigenin-labeled probe.
6. Incubate the blot with probe for a minimum of 1 hour at 42°C, rotating.
7. After hybridization, decant probe into sink.
8. Turn oven temperature down to 27°C. *Remaining steps are performed at room temperature in hybridization oven.* Ice may be added to bottom tray to lower temperature rapidly.
9. Wash the blot with Southern hybridization wash solution from the carboy (not prewarmed) two times for 5 minutes each at room temperature, rotating. Fill bottle half full for each wash. Discard washing solution in sink.
10. Rinse blot for 1 to 2 minutes in 10 mL (20 mL for large blots) of maleic acid buffer, 1X (Buffer 1), rotating. Discard buffer in sink. Pour off any water in tray if ice was added to lower oven temperature to room temperature.
11. Add 1X blocking solution (Buffer 1 + blocking solution) 5 mL/bottle (10 mL for large blots) and incubate membrane, rotating for 20 minutes.
12. Dilute antibody solution (1X blocking solution + Antidig antibody). Spin antibody (2 minutes maximum speed) to precipitate particulate. DO NOT VORTEX OR MIX VIAL OF ANTIBODY. Determine amount of antibody solution needed. Need 5 mL/blot. Add 0.5 μL anti-digoxigenin-alkaline phosphatase per 5 mL of blocking solution in 50-mL tube. Vortex the 50-mL tube to mix. Incubate blot in 5 mL of diluted antibody conjugate solution (or 10 mL for large blot) for 30 minutes, rotating.
13. Fill bottles half full with 1X washing buffer (Buffer 1 + Tween 20) and wash blots twice, rotating 15 minutes each time.
14. Make 1X detection buffer in 50-mL tube. Pour contents into clear plastic box. Incubate blots face down for at least 2 minutes in detection buffer.
15. Make 5 mL of substrate: To do this dilute CDP-Star 1:100 in detection buffer. Add 50 μL CDP Star to 15-mL tube with 5 mL 1X detection buffer, and mix thoroughly. Pour 5 mL of substrate into hard plastic lid of plastic box.
16. Incubate blots, one at a time, face down for 1 to 3 minutes. Drain excess substrate off blot and place in plastic document protector. Tape edges (with autoclave tape) closed to keep membrane moist.
17. Turn oven to 37°C. Incubate blots at room temperature for approximately 10 minutes; then place in oven at 37°C for 15 to 20 minutes.
18. Place the membrane(s) in a film cassette with intensifying screens and a piece of Kodak X-OMAT AR film. Expose to film for 10 minutes at room temperature. Develop film using the automatic processor. Exposure time may be lengthened or shortened depending on the signal intensity desired.

PROCEDURE NOTES

To clean hybridization bottles, remove O-ring from cap assembly and rinse. Dry before reassembling cap assembly.

The procedure for removing the probe from Southern blot is as follows:

1. Wash the membrane in water for 1 minute.
2. Incubate the membranes twice for 10 minutes in 10 mL of alkaline probe-stripping solution at 37°C (alkaline probe-stripping solution: 0.4N NaOH, 0.1% SDS).
3. Rinse the membranes thoroughly in 2X SSC.
4. Membranes may be re-probed, beginning with the pre-hybridization step.

SOP 13

RT-PCR-β_2-MICROGLOBULIN (HUMAN RNA CONTROL)

PCR/SOUTHERN BLOT PROCEDURE

PRINCIPLE

RT PCR is performed on a control gene to assess the integrity of the sample RNA. The β_2-microglobulin primers span intron 2 of the gene, which is highly expressed in almost all nucleated cells. The 158 base-pair product is separated by agarose gel electrophoresis, Southern blotted, and probed with a specific digoxigenin-labeled oligonucleotide.

SPECIMEN (see SOP 1)

REAGENTS, SUPPLIES, AND EQUIPMENT

ALWAYS WEAR GLOVES WHEN HANDLING REAGENTS. FOLLOW PROCEDURES FOR AVOIDING CONTAMINATION OF PCR REACTIONS!! (SEE SOP 2.)

The primers and probes for β_2-microglobulin were selected from published sequences. Reverse transcriptase (RT), Taq polymerase, and PCR primers and all RT-PCR reagents, except $MgCl_2$, are stored in the RNA freezer in the PCR setup room. $MgCl_2$ is stored in the RNA refrigerator in the PCR setup area. RNA extracts and actin positive controls are kept in the −70° C freezer in the hall for long-term storage (more than 1 week). RNA extracts are kept at −20° C for up to 1 week. Probes for β_2-microglobulin are kept in the freezer in the post-PCR room. Aliquots of reagents and standards are stored in microcentrifuge tubes (1.5 and 0.5 mL). Do not put unused aliquots back in tubes or containers. Throw them away.

The usual source of a reagent is indicated in BRACKETS []: Fisher[FI], PerkinElmer[PE], Promega [PR], etc. Homemade reagents are abbreviated [MDL] and have been quality control tested before use. An asterisk [*] is used when the source varies.

Cutting Blocks (see SOP 3)

RNA Extraction (see SOP 5)

RT-Polymerase Chain Reaction

REAGENTS

HPLC-grade water [FI]
First strand buffer (5X) [BRL]
DTT (0.1 mol/L) [BRL]
PCR buffer II (10X) [PE]
dNTP: 2.5 mmol/L each [PR][MDL]

1. To prepare, first make a 10 mmol/L solution from a 100-mmol/L stock (1:10 dilution) of each dNTP (dATP, dCTP, dGTP, and dTTP) as follows. To four microcentrifuge tubes, add 900 μL of water, then add 100 μL of dNTP (100 mmol/L). Mix well.
2. Next, mix equal volumes of each 10 mmol/L solution to make each dNTP 2.5 mmol/L in the final mix.
3. Aliquot and label tubes. Store in DNA freezer.

MMLV reverse transcriptase: 200U/μL [BRL]
Taq polymerase (5 U/μL) [PE]
$MgCl_2$ (25 mmol/L) [PE]

PRIMERS [BRL]

Primers are stored in the RNA freezer in a working dilution of 15 μmol/L.

REVERSE TRANSCRIPTASE PRIMER

BM3 5′-CCT CCA TGA TGC TGC TTA CAT GTC (1023–046)

PCR PRIMER

BM5 5′-CTT GTC TTT CAG CAA GGA CTG G (274–295)

REVERSE TRANSCRIPTASE MASTER MIX

The volumes per 20-μL reaction with 5-μL sample are as follows:

4 μL	5X first strand buffer
2 μL	DTT (0.01 mol/L)
1.6 μL	dNTPs (200 μmol/L final concentration in room temperature)
6.1 μL	water
13.7 μL	total volume per sample

One microliter of the BM3 RT primer (15 μM working dilution, final concentration = 300 nmol/L) and 0.3 μL of MMLV-RT (1.2 U/reaction) is added to the RT master mix before use.

PCR-RNA MASTER MIX (UPPER MIX)

The volumes to prepare 30 μL of reaction mix are as follows:

3 μL	10X PCR buffer II
2 μL	Mg^{2+} (2.2 mmol/L final concentration)
23.7 μL	water
28.7 μL	total volume per sample

One microliter of BM5 primer 1 (15 μmol/L) and 0.3 μL Taq polymerase (1.25 U/reaction) is added to the PCR-RNA master mix before use.

SUPPLIES AND EQUIPMENT

Microcentrifuge tubes (1.5 mL and 0.5 mL)
Aerosol-resistant pipette tips (ART tips)
Disposable gloves
Extra-fine-tip permanent marker and racks
Pipetters
Microcentrifuge (reserved for pre-PCR use only)
PerkinElmer Thermal Cycler Model 9600
Vortexer

Agarose Gel Electrophoresis (see SOP 6)

All reagents are in the post-PCR room. Use 2.5% agarose.

Southern Blotting of PCR Products (see SOP 9)

End-Labeling Oligonucleotide Probes (see SOP 7)

Oligonucleotide probes are stored in the post-PCR room freezer in a working dilution of 15 μmol/L.

β_2-MICROGLOBULIN PROBE
BMP1 5′-AGT ATG CCT GCC GTG TGA ACC ATG (345–368)

Hybridization and Washing Southern Blots (see SOP 12)

Exposing and Developing Film (see SOP 11)

QUALITY CONTROL

Positive Assay Control

The positive control is an RNA lysate of K562. The amplified product is 158 base pairs.

Negative Assay Controls

WATER CONTROL. An RT-PCR reaction mix containing water as the sample tested is set up first in the RT-PCR run, before patient samples, to assess the purity of the reagents.

LYSATE CONTROL. A lysate (no RNA template) prepared in parallel to patient samples should give no detectable band, indicating that the tube was not contaminated with patient RNA during extraction.

Amplification Control

β_2-Microglobulin serves as a control gene for the assessment of RNA integrity. The amplified β_2-microglobulin product is 158 base pairs.

Contamination Control

A negative control PCR reaction containing water as the sample tested is also set up last in the PCR run, after the positive control. This reaction assesses the overall quality of the assay setup procedure in avoiding carryover contamination from a positive to an adjacent negative sample.

Assay Controls

Run positive control and negative controls along with patient samples.

Positive controls are tested at two concentrations: 1 μL and 5 μL of the 1:100 dilution of a K562 lysate.

A water control (5 μL water), 5 μL of lysate control (an empty tube that was treated with the same reagents used during the preparation of the patient RNA extracts), and a contamination control (5 μL water) at the end of each run serve as negative controls.

Patient samples are tested at one concentration: 5 μL of the undiluted extract.

The current master mix lot, containing all reaction components except RNA, enzymes, and β_2-microglobulin-specific primers, is prepared and tested in advance with positive and negative controls.

PROCEDURE

FOLLOW PROCEDURES FOR AVOIDING CONTAMINATION OF PCR REACTIONS!! (See SOP 2.)

Cutting Blocks (see SOP 3)

RNA Extraction (see SOP 5)

RT-Polymerase Chain Reaction (RT-PCR)

Use PerkinElmer Thermal Cycler Model 9600.

1. Determine the number of samples to be assayed (one dilution of each patient extract, a water control, at least one lysate control, and two positive controls). Prepare enough reagents for 2 additional assays; two plus the number of samples and controls = N. Remove the appropriate number of master mix aliquots for the setup. Aliquots of master mix are sufficient for 12 assays. Record the master mix lot numbers on the worksheet. The reverse transcriptase (RT) master mix is aliquotted with 13.7 μL per sample; the PCR-RNA master mix is aliquotted with 28.7 μl per sample. Calculate the amount of RT master mix needed by multiplying N × 13.7 μL. Calculate the amount of PCR-RNA master mix by multiplying N × 28.7 μL.
2. Number the side of each MicroAmp tube, consecutively, with an extra-fine-point permanent marker. Record assay number and identity of sample (MDL#, control) on worksheet.
3. Add 0.3 μL × N MMLV and 1 μL × N BM3 RT primer to 13.7 μL of the RT master mix (0.3 μL + 1 μL + 13.7 μL = 15 μL). Tap tube gently to mix. Store on ice until use.
4. Add 0.3 μl × N Taq polymerase and 1 μL × N BM5 primer to N × 28.7 μL of the PCR master mix (0.3 μL + 1 μL + 28.7 μL = 30 μL). Tap tube gently to mix. Store the master mixes on ice until use.
5. Add 15 μL RT master mix to each reaction tube. Cap tubes.
6. Add 5 μL water to water control and 4 μL water to the positive control that will contain 1 μL of extract.
7. Add 5 μL of the negative control lysate to the negative lysate control.
8. Add sample to each tube (5 μL of the undiluted extract). The final volume of the RT reaction is 20 μL.
9. After all samples have been added, add controls to appropriate tube. For the positive controls, add 1 μL and 5 μL of the 1:100 dilution of K562 RNA lysate.
10. Add 5 μL of water to the contamination control.
11. Place in PerkinElmer Thermal Cycler Model 9600 and incubate at 37°C for 1 hour (Program 29).
12. Remove tubes from thermal cycler and place in racks with at least one space between each tube.
13. Add 30 μL PCR-RNA master mix to each reaction tube. Cap tubes.
14. Place in thermal cycler and cycle on Program 28 at the times and temperatures below:

    Initial step: 5 min 94°C
    40 cycles of: 1 min 94°C
    1 min 55°C
    1 min 72°C
    Final step: 5 min 72°C
15. Remove tube from thermal cycler and place in refrigerator in post-PCR room for analysis by gel electrophoresis.

Agarose Gel Electrophoresis (see SOP 6)

All reagents are in the post-PCR room. The 158-base-pair product is resolved on 2.5% agarose (2% LMP, 0.5% agarose) in 1X TBE.

Southern Blotting (see SOP 9)

Labeling Oligonucleotide Probes (see SOP 7)

Hybridization and Washing Southern Blots (see SOP 12)

Exposing and Developing Film (see SOP 11)

If there is a negative signal for the actin gene, the viral assay is reported as indeterminate.

REPORTING RESULTS

A positive result for β_2-microglobulin is reported if a positive signal is seen with the specific probe and the patient sample, provided all the appropriate controls are working. If not, repeat the assay.

PROCEDURE NOTES

Avoid freeze/thawing the sample too often. The sample may be heated to 90°C before the RT reaction.

REFERENCE

The assay was developed in the MDL.

Gussow D, Rein R, Ginjaar I, et al: The human β_2-microglobulin gene. J Immunol 1987;139:3132–3138.

SOP 14

PCR PROCEDURE: *ERBB2* (DNA CONTROL)

PRINCIPLE

PCR is performed on a control gene to assess the integrity of the DNA lysate extracted from paraffin-embedded tissue. The primer set for *ERBB2*, a single-copy gene in the human genome, gives rise to a 241-base pair amplified product. The sequence of the *ERBB2* primers corresponds to nucleotides 929 to 948 (exon 2) and 1150 to 1170 (exon 3) of the ERBB2 gene.

SPECIMEN—SEE SOP 1

REAGENTS—SPECIAL SUPPLIES AND EQUIPMENT

ALWAYS WEAR GLOVES WHEN HANDLING REAGENTS. FOLLOW PROCEDURES FOR AVOIDING CONTAMINATION OF PCR REACTIONS!! SEE SOP 2

The primers and a probe for a segment of the *ERBB2* gene were selected based on a published partial sequence for the gene.

ERBB2 primers and the *ERBB2* positive control (Raji) are kept in the DNA freezer in the PCR setup room. *ERBB2* probes are in the post-PCR freezer. Aliquots of reagents and standards are stored in Eppendorf tubes (1.5 and 0.5 mL). *Do not put unused aliquots back in tubes or containers. Throw them away.*

The usual source of a reagent is indicated in BRACKETS [ ]. Fisher [FI], Perkin Elmer [PE], Promega [PR], etc. Homemade reagents are abbreviated [MDL] and have been quality control tested before use. An [*] is used when the source varies.

Cutting Blocks—SEE SOP 3

DNA Extraction—SEE SOP 4

Polymerase Chain Reaction (PCR)

Extracts and most PCR reagents are stored in the PCR setup DNA freezer. Mg^{2+} is stored in the PCR setup room RNA refrigerator.

REAGENTS

HPLC-grade water [FI]
PCR buffer II (10X) [PE]
dNTP—2.5 mM each [PR]

1. To prepare dNTP, first make a 10 mM solution from a 100 mM stock of each dNTP (dATP, dCTP, dGTP, and dTTP). To make 1 mL of a 10 mM solution, add 900 μL of water and 100 μL of each dNTP (100 mM) to four microcentrifuge tubes and mix well.
2. Next, mix equal volumes of each 10 mM solution to make each dNTP 2.5 mM in the final mix.
3. Aliquot and label tubes. Store in DNA freezer.

Taq polymerase (5 Units/μL) [PE]
$MgCl_2$ (25 mM) [PE] Refrigerator

PRIMERS

ERBB2-S sense primer-1:
5′-GGG AAA ACC GCG GAC GCC TG-3′

ERBB2-A antisense primer-2:
5′-GTC CCT GTG TAC GAG CCG CAC-3′

Primers are stored in the freezer in a working dilution of 5 μM.

MASTER MIX

NOTE: Use a master mix. The same master mix is used for *ERBB2*, EBV, and HIV assays. Refer to SOP 13 for additional information on master mixes and then set-up. The master mixes for *ERBB2* do not contain the primers or Taq polymerase.

The volume per 50 μL reaction with 5 μL sample is as follows:

5.0 μL	10X PCR Buffer II
4.0 μL	dNTP Mix I (200 μM final concentration)
3.4 μL	25 mM $MgCl_2$ (2.5 mM final concentration)
30.3 μL	HPLC water
42.7 μL	

Add 0.3 μL × N Taq polymerase and 1 μL each of *ERBB2*-S and *ERBB2*-A immediately before use.

SUPPLIES

Microcentrifuge tubes (1.5 mL and 0.5 mL)
Aerosol resistant pipette tips (ART tips)
Disposable gloves
Extra fine point permanent marker and racks

EQUIPMENT

Pipetters
Microcentrifuge (reserved for pre-PCR use only)
Thermal Cycler (model 9600)

Agarose Gel Electrophoresis—See SOP 6

All reagents are in the post-PCR room. The 241-bp product is resolved on 2.5% agarose (2% LMP, 0.5% agarose) in 1X TBE.

Southern Blotting of PCR Products—SEE SOP 9

End Labeling Oligonucleotide Probes—SEE SOP 7

ERBB2 OLIGO Probe:
5′-GGA CCT GCT GAA CTG GTG TAT GCA GAT TGC C-3′

Oligonucleotides for probes are stored in the post-PCR room freezer in a working dilution of 15 μmol/L.

Hybridization and Washing Southern Blots—SEE SOP 10

Exposing and Developing Film—SEE SOP 11

QUALITY CONTROL

Several types of positive and negative controls are run with each assay as controls for test performance. The placement of the controls within an assay is crucial to the detection of contamination at each step in the test system.

Positive Assay Control: The *ERBB2* positive control is a DNA lysate prepared from a paraffin-embedded sample of the EBV-containing Burkitt's lymphoma cell line (Raji) as described in SOP 4. The amplified *ERBB2* product is 241 base pairs. The amount of *ERBB2* template added per assay is at a level low enough so as not to serve as a source of cross-over contamination.

Negative Assay Controls: A negative control is used to control for each step in the test sample: lysate preparation, reagent mix preparation, and carryover contamination from sample to sample in the assay setup procedure.

1. **Water control**: A PCR reaction mix containing water as the sample tested is set up as first in the PCR run, before patient samples, to assess the purity of the assay reagents.
2. **Lysate control**: A lysate (no DNA template) prepared in parallel with patient samples should give no detectable band, indicating that the tube was not contaminated with DNA during lysate preparation.
3. **Contamination Control**: A negative control PCR reaction containing water as the sample tested is also set up last in the PCR run, after the positive control. This reaction assesses the overall quality of the assay set-up procedure in avoiding carryover contamination from a positive to an adjacent negative sample.

ASSAY CONTROLS

Run positive control and negative controls along with patient samples.

The positive control is tested at one concentration: 1 μL of the undiluted Raji cell lysate.

A water control (5 μL water) and 1 μL of lysate controls (an empty tube that was treated with the same reagents used during the preparation of the patient DNA lysates) serve as negative controls.

Patient samples are tested at three concentrations: 1 μL of a 1:5 dilution (1:5) of tissue lysate, 1 μL of the undiluted lysate (1X) and 5 μL of the undiluted lysate (5X).

AMPLIFICATION CONTROL

Paraffin-embedded tissues may contain inhibitors of PCR or fixatives that severely compromise nucleic acid integrity. *ERBB2* serves as a control gene to assess whether amplifiable nucleic acid is present in the sample.

The current Master Mix lot, containing all reaction components except DNA, Taq polymerase and *ERBB2*-specific primers, is prepared and tested in advance with positive and negative controls.

PROCEDURE—STEPWISE

FOLLOW PROCEDURES FOR AVOIDING CONTAMINATION OF PCR REACTIONS!! See SOP 2

Cutting blocks—See SOP 3

Preparation of DNA Lysates—See SOP 4

Polymerase Chain Reaction (PCR). Use Perkin Elmer Model 9600 Thermal Cycler

1. Determine the number of samples to be assayed (3 dilutions of each patient lysate, a water control, one lysate control, two positive controls, and a contamination control). Prepare enough reagents for 2 additional assays; two plus the number of samples and controls = N. Remove the appropriate number of master mix aliquots for the setup. Aliquots of master mix are sufficient for 12 assays. Record the master mix lot numbers on the worksheet. The master mix is aliquotted with 42.7 mL per reaction.
2. Number the top of each 0.5 mL microcentrifuge reaction tube, consecutively, with an extra fine point permanent marker. Record assay number and identity of sample (MDL#, control) on worksheet.
3. Add 42.7 μL $\times$ N of the master mix to a labeled 1.5 mL tube. Use a larger tube for total volumes_ 1.5 mL. Add 0.3 μL $\times$ N Taq polymerase, 1 μL $\times$ N of *ERBB2*-S, and 1 μL $\times$ N of *ERBB2*-A to the Master Mix (0.3 μL + 1 μL + 1 μL + 42.7 μL = 45 μL). For total volumes $<$ 0.5 mL tap tube gently to mix. For total volumes $>$ 0.5 mL, invert. Store on ice until use.
4. Add master mix to each reaction tube (45 L). Cap tubes.
5. Add 5 μL water to water control, 4 μL water to 1:5 tubes and 1X tubes to give a combined volume of water and patient sample equal to 5 μL.
6. Add 1 μL of the negative control lysate (without DNA template) to the negative lysate control tube.
7. Make dilutions of patient samples and add 1 μL of a 1:5 dilution to the 1:5 tube. Add 1 μL of the undiluted lysate to the 1× tube. Add 5 μL of the undiluted lysate to the 5× tube.
8. Add positive control Raji cell lysate to appropriate tube after all samples have been prepared: 1 μL of the undiluted Raji cell lysate. The setup order is (1) water, (2) lysate control, (3) patient samples, (4) positive controls, and (5) contamination control.
9. Add 5 μL water to the contamination control.
10. Place in Thermal Cycler (Perkin Elmer Model 9600) with times and temperatures set as follows:

Initial step:	5 min 94°C
40 cycles of:	1 min 94°C
	1 min 55°C
	1 min 72°C
Final step:	5 min 72°C

11. Remove sample tray from Thermal Cycler and place tubes in rack in refrigerator in post-PCR room for analysis by gel electrophoresis.

AGAROSE GEL ELECTROPHORES—See SOP 6

All reagents are in the post-PCR room. The 241-bp product is resolved on 2.5% agarose (2% low melting point, 0.5% agarose) in 1× TBE.

Southern Blotting—See SOP 9

Labelling Oligonucleotide Probes—See SOP 7

Hybridization and Washing Southern Blots—See SOP 12

Exposing and Developing Film—See SOP 11

REPORTING RESULTS

A positive result for the *ERBB2* gene is reported if a positive signal is seen in at least two of three dilutions.

If there is a positive signal in only one of three dilutions, repeat the assay. A negative result for the *ERBB2* gene is reported if no signal is seen in at least two of three dilutions of the repeated assay.

REFERENCES

Wright, CF, AH Reid, MM Tsai, et al: Detection of Epstein-Barr virus sequences in Hodgkin's disease by the polymerase chain reaction. Am J Pathol 1991;139:393–397.

SOP 15

PREPARATION OF BUFFERS FOR JC VIRUS IN SITU HYBRIDIZATION

BUFFERS

200 mmol/L EDTA: pH 8.0

Ethylenediaminetetraacetic acid (EDTA), disodium, dihydrate
Sigma No. E-5134 Formula WT. 372.2
Mix 37.22 g of EDTA in 400 mL quality water.
Adjust pH to 8.0 with 1.0N NaOH.
Add enough quality water to make a final volume of 500 mL.
Filter through a 0.2-μmol/L filter.

10% SDS: (W/V)

Sodium dodecyl sulfate (SDS)
Bio-Rad No. 161-0301 Formula WT. 288.38
Mix 10 g SDS into 100 mL of water.

Phosphate Buffered Saline (PBS): pH 7.4

Dulbecco's Phosphate Buffered Saline (DPBS) 10X (w/o calcium chloride and magnesium chloride)

0.07 mol/L dibasic sodium phosphate (Na_2HPO_4)
0.03 mol/L monobasic sodium phosphate ($NaHPO_4$)
1.5 mol/L sodium chloride (NaCl) Gibco No. 310-4200A 10X liquid

PBSE = 1× PBS + 5 mmol/L EDTA in 500 mL

For 1X PBSE, mix:

- 437.5 mL quality water
- 50 mL 10X DPBS
- 12.5 mL 200 mmol/L EDTA

Filter.
Check pH.

Saline Sodium Citrate (SSC): pH 7.0

Saline-Sodium Citrate Buffer (SSC) 20X

0.3 mol/L Citric acid trisodium
3.0 mol/L Sodium chloride (NaCl)
Sigma No. S-6639 20X liquid

2X SSC
Mix 9 parts quality water with 1 part 20X SSC.
Filter.
Check pH.

0.2X SSC
Mix 99 parts quality water with 1 part 20X SSC.
Filter.
Check pH.

SOP 16

PREPARATION OF PROTEINASE K SOLUTION

PRINCIPLE

Because the biotin-labeled gene probes are large (100 to 2000 base pairs long), the tissue requires enzymatic permeabilization for maximum signal. This is far and away the trickiest and most crucial step when using large probes. The tissues are presented to the enzyme in a dry state to help adherence. The addition of EDTA helps to inhibit endogenous nucleases found in the enzyme preparation. Drying the tissue before and after the digestion ensures maximum control of the enzyme.

MATERIALS AND METHODS

Protease type XXVIII (proteinase K)
Sigma No. P-4914

0.125 mg of proteinase K is diluted in each milliliter of PBSE. The solution is warmed to 37°C until use. Incubate at 37°C for 5 to 10 minutes.

SOP 17

PREPARATION OF HYDROGEN PEROXIDE SOLUTION

PRINCIPLE

This procedure removes endogenous peroxide, which would add to the background in the tissue sections. Endogenous peroxide activity if not quenched would add to the overall staining of the tissue.

MATERIALS AND METHODS

Hydrogen peroxide 30%
Fisher Scientific No. H325-500
Store at 4°C.

The working dilution of hydrogen peroxide for this procedure is 3% (v/v). Therefore, a 1:10 dilution of the stock hydrogen peroxide is made in PBSE.

SOP 18

PREPARATION OF DNA PROBE (JC VIRUS)

PRINCIPLE

Labeled probes are specific DNA sequences labeled with a modified nucleotide and can be used for positive identification of pathogens and DNA sequences. These probes can be used in a variety of formats based on hybridization to complementary nucleic acid sequences. The hybridized DNA probe is detected by its interaction with a biotin-binding protein, such as streptavidin, and consequently visualized by a color-enhanced enzyme such as AEC.

The name of reagent, amount, concentration, lot number, expiration, date, and optimal dilution is entered in the log for the ultra-low freezer. Some of the DNA probes are very expensive or difficult to produce. These DNA sequences are well preserved at −70°C and have been shown to retain reactivity for an indefinite period of time. In fact, some of the DNA probes obtained commercially do not include an expiration date. If stored frozen, these reagents should be reliable for quite some time, and purchase of new probes can be delayed until supplies are sufficiently low. Because control slides are performed with each run, a written record exists as to reagent performance. These reagents are closely monitored for their reliability. The use of outdated probes and new lots of probe will be compared with existing lots to determine strength and the results will be stored in the Laboratory Lab Book.

MATERIALS AND METHODS

JC Virus Positive Probe

From a 4-kb fragment of JC virus DNA cloned into the *Eco*R1 site of pBR322
Enzo Diagnostics No. BP-847
Concentration: 20 μg/mL
Quantity: 1.6 μg
Fragment size: 200 to 2000 base pairs, as estimated by gel electrophoresis

pBR322 Negative Probe

Grown in *Escherichia coli* HB101, extracted by standard molecular procedures and purified by isopyknic banding in CsCl gradient.
Enzo Diagnostics No. BP-841
Concentration: 25 μg/mL
Quantity: 2.5 μg
Fragment size: 200 to 2000 base pairs, as estimated by gel electrophoresis

Carrier DNA

Salmon sperm DNA supplied at 10 mg/mL
Enzo Diagnostics
One vial is supplied with each vial of DNA probe.
Used in in situ hybridization as a blocking agent. Remove desired amount from freezer and boil for 10 minutes; quickly cool and add to DNA probe mixture at 100 μg/mL of hybridization solution.

Dextran Sulfate 50% Solution (w/v)

Sigma No. D-7140 Mol. wt. 500,000
Diluted in quality water with long mixing and possibly sonication to drive it into solution. The 50% solution is very heavy with a "syrupy" texture and light brown color.

Deionized Formamide

Sigma No. F-7503
Concentrations of 40% to 50% are used in in situ hybridization. Each 1% formamide lowers the TM (melting temperature of DNA) by 0.7%. Commercial preparations of this chemical usually contain salt impurities as well as hydrolysis products, ammonium formate, NH^{4+}, and formic acid. The formamide should have a conductivity below 40 μS, and a 50% solution of it should have a pH below 7.5. The formamide can be cleaned by stirring 1 L with 10 g of Norite A (Fisher Scientific) and 50 g of mixed bed resin (AG501- X8[d], 20–50 mesh, Biorad) at 4°C for 2 hours. Filter twice through Whatman #1 filter paper. Store aliquots at −70°C.

PREPARATION OF HYBRIDIZATION MIXTURE

Deionized formamide pH 6.8 to 7.2 50 μL
50% Dextran sulfate 20 μL
20X SSC 10 μL
JC Virus Probe 20 μL
Carrier DNA 4 μL

This mixture is stable for 12+ months at 4°C. This is enough for five samples of 20 mm × 20 mm.

SOP 19

PREPARATION OF BIOTINYL TYRAMIDE

PRINCIPLE

This technique is a post-hybridization amplification system for the increased sensitivity of this in situ hybridization technique. It is known as the Tyramide Signal Amplification (TSA) and is also identified as a CARD (CAtylzed Reporter Deposition) system. This detection system is based on the enzymatic proximal deposition of labeled (i.e., biotinylated) tyramide molecules by peroxidase activity. The increased signal amplification is the result of the high affinity for the horseradish-biotin complex integrated into the DNA probe site. The hybridized probe is then visualized by the enzyme-mediated deposition of a chromagen reporter molecule, AEC.

MATERIALS AND METHODS

Tyramide Signal Amplification (TSA) NEN Life Sciences, NEL730

The biotinyl tyramide is mixed with an amplification buffer (vendor supplied) at 1:100. The staining time is 3 to 10 minutes at room temperature followed by three washes in vendor-supplied buffer consisting of 0.1 mol/L TRIS-HCl, pH 7.5, 0.15 mol/L NaCl, and 0.05% Tween 20 for 5 minutes each.

SOP 20

PREPARATION OF DETECTION COMPLEX

PRINCIPLE

Detection is based on the binding between the biotin of the probe and avidin, a biotin-binding protein. The detection complex is streptavidin peroxidase with a high affinity for the biotin integrated into the DNA probe.

MATERIALS AND METHODS

Horseradish Peroxidase-Streptavidin (HRP-SA) Amersham No. RPN.1231

The HRP-SA is mixed with phosphate-buffered iodine at 1:400 for proper dilution in this procedure. The staining time is 15 minutes at 37° C.

SOP 21

PREPARATION OF CHROMAGEN

PRINCIPLE

The chromagen used in this assay is AEC. It has the ability to turn color (red) in the presence of horseradish peroxidase, which is deposited by the detection complex. Chromogenic substrates, when oxidized, form colored compounds. Horseradish peroxidase is used to develop the chromogen in the presence of H_2O_2. During this development, the soluble chromagen becomes insoluble and visible.

MATERIALS AND METHODS

Peroxidase Chromagen Kit
3-Amino-9-Ethyl Carbazole) 20 mg/mL in dimethylformamide
Biomeda Corp. No. S01

1. Transfer 5 mL of distilled water to empty bottle labeled Working Reagent (red bottle #3).
2. Add 2 drops of chromagen buffer (bottle 3A).
3. Add 1 drop of concentrated chromagen (bottle 3B).
4. Mix quickly.
5. Add 1 drop of 2% hydrogen peroxide (bottle 3C).
6. Mix.
7. Place nozzle on bottle and cap.
8. Store away from direct sunlight until used.

INDEX

Note: Page numbers followed by f refer to illustrations; page numbers followed by t refer to tables.

M

N

Q

R

S